KT-477-870

ANTI...

ESSENTIALS

Edited by

Burke A. Cunha, MD, MACP

Chief, Infectious Disease Division
Winthrop-University Hospital
Mineola, New York
Professor of Medicine
State University of New York
School of Medicine
Stony Brook, New York

2013

JONES & BARTLETT
LEARNING

World Headquarters
Jones & Bartlett Learning
5 Wall Street
Burlington, MA 01803
978-443-5000
info@jblearning.com
www.jblearning.com

Jones & Bartlett Learning books and products are available through most bookstores and online booksellers. To contact Jones & Bartlett Learning directly, call 800-832-0034, fax 978-443-8000, or visit our website at www.jblearning.com.

Substantial discounts on bulk quantities of Jones & Bartlett Learning publications are available to corporations, professional associations, and other qualified organizations. For details and specific discount information, contact the special sales department at Jones & Bartlett Learning via the above contact information or send an email to specialsales@jblearning.com

The authors, editor, and publisher have made every effort to provide accurate information. However, they are not responsible for errors, omissions, or for any outcomes related to the use of the contents of this book and take no responsibility for the use of the products and procedures described. Treatments and side effects described in this book may not be applicable to all people; likewise, some people may require a dose or experience a side effect that is not described herein. Drugs and medical devices are discussed that may have limited availability controlled by the Food and Drug Administration (FDA) for use only in a research study or clinical trial. Research, clinical practice, and government regulations often change the accepted standard in this field. When consideration is being given to use of any drug in the clinical setting, the healthcare provider or reader is responsible for determining FDA status of the drug, reading the package insert, and reviewing prescribing information for the most up-to-date recommendations on dose, precautions, and contraindications, and determining the appropriate usage for the product. This is especially important in the case of drugs that are new or seldom used.

Production Credits
Senior Acquisitions Editor: Nancy Anastasi Duffy
Senior Production Editor: Daniel Stone
V.P., Manufacturing and Inventory Control: Therese Connell
Composition: diacriTech, Chennai, India
Cover Design: Scott Moden
Printing and Binding: Cenveo
Cover Printing: Cenveo

ISBN-13: 978-1-284-02798-3

6048

Printed in the United States of America
17 16 15 14 13   10 9 8 7 6 5 4 3 2 1

ABOUT THE EDITOR

Burke A. Cunha, MD, MACP, is Chief, Infectious Disease Division at Winthrop-University Hospital, Mineola, New York; Professor of Medicine, State University of New York School of Medicine, Stony Brook, New York; and is one of the world's leading authorities on infectious diseases. During his career, he has written/edited 1225 articles, 193 book chapters, and 30 books on infectious diseases. He has received numerous teaching awards, including the Aesculapius Award for teaching excellence and the Spatz Award for clinical excellence and teaching excellence. Dr. Cunha is a Fellow of the Infectious Disease Society of America, American Academy of Microbiology, American College of Clinical Pharmacology, Surgical Infection Society, American College of Chest Physicians and Society of Hospital Epidemiologists of America. He has had a long interest in clinical syndromic diagnosis, diagnostic reasoning, antimicrobial therapy and resistance, atypical pneumonias, surgical infections, infections in compromised hosts, zoonoses, FUOs, meningitis and encephalitis, endocarditis, and nosocomial infections. Dr. Cunha is a Master of the American College of Physicians, awarded for lifetime achievement as a master clinician and master teacher.

DEDICATION

for
Marie

**"Grace in her steps,
Heaven in her eye,
In every gesture, dignity and love"**

Milton

TABLE OF CONTENTS

Table of Contents

EDITORS

Burke A. Cunha, MD, MACP
Editor

Cheston B. Cunha, MD
Associate Editor

CONTRIBUTORS

Burke A. Cunha, MD, MACP
Chief, Infectious Disease Division
Winthrop-University Hospital
Mineola, New York
Professor of Medicine
State University of New York
School of Medicine
Stony Brook, New York
*All chapters except HIV Infection &
Pediatric ID*

Edward J. Bottone, PhD
Professor of Medicine
Professor of Microbiology
Professor of Pathology
Mount Sinai
School of Medicine
New York, New York
*Medical Microbiology; Parasites,
Fungi, Unusual Organisms*

John L. Brusch, MD
Associate Chief of Medicine
Cambridge Health Alliance
Infectious Disease Service
Cambridge Health Alliance
Medical Director, Somerville Hospital
Assistant Professor of Medicine
Harvard Medical School
Boston, Massachusetts
Endocarditis: Therapy & Prophylaxis

Daniel Caplivski, MD
Infectious Disease Division
Assistant Professor of Medicine
Mt. Sinai School of Medicine
New York, New York
Fungal Stain Atlas

Cheston B. Cunha, MD
Infectious Disease Division
Rhode Island Hospital and The Miriam Hospital
Alpert School of Medicine, Brown University
Providence, Rhode Island
*Infectious Disease Differential Diagnosis
Overview of Antimicrobial Therapy
Empiric Therapy Based of Clinical Syndromes
Antimicrobial Drug Summaries*

Dennis J. Cleri, MD
St. Francis Medical Center
Professor of Medicine
Seton Hall University
School of Graduate Medical Education
Trenton, New Jersey
Bioterrorism

Staci A. Fischer, MD
Director, Transplant Infectious Diseases
Rhode Island Hospital
Associate Professor of Medicine
Alpert School of Medicine, Brown University
Providence, Rhode Island
Transplant Infections: Therapy & Prophylaxis

Pierce Gardner, MD
Senior Advisor, Clinical Research and Training
National Institutes of Health
John E. Fogarty International Center for
Advanced Study in the Health Sciences
Bethesda, Maryland
Prophylaxis and Immunization

Arthur Gran, MD
Infectious Disease Division
Winthrop-University Hospital
Mineola, New York

State University of New York
School of Medicine
Stony Brook, New York
Antimicrobial Drug Summaries

Jean E. Hage, MD
Infectious Disease Division
Winthrop-University Hospital
Mineola, New York
State University of New York
School of Medicine
Stony Brook, New York
*Empiric Therapy of Clinical Syndromes;
Prophylaxis & Immunization;
Parasitic & Fungi; Unusual Organisms;
Antimicrobial Drug Summaries*

Mark H. Kaplan, MD
Professor of Medicine
Infectious Diseases
University of Michigan School of Medicine
Ann Arbor, Michigan
HIV Drug Summaries

Douglas S. Katz, MD
Vice Chair for Clinical Research and
Education
Director, Body CT
Winthrop-University Hospital
Mineola, New York
Professor of Clinical Radiology
State University of New York School of
Medicine
Stony Brook, New York
Chest X-ray Atlas

Raymond S. Koff, MD
Clinical Professor of Medicine
University of Connecticut School of Medicine
Farmington, Connecticut
Viral Hepatitis: Therapy & Prophylaxis

Leonard R. Krilov, MD
Chief, Pediatric Infectious Disease Division
Winthrop-University Hospital
Mineola, New York
Professor of Pediatrics
State University of New York

School of Medicine
Stony Brook, New York
Pediatric Infectious Diseases

David W. Kubiak, PharmD
Infectious Disease Clinical Pharmacist
Brigham and Women's Hospital
Boston, Massachusetts
Antiretroviral Drug Summaries

George H. McCracken, Jr., MD
Distinguished Professor of Pediatric Infectious
Disease and the Sarah M. and Charles E. Seay
Chair in Pediatric Infectious Disease
University of Texas Southwestern Medical Center
Dallas, Texas
Pediatric Infectious Diseases

James H. McGuire, MD
Master Clinician
Division of Infectious Diseases
Brigham and Women's Hospital
Professor of Medicine
Harvard Medical School
Boston, Massachusetts
Parasites, Fungi, Unusual Organisms

Nardeen Mickail, MD
Infectious Disease Division
Winthrop-University Hospital
Mineola, New York
State University of New York
School of Medicine
Stony Brook, New York
Antimicrobial Drug Summaries

Robert Moore, MD
Chairman, Department of Radiology
Stony Brook University Hospital
Professor of Radiology
State University of New York School
of Medicine
Stony Brook, New York
Chest X-ray Atlas

Sigridh Muñoz-Gomez, MD
Infectious Disease Division
Winthrop-University Hospital
Mineola, New York
State University of New York

School of Medicine
Stony Brook, New York
Antimicrobial Drug Summaries

Ronald L. Nichols, MD
William Henderson Professor of Surgery
Professor of Microbiology and Immunology
Tulane University School of Medicine
New Orleans, Louisiana
*Surgical Antimicrobial Prophylaxis
and Therapy*

Genovefa Papanicolaou, MD
Attending Physician, Infectious Disease Service
Memorial Sloan Kettering Cancer Center
Associate Professor of Medicine
Weill Cornell Medical College
New York, New York
Transplant Infections: Therapy & Prophylaxis

Michael F. Rein, MD
Professor of Medicine (Emeritus)
University of Virginia Health System
Charlottesville, Virginia
Sexually Transmitted Diseases

John H. Rex, MD
Adjunct Professor of Medicine
University of Texas Medical School
Houston, Texas
Vice-President and Medical Director
for Infection
AstraZeneca Pharmaceuticals
Macclesfield, UK
Antifungal Therapy

Paul E. Sax, MD
Clinical Director, Division of Infectious Diseases
and HIV Program
Division of Infectious Diseases
Brigham and Women's Hospital
Associate Professor of Medicine
Harvard Medical School
Boston, Massachusetts
HIV Infection

David Schlossberg, MD
Tuberculosis Control Program
Philadelphia Department of Health
Professor of Medicine
Temple University School of Medicine
Philadelphia, Pennsylvania
Tuberculosis

Paul E. Schoch, PhD
Director, Clinical Microbiology Laboratory
Winthrop-University Hospital
Mineola, New York
*Medical Microbiology and Gram
Stains Atlas*

Daniel S. Siegal, MD
Department of Radiology
Mount Auburn Hospital
Harvard Medical School
Boston, Massachusetts
Chest X-ray Atlas

Stephanie Strollo, MD
Infectious Disease Division
Winthrop-University Hospital
Mineola, New York
State University of New York
School of Medicine
Stony Brook, New York
*Initial Therapy of Isolates Pending
Susceptibility Testing*

Uzma Syed, DO
Infectious Disease Division
Winthrop-University Hospital
Mineola, New York
State University of New York
School of Medicine
Stony Brook, New York
*Initial Therapy of Isolates Pending
Susceptibility Testing*

Damary C. Torres, PharmD
Clinical Pharmacy Specialist
Winthrop-University Hospital
Mineola, New York
Associate Clinical Professor of Pharmacy
College of Pharmacy, St. John's University
Queens, New York
Antimicrobial Drug Summaries

Kenneth F. Wagner, DO
Infectious Disease Consultant
National Naval Medical Center
Associate Professor of Medicine
Uniformed Services, University of
the Health Sciences
F. Edward Hebert School of Medicine
Bethesda, Maryland
Parasites, Fungi, Unusual Organisms

ACKNOWLEDGMENTS

To accomplish the task of presenting the data compiled in this reference, a small, dedicated team of professionals was assembled. This team focused their energy and discipline for many months into typing, revising, designing, illustrating, and formatting the many chapters that make up this text. I wish to acknowledge Monica Crowder Kaufman and Rebecca Smith for their important contribution. I would also like to thank the many contributors who graciously contributed their time and energy; and Mark Freed, MD, past President and Editor-in-Chief of Physicians' Press, for his vision, commitment, and guidance.

Burke A. Cunha, MD

NOTICE

Antibiotics Essentials has been developed as a concise, practical, and authoritative guide for the treatment of infectious diseases. Aside from Chapter 7, Pediatric Infectious Diseases, the book pertains to the treatment of infectious diseases and use of antimicrobial agents in adults. The clinical recommendations set forth in this book are those of the authors and are offered as general guidelines, not specific instructions for individual patients. Clinical judgement should always guide the physician in the selection, dosing, and duration of antimicrobial therapy for individual patients. **Not all recommendations in this book are approved indications by the U.S. Food and Drug Administration, and antimicrobial recommendations are not limited to indications in the package insert. The use of any drug should be preceded by careful review of the package insert, which provides indications and dosing approved by the U.S. Food and Drug Administration**. The information provided in this book is essential not exhaustive, and the reader is referred to other medical references and the manufacturer's product literature for further information. *Clinical use of the information provided and any consequences that may arise from its use is the responsibility of the prescribing physician. The authors, editors, and publisher do not warrant or guarantee the information herein contained and do not assume and expressly disclaim any liability for errors or omissions or any consequences that may occur from use of this information.*

BASIS OF RECOMMENDATIONS

The therapeutic recommendations in Antibiotic Essentials are based on the contributor's clinical expertise and experience as well as the literature and clinical guidelines.

ABBREVIATIONS

3TC	lamivudine	ddI	didanosine
ABC	abacavir	DFA	direct fluorescent antibody
ABE	acute bacterial endocarditis	DI	diabetes insipidus
ABM	acute bacterial meningitis	DIC	disseminated intravascular coagulation
ADA	adenosine deaminase	DLV	delavirdine
AFB	acid fast bacilli	DM	diabetes mellitus
AIH	autoimmune lupoid hepatitis	DOT	directly observed therapy
AIHA	autoimmune hemolytic anemia	DRV	darunavir
AML	acute myelogenous leukemia	e.g.	for example
ANA	antinuclear antibody	EBV	Ebstein-Barr virus
ARDS	adult respiratory distress syndrome	EEE	Eastern equine encephalitis
ATV	atazanavir	EEG	electroencephalogram
A-V	atrio-ventricular	EFV	efavirenz
β-lactams	penicillins, cephalosporins, cephamycins (not monobactams or carbapenems)	EIA	enzyme immunoassay
		ELISA	enzyme-linked immunosorbent assay
		EM	erythema migrans
BAL	bronchoalveolar lavage	EMB	ethambutol
BMT	bone marrow transplant	ENF	enfuvirtide
BPH	benign prostatic hypertrophy	Enterobacteriaceae:	Citrobacter, Edwardsiella, Enterobacter, E. coli, Klebsiella, Proteus, Providencia, Shigella, Salmonella, Serratia, Hafnia, Morganella, Yersinia
CAB	catheter associated bacteriuria		
CABG	coronary artery bypass grafting		
CAC	catheter associated candiduria		
CAH	chronic active hepatitis		
CA-MRSA	community-acquired MRSA (see p. 14)	ESBLs	extended spectrum β-lactamases
CAP	community-acquired pneumonia	esp	especially
CD₄	CD₄ T-cell lymphocyte	ESR	erythrocyte sedimentation rate
CE	California encephalitis virus	ESRD	end-stage renal disease
CFS	chronic fatigue syndrome	ET	endotracheal
CGD	chronic granulomatous disease	ETR	etavirine
CIE	counter-immunoelectrophoresis	FTA-ABS	fluorescent treponemal antibody absorption test
CLL	chronic lymphocytic leukemia		
CML	chronic myelogenous leukemia	FPV	fosamprenavir
CMV	Cytomegalovirus	FTC	emtricitabine
CNS	central nervous system	FUO	fever of unknown origin
CO-MRSA	community-onset MRSA (see p. 16)	G6PD	glucose-6-phosphate dehydrogenase
CoNS	coagulase-negative staphylococci	GC	gonococcus/gonorrhea
CPH	chronic persistent hepatitis	GCA	giant cell arteritis
CPK	creatine phosphokinase	GI	gastrointestinal
CrCl	creatinine clearance	gm	gram
CSD	cat scratch disease	GU	genitourinary
CSF	cerebrospinal fluid	GVHD	graft versus host disease
CT	computerized tomography	HA-MRSA	hospital-acquired MRSA
CVA	costovertebral angle	HAP	hospital-acquired pneumonia
CVC	central venous catheter	HAV	hepatitis A virus
CVID	common variable immune deficiency	HBcAb	hepatitis B core antibody
CVVH	continuous veno venous hemo filtration	HBoV	human bocavirus
		HBsAg	hepatitis B surface antigen
CXR	chest x-ray	HBV	Hepatitis B virus
d4T	stavudine		
ddC	zalcitabine		

HCV	hepatitis C virus
HD	hemodialysis
HDV	hepatitis D virus
HEV	hepatitis E virus
HFHD	high flux hemodialysis
HFV	hepatitis F virus
HFM	hand foot mouth disease
HGA	human granulocytic anaplasmosis
HGE	human granulocytic ehrlichiosis
HHV-6,7,8	human Herpes virus 6,7,8
HME	human monocytic ehrlichiosis
HMPV	human metapneumovirus
HPS	Hanta virus pulmonary syndrome
HPV	human papilloma virus
HTLV-1	human T-cell leukemia virus
HRIG	human rabies immune globulin
HSV	herpes simplex virus
I & D	incision and drainage
IDV	indinavir
IFA	immunofluorescent antibody
IgA	immunoglobulin A
IgG	immunoglobulin G
IgM	immunoglobulin M
INH	isoniazid
IP	intraperitoneal
IT	intrathecal
ITP	idiopathic thrombocytopenic purpura
IV	intravenous
IV/PO	IV or PO
IVDA	intravenous drug abuser
JE	Japanese encephalitis
kg	kilogram
L	liter
LCM	lymphocytic choriomeningitis
LDH	lactate dehydrogenase
LFTs	liver function tests
LGV	lymphogranuloma venereum
LPV/r	lopanavir/ritonavir
MAI	Mycobacterium avium-intracellulare
mcg	microgram
mcL	microliter
MDR	multidrug resistant
MDRSP	multidrug-resistant S. pneumoniae
mg	milligram
mL	milliliter
MIC	minimum inhibitory concentration
min	minute
MMR	measles, mumps, rubella
MRI	magnetic resonance imaging
MRSA	methicillin-resistant S. aureus
MRSE	methicillin-resistant S. epidermidis
MS	multiple sclerosis
MSSA	methicillin-sensitive S. aureus
MSSE	methicillin-sensitive S. epidermidis
MTT	methyltetrathiazole
MU	million units
MVC	maraviroc
MVP	mitral valve prolapse
NFV	nelfinavir
NHAP	nursing home acquired pneumonia
NNRTI	non-nucleoside reverse transcriptase inhibitor
NP	nosocomial pneumonia
NRTI	nucleoside reverse transcriptase inhibitor
NSAIDS	nonsteroidal anti-inflammatory drugs
NVP	nevirapine
OI	opportunistic infection
PAN	polyarteritis nodosa
PBC	primary biliary cirrhosis
PBS	protected brush specimen
PCEC	purified chick embryo cells
PCN	penicillin
PCP	Pneumocystis (carinii) jiroveci pneumonia
PCR	polymerase chain reaction
PD	peritoneal dialysis
PDA	patent ductus arteriosus
PE	Powassan encephalitis
PEP	post-exposure prophylaxis
PI	protease inhibitor
PID	pelvic inflammatory disease
PML	progressive multifocal leukoencephalopathy
PMN	polymorphonuclear leucocytes
PO	oral
PPD	tuberculin skin test
PPIs	proton pump inhibitors
PPNG	penicillinase-producing N. gonorrhoeae
PTBM	partially treated bacterial meningitis
PVE	prosthetic valve endocarditis
PVL	Panton-Valentine leukocidin
PZA	pyrazinamide
q__d	every __ days
q__h	every __ hours
q month	once a month
q week	once a week
RA	rheumatoid arthritis
RAL	raltegravir
RBC	red blood cells
RE	regional ileitis (Crohn's disease)
RMSF	rocky mountain spotted fever
RSV	respiratory syncytial virus
RTV	ritonavir
RUQ	right upper quadrant
RVA	rabies vaccine absorbed
SARS	severe acute respiratory syndrome

SBE	subacute bacterial endocarditis
SCID	severe combined immune deficiency
SGOT/SGPT	serum transaminases
SLE	systemic lupus erythematosus
St. LE	Saint Louis encephalitis
SOT	solid organ transplant
sp.	species
SPB	spontaneous bacterial peritonitis
SPEP	serum protein electrophoresis
SQ	subcutaneous
SQV	saquinavir
STD	sexually transmitted diseases
TA	temporal arteritis
TAH/BSO	total abdominal hysterectomy/bilateral salpingoopherectomy
TB	M. tuberculosis
TDF	tenofovir disoproxil fumarate
TEE	transesophageal echocardiogram
TEN	toxic epidermal necrolysis
TID	three times per day
TMP	trimethoprim
TMP–SMX	trimethoprim-sulfamethoxazole
TPN	total parenteral nutrition
TPV	tipranavir

TRNG	tetracycline-resistant N.gonorrhoeae
TSS	toxic shock syndrome
TTE	transthoracic echocardiogram
TTP	thrombotic thrombocytopenic purpura
TURP	transurethral resection of prostate
UC	ulcerative colitis
UTI	urinary tract infection
VA	ventriculoatrial
VAP	ventilator-associated pneumonia
VCA	viral capsid antigen
VEE	Venezuelan equine encephalitis virus
VISA	vancomycin-intermediate S. aureus
VLM	visceral larval migrans
VP	ventriculoperitoneal
VRE	vancomycin-resistant enterococci
VRSA	vancomycin-resistant S. aureus
VSE	vancomycin-sensitive enterococci
VZV	Varicella zoster virus
WBC	white blood cells
WEE	western equine encephalitis
WNE	west nile encephalitis
XMRV	xenotropic murine leukemia related virus
yrs	years
ZDV	zidovudine

Chapter 1

Overview of Antimicrobial Therapy

Burke A. Cunha, MD
Jean E. Hage, MD
Paul E. Schoch, PhD
Cheston B. Cunha, MD
Edward J. Bottone, PhD
Demary C. Torres, Pharm D

Overview of Antimicrobial Therapy

Despite the ability of antimicrobial therapy to prevent/control infection, prescribing errors are common, including treatment of colonization, suboptimal empiric therapy, inappropriate combination therapy, dosing and duration errors, and mismanagement of apparent antibiotic failure. Inadequate consideration of antibiotic resistance potential, tissue penetration, drug interactions, and side effects, limit the effectiveness of antimicrobial therapy. *Antibiotic Essentials* is a concise, practical, and authoritative guide to the treatment and prevention of infectious diseases commonly encountered.

FACTORS IN ANTIBIOTIC SELECTION

A. **Spectrum.** Antibiotic spectrum refers to the range of microorganisms an antibiotic is usually effective against, and is the basis for empiric antibiotic therapy (Chapter 2). Antibiotics with "concentration-dependent" kinetics, e.g., quinolones, aminoglycosides display increasing killing with increasing concentrations above MIC of organism; antibiotics with "time-dependent" kinetics, e.g., β-lactams do not.

B. **Tissue Penetration.** Antibiotics that are effective against a microorganism in vitro but unable to reach the site of infection are of little or no benefit to the host. Antibiotic tissue penetration depends on properties of the antibiotic, e.g., lipid solubility, molecular size and tissue, e.g., adequacy of blood supply, presence of inflammation. Antibiotic tissue penetration is rarely problematic in acute infections due to increased microvascular permeability from local release of chemical inflammatory mediators. In contrast, chronic infections, e.g., chronic pyelonephritis, chronic prostatitis, chronic osteomyelitis and infections caused by intracellular pathogens often rely on chemical properties of an antibiotic, e.g., high lipid solubility, small molecular size for adequate tissue penetration. Antibiotics cannot be expected to eradicate organisms from areas that are difficult to penetrate or have impaired blood supply, such as abscesses, which usually require surgical drainage for cure. In addition, implanted foreign materials associated with infection usually need to be removed for cure, since microbes causing infections associated with prosthetic joints, shunts, and intravenous lines produce a slime/biofilm on plastic/metal surfaces that permits organisms to survive despite antimicrobial therapy.

C. **Antibiotic Resistance.** Bacterial resistance to antimicrobial therapy may be classified as natural/intrinsic or acquired, and as relative or absolute. Pathogens not covered by the usual spectrum of an antibiotic are termed *naturally/intrinsically* resistant, e.g., 25% of S. pneumoniae are naturally resistant to macrolides; *acquired* resistance refers to a previously susceptible pathogen that is no longer susceptible to an antibiotic, e.g., ampicillin-resistant H. influenzae. Organisms with *intermediate level (relative)* resistance manifests as an increase in minimum inhibitory concentrations (MICs), but are susceptible at achievable serum/tissue concentrations, e.g., penicillin-resistant S. pneumoniae. In contrast, organisms with *high level (absolute)* resistance manifests as a sudden increase in MICs during therapy, and cannot be overcome by higher-than-usual antibiotic doses, e.g., gentamicin-resistant P. aeruginosa. Most acquired antibiotic resistance is *agent-specific*, not a class specific, and is usually limited to one or two species. Resistance is *not* related, per se, to volume or duration of use. Some antibiotics have little resistance potential i.e., "low resistance" potential even when used in high volume; other antibiotics can induce resistance, e.g., "high resistance" potential with little use.

Successful antibiotic resistance control strategies include eliminating antibiotics from animal feeds, microbial surveillance to detect resistance problems early, infection control precautions to limit/contain spread of clonal resistant species, restricted hospital formulary i.e., controlled use of high resistance potential antibiotics, and preferential use of "low resistance" potential antibiotics by clinicians. Unsuccessful strategies include rotating formularies, restricted use of certain antibiotic classes, e.g., 3rd generation cephalosporins, fluoroquinolones, and use of combination therapy. In choosing between similar antibiotics, try to select an antibiotic with "low resistance" potential. Some antibiotics, e.g., ceftazidime are also associated with increased prevalence of methicillin-resistant S. aureus (MRSA); other antibiotics, e.g., vancomycin are associated with increased prevalence of vancomycin-resistant enterococci (VRE).

The antibiotic Resistance Potential of each antibiotic is included in each Drug Summary (see chapter 11).

D. Safety Profile. Whenever possible, avoid antibiotics with serious/frequent side effects.

E. Cost. Switching early from IV to PO antibiotics is the single most important cost saving strategy in hospitalized patients, as the institutional cost of IV administration (~$10/dose) may exceed the cost of the antibiotic itself. Antibiotic costs can also be minimized by using antibiotics with long half-lives, and by choosing monotherapy over combination therapy. Other factors adding to the cost of antimicrobial therapy include the need for an obligatory second antimicrobial agent, antibiotic side effects, e.g., diarrhea, cutaneous reactions, seizures, phlebitis, and outbreaks of resistant organisms, which require cohorting and prolonged hospitalization.

FACTORS IN ANTIBIOTIC DOSING

"Usual antibiotic dose" assumes normal renal and hepatic function. Patients with significant renal insufficiency and/or hepatic dysfunction may require dosage reduction in antibiotics metabolized/eliminated by these organs (Table 1.1). Specific dosing recommendations based on the degree of renal and hepatic insufficiency are detailed (see Chapter 11).

A. Renal Insufficiency. Since most antibiotics eliminated by the kidneys have a wide "toxic-to-therapeutic ratio," dosing strategies are frequently based on formula-derived estimates of creatinine clearance (Table 1.1), rather than precise quantitation of glomerular filtration rates. Dosage adjustments are especially important for antibiotics with narrow toxic-to-therapeutic ratios, and for patients who are receiving other nephrotoxic medications or have preexisting renal disease.

Table 1.1. Dosing Strategies in Hepatic/Renal Insufficiency*

Hepatic Insufficiency
* Decrease total daily dose of hepatically-eliminated antibiotic by 50% in presence of clinically severe liver disease.
* **Alternative: Use antibiotic eliminated/inactivated by the renal route in usual dose.**

Renal Insufficiency (Examples)
* If creatinine clearance ~ 40–60 mL/min, decrease dose of renally-eliminated antibiotic by 50% and maintain the usual dosing interval.
* If creatinine clearance ~10–40 mL/min, decrease dose of renally-eliminated antibiotic by 50% and double the dosing interval.
* **Alternative: Use antibiotic eliminated/inactivated by the hepatic route in usual dose.**

Major Route of Elimination			
Hepatobiliary		**Renal**	
Chloramphenicol	Pyrazinamide	Most β-lactams	Amantadine
Cefoperazone	Linezolid	Aminoglycosides	Rimantadine
Ceftriaxone†	Itraconazole	TMP–SMX	Acyclovir
Doxycycline	Caspofungin	Aztreonam	Valacyclovir
Minocycline	Micafungin	Carbapenems	Famciclovir
Telithromycin	Anidulafungin	Polymyxin B	Valganciclovir
Moxifloxacin	Ketoconazole	Colistin	Oseltamavir
Macrolides	Voriconazole	Ciprofloxacin	Peramavir
Nafcillin	Posaconazole	Levofloxacin	Zanamavir
Clindamycin		Gatifloxacin	Tetracycline
Metronidazole		Gemifloxacin	Oxacillin
Tigecycline		Flucytosine	Daptomycin
Quinupristin/dalfopristin		Fluconazole	Telavancin
Isoniazid		Amphotericin	Ceftaroline fosamil
Ethambutol		Vancomycin	Fosfomycin
Rifampin		Nitrofurantoin	Cycloserine

*   See individual drug summaries in Chapter 11 for specific dosing recommendations. Creatinine clearance (CrCl) is used to assess renal function and can be estimated by the following formula: CrCl (mL/min) = [(140 – age) × weight (kg)] / [72 × serum creatinine (mg/dL)]. Multiply by 0.85 if female. It is important to recognize that due to age-dependent declines in renal function, elderly patients with "normal" serum creatinines may have CrCls requiring dosage adjustment. For example, a 70-year-old, 50-kg female with a serum creatinine of 1.2 mg/dL has an estimated CrCl of 34 mL/min.

†   ~⅓ eliminated renally.

1. **Initial and Maintenance Dosing in Renal Insufficiency.** For drugs eliminated by the kidneys, **the initial dose is unchanged**, and the **maintenance dose/dosing interval are modified in proportion to the degree of renal insufficiency (CrCl)**. Dosing adjustment problems in renal insufficiency can be circumvented by selecting an antibiotic with a similar spectrum that is eliminated by the hepatic route.

2. **Aminoglycoside Dosing.** Single daily dosing—adjusted for the degree of renal insufficiency after the loading dose is administered–has virtually eliminated the nephrotoxic potential of aminoglycosides, and is recommended for all patients,

including the critically ill (a possible exception is enterococcal endocarditis, where gentamicin dosing every 8 hours may be preferable). Aminoglycoside-induced tubular dysfunction is best assessed by quantitative renal tubular cast counts in urine, which more accurately reflect aminoglycoside nephrotoxicity than serum creatinine.

B. Hepatic Insufficiency. Antibiotic dosing for patients with hepatic dysfunction is problematic, since there is no hepatic counterpart to the serum creatinine to accurately assess liver function. In practice, antibiotic dosing is based on clinical assessment of the severity of liver disease. For practical purposes, dosing adjustments are usually not required for mild or moderate hepatic insufficiency. For severe hepatic insufficiency, dosing adjustments are usually made for antibiotics with hepatotoxic potential (Chapter 9). Relatively few antibiotics depend solely on hepatic inactivation/elimination, and dosing adjustment problems in these cases can be circumvented by selecting an appropriate antibiotic eliminated by the renal route.

C. Combined Renal and Hepatic Insufficiency. There are no good dosing adjustment guidelines for patients with hepatorenal insufficiency. If renal insufficiency is worse than hepatic insufficiency, antibiotics eliminated by the liver are often administered at half the total daily dose. If hepatic insufficiency is more severe than renal insufficiency, renally eliminated antibiotics are usually administered and dosed in proportion to renal function.

D. Mode of Antibiotic and Excretion/Excretory Organ Toxicity. The mode of elimination/excretion does not predispose to excretory organ toxicity per se, e.g., nafcillin (hepatically eliminated) is not hepatotoxic.

MICROBIOLOGY AND SUSCEPTIBILITY TESTING

A. Overview. In vitro susceptibility testing provides information about microbial sensitivities of a pathogen to various antibiotics and is useful in guiding therapy. Proper application of microbiology and susceptibility data requires careful assessment of the in vitro results to determine if they are consistent with the clinical context; if not, the clinical impression usually should take precedence.

B. Limitations of Microbiology Susceptibility Testing
1. ***In vitro* data do not differentiate between colonizers and pathogens.** Before responding to a culture report from the microbiology laboratory, it is important to determine whether the organism is a pathogen or a colonizer in the clinical context. As a rule, colonization should not be treated.

2. ***In vitro* data do not necessarily translate into *in vivo* efficacy.** Reports which indicate an organism is "susceptible" or "resistant" to a given antibiotic in vitro do not necessarily reflect in vivo activity. Table 1.2 lists antibiotic-microorganism combinations for which susceptibility testing is usually unreliable.

3. **In vitro susceptibility testing is dependent on the microbe, methodology, and antibiotic concentration.** *In vitro* susceptibility testing by the microbiology laboratory *assumes* the isolate was recovered from *blood*, and is being exposed to *serum* concentrations of an antibiotic given in the *usual* dose. Since some body sites e.g., bladder, urine contain higher antibiotic concentrations than found in serum, and other body sites e.g., CSF contain lower antibiotic concentrations than found in serum, *in vitro* data may be misleading for non-bloodstream infections. For example, a Klebsiella pneumoniae isolate obtained from the CSF may be reported as "sensitive" to cefazolin even though cefazolin does not penetrate the CSF. Likewise, E. coli and Klebsiella urinary isolates are often reported as "resistant" to ampicillin/sulbactam despite *in vivo* efficacy, due to high antibiotic concentrations in the urinary tract. Antibiotics should be prescribed at the usual recommended doses; attempts to lower cost by reducing dosage may decrease antibiotic efficacy e.g., cefoxitin 2 gm IV inhibits ~ 85% of B. fragilis isolates, whereas 1 gm IV inhibits only ~ 20% of strains.

Table 1.2. Antibiotic-Organism Combinations for Which *in Vitro* Susceptibility Testing Does Not Predict *in Vivo* Effectiveness[1]

Antibiotic	"Susceptible" Organism
Penicillin	H. influenzae, Yersinia pestis
TMP–SMX	Klebsiella, Enterococci, Bartonella
Polymyxin B	Proteus, Salmonella
Imipenem	Stenotrophomonas maltophilia[2]
Gentamicin	Mycobacterium tuberculosis
Vancomycin	Erysipelothrix rhusiopathiae
Aminoglycosides	Streptococci, Salmonella, Shigella
Clindamycin	Fusobacteria, Clostridia, enterococci, Listeria
Macrolides	P. multocida
1st, 2nd generation cephalosporins	Salmonella, Shigella, Bartonella
3rd, 4th generation cephalosporins[4]	Enterococci, Listeria, Bartonella
All antibiotics	MRSA[3]

1. *In vitro* susceptibility *does not* predict *in vivo* activity; susceptibility data cannot be relied upon to guide therapy for antibiotic-organism combinations in this table.
2. Formerly Pseudomonas.
3. In spite of apparent *in vitro* susceptibility of antibiotics against MRSA, only vancomycin, minocycline, quinupristin/dalfopristin, linezolid, daptomycin, ceftaroline fosamil (ABSSSI only), telavancin, and tigecycline are effective *in vivo*.
4. Cefoperazone is the only cephalosporin with clinically useful anti-enterococcal activity against E. faecalis (VSE), *not* E. faecium (VRE).

4. **Unusual susceptibility patterns.** Organisms have predictable susceptibility patterns to antibiotics. When an isolate has an unusual susceptibility pattern (i.e., isolate of a species is inconsistent with its usual susceptibility pattern) (Table 1.3), further testing should be performed by the microbiology laboratory. Expanded susceptibility testing may be warranted.

Table 1.3. Unusual Susceptibility Patterns Requiring Further Testing

Organism	Unusual Susceptibility Patterns	Usual Susceptibility Patterns
Neisseria meningitidis	Penicillin resistant	Penicillin susceptible
Staphylococci	Vancomycin/clindamycin resistant; erythromycin susceptible	Vancomycin susceptible
Viridans streptococci	Vancomycin intermediate/resistant	Vancomycin susceptible
S. pneumoniae	Vancomycin intermediate/resistant	Vancomycin susceptible
β-hemolytic streptococci	Penicillin intermediate/resistant	Penicillin susceptible
Enterobacteriaceae	Imipenem resistant	Imipenem susceptible
E. coli, P. mirabilis, Klebsiella	Cefoxitin/cefotetan resistant	2nd generation cephalosporin susceptible
Enterobacter, Serratia	Ampicillin/cefazolin susceptible	Ampicillin/cefazolin resistant
Morganella, Providencia	Ampicillin/cefazolin susceptible	Ampicillin/cefazolin resistant
Klebsiella	Cefotetan susceptible; ceftazidime resistant	Cefotetan resistant; ceftazidime susceptible
P. aeruginosa	Amikacin resistant; gentamicin/ tobramycin susceptible	Amikacin susceptible; gentamicin/ tobramycin resistant
Stenotrophomonas maltophilia	TMP–SMX resistant; imipenem susceptible	TMP–SMX susceptible

Isolates with unusual susceptibility patterns require further testing by the microbiology laboratory to verify the identity of the isolate and characterize resistance mechanism. Expanded susceptibility testing is indicated.

Table 1.4. Susceptibility Patterns of Multi-Drug Resistant Organisms (MDROs) and Extended-Spectrum β-Lactamase (ESBL) Organisms*

MDROs & ESBL Resistance Profiles

Resistance Profiles
- MDRO Acinetobacter sp. **resistant to ciprofloxacin and amikacin and ceftazidime**
- MDRO *Pseudomonas aeruginosa* **resistant to amikacin and meropenem**
- ESBL *Klebsiella oxytoca* **resistant to ceftazidime**
- ESBL *Klebsiella pneumoniae* **resistant to ceftazidime**
- ESBL *Enterobacter sp.* **resistant to ceftazidime**
- ESBL *Escherichia coli* **resistant to ceftazidime**
- ESBL *Proteus mirabilis* **resistant to ceftazidime**

* Most common ESBL producing organisms *Klebsiella, Enterobacter, E. coli.*

C. **Susceptibility Breakpoints for Streptococcus pneumoniae.** Because antibiotic susceptibility is, in part, concentration related, the Clinical and Laboratory Standards Institute (CLSI), formerly the National Committee for Clinical Laboratory Standards (NCCLS), has revised its breakpoints for S. pneumoniae susceptibility testing, which differentiate between meningeal and non-meningeal sites of pneumococcal infection (Table 1.5).

Table 1.5. CLSI Susceptibility Breakpoints for Streptococcus pneumoniae*

Antibiotic	MIC (mcg/mL)		
	Sensitive	Intermediate	Resistant
Amoxicillin (non-meningitis)	≤ 2	4	≥ 8
Amoxicillin-clavulanic acid (non-meningitis)	≤ 2/1	4/2	≥ 8/4
Penicillin (meningitis)	≤ 0.06	–	≥ 0.12
Penicillin (non-meningitis)	≤ 2	4	≥ 8
Azithromycin	≤ 0.5	1	≥ 2
Clarithromycin/erythromycin	≤ 0.25	0.5	≥ 1
Doxycycline/tetracycline	≤ 2	4	≥ 8
Telithromycin	≤ 1	2	≥ 4
Cefaclor	≤ 1	2	≥ 4
Cefdinir/cefpodoxime	≤ 0.5	1	≥ 2
Cefprozil	≤ 2	4	≥ 8
Cefuroxime axetil (oral)	≤ 1	2	≥ 4
Loracarbef	≤ 2	4	≥ 8
Cefepime (non-meningitis)	≤ 1	2	≥ 4

Table 1.5. CLSI Susceptibility Breakpoints for Streptococcus pneumoniae* (cont'd)

Antibiotic	MIC (mcg/mL)		
	Sensitive	Intermediate	Resistant
Cefepime (meningitis)	≤ 0.5	1	≥ 2
Cefotaxime (non-meningitis)	≤ 1	2	≥ 4
Cefotaxime (meningitis)	≤ 0.5	1	≥ 2
Ceftriaxone (non-meningitis)	≤ 1	2	≥ 4
Ceftriaxone (meningitis)	≤ 0.5	1	≥ 2
Imipenem	≤ 0.12	0.25–0.5	≥ 1
Meropenem	≤ 0.25	0.5	≥ 1
Ertapenem	≤ 1	2	≥ 4
Vancomycin	≤ 1	–	–
Moxifloxacin	≤ 1	2	≥ 4
Levofloxacin	≤ 2	4	≥ 8
TMP–SMX	≤ 0.5/9.5	1/19–2/38	≥ 4/78
Chloramphenicol	≤ 4	–	≥ 8
Clindamycin	≤ 0.25	0.5	≥ 1
Linezolid	≤ 2	–	–
Rifampin	≤ 1	2	≥ 4

CLSI = Clinical and Laboratory Standards Institute (formerly NCCLS = National Committee for Clinical Laboratory Standards) M100–S20 (2010).

* *Testing Conditions:* Medium: Mueller-Hinton broth with 2.5% lysed horse blood (cation-adjusted). Inoculum: colony suspension. Incubation: 35°C (20–24 hours).

D. Summary. In vitro susceptibility testing is useful in most situations, but should not be followed blindly. Many factors need to be considered when interpreting in vitro microbiologic data, and infectious disease consultation is recommended for all but the most straightforward susceptibility interpretation problems. IV-to-PO switch changes using antibiotics of the same or other antibiotic class is best made when the oral antibiotic can achieve similar blood/tissue levels as the IV antibiotic. For example, IV-to-PO switch from cefazolin 1 gm (IV) to cephalexin 500 mg (PO) may not be effective against all pathogens at all sites, since cephalexin 500 mg (PO) achieves much lower serum concentrations compared to cefazolin 1 gm (IV) (16 mcg/mL vs. 200 mcg/mL).

OTHER CONSIDERATIONS IN ANTIMICROBIAL THERAPY

A. **Bactericidal vs. Bacteriostatic Therapy.** For most infections, bacteriostatic and bactericidal antibiotics inhibit/kill organisms at the same rate, and **should not be a factor in antibiotic selection**. Bactericidal antibiotics have an advantage in certain infections, such endocarditis, meningitis, and febrile leukopenia, but there are exceptions even in these cases.

B. **Monotherapy vs. Combination Therapy. Monotherapy is preferred to combination therapy for nearly all infections.** In addition to cost savings, monotherapy results in less chance of medication error and fewer missed doses/drug interactions. Combination therapy may be useful for drug synergy or for extending spectrum beyond what can be obtained with a single drug. However, since drug synergy is difficult to assess and the possibility of antagonism always exists, antibiotics should be combined for synergy if synergy is based on actual testing. Combination therapy is not effective in preventing antibiotic resistance, except in very few situations (Table 1.6).

Table 1.6. Combination Therapy and Antibiotic Resistance

Examples of Antibiotic Combinations That Prevent Resistance
Anti-pseudomonal penicillin (carbenicillin) + aminoglycoside (gentamicin, tobramycin, amikacin)
Rifampin + other TB drugs (INH, ethambutol, pyrazinamide)
5-flucytosine + amphotericin B

Examples of Antibiotic Combinations That Do Not Prevent Resistance*
TMP–SMX
Aztreonam + ceftazidime
Cefepime + ciprofloxacin
Aminoglycoside + imipenem
Most other antibiotic combinations

---

*   These combinations are often prescribed to prevent resistance when, in actuality, they do not.

C. **Intravenous vs. Oral Switch Therapy.** Patients admitted to the hospital are usually started on IV antibiotic therapy, then switched to equivalent oral therapy after clinical improvement/defervescence (usually within 72 hours). **Advantages of early IV-to-PO switch programs include reduced cost, early hospital discharge, less need for home IV therapy, and virtual elimination of IV line infections**. Drugs well-suited for IV-to-PO switch or for treatment entirely by the oral route include doxycycline, minocycline, clindamycin, metronidazole, chloramphenicol, amoxicillin, trimethoprim-sulfamethoxazole, quinolones, and linezolid.

Most infectious diseases should be treated orally unless the patient is critically ill, cannot take antibiotics by mouth, or there is no equivalent oral antibiotic. If the patient is able to take/absorb oral antibiotics, there is no difference in clinical outcome using equivalent IV or PO antibiotics. It is more important to think in terms of antibiotic spectrum, bioavailability and tissue penetration, rather than route of administration. **Nearly all non-critically ill patients should be treated in part or entirely with oral antibiotics.** When switching from IV to PO therapy, **the oral antibiotic chosen should have the same spectrum/degree of activity against the presumed/known pathogen and achieve the same blood and tissue levels as the equivalent IV antibiotic** (Table 1.7).

Table 1.7. Bioavailability of Oral Antimicrobials

Bioavailability	Antimicrobials		
Excellent[1] (> 90%)	Amoxicillin Cephalexin Cefprozil Cefadroxil Clindamycin Quinolones	TMP TMP–SMX Doxycycline Minocycline Chloramphenicol Metronidazole	Linezolid Fluconazole Voriconazole Rifampin Isoniazid Pyrazinamide Cycloserine
Good[2] (60–90%)	Cefixime Cefpodoxime Ceftibuten Cefuroxime	Valacyclovir Famciclovir Valganciclovir Macrolides Cefaclor Nitrofurantoin	Ethambutol 5-Flucytosine Posaconazole Itraconazole (solution) Nitazoxanide (with food)
Poor[3] (< 60%)	Vancomycin Acyclovir	Cefdinir Cefditoren	Nitazoxanide (without food) Fosfomycin

1. Oral administration results in *equivalent blood/tissue levels* as the same dose given IV (PO = IV).
2. Oral administration results in *lower but effective blood/tissue levels* than the same dose given IV (PO < IV).
3. Oral administration results in *suboptimal blood/tissue levels*.

D. Duration of Therapy. Most bacterial infections in normal hosts are treated with antibiotics for 1–2 weeks. The duration of therapy may need to be extended in patients with impaired immunity e.g., diabetes, SLE, alcoholic liver disease, neutropenia, diminished splenic function, etc., chronic bacterial infections e.g., endocarditis, osteomyelitis, chronic viral and fungal infections, or certain bacterial intracellular pathogens (Table 1.8). Infections such as HIV may require life-long therapy. Antibiotic therapy should ordinarily not be continued for more than 2 weeks, even if low-grade fevers persist (Table 1.8). Prolonged therapy offers no benefit, and increases the risk of adverse side effects, drug interactions, and superinfections.

Table 1.8. Infectious Diseases Requiring Prolonged Antimicrobial Therapy

Therapy	Infectious Diseases
3 weeks	Lymphogranuloma venereum (LGV), syphilis (late latent), H. pylori, chronic prostatitis
4 weeks	Chronic otitis media, chronic sinusitis, acute osteomyelitis, chronic pyelonephritis, brain abscess, SBE
4–6 weeks	Acute bacterial endocarditis (S. aureus, listeria, enterococcal), chronic osteomyelitis[4]
3 months	Lung abscess[1], meliodosis, bartonella
6 months	Pulmonary TB, extrapulmonary TB, actinomycosis[2], nocardia[3], prosthetic-related infections[5]
12 months	Whipple's disease
> 12 months	Lepromatous leprosy, HIV, Q fever (SBE/PVE)

1. Treat until resolved or until chest x-ray is normal/nearly normal and remains unchanged.
2. May require longer treatment; treat until resolved.
3. May require longer treatment in compromised hosts.
4. Adequate surgical debridement is required for cure.
5. Implanted foreign materials associated with infection (prosthetic valves, vascular grafts, joint replacements, hemodialysis shunts) should be removed as soon as possible after diagnosis. If removal is not feasible, then chronic suppressive therapy may be attempted, although clinical failure is the rule.

EMPIRIC ANTIBIOTIC THERAPY

Microbiology susceptibility data are not ordinarily available prior to initial treatment with antibiotics. Empiric therapy is based on directing coverage against the most likely pathogens, and takes into consideration drug allergy history, hepatic/renal function, possible antibiotic side effects, resistance potential, and cost. If a patient is moderately or severely ill, empiric therapy is usually initiated intravenously. Patients who are mildly ill, whether hospitalized or ambulatory, may be started on oral antibiotics with high bioavailability. Cultures of appropriate clinical specimens e.g., blood, sputum, urine should be obtained prior to starting empiric therapy to provide bacterial isolates for in vitro susceptibility testing. Empiric therapy for common infectious diseases is described in Chapter 2.

ANTIBIOTIC FAILURE

There are many possible causes of *apparent* antibiotic failure, including drug fever, antibiotic-unresponsive infections, and febrile noninfectious diseases. The most common error in the management of apparent antibiotic failure is changing/adding additional antibiotics instead of determining the cause (Tables 1.9, 1.10).

Table 1.9. Causes of Apparent/Actual Antibiotic Failure

Microbiologic Factors
- *In vitro* susceptibility but ineffective *in vivo*
- Antibiotic tolerance with gram-positive cocci
- Treating colonization (not infection)

Antibiotic Factors
- Inadequate coverage/spectrum
- Inadequate antibiotic blood levels
- Inadequate antibiotic tissue levels
- Decreased antibiotic activity in tissue
- Drug-drug interactions
    - Antibiotic inactivation
    - Antibiotic antagonism

Antibiotic Penetration Problems
- Undrained abscess
- Foreign body-related infection
- Protected focus e.g., cerebrospinal fluid
- Organ hypoperfusion/diminished blood supply
    - Chronic osteomyelitis
    - Chronic pyelonephritis

Noninfectious Diseases
- Medical disorders mimicking infection e.g., SLE
- Drug fever

Antibiotic-unresponsive Infectious Diseases
- Viral infections
- Fungal infections

Table 1.10. Clinical Features of Drug Fever

History

Many but not all individuals are atopic

Patients have been on a sensitizing medication for days or years "without a problem"

Physical exam

Relative bradycardia (see p. 14)

Fevers may be low- or high-grade, but usually range between 102°–104°F and may exceed 106°F

Patient appears "inappropriately well" for degree of fever

Laboratory tests

Elevated WBC count (usually with left shift)

Eosinophils almost always present, but eosinophilia is uncommon

Elevated erythrocyte sedimentation rate in majority of cases

Early, transient, mild elevations of serum transaminases (common)

Negative blood cultures (excluding contaminants)

Relative Bradycardia*
Temperature-Pulse Relationships

Temperature	Appropriate Pulse Response (beats/min)	If Relative Bradycardia Pulse (beats/min)
106°F (41.1°C)	150	< 140
105°F (40.6°C)	140	< 130
104°F (40.7°C)	130	< 120
103°F (39.4°C)	120	< 110
102°F (38.9°C)	110	< 100

*   Relative bradycardia refers to heart rates that are inappropriately slow relative to body temperature (pulse
    must be taken simultaneously with temperature elevation). Applies to adult patients with temperature
    ≥ 102°F; does not apply to patients with second/third-degree heart block, pacemaker-induced rhythms,
    or those taking beta-blockers, diltiazem, or verapamil.

METHICILLIN-RESISTANT STAPHYLOCOCCUS AUREUS (MRSA)

MRSA infections occur most commonly in hospitals and healthcare settings, e.g., nursing
homes, dialysis centers but can occur in the community setting as well. MRSA infections
are classified as hospital-acquired (HA-MRSA), community-onset (CO-MRSA), or community-
acquired (CA-MRSA), which has implications for therapy (Table 1.11).

Table 1.11. Classification of MRSA Infections

MRSA Strain	Epidemiology & Microbiology	Therapy
Hospital *acquired* MRSA (HA-MRSA)*	Strains *originate within the hospital*, have SCC *mec* I,II,III genes, PVL+ (rare), and elaborate several S. aureus toxins.	Resistant to most antibiotics. Only vancomycin, quinupristin/ dalfopristin, minocycline, linezolid, tigecycline, or daptomycin are *reliably* effective.
Community *onset* MRSA (CO-MRSA)*	Strains *originate in the hospital and later present from community*, have SCC *mec* I,II,III genes, PVL+ (rare) and elaborate several S. aureus toxins.	CO-MRSA strains are have the *same antibiotic susceptibility* as HA-MRSA strains and *should be treated as HA-MRSA.*

PVL = Panton-Valentine Leukocidin.
*CO-MRSA = HA-MRSA.

Table 1.11. Classification of MRSA Infections (cont'd)

MRSA Strain	Epidemiology & Microbiology	Therapy
Community *acquired* MRSA (CA-MRSA)	*Only* MRSA infections "from the community" presenting as *severe pyomyositis or severe/ necrotizing community acquired MRSA pneumonia (with influenza)* should be considered as potentially due to CA-MRSA. *All other MRSA infections from the community should be clinically considered as CO-MRSA.* SCC *mec* IV, V genes. PVL+, (common). CA-MRSA PVL - Strains are *clinically indistinguishable* from MSSA or CO-MRSA. Elaborate the usual *S.aureus* toxins plus 18 other toxins.	CA-MRSA strains are susceptible to clindamycin, TMP–SMX, and doxycycline. Antibiotics used to treat CO-MRSA/HA-MRSA are also effective against CA-MRSA, but *not* vice versa.

PVL. = Panton-Valentine Leukocidin.
*CO-MRSA = HA-MRSA.
Adapted from: Cunha BA. Clinical Manifestations and Antimicrobial Therapy of Methicillin Resistant Staphylococcus aureus (MRSA). Clin Microbiol Infect 11:33–42, 2005 and Cunha BA: Simplified Clinical Approach to Community acquired MRSA (CA-MRSA) Infections. Journal of Hospital Infection 68:271–273, 2008.

PITFALLS IN ANTIBIOTIC PRESCRIBING

- **Use of antibiotics *to treat colonization or noninfectious/antibiotic-unresponsive infectious diseases.***

- **Overuse of combination therapy**. *Monotherapy is preferred over combination therapy unless compelling reasons prevail*, such as drug synergy or extended spectrum beyond what can be obtained with a single drug. *Monotherapy reduces the risk of drug interactions and side effects, and is usually less expensive.*

- **Use of antibiotics for persistent fevers**. For patients with persistent fevers on an antimicrobial regimens that appears to be failing, it is important to reassess the patient rather than add additional antibiotics. Causes of prolonged fevers include undrained septic foci, noninfectious medical disorders, and drug fevers. *Undiagnosed causes of leukocytosis/low-grade fevers should not be treated with prolonged courses of antibiotics.*

- **Inadequate surgical therapy**. Infections involving infected prosthetic materials or fluid collections e.g., abscesses often require surgical therapy for cure. *For infections such as chronic osteomyelitis, surgery is the only way to cure the infection*; antibiotics are useful only for suppression or to prevent local infectious complications.

- **Home IV therapy**. There is *less need to use home IV therapy given the vast array of excellent oral antibiotics* e.g., doxycycline, minocycline, quinolones, TMP–SMX, linezolid available.

REFERENCES AND SUGGESTED READINGS

Bosso JA, Mauldin PD, Salgado CD. The association between antibiotic use and resistance: the role of secondary antibiotics. Eur J Clin Microbiol. Infect Dis. 29:1125–1192, 2010.

Cunha BA. Oral Antibiotic Therapy of Serious Systemic Infections. Med Clin N Am 90:1197–1222, 2006.

Cunha BA. Pseudomonas aeruginosa: Resistance and therapy. Semin Respir Infect 17:231–9, 2002.

Cunha BA. Clinical relevance of penicillin-resistant Streptococcus pneumoniae. Semin Respir Infect 17:204–14, 2002.

Cunha BA. Effective antibiotic resistance and control strategies. Lancet 357:1307–1308, 2001.

Cunha BA. The significance of antibiotic false sensitivity testing with in vitro testing. J Chemother 9:25–33, 1997.

Cunha BA, Ortega A. Antibiotic failure. Medical Clinics of North America 79:663–672, 1995.

Empey KM, Rapp RP, Evans ME. The effect of an antimicrobial formulary change on hospital resistance patterns. Pharmacotherapy 22:81–7, 2002.

Endimiani A, Perez F, Bajaksouzian S, et al. Evaluation of updated interpretive criteria for categorizing Klebsiella pneumoniae with reduced carbapenem susceptibility. J Clin Microbiol. 48:4417–4425, 2010.

Hicks LA, Monnet DL, Roberts RM. Increase in pneumococcus macrolide resistance, USA. Emerg. Infect. Dis. 16:896–897, 2010.

Johnson DH, Cunha BA. Drug fever. Infectious Disease Clinics of North America 10:85–91, 1996.

Jorgensen JH, Ferraro MJ. Antimicrobial susceptibility testing: a review of general principles and contemporary practices. Clin Infect Dis 49:1749–1755, 2009.

Leekha S, Terrell CL, Edson RS. General principles of antimicrobial therapy. Mayo Clin. Proc. 86:156–167, 2011.

Patel SM, Saravolatz LD. Monotherapy versus combination therapy. Med Clin N Am 90:1183–95, 2006.

Riou M, Carbonnelle S, Avrain L, et al. In vivo development of an antimicrobial resistance in Pseudomonas aeruginosa strains isolated from the lower respiratory tract of intensive care unit patients with nosocomial pneumonia and receiving antipseudomonal therapy. Int J. Antimicrobial Agents. 36:513–522, 2010.

Schlossberg D. Clinical approach to antibiotic failure. Med Clin N Am 90:1265–77, 2006.

Tenover FC, Moellering RC. The rationale for revising the clinical and laboratory standards institute vancomycin minimal inhibitory concentration interpretive criteria for Staphylococcus aureus. Clinical Infect Dis 44:1208–1215, 2007.

Weinstein MP, Klugman KP, Jones RN. Rationale for revised penicillin susceptibility breakpoints versus Streptococcus pneumoniae: coping with antimicrobial susceptibility in an era of resistance. Clin Infect Dis 48:1596–1600, 2009.

TEXTBOOKS

Anaissie EJ, McGinnis MR, Pfaller MA (eds). Clinical Mycology. Churchill Livingstone, New York, 2003.

Baddour L,Gorbach SL (eds). Therapy of Infectious Diseases. Saunders, Philadelphia, 2003.

Bryskier A (ed). Antimicrobial Agents. ASM Press, Washington, D.C., 2005.

Chadwick DJ, Goode J (eds). Antibiotic Resistance: Origins, Evolution, Selection and Spread. John Wiley & Sons, New York, 1997.

Cohen J, Powderly WG. Infectious Diseases (2nd ed.). Philadelphia: Elsevier, 2004.

Finch RG, Greenwood D, Norrby SR, Whitley RJ (eds). Antibiotic and Chemotherapy, 8th Edition. Churchill Livingstone, Edinburgh, 2003.

Gorbach SL, Bartlett JG, Blacklow NR (eds). Infectious Diseases, 3rd Edition. Philadelphia, Lippincott, Williams & Wilkins, 2004.

Grayson ML (ed). Kucers' The Use of Antibiotics, 6th Edition, ASM Press, Washington, DC, 2010.

Mandell GL, Bennett JE, Dolin R (eds). Mandell, Douglas, and Bennett's Principles and Practice of Infectious Diseases, 7th Edition. Philadelphia Elsevier Churchill Livingstone, 2010.

O'Grady F, Lambert HP, Finch RG, Greenwood D (eds). Antibiotic and Chemotherapy, 2nd Edition. Churchill Livingston, New York, 1997.

Ristuccia AM, Cunha BA (eds). Antimicrobial Therapy. Raven Press, New York, 1984.

Scholar EM Pratt WB (eds). The Antimicrobial Drugs, 2nd Edition, Oxford University Press, New York, 2000.

Schlossberg D (ed). Clinical Infectious Disease. Cambridge University Press, Cambridge, 2008.

Yoshikawa TT, Rajagopalan S (eds). Antibiotic Therapy for Geriatric Patients. Taylor & Francis, New York, 2006.

Yu V, Edwards G, McKinnon PS, Peloquin C, Morse G (eds). Antimicrobial Therapy and Vaccines, Volume II: Antimicrobial Agents, 2nd Edition. Esun Technologies, Pittsburgh, 2005.

Chapter 2

Empiric Therapy Based on Clinical Syndrome

Burke A. Cunha, MD, John L. Brusch, MD, Ronald L. Nichols, MD
Genovefa Papanicolaou, MD, Jean E. Hage, MD
Raymond S. Koff, MD, John H. Rex, MD, Dennis J. Cleri, MD
Cheston B. Cunha, MD, Staci A. Fischer, MD
David Schlossberg, MD

This chapter is organized by clinical syndrome, patient subset, and in some cases, specific organism. Clinical summaries immediately follow each treatment grid. Unless otherwise specified, **this chapter pertains to infectious diseases and antimicrobial agents in adults. For pediatric infectious diseases and antimicrobial therapy see chapter 7.** Therapeutic recommendations are based on antimicrobial effectiveness, reliability, cost, safety, and resistance potential. The antimicrobial dosages in this section represent the usual dosages for normal renal and hepatic function in adults. For any treatment category (i.e., preferred IV therapy, alternate IV therapy, PO therapy), *in any given grid category drugs listed are equivalent alternatives and not ranked.* Dosage adjustments, side effects, drug interactions, and other important prescribing information are described in the individual drug summaries in Chapter 11. Use of any drug should be preceded by careful review of the package insert, which provides indications and dosing approved by the U.S. Food and Drug Administration. *"IV-to-PO Switch"* in the last column of the shaded title bar in each treatment grid indicates the clinical syndrome should be treated either by IV therapy alone or IV followed by PO therapy, but *not* by PO therapy alone. *"PO Therapy or IV-to-PO Switch"* indicates the clinical syndrome can be treated by IV therapy alone, PO therapy alone, or IV followed by PO therapy (unless otherwise indicated in the footnotes under each treatment grid). Most patients on IV therapy should be switched to PO equivalent therapy after clinical improvement.

Empiric Therapy of CNS Infections

Acute Bacterial Meningitis (ABM) (see Color Atlas for CSF Gram stains)

Subset	Usual Pathogens	Preferred IV Therapy	Alternate IV Therapy	IV-to-PO Switch
Normal host	N. meningitidis H. influenzae S. pneumoniae	Ceftriaxone 2 gm (IV) q12h × 2 weeks	Meropenem 2 gm (IV) q8h × 2 weeks **or** Cefotaxime 3 gm (IV) q6h × 2 weeks **or** Ceftizoxime 3 gm (IV) q6h × 2 weeks	Chloramphenicol 500 mg (PO) q6h × 2 weeks
Elderly or malignancy	Listeria monocytogenes plus usual meningeal pathogens in normal hosts	Before culture results Ceftriaxone 2 gm (IV) q12h × 3 weeks **plus** Ampicillin 2 gm (IV) q4h × 3 weeks After culture results *Listeria present* Ampicillin 2 gm (IV) q4h × 3 weeks *Listeria not present* Treat as normal host	After culture results *Listeria present* TMP–SMX 5 mg/kg (IV) q6h × 3 weeks **or** Meropenem 2 gm (IV) q8h × 3 weeks **or** Chloramphenicol 500 mg (IV) q6h × 3 weeks **or** Linezolid 600 mg (IV) q12h × 3 weeks *Listeria not present* Treat as for normal host, above	For Listeria meningitis only TMP–SMX 5 mg/ kg (PO) q6h × 3 weeks **or** Chloramphenicol 500 mg (PO) q6h × 3 weeks **or** Linezolid 600 mg (PO) q12h × 3 weeks For usual meningeal pathogens Chloramphenicol 500 mg (PO) q6h × 3 weeks

Acute Bacterial Meningitis (ABM) (cont'd) (see Color Atlas for CSF Gram stains)

Subset	Usual Pathogens	Preferred IV Therapy	Alternate IV Therapy	IV-to-PO Switch
CNS shunt infections (VA shunts) (Treat initially for MSSA; if later identified as MRSA, MSSE, or MRSE, treat accordingly)	S. aureus S. epidermidis (coagulase-negative staphylococci) CoNS	<u>MSSA/MSSE</u> Cefotaxime 3 gm (IV) q6h* **or** Ceftizoxime 3 gm (IV) q6h* <u>MRSA/MRSE</u> Linezolid 600 mg (IV) q12h*	<u>MSSA/MSSE</u> Cefepime 2 gm (IV) q8h* **or** Meropenem 2 gm (IV) q8h* <u>MRSA/MRSE</u> Vancomycin 2 gm (IV) q12h* **plus** 20 mg (IT) q24h until shunt removal	<u>MSSE/MRSE</u> Linezolid 600 mg (PO) q12h* <u>MSSA/MRSA</u> Minocycline 100 mg (PO) q12h* **or** Linezolid 600 mg (PO) q12h*
CNS shunt infections (VP shunts)	E. coli K. pneumoniae Enterobacter S. marcescens	Ceftriaxone 2 gm (IV) q12h × 2 weeks after shunt removal	TMP–SMX 5 mg/kg (IV) q6h × 2 weeks after shunt removal	TMP–SMX 5 mg/kg (PO) q6h × 2 weeks after shunt removal
	MDR P. aeruginosa	Meropenem 2 gm (IV) q8h ± Colistin 1.7 mg/kg (IV) q8h **plus** Colistin 10 mg (IT) q24h × 2 weeks after shunt removal	Meropenem 2 gm (IV) q8h ± Amikacin 1 gm (IV) q24h **plus** Amikacin 10 mg (IT) q24h × 2 weeks after shunt removal	
	MDR Acinetobacter baumanii	Meropenem 2 gm (IV) q8h **or** Ampicillin/sulbactam 4.5 gm (IV) q6h ± Colistin 1.7 mg/kg (IV) q8h **plus** Colistin 10 mg (IT) q12h × 2 weeks after shunt removal	Meropenem 2 gm (IV) q8h **plus** Ampicillin/sulbactam 4.5 gm (IV) q6h × 2 weeks after shunt removal	

MSSA/MRSA = methicillin-sensitive/resistant S. aureus; MSSE/MRSE = methicillin-sensitive/resistant S. epidermidis. Duration of therapy represents total time IV or IV + PO. Most patients on IV therapy able to take PO meds should be switched to PO therapy after clinical improvement.

MDR = multidrug-resistant. Duration of therapy represents total time IV or IV + PO. Most patients on IV therapy able to take PO meds should be switched to PO therapy after clinical improvement.

*   Treat for 1 week after shunt removal.

Clinical Presentation: Abrupt onset of fever, headache, stiff neck.
Diagnosis: CSF gram stain/culture.

Acute Bacterial Meningitis (Normal Hosts)

Diagnostic Considerations: Gram stain of centrifugated CSF is still the best diagnostic test. CSF antigen/CIE are unhelpful in establishing the diagnosis (many false-negatives). Blood cultures are positive for ABM pathogen in 80–90%. Typical CSF findings include a WBC count of 100–5000 cells/mm³, elevated opening pressure, elevated protein and lactic acid levels (> 4–6 mmol/L), and a positive CSF gram stain. If the WBC is extremely high (> 20,000 cells/mm³), suspect brain abscess with rupture into the ventricular system, and obtain a CT/MRI to confirm. S. pneumoniae meningitis is associated with cranial nerve abnormalities, mental status changes, and neurologic sequelae. With H. influenzae or S. pneumoniae meningitis, obtain a head CT/MRI to rule out other CNS pathology.
Pitfalls: If ABM is suspected, always perform lumbar puncture (LP) *before* obtaining a CT scan, since early antibiotic therapy is critical to prognosis. A CT/MRI should be obtained before LP *only* if a mass lesion/suppurative intracranial process is of primary concern, after blood cultures have been drawn. A stiff neck on physical examination has limited diagnostic value in the elderly, since nuchal rigidity may occur without meningitis (e.g., cervical arthritis) and meningitis may occur without nuchal rigidity. Recurrence of fever during the first week of H. influenzae meningitis is commonly due to subdural effusion, which usually resolves spontaneously over several days. Meningococcal meningitis may occur with or without meningococcemia. On gram stain, S. pneumoniae may be mistaken for H. influenzae, and Listeria may be mistaken for S. pneumoniae. Meningococcal meningitis may occur in those who received the meningococcal vaccine especially serogroup B not in meningococcal vaccine.
Therapeutic Considerations: Do not reduce meningeal antibiotic dosing as the patient improves. Repeat LP if the patient is not responding to antibiotics after 48 hours; lack of response may be due to therapeutic failure, relapse, or a Noninfectious CNS disorder. For S. pneumoniae meningitis, obtain penicillin MICs on all CSF isolates. Penicillin-resistant strains are susceptible to meningeal doses of beta-lactam antibiotics (e.g., ceftriaxone). All but the most highly penicillin-resistant pneumococci are still effectively treated with meningeal doses of beta-lactams. Highly resistant pneumococcal strains (rare in the CSF) may be treated for 2 weeks with meropenem 2 gm (IV) q8h, or, linezolid 600 mg (IV) q12h. Dexamethasone 0.15 mg/kg (IV) q6h × 4 days may be given to children with ABM to reduce the incidence/severity of neurologic sequelae, although the value of steroids in adult ABM is unclear; if used, give dexamethasone 30 minutes *before* the initial antibiotic dose.
Prognosis: Often fatal without treatment. Case-fatality rates in treated adults are 10–20%. Neurological deficits on presentation are associated with a poor prognosis. Permanent neurological deficits are more frequent with S. pneumoniae than H. influenzae, even with prompt therapy. In meningococcal meningitis with meningococcemia, prognosis is related to the number of petechiae, with few or no neurological deficits in survivors.

Acute Bacterial Meningitis (Elderly Malignancy)

Diagnostic Considerations: Diagnosis by CSF gram stain/culture. ABM pathogens include usual pathogens in normal hosts plus Listeria monocytogenes, a gram-positive, aerobic, bacillus. Listeria is the most common ABM pathogen in patients with malignancies, and is a common pathogen in the elderly. With Listeria meningitis, CSF cultures are positive in 100%, but CSF gram stain is negative in 50%. Meningeal carcinomatosis is suggested by multiple cranial nerve abnormalities.

Pitfalls: "Diphtheroids" isolated from CSF should be speciated to rule out Listeria. Listeria are motile and hemolytic on blood agar plate, diphtheroids are not.

Therapeutic Considerations: Elderly patients and cancer patients with ABM require empiric coverage of Listeria plus other common pathogens in normal hosts (N. meningitidis, H. influenzae, S. pneumoniae). Third-generation cephalosporins are not active against Listeria.

Prognosis: Related to underlying health of host.

Acute Bacterial Meningitis (CNS Shunt Infections)

Diagnostic Considerations: Diagnosis by CSF gram stain/culture. S. epidermidis meningitis usually occurs only with infected prosthetic implant material (e.g., CNS shunt).

Pitfalls: Blood cultures are usually negative for shunt pathogens. CSF P. acnes cultures usually represent skin contamination. P. acnes is rarely a CNS shunt pathogen.

Therapeutic Considerations: 15% of S. epidermidis strains are resistant to nafcillin/clindamycin. In addition to systemic antibiotics in meningeal doses, adjunctive intraventricular/intrathecal antibiotics are sometimes given to control shunt infections before shunt removal. If vancomycin is used to treat CNS S. aureus (MSSA/MRSA) infection, I.T. dosing needed in addition to IV therapy.

Prognosis: Good if prosthetic material is removed.

Acute Nonbacterial Meningitis/Chronic Meningitis

Subset	Usual Pathogens	Preferred IV Therapy	Alternate IV Therapy	PO Therapy or IV-to-PO Switch
Viral (aseptic)	EBV, LCM, Parvo B19, mumps, Enteroviruses, WNE. No effective therapy for most. For HIV (see Chapter 5)			
	HSV-1 HSV-2	<u>IV Therapy:</u> Acyclovir 10 mg/kg (IV) q8h × 10 days **or** Ganciclovir 5 mg/kg (IV) q12h × 10 days. IV → PO: Valacyclovir 1 gm (PO) q8h × 10 days		
	VZV	Acyclovir 10 mg/kg (IV) q8h × 10 days. IV → PO: Valacyclovir 2 gm (PO) q6h × 10 days		
	HHV-6	<u>Ganciclovir:</u> 5 mg/kg (IV) of 12h × 2 weeks **or** Foscarnet 90 mg/kg (IV) q12h × 2 weeks		
Primary amebic meningo-encephalitis	Naegleria fowleri	Amphotericin B deoxycholate 1 mg/kg (IV) q24h until cured **plus** Amphotericin B deoxycholate 1 mg into ventricles via Ommaya reservoir q24h until cured		
Lyme neuro-borreliosis	Borrelia burgdorferi	Ceftriaxone 1 gm (IV) q12h × 2 weeks **or** Minocycline 100 mg (IV) q12h × 2 weeks **or** Doxycycline 200 mg (IV) q12h × 3 days, then 100 mg (IV) q12h × 11 days		Minocycline 100 mg (PO) q12h × 2 weeks **or** Doxycycline 200 mg (PO) q12h × 3 days, then 100 mg (PO) q12h × 11 days (loading dose not needed PO if given IV with same drug)

Acute Nonbacterial Meningitis/Chronic Meningitis (cont'd)

Subset	Usual Pathogens	Preferred IV Therapy	Alternate IV Therapy	PO Therapy or IV-to-PO Switch
Granulomatous amebic meningoencephalitis	Acanthamoeba	No proven treatment (amphotericin B, fluconazole, ketoconazole, itraconazole, flucytosine, rifampin, isoniazid, aminoglycosides, sulfonamides, pentamidine mostly with little success. Success reported in transplant recipient with IV pentamidine followed by itraconazole, and in AIDS patient with ketoconazole plus flucytosine)		
Neurobrucellosis	Brucella sp.	Ceftriaxone 2 gm (IV) q12h **plus** Doxycycline 100 mg (PO) q12h **plus** Rifampin 600 mg (PO) q24h × 4 weeks, then Doxycycline **plus** Rifampin (same doses) × 4 weeks		
TB	M. tuberculosis	INH 300 mg (IV/PO) q24h × 6 months **plus** Rifampin 600 mg (IV/PO) q24h × 6 months **plus** PZA 25 mg/kg (PO) q24h × 2 months **plus** EMB 15 mg/kg (PO) q24h (until susceptibilities known)		
		Begin with 4 drugs, as for pulmonary TB, but extend treatment for 9–12 months. Corticosteroids tapered over 1–2 months is helpful. If resistance is demonstrated or suspected, ID consultation is advised		
Fungal *Non-HIV*	Cryptococcus neoformans	Amphotericin B 0.7–1 mg/kg (IV) q24h × 2–6 weeks* **plus** Flucytosine 25 mg/kg (PO) q6h × 6 weeks*, **followed by** Fluconazole 800 mg (IV or PO) × 1 dose, then 400 mg (PO) q24h × 10 weeks*	Liposomal amphotericin B (AmBisome) 6 mg/kg (IV) q24h × 6–10 weeks† **or** Fluconazole 800 mg (IV or PO) × 1 dose, then 400 mg (PO) q24h × 10 weeks*	<u>PO therapy alone</u> Fluconazole may be given PO*
HIV	Cryptococcus neoformans (see p. 329) Blastomyces dermatitidis (see p. 269)			
Chronic meningitis	Coccidioidomycosis (see p. 271), Histoplasmosis (see p. 269), Neurocysticercosis (see p. 262)			Do not treat empirically

Duration of therapy represents total time PO (for TB), IV, or IV + PO.

*   The 6-week amphotericin B deoxycholate plus flucytosine regimen is the classical approach to achieving a durable cure. Anecdotal data suggest that a shorter course followed by Fluconazole × 10 weeks (or longer) may be successful. ID consultation is advised.

†   Other lipid-associated Amphotericin B formulations at 3–5 mg/kg (IV) q24h may also be used (p. 525).

‡   Levofloxacin 500 mg or Moxifloxacin 400 mg.

Viral (Aseptic) Meningitis

Clinical Presentation: Headache, low-grade fever, mild meningismus, photophobia.

Diagnostic Considerations: Diagnosis by specific serological tests/viral culture. HSV-2 genital infections are often accompanied by mild CNS symptoms, which usually do not require anti-viral therapy. HSV-1 causes a variety of CNS infections, including meningitis, meningoencephalitis, and encephalitis (most common; see p. 25). HSV HHV-6, and WNE meningitis is indistinguishable clinically from other causes of viral meningitis. EBV meningitis is usually associated with clinical/laboratory features of EBV infectious mononucleosis; suspect the diagnosis in a patient with a positive mono-spot and unexplained meningoencephalitis. VZV meningitis is typically associated with cutaneous vesicular lesions (H. zoster), and usually does not require additional therapy beyond that given for shingles. LCM meningitis begins as a "flu-like" illness usually in the fall after hamster contact, and may have low CSF glucose. Enterovirus meningitis is often associated with a maculopapular rash, non-exudative pharyngitis, diarrhea, and rarely low CSF glucose. Aseptic meningitis due to mumps may present without parotid swelling ± acute deafness. Drug induced aseptic meningitis may have eosinophils in the CSF and little/no fever.

Pitfalls: Consider NSAIDs, TMP–SMX, and IV immunoglobulin as causes of drug induced aseptic meningitis.

Therapeutic Considerations: Treat specific pathogen.

Prognosis: Without neurological deficits, full recovery is the rule.

Primary Amebic Meningoencephalitis (PAM) (Naegleria fowleri)

Clinical Presentation: Acquired by freshwater exposure containing the protozoa, often by jumping into a lake/pool. Affects healthy children/young adults. Organism penetrates cribriform plate and enters CSF. Symptoms occur within 7 days of exposure and may be indistinguishable from fulminant bacterial meningitis, including headache, fever, anorexia, vomiting, signs of meningeal inflammation, altered mental status, coma. May complain of unusual smell/taste sensations early in infection. CSF has RBCs and very low glucose.

Diagnostic Considerations: Diagnosis by demonstrating organism in CSF. Worldwide distribution. Free-living freshwater amoeba flourish in warmer climates. Key to diagnosis rests on clinical suspicion based on history of freshwater exposure in previous 1–2 weeks.

Pitfalls: CSF findings resemble bacterial meningitis, but RBCs present.

Therapeutic Considerations: Often fatal despite early treatment.

Prognosis: Frequently fatal.

Granulomatous Amebic Meningoencephalitis (Acanthamoeba sp.)

Clinical Presentation: Insidious onset with focal neurologic deficits ± mental status changes, seizures, fever, headache, hemiparesis, meningismus, ataxia, visual disturbances. May be associated with Acanthamoeba keratoconjunctivitis, skin ulcers, or disseminated disease. Usually seen only in immunocompromised/debilitated patients.

Diagnostic Considerations: Diagnosis by demonstrating organism in brain biopsy specimen. CT/MRI shows mass lesions. "Stellate cysts" characteristic of Acanthamoeba. Worldwide distribution. Strong association with extended wear of contact lenses. Differentiate from N. fowleri by culture.

Pitfalls: Not associated with freshwater exposure, unlike primary amebic meningoencephalitis (Naegleria fowleri). Resembles subacute/chronic meningitis. No trophozoites in CSF. Skin lesions may be present for months before onset of CNS symptoms.

Therapeutic Considerations: No proven treatment. Often fatal despite early treatment.
Prognosis: Usually fatal.

Neuroborreliosis (CNS Lyme Disease)

Clinical Presentation: May have mild neck stiffness not frank nucal rigidity. Low grade fever < 102°F usually ~ 100–101°F. Recent tick exposure. Often without rash. Sore throat in some, WBC count WNL, mildly ↑ AST/ALT in some.

Diagnostic Considerations: Diagnosed by demonstrating B. burgdorferi antibody production in the CNS. A CSF-to-serum IgM Lyme titer ratio > 1:1 is diagnostic.

Pitfalls: If CNS symptoms present with acute Lyme disease, rash may be absent and serology may be negative early. Neuroborreliosis cannot be reliably diagnosed using CSF-to-serum IgM if antibiotics given before the LP (antibiotics change the ratio and render it useless).

Therapeutic Considerations:

Prognosis: Related to underlying health of host. Prognosis with neuroborreliosis is good even with delayed treatment.

TB Meningitis (Mycobacterium tuberculosis)

Clinical Presentation: Subacute onset of nonspecific symptoms. Fever usually present ± headache, nausea, vomiting. Acute presentation and cranial nerve palsies uncommon.

Diagnostic Considerations: Diagnosis by CSF AFB smear/culture; PCR of CSF is specific but not very sensitive. CSF may be normal but usually shows a mild lymphocytic pleocytosis, ↓ glucose, ↑ protein, and few RBCs. Adenosine deaminase (ADA) levels ↑.

Pitfalls: CSF may have PMN predominance early, before developing typical lymphocytic predominance. Eosinophils in CSF is not a feature of TB, and should suggest another diagnosis. Chest x-ray, PPD, and CSF smear/culture may be negative. ADA levels more highly elevated in TB than in ABM, listeria, neurobrucellosis.

Therapeutic Considerations: Dexamethasone 4 mg (IV or PO) q6h × 4–8 weeks is useful to reduce CSF inflammation if given early. Proteinaceous TB exudates may obstruct ventricles and cause hydrocephalus, which is diagnosed by CT/MRI and may require shunting.

Prognosis: Poor prognostic factors include delay in treatment, neurologic deficits, or hydrocephalus.

Fungal (Cryptococcal) Meningitis (Cryptococcus neoformans)

Clinical Presentation: Insidious onset of nonspecific symptoms. Headache most common. Chronic cases may have CNS symptoms for weeks to months with intervening asymptomatic periods. Acute manifestations are more common in AIDS, chronic steroid therapy, lymphoreticular malignancies. 50–80% of patients are abnormal hosts.

Diagnostic Considerations: C. neoformans is the most common cause of fungal meningitis, and the only encapsulated yeast in the CSF to cause meningitis. Diagnosis by CSF India ink preparations showing encapsulated yeasts/cryptococcal latex antigen by latex agglutination/culture. Rule out HIV and other underlying immunosuppressive diseases.

Pitfalls: False + crytococcal antigen may occur with BBL Port-A-Cul transport vials. CSF latex antigen titer may not return to zero. Continue treatment until titers decline/do not decrease further, and until CSF culture is negative for cryptococci. India ink preparations showing encapsulated yeasts of CSF are useful for initial infection, but should not be relied on to diagnose recurrent episodes, since smears may be positive despite negative CSF cultures (dead cryptococci may remain in CSF for years). Diagnosis of recurrences rests on CSF culture.

Therapeutic Considerations: Treat until CSF is sterile or CSF latex antigen titer is zero or remains near zero on serial lumbar punctures. After patient defervesces on amphotericin B/5FC, switch to oral fluconazole × 10 weeks. Lipid amphotericin may be used if amphotericin B cannot be tolerated. HIV patients require life-long suppressive therapy with fluconazole 200 mg (PO) q24h. Expert consultation is strongly advised.

Prognosis: Good. Poor prognostic factors include no CSF pleocytosis, many organisms in CSF, and altered consciousness on admission.

Encephalitis

Subset	Usual Pathogens	IV-to-PO Switch		
Herpes simplex	HSV-1 HSV-2	<u>IV Therapy:</u> Acyclovir 10 mg/kg (IV) q8h × 10 days **or** Ganciclovir 5 mg/kg (IV) q12h × 10 days. IV → PO: Valacyclovir 1 gm (PO) q8h × 10 days		
Herpes zoster (VZV)	VZV	Acyclovir (IV) q8h 10 mg/kg × 10 days. IV → PO: Valacyclovir 2 gm (PO) q6h × 10 days		
	HHV-6	Ganciclovir 5 mg/kg (IV) q12h × 2 weeks **or** Foscarnet 90 mg/kg (IV) q12h × 2 weeks		
Arbovirus	<u>Mosquito borne:</u> California encephalitis (CE), Western equine encephalitis (WEE), Venezuelan equine encephalitis (VEE), Eastern equine encephalitis (EEE), St. Louis encephalitis (St. LE), Japanese encephalitis (JE), West Nile encephalitis (WNE) <u>Tick borne:</u> Powassan (PE), TBE (RSSE/CCE) <u>IV/PO Therapy:</u> None			
Mycoplasma	M. pneumoniae	Doxycycline 200 mg (IV) q12h × 3 days, then 100 mg (IV) q12h × 2 weeks	Minocycline 100 mg (IV) q12h × 2 weeks	Doxycycline 200 mg (PO) q12h × 3 days, then 100 mg (PO) q12h × 2 weeks* **or** Minocycline 100 mg (PO) q12h × 2 weeks
Listeria	L. monocytogenes	Treat as for Listeria meningitis (see p. 18) but treat for 6–8 weeks		
HIV	see Chapter 5 (p. 304)			
Transplants, HIV	CMV HHV-6 Toxoplasma gondii	Transplants (see p. 160) HIV (see p. 304)		

Duration of therapy represents total time IV or IV + PO. Most patients on IV therapy able to take PO meds should be switched to PO therapy after clinical improvement.
* Loading dose is not needed PO if given IV with the same drug.

Herpes Encephalitis (HSV-1)

Clinical Presentation: Acute onset of fever and change in mental status without nuchal rigidity.

Diagnostic Considerations: EEG is best early (< 72 hours) presumptive test, showing unilateral temporal lobe abnormalities. Brain MRI is abnormal before CT scan, which may require several days before a temporal lobe focus is seen. Definitive diagnosis is by CSF PCR for HSV-1 DNA. Usually presents as encephalitis or meningoencephalitis; presentation as meningitis alone is uncommon. Profound decrease in sensorium is characteristic of HSV meningoencephalitis. CSF may have PMN predominance and low glucose levels, unlike other viral causes of meningitis.

Pitfalls: In normal hosts, HHV-6 may mimic HSV-1 encephalitis with a frontal/temporal focus on EEG.

Therapeutic Considerations: HSV is one of the treatable causes of viral encephalitis in normal hosts. Treat as soon as possible, since neurological deficits may be mild and reversible early on, but severe and irreversible later.

Prognosis: Related to extent of brain injury and early anti-HSV therapy.

Arboviral Encephalitis

Clinical Presentation: Acute onset of fever, headache, change/decrease in mental status days to weeks after insect bite (e.g., mosquito/tick). WNE is suggested by encephalitis ± with highly elevated ferritin levels ± new onset tremors or flaccid paralysis. EEG: diffuse slowing ± ↑ activity basal ganglia/thalamus. Prognosis ~ severity of neurologic deficits and degree/duration of relative lymphopenia/ferritin levels.

Diagnostic Considerations: Diagnosis by specific arboviral serology.

Pitfalls: Usually occurs in summer/fall. SIADH common, may occur.

Therapeutic Considerations: Only supportive therapy is available at present.

Prognosis: Permanent neurological deficits are common, but not predictable. May be fatal.

Mycoplasma Encephalitis

Clinical Presentation: Acute onset of fever and change in mental status without nuchal rigidity.

Diagnostic Considerations: Diagnosis suggested by CAP with sore throat, otitis, E. multiforme, soft stools/diarrhea—with elevated IgM mycoplasma titers, and very high (≥ 1:1024) cold agglutinin titers. CSF shows mild mononucleosis/pleocytosis and normal/low glucose.

Pitfalls: CNS findings may overshadow pulmonary findings.

Therapeutic Considerations: Macrolides not effective for CNS infection. Doxycycline rapidly ↓ mycoplasma shedding in oropharyngeal secretions (vs. prolonged shedding with macrolides).

Prognosis: With early treatment, prognosis is good without neurologic sequelae.

Listeria Encephalitis

Clinical Presentation: Fever/mental confusion (encephalitis/cerebritis) ± nuchal rigidity (meningo-encephalitis).

Diagnostic Considerations: Diagnosis by LP. Suspect Listeria if CSF with "purulent profile" plus RBCs. Listeria seen on Gram stain of CSF in 50%; but culture positive in 100%.

Pitfalls: Not to be confused with other gram-positive bacilli (skin contaminants) isolated from CSF (diphtheroids). Listeria are motile and hemolytic on blood agar.

Therapeutic Considerations: 3rd generation cephalosporins not active against Listeria. In penicillin-tolerant patients, use meningeal dose ampicillin (not penicillin).

Prognosis: Good with early/adequate treatment. Related to degree of T lymphocyte dysfunction.

CMV Encephalitis (see p. 329)

Toxoplasma Encephalitis (see p. 331)

Brain Abscess/Subdural Empyema/Cavernous Vein Thrombosis/Intracranial Suppurative Thrombophlebitis

Subset	Usual Pathogens	Preferred IV Therapy	Alternate IV Therapy	IV-to-PO Switch
Brain Abscess (Single Mass Lesion)				
Open trauma	S. aureus (MSSA) Entero-bacteriaceae P. aeruginosa	Meropenem 2 gm (IV) q8h × 2 weeks **or** Cefepime 2 gm (IV) q8h × 2 weeks	Not applicable	
Neurosurgical procedure (Treat initially for MSSA; if later identified as MRSA, MSSE, or MRSE, treat accordingly)	S. aureus S. epidermidis (CoNS)	MSSA Nafcillin 2 gm (IV) q4h × 2 weeks **or** MRSA/MSSE/MRSE Linezolid 600 mg (IV) q12h × 2 weeks **or** Minocycline 100 mg (IV) q12h × 2 weeks		MSSA/MRSA/ MSSE/MRSE Linezolid 600 mg (PO) q12h × 2 weeks **or** Minocycline 100 mg (PO) q12h × 2 weeks
Mastoid/otitic source	Enterobacter Proteus	Treat the same as for open trauma (see above)		
Dental source	Oral anaerobes Actinomyces	Ceftriaxone 2 gm (IV) q12h × 2 weeks **plus** Metronidazole 500 mg (IV) q12h × 2 weeks	Ceftizoxime 3 gm (IV) q6h × 2 weeks	
Subdural empy-ema/sinus source	Oral anaerobes H. influenzae	Treat the same as for dental source (see above)		
Cardiac source (ABE; right-to-left shunt)	S. aureus (MSSA) S. pneumoniae H. influenzae	Ceftriaxone 2 gm (IV) q12h × 2 weeks **or** Meropenem 2 gm (IV) q8h × 2 weeks		
	S. aureus (MRSA)	Linezolid 600 mg (IV) q12h × 2 weeks **or** Vancomycin 2 gm (IV) q12h × 2 weeks **or** Minocycline 100 mg (IV) q12h × 2 weeks	Linezolid 600 mg (PO) q12h × 2 weeks **or** Minocycline 100 mg (PO) q12h × 2 weeks	

Brain Abscess/Subdural Empyema/Cavernous Vein Thrombosis/Intracranial Suppurative Thrombophlebitis (cont'd)

Subset	Usual Pathogens	Preferred IV Therapy	Alternate IV Therapy	IV-to-PO Switch
Brain Abscess (Single Mass Lesion)				
Pulmonary source	Oral anaerobes Actinomyces	Ceftriaxone 2 gm (IV) q12h × 2 weeks **plus** Metronidazole 500 mg (IV) q12h × 2 weeks	Ceftizoxime 3 gm (IV) q6h × 2 weeks	

MSSA/MRSA = methicillin-sensitive/resistant S. aureus; MSSE/MRSE = methicillin-sensitive/resistant S. epidermidis. Duration of therapy represents total time IV or IV + PO. Most patients on IV therapy able to take PO meds should be switched to PO therapy after clinical improvement.

Clinical Presentation: Variable presentation, with fever, change in mental status, cranial nerve abnormalities ± headache.

Diagnostic Considerations: Diagnosis by CSF gram stain/culture. If brain abscess is suspected, obtain head CT/MRI. Lumbar puncture may induce herniation.

Pitfalls: CSF analysis is negative for bacterial meningitis unless abscess ruptures into ventricular system.

Therapeutic Considerations: Treatment with meningeal doses of antibiotics is required. Large single abscesses may be surgically drained; multiple small abscesses are best treated medically.

Prognosis: Related to underlying source and health of host.

Brain Abscess (Mastoid/Otitic Source)

Diagnostic Considerations: Diagnosis by head CT/MRI demonstrating focus of infection in mastoid.

Pitfalls: Rule out associated subdural empyema.

Therapeutic Considerations: ENT consult for possible surgical debridement of mastoid.

Prognosis: Good. May require mastoid debridement for cure.

Brain Abscess (Dental Source)

Diagnostic Considerations: Diagnosis by Panorex x-rays/gallium scan of jaw demonstrating focus in mandible/erosion into sinuses.

Pitfalls: Apical root abscess may not be apparent clinically.

Therapeutic Considerations: Large single abscess may be surgically drained. Multiple small abscesses are best treated medically. Treat until lesions on CT/MRI resolve or do not become smaller on therapy.

Prognosis: Good if dental focus is removed.

Brain Abscess (Subdural Empyema/Sinus Source)

Diagnostic Considerations: Diagnosis by sinus films/CT/MRI to confirm presence of sinusitis/bone erosion (cranial osteomyelitis/epidural abscess). Usually from paranasal sinusitis.

Pitfalls: Do not overlook underlying sinus infection, which may need surgical drainage.
Therapeutic Considerations: Obtain ENT consult for possible surgical debridement of sinuses.
Prognosis: Good prognosis if sinus is drained.

Brain Abscess (Cardiac Source; Acute Bacterial Endocarditis)

Diagnostic Considerations: Blood cultures often positive if brain abscess due to acute bacterial endocarditis (ABE) pathogen. Head CT/MRI shows multiple mass lesions.
Pitfalls: Do not overlook right-to-left cardiac shunt (e.g., patent foramen ovale, atrial septal defect) as source of brain abscess. Cerebral embolization results in aseptic meningitis in SBE, but septic meningitis/brain abscess in ABE (due to high virulence of pathogens).
Therapeutic Considerations: Multiple lesions suggest hematogenous spread. Use susceptibility of blood culture isolates to determine coverage. Meningeal doses are the same as endocarditis doses.
Prognosis: Related to location/size of CNS lesions and extent of cardiac valvular involvement.

Brain Abscess (Pulmonary Source)

Diagnostic Considerations: Diagnosis suggested by underlying bronchiectasis, empyema, cystic fibrosis, or lung abscess in a patient with a brain abscess.
Pitfalls: Brain abscesses are most often due to chronic suppurative lung disease (e.g., bronchiectasis, lung abscess/empyema), not chronic bronchitis/AECB. If patient doesn't have a cardiopulmonary disorder predisposing to brain abscess, look for a clinically silent dental (apical root) abscess by gallium scan of jaws/Panorex dental x-rays.
Therapeutic Considerations: Lung abscess may need surgical drainage.
Prognosis: Related to extent/location of CNS lesions, drainage of lung abscess/empyema, and control of lung infection.

Empiric Therapy of HEENT Infections

Facial/Periorbital Cellulitis

Subset	Usual Pathogens	Preferred IV Therapy	Alternate IV Therapy	PO Therapy or IV-to-PO Switch
Facial cellulitis	Group A streptococci H. influenzae	Ceftriaxone 1 gm (IV) q24h × 2 weeks **or** Cefotaxime 2 gm (IV) q6h × 2 weeks **or** Ceftizoxime 2 gm (IV) q8h × 2 weeks	Respiratory quinolone* (IV) q24h × 2 weeks	Any oral 2nd or 3rd gen. cephalosporin × 2 weeks **or** Respiratory quinolone* (PO) q24h × 2 weeks

Duration of therapy represents total time IV, PO, or IV + PO. Most patients on IV therapy able to take PO meds should be switched to PO therapy soon after clinical improvement (usually < 72 hours).
*   Levofloxacin 500 mg or Moxifloxacin 400 mg.

Clinical Presentation: Acute onset of warm, painful, facial rash without discharge, swelling, pruritus.

Diagnostic Considerations: Diagnosis by clinical appearance. May spread rapidly across face. Purplish hue suggests H. influenzae.

Pitfalls: If periorbital cellulitis, obtain head CT/MRI to rule out underlying sinusitis/CNS involvement. If secondary to an abrasion after contact with a saliva-contaminated surface, consider Herpes gladiatorum; lesions are painful/edematous and do not respond to antibiotic therapy for cellulitis.

Therapeutic Considerations: May need to treat × 3 weeks in compromised hosts (chronic steroids, diabetics, SLE, etc.).

Prognosis: Good with early treatment; worse if underlying sinusitis/CNS involvement.

Bacterial Sinusitis

Subset	Usual Pathogens	IV Therapy (Hospitalized)	PO Therapy or IV-to-PO Switch (Ambulatory)
Acute	S. pneumoniae H. influenzae M. catarrhalis	Respiratory quinolone† (IV) q24h × 1–2 weeks **or** Ceftriaxone 1 gm (IV) q24h × 1–2 weeks **or** Doxycycline 200 mg (IV) q12h × 3 days, then 100 mg (IV) q12h × 11 days	Respiratory quinolone† (PO) q24h × 1–2 weeks **or** Amoxicillin/clavulanic acid XR 2 tablets (PO) q12h × 10 days **or** Doxycycline 200 mg (PO) q12h × 3 days, then 100 mg (PO) q12h × 11 days* **or** Cephalosporin‡ (PO) × 2 weeks **or** Clarithromycin XL 1 gm (PO) q24h × 2 weeks
Chronic	Same as acute + oral anaerobes	Requires prolonged antimicrobial therapy (2–4 weeks)	

Duration of therapy represents total time IV, PO, or IV + PO in adults. Most patients on IV therapy able to take PO meds should be switched to PO therapy soon after clinical improvement (usually < 72 hours). See Chapter 7 for pediatric therapy.

*   Loading dose is not needed PO if given IV with the same drug.
†   Moxifloxacin 400 mg × 7 days or Levofloxacin 750 mg × 5 days.
‡   Cefdinir 300 mg q12h or Cefditoren 400 mg q12h or Cefixime 400 mg q12h or Cefpodoxime 200 mg q12h.

Acute Bacterial Sinusitis

Clinical Presentation: Nasal discharge and cough frequently with headache, facial pain, and low-grade fever lasting > 10–14 days. Can also present acutely with high fever (≥ 104°F) and purulent nasal discharge ± intense headache lasting for ≥ 3 days. Other manifestations depend on the affected sinus: <u>maxillary sinus</u>: percussion tenderness of molars; maxillary toothache; local extension may cause osteomyelitis of facial bones with proptosis, retroorbital cellulitis, ophthalmoplegia; direct intracranial extension is rare; <u>frontal sinus</u>: prominent headache; intracranial extension may cause epidural/brain abscess, meningitis, cavernous sinus/superior sagittal sinus thrombosis; orbital extension may cause periorbital cellulitis; <u>ethmoid sinus</u>: eyelid edema and prominent tearing; extension may cause retroorbital pain/periorbital cellulitis and/or cavernous sinus/superior sagittal sinus thrombosis; <u>sphenoid sinus</u>: severe headache; extension into cavernous sinus may cause meningitis, cranial nerve paralysis [III, IV, VI], temporal lobe abscess, cavernous sinus thrombosis). Cough and nasal discharge are prominent in children.

Diagnostic Considerations: Diagnosis by sinus x-rays or CT/MRI showing complete sinus opacification, air-fluid levels, mucosal thickening. Consider sinus aspiration in immunocompromised hosts or treatment failures. In children, acute sinusitis is a clinical diagnosis; imaging studies are not routine.

Pitfalls: May present as periorbital cellulitis (obtain head CT/MRI to rule out underlying sinusitis). If CT/MRI demonstrates "post-septal" involvement, treat as acute bacterial meningitis. In children, transillumination, sinus tenderness to percussion, and color of nasal mucus are not reliable indicators of sinusitis.

Therapeutic Considerations: Treat for full course to prevent relapses/complications. Macrolides and TMP–SMX may predispose to drug-resistant S. pneumoniae (DRSP), and ≥ 30% of S. pneumoniae are naturally resistant to macrolides. Consider local resistance rates before making empiric antibiotic selections.

Prognosis: Good if treated for full course. Relapses may occur with suboptimal treatment. For frequent recurrences, consider radiologic studies and ENT consultation.

Chronic Bacterial Sinusitis

Clinical Presentation: Generalized headache, fatigue, nasal congestion, post-nasal drip lasting > 3 months with little/no sinus tenderness by percussion. Local symptoms often subtle. Fever is uncommon.

Diagnostic Considerations: Sinus films and head CT/MRI are less useful than for acute sinusitis (chronic mucosal abnormalities may persist after infection is treated). Many cases of chronic maxillary sinusitis are due to a dental cause; obtain odontogenic x-rays if suspected.

Pitfalls: Clinical presentation is variable/nonspecific. Malaise and irritability may be more prominent than local symptoms. May be mistaken for allergic rhinitis. Head CT/MRI can rule out sinus tumor.

Therapeutic Considerations: Therapeutic failure/relapse is usually due to inadequate antibiotic duration, dose, or tissue penetration. Treat for full course. If symptoms persist after 4 weeks of therapy, refer to ENT for surgical drainage procedure.

Prognosis: Good if treated for full course. Relapses may occur with suboptimal treatment. For frequent recurrences, consider radiologic studies and ENT consultation.

Keratitis

Subset	Pathogens	Topical Therapy
Bacterial	S. aureus S. pneumoniae Bacillus cereus M. catarrhalis P. aeruginosa	Antibacterial eyedrops (ciprofloxacin, ofloxacin, or tobramycin/bacitracin/polymyxin B) hourly while awake × 2 weeks
Viral	HSV-1	Trifluridine 1% solution 1 drop hourly while awake × 2 days, then 1 drop q6h × 14–21 days **or** viral ophthalmic topical ointment (e.g., vidarabine) at bedtime × 14–21 days

Keratitis (cont'd)

Subset	Pathogens	Topical Therapy
Amebic	Acanthamoeba	Propamidine (0.1%), neomycin, gramicidin, or polymyxin B eyedrops hourly while awake × 1–2 weeks **or** polyhexamethylene biguanide (0.02%) eyedrops hourly while awake × 1–2 weeks **or** chlorhexidine (0.02%) eyedrops hourly while awake × 1–2 weeks

Clinical Presentation: Corneal haziness, infiltrates, or ulcers.
Diagnosis: Appearance of corneal lesions/culture.

Bacterial Keratitis
Diagnostic Considerations: Usually secondary to eye trauma. Always obtain ophthalmology consult.
Pitfalls: Be sure to culture ulcer. Unusual organisms are common in eye trauma.
Therapeutic Considerations: Treat until lesions resolve. Ointment easier/lasts longer than solutions. Avoid topical steroids.
Prognosis: Related to extent of trauma/organism. S. aureus, B. cereus, P. aeruginosa have worst prognosis.

Viral Keratitis (HSV-1)
Diagnostic Considerations: "Dendritic" corneal ulcers characteristic. Obtain ophthalmology consult.
Pitfalls: Small corneal ulcers may be missed without fluorescein staining.
Therapeutic Considerations: Treat until lesions resolve. Oral acyclovir is not needed. Avoid ophthalmic steroid ointment.
Prognosis: Good if treated early (before eye damage is extensive).

Amebic Keratitis (Acanthamoeba)
Diagnostic Considerations: Usually associated with extended use of soft contact lenses. Corneal scrapings are positive with calcofluor staining. Acanthamoeba keratitis is painful with typical circular, hazy, corneal infiltrate. Always obtain ophthalmology consult.
Pitfalls: Do not confuse with HSV-1 dendritic ulcers. Avoid topical steroids.
Therapeutic Considerations: If secondary bacterial infection, treat as bacterial keratitis.
Prognosis: No good treatment. Poor prognosis.

Conjunctivitis

Subset	Usual Pathogens	PO/Topical Therapy
Bacterial	M. catarrhalis H. influenzae S. pneumoniae N. meninsititis N. gonorrhea	Antibacterial eyedrops (ciprofloxacin, ofloxacin, moxifloxacin, or tobramycin/bacitracin/polymyxin B) q12h × 1 week plus antibacterial ointment (same antibiotic) at bedtime × 1 week

Conjunctivitis (cont'd)

Subset	Usual Pathogens	PO/Topical Therapy
Viral	Adenovirus	Not applicable
	VZV	Valacyclovir 1 gm (PO) q8h × 10–14 days **or** Famciclovir 500 mg (PO) q8h × 10–14 days
Chlamydial	C. trachomatis (trachoma)	Doxycycline 100 mg (PO) q12h × 1–2 weeks **or** Azithromycin 1 gm (PO) × 1 dose

Bacterial Conjunctivitis
Clinical Presentation: Profuse, purulent exudate from conjunctiva.
Diagnostic Considerations: Reddened conjunctiva; culture for specific pathogen.
Pitfalls: Do not confuse with allergic conjunctivitis, which itches and has a clear discharge.
Therapeutic Considerations: Obtain ophthalmology consult. Ointment lasts longer in eye than solution. Do not use topical steroids without an antibacterial.
Prognosis: Excellent when treated early, with no residual visual impairment.

Viral Conjunctivitis
Adenovirus
Clinical Presentation: Reddened conjunctiva, watery discharge, negative bacterial culture.
Diagnostic Considerations: Diagnosis by cloudy/steamy cornea with negative bacterial cultures. Clue is punctate infiltrates with a cloudy cornea. Extremely contagious; careful handwashing is essential. Obtain viral culture of conjunctiva for diagnosis.
Pitfalls: Pharyngitis a clue to adenoviral etiology (pharyngoconjunctival fever).
Therapeutic Considerations: No treatment available. Usually resolves in 1–2 weeks.
Prognosis: Related to degree of corneal haziness. Severe cases may take weeks to clear.

VZV Ophthalmicus
Diagnostic Considerations: Vesicles on tip of nose predict eye involvement.
Pitfalls: Do not miss vesicular lesions in external auditory canal in patients with facial palsy (Ramsey-Hunt Syndrome).
Therapeutic Considerations: Obtain ophthalmology consult. Topical steroids may be used if given with anti-VZV therapy.
Prognosis: Good if treated early with systemic antivirals.

Trachoma (C. trachomatis) Conjunctivitis
Diagnostic Considerations: Diagnosis by direct fluorescent antibody (DFA)/culture of conjunctiva.
Pitfalls: Do not confuse bilateral, upper lid, granular conjunctivitis of Chlamydia with viral/bacterial conjunctivitis, which involves both upper and lower eyelids.
Therapeutic Considerations: Ophthalmic erythromycin treatment is useful for neonates. Single-dose azithromycin may be associated with recurrence.
Prognosis: Excellent with early treatment.

Chorioretinitis

Subset	Usual Pathogens	Preferred IV Therapy	Alternate IV Therapy	PO Therapy or IV-to-PO Switch
Viral	CMV	See p. 327		
Fungal†	Candida albicans	Fluconazole 800 mg (IV) × 1 dose, then 400 mg (IV) q24h × 2 weeks‡ **or** Voriconazole 6 mg/kg (IV) q12h × 1 day, then 4 mg/kg (IV) q12h × 2 weeks‡	Amphotericin B 0.6 mg/kg (IV) q24h for total of 1 gm **or** Lipid amphotericin (p. 525) (IV) q24h × 3 weeks‡	Fluconazole 800 mg (PO) × 1 dose, then 400 mg (PO) q24h × 2 weeks*‡
Protozoal	Toxoplasma gondii	IV Therapy Not applicable	PO Therapy Pyrimethamine 75 mg (PO) × 1 dose, then 25 mg (PO) q24h × 6 weeks **plus either** Sulfadiazine 1 gm (PO) q6h × 6 weeks **or** Clindamycin 300 mg (PO) q8h × 6 weeks	

Duration of therapy represents total time IV, PO, or IV + PO. Most patients on IV therapy able to take PO meds should be switched to PO therapy after clinical improvement.

† Treat IV or IV-to-PO switch.

* Loading dose is not needed PO if given IV with the same drug.

‡ Duration of therapy is approximate and should be continued until resolution of infection. Close follow-up with an ophthalmologist is required.

CMV Chorioretinitis (see p. 327)

Candida Chorioretinitis
Clinical Presentation: Small, raised, white, circular lesions on retina.
Diagnostic Considerations: Fundus findings similar to white, raised colonies on blood agar plates.
Pitfalls: Candida endophthalmitis signifies invasive/disseminated candidiasis.
Therapeutic Considerations: Treat as disseminated candidiasis.
Prognosis: Good with early treatment.

Toxoplasma Chorioretinitis
Clinical Presentation: Grey/black pigmentation of macula.
Diagnostic Considerations: Diagnosis by IgM IFA toxoplasmosis titers.
Pitfalls: Unilateral endophthalmitis usually indicates acquired toxoplasmosis; congenital toxoplasmosis is usually bilateral.
Therapeutic Considerations: Obtain ophthalmology consult. Treat only acute/active toxoplasmosis with visual symptoms; do not treat chronic chorioretinitis. Add folinic acid 10 mg (PO) q24h to prevent folic acid deficiency.
Prognosis: Related to degree of immunosuppression.

Endophthalmitis

Subset	Usual Pathogens	Preferred IV Therapy	Alternate IV Therapy	PO Therapy or IV-to-PO Switch
Bacterial (Treat initially for MSSA; if later identified as MRSA or S. epidermidis, treat accordingly)	Streptococci H. influenzae S. aureus (MSSA)	**Intravitreal injection:** Cefepime 2.25 mg/0.1 mL sterile saline × 1 dose; repeat × 1 if needed in 2–3 days **plus** **Subconjunctival injection:** Cefepime 100 mg/0.5 mL sterile saline q24h × 1–2 weeks **plus** Levofloxacin 500 mg (IV/PO) q12h × 1–2 weeks		
	S. aureus (MRSA) S. epidermidis (CoNS)	**Intravitreal injection:** Vancomycin 1 mg/0.1 mL sterile saline × 1 dose; repeat × 1 if needed in 2–3 days **plus Subconjunctival injection:** Vancomycin 2.5 mg/0.5 mL sterile saline q24h × 1–2 weeks **plus** Linezolid 600 mg (IV/PO) q12h × 1–2 weeks		
Fungal‡	C. albicans	Fluconazole 800 mg (IV) × 1 dose, then 400 mg (IV) q24h × 2 months	Voriconazole (see "usual dose," p. 714) × 2 months	Fluconazole (same as IV dose) **or** Voriconazole (see p. 714) × 2 months
	A. fumigatus A. flavus	Amphotericin B (intravitreal) 10 mcg (in 0.1 mL of saline) q2–3 days	Voriconazole (see "usual dose," p. 714) × 2 months	Voriconazole (see "usual dose," p. 714) × 2 months
TB	M. tuberculosis	Treat the same as for TB pneumonia (see p. 53)		
Infected lens implant* (Treat initially for MSSA; if later identified as MRSA, treat accordingly)	Entero-bacteriaceae S. aureus (MSSA)	Meropenem 1 gm (IV) q8h × 2 weeks **or** Cefepime 2 gm (IV) q8h × 2 weeks	Chloramphenicol 500 mg (IV) q6h × 2 weeks	Chloramphenicol 500 mg (PO) q6h × 2 weeks
	S. aureus (MRSA)	Linezolid 600 mg (IV) q12h × 2 weeks	Minocycline 100 mg (IV) q12h × 2 weeks	Linezolid 600 mg (PO) q12h × 2 weeks **or** Minocycline 100 mg (PO) q12h × 2 weeks

MSSA/MRSA = methicillin-sensitive/resistant S. aureus. Duration of therapy represents total time IV, PO, or IV + PO. Most patients on IV therapy able to take PO meds should be switched to PO therapy after clinical improvement (usually < 72 hours).

* Treat only IV or IV-to-PO switch.

‡ Duration of therapy is approximate and should be continued until resolution of disease. Close follow-up with an ophthalmologist is required.

Bacterial Endophthalmitis

Clinical Presentation: Ocular pain/sudden vision loss.

Diagnosis: Post-op endophthalmitis occurs 1–7 days after surgery. Hypopyon seen in anterior chamber.

Pitfalls: Delayed-onset endophthalmitis may occur up to 6 weeks post-op. White intracapsular plaque is characteristic.

Therapeutic Considerations: Use steroids (dexamethasone 0.4 mg/0.1 mL intravitreal and 10 mg/1 mL subconjunctival) with antibiotics in post-op endophthalmitis. Also use systemic antibiotics for severe cases. Vitrectomy is usually necessary.

Prognosis: Related to pathogen virulence.

Fungal Endophthalmitis

Clinical Presentation: Slow deterioration in visual acuity ± eye pain. N fever. Antecedent/concomitant TPN, central IV line, prolonged antibiotic/immunosuppressive therapy, steroids, IVDA, or post-cataract surgery.

Diagnostic Considerations: Blood cultures frequently positive in Candida endophthalmitis. Small/round white lesions near retinal vessels. Cultures of aqueous/vitreous humors diagnostic.

Pitfalls: Symptoms develop insidiously with little/no eye pain or fever. Blood cultures negative with Aspergillus endophthalmitis.

Therapeutic Considerations: Penetration of antibiotic into vitreous humor requires high lipid solubility and inflammation. IV/intravitreous/subconjunctival antimicrobial choice depends on physiochemical properties of drug selected. Vitrectomy preferred by some.
If using intravitreal amphotericin B, there is no benefit in adding systemic IV therapy. Voriconazole penetrates CSF/eye, but clinical experience is limited. Based on limited data, caspofungin appears to have poor penetration into the vitreous and should not be relied upon to treat fungal endophthalmitis.

Prognosis: Best results with vitrectomy plus intravitreal antifungal therapy.

Tuberculous (TB) Endophthalmitis

Clinical Presentation: Raised retinal punctate lesions ± visual impairment.

Diagnostic Considerations: Signs of extraocular TB are usually present. Confirm diagnosis of miliary TB by liver/bone biopsy.

Pitfalls: TB endophthalmitis is a sign of disseminated TB.

Therapeutic Considerations: Treat as disseminated TB. Systemic steroids may be used if given with anti-TB therapy.

Prognosis: Related to degree of immunosuppression.

Infected Lens Implant

Diagnostic Considerations: Diagnosis by clinical appearance and culture of anterior chamber. Obtain ophthalmology consult.

Pitfalls: Superficial cultures are inadequate. Anterior chamber aspirate may be needed for culture.

Therapeutic Considerations: Infected lens must be removed for cure.

Prognosis: Good with early lens removal and recommended antibiotics.

External Otitis

Subset	Usual Pathogens	Preferred IV Therapy	Alternate IV Therapy	Topical Therapy or IV-to-PO Switch
Benign	P. aeruginosa	Use otic solutions only (ofloxacin 0.3%, tobramycin, polymyxin B); apply ear drops q6h × 1 week		
Malignant	P. aeruginosa	**One "A" drug ± one "B" drug:** **"A" drugs:** Meropenem 1 gm (IV) q8h **or** Cefepime 2 gm (IV) q8h **or** Piperacillin 4 gm (IV) q8h × 4–6 weeks **"B" drugs:** Ciprofloxacin 400 mg (IV) q8h **or** Levofloxacin 750 mg (IV) q24h × 4–6 weeks **or** Amikacin 1 gm (IV) q24h × 4–6 weeks		Ciprofloxacin 750 mg (PO) q12h **or** Levofloxacin 750 mg (PO) q24h × 4–6 weeks

Duration of therapy represents total time topically (benign), or IV + PO (malignant). Most patients on IV therapy able to take PO meds should be switched to PO therapy soon after clinical improvement (usually < 72 hours).

Benign External Otitis (Pseudomonas aeruginosa)

Clinical Presentation: Acute external ear canal drainage without perforation of tympanic membrane or bone involvement.

Diagnostic Considerations: Diagnosis suggested by external ear drainage after water exposure. Usually acquired from swimming pools ("swimmers ear"). Not an invasive infection.

Pitfalls: Be sure external otitis is not associated with perforated tympanic membrane, which requires ENT consultation and systemic antibiotics.

Therapeutic Considerations: Treat topically until symptoms/infection resolve.

Prognosis: Excellent with topical therapy.

Malignant External Otitis (Pseudomonas aeruginosa)

Clinical Presentation: External ear canal drainage with bone involvement.

Diagnostic Considerations: Diagnosis by demonstrating P. aeruginosa in soft tissue culture from ear canal plus bone/cartilage involvement on x-ray. Usually affects diabetics. CT/MRI of head shows bony involvement of external auditory canal.

Pitfalls: Rare in non-diabetics.

Therapeutic Considerations: Requires surgical debridement plus antibiotic therapy for cure.

Prognosis: Related to control of diabetes mellitus.

Acute Otitis Media

Subset	Usual Pathogens	IM Therapy	PO Therapy
Initial uncomplicated bacterial infection	S. pneumoniae H. influenzae M. catarrhalis	Ceftriaxone 50 mg/kg (IM) × 1 dose	Amoxicillin 1 gm or 10 mg/kg (PO) q8h × 10 days **or** Clarithromycin 7.5 mg/kg (PO) q12h × 10 days **or** Azithromycin 10 mg/kg (PO) × 1 dose, then 5 mg/kg (PO) q24h × 4 days
Treatment failure or resistant organism*	MDRSP β-lactamase positive H. influenzae	Ceftriaxone 50 mg/kg (IM) q24h × 3 doses	Amoxicillin/clavulanic acid ES-600 90 mg/kg/day (PO) in 2 divided doses × 10 days† **or** Cephalosporin† (PO) × 10 days

MDRSP = multidrug-resistant S. pneumoniae. Pediatric doses are provided; acute otitis media is uncommon in adults. For chronic otitis media, prolonged antimicrobial therapy is required.

*   Treatment failure = persistent symptoms and otoscopy abnormalities 48–72 hours after starting initial antimicrobial therapy. For risk factors for MDRSP, see Therapeutic Considerations.

†   ES-600 = 600 mg amoxicillin/5 mL. Cephalosporins: Cefuroxime axetil 15 mg/kg (PO) q12h or Cefdinir 7 mg/kg (PO) q12h or 14 mg/kg (PO) q24h or Cefpodoxime 5 mg/kg (PO) q12h may be used.

Acute Otitis Media

Clinical Presentation: Fever, otalgia, hearing loss. Nonspecific presentation is more common in younger children (irritability, fever). Key to diagnosis is examination of the tympanic membrane. Uncommon in adults.

Diagnostic Considerations: Diagnosis is made by finding an opaque, hyperemic, bulging tympanic membrane with loss of landmarks and decreased mobility on pneumatic otoscopy.

Pitfalls: Failure to remove cerumen (inadequate visualization of tympanic membrane) and reliance on history of ear tugging/pain are the main factors associated with overdiagnosis of otitis media. Otitis media with effusion (i.e., tympanic membrane retracted or in normal position with decreased mobility or mobility with negative pressure; fluid present behind the drum but normal in color) usually resolves spontaneously and should not be treated with antibiotics.

Therapeutic Considerations: Risk factors for infection with MDRSP S. pneumoniae include antibiotic therapy in past 30 days, failure to respond within 48–72 hours of therapy, day care attendance, and antimicrobial prophylaxis. Macrolides and TMP–SMX may predispose to DRSP, and 25% of S. pneumoniae are naturally resistant to macrolides.

Prognosis: Excellent, but tends to recur. Chronic otitis, cholesteatomas, mastoiditis are rare complications. Tympanostomy tubes/adenoidectomy for frequent recurrences of otitis media are the leading surgical procedures in children.

Mastoiditis

Subset	Usual Pathogens	Preferred IV Therapy	Alternate IV Therapy	PO Therapy or IV-to-PO Switch
Acute	S. pneumoniae H. influenzae S. aureus (MSSA)	Ceftriaxone 1–2 gm (IV) q24h × 2 weeks **or** Cefotaxime 2 gm (IV) q6h × 2 weeks **or** Cefepime 2 gm (IV) q12h × 2 weeks	Moxifloxacin 400 mg (IV) q24h × 2 weeks **or** Levofloxacin 500 mg (IV) q24h × 2 weeks	Moxifloxacin 400 mg (PO) q24h × 2 weeks **or** Levofloxacin 500 mg (PO) q24h × 2 weeks
Chronic	S. pneumoniae H. influenzae P. aeruginosa S. aureus (MSSA) Oral anaerobes	Meropenem 1 gm (IV) q8h × 4 weeks **or** Cefepime 2 gm (IV) q8h × 4 weeks	Moxifloxacin 400 mg (IV) × 4–6 weeks **or** Levofloxacin 750 mg (IV) q24h	Moxifloxacin 400 mg (PO) × 4–6 weeks

Duration of therapy represents total time IV, PO, or IV + PO. Most patients on IV therapy able to take PO meds should be switched to PO therapy soon after clinical improvement (usually < 72 hours).

Acute Mastoiditis
Clinical Presentation: Pain/tenderness over mastoid with fever.
Diagnostic Considerations: Diagnosis by CT/MRI showing mastoid involvement.
Pitfalls: Obtain head CT/MRI to rule out extension into CNS presenting as acute bacterial meningitis.
Prognosis: Good if treated early.

Chronic Mastoiditis
Clinical Presentation: Subacute pain/tenderness over mastoid with low-grade fever.
Diagnostic Considerations: Diagnosis by CT/MRI showing mastoid involvement. Rarely secondary to TB (diagnose by AFB smear/culture of bone biopsy or debrided bone).
Pitfalls: Obtain head CT/MRI to rule out CNS extension.
Therapeutic Considerations: Usually requires surgical debridement for cure. Should be viewed as chronic osteomyelitis. If secondary to TB, treat as skeletal TB.
Prognosis: Progressive without surgery. Poor prognosis with associated meningitis/brain abscess.

Suppurative Parotitis

Subset	Usual Pathogens	Preferred IV Therapy	Alternate IV Therapy	PO Therapy or IV-to-PO Switch
Parotitis (bacterial)	S. aureus (MSSA) Entero-bacteriaceae Oral anaerobes	Meropenem 1 gm (IV) q8h × 2 weeks **or** Quinolone* (IV) q24h × 2 weeks	Ceftriaxone 1 gm (IV) q24h × 2 weeks **or** Ceftizoxime 2 gm (IV) q8h × 2 weeks	Quinolone* (PO) q24h × 2 weeks

Duration of therapy represents total time IV, PO, or IV + PO. Most patients on IV therapy able to take PO meds should be switched to PO therapy soon after clinical improvement (usually < 72 hours).
* Levofloxacin 500 mg or Moxifloxacin 400 mg.

Clinical Presentation: Unilateral parotid pain/swelling with discharge from Stensen's duct ± fever.
Diagnostic Considerations: Diagnosis by clinical presentation, ↑ amylase, CT/MRI demonstrating stone in parotid duct/gland involvement.
Pitfalls: Differentiate from unilateral mumps by purulent discharge from Stensen's duct.
Therapeutic Considerations: If duct is obstructed, remove stone.
Prognosis: Good with early therapy/hydration.

Pharyngitis

Subset	Usual Pathogens	PO Therapy
Bacterial	Group A streptococci	Amoxicillin 1 gm (PO) q8h × 7–10 days **or** Cefprozil 500 mg (PO) q12h × 7–10 days **or** Clindamycin 300 mg (PO) q8h × 7–10 days **or** Clarithromycin XL 1 gm (PO) q24h × 7–10 days **or** Azithromycin 500 mg (PO) × 1 dose, then 250 mg (PO) q24h × 4 days
Membranous	Arcanobacterium (Corynebacterium) hemolyticum	Doxycycline 100 mg (IV or PO) q12h × 1–2 weeks **or** Clarithromycin XL 1 gm (PO) q24h × 1–2 weeks **or** Azithromycin 500 mg (IV or PO) × 1 dose then 250 mg (IV or PO) q24h × 1–2 weeks **or** Cephalosporin (IV or PO) × 1–2 wks
	C. diphtheriae C. ulcerans	Diphtheria antitoxin (see p. 170) ± penicillin or macrolide
Viral	Respiratory viruses, EBV, CMV, HHV-6	Not applicable. EBV/CMV do not cause primary pharyngitis, but pharyngitis part of infectious mononucleosis syndrome, along with hepatitis and lymph node involvement. Viral hepatitis (see pp. 97–98)

Pharyngitis (cont'd)

Subset	Usual Pathogens	PO Therapy
Other	M. pneumoniae C. pneumoniae	Respiratory quinolone* (PO) q24h × 1 week **or** Doxycycline 100 mg (PO) q12h × 1 week **or** Clarithromycin XL 1 gm (PO) q24h × 1 week **or** Azithromycin 500 mg (PO) × 1 dose, then 250 mg (PO) q24h × 4 days

Chronic fatigue syndrome.†

* Levofloxacin 500 mg or Moxifloxacin 400 mg.
† Not a cause of pharyngitis, pathogen unknown (not EBV) but may be caused by xenotropic murine leukemia related virus (XMRV). For therapeutic considerations (see p. 43).

Bacterial Pharyngitis

Clinical Presentation: Acute sore throat with fever, bilateral anterior cervical adenopathy, and elevated ASO titer. No hoarseness.

Diagnostic Considerations: Diagnosis of Group A streptococcal pharyngitis by elevated ASO titer after initial sore throat and positive throat culture. Rapid strep tests unnecessary, since delay in culture results (~1 week) still allows adequate time to initiate therapy and prevent acute rheumatic fever. Group A streptococcal pharyngitis is rare in adults > 30 years.

Pitfalls: Gram stain of throat exudate differentiates Group A streptococcal colonization (few or no PMNs) from infection (many PMNs) in patients with a positive throat culture or rapid strep test. Neither throat culture nor rapid strep test alone differentiates colonization from infection.

Therapeutic Considerations: Benzathine penicillin 1.2 mu (IM) × 1 dose can be used as an alternative to oral therapy. Penicillin, erythromycin, and ampicillin fail in 15% of cases due to poor penetration into oral secretions or beta-lactamase producing oral organisms.

Prognosis: Excellent. Treat within 10 days to prevent acute rheumatic fever.

Membranous Pharyngitis

Clinical Presentation: A. hemolyticum presents with a scarlet fever-like rash and membranous pharyngitis. C. diphtheriae pharyngitis has no fever/rash.

Diagnostic Considerations: Diagnosis by throat culture/recovery of organism in patients with scarlatiniform rash.

Pitfalls: A. hemolyticum must be differentiated from C. diphtheriae on culture.

Therapeutic Considerations: For A. hemolyticum, doxycycline or erythromycin are more active than beta-lactams. Penicillin or macrolides are preferred for C. diphtheriae. C. diphtheriae should be treated with antitoxin ASAP since antibiotic therapy is adjunctive.

Prognosis: Related to degree of airway obstruction. Good with early treatment of A. hemolyticum. Diphtheria prognosis related to early antitoxin treatment and to presence/severity of toxic myocarditis.

Viral Pharyngitis

Clinical Presentation: Acute sore throat. Other features depend on specific pathogen.

Diagnostic Considerations: Most cases of viral pharyngitis are caused by respiratory viruses, and are frequently accompanied by hoarseness, but not high fever, pharyngeal exudates, palatal petechiae, or posterior cervical adenopathy. Other causes of viral pharyngitis (EBV, CMV, HHV-6) are usually associated with posterior cervical adenopathy and ↑ SGOT/SGPT. EBV mono may present with exudative or non-exudative pharyngitis, and is diagnosed by negative ASO titer with a positive mono spot test or elevated EBV IgM viral capsid antigen (VCA) titer. Before mono spot test turns positive (may take up to 8 weeks), a presumptive diagnosis of EBV mono can be made by ESR and SGOT, which are elevated in EBV and normal in Group A streptococcal pharyngitis. If EBV mono spot is negative, retest weekly × 8 weeks; if still negative, obtain IgM CMV/toxoplasmosis titers to diagnose the cause of "mono spot negative" pharyngitis.

Pitfalls: 30% of patients with viral pharyngitis have Group A streptococcal colonization. Look for viral features to suggest the correct diagnosis (leukopenia, lymphocytosis, atypical lymphocytes).

Therapeutic Considerations: Symptomatic care only. Short-term steroids should only be used in EBV infection if airway obstruction is present/imminent. Since 30% of patients with viral pharyngitis are colonized with Group A streptococci, do not treat throat cultures positive for Group A streptococci if non-streptococcal pharyngitis features are present (e.g., bilateral posterior cervical adenopathy).

Prognosis: Related to extent of systemic infection. Post-viral fatigue is common. CMV may remain active in liver for 6–12 months with mildly elevated serum transaminases.

Mycoplasma/Chlamydophilia (Chlamydia) Pharyngitis

Clinical Presentation: Acute sore throat ± laryngitis. Usually non-exudative.

Diagnostic Considerations: Diagnosis by elevated IgM M. pneumoniae or C. pneumoniae titers. Consider diagnosis in patients with non-exudative pharyngitis without viral or streptococcal pharyngitis. Mycoplasma pharyngitis is often accompanied by otitis/bullous myringitis.

Pitfalls: Patients with C. pneumoniae frequently have laryngitis, which is not a feature of EBV, CMV, Group A streptococcal, or M. pneumoniae pharyngitis.

Therapeutic Considerations: Treatment of C. pneumoniae laryngitis results in rapid (~ 3 days) return of normal voice, which does not occur with viral pharyngitis.

Prognosis: Excellent.

Chronic Fatigue Syndrome (CFS)

Clinical Presentation: Fatigue > 1 year with cognitive impairment and no pharyngitis.

Diagnostic Considerations: Rule out other causes of chronic fatigue (cancer, adrenal/thyroid disease, etc.) before diagnosing CFS. HHV-6/Coxsackie B titers are usually elevated. Some have ↓ natural kill (NK) cells/activity. ESR ~ 0. Crimson crescents in the posterior pharynx are common.

Pitfalls: ↑ VCA IgG EBV titers is common in CFS, but EBV does not cause CFS. Do not confuse CFS with fibromyalgia, which has muscular "trigger points" and no cognitive impairment. CFS and fibromyalgia may coexist. In presumed CFS, if there is pharyngitis or if the ESR is elevated, consider an alternate diagnosis.

Therapeutic Considerations: No specific therapy is available. Patients with ↓ NK cells may benefit from β-carotene 50,000 U (PO) q24h × 3 weeks. Patients with ↑ C. pneumoniae IgG titers may benefit from doxycycline 100 mg (PO) q24h × 3 weeks.

Prognosis: Cyclical illness with remissions (precipitated by exertion, stress, or sleep lack). Avoid exercise.

Thrush (Oropharyngeal Candidiasis)

Subset	Pathogens	PO Therapy
Fungal	C. albicans	Fluconazole 200 mg (PO) × 1 dose, then 100 mg (PO) q24h ×† weeks **or** Posaconazole 100 mg (PO) q12h × 1 day, then 100 mg (PO) q24h × 13 days **or** Clotrimazole 10 mg troches (PO) 5x/day ×† weeks **or** Itraconazole 200 mg (PO) q24h ×† weeks
	Fluconazole-resistant Candida species	Posaconazole 400 mg (PO) q12h ×† weeks* **or** Voriconazole 200 mg (PO) q12h ×† weeks* **or** Caspofungin 70 mg (IV) × 1, then 50 mg (IV) q24h ×† weeks* **or** Itraconazole 200 mg (PO) q12h ×† weeks*

* Duration of therapy depends on underlying disease and clinical response.
† See Fluconazole unresponsive esophagitis (see p. 612).

Thrush (Oropharyngeal Candidiasis)

Clinical Presentation: White coated tongue or oropharynx. White adherent plaques may be on any part of the oropharynx.

Diagnostic Considerations: Gram stain/culture of white plaques demonstrates yeasts (Candida). Culture and susceptibility testing of causative fungus is useful in analyzing failure to respond to therapy.

Pitfalls: Lateral, linear, white, striated tongue lesions may resemble thrush but really represent hairy leukoplakia. Hairy leukoplakia should suggest HIV. Thrush may occur in children, alcoholics, diabetics, those receiving steroids/antibiotic therapy, or HIV.

Therapeutic Considerations: Almost all infections are caused by C. albicans, a species that is usually susceptible to fluconazole. Fluconazole-unresponsive infections may be caused by infection with fluconazole-resistant C. albicans (most common explanation), infection with a fluconazole-resistant non-albicans species (rare), noncompliance with therapy (common), or drug interactions (e.g., concomitant usage of rifampin, which markedly reduced azole blood levels). For suspected fluconazole-resistance, a trial with another azole is appropriate as cross-resistance is not universal.

Prognosis: Non-HIV patients respond well to therapy, particularly when the predisposing factor is eliminated/decreased (i.e., antibiotics discontinued, steroids reduced, etc.). HIV patients may require longer courses of therapy and should be treated until cured. Relapse is frequent in HIV patients, and institution of effective antiretroviral therapy is the most effective general strategy.

Mouth Ulcers/Vesicles

Subset	Usual Pathogens	Preferred IV Therapy	Alternate IV Therapy	PO Therapy or IV-to-PO Switch
Vincent's angina	Borrelia Fusobacterium	Clindamycin 600 mg (IV) q8h × 2 weeks	Ceftizoxime 2 gm (IV) q8h × 2 weeks **or** Any β-lactam (IV) × 2 weeks	Clindamycin 300 mg (PO) q8h × 2 weeks **or** Amoxicillin/clavulanic acid 500/125 mg (PO) q8h × 2 weeks
Ludwig's angina	Group A streptococci	Clindamycin 600 mg (IV) q8h × 2 weeks	Ceftizoxime 2 gm (IV) q8h × 2 weeks **or** Any β-lactam (IV) × 2 weeks	Clindamycin 300 mg (PO) q8h × 2 weeks **or** Amoxicillin/clavulanic acid 500/125 mg (PO) q8h × 2 weeks
Stomatitis	Normal mouth flora	Not applicable		
Herpangina	Coxsackie A virus	Not applicable		
Herpes gingivo-stomatitis	HSV-1	<u>PO Therapy</u> Valacyclovir 500 mg (PO) q12h × 1 week **or** Famciclovir 500 mg (PO) q12h × 1 week **or** Acyclovir 400 mg (PO) 5x/day × 1 week		
Herpes labialis (cold sores/ fever blisters)	HSV-1 (recurrent)	<u>PO Therapy</u> Valacyclovir 2 gm (PO) q12h × 1 day (2 doses) started at onset of symptoms (tingling/burning) Acyclovir 400 mg (PO) 5x/day × 1 week **or** Famciclovir 500 mg (PO) q12h × 1 week <u>Topical Therapy</u> Penciclovir 1% cream q2h while awake × 4 days **or** Acyclovir 5% cream 5x/d × 4 days		
Aphthous ulcers	Normal mouth flora	Not applicable		

Duration of therapy represents total time IV, PO, or IV + PO. Most patients on IV therapy able to take PO meds should be switched to PO therapy soon after clinical improvement (usually < 72 hours).

Vincent's Angina (Borrelia/Fusobacterium)

Clinical Presentation: Painful/bleeding gums without fever.

Diagnostic Considerations: Foul breath, poor dental hygiene/pyorrhea.

Pitfalls: Do not attribute foul breath to poor dental hygiene without considering other serious causes (e.g., lung abscess, renal failure).

Therapeutic Considerations: After control of acute infection, refer to dentist.

Prognosis: Excellent with early treatment.

Ludwig's Angina (Group A streptococci)

Clinical Presentation: Painful floor of mouth with fever.

Diagnostic Considerations: Elevated floor of mouth is diagnostic. Massive neck swelling may be present.

Pitfalls: C_{1q} deficiency has perioral/tongue swelling, but no fever or floor of mouth elevation. Rarely, Ludwig's, angina may be due to F. necrophorum.

Therapeutic Considerations: Surgical drainage is not necessary. May need airway emergently; have tracheotomy set at bedside.

Prognosis: Early airway obstruction has adverse impact on prognosis.

Stomatitis (normal mouth flora)

Clinical Presentation: Painful mouth ulcers with fever.

Diagnostic Considerations: Diagnosis based on clinical appearance.

Pitfalls: Do not miss a systemic cause (e.g., acute leukemia).

Therapeutic Considerations: Painful; treat symptomatically.

Prognosis: Related to severity of underlying systemic disease.

Herpangina (Coxsackie A virus)

Clinical Presentation: Painful mouth ulcers/vesicles with fever.

Diagnostic Considerations: Ulcers located posteriorly in pharynx. No gum involvement or halitosis.

Pitfalls: Do not confuse with anterior vesicular lesions of HSV.

Therapeutic Considerations: No good treatment available. Usually resolves spontaneously in 2 weeks.

Prognosis: Good, but may be recurrent.

Herpes Gingivostomatitis (HSV-1)

Clinical Presentation: Painful gums with fever.

Diagnostic Considerations: Anterior ulcers in pharynx. Associated with bleeding gums, not halitosis.

Pitfalls: Do not miss a systemic disease associated with bleeding gums (e.g., acute myelogenous leukemia). Periodontal disease is not usually associated with oral ulcers.

Therapeutic Considerations: Oral analgesic solutions may help in swallowing.

Prognosis: Excellent with early treatment.

Herpes Labialis (Cold Sores/Fever Blisters) (HSV-1)

Clinical Presentation: Painful vesicles along vermillion border of upper or lower lip with fever.

Diagnostic Considerations: Caused by recurrent HSV-1 infection, which appears as painful vesicular lesions on/near the vermillion border of lips. Attacks may be triggered by stress, sun exposure, menstruation, and often begin with pain or tingling before vesicles appear. Vesicles crust over and attacks usually resolve by 1 week. "Fever blisters" are not triggered by temperature elevations per se, but may accompany malaria, pneumococcal/meningococcal meningitis. Diagnosis is clinical.

Pitfalls: Do not confuse with perioral impetigo; impetigo has crusts (not vesicles), is itchy (not painful), and does not involve the vermillion border of the lips.

Therapeutic Considerations: Treatment is not always needed. If valacyclovir if used, it should be started when pain/tingling appear to decrease symptoms/vesicles/duration of attack. Valacyclovir is of no proven value once vesicles have appeared. Non-prescription topical products (docosanol 10%, tetracaine cream) may decrease pain/itching. Once-daily suppressive therapy may be considered for frequent recurrences or during times of increased risk (e.g., sun exposure). Sun screen may be helpful.

Prognosis: Tends to be recurrent in normal hosts. May be severe in compromised hosts.

Aphthous Ulcers (normal mouth flora)

Clinical Presentation: Painful mouth ulcers/vesicles without fever.

Diagnostic Considerations: Usually an isolated finding. Ulcers are painful.

Pitfalls: May be a clue to systemic disorder, e.g., Behcet's syndrome. Mouth ulcers in SLE are painless.

Therapeutic Considerations: Usually refractory to all treatment and often recurrent. Steroid ointment (Kenalog) may be helpful.

Prognosis: Good, but tends to recur.

Deep Neck Infections, Lemierre's Syndrome, Severe Dental Infections

Subset	Usual Pathogens	Preferred IV Therapy	Alternate IV Therapy	IV-to-PO Switch
Deep neck infections (lateral pharyngeal, retro-pharyngeal, space)	Oral anaerobes Oral streptococci	Meropenem 1 gm (IV) q8h × 2 weeks **or** Tigacycline 100 mg (IV) × 1 dose, then 100 mg (IV) q24h or 50 mg (IV) q12h × 2 weeks **or** Piperacillin 4 gm (IV) q8h × 2 weeks	Clindamycin 600 mg (IV) q8h × 2 weeks **or** Ceftizoxime 2 gm (IV) q8h × 2 weeks **or** Ertapenem 1 gm (IV) q24h × 2 weeks	Clindamycin 300 mg (PO) q8h × 2 weeks **or** Doxycycline 200 mg (PO) q12h × 3 days, then 100 mg (PO) q12h × 11 days*
Lemierre's Syndrome	Fusobacterium necrophorum	Treat as deep neck infection, see above		
Severe dental infections	Oral anaerobes Oral streptococci	Clindamycin 600 mg (IV) q8h × 2 weeks **or** Piperacillin 4 gm (IV) q8h × 2 weeks	Ertapenem 1 gm (IV) q24h × 2 weeks **or** Meropenem 1 gm (IV) q8h × 2 weeks	Clindamycin 300 mg (PO) q8h × 2 weeks **or** Doxycycline 200 mg (PO) q12h × 3 days, then 100 mg (PO) q12h × 11 days*

Duration of therapy represents total time IV or IV + PO. Most patients on IV therapy able to take PO meds should be switched to PO therapy after clinical improvement.

* Loading dose is not needed PO if given IV with the same drug.

Deep Neck Infections
(lateral pharyngeal, retropharyngeal,)

Diagnostic Considerations: Lateral pharyngeal space infection: Anterior → fever/chills, trismus, dysphagia, swelling or angle of mandible, ± parotid swelling, and bulging of lateral pharyngeal wall. Posterior pharyngeal space infection → bacteremic septic, no trismus/pain, and no pharyngeal wall bulging. Retropharyngeal space infection: fever/chills, dysphagia, dyspnea, ± mucal rigidity, esophageal regurgitation, and bulging of posterior pharyngeal wall.

Pitfalls: Retropharyngeal "danger space" infection may extend to mediastinum and present as mediastinitis.

Therapeutic Considerations: Obtain ENT consult for surgical drainage.

Prognosis: Worst prognosis with posterior lateral and retropharyngeal space infections.

Lemierre's Syndrome

Clinical Presentation: Severe sore throat with fever, toxemic appearance, and tenderness over jugular vein. Jugular vein septic thrombophlebitis and septic pulmonary emboli.

Diagnostic Considerations: May present as multiple septic pulmonary emboli. Usually follows recent dental infection. Jugular vein tenderness diagnostic. Blood cultures positive for F. necrophorum or F. nucleatum; rarely MSSA/MRSA.

Pitfalls: Suspect Lemierre's syndrome in patients with concurrent/antecedent dental/oropharyhngeal infection with severe sore throat and jugular vein tenderness.

Therapeutic Considerations: If unresponsive to antibiotic therapy, may need venotomy.

Prognosis: Good with prompt treatment. May be more severe with concurrent M. pneumoniae or EBV pharyngitis.

Severe Dental Infections

Diagnostic Considerations: Obtain CT/MRI of jaws to rule out osteomyelitis or abscess.

Pitfalls: Chronic drainage in a patient with an implant is diagnostic of chronic osteomyelitis/abscess until proven otherwise.

Therapeutic Considerations: Abscesses should be drained for cure.

Prognosis: Poor prognosis and recurrent without adequate surgical drainage.

Epiglottitis

Subset	Usual Pathogens	Preferred IV Therapy	Alternate IV Therapy	IV-to-PO Switch
Epiglottitis	S. pneumoniae H. influenzae Respiratory viruses	Ceftriaxone 1 gm (IV) q24h × 2 weeks **or** Ceftizoxime 2 gm (IV) q8h × 2 weeks	Ertapenem 1 gm (IV) q24h × 2 weeks **or** Meropenem 1 gm (IV) q8h × 2 weeks **or** Moxifloxacin 400 mg (IV) q24h × 2 weeks **or** Levofloxacin 500 mg (IV) q24h × 2 weeks	Moxifloxacin 400 mg (PO) q24h × 2 weeks **or** Levofloxacin 500 mg (PO) q24h × 2 weeks **or** Cefprozil 500 mg (PO) q12h × 2 weeks

Duration of therapy represents total time IV or IV + PO. Most patients on IV therapy able to take PO meds should be switched to PO therapy after clinical improvement.

Clinical Presentation: Stridor with upper respiratory infection.

Diagnostic Considerations: Lateral film of neck shows epiglottic edema. Neck CT/MRI may help if neck films are non-diagnostic.

Pitfalls: Do not attempt to culture the epiglottis (may precipitate acute upper airway obstruction).

Therapeutic Considerations: Treat empirically as soon as possible. Obtain ENT consult.

Prognosis: Early airway obstruction is associated with an adverse prognosis.

Empiric Therapy of Lower Respiratory Tract Infections

Acute Bacterial Exacerbation of Chronic Bronchitis (AECB)

Subset	Pathogens	PO Therapy
AECB	S. pneumoniae H. influenzae M. catarrhalis	Respiratory quinolone* (PO) q24h × 5 days **or** Amoxicillin/clavulanic acid 500/125 mg (PO) q12h × 5 days **or** Clarithromycin XL 1 gm (PO) q24h × 5 days **or** Doxycycline 100 mg (PO) q12h × 5 days **or** Azithromycin 500 mg (PO) × 3 days

*   Moxifloxacin 400 mg or Levofloxacin 500 mg.

Clinical Presentation: Productive cough and negative chest x-ray in a patient with chronic bronchitis.

Diagnostic Considerations: Diagnosis by productive cough, purulent sputum, and chest x-ray negative for pneumonia. H. influenzae is relatively more common than other pathogens.

Pitfalls: Do not obtain sputum cultures in chronic bronchitis; cultures usually reported as normal/mixed flora and should not be used to guide therapy.

Therapeutic Considerations: Treated with same antibiotics as for community-acquired pneumonia, since pathogens are the same (even though H. influenzae is relatively more frequent). Respiratory viruses/C. pneumoniae may initiate AECB, but is usually followed by bacterial infection, which is responsible for symptoms and is the aim of therapy. Bronchodilators are helpful for bronchospasm. Macrolide-resistant S. pneumoniae is an important clinical problem (prevalence ≥ 30%).

Prognosis: Related to underlying cardiopulmonary status.

Mediastinitis

Subset	Usual Pathogens	IV Therapy	IV-to-PO Switch
Following esophageal perforation or thoracic surgery	Oral anaerobes	Preferred: Piperacillin 4 gm (IV) q8h × 2 wks **or** Ampicillin/sulbactam 3 gm (IV) q6h × 2 wks Alternate: Meropenem 1 gm (IV) q8h × 2 weeks or Ertapenem 1 gm (IV) q24h × 2 weeks	Amoxicillin/clavulanic acid 500/125 mg (PO) q8h × 2 weeks **or** Respiratory quinolone* (PO) q24h × 2 weeks

Duration of therapy represents total time IV or IV + PO. Most patients on IV therapy able to take PO meds should be switched to PO therapy after clinical improvement.
* Moxifloxacin 400 mg or Levofloxacin 500 mg.

Diagnostic Considerations: Chest x-ray usually shows perihilar infiltrate in mediastinitis. Pleural effusions from esophageal tears have elevated amylase levels.
Pitfalls: Do not overlook esophageal tear in mediastinitis with pleural effusions.
Therapeutic Considerations: Obtain surgical consult if esophageal perforation is suspected.
Prognosis: Related to extent, location, and duration of esophageal tear/mediastinal infection.

Community-Acquired Pneumonia (CAP) (see Color Atlas for Sputum Gram stains and Chapter 8 for Differential Diagnosis of CXR patterns)

Subset	Usual Pathogens*	Alternate IV Therapy	PO Therapy or IV-to-PO Switch
Pathogen unknown	S. pneumoniae¶ H. influenzae M. catarrhalis B. pertussis Legionella sp. Mycoplasma pneumoniae Chlamydophilia (Chlamydia) pneumoniae	Respiratory quinolone† (IV) q24h **or** **combination therapy with** Ceftriaxone 1 gm (IV) q24h × 1–2 week **plus either** Doxycycline‡ (IV) × 1–2 weeks **or** Azithromycin 500 mg (IV) q24h × 1–2 weeks (minimum 2 doses before switching to PO therapy)	Respiratory quinolone† (PO) q24h **or** Doxycycline‡ (PO) × 1–2 weeks **or** Macrolide††¶ (PO) q24h × 1–2 weeks

Duration of therapy represents total time IV or IV, PO, or IV + PO. Most patients on IV therapy able to take PO meds should be switched to PO therapy after clinical improvement.
* Compromised hosts may require longer courses of therapy.
† Moxifloxacin 400 mg × 1–2 weeks or Levofloxacin 750 mg × 5 days (or 500 mg × 1–2 weeks).
†† Azithromycin 500 mg or Clarithromycin XL 1 gm.
¶ Macrolide monotherapy should be avoided in areas where *macrolide-resistant S. pneumoniae (MRSP) or multidrug-resistant S. pneumoniae (MDRSP)* strains are prevalent.
‡ Doxycycline 200 mg (IV or PO) q12h × 3 days, then 100 mg (IV or PO) q12h × 4–11 days.

Community-Acquired Pneumonia (CAP) (cont'd)

Subset	Usual Pathogens*	Preferred IV Therapy	Alternate IV Therapy	PO Therapy or IV-to-PO Switch
Typical bacterial pathogens	S. pneumoniae¶ H. influenzae M. catarrhalis	Respiratory quinolone† (IV) q24h × 1–2 weeks **or** Ceftriaxone 1 gm (IV) q24h × 1–2 wks **or** Tigecycline** 100 mg (IV) × 1 dose, then 50 mg (IV) q12h × 1–2 weeks	Doxycycline‡ (IV) × 1–2 weeks **or** Ertapenem 1 gm (IV) q24h × 1–2 weeks **or** Ceftaroline fosamil*** 600 mg (IV) q12h × 5–7 days	(see unknown pathogen) **or** Amoxicillin/ clavulanic acid XR 2 tablets (PO) q12h × 7–10 days **or** Cefprozil 500 mg (PO) q12h × 1–2 weeks
	K. pneumoniae*	Meropenem 1 gm (IV) q8h × 2 weeks **or** Ertapenem 1 gm (IV) q24h × 2 weeks **or** Respiratory quinolone§ (IV) q24h × 2 weeks	Ceftaroline fosamil*** 600 mg (IV) q12h × 5–7 days **or** Ceftriaxone 1 gm (IV) q24h × 2 weeks **or** Doripenem 1 gm (IV) q8h¶¶	Respiratory quinolone§ (PO) q24h × 2 weeks
	MDR K. pneumoniae	Tigecycline 200 mg¶ (IV) × 1 dose, then 100 mg (IV) q24h × 1–2 weeks**	Colistin 80 mg or 1.7 mg/kg (IV) q8h¶¶ ± Rifampin 300 mg (PO) q12h¶¶ **or** Polymyxin B 1–1.25 mg/kg (IV) q12h¶¶¥	None

* Compromised hosts may require longer courses of therapy.
† Moxifloxacin 400 mg × 1–2 weeks or Levofloxacin 750 mg × 5 days (or 500 mg × 1–2 weeks).
§ Moxifloxacin 400 mg or Levofloxacin 500 mg.
¥ 1 mg Colistin = 12,500 IU; 1 mg Polymyxin B = 10,000 IU.
‡ Doxycycline 200 mg (IV or PO) q12h × 3 days, then 100 mg (IV or PO) q12h × 4–11 days.
** Tigecycline indicated for S. pneumoniae, H. influenzae, and Legionella CAP.
¶ Higher than usual doses of tigecycline may be necessary for susceptible MDR GNBs.
¶¶ Treat until cured.
*** Ceftaroline fosamil indicated for CABP caused by S. pneumoniae, S. aureus (methicillin susceptible isolates only), H. influenzae, K. Pneumoniae, K. oxytoca, and E. coli.

Community-Acquired Pneumonia (CAP)

Subset	Usual Pathogens*	Preferred IV Therapy	Alternate IV Therapy	PO Therapy or IV-to-PO Switch
Atypical pathogens *Zoonotic*	C. psittaci (psittacosis) Coxiella burnetii (Q fever) Francisella tularensis (tularemia)	Doxycycline 200 mg (IV) q12h × 3 days, then 100 mg (IV) q12h × 2 weeks	Respiratory quinolone† (IV) q24h × 2 weeks	Doxycycline 200 mg (PO) q12h × 3 days, then 100 mg (PO) q12h × 11 days **or** Quinolone† (PO) q24h × 2 weeks
Non-zoonotic	Legionella sp.‡ Mycoplasma ÷pneumoniae‡ C. pneumoniae‡	Moxifloxacin 400 mg (IV) q24h × 1–2 weeks **or** Levofloxacin 500 mg (IV) q24h × 1–2 weeks **or** Tigecycline 100 mg (IV) × 1 dose, then 50 mg (IV) q12h × 1–2 weeks**	Doxycycline 200 mg (IV) q12h × 3 days, then 100 mg (IV) q12h × 4–11 days **or** Azithromycin 500 mg (IV) q24h × 1–2 weeks (minimum of 2 doses before switching to PO therapy)	Respiratory quinolone† (PO) q24h × 1–2 weeks **or** Doxycycline 200 mg (PO) q12h × 3 days, then 100 mg (PO) q12h × 4–11 days **or** Azithromycin 500 mg (PO) q24h × 1–2 weeks **or** Clarithromycin XL 1 gm (PO) q24h × 1–2 weeks
	CMV	Valganciclovir 900 mg (PO) q12h until cured		
Influenza (*mild or moderate without bacterial CAP*)	Influenza A Human Seasonal Swine influenza (H_1N_1)	Oseltamivir (Tamiflu) 75 mg (PO) q24h × 5 days	Zanamivir (Relenza) 10 mg (2 puffs via oral inhaler) q12h × 5 days	Oseltamivir may be ineffective against human seasonal influenza/avian influenza (H_5N_1), but appears effective against swine influenza (H_1N_1)

* Compromised hosts may require longer courses of therapy.
† Moxifloxacin 400 mg or Levofloxacin 500 mg.
‡ May require prolonged therapy: Legionella (2–3 weeks); Mycoplasma (2 weeks); Chlamydia (2 weeks).
** Tigecycline indicated for Legionella CAP.

Community-Acquired Pneumonia (CAP) (cont'd)

Subset	Usual Pathogens*	Preferred IV Therapy	Alternate IV Therapy	PO Therapy or IV-to-PO Switch
Influenza (*severe with simultaneous CAP*)§	Influenza A Human seasonal Swine influenza (H_1N_1)	Oseltamivir (Tamiflu) 75 mg (PO) q12h × 5 days¶ **plus either** Rimantadine 100 mg (PO) q12h × 7–10 days¶¶ **or** Amantadine 200 mg (PO) q24h × 7–10 days¶¶		Start treatment as soon as possible after onset of symptoms, preferably within 2 days. Rimantadine/ amantadine inactive against Influenza B.
Influenza (*with subsequent bacterial CAP*)	S. pneumoniae H. influenzae	Quinolone‡ (IV) q24h × 2 weeks **plus either** Nafcillin 2 gm (IV) q4h × 2 weeks **or** Clindamycin 600 mg (IV) q8h × 2 weeks	Ceftriaxone 1 gm (IV) q24h × 2 wks **plus either** Vancomycin 1 gm (IV) q12h × 2 weeks **or** Linezolid 600 mg (IV) q12h × 2 weeks	Quinolone‡ (PO) q24h × 2 weeks
		Plus influenza therapy (see preceeding page)		
Chickenpox pneumonia	VZV	Acyclovir 5–10 mg/kg (IV) q8h × 10 days		Valacyclovir 1–2 gm (PO) q8h × 10 days

Duration of therapy represents total time IV or IV, PO, or IV + PO.

* Compromised hosts predisposed to organisms listed, but may be infected by usual pathogens in normal hosts.

¶ Although resistance common, these drugs may improve oxygenation in severe cases of influenza A, on ventilatory support.

Serious neuropsychiatric symptoms (delirium/behavioral abnormalities, panic attacks, convulsions) may occur in some children and adults. See drug summary for details.

‡ May require prolonged therapy: Legionella (2–3 weeks); Mycoplasma (2 weeks); Chlamydia (2 weeks).

§ If CXR shows multiple rapidly cavitating infiltrates < 72 hours, begin empiric anti-MSSA/CA-MRSA therapy with anti-influenza therapy.

¶¶ Although resistance common, may improve oxygenation in severe influenza A.

Community-Acquired Pneumonia (CAP) (cont'd)

Subset	Usual Pathogens*	Preferred IV Therapy	Alternate IV Therapy	PO Therapy or IV-to-PO Switch
Aspiration	Oral anaerobes S. pneumoniae H. influenzae M. catarrhalis	Ceftriaxone 1 gm (IV) q24h × 2 weeks **or** Quinolone‡ (IV) q24h × 2 weeks	Doxycycline 200 mg (IV) q12h × 3 days, then 100 mg (IV) q12h × 11 days	Respiratory quinolone‡ (PO) q24h × 2 weeks **or** Doxycycline 200 mg (PO) q12h × 3 days, then 100 mg (PO) q12h × 4–11 days** **or** Amoxicillin/clavulanic acid XR 2 tablets (PO) q12h × 2 weeks
Tuberculosis (TB)	M. tuberculosis	INH 300 mg (PO) q24h (and pyridoxine 50 mg (PO) q24h) × 6 months **plus** RIF 600 mg (PO) q24h × 6 months **plus** PZA 25 mg/kg (PO) q24h × 2 months **plus** EMB 15 mg/kg (PO) q24h (until susceptibilities known)††			
MDR-TB	M. tuberculosis	Bedaquiline (Sirturo) 400 mg (PO) q24h (D.O.T.) × 2 weeks, then 200 mg (PO) 3 × per week × 22 weeks*.			
Non-tuberculous (atypical tuberculosis) Mycobacteria	Mycobacterium avium-intracellulare (MAI)	<u>Treat for 12 months after sputum negative for MAI:</u> EMB 15 mg/kg (PO) q24h **plus either** Clarithromycin 500 mg (PO) q12h **or** Azithromycin 500 mg (PO) q24h **plus either** (Rifampin or Rifabutin). May substitute a quinolone (PO)‡ q24h for rifamycin			
	M. kansasii	<u>Preferred therapy</u> RIF 600 mg (PO) q24h **plus** INH 300 mg (PO) q24h **plus** pyridoxine 50 mg (PO) q24h **plus** EMB 15 mg/kg (PO) q24h. Treat × 12 months after negative sputum <u>Alternate therapy</u> RIF 600 mg (PO) thrice weekly **or** daily **plus** EMB 15 mg/kg (PO) thrice weekly **or** daily **plus** clarithromycin 500–1000 mg (PO) thrice weekly **or** daily. Treat × 12 months after negative sputum			

*   May be used in adults as part of a multidrug TB regimen (>3 drugs). Take with food. Side effects include nausea, headache, arthralgias, QT_c prolongation.

‡   Moxifloxacin 400 mg or Levofloxacin 500 mg.

†† If isolate is sensitive, discontinue EMB and continue as above to complete 6 months. If INH-resistant, continue EMB, RIF and PZA to complete 6 months. If any other resistance is present (MDR-TB), obtain infectious disease or pulmonary consult.

Community-Acquired Pneumonia (CAP) (cont'd)

Subset	Usual Pathogens*	Preferred IV Therapy	Alternate IV Therapy	PO Therapy or IV-to-PO Switch
Chronic alcoholics	K. pneumoniae S. pneumoniae H. influenzae M. catarrhalis	Meropenem 1 gm (IV) q24h × 2 weeks **or** Ertapenem 1 gm (IV) q24h × 2 weeks **or** Tigacycline 100 mg (IV) × 1, then 50 mg (IV) q12h **or** 100 mg (IV) q24h × 2 weeks	Ceftriaxone 1 gm (IV) q24h × 2 weeks **or** Quinolone‡ (IV) q24h × 2 weeks	Respiratory quinolone (PO) q24h × 2 weeks
	MDR K. pneumoniae	Tigecycline 200 mg (IV) × 1 dose, 100 mg (IV) q24h × 1–2 weeks**	Doripenem 1gm (IV) q8h¶ **or** Colistin 80 mg or 1.7 mg/kg (IV) q8h¶ ± Rifampin 300 mg (PO) q12h¶ **or** Polymyxin B 1–1.25 mg/kg (IV) q12h¶¥	None
Bronchiectasis, cystic fibrosis	S. maltophilia B. cepacia Alcaligenes xyloxidans	<u>Preferred</u>: TMP–SMX 2.5 mg/kg (IV) q6h¶ **or** Minocycline 100 mg (IV) q12h¶ <u>Alternate</u>: Doxycycline 100 mg (IV) q12h¶		TMP–SMX 1 SS tablet (PO) q6h¶ **or** Minocycline 100 mg (PO) q12h¶ **or** Respiratory quinolone‡ (PO) q24h
	P. aeruginosa	Meropenem 2 gm (IV) q8h¶	Levofloxacin 750 mg (IV) q24h¶ **or** Cefepime 2 gm (IV) q8h¶ ± Amikacin 1 gm (IV) q24h¶	Levofloxacin 750 mg (PO) q24h¶ **or** Ciprofloxacin 750 mg (PO) q12h
	MDR P. aeruginosa	Doripenem 1gm (IV) q8h¶ **or** Colistin 80 mg or 1.7 mg/kg (IV) q8h¶	Polymyxin B 1–1.25 mg/kg (IV) q12h¶¥	None

CO/CA-MRSA = community-onset/community-acquired methicillin-resistant S. aureus (see pp. 14–15). Duration of therapy represents total time IV or IV, PO, or IV + PO.

*   Compromised hosts predisposed to organisms listed but may be infected by usual pathogens in normal hosts.

¶   Treat until cured.

‡   Moxifloxacin 400 mg or Levofloxacin 500 mg.

** Tigecycline indicated for S. pneumoniae (PCN sensitive), H. influenzae (β-lactamase –), and Legionella CAP.

¥   Colistin 1 mg = 12,500 IU; Polymyxin B 1 mg = 10,000 IU.

Community-Acquired Pneumonia (CAP) (cont'd)

Subset	Usual Pathogens*	Preferred IV Therapy	Alternate IV Therapy	PO Therapy or IV-to-PO Switch
Chronic steroid therapy†	Aspergillus sp.	Voriconazole (see "usual dose," p. 714)¶	Lipid ampho-tericin (p. 525)¶ **or** Caspofungin 70 mg (IV) × 1 then 50 mg (IV) q24h¶ **or** amphotericin B 1–1.5 mg/kg (IV) q24h¶	Voriconazole (see "usual dose," p. 714)¶ **or** Posaconazole 200 mg q6h initially, then 400 mg q12h when stabilized¶ **or** Itraconazole 200 mg (IV) q12h × 2 days then 200 mg (PO) q12h**¶
	P. (carinii) jiroveci (PCP)	TMP–SMX 5 mg/kg (IV) q6h × 3 weeks‡	Pentamidine 4 mg/kg (IV) q24h × 3 weeks‡	TMP–SMX 5 mg/kg (PO) q6h × 3 weeks **or** Atovaquone 750 mg (PO) of q12h **or** Dapsone 100 mg (PO) of q24h
	CMV	Valganciclovir 900 mg (PO) q12h until cured		
HIV	Typical/atypical CAP pathogens	see pp. 50–51		
	P. (carinii) jiroveci (PCP)	see p. 325		
Other pathogens	For Crytococcus neoformans, Blastomyces, Histoplasma, Coccidioides, Paracoccidioides, Actinomyces, Nocardia, Pseudallescheria boydii, Sporothrix, Mucor (see pp. 267–269).			

¶   Treat until cured.
†   Treat IV or IV-to-PO switch.
*   Compromised hosts predisposed to organisms listed, but may be infected by usual pathogens of normal hosts.
** Loading dose is not needed PO if given IV with the same drug.
‡   Steroid dosage: prednisone 40 mg (PO) q12h on days 1–5, then 40 mg (PO) q24h on days 6–10, then 20 mg (PO) q24h on days 11–21. Methylprednisolone (IV) can be substituted at 75% of prednisone dose.
†† Moxifloxacin 400 mg or Levofloxacin 500 mg.

Clinical Presentation: Fever, cough, respiratory symptoms, chest x-ray consistent with pneumonia. Typical CAPs present only with pneumonia without extrapulmonary findings.

Diagnosis: Identification of organism on sputum gram stain/culture. Same organism is found in blood if blood cultures are positive. Also see Chapter 8 for typical chest x-ray patterns.

Community-Acquired Pneumonia (Typical Bacterial Pathogens)

Diagnostic Considerations: Sputum is useful if a single organism predominates and is not contaminated by saliva. Purulent sputum, pleuritic chest pain, pleural effusion favor typical pathogens.

Pitfalls: Obtain chest x-ray to verify the diagnosis and rule out noninfectious mimics (e.g., heart failure).

Therapeutic Considerations: Do not switch to narrow-spectrum antibiotic after organism is identified on gram stain/blood culture. Pathogen identification is important for prognostic and public health reasons, not for therapy. Severity of CAP is related to the degree of cardiopulmonary/immune dysfunction and impacts the length of hospital stay, not the therapeutic approach or antibiotic choice.

Prognosis: Related to cardiopulmonary status and splenic function.

Community-Acquired Pneumonia (Pertussis)

Clinical Presentation: Rhinorrhea over 1–2 weeks (catarrhal stage) progressing to paroxysms of cough (paroxysmal stage) lasting 2–4 weeks, often without a characteristic inspiratory whoop, followed by a convalescent stage lasting 1–2 weeks during which cough paroxysms decrease in frequency/severity. Fever is low grade or absent. In children < 6 months, whoop is frequently absent and apnea may occur. Older children/adults may present with persistent cough (without whoop) lasting 2–6 weeks.

Diagnostic Considerations: A positive PCR or DFA for Bordetella pertussis from a nasopharyngeal swab (NP). May be cultured by beside inoculation from NP swab of Bordet-Gengou media. "Shaggy heart" on chest x-ray is characteristic. The only CAP with lymphocytosis > 60%.

Pitfalls: Consider pertussis in older children and adults with prolonged coughing. Hoarseness uncommon, but may be misleading by mimicing viral laryngitis or C. pneumoniae.

Therapeutic Considerations: By the paroxysmal stage, antibiotics have minimal effect on the course of the illness but are indicated to decrease transmission.

Prognosis: Good, despite the prolonged course.

Community-Acquired Pneumonia (Atypical Pathogens)

Clinical Presentation: CAP with extra-pulmonary symptoms, signs, or laboratory abnormalities.

Diagnosis: Confirm by specific serological tests.

Legionnaire's Disease (Legionnaire sp.)

Legionella organisms live in a fresh water environment and survive in a symbiotic relationship with freshwater amoeba. Legionella infection may be introduced into humans via droplet aerosolization of Legionella-contaminated water supplies (e.g., cooling towers, water systems, whirlpools, showers, air conditioners, respiratory therapy devices). Legionnaires' disease can occur in isolated cases or in outbreaks (community-acquired or nosocomial). Legionella has a seasonal predisposition and is most common in the fall/winter. Legionella is rare in young children, uncommon in young adults, and is most common in adult/elderly patients. Individuals with impaired cell-mediated immunity (↓ T-lymphocyte function) are most susceptible, but normal hosts can be infected as well.

Clinical Presentation: In normal hosts Legionella CAP is usually more severe than M. pneumoniae or C. pneumoniae CAP onset is usually acute, with high fever (≥ 102°F) and relative bradycardia. Myalgias and chills are not uncommon. Like other atypical pneumonias, Legionella is characterized by its pattern of extra-pulmonary manifestations (Tables 2.1), which is the key to presumptive clinical diagnosis. On chest x-ray, Legionella is suggested not by the appearance of the infiltrate, which can be variable, but by its rapid, asymmetric progression. With Legionella CAP, bilateral involvement is usual, consolidation/pleural effusion are not uncommon, and cavitation is rare. Legionella testing is in CAP patients with fever ≥ 102°F plus relative bradycardia (if not on verapamil, diltiazem or beta-blockers or have arrhythmias/heart block), mental confusion, watery diarrhea, abdominal pain, relative lymphopenia ↑ ESR/CRP, mild/transient ↑ SGOT/SGPT, early/transient ↓ serum phosphorus, ↑ ferritin levels (> 2 × n) ↑ CPK, and microscopic hematuria.

Diagnostic Considerations: Lack of response to beta-lactam therapy in a CAP patient should also suggest the possibility of Legionella and prompt specific testing. The diagnosis is confirmed by Legionella DFA of sputum/respiratory secretions, Legionella IGA titers (a single titer ≥ 1:256 or ≥ 4 fold increase between acute and convalescent titers) is diagnostic. Legionella may also be cultured on BCYE agar from sputum respiratory secretions, pleural effusion, or lung tissue. Legionella pneumophila (serotypes 01-06) may also be diagnosed by urinary antigen test.

Pitfalls: As no individual finding is pathognomonic the constellation of signs/symptoms of Leogionella CAP are often overlooked and the pattern of extrapulmonary organ involvement differentiates Legionella from other causes of CAP. Hyponatremia is common but nonspecific. Decreased serum phosphorus is a less common but more specific for Legionella. Findings suggestive of an alternate (non-Legionella) cause of CAP include ↑ cold agglutinin titer, normal SGOT/SGPT, normal serum phosphorus, normal CPK level, upper respiratory tract involvement (non-exudative pharyngitis, laryngitis, otitis). Legionella DFA of sputum/respiratory secretions is positive early and rapidly becomes negative with treatment. IFA serological testing, as with other pathogens, may be negative if ordered too early (usually at the time of presentation), and antimicrobial therapy may eliminate/blunt IFA titers and making confirmation of the diagnosis (serologically) difficult/impossible. Legionella urinary antigen testing is useful but has limitations, as it is not always positive when the patient presents, and detects only Legionella pneumophila (serotypes 01-06) and not other Legionella species.

Therapeutic Considerations: Antimicrobial agents with a high degree of anti-Legionella activity are quinolones, doxycycline, and macrolides. Rifampin has in vitro anti-Legionella activity, but as part of combination therapy (erythromycin + rifampin) has not been shown to offer any advantage over well selected monotherapy (quinolone, doxycycline). Legionella does not respond to beta-lactams and only somewhat to erythromycin. Patients treated with a quinolone, tigacycline, or doxycycline typically defervesce slowly (5–7 days). Therapy is usually continued for 2–3 weeks depending upon clinical severity/host factors.

Prognosis: In immunocompetent hosts with good cardiopulmonary function, prognosis is good. Prognosis is guarded in elderly hosts with impaired CMI (HIV, organ transplants, corticosteroid therapy) and in those severe cardiopulmonary disease (CAD, valvular heart disease, COPD, chronic bronchiectasis).

Mycoplasma pneumoniae

Epidemiology: M. pneumoniae primarily affects young adults and the elderly. M. pneumoniae is spread from person-to-person via aerosolized droplets.

Clinical Presentation: Onset is subacute with a characteristic dry/nonproductive cough that lasts for weeks, low-grade fever (< 102°F) /chills, and mild myalgias. As with other atypical CAPs, M. pneumoniae is characterized by its pattern of extrapulmonary organ involvement, which may include sore throat (non-exudative pharyngitis), bullous myringitis, otitis media, and/or watery loose stools/diarrhea (Table 2.1). Features that argue against the diagnosis of M. pneumoniae CAP include high fevers (> 102°F), relative bradycardia, laryngitis, abdominal pain, ↑ SGOT/SGPT, low serum phosphorus, or renal abnormalities. Chest x-ray typically shows ill-defined unilateral infiltrates without pleural effusion, consolidation or cavitation. M. pneumoniae may present as severe CAP in compromised hosts, the elderly, and those with advanced COPD.

Diagnostic Considerations: M. pneumoniae testing is recommended for patients with otherwise unexplained protracted nonproductive cough, low-grade fevers, loose stools/watery diarrhea, and an ill-defined infiltrate on chest x-ray. Cold agglutinin titers are elevated early/transiently (75%) and provide a rapid presumptive diagnosis; titers ≥ 1:64 are due to M. pneumoniae. An elevated M. pneumoniae IgM ELISA titer suggests acute infection, but an elevated IgG titer indicates only past exposure; M. pneumoniae may be cultured from respiratory secretions on viral media (requires 1–2 weeks for growth).

Pitfalls: A dry, nonproductive cough also suggests an ILI or C. pneumoniae. Before ascribing E. multiforme to M. pneumoniae, be sure that it is not due to other causes (e.g., drug induced). Features that argue against the diagnosis of M. pneumoniae include temperature > 102°F, relative bradycardia, moderate/large pleural effusion, consolidation/cavitation, otherwise unexplained abdominal pain, ↑ SGOT/SGPT or low serum phosphorus. Suspect M. pneumoniae in chronic dry cough/new onset asthma.

Therapeutic Considerations: Doxycycline, macrolides, quinolones, or tigacycline result in rapid clinical response: in < 72 hours, but dry cough usually persists for weeks. Because Mycoplasma organisms reside on/in the bronchial epithelium, antimicrobial therapy should be continued for 2 weeks to eliminate carriage from oropharyngeal secretions and reduce the risk of transmission via aerosolized droplets.

Prognosis: M. pneumoniae is usually a mild, self-limiting illness in immunocompetent adults. M. pneumoniae may be severe in compromised hosts, the elderly, and those with advanced lung disease. Patients with M. pneumoniae and meningoencephalitis (headaches/stiff neck, mental confusion, very high cold agglutinin titers [often ≥ 1:1024]) have a good prognosis. M. pneumoniae may be complicated by transverse myelitis, brain stem/cerebellar ataxia, or Guillain-Barré syndrome after M. pneumoniae some patients develop permanent asthma.

Chlamydophilia (Chlamydia) pneumoniae

Epidemiology: C. pneumoniae is may occur as sporadic cases part of an outbreak NHAP. C. pneumoniae is spread from person-to-person via aerosolized droplets. C. pneumoniae has no seasonal predisposition. Some patients with C. pneumoniae CAP develop permanent asthma.

Clinical Presentation: C. pneumoniae presents as a "mycoplasma-like" illness. Like other atypical CAPs, C. pneumoniae CAP is characterized by extra-pulmonary findings, particularly nasal discharge, sore throat, and hoarseness (Table 2.1). Temperature is usually ≤ 102°F. Chest x-ray findings typically show a unilateral ill-defined infiltrate without consolidation, cavitation, or pleural effusion. C. pneumoniae testing is recommended in a patient with a "mycoplasma-like" illness and hoarseness.

Diagnostic Considerations: The diagnosis of C. pneumoniae CAP requires a single IgM titer of ≥ 1:16 or an IgG titer > 1:512 (ELISA or MIF). C. pneumoniae may be cultured from respiratory secretions using viral culture media.

Pitfalls: IgG titers indicate past exposure, not current infection. ↑ IgM and ↑ IgG titers may be delayed for more than 3 and 6 weeks, respectively. False negatives may occur if IgM titers are obtained too early. Recovery of C. pneumoniae from respiratory secretions does not differentiate carriage from infection. In a CAP patient with otherwise unexplained wheezing should suggest the possibility of C. Pneumoniae.

Therapeutic Considerations: Doxycycline, or quinolones are effective. C. pneumoniae is sensitive to erythromycin in vitro, but erythromycin is often ineffective in vivo. C. pneumoniae also responds to newer macrolides.

Prognosis: C. pneumoniae CAP is usually a mild/moderate pneumonia with an excellent prognosis. Severe CAP may occur in compromised hosts, the elderly, or those with severe lung disease some develop permanent asthma.

Table 2.1. Diagnostic Features of Non-zoonotic Atypical Pneumonias

Key Characteristics	Mycoplasma pneumoniae	Legionnaires' Disease	C. pneumoniae
Symptoms			
Mental confusion	$-^\dagger$	+	–
Prominent headache	–	±	–
Meningismus	–	–	–
Myalgias	±	±	±
Ear pain	+	–	±
Pleuritic pain	–	±	–
Abdominal pain	–	±	–
Loose stools/watery diarrhea	±	±	–
Signs			
Rash	± a	–	–
Non-exudative pharyngitis	+	–	+
Hemoptysis	–	+	–
Wheezing	–	–	+
Lobar consolidation	–	+	–
Cardiac involvement	± b	– c	–
Splenomegaly	–	–	–
Relative bradycardia	–	+	–
Laboratory Abnormalities			
WBC count	↑/N	↑	N
Acute thrombocytosis	±	–	–
Hyponatremia	–	+	–
Hypophosphatemia	–	+	–
↑ AST/ALT (SGOT/SGPT)	–	+	–
↑ CPK	–	+	–
↑ CRP (> 30)	–	+	–
↑ Ferritin (> 2 x n)	–	+	–
↑ Cold agglutinins (≥ 1:64)	+	–	–
Microscopic hematuria	–	±	–
Chest X-Ray			
Infiltrate	Patchy	Patchy or consolidation	Circumscribed lesions
Bilateral hilar adenopathy	–	–	–
Pleural effusion	± (small)	±	–

ALT = alanine aminotransferase; AST = aspartate aminotransferase; N = normal; WBC = white blood cell.
+ = usually present; ± = sometimes present; – = usually absent.
↑ = increased; ↓ = decreased; ↑↑↑ = markedly increased.
a = erythema multiforme; b = myocarditis, heart block, or pericarditis; c = unless endocarditis.
† = mental confusion only if meningoencephalitis.
†† = often not be positive early, but antigenuria persists for weeks. Useful only to diagnose L. pneumophila (serogroups 01-06), not other species/serogroups.

Zoonotic Atypical Pneumonia (see Chapter 8 for Differential Diagnosis of Chest X-Ray patterns)

Subset	Usual Pathogens*	Preferred IV Therapy	Alternate IV Therapy	PO Therapy or IV-to-PO Switch
Zoonotic pathogens (zoonotic vector)	C. psittaci (psittacosis) Coxiella burnetii (Q fever) Francisella tularensis (tularemia)	Doxycycline 200 mg (IV) q12h × 3 days, then 100 mg (IV) q12h × 11 days	Levofloxacin 500 mg (IV) × 2 weeks **or** Moxifloxacin 400 mg (IV) × 2 weeks	Doxycycline 200 mg (PO) q12h × 3 days, then 100 mg (PO) q12h × 11 days† **or** Levofloxacin 500 mg (PO) × 2 weeks **or** Moxifloxacin 400 mg (PO) × 2 weeks

Duration of therapy represents total time IV, PO, or IV + PO.
*   Compromised hosts may require longer courses of therapy.
†   Loading dose is not needed PO if give IV with the same drug.

Clinical Presentation: CAP with extrapulmonary symptoms, signs, or laboratory abnormalities (Table 2.2).

Diagnostic Considerations: Zoonotic contact history is key to presumptive diagnosis: psittacosis (parrots and psittacine birds); Q fever (sheep, parturient cats); tularemia (rabbit, deer, deer fly bite). The diagnosis is confirmed by specific serological testing. Zoonotic CAP with splenomegaly/relative bradycardia suggests Q fever or psittacosis.

Pitfalls: Organisms are difficult/dangerous to grow. Do not culture. Use serological tests for diagnosis. The diagnosis of acute Q fever is by demonstrating elevated IgG (phase II) C. burnetii titers. Most patients with acute Q fever do not become chronic e.g., Q fever SBE. The diagnosis of chronic Q fever is made by demonstrating elevated IgG (phase I) titers ≥ 1:1024 at 6 months following acute Q fever. C. burnetii (Q fever) titers may cross react with Bartonella titers.

Therapeutic Considerations: Q fever endocarditis requires prolonged therapy.

Prognosis: Good except for Q fever with complications, e.g., myocarditis, SBE.

Table 2.2. Diagnostic Features of Zoonotic Atypical Pneumonias

Key Characteristics	Psittacosis	Q Fever	Tularemia
Symptoms			
Mental confusion	−	±	−
Prominent headache	+	+	+
Meningismus	−	−	−
Myalgias	+	+	+
Ear pain	−	−	−
Pleuritic pain	±	±	+
Abdominal pain	−	−	−
Diarrhea	−	−	−
Signs			
Rash	± a	−	−
Nonexudative pharyngitis	−	−	±
Hemoptysis	−	−	±
Lobar consolidation	+	+	+
Cardiac involvement	± b	± c	−
Splenomegaly	±	+	−
Relative bradycardia	±	±	−
Chest X-Ray			
Infiltrate	Patchy consolidation	"Round" infiltrates or consolidation	"Ovoid infiltrates"
Bilateral hilar adenopathy	−	−	±
Pleural effusion	−	−	Bloody
Laboratory Abnormalities			
WBC count	↓	↑/N	↑/N
Acute thrombocytosis	−	+	−
Hyponatremia	±	±	±
Hypophosphatemia	−	−	−
↑ AST/ALT (SGOT/SGPT)	+	+	−
↑ Cold agglutinins	−	±	−
Anti-smooth muscle antibodies (anti-SMA)	−	±	−
Microscopic hematuria	−	−	−

ALT = alanine aminotransferase; AST = aspartate aminotransferase; N = normal; WBC = white blood cell.
+ = usually present; ± = sometimes present; − = usually absent.
↑ = increased; ↓ = decreased; ↑↑↑ = markedly increased.
a = Horder's spots (facial spots, resemble the abdominal rash of typhoid fever (rose spots); b = Mycocarditis;
c = Endocarditis.

Zoonotic Infections (Severe Acute Respiratory Syndrome; SARS)

Presentation: Fever, dry cough, myalgias, diarrhea in some. Auscultation of the lungs resembles viral influenza (i.e., quiet, no rales). Biphasic infection: fever decreases after few days, patient improves, then fever recurs in a few days and patients become short of breath/hypoxic. Chest x-ray shows bilateral interstitial (diffuse) infiltrates. WBC and platelet counts are usually normal or slightly decreased. Relative lymphopenia present early. Mild increases in SGOT/SGPT, LDH, CPK are common.

Diagnostic Considerations: Diagnosis by viral isolation or specific SARS serology. Important to exclude influenza A, Legionnaires' disease and tularemic pneumonia.

Pitfalls: Should not be confused with viral influenza (a 3-day illness). Patients with SARS deteriorate during week 2 when influenza patients are recovering. Early, chest x-ray in SARS has discrete infiltrates (unlike influenza unless superimposed CAP) that may be ovoid. Late, ARDS on chest x-ray.

Therapeutic Considerations: Most patients are severely hypoxemic and require oxygen/ventilatory support. In a preliminary study, some patients benefitted from corticosteroids (pulse-dosed methylprednisolone 500 mg [IV] q24h × 3 days followed by taper/step down with prednisone [PO] to complete 20 days) plus Interferon alfacon-1 (9 mcg [SQ] q24h × at least 2 days, increased to 15 mcg/d if no response) × 8–13 days. Ribavirin of no benefit.

Prognosis: Related to underlying cardiopulmonary/immune status/ARDS. Frequently fatal.

Pitfalls: Failure to respond to beta-lactams should suggest diagnosis of atypical CAP.

Therapeutic Considerations: Treat Legionella × 4 weeks. Treat Mycoplasma or Chlamydia × 2 weeks.

Prognosis: Related to severity of underlying cardiopulmonary disease.

Avian Influenza (Influenza A (H$_5$N$_1$)

Clinical Presentation: Influenza following close contact with infected poultry. Recent outbreaks in humans in Asia. Human-to-human transmission reported. Often fulminant respiratory illness rapidly followed by ARDS/death.

Diagnostic Considerations: Often acute onset of severe influenza illness ± diarrhea/conjunctival suffusion with leukopenia, lymphopenia, mildly ↑ serum transaminases and ↑ LDH. Diagnosis by hemagglutin-specific RT-PCR for avian influenza or culture of respiratory secretions.

Pitfalls: Although avian influenza is caused by influenza A virus, the hemagglutinin inhibition serological test used to diagnose influenza A is insensitive to avian hemagglutinin, resulting in negative testing.

Therapeutic Considerations: Antivirals must be given early to be effective. Avian influenza strains may be resistant to oseltamivir and amantadine/rimantadine. Oseltamivir 150 mg dose may be more effective than 75 mg dose. Even if resistant, amantadine/rimantadine should be given to increase peripheral airway dilatation/oxygenation.

Prognosis: Often fulminant with ARDS/death. Unlike human/swine influenza, avian influenza is often rapidly/highly lethal but *not* complicated by MSSA/MRSA CAP.

Human/Seasonal Influenza (types A/B)

Clinical Presentation: Acute onset of fever, headache, myalgias/arthralgias, sore throat, prostration, dry cough. Myalgias most pronounced in lower back/legs. Eye pain is common. Rapid high fever initially, which decreases in 2–3 days. Severity ranges from mild flu to life-threatening pneumonia. Chest x-ray in early influenza is normal/near normal without focal/segmental infiltrates or pleural effusion.

Diagnostic Considerations: Mild cases with headache, sore throat, and rhinorrhea resemble the common cold/respiratory viruses (influenza-like illnesses) and can be caused by type A or B. Severe flu is usually due to type A. Rapid diagnosis by DFA of respiratory secretions (nasopharyngeal swabs). Influenza virus may be cultured in viral media from respiratory secretions and typed.

Pitfalls: Influenza pneumonia has no chest auscultatory findings and the chest x-ray is normal/near normal. Severe influenza pneumonia is accompanied by an oxygen diffusion defect (↑ A-a gradient), and patients are hypoxemic/cyanotic. Pleuritic chest pain may be present Influenza can invade the intercostal muscles to mimic pleuritic chest pain. Infiltrates on chest x-ray with viral pneumonia indicate simultaneous/subsequent bacterial CAP. If CAP presents with fulminant/severe necrotizing pneumonia in a normal host. Ask about antecedent "flu/flu-like illness".

Therapeutic Considerations: Mild/moderate influenza can be treated with neuraminidase inhibitors (Tamiflu/Relenza), which reduce symptoms by 1–2 days. Start treatment within 2 days of symptom onset. Reduce the dose of Tamiflu to 75 mg (PO) q48h for CrCl 10–30 cc/min. Relenza is generally not recommended for patients with underlying COPD/asthma (increased risk of bronchospasm) and should be discontinued if bronchospasm or a decline in respiratory function occurs. For severe influenza/pneumonia, treat with rimantadine or amantadine, which may increase peripheral airway dilatation/oxygenation. Reduce the dose of rimantadine to 100 mg (PO) q24h in the elderly, severe liver dysfunction, or CrCl < 10 cc/min. Flu with simultaneousbacterial CAP is often due to MSSA/MRSA and subsequent post-influenza CAP usually due to S. pneumoniae or H. influenzae (see p. 52).

Prognosis: Good for mild/moderate flu. Severe flu may be fatal due to influenza pneumonia with profound hypoxemia. Prognosis is worse if presents with simultaneous MSSA/MRSA. Influenza with necrotizing community-acquired (CA) MSSA/MRSA CAP is frequently fatal. Prognosis is worst for CA-MRSA Panton-Valentine Leukocidin (PVL)-positive strains. Dry cough/fatigue may persist for weeks after influenza.

Table 2.3. The 3 Clinical Presentations of Influenza A Pneumonia in Adults

Clinical features at time of onset	Severity	Usual Pathogens
• Influenza pneumonia (**no focal/lobar infiltrates**)	Mild → *rarely fatal*	Influenza (human, swine†)
• Influenza pneumonia **plus** bacterial CAP (**with multiple rapidly cavitating infiltrates**)	Severe → *often rapidly fatal*	Influenza (human, swine *not* avian) **plus** MSSA/CA-MRSA*
• Influenza pneumonia **plus** bacterial CAP (**followed by non-cavitating focal/lobar infiltrates** (after ~1 week of improvement))	Mild/moderate → *rarely fatal* (unless underlying cardiopulmonary disease/Immunodeficiency)	S. pneumoniae, H. influenzae

† Avian influenza (H_5N_1) often rapidly fatal in young/healthy adults.
* CA-MRSA PVL + strains usually virulent/lethal.

Swine Influenza (H_1N_1) Pneumonia

Clinical Presentation: Swine influenza (H_1N_1) may present ranging from a mild illness with fever, cough, and loose stool/diarrhea to severe viral pneumonia requiring ventilation that may rapidly progress to ARDS/death. Because the clinical presentation resembles that of human seasonal influenza, patients with swine influenza (H_1N_1) pneumonia as well as other viral pneumonias typically present as influenza-like illnesses (ILIs). Unlike human seasonal influenza, swine influenza (H_1N_1) pneumonia affects primarily young healthy adults. As with human seasonal influenza, swine influenza (H_1N_1) may affect children, pregnant females, and the elderly with co-morbid conditions. In admitted adults, swine influenza (H_1N_1) pneumonia typically presents with high fevers > 102°F often with shaking chills and myalgias. Patients may also complain of headache or sore throat. Dry cough is characteristic but a mildly productive cough with thin mucoid sputum is also common. Patients are variably short of breath. Conjunctival suffusion is rare. Lungs are clear to auscultation. Patients often have loose stools/diarrhea but not abdomi-nal pain. Swine influenza (H_1N_1) pneumonia clinically resembles human sea-sonal influenza, avian influenza, CMV or adenoviral CAP. CXR early (< 48 hours) typically is clear or may show accentuated bibasilar lung markings resembling basilar atelectasis. CXR later (> 48 hours) typically shows bilateral patchy interstitial infiltrates. Consolidation may occur later, but cavitations or moderate/large pleural effusions are not features. Degree of hypoxemia is related to the severity of pneumonia. In adults, nonspecific laboratory clues include otherwise unexplained relative lymphopenia thrombocytopenia elevated CPKs or mildly elevated serum transaminases (SGOT/SGPT). Atypical lym-phocytes are not present in adults. Unlike in human seasonal and avian influenza (H_5N_1), leukopenia is uncommon in swine influenza (H_1N_1) pneumonia in adults. Serum LDH is variably elevated. Elevated cold agglutinin titers are not elevated. Nosocomial transmission may occur.

Diagnostic Considerations: Definitive diagnosis is by RT-PCR of oropharyngeal/respiratory secretions/lung. Rapid influenza diagnostic screening tests (RIDTs), if positive, correlate well with RT-PCR positivity. However, ~30% of (RIDTs) are false negative. Therefore, negative (RIDTs) does not rule out swine influ-enza (H_1N_1). Respiratory fluorescent antibody (FA) viral testing may or may not be positive. Discordant testing results with rapid influenza A, respiratory FA viral panel, and RT-PCR may be due to variability of specimens rather than differences in test sensitivity/specificity. All diagnostic tests may be negative in autopsy proven cases of swine influenza (H_1N_1) pneumonia whose lungs are RT-PCR positive.

Pitfalls: Since swine influenza (H_1N_1) pneumonia presents as an ILI, care must be taken to rule out other viral pneumonias as well as mimics of viral pneumonia. During the swine influenza (H_1N_1) pandemic, the most frequent diagnostic error was to assume a negative RIDT was predictive of a negative RT-PCR for H_1N_1. In adults with ILIs and negative RIDTs, clinical criteria are helpful in iden-tifying swine influenza (H_1N_1) pneumonia (Table 2.3). The CXR is important in identifying possible mimics of swine flu. While human seasonal influenza may present simultaneously with MSSA/MRSA CAP or subsequently after an interval (5–7 days) of improvement with *S. pneumoniae* or *H. influenzae* CAP, this and has been uncommon with swine influenza (H_1N_1) pneumonia and has not been a complication of avian influenza (H_5N_1) pneumonia. Swine influenza (H_1N_1) pneumonia on CXR appears initially with clear lung fields and with subsequent bilateral patchy infiltrates. Cold agglutinins and atypical lymphocytes may occur in pediatric cases but in adults should suggest an alternate diagnosis, e.g., adenoviral or CMV pneumonia. Diagnostic tests for swine influenza (H_1N_1) pneumonia may all be negative. In some autopsy proven cases of swine influenza (H_1N_1) pneumonia with negative tests have had positive RT-PCR for H_1N_1 in lung.

Therapeutic Considerations: Swine influenza (H_1N_1) appears to respond to oseltamivir. There are no benefits to steroids. Although amantadine or rimantadine are ineffective against swine influ-enza (H_1N_1), patients who are severely hypoxemic may benefit from amantadine or rimantadine by increasing peripheral airway dilatation/oxygenation. If the CXR in swine influenza (H_1N_1) pneumonia has no lobar/focal infiltrates, there is no need to treat with empiric antimicrobial therapy. Swine influenza (H_1N_1) pneumonia with multiple lobar/focal infiltrates that rapidly cavitate (< 72 hours) empiric anti-MSSA/CA-MRSA therapy should be given with oseltamivir. For patients with swine influ-enza (H_1N_1) pneumonia that improves and after 5–7 days re-present with focal segmental/lobar (non-cavitating) infiltrates, treat as for typical CAP to cover S. pneumoniae or H. influenzae.

In patients unable to take oval oseltamivir, IV peramivir may be given. (See p. 665 for dosing recommendations.)

Prognosis: In immuncompetent adults, prognosis is related to severity of swine influenza (H_1N_1) pneumonia. With swine influenza (H_1N_1), prognosis is directly related to the severity of pneumonia (associated oxygen diffusion defect) i.e., degree/duration of severe hypoxemia. Prognosis is worst with simultaneous MSSA/MRSA CAP, but is not worse with subsequent S. pneumoniae or H. influenzae CAP.

Table 2.4. Rapid Clinical Diagnosis of Swine Influenza (H_1N_1) Pneumonia in Hospitalized Adults with Negative Rapid Influenza Diagnostic Tests (RIDTs): Diagnostic Swine Influenza Triad

Probable Swine Influenza (H_1N_1) Pneumonia (Clinical Criteria) Diagnosis
ILI with dry cough, temperature > 102°F and myalgias with a CXR without focal/segmental lobar infiltrates with negative RIDTs* *plus any 3 of the following*§:

- Relative lymphopenia[†]
- Thrombocytopenia[†]
- Elevated SGOTs/SGPTs[†]
- Elevated CPKs[†]

* Diagnostic tests negative for other viral CAP pathogens (CMV, SARS, HPS, RSV, metapneumoviruses, parainfluenza viruses, adenoviruses).
§ Present during first 3 days of hospitalization.
† Otherwise unexplained.

Aspiration Pneumonia

Diagnostic Considerations: Sputum not diagnostic. No need for transtracheal aspirate culture.
Pitfalls: Lobar location varies with patient position during aspiration.
Therapeutic Considerations: Oral anaerobes are sensitive to all beta-lactams and most antibiotics used to treat CAP. Additional anaerobic (B. fragilis) coverage is not needed.
Prognosis: Related to severity of CNS/esophageal disease.

CAP in HIV (*Sputum Negative for AFB*) (PCP see p. 325)

Clinical Presentation: Bacterial CAP in HIV patient with focal infiltrate(s) and normal/slightly depressed CD_4.
Diagnostic Considerations: Diagnosis by sputum gram stain/culture ± positive blood cultures (bacterial pathogens) or Legionella/Chlamydia serology (atypical pathogens). S. pneumoniae and H. influenzae are particularly common.
Pitfalls: Atypical chest x-ray appearance is not uncommon. Treat syndrome of CAP, not chest x-ray. Bacterial CAP (focal/segmental infiltrates) in HIV does not resemble PCP (bilateral patchy interstitial infiltrates). PCP presents with profound hypoxemia and ↑ LDH/↑ β-glucan levels.
Therapeutic Considerations: R/O TB/MAI with negative sputum AFB stain. If AFB negative, treat same as bacterial CAP in normal hosts.
Prognosis: Same as bacterial CAP in normal hosts.

Tuberculous (TB) Pneumonia

Clinical Presentation: Community-acquired pneumonia with single/multiple infiltrates.
Diagnostic Considerations: Diagnosis by sputum AFB smear/culture. Primary TB is lower lobe usually with a pleural effusion. Reactivation TB is usually bilateral/apical ± old, healed Ghon complex; cavitation/fibrosis are common, but adenopathy or pleural effusions uncommon. TB reactivation ↑ with steroids, immunosuppressive drugs, HIV, gastorectomy, jejunoileal bypass, silicosis, DM, CRI, advanced age.

Pitfalls: Primary TB may present as CAP and improve transiently with quinolone therapy. Primary TB patients with large pleural effusion usually anergic.

Therapeutic Considerations: Usually sputum becomes smear negative in 1–2 weeks of therapy.

Prognosis: Related to underlying health status.

Mycobacterium avium-intracellulare (MAI) Pneumonia

Clinical Presentation: Community-acquired pneumonia in normal hosts or immunosuppressed/HIV patient with focal single/multiple infiltrates indistinguishable from TB.

Diagnostic Considerations: Diagnosis by AFB culture. In HIV, MAI may disseminate, resembling miliary TB. MAI typically lingular with "tree in bud" appearance on chest CT. BHA more frequent than with TB.

Pitfalls: May mimic reactivation TB. Must differentiate TB from MAI by AFB culture, since therapy for MAI differs from TB.

Therapeutic Considerations: Should be treated until sputum cultures are negative × 1 year.

Prognosis: Good in normal hosts. In HIV related to degree of immunosuppression/CD_4 count.

Mycobacterium kansasii Pneumonia

Clinical Presentation: Subacute CAP resembling reactivation TB.

Diagnostic Considerations: Chest x-ray infiltrates/lung disease plus M. kansasii in a single sputum specimen. M. kansasii can cause disseminated infection, like TB, and is diagnosed by culturing M. kansasii from sputum, blood, liver, or bone marrow.

Pitfalls: M. kansasii in sputum with a normal chest x-ray and no symptoms does not indicate infection.

Therapeutic Considerations: Should be treated until sputum cultures are negative × 1 year.

Prognosis: Good in normal hosts. May be rapidly progressive/fatal without treatment in HIV patients.

Pneumonia in Chronic Alcoholics

Diagnostic Considerations: Klebsiella pneumoniae usually occurs only in chronic alcoholics, and is characterized by blood-flecked "currant jelly" sputum and cavitation (typically in 3–5 days).

Pitfalls: Suspect Klebsiella in "pneumococcal" pneumonia that cavitates. Empyema is more common than pleural effusion.

Therapeutic Considerations: Monotherapy with newer anti-Klebsiella agents, e.g., 3rd GC, carbapenems, colistin, tigacycline, are as effective or superior to "double-drug" therapy with older agents.

Prognosis: Related to degree of hepatic/splenic dysfunction.

Influenza Pneumonia

Diagnostic Considerations: S. aureus pneumonia or Legionnaire's disease may present *concurrently* with influenza pneumonia. MSSA/MRSA CAP is characterized by cyanosis and rapid cavitation < 72 hrs. Do not diagnose staphylococcal pneumonia without these findings.

Pitfalls: Following clinical improvement after ~1 week bacterial CAP due to S. pneumoniae or H. influenzae may follow viral influenza pneumonia.

Therapeutic Considerations: No need to cover MRSA for post-viral influenza bacterial CAP. Treat for typical bacterial CAP. Due to S. pneumoniae or H. influenzae.

Prognosis: Related to severity of influenza pneumonia and host factors, e.g., cardiopulmonary disease.

Bronchiectasis/Cystic Fibrosis

Diagnostic Considerations: Cystic fibrosis/bronchiectasis is characterized by viscous secretions ± low grade fevers; less commonly may present as lung abscess. Onset of pneumonia/lung abscess heralded by cough/decrease in pulmonary function.

Pitfalls: Sputum colonization is common (e.g., S. maltophilia, B. cepacia, P. aeruginosa); may not reflect pathogens.

Therapeutic Considerations: Important to select antibiotics with low resistance potential and good penetration into respiratory secretions (e.g., quinolones, meropenem).

Prognosis: Related to extent of underlying lung disease/severity of infection.

Pneumonia in Organ Transplants

Clinical Presentation: CAP with perihilar infiltrates and hypoxemia.

Diagnostic Considerations: CMV is diagnosed by stain/culture of lung biopsy.

Therapeutic Considerations: Treat as CMV pneumonia if CMV is predominant pathogen on lung biopsy. CMV may progress despite ganciclovir therapy.

Prognosis: Related to degree of immunosuppression.

Pneumonia in Chronic Steroid Therapy

If fungal infection is suspected, obtain lung biopsy to confirm diagnosis/identify causative organism. Non-responsiveness to appropriate antibiotics should suggest fungal infection. Avoid empirically treating fungi; due to the required duration of therapy, it is advantageous to confirm the diagnosis by lung biopsy first. Prognosis related to degree of immunosuppression.

Acute Aspergillus Pneumonia

Clinical Presentation: Chest x-ray shows progressive necrotizing pneumonia (bilateral in half) unresponsive to antibiotics. Characteristic of early Apsergillus pneumonia is the "halo sign". A few days later the halo decreases in size. After a week after the appearance of the halo sign, the "air crescent sign" is typically present. Usually seen only in compromised hosts.

Diagnostic Considerations: Diagnosis by lung biopsy (not broncho-alveolar lavage) demonstrating hyphae invading lung parenchyma/blood vessels. Usually occurs only in patients on chronic steroids, cancer chemotherapy, organ transplants, leukopenic compromised hosts, or with chronic granulomatous disease (CGD). Apsergillus galactomannan (GM) may XR with Geotrichum, Blastomyces, Penicillium, or Alternaria. ↑ GM levels with cyclophosphamide and if enteritis/colitis (↑ absorption of GM).

Pitfalls: Invasive Aspergillus pneumonia does not occur in normal/non-immunosuppressed hosts. ↑ β-glucan levels like PCP, but unlike PCP not ↑ LDH levels.

Prognosis: Cavitation is a good prognostic sign. Prognosis related to degree of immunosuppression.

Lung Abscess/Empyema

Subset	Usual Pathogens	Preferred IV Therapy	Alternate IV Therapy	PO Therapy or IV-to-PO Switch
Lung abscess/ empyema	Oral anaerobes S. aureus K.pneumoniae S. pneumoniae	Clindamycin 600 mg (IV) q8h* **or** Piperacillin/ tazobactam 3.375 gm (IV) q8h*	Meropenem 1 gm (IV) q8h* **or** Ertapenem 1 gm (IV) q24h*	Clindamycin 300 mg (PO) q8h* **or** Quinolone† (PO) q24h*

Bronchiectasis, cystic fibrosis (P. aeruginosa): see p. 54

* Treat until resolved. Duration of therapy represents total time IV, PO, or IV + PO. Most patients on IV therapy able to take PO meds should be switched to PO therapy soon after clinical improvement (usually < 72 hours).

† Moxifloxacin 400 mg or Levofloxacin 500 mg.

Clinical Presentation: Lung abscess presents as single/multiple cavitary lung lesion(s) with fever. Empyema presents as persistent fever/pleural effusion without layering on lateral decubitus chest x-ray.

Diagnostic Considerations: In lung abscess, plain film/CT scan demonstrates cavitary lung lesions appearing > 1 week after pneumonia. Most CAPs are not associated with pleural effusion, and few develop empyema. In empyema, pleural fluid pH is ≤ 7.2; culture purulent exudate for pathogen.

Pitfalls: Pleural effusions secondary to CAP usually resolve rapidly with treatment. Suspect empyema in patients with persistent pleural effusions with fever.

Therapeutic Considerations: Chest tube/surgical drainage needed for empyema. Treat lung abscess until it resolves (usually 3–12 months).

Prognosis: Good if adequately drained.

Nursing Home-Acquired Pneumonia (NHAP)

Subset	Usual Pathogens*	Preferred IV Therapy	Alternate IV Therapy	PO Therapy or IV-to-PO Switch
Nursing home-acquired pneumonia (NHAP)	H. influenzae S. pneumoniae M. catarrhalis	Ceftriaxone 1 gm (IV) q24h × 2 weeks **or** Respiratory quinolone†† (IV) q24h × 2 weeks **or** Doxycycline 200 mg (IV) q12h × 3 days; then 100 mg (IV) q12h × 2 weeks	Ertapenem 1 gm (IV) q24h × 2 weeks **or** Cefepime 2 gm (IV) q12h × 2 weeks	Respiratory quinolone†† (PO) q24h × 2 weeks **or** Doxycycline 200 mg (PO) q12h × 3 days, then 100 mg (PO) q12h × 11 days

Diagnostic Considerations: Difficult to obtain sputum in elderly/debilitated patients. H. influenzae is common; K. pneumoniae is uncommon in non-alcoholics, even in this population.

Pitfalls: Resembles community-acquired pneumonia in terms of pathogens and length of hospital stay, not nosocomial pneumonia.

Therapeutic Considerations: Treat as community-acquired pneumonia, not nosocomial pneumonia. No need to cover P. aeruginosa or GNBs.

Prognosis: Related to underlying cardiopulmonary status.

Nosocomial Pneumonia (NP) / Hospital-Acquired Pneumonia (HAP) / Ventilator-Associated Pneumonia (VAP)§

Subset	Usual Pathogens	Preferred IV Therapy	Alternate IV Therapy	IV-to-PO Switch
Empiric therapy	P. aeruginosa* E. coli K. pneumoniae S. marcescens (S. aureus)†	Meropenem 1 gm (IV) q8h × 1–2 weeks **or** Doripenem 1 gm (IV) q8h × 2 weeks **or** Levofloxacin 750 mg (IV) q24h × 1–2 weeks **or** Piperacillin/tazobactam 4.5 gm (IV) q6h **plus** amikacin 1 gm (IV) q24h × 1–2 wks		Levofloxacin 750 mg (PO) q24h × 1–2 weeks **or** Ciprofloxacin 750 mg (PO) q12h × 1–2 weeks

*   For *confirmed* P. aeruginosa NP/VAP, combination therapy *preferred*.

†   **MSSA/MRSA are common colonizers of respiratory secretions. In ventilated patients with fever, leukocytosis, and infiltrates on CXR, are *not* diagnostic of MSSA/MRSA NP/HAP/VAP. MSSA/MRSA NP/HAP/VAP is clinically distinctive and rare.**

§   Treat aspiration NP same as NP/VAP. Anerobes not pathogens in aspiration NP.

Nosocomial Pneumonia (NP) / Hospital-Acquired Pneumonia (HAP) / Ventilator-Associated Pneumonia (VAP) (cont'd)

Subset	Usual Pathogens	Preferred IV Therapy	Alternate IV Therapy	IV-to-PO Switch
Specific therapy	P. aeruginosa*‡	Meropenem 1 gm (IV) q8h × 2 weeks **or** Doripenem 1 gm (IV) q8h × 2 weeks† **plus either** Levofloxacin 750 mg (IV) q24h × 2 weeks **or** Ciprofloxacin 400 mg (IV) q8h × 2 weeks **or** Amikacin 1 gm (IV) q24h × 2 weeks		Levofloxacin 750 mg (PO) q24h × 2 weeks **or** Ciprofloxacin 750 mg (PO) q12h × 2 weeks
	MDR Klebsiella or MDR Acinetobacter	Meropenem 1 gm (IV) q8h × 2 weeks **or** Doripenem 1 gm (IV) q8h × 2 weeks† **or** Tigacycline 200 mg (IV) × 1 dose, then 100 mg (IV) q24h × 2 weeks¶		
	MDR P. aeruginosa	Doripenem 1 gm (IV) q8h × 2 weeks† **or** Colistin 1.7 mg/kg (IV) q8h × 2 weeks **or** Polymyxin B 1–1.25 mg/kg (IV) q12h × 2 weeks **or** Meropenem 1 gm (IV) q8h × 2 weeks§		
	HSV-1**	Acyclovir 10 mg/kg (IV) q8h × 10 days		Valacyclovir 1 gm (PO) q8h × 10 days

* **For empiric P. aeruginosa coverage, monotherapy sufficient.** For *proven* P. aeruginosa NP/VAP, *combination therapy preferred.*

‡ P. aeruginosa NP/VAP shows multiple infiltrates with rapid cavitation in <72 h on CXR ± otherwise unexplained blood cultures for P. aeruginosa (BCs negative with inhalation acquired P. aeruginosa VAP and BCs + with in hematogenously acquired P. aeruginosa NP/VAP).

† Give as a 4 hour infusion.

** Presents late in course of VAP as "failure to wean", does *not* present as early VAP.

§ If susceptible.

¶ Higher than usual doses of tigacycline may be necessary for susceptible MDR GNBs.

Clinical Presentation: Pulmonary infiltrate compatible with a bacterial pneumonia occurring ≥ 1 week in-hospital ± fever/leukocytosis.

Diagnostic Considerations: CXR infiltrates with leukocytosis and fever are nonspecific/nondiagnostic of NP/VAP. Definitive diagnosis by lung biopsy. P. aeruginosa is a common colonizer in ventilated patients. P. aeruginosa VAP manifests as a necrotizing pneumonia with rapid cavitation (< 72 hours), microabscesses, and blood vessel invasion. S. aureus (MSSA/MRS) NP/VAP is very rare despite being cultured from 25% of ET tube BAL or respiratory secretions. Acinetobacter/ Legionella NP/VAP usually occur in outbreaks.

Pitfalls: No rationale for covering non-pulmonary pathogens colonizing respiratory secretions in ventilated patients (Enterobacter, B. cepacia, S. maltophilia, Citrobacter, Flavobacterium, Enterococci); these organisms rarely if ever cause NP/VAP. Semi-quantitative BAL/protected brush specimens may reflect airway colonization. Even tissue biopsy is needed for definitive diagnosis of P. aeruginosa NP/VAP. MSSA/MRSA are common colonizers of respiratory secretions and are not uncommon pathogens causing tracheobronchitis in ventilated patients. MSSA/MRSA necrotizing/rapidly cavitating NP/VAP is rare.

Therapeutic Considerations: NP (HAP/VAP) is defined as pneumonia acquired > 5 hospital days. So called "early" NP occurring < 5 days of hospitalization, which may be due to S. pneumoniae (including DRSP strains) or H. influenzae, actually represents CAP that manifests early after hospital admission. Empiric therapy recommendations (p. 68) cover "early" and "late" NP/VAP pathogens. Monotherapy is as effective as combination therapy for non-P. aeruginosa NP/VAP, but 2-drug therapy is recommended for confirmed P. aeruginosa NP/VAP. If MSSA/MRSA necrotizing/rapidly cavitating NP/VAP present, may be treated with vancomycin, quinupristin/dalfopristin or linezolid (see drug summaries in Chapter 11). After 2 weeks of appropriate antibiotic therapy, nonprogressive/stable pulmonary infiltrates with fever and leukocytosis are usually due to a noninfectious cause, rather than persistent infection. Treat aspiration NP/VAP the same as NP/VAP since anaerobes are not pathogens in NP/VAP.

Prognosis: Related to underlying cardiopulmonary status.

Empiric Therapy of Cardiovascular Infections

Native Valve Subacute Bacterial Endocarditis (SBE)

Subset	Usual Pathogens	Preferred IV Therapy	Alternate IV Therapy	PO Therapy or IV-to-PO Switch
No obvious source or oral	Viridans streptococci*[†] Group B, C, G streptococci, S. bovis (PCN MIC < 0.12 mcg/ml)	Ceftriaxone 2 gm (IV) q24h × 2 weeks*[‡] **plus** Gentamicin 240 mg or 3 mg/kg (IV) q24h × 2 weeks* **or** **monotherapy with** Ceftriaxone 2 gm (IV) q24h × 4 weeks	Penicillin G 3 mu (IV) q4h × 2 weeks*[‡] **plus** Gentamicin 240 mg or 3 mg/kg (IV) q24h × 2 weeks* **or** Vancomycin 1 gm (IV) q12h × 2 weeks **or** Linezolid 600 mg (IV) q12h × 4 weeks	Linezolid[§] 600 mg (PO) q12h × 4–6 weeks **or** Amoxicillin[§] 1 gm (PO) q8h × 4–6 weeks

*   If *relatively* PCN resistant (MIC 0.12–0.5 mcg/ml) or if *no intra/extra cardiac complications* treat × 4 weeks.
†   S. mitis (S. mitior), S. oralis, S. gordonii, S. parasanguis, S. sanguis, S. mutans, S. sobrinus, S. thermophilus, S. angiosus, S. milleri, S. intermedius, S. constellatus.
‡   In PCN allergic patients, Vancomycin 1 gm (IV) q12h × 2 weeks.
§   IV therapy preferred. PO therapy if no IV access or if patient not a surgical candidate.

Native Valve Subacute Bacterial Endocarditis (SBE) (cont'd)

Subset	Usual Pathogens	Preferred IV Therapy	Alternate IV Therapy	PO Therapy or IV-to-PO Switch
	Nutritionally- variant streptococci (NVS) pyridoxal B$_6$ dependent streptocci‡	As above, but treat × 6 weeks	As above, but treat × 6 weeks	As above§, but treat × 6 weeks
	Listeria monocytogenes	Ampicillin 2 gm (IV) q4h × 4–6 weeks **or** TMP-SMX 5 mg/kg (IV) q6h	Meropenem 1 gm (IV) q8h × 4–6 weeks	Amoxicillin§ 1 gm (PO) q8h × 4–6 weeks **or** Linezolid§ 600 mg (PO) q12h × 4–6 weeks
GI/GU source likely (Treat initially for E. faecalis (VSE); if later identified as E. faecium (VRE), treat accordingly)	E. faecalis (VSE)†	Ampicillin in 2 gm (IV) q4h × 4–6 weeks **plus** Gentamicin 1 mg/kg (IV) or 80 mg (IV) q8h × 4–6 weeks	Vancomycin 1 gm or 15 mg/kg (IV) q12h × 4–6 weeks **plus** Gentamicin 240 mg or 3 mg/kg (IV) q24h × 2 weeks	Amoxicillin§ 1 gm (PO) q8h × 4–6 weeks **or** Linezolid§ 600 mg (PO) q12h × 4–6 weeks
	E. faecium (VRE)†	Linezolid 600 mg (IV) q12h × ≥ 8 weeks **or** Quinupristin/dalfopristin 7.5 mg/kg (IV) q8h × ≥ 8 weeks		Linezolid§ 600 mg (PO) q12h × ≥ 8 weeks
GI source	S. (bovis) gallolyticus (Non-enterococcal group D streptococci)	Treat the same as "no obvious source" subset (see p. 70)		

VRE = vancomycin-resistant enterococci. Duration of therapy represents total time IV, PO, or IV + PO.
†   Symptoms < 3 months → treat × 4 weeks.
    Symptoms > 3 months → treat × 6 weeks.
‡   *NVS (nutritionally variant streptococci) include: Abiotrophia defectivus, Granulicata adjacens/elegans.*
§   IV therapy preferred. PO therapy if no IV access or if patient not a surgical candidate.

Native Valve Subacute Bacterial Endocarditis (SBE) (cont'd)

Subset	Usual Pathogens	Preferred IV Therapy	Alternate IV Therapy	PO Therapy or IV-to-PO Switch
"Culture negative" SBE*	Pathogen unknown (Abiotrophia, enterococci)	Ampicillin/ Sulbactam 3 gm (IV) q6h × 4–6 weeks **plus** Gentamicin§ 240 mg or 3 mg/ kg (IV) q24h × 2 weeks	Quinolone† (IV) q24h × 4–6 weeks	Quinolone†§ (PO) q24h × 4–6 weeks
	Hemophilus sp. Actinobacillus actinomycetem- comitans Cardiobacterium hominis Eikenella corrodens Kingella kingae (HACEK organisms)	Ceftriaxone 2 gm (IV) q24h × 4–6 weeks **or** Any 3rd generation cephalosporin (IV) × 4–6 weeks **or** Cefepime 2 gm (IV) q12h × 4–6 weeks	Ampicillin 2 gm (IV) q4h × 4–6 weeks **plus** Gentamicin§ 240 mg or 3 mg/ kg (IV) q24h × 2 weeks **or monotherapy with** Ampicillin/ Sulbactam 3 gm (IV) q6h × 4–6 weeks **or** Quinolone† (IV) q24h × 4–6 weeks	Quinolone†§ (PO) q24h × 4–6 weeks
	Legionella Chlamydophilia (Chlamydia) psittaci	Doxycycline** 200 mg (IV) q12h × 3 days, then 100 mg (IV) q12h × 3 months	Quinolone† (IV) q24h × 3 months	Doxycycline**§ 200 mg (PO) q12h × 3 days, then 100 mg (PO) q12h × 3 months
	Coxiella burnetii (Q fever)	Doxycycline** 200 mg (IV/PO) q12h × 3 days, then 100 mg (PO) q12h × 24 months **plus** Hydroxchloroquin 200 mg (PO) q8h × 24 months		

* Slow growing/fastidious organisms may require ↑ CO_2 and prolonged incubation.
† Levofloxacin 500 mg or Moxifloxacin 400 mg.
** Loading dose is not needed PO if given IV with the same drug.
§ IV therapy preferred. PO therapy if no IV access or if patient not a surgical candidate.

Native Valve Subacute Bacterial Endocarditis (SBE) (cont'd)

Subset	Usual Pathogens	Preferred IV Therapy	Alternate IV Therapy	PO Therapy or IV-to-PO Switch
Brucella SBE†	Brucella melitensis, abortus, canis, suis	Doxycycline 200 mg** (IV) q12h × 3 days, then 100 mg (PO) q12h × ≥ 6 weeks **plus** Rifampin 300 mg (PO) q8h × ≥ 6 weeks **plus** Gentamicin§§ 3 mg/kg (IV) q24h × ≥ 6 weeks		

† Levofloxacin 500 mg or Moxifloxacin 400 mg.
** Loading dose is not needed PO if given IV with the same drug or if patient not a surgical candidate.
§§ May be given as a once daily dose or given as divided doses q8h.

Native Valve SBE

Clinical Presentation: Subacute febrile illness ± localizing symptoms/signs in a patient with a heart murmur. Peripheral manifestations are commonly absent with early diagnosis/treatment.
Diagnosis: High grade/continuous bacteremia (due to a endocarditis pathogen) plus vegetation on TTE/TEE is diagnostic.

SBE (No Obvious Source)

Diagnostic Considerations: Most common pathogen is viridans streptococci. Source is usually the mouth, although oral/dental infection is usually inapparent clinically.
Pitfalls: Vegetations without positive blood cultures or peripheral manifestations of SBE are not diagnostic of endocarditis. SBE vegetations may persist after antibiotic therapy, but are sterile.
Therapeutic Considerations: In penicillin-allergic (anaphylactic) patients, vancomycin may be used alone or in combination with gentamicin. Follow ESR weekly to monitor antibiotic response. No need to repeat blood cultures unless patient has persistent fever or is not responding clinically. Two-week treatment is acceptable for uncomplicated viridans streptococcal SBE. Treat nutritionally-variant streptococci (NVS) (B₆/pyridoxal dependent streptococcus) same as viridans streptococcal SBE.
Prognosis: Related to extent of embolization/severity of heart failure.

SBE (GI/GU Source Likely)

Diagnostic Considerations: Commonest pathogens from GI/GU source are Enterococci (especially) E. faecalis. If S. bovis, look for GI polyp, tumor source. Enterococcal SBE commonly follows GI/GU instrumentation.
Pitfalls: Low back pain prominent with enterococcal/S. bovis SBE, S. bovis associated with CNS embolization, Vertebral osteomyelitis, and large valvular vegetations.
Therapeutic Considerations: For penicillin-allergic patients, use vancomycin plus gentamicin. Vancomycin alone is inadequate for enterococcal (E. faecalis) SBE. Treat enterococcal PVE the same as for native valve enterococcal SBE. Treat S. bovis SBE the same as S. viridans SBE.
Prognosis: Related to extent of embolization.

"Culture Negative" SBE (Culturable Pathogens)

Diagnostic Considerations: Culture of organisms may require enhanced CO_2/special media (Castaneda vented bottles) and prolonged incubation (2–4 weeks). True "culture negative" SBE is rare, and is characterized by peripheral signs of SBE, a murmur, vegetation (by TTE/TEE), and negative blood cultures.

Pitfalls: Most cases of "culture negative" SBE are not, in fact, culture negative SBE, but are due to slow growing organisms. Vegetations may not be visible by TTE/TEE with Q fever SBE.

Therapeutic Considerations: Follow clinical improvement with serial ESRs, which should return to pretreatment levels with therapy. Serial TTEs/TEEs show decreasing vegetation size during effective therapy. Sterile vegetations may persist after antibiotic therapy.

Prognosis: Related to extent of embolization.

"Culture Negative" SBE Non–Culturable/(Serologically Diagnosed Pathogens)

Diagnostic Considerations: Diagnosis by specific serology. Large vessel emboli suggests culture negative SBE in patients with negative blood cultures but signs of SBE, e.g., splenomegaly/peripheral manifestation's.

Pitfalls: Do not diagnose culture negative SBE in patients with a heart murmur and negative blood cultures if peripheral SBE manifestations are absent. Vegetations may not be visible on TTE/TEE in Q fever SBE. The diagnosis of chronic Q fever is made by demonstrating elevated IgG (phase I) titers ≥ 1:1024 at 6 months following acute Q fever. Since Bartonella titers may cross react with C. burnetii (Q fever) titers and vice versa, an elevation of either titer may be a clue to the other and should prompt testing for both.

Therapeutic Considerations: Treatment is based on specific organism identified by diagnostic tests.

Prognosis: Related to extent of embolization/severity of heart failure.

Native Valve Acute Bacterial Endocarditis (ABE)

Subset	Usual Pathogens	Preferred IV Therapy	Alternate IV Therapy	IV-to-PO Switch Therapy
Normal hosts* (Treat initially for MRSA; if later identified as MSSA, treat accordingly)	S. aureus (MRSA)	Daptomycin 6 mg/kg (IV) q24h × 4–6 weeks **or** Linezolid 600 mg (IV) q24h × 4–6 weeks **or** Vancomycin 1 gm or 15 mg/kg (IV) q12h × 4–6 weeks	Linezolid 600 mg (PO) q12h × 4–6 wks **or** Minocycline 100 mg (PO) q12h × 4–6 wks
	S. aureus (MSSA)	Nafcillin 2 gm (IV) q4h × 4–6 weeks **or** Cefazolin 1 gm (IV) q8h × 4–6 weeks	Linezolid 600 mg (PO) q12h × 4–6 wks **or** Cephalexin 1 gm (PO) q6h × 4–6 weeks

MRSA/MSSA = methicillin-resistant/sensitive S. aureus. Duration of therapy represents total time IV, PO, or IV + PO.
*   Treat IV or with IV-to-PO switch therapy or if patient not a surgical candidate.

Native Valve Acute Bacterial Endocarditis (ABE) (cont'd)

Subset	Usual Pathogens	Preferred IV Therapy	Alternate IV Therapy	IV-to-PO Switch Therapy
IV drug abusers (IVDAs)† (Treat as MRSA before culture results; treat according to pathogen after culture results)	S. aureus (MRSA)	<u>Before culture results</u> Meropenem 1 gm (IV) q8h **plus** Vancomycin 1 gm or 15 mg/kg (IV) q12h	<u>After culture results</u> Daptomycin 6–12mg/kg (IV) q24h × 6 weeks **or** Linezolid 600 mg (IV) q12h × 6 weeks **or** Vancomycin 1 gm or 15 mg/kg (IV) q12h × 6 weeks	<u>After culture results</u> Linezolid 600 mg (PO) q12h × 4–6 weeks **or** Minocycline† 100 mg (PO) q12h × 4–6 weeks
	S. aureus (MSSA)	<u>Before culture results</u> Meropenem 1 gm (IV) q8h	<u>After culture results</u> Nafcillin 2 gm (IV) q4h × 4–6 weeks **or** Cefazolin 1 gm (IV) q8h × 4–6 weeks **or** Daptomycin 6 mg/kg (IV) q24h × 4–6 weeks **or** Linezolid 600 mg (IV) q12h × 4–6 weeks **or** any carbapenem (IV) × 4–6 weeks	<u>After culture results</u> Linezolid 600 mg (PO) q12h × 4–6 weeks **or** Cephalexin 1 gm (PO) q6h × 4–6 weeks
	P. aeruginosa* S. marcesens Aerobic GNBs	<u>Before culture results</u> Meropenem 1 gm (IV) q8h **or** Piperacillin 4 gm (IV) q6h	<u>After culture results</u> One "A" drug ± one "B" drug **"A" Drugs** Meropenem 1 gm (IV) q8h × 4–6 weeks **or** Doripenem 1 gm (IV) q8h × 4–6 weeks <u>**"B" Drugs**</u> Amikacin 500 mg or 15 mg/kg (IV) q24h × 4–6 weeks **or** Aztreonam 2 gm (IV) q8h × 4–6 weeks	None

MRSA/MSSA = methicillin-resistant/sensitive S. aureus. Duration of therapy represents total time IV, PO, or IV + PO.

*   Treat IV or with IV-to-PO switch therapy or if patient not a surgical candidate.

†   *MSSA/MRSA TV ABE may be treated IV/PO × 2 weeks if no intra-cardiac or CNS complications.* Pulmonary septic emboli are a feature of *right sided* ABE e.g., TV and are *not*, per se, an extracardiac complication.

Acute Bacterial Endocarditis (ABE)

Diagnostic Considerations: Clinical criteria for MRSA/MSSA ABE: continuous/high-grade bacteremia (repeatedly 3/4 or 4/4 positive blood cultures), fever (temperature usually ≥ 102°F), no, new or changing murmur, and vegetation by transesophageal/transthoracic echocardiogram.

Pitfalls: Obtain a baseline TTE for comparative purposes should ABE be complicated by valve destruction, heart failure or ring/perivalvular abscess. Obtain infectious disease and cardiology consultations. In MSSA/MRSA ABE patients initially treated with vancomycin, resistance to deptomycin may occur during therapy.

Therapeutic Considerations: Treat for 4–6 weeks. Follow teichoic acid antibody titers weekly in S. aureus ABE, which fall (along with the ESR) with effective therapy. If MSSA/MRSA ABE unresponsive (persistent high grade bacteremia) to appropriate antibiotic therapy or if a myocardial/paravalvular abscess present that cannot be surgically drained, "high dose" daptomycin 12 mg/kg (IV) q24h may be effective. With daptomycin resistant MSSA/MRSA strains, Quinupristin dalfopristin 7.5 mg/kg (IV) q8h may be effective.

Prognosis: Related to extent of embolization/severity of valve destruction/heart failure.

Acute Bacterial Endocarditis (IVDAs)

Diagnostic Considerations: Clinically IVDAs with S. aureus usually have relatively mild ABE, permitting oral treatment.

Pitfalls: IVDAs with new aortic or tricuspid regurgitation should be treated IV ± valve replacement.

Therapeutic Considerations: After pathogen is isolated, may switch from IV to PO regimen to complete treatment course.

Prognosis: Prognosis is better than ABE in normal hosts if not complicated by abscess, valve regurgitation, or heart failure.

Prosthetic Valve Endocarditis (PVE)

Subset	Usual Pathogens	Before Culture Results	After Culture Results
Early PVE (< 60 days post-PVR)	S. aureus (MSSA/MRSA) S. epidemidis (CoNS) Enterobacteriaceae	Vancomycin 1 gm or 15 mg/kg (IV) q12h **plus** Gentamicin§§ 240 mg or 3 mg/kg (IV) q24h	<u>MSSA/Enterobacteriaceae</u> Meropenem 1 gm (IV) q8h × 6 weeks <u>MSSA/MRSA†</u> Daptomycin 6 mg/kg (IV) q24h × 6 weeks **or** Linezolid 600 mg (IV or PO) q12h × 6 weeks **or** Vancomycin 1 gm or 15 mg/kg (IV) q12h × 6 weeks
	Candida species§	Mycafungin 150 mg or 3 mg/kg (IV) q24h	Lipid amphotericin 3–5 mg/kg (IV) q24h × 6 weeks **plus** 5-FC 25 mg/kg (PO) q6h × 6 weeks

MSSA/MRSA = methicillin-sensitive/resistant S. aureus. Duration of therapy represents total time IV or IV + PO.

†   MRSA drugs also effective against MSSA.

§   Value removal usually needed for cure.

§§ May be given as a once daily dose or given as divided doses q8h.

Prosthetic Valve Endocarditis (PVE) (cont'd)

Subset	Usual Pathogens	Before Culture Results	After Culture Results
Late PVE (> 60 days post-PVR)	Viridans streptococci S. epidermidis (CoNS)	Vancomycin 1 gm or 15 mg/kg (IV) q12h **plus** Gentamicin§§ 240 mg or 3 mg/kg (IV) q24h	<u>Viridans streptococci</u> Ceftriaxone 2 gm (IV) q24h × 6 weeks ***plus*** Rifampin 300 mg (PO) q8h × 6 weeks **or** Meropenem 1 gm (IV) q8h × 6 weeks ***plus*** Rifampin 300 mg (PO) q8h × 6 weeks **or** Ertapenem 1 gm (IV) q24h × 6 weeks ***plus*** Rifampin 300 mg (PO) q8h × 6 weeks <u>CoNS</u> Linezolid 600 mg (IV or PO) q12h × 6 weeks ***plus*** Rifampin 300 mg (PO) q8h × 6 weeks **or** Vancomycin 1 gm or 15 mg/kg (IV) q12h × 6 weeks ***plus*** Rifampin 300 mg (PO) q8h × 6 weeks

MSSA/MRSA = methicillin-sensitive/resistant S. aureus; MSSE/MRSE = methicillin-sensitive/resistant S. epidermidis. Duration of therapy represents total time IV or IV + PO.
§§ May be given as a once daily dose or given as divided doses q8h.

Clinical Presentation: Prolonged fevers and chills following prosthetic valve replacement (PVR).
Diagnosis: High-grade blood culture positivity (3/4 or 4/4) with endocarditis pathogen and no other source of infection.

Early PVE (< 60 days post-PVR)
Diagnostic Considerations: Blood cultures persistently positive. Temperature usually ≤ 102°F.
Pitfalls: Obtain baseline TTE/TEE. Premature closure of mitral leaflet is early sign of impending aortic valve regurgitation.
Therapeutic Considerations: Patients improve clinically on treatment, but prosthetic valve removal may be necessary for cure.
Prognosis: Related to extent of embolization/severity of heart failure.

Late PVE (> 60 days post-PVR)
Pitfalls: Culture of removed valve may be negative, but valve gram stain will be positive.
Therapeutic Considerations: Clinically, late PVE resembles viridans streptococcal SBE. Patients improve clinically on treatment, but prosthetic valve removal may be necessary for cure.
Prognosis: Related to extent of embolization/severity of heart failure.

Pericarditis/Myocarditis

Subset	Usual Pathogens	Preferred Therapy
Diptheritic myocarditis	C. diphtheriae	Treat same as diphtheriae (see p. 170)
Viral	Coxsackie, influenza	No treatment for Coxsackie, for influenza therapy
Lyme myocarditis	B. burgdorferi	Ceftriaxone 2 gm (IV) q24h × 2 weeks **or** Doxycycline 100 mg (IV) q12h × 2 weeks
TB pericarditis	M. tuberculosis	Treat same as pulmonary TB (see p. 53). Add a tapering dose of corticosteroids × 4–8 weeks
Suppurative pericarditis	S. pneumoniae S. aureus	Treat same as lung abscess/empyema (see p. 67)

Clinical Presentation: Viral pericarditis presents with acute onset of fever/chest pain (made worse by sitting up) following a viral illness. TB pericarditis is indolent in presentation, with ↑ jugular venous distension (JVD), pericardial friction rub (40%), paradoxical pulse (25%), and chest x-ray with cardiomegaly ± left-sided pleural effusion. Suppurative pericarditis presents as acute pericarditis (patients are critically ill). Develops from contiguous (e.g., pneumonia) or hematogenous spread e.g., S. aureus bacteremia. Viral myocarditis presents with heart failure, arrhythmias ± emboli.

Diagnostic Considerations: Pericarditis/effusion manifests cardiomegaly with decreased heart sounds ± tamponade. Diagnosis by culture/biopsy of pericardial fluid or pericardium for viruses, bacteria, or acid-fast bacilli (AFB). Diagnosis of myocarditis is clinical ± myocardial biopsy.

Pitfalls: Consider other causes of pericardial effusion (malignancy, esp. if bloody effusion, uremia, etc). Otherwise unexplained tachycardia should suggest myocarditis until proven otherwise. Rule out treatable non-viral causes of myocarditis e.g., RMSF, Lyme, diphtheria. Suspect Lyme disease in any person without heart disease with exposure to endemic area who presents with otherwise unexplained heart block. Lyme IgM titers may be negative early when patients present with heart block.

Therapeutic Considerations: No specific treatment for viral myocarditis/pericarditis. TB pericarditis is treated the same as pulmonary TB ± pericardiectomy. Suppurative pericarditis is treated the same as lung abscess plus surgical drainage (pericardial window). Heart block in Lyme disease rapidly reverses with therapy, but a temporary pacemaker may be needed until heart block is reversed.

Prognosis: For viral pericarditis, the prognosis is good, but viral myocarditis may be fatal. For TB pericarditis, the prognosis is good if treated before constrictive pericarditis/adhesions develop. Suppurative pericarditis is often fatal without early pericardial window/antibiotic therapy. With Lyme myocarditis/heart block, prognosis is good if treatment is started early when diagnosis is suspected.

Central Venous Catheter (CVC) and Pacemaker/Lead Infections

Subset	Usual Pathogens	Preferred IV Therapy	Alternate IV Therapy	IV-to-PO Switch
CVC (temporary) Infections* _Bacterial_ (Treat initially for MSSA; if later identified as MRSA, treat accordingly)	S. aureus (MSSA) Aerobic GNBs	Meropenem 1 gm (IV) q8h** **or** Cefepime 2 gm (IV) q12h**	Ceftizoxime 2 gm (IV) q8h** **or** Cefotaxime 2 gm (IV) q6h**	Quinolone‡ (PO) q24h**†
	S. aureus (MRSA/MSSA§)	Daptomycin 6 mg/kg (IV) q24h** **or** Linezolid 600 mg (IV) q12h** **or** Vancomycin 1 gm or 15 mg/kg (IV) q12h**		Linezolid 600 mg (PO) q12h**† **or** Minocycline 100 mg (PO) q12h**†
Candida¶ (Treat initially for C. albicans; if later identified as non-albicans Candida, treat accordingly).	C. albicans	Treat the same as for Candidemia (p. 153)		
	Non-albicans Candida	Treat the same as for Candidemia (p. 153)		
CVC (semi-permanent Hickman/ Broviac/Tessio) Infections* _Bacterial_	S. aureus (MSSA/MRSA)	Daptomycin 6 mg/kg (IV) q24h** **or** Linezolid 600 mg (IV) q12h** **or** Vancomycin 1 gm or 15 mg/kg (IV) q12h**		Linezolid 600 mg (PO) q12h**† **or** Minocycline 100 mg (PO) q12h**†

MSSA/MRSA = methicillin-sensitive/resistant S. aureus.

†   IV therapy preferred. PO therapy if no IV access

‡   Levofloxacin 500 mg or Moxifloxacin 400 mg.

*   If clinically possible, CVC should be removed if CVC suspected source of bacteremia in a septic patient. If high grade/sustained bacteremia obtain TTE/TEE to rule out ABE.

**   Treat × 2 weeks after CVC removal if no ABE.

¶   For candidemia not associated with CVCs, (see pp. 153–154).

§   MRSA drugs also effective against MSSA.

Central Venous Catheter (CVC) and Pacemaker/Lead Infections (cont'd)

Subset	Usual Pathogens	Preferred IV Therapy	Alternate IV Therapy	IV-to-PO Switch
	S. epidermidis (CoNS)	Daptomycin 6 mg/kg (IV) q24h** or Linezolid 600 mg (IV) q12h** or Vancomycin 1 gm or 15 mg/kg (IV) q12h**		Linezolid 600 mg (PO) q12h**†
Pacemaker wire/generator infection (Treat initially for S. aureus; if later identified as S. epidermidis, treat accordingly)	S. aureus (MSSA/MRSA)	Daptomycin 6 mg/kg (IV) q24h†§ or Linezolid 600 mg (IV) q12h†§ or Vancomycin 1 gm or 15 mg/kg (IV) q12h†		Linezolid 600 mg (PO) q12h†§* or Minocycline 100 mg (PO) q12h†§*
	S. epidermidis (CoNS)	Daptomycin 6 mg/kg (IV) q24h† or Linezolid 600 mg (IV) q12h† or Vancomycin 1 gm or 15 mg/kg (IV) q12h†		Linezolid 600 mg (PO) q12h†*

MSSA/MRSA = methicillin-sensitive/resistant S. aureus; MSSE/MRSE = methicillin-sensitive/resistant S. epidermidis.

† IV therapy preferred. PO therapy if no IV access.

** Treat × 2 weeks after CVC removal if no IE.

* Treat × 2 weeks after wire/generator removal if no IE.

§ Obtain teichoic acid antibody titers after 2 weeks. If titers are < 1:2, 2 weeks of therapy is sufficient. If titers are > 1:2, rule out endocarditis and complete 4–6 weeks of therapy.

Central Venous Catheter (CVC) and Pacemaker/Lead Infections (cont'd)

Subset	Usual Pathogens	Preferred IV Therapy	Alternate IV Therapy	IV-to-PO Switch
Septic thrombophlebitis (Treat initially for MSSA; if later identified as MRSA, treat accordingly)	S. aureus (MSSA)	Nafcillin 2 gm (IV) q4h × 2 weeks* **or** Linezolid 600 mg (IV) q12h × 2 weeks* **or** Meropenem 1 gm (IV) q8h × 2 weeks*	Ceftizoxime 2 gm (IV) q8h × 2 weeks* **or** Cefotaxime 2 gm (IV) q6h × 2 weeks*	Linezolid 600 mg (PO) q12h × 2 weeks*† **or** Clindamycin 300 mg (PO) q8h × 2 weeks*† **or** Cephalexin 1 gm (PO) q6h × 2 weeks*†
	S. aureus (MRSA)	Linezolid 600 mg (IV) q12h × 2 weeks* **or** Vancomycin 1 gm or 15 mg/kg (IV) q12h × 2 weeks* **or** Minocycline 100 mg (IV) q12h × 2 weeks*		Linezolid 600 mg (PO) q12h × 2 weeks*† **or** Minocycline 100 mg (PO) q12h × 2 weeks*†

MSSA/MRSA = methicillin-sensitive/resistant S. aureus. Duration of therapy represents total time IV or IV + PO. Most patients on IV therapy able to take PO meds should be switched to PO therapy after clinical improvement.

* Obtain teichoic acid antibody titers after 2 weeks. If titers are < 1:2, 2 weeks of therapy is sufficient. If titers are ≥ 1:2, TTE/TEE to rule out ABE and complete 4–6 weeks of therapy.

† IV therapy preferred. PO therapy if no IV access.

CVC (Temporary) Infections

Clinical Presentation: Temperature ≥ 102°F ± IV site erythema.

Diagnostic Considerations: Diagnosis by semi-quantitative catheter tip culture with ≥ 15 colonies plus blood cultures with same pathogen. If no other explanation for fever and line has been in place ≥ 7 days, remove line and obtain semi-quantitative catheter tip culture. Suppurative thrombophlebitis presents with hectic/septic fevers and pus at IV site ± palpable venous cord.

Pitfalls: Temperature ≥ 102°F with IV line infection, in contrast to phlebitis.

Therapeutic Considerations: Line removal is usually curative, but antibiotic therapy is usually given for 1 week after IV line removal for gram-negative bacilli or 2 weeks after IV line removal for S. aureus (MSSA/MRSA). Antifungal therapy is usually given for 2 weeks after IV line removal for Candidemia.

Prognosis: Good if line is removed before endocarditis/metastatic spread.

CVC (Semi-Permanent) Hickman/Broviac Infections

Clinical Presentation: Fever ± IV site erythema.

Diagnostic Considerations: Positive blood cultures plus gallium scan pickup on catheter is diagnostic.

Pitfalls: Antibiotics will lower temperature, but patient will usually not be afebrile without line removal.

Therapeutic Considerations: Lines usually need to be removed for cure. Rifampin 600 mg (PO) q24h may be added to IV/PO regimen if pathogen is S. aureus.

Prognosis: Good with organisms of low virulence.

Pacemaker/Lead Infections

Clinical Presentation: Persistently positive blood cultures without endocarditis in a pacemaker patient.

Diagnostic Considerations: Positive blood cultures with gallium scan pickup on wire/pacemaker generator is diagnostic. Differentiate wire from pacemaker pocket infection by chest CT/MRI.

Pitfalls: Positive blood cultures are more common in wire infections than pocket infections. Blood cultures may be negative in both, but more so with pocket infections.

Therapeutic Considerations: Wire alone may be replaced if infection does not involve pacemaker generator. Replace pacemaker generator if involved; wire if uninvolved can usually be left in place.

Prognosis: Good if pacemaker wire/generator replaced before septic complications develop.

Septic Thrombophlebitis

Clinical Presentation: Temperature ≥ 102°F with local erythema and signs of sepsis.

Diagnostic Considerations: Palpable venous cord and pus at IV site when IV line is removed.

Pitfalls: Suspect diagnosis if persistent bacteremia and no other source of infection in a patient with a peripheral IV.

Therapeutic Considerations: Remove IV catheter. Surgical venotomy is usually needed for cure.

Prognosis: Good if removed early before septic complications develop.

Vascular Graft Infections

Subset	Usual Pathogens	Preferred IV Therapy	Alternate IV Therapy	IV-to-PO Switch
AV graft/shunt infection (Treat initially for MRSA, etc.; if later identified as MSSA, treat accordingly)	S. aureus (MRSA)	Daptomycin*†§ 6 mg/kg (IV) q24h **plus** Rifampin 300 mg (PO) q8h **or** Linezolid†§ 600 mg (IV) q12h **plus** Rifampin†§ 300 mg (PO) q8h	Vancomycin*†§ 1 gm or 15 mg/kg (IV) q12h **plus** Rifampin 300 mg (PO) q8h **or** Minocycline†§ 100 mg (IV) q12h **plus** Rifampin†§ 300 mg (PO) q8h	Linezolid†§ 600 mg (PO) q12h **plus** Rifampin 300 mg (PO) q8h **or** Minocycline†§ 100 mg (PO) q12h **plus** Rifampin†§ 300 mg (PO) q8h

MRSA/MSSA = methicillin-resistant/sensitive S. aureus. Duration of therapy represents total time IV or IV + PO. Most patients on IV therapy able to take PO meds should be switched to PO therapy after clinical improvement.

*   Follow with maintenance dosing for renal failure (CrCl < 10 mL/min) and type of dialysis.

†   If ABE not present, treat for 2 weeks after graft is removed/replaced. If ABE present, treat for 6 weeks.

§   IV therapy preferred. PO therapy if no IV access.

Vascular Graft Infections (cont'd)

Subset	Usual Pathogens	Preferred IV Therapy	Alternate IV Therapy	IV-to-PO Switch
	S. aureus (MSSA)	Nafcillin 3 gm (IV) q12h†	Vancomycin 1 gm or 15 mg/kg (IV) q12h*†	Moxifloxacin 400 mg (IV or PO) q24h*†§
	E. faecalis (VSE) Aerobic GNBs	Ampicillin 2 gm (IV) q4h*† **plus** Gentamicin 240 mg or 3 mg/kg (IV) q24h*†	Vancomycin 1 gm or 15 mg/kg (IV) q24h† **plus** Gentamicin 120 mg or 3 mg/kg (IV) q24h*†	
Aortic graft infection	S. aureus (MSSA) Aerobic GNBs P. aeruginosa	Meropenem 1 gm (IV) q8h†** **or** Cefepime 2 gm (IV) q12h†**	Piperacillin 4 gm (IV) q8h† **or** Moxifloxacin 400 mg (IV) q24h†	Moxifloxacin 400 mg (PO) q24h† Levofloxacin 750 mg (PO) q24h†

MRSA/MSSA = methicillin-resistant/sensitive S. aureus. Duration of therapy represents total time IV or IV
* Follow with maintenance dosing for renal failure (CrCl < 10 mL/min) and type of dialysis.
** Depending on susceptibilities.
† If ABE not present, treat for 2 weeks after graft is removed/replaced. If graft not removable/replaceable, treat for 6 weeks.
§ IV therapy preferred. PO therapy if no IV access.

AV Graft Infection
Clinical Presentation: Persistent fever/bacteremia without endocarditis in a patient with an AV graft on hemodialysis.
Diagnostic Considerations: Diagnosis by persistently positive blood cultures and gallium scan pickup over infected AV graft. Gallium scan will detect deep AV graft infection not apparent on exam.
Pitfalls: Antibiotics will lower temperature, but patient will usually not become afebrile without AV graft replacement.
Therapeutic Considerations: Graft usually must be removed for cure. MRSA is a rare cause of AV graft infection; if present, treat with linezolid 600 mg (IV or PO) q12h until graft is removed/replaced.
Prognosis: Good if new graft does not become infected at same site.

Aortic Graft Infection
Clinical Presentation: Persistently positive blood cultures without endocarditis in a patient with an aortic graft.
Diagnostic Considerations: Diagnosis by positive blood cultures plus gallium scan pickup over infected aortic graft or abdominal CT/MRI scan.
Pitfalls: Infection typically occurs at anastomotic sites.

Therapeutic Considerations: Graft must be removed for cure. Operate as soon as diagnosis is confirmed (no value in waiting for surgery). MRSA is a rare cause of AV graft infection; if present, treat with linezolid 600 mg (IV or PO) q12h until graft is replaced.

Prognosis: Good if infected graft is removed before septic complications develop.

Empiric Therapy of GI Tract Infections

Esophagitis

Subset	Usual Pathogens	Preferred IV Therapy	Alternate IV Therapy	PO Therapy or IV-to-PO Switch
Fungal	Candida albicans	Fluconazole 200 mg (IV or PO) × 1 dose, then 100 mg (IV or PO) q24h × 2–3 weeks	Micafungin 150 mg (IV) q24h × 2–3 weeks **or** Caspofungin 50 mg (IV) q24h × 2–3 weeks **or** Anidulafungin 100 mg (IV or PO) × 1 dose then 50 mg (IV) q24h × 2–3 weeks **or** Amphotericin B deoxycholate 0.5 mg/kg (IV) q24h × 2–3 weeks **or** Itraconazole 200 mg (IV) q12h × 2 days, then 200 mg (IV) q24 h × 2–3 weeks	Fluconazole 200 mg (PO) × 1 dose, then 100 mg (PO) q24h × 2–3 weeks* **or** Posaconazole 100 mg (PO)q12h × 1 day, then 100 mg (PO) q24h × 2 weeks **or** Itraconazole 200 mg (PO) solution q24h × 2–3 weeks
Viral	HSV-1	Acyclovir 5 mg/kg (IV) q8h × 3 weeks	Valacyclovir 500 mg (PO) q12h × 3 weeks **or** Famciclovir 500 mg (PO) q12h × 3 weeks	
	CMV	Ganciclovir 5 mg/kg (IV) q12h × 3 weeks	Valganciclovir 900 mg (PO) q12h × 3 weeks	

Duration of therapy represents total time IV, PO, or IV + PO. Most patients on IV therapy able to take PO meds should be switched to PO therapy soon after clinical improvement (usually < 72 hours).

*   Loading dose is not needed PO if given IV with the same drug.

Clinical Presentation: Pain on swallowing.

Diagnosis: Stain/culture for fungi/HSV/CMV on biopsy specimen.

Fungal (Candida) Esophagitis

Diagnostic Considerations: Rarely if ever in normal hosts. Often (but not always) associated with Candida in mouth. If patient is not alcoholic or diabetic and is not receiving antibiotics, test for HIV.

Pitfalls: Therapy as a diagnostic trial is appropriate. Suspect CMV-related disease and proceed to endoscopy if a patient with a typical symptom complex fails to respond to antifungal therapy.

Therapeutic Considerations: In normal hosts, treat for 1 week after clinical resolution. HIV patients respond more slowly than normal hosts and may need higher doses/treatment for 2–3 weeks after clinical resolution (p. 336).
Prognosis: Related to degree of immunosuppression.

Viral Esophagitis
Diagnostic Considerations: Rarely in normal hosts. May occur in the immunosuppressed.
Pitfalls: Viral and non-viral esophageal ulcers look similar; need biopsy for specific viral diagnosis.
Therapeutic Considerations: In normal hosts, treat for 2–3 weeks after clinical resolution. HIV patients respond more slowly and may need treatment for weeks after clinical resolution.
Prognosis: Related to degree of immunosuppression.

Peptic Ulcer Disease (H. pylori)

Triple Therapy	Quadruple Therapy	Sequential Therapy
PPI + amoxicillin 1 gm (PO) q12h **plus either** clarithromycin 500 mg (PO) q12h **or** tinidazole (or metronidazole) 500 mg (PO) q12h all × 2 weeks	PPI + metronidazole 500 mg (PO) q12h + doxycycline 100 mg (PO) q12h + bismuth subsalicylate 525 mg tabs (PO) q6h all × 2 weeks	*5 days:* PPI + amoxicillin 1 gm (PO) q12h; *next 5 days:* PPI **plus** either clarithromycin 500 (PO) q12h **or** levofloxacin 500 mg (PO) q24h

Diagnostic Considerations: Invasive: rapid urease test, histology, culture. **Noninvasive:** serum ELISA test, urea breath test, stool (monoclonal antibody) antigen test.
Pitfalls: *False negative H. pylori tests with antibiotics, bismuth, PPIs.*
Therapeutic Considerations: See above grid. **Therapeutic failure:** *substitute* bismuth (for amoxicillin) or *substitute* nitazoxanide 1 gm (PO) q12h (for clarithromycin, metronidazole or tinidazole) all × 2 weeks. *1 week of therapy often fails.*
Tests of Cure: Urea breath test → 4–6 weeks post-therapy. Stool antigen test → 6–8 weeks post-therapy. *Stop PPIs 2 weeks before re-testing.*

Gastric Perforation

Subset	Usual Pathogens	Preferred IV Therapy	Alternate IV Therapy	IV-to-PO Switch
Gastric perforation	Oral anaerobes	Cefazolin 1 gm (IV) q8h × 1–3 days	Any beta-lactam (IV) × 1–3 days	Amoxicillin 1 gm (PO) q8h × 1–3 days **or** Cephalexin 500 mg (PO) q6h × 1–3 days **or** Quinolone* (PO) q24h × 1–3 days

* Levofloxacin 500 mg or Moxifloxacin 400 mg.

Clinical Presentation: Presents acutely with fever and peritonitis.
Diagnostic Considerations: Obtain CT/MRI of abdomen for perforation/fluid collection.
Pitfalls: No need to cover B. fragilis with perforation of stomach/small intestine.
Therapeutic Considerations: Obtain surgical consult for possible repair.
Prognosis: Good if repaired.

Infectious Diarrhea/Typhoid (Enteric) Fever

Subset	Usual Pathogens	Preferred Therapy	Alternate Therapy
Acute watery diarrhea	E. coli (ETEC, EHEC) Campylobacter Yersinia Salmonella Vibrio sp.	Quinolone[†] (IV or PO) × 5 days	Doxycycline 100 mg (IV or PO) q12h × 5 days **or** TMP–SMX 1 DS tablet (PO) q12h × 5 days
C. difficile diarrhea/ colitis	Clostridium difficile	**Diarrhea** [†§] **Initial episode:** Vancomycin 250 mg (PO) q6h × 7–10 days* (If no improvement in 3 days, ↑ dose to 500 mg (PO) q6h × 7 days)** **Relapse:** Vancomycin 500 mg (PO) q6h × 14 days** **Recurrence:**[††] Vancomycin 500 mg (PO) q6h × 1 month (**do not taper vancomycin dose**). If another recurrence, *re-treat* with Vancomycin 500 mg (PO) q6h × *2 months*. If another recurrence, *re-treat* with Vancomycin 500 mg (PO) q6h × *3 months*. If dose not tapered and if no colitis, **this regimen will not fail!** If diarrhea continues, rule out C. difficile *colitis* or look for alternate diagnosis.	**Diarrhea** **Initial episode:** Nitazoxanide 500 mg (PO) q12h × 7–10 days **or** Metronidazole 250 mg (PO) q6h × 7–10 days* **Relapse:** Nitazoxanide 500 mg (PO) q12h × 7–10 days **Recurrence:** Nitazoxanide 500 mg (PO) q12h × 7–10 days **or** Rifaximin 400 mg (PO) q8h × 10 days **or** Fidoxamicin 200 mg (PO) q12h × 10 days

*　　**Treatment failure common with Vancomycin 125 mg (PO) q6h and with Metronidazole at any dose, (Flagyl frequently fails!).**

**　*If no improvement after 3 days with Vancomycin 500 mg (PO) q6h, **rule out** colitis with abdominal CT scan. If abdominal CT scan shows **colitis** treat as C. difficile **colitis**.*

†　　When treating C. difficile diarrhea or colitis, ***discontinue antibiotics with a high C. difficile potential***, e.g., cilndamycin, ciprofloxacin, α-lactams (*excluding* ceftriaxone).
　　Patients being treated with levofloxacin or moxifloxacin *should not concurrently be taking PPIs.* Either discontinue PPI or switch to a H₂ blocker during quinolone therapy.

††　**Avoid C. difficile "prophylaxis."** Do *not* treat **"history of C. difficile."** Instead, *repeat C. difficile stool PCR to verify diagnosis*. Treat C. difficile diarrhea **only if** PCR + for C. difficile.

§　　**Avoid anti-spasmatics in C. difficile diarrhea;** use may result in C. difficile **colitis**.

§§　Colectomy may be lifesaving in severe C. difficile pancolitis.

Infectious Diarrhea/Typhoid (Enteric) Fever (cont'd)

Subset	Usual Pathogens	Preferred Therapy	Alternate Therapy
		Colitis **Initial episode:** Metronidazole 1 gm (IV) q24h until cured **plus** Ertapenem 1 gm (IV) 124h (until associated peritonitis component resolves) **Severe Pancolitis:**[§§] Metronidazole 500 mg (IV/PO) q6h–8h until cured **plus** Nitazoxanide 500 mg (PO) q12h × until cured **plus** Tigacycline 200 mg (IV) × 1 dose, then, 100 mg (IV) q24h until cured **Relapse or Recurrence:** Re-treat with Metronidazole 500 mg (IV/PO) q6–8h until cured	**Colitis** **Initial Episode:** Metronidazole 250 mg (PO) q6h until cured **plus** Tigacycline 200 mg (IV) × 1 dose, then 100 mg (IV) q24h until cured **or** Nitazoxanide 500 mg (PO) q12h until cured **Relapse or Recurrence:** Nitazoxanide 500 mg (PO) q12h until cured
Cytomegalo-virus colitis	CMV	Valganciclovir 900 mg (PO) q12h × 21 days; for HIV, see p. 334	

§ Colectomy may be lifesaving in severe C. difficile pancolitis.

Infectious Diarrhea/Typhoid (Enteric) Fever (cont'd)

Subset	Usual Pathogens	Preferred Therapy	Alternate Therapy
Typhoid (enteric) fever	Salmonella typhi/ paratyphi	Quinolone[†] (IV or PO) × 10–14 days **or** TMP–SMX 5 mg/kg (IV or PO) q6h × 10–14 days	Chloramphenicol 500 mg (IV or PO) q6h × 10–14 days **or** any 3rd gen cephalosporin (IV or PO) × 10–14 days **or** Azithromycin 1 gm (PO) q24h × 5 days
Chronic watery diarrhea	Giardia lamblia*	Tinidazole 2 gm (PO) × 1 dose **or** Nitazoxanide 500 mg (PO) q12h × 3 days **or** Metronidazole 2 gm (PO) q24h × 3 days	Albendazole 400 mg (PO) q24h × 5 days **or** Quinacrine 100 mg (PO) q8h × 5 days
	Cryptosporidia*	Nitazoxanide 500 mg (PO) q12h × 5 days[§]	Paromomycin 500–750 mg (PO) q8h until response **or** Azithromycin 600 mg (PO) q24h × 4 weeks
	Isospora* Cyclospora*	TMP–SMX 1 DS tablet (PO) q12h × 10 days[‡]	
Acute dysentery	Entamoeba histolytica	<u>Preferred therapy:</u> Metronidazole 750 mg (PO) q8h × 10 days **followed by either** Iodoquinol 650 mg (PO) q8h × 20 days **or** Paromomycin 500 mg (PO) q8h × 7 days <u>Alternate therapy:</u> Tinidazole 1 gm (PO) q12h × 3 days	
	Shigella	Quinolone[†] (IV or PO) × 3 days	TMP–SMX 1 DS tablet (PO) q12h × 3 days **or** Azithromycin 500 mg (IV or PO) q24h × 3 days

Duration of therapy represents total time IV, PO, or IV + PO. Most patients on IV therapy able to take PO meds should be switched to PO therapy soon after clinical improvement (usually < 72 hours).

*   May also present as acute watery diarrhea.

†   Ciprofloxacin 400 mg (IV) or 500 mg (PO) q12h or Levofloxacin 500 mg (IV or PO) q24h or Moxifloxacin 400 mg (IV or PO) q24h.

§   Longer duration of therapy may be needed in immunosuppressed patients (treat until cured).

Acute Watery Diarrhea

Clinical Presentation: Acute onset of watery diarrhea without blood/mucus.

Diagnostic Considerations: Diagnosis by culture of organism from stool specimens.

Pitfalls: Recommended antibiotics are active against most susceptible enterotoxigenic bacterial pathogens causing diarrhea, but not viruses/parasites. Concomitant transient lactase deficiency may prolong diarrhea if dairy products are taken during an infectious diarrhea.

Therapeutic Considerations: Avoid norfloxacin and ciprofloxacin due to resistance potential. V. cholerae may be treated with a single dose of any oral respiratory quinolone or doxycycline.

Prognosis: Excellent. Most recover with supportive treatment.

Clostridium difficile Diarrhea/Colitis

Clinical Presentation: Voluminous watery diarrhea following exposure to C. difficile contaminated fomites, exposure to patients with C. difficile, recent cancer chemotherapy or antibiotic therapy with some, *but not most*, antibiotics. Most often associated with clindamycin, ciprofloxacin, and β-lactams (excluding ceftriaxone).

Diagnostic Considerations: Watery diarrhea with positive C. difficile stool toxin. A single positive PCR C. difficile stool toxin test is sufficiently sensitive/specific for diagnosis (endpoint is end of diarrhea, not stool toxin negativity); *If negative, no need to retest*. If C. difficile colitis suspected in C. difficile positive patients with fever/prominent leukocytosis/abdominal pain, confirm diagnosis by abdominal CT scan.

Pitfalls: C. difficile colitis is suggested by the presence of otherwise unexplained leukocytosis, ↑ ESR, abdominal pain and often temperature > 102°F; confirm diagnosis with CT/MRI of abdomen. Virulent strains of C. difficile may present with colitis with temperature ≤ 102°F, leukocytosis (often very high, i.e., 25–50 K/mm³), and little/no abdominal pain; confirm diagnosis with CT/MRI of abdomen. Radiographically C. difficile colitis typically is a pancolitis. Segmental colitis suggests a non-C. difficile etiology, i.e., ischemic colitis. C. difficile toxin test may remain positive in stools following resolution of diarrhea; In patients receiving enteral feeds, diarrhea is likely due to enteral feeds (high infusion rates/high osmotic loads) rather than C. difficile. Norovirus diarrhea may mimic C. difficile diarrhea or concurrent outbreaks may occur. Vancomycin may be *ineffective* in C. difficile *colitis*.

Therapeutic Considerations: For **C. difficile diarrhea** oral vancomycin or nitazoxanide are preferred; *Flagyl frequently fails*. Rifaxamin and Fidaxomycin have no advantage over vancomycin. With effective therapy, C. difficile diarrhea begins to improve (≤ 3 days) and usually resolves by 5–7 days, although some patients require 10 days of therapy. If no improvement with vancomycin 250 mg (PO) q6h, ↑ dose to 500 mg (PO) q6h or use nitazoxanide. *Do not treat C. difficile negative diarrhea with oral vancomycin or metronidazole.* For **C. difficle colitis**, treat until colitis resolves (follow with serial ESRs/abdominal and or CT scans). Add aerobic GNB coverage for microscopic/gross peritonitis with ESRs ertapenem. Tigacycline highly effective monotherapy for C. difficile colitis; and also provides anti-B fragilis coverage (for associated microscopic/clinical peritonitis). **Avoid** anti-motility agents, e.g., *loperamide with C. difficile diarrhea which may result in C. difficile colitis/toxic megacolon.*

Prognosis: Prognosis with C. difficile diarrhea is excellent. C. difficile colitis prognosis is related to strain virulence/and extent of the colitis.

Typhoid (Enteric) Fever (Salmonella typhi/Paratyphi)

Clinical Presentation: High fevers (> 102°F) increasing in a stepwise fashion accompanied by relative bradycardia (without chills) with watery diarrhea/constipation, headache, anorexia, abdominal pain, dry cough/sore throat, tender hepatomegaly, ± Rose spots. Dull mental affect ("apathetic facies") peculiar to typhoid fever. Thrombocytopenia should suggest another diagnosis eg. malaria or viral coinfection eg. dengue.

Diagnostic Considerations: Most community-acquired watery diarrheas are not accompanied by temperatures > 102°F and relative bradycardia. Diagnosis is confirmed by demonstrating Salmonella in blood, bone marrow, Rose spots, or stool cultures. Culture of bone marrow is the quickest/most reliable method of diagnosis. WBC count is usually low/low normal. Leukocytosis should suggest another diagnosis or bowel perforation, which may occur during 2nd week of typhoid fever.

Pitfalls: Rose spots are few/difficult to see and not present in all cases. Typhoid fever usually presents with constipation, not diarrhea. Severe rigors not a feature of typhoid fever. If present, consider malaria.

Therapeutic Considerations: 2nd generation cephalosporins, aztreonam, and aminoglycosides are ineffective. Since Salmonella strains causing enteric fever are intracellular pathogens, treat for a full 2 weeks to maximize cure rates/minimize relapses. Treat relapses with the suggested antibiotics × 2–3 weeks. Salmonella excretion into feces usually persists < 3 months. Persistent excretion > 3 months suggests a carrier state—rule out hepatobiliary/urinary calculi.

Prognosis: Good if treated early. Poor with late treatment/bowel perforation.

Chronic Watery Diarrhea

Clinical Presentation: Watery diarrhea without blood/mucus lasting > 1 month.

Diagnostic Considerations: Diagnosis by demonstrating organisms/cysts in stool specimens. Multiple fresh daily stool samples often needed for diagnosis especially for protozoan parasites.

Pitfalls: Concomitant transient lactase deficiency may prolong diarrhea if dairy products are consumed during an infectious diarrhea.

Therapeutic Considerations: Cryptosporidia and Isospora are being recognized increasingly in acute/chronic diarrhea in normal hosts.

Prognosis: Excellent in well-nourished patients. Untreated patients may develop malabsorption.

Giardia lamblia

Clinical Presentation: Acute/subacute onset of diarrhea, abdominal cramps, bloating, flatulence. Incubation period 1–2 weeks. Malabsorption may occur in chronic cases. No eosinophilia.

Diagnostic Considerations: Diagnosis by demonstrating trophozoites or cysts in stool/antigen detection assay. If stool exam and antigen test are negative and Giardiasis is suspected, perform "string test"/duodenal aspirate and biopsy.

Pitfalls: Cysts intermittently excreted into stool. Usually need multiple stool samples for diagnosis. Often accompanied by transient lactase intolerance.

Therapeutic Considerations: Nitazoxanide effective therapy. Diarrhea may be prolonged if milk (lactose-containing) products are ingested after treatment/cure. May need repeat courses of therapy.

Prognosis: Related to severity of malabsorption and health of host.

Cryptosporidia

Clinical Presentation: Acute/subacute onset of diarrhea. Usually occurs in HIV patients with CD_4 counts < 200. Biliary cryptosporidiosis is seen only in HIV; may present as acalculous cholecystitis or sclerosing cholangitis with RUQ pain, fever, ↑ alkaline phosphatase, but bilirubin is normal.

Diagnostic Considerations: Diagnosis by demonstrating organism in stool/intestinal biopsy specimen. Cholera-like illness in normal hosts. Chronic watery diarrhea in compromised hosts.

Pitfalls: Smaller than Cyclospora. Oocyst walls are smooth (not wrinkled) on acid fast staining.

Therapeutic Considerations: Nitazoxanide effective therapy.

Prognosis: Related to adequacy of fluid replacement/underlying health of host.

Cyclospora

Clinical Presentation: Acute/subacute onset of diarrhea. Incubation period 1–14 days.

Diagnostic Considerations: Diagnosis by demonstrating organism in stool/intestinal biopsy specimen. Clinically indistinguishable from cryptosporidial diarrhea (intermittent watery diarrhea without blood or mucus). Fatigue/weight loss common.

Pitfalls: Oocysts only form seen in stool and are best identified with modified Kinyoun acid fast staining. Acid fast fat globules stain pink with acid fast staining. "Wrinkled wall" oocysts are characteristic of Cyclospora, not Cryptosporidia. Oocysts are twice the size of similar appearing Cryptosporidia (~ 10 μm vs. 5 μm).

Therapeutic Considerations: Nitazoxanide effective therapy.

Prognosis: Related to adequacy of fluid replacement/underlying health of host.

Acute Dysentery

Entamoeba histolytica

Clinical Presentation: Acute/subacute onset of bloody diarrhea/mucus. Fecal WBC/RBCs due to mucosal invasion. E. histolytica may also cause chronic diarrhea. Colonic ulcers secondary to E. histolytica are round and may form "collar stud" abscesses.

Diagnostic Considerations: Diagnosis by demonstrating organism/trophozoites in stool/intestinal biopsy specimen. Serology is negative with amebic dysentery, but positive with extra-intestinal forms. Test to separate E. histolytica from non-pathogenic E. dispar cyst passers. On sigmoidoscopy, ulcers due to E. histolytica are round with normal mucosa in between, and may form "collar stud" abscesses. In contrast, ulcers due to Shigella are linear and serpiginous without normal intervening mucosa. Bloody dysentery is more subacute with E. histolytica compared to Shigella.

Pitfalls: Intestinal perforation/abscess may complicate amebic colitis. Rule out infectious causes of bloody diarrhea with mucus before diagnosing/treating inflammatory bowel disease (IBD). Obtain multiple stool cultures for bacterial pathogens/parasites. Do not confuse E. histolytica in stool specimens with E. hartmanni, a non-pathogen protozoa similar in appearance but smaller in size.

Therapeutic Considerations: E. histolytica cyst passers should be treated, but metronidazole is ineffective against cysts. Recommended antibiotics treat both luminal and hepatic E. histolytica. Use paromomycin 500 mg (PO) q8h × 7 days for asymptomatic cysts.

Prognosis: Good if treated early. Related to severity of dysentery/ulcers/extra-intestinal amebiasis.

Shigella

Clinical Presentation: Acute onset of bloody diarrhea/mucus.

Diagnostic Considerations: Diagnosis by demonstrating organism in stool specimens. Shigella ulcers in colon are linear, serpiginous, and rarely lead to perforation.

Therapeutic Considerations: Shigella dysentery is more acute/fulminating than amebic dysentery. Shigella has no carrier state, unlike Entamoeba.

Prognosis: Good if treated early. Severity of illness related to Shigella species: S. dysenteriae (most severe) > S. flexneri > S. boydii/S. sonnei (mildest).

Cholecystitis

Subset	Usual Pathogens	Preferred IV Therapy	Alternate IV Therapy	PO Therapy or IV-to-PO Switch
Normal host	E. coli Klebsiella E. faecalis (VSE)	Meropenem 1 gm (IV) q8h* **or** Piperacillin/tazobactam 3.375 gm (IV) q6h* **or** Tigacyline 100 mg (IV) × 1 dose, then 50 mg (IV) q12h*	Cefazolin 1 gm (IV) q8h* ± Ampicillin 1 gm (IV) q6h* **or** Quinolone‡ (IV)*	Quinolone‡ (PO)*
Emphy-sematous cholecystitis†	Clostridium perfringens E. coli	Meropenem 1 gm (IV) q8h¶ **or** Piperacillin/tazobactam 3.375 gm (IV) q6h¶	Ertapenem 1 gm (IV) q24h¶ **or** Ticarcillin/ clavulanate 3.1 gm (IV) q6h¶	Clindamycin 300 mg (PO) q8h¶

Duration of therapy represents total time IV, PO, or IV + PO. Most patients on IV therapy able to take PO meds should be switched to PO therapy after clinical improvement.

†   Treat only IV or IV-to-PO switch.

‡   Ciprofloxacin 400 mg (IV) or Levofloxacin 500 mg (IV or PO) q24h or Moxifloxacin 400 mg (IV or PO) q24h.

*   If no cholecystectomy, treat × 5–7 days. If cholecystectomy is performed, treat × 3–4 days post-operatively.

¶   Treat × 4–7 days after cholecystectomy.

Cholecystitis

Clinical Presentation: RUQ pain, fever usually ≤ 102°F, positive Murphy's sign, no percussion tenderness over right lower ribs.

Diagnostic Considerations: Diagnosis by RUQ ultrasound/positive HIDA scan.

Pitfalls: No need to cover B. fragilis.

Therapeutic Considerations: Obtain surgical consult for possible cholecystectomy.

Prognosis: Related to cardiopulmonary status.

Emphysematous Cholecystitis

Clinical Presentation: Clinically presents as cholecystitis. Usually in diabetics.

Diagnostic Considerations: RUQ/gallbladder gas on flat plate of abdomen.

Pitfalls: Requires immediate cholecystectomy.

Therapeutic Considerations: Usually a difficult/prolonged post-op course.

Prognosis: Related to speed of gallbladder removal.

Cholangitis

Subset	Usual Pathogens	Preferred IV Therapy	Alternate IV Therapy	IV-to-PO Switch
Normal host	E. coli Klebsiella E. faecalis (VSE)	Meropenem 1 gm (IV) q8h* **or** Tigecycline 200 mg (IV) × 1 dose, then 100 mg (IV) q24h* **or** Piperacillin/tazobactam 3.375 gm (IV) q6h*	Ampicillin/sulbactam 3 gm (IV) q6h* **or** Cefoperazone 2 gm (IV) q12h* **or** Doripenem 1 gm (IV) q8h	Ciprofloxacin 500 mg (PO) q12h* **or** Levofloxacin 500 mg (PO) q24h* **or** Moxifloxacin 400 mg (PO) q24h*

Duration of therapy represents total time IV or IV + PO. Most patients on IV therapy able to take PO meds should be switched to PO therapy after clinical improvement.

* Treat until resolved (usually 5–7 days).

Clinical Presentation: RUQ pain, fever > 102°F, positive Murphy's sign, percussion tenderness over right lower ribs.

Diagnostic Considerations: Obstructed common bile duct on ultrasound/CT/MRI of abdomen.

Pitfalls: Charcot's triad (fever, RUQ pain, jaundice) is present in only 50%.

Therapeutic Considerations: Obtain surgical consult to relieve obstruction. Continue antibiotics for 4–7 days after obstruction is relieved.

Prognosis: Related to speed of surgical relief of obstruction.

Gallbladder Wall Abscess/Perforation

Subset	Usual Pathogens	Preferred IV Therapy	Alternate IV Therapy	IV-to-PO Switch
Gallbladder wall abscess/ perforation	E. coli Klebsiella E. faecalis (VSE)	Piperacillin/ tazobactam 3.375 gm (IV) q6h* **or** Tigecycline 100 mg (IV) × 1 dose, then 50 mg (IV) q12h* **or** Meropenem 1 gm (IV) q8h*	Ampicillin/ sulbactam 3 gm (IV) q6h* **or** Cefoperazone 2 gm (IV) q12h* **or** Doripenem 1 gm (IV) q8h	Ciprofloxacin 500 mg (PO) q12h* **or** Levofloxacin 500 mg (PO) q24h* **or** Moxifloxacin 400 mg (PO) q24h*

Duration of therapy represents total time IV or IV + PO.

* Treat until resolved (usually 1–2 weeks).

Clinical Presentation: RUQ pain, fever ≤ 102°F, positive Murphy's sign, no percussion tenderness over right lower ribs.

Diagnostic Considerations: Diagnosis by CT/MRI of abdomen. Bile peritonitis is common.

Pitfalls: Bacterial peritonitis may be present.

Therapeutic Considerations: Obtain surgical consult for possible gallbladder removal. Usually a difficult and prolonged post-op course.

Prognosis: Related to removal of gallbladder/repair of perforation.

Acute Pancreatitis

Subset	Usual Pathogens	Preferred IV Therapy	Alternate IV Therapy	IV-to-PO Switch
Edematous pancreatitis	None	Not applicable	Not applicable	Not applicable
Hemorrhagic/ necrotizing pancreatitis	Aerobic GNBs B. fragilis	Meropenem 1 gm (IV) q8h* **or** Ertapenem 1 gm (IV) q24h*	Piperacillin 4 gm (IV) q8h* **or** Ampicillin/sulbactam 1.5 gm (IV) q6h* **or** Ticarcillin/ clavulanate 3.1 gm (IV) q6h*	Clindamycin 300 mg (PO) q8h* **plus** Levofloxacin 500 mg (PO) q24h* **or monotherapy with** Moxifloxacin 400 mg (PO) q24h*

Duration of therapy represents total time IV or IV + PO and varies depending on the clinical response. Most patients on IV therapy able to take PO meds should be switched to PO therapy after clinical improvement.
* Treat until resolved (usually 1–2 weeks).

Edematous Pancreatitis
Clinical Presentation: Sharp abdominal pain with fever ≤ 102°F ± hypotension.
Diagnostic Considerations: Diagnosis by elevated serum amylase and lipase levels with normal methemalbumin levels. May be drug-induced (e.g., steroids).
Pitfalls: Amylase elevation alone is not diagnostic of acute pancreatitis.
Therapeutic Considerations: NG tube is not needed. Aggressively replace fluids.
Prognosis: Good with adequate fluid replacement.

Hemorrhagic/Necrotizing Pancreatitis
Clinical Presentation: Sharp abdominal pain with fever ≤ 102°F ± hypotension. Grey-Turner/ Cullen's sign present in some.
Diagnostic Considerations: Mildly elevated serum amylase and lipase levels with high methemalbumin levels.
Pitfalls: With elevated lipase, amylase level is inversely related to severity of disease.
Therapeutic Considerations: Obtain surgical consult for possible peritoneal lavage as adjunct to antibiotics. Serum albumin/dextran are preferred volume expanders.
Prognosis: Poor with hypocalcemia or shock.

Pancreatic Abscess/Infected Pancreatic Pseudocyst

Subset	Usual Pathogens	Preferred IV Therapy	Alternate IV Therapy	IV-to-PO Switch
Infected pancreatic pseudocyst/ pancreatic abscess	Aerobic GNBs B. fragilis	Meropenem 1 gm (IV) q8h* **or** Piperacillin/ tazobactam 3.375 gm (IV) q6h* **or** Ertapenem 1 gm (IV) q24h*	Ampicillin/sulbactam 1.5 gm (IV) q6h* **or** Ticarcillin/ clavulanate 3.1 gm (IV) q6h* **or** Doripenem 1 gm (IV) q8h	Moxifloxacin 400 mg (PO) q24h* **or combination therapy with** Clindamycin 300 mg (PO) q8h* **plus** Quinolone† (PO)*

Duration of therapy represents total time IV or IV + PO.
†   Ciprofloxacin 500 mg q12h or Levofloxacin 500 mg q24h.
*   Treat until resolved.

Clinical Presentation: Follows acute pancreatitis or develops in a pancreatic pseudocyst. An infected pancreatic pseudocyst is an abscess equivalent. Fevers usually ≥ 102°F.
Diagnostic Considerations: CT/MRI of abdomen demonstrates pancreatic abscess.
Pitfalls: Peritoneal signs are typically absent.
Prognosis: Related to size/extent of abscess and adequacy of drainage.

Liver Abscess

Subset	Usual Pathogens	Preferred IV Therapy	Alternate IV Therapy	PO Therapy or IV-to-PO Switch
Liver abscess	Aerobic GNBs Enterococci (VSE) B. fragilis	Piperacillin/ tazobactam 3.375 gm (IV) q6h* **or** Tigecycline 100 mg (IV) × 1 dose, then 50 mg (IV) q12h* **or** Meropenem 1 gm (IV) q8h* **or**	Quinolone† (IV)* **plus either** Metronidazole 1 gm (IV) q24h* **or** Clindamycin 600 mg (IV) q8h* Moxifloxacin 400 mg (IV) q24h* **or** Sulbactam/ampicillin 3 gm (IV) q6h	Amoxicillin/clavulanic acid 875/125 mg (PO) q12h* **or** Moxifloxacin 400 mg (PO) q24h* **or combination therapy with** Quinolone† (PO)* **plus either** Metronidazole 500 mg (PO) q12h* **or** Clindamycin 300 mg (PO) q8h*
	E. histolytica	See p. 274		

Duration of therapy represents total time IV, PO, or IV + PO.
*   Treat until abscess(es) are no longer present or stop decreasing in size on serial CT scans.
†   Ciprofloxacin 400 mg (IV) or 500 mg (PO) q12h or Levofloxacin 500 mg (IV or PO) q24h.

Liver Abscess (cont'd)

Clinical Presentation: Fever, RUQ tenderness, negative Murphy's sign, and negative right lower rib percussion tenderness.

Diagnostic Considerations: Diagnosis by CT/MRI scan of liver and aspiration of abscess. CT shows multiple lesions in liver. Source is usually either the colon (diverticulitis or diverticular abscess with portal pyemia) or retrograde infection from the gallbladder (cholecystitis or gallbladder wall abscess).

Pitfalls: Bacterial abscesses are usually multiple and involve multiple lobes of liver; amebic abscesses are usually solitary and involve the right lobe of liver.

Therapeutic Considerations: Liver laceration/trauma usually requires ~ 2 weeks of antibiotics.

Prognosis: Good if treated early.

Hepatosplenic Candidiasis

Subset	Usual Pathogens	Preferred IV Therapy	Alternate IV Therapy	IV-to-PO Switch
Hepato-splenic candidiasis	Candida albicans	Fluconazole 800 mg (IV) × 1 dose, then 400 mg (IV) q24h × 2–4 weeks **or** Micafungin 100 mg (IV) q24h × 2–4 weeks **or** Caspofungin 70 mg (IV) × 1 dose, then 50 mg (IV) q24h × 2–4 weeks	Ambisome (L-Amb) (p. 540) (IV) q24h × 2–4 weeks **or** Amphotericin B 0.7 mg/kg (IV) q24h × 2–4 weeks	Fluconazole 800 mg (PO) × 1 dose, then 400 mg (PO) q24h × 2–4 weeks* **or** Itraconazole 200 mg (PO) solution q12h × 2–4 weeks

Duration of therapy represents total time IV or IV + PO. Most patients on IV therapy able to take PO meds should be switched to PO therapy after clinical improvement.
* Loading dose is not needed PO if given IV with the same drug.

Clinical Presentation: New high spiking fevers with RUQ/LUQ pain after 2 weeks in a patient with afebrile leukopenia.

Diagnostic Considerations: Diagnosis by abdominal CT/MRI showing mass lesions in liver/spleen.

Pitfalls: Do not overlook RUQ tenderness and elevated alkaline phosphatase in leukopenic cancer patients as a clue to the diagnosis.

Therapeutic Considerations: Treat until liver/spleen lesions resolve. Should be viewed as a form of disseminated disease.

Prognosis: Related to degree/duration of leukopenia.

Granulomatous Hepatitis (BCG)

Subset	Pathogen	Preferred Therapy
BCG hepatitis	Bacille Calmette-Guérin (BCG)	INH 300 mg (PO) q24h × 6 months + rifampin 600 mg (PO) q24h × 6 months

Clinical Presentation: Fever, chills, anorexia, weight loss, hepatomegaly ± RUQ pain days to weeks after intravesicular BCG for bladder cancer.

Diagnostic Considerations: ↑ alkaline phosphatase > ↑ SGOT/SGPT. Liver biopsy is negative for AFB/positive for granulomas.

Pitfalls: Exclude other causes of hepatomegaly.

Therapeutic Considerations: INH plus rifampin × 6 months is curative.

Prognosis: Excellent with early treatment.

Leptospirosis

Clinical Presentation: After incubation period of 1–2 weeks, abrupt onset of fever, no chills, severe headache, conjunctival suffusion, meningismus, dry cough, intense myalgias (gastroc myalgias/tenderness) ± abdominal pain. 1st (leptospiremic) phase (4–9 days); 2nd (immune) phase (6–12 days). Leukocytosis with no thrombocytopenia usual. Hepatic (↑ bilirubin/transaminases) and renal (azotemia, proteinuria, sterile, pyuria) involvement. Meningitis (early) → ABM with CSF + for leptospires; meningitis (late) → aseptic meningitis CSF–for leptospires. Progressive vomiting, epistaxis, jaundice/hepatosplenomegaly only with Weil's syndrome (icteric leptospirosis). Intense myalgias with hepatic and renal involvement should suggest leptospirosis.

Diagnostic Considerations: Recent occupational or contaminated water (rat urine) exposure. Leptospiruria (after 2 weeks) seen in dark-field of urine. BCs + early (– late); UCs + late. Leptospires die rapidly in acid urine (add buffered saline before culture). Diagnosis by blood/urine culture or ↑ MAT IgM titers (after 1 week). Antibiotic therapy may blunt, delay or abort titer rise.

Pitfalls: Like influenza (headache, sore throat, myalgias), patients can recall exact hour of onset. Unlike influenza, no chills but conjunctival suffusion. CXR–in influenza (early) but CXR often + in leptospirosis. Differentiate from viral hepatitis (< 102°F, no conjunctival suffusion, leukopenia, highly ↑ transaminases, no renal involvement). Differentiate from EBV, CMV, HSV hepatitis by + atypical lymphocytes (– with leptospirosis) and specific serologies. Like aseptic (viral) meningitis (normal glucose, WBCs < 500/hpf). Only ID with CSF bilirubin > serum. Clinically irrelevant serologic XR with Borrelia/treponeme titers.

Therapeutic Considerations: penicillin or doxycycline (± Jarisch-Herxheimer reaction)

Prognosis: Excellent if treated early, 5–40% mortality for Weil's syndrome and elderly.

Viral Hepatitis

Subset	Pathogens	Therapy
Acute		HAV (none); HBV (consider nucleos(t)ides for HBV-acute liver failure); HCV (consider pegylated interferon +/– ribavirin if no viral clearance after 12–16 weeks); HDV (none); HEV (consider ribavirin fir severe hepatitis)
Chronic	HBV	<u>Preferred:</u> Tenofovir 300 mg (PO) **or** Entecavir 0.5 mg (PO) q24h × ≥ 12 months For lamivudine resistant strains use **either** Entecavir 1.0 mg q24h **or** Pegylated interferon alfa-2a 180 mcg (SQ)/ week *without* ribavirin × 12 months <u>Alternate:</u> Telbivudine 600 mg (PO) q24h **or** Adefovir 10 mg (PO) q24h **or** Lamivudine 100 mg (PO) for × ≥ 12 months

Viral Hepatitis (cont'd)

Subset	Pathogens	Therapy
	HCV	**Genotype 1** <u>Preferred</u>: Triple therapy × 12 weeks with telaprevir 750 mg (PO) 7–9 (with food) **plus** pegylated interferon alfa-2a/2b 180 mcg/week (SQ) **and** weight-based ribavirin 1000 mg (<75 kg body weight) **or** 1200 mg (>75 kg body weight) (PO) in divided doses, **then** continue pegylated interferon **plus** ribavirin × 12 or 36 more weeks depending on viral clearance at weeks 4 and 12. Treatment duration for naïve patients and relapsers: 24 weeks total. **For prior null or partial responders,** treatment duration 48 weeks. **Genotype 1** <u>Alternate</u>: Pegylated interferon **and** ribavirin (as above) × 4 weeks, followed by triple therapy *with the addition* of boceprevir 800 mg (PO) 7–9 (with food) × either 28 or 48 weeks dependent on virologic clearance at week 8 and 24 in naïve patients. **For prior relapsers or partial responders** total treatment duration 36 or 48 weeks (dependent on viral clearance at weeks 8 and 24). **Genotype 4, 5, 6:** Treat with pegylated interferon and ribavirin as for genotype 1 (see above) but *without telaprevir or boceprevir.* **Genotype 2 or 3:** Peginterferon alfa-2a 180 mcg/week (SQ) **plus** 800 mg (PO) ribavirin in divided doses for 24 weeks *without telaprevir or boceprevir*
	HDV	Prolonged therapy with pegylated interferon alfa-2a *without* ribavirin as for chronic hepatitis B (see above)
	HEV	Ribavirin 600–1200 mg daily × 12 weeks or pegylated interferon weekly × 12 weeks +/− ribavirin

Adapted from Koff R.S. Hepatitis Essentials. Jones & Bartlett, Sudbury, MA; 2011.
*   For genotype 1, 1.0 mcg/kg was as effective as 1.5 mcg/kg.

Acute Viral Hepatitis
Clinical Presentation: Asymptomatic or anorexia, malaise, nausea, serum-sickness like syndrome, ± jaundice, dark urine.
Diagnostic Considerations: Diagnosis by presence in HAV of IgM anti-HAV or in HBV of HBsAg and IgM anti-HBc or in HCV of anti-HCV and HCV RNA or in HDV of HBsAg, anti-HDV and HDV RNA or in HEV of anti-HEV and HEV RNA, with markedly elevated serum aminotransferases (ALT > 400). Serum alkaline phosphatase normal/mildly elevated; albumin normal or mildly depressed; INR normal or minimally elevated.
Pitfalls: Rule out other hepatitis-causing agents (EBV, CMV, HSV, etc) and drug-induced liver injury if serologic tests for HAV, HBV, HCV, HDV, and HEV are negative.
Therapeutic Considerations: For patients who develop encephalopathy and/or a prolonged INR (acute liver failure) admit to liver transplantation center.
Prognosis: Hepatitis A generally self-limited; Hepatitis B, C, D and rarely E may progress to chronic hepatitis/cirrhosis/hepatocellular carcinoma.

EBV/CMV Hepatitis

Clinical Presentation: Similar to acute viral hepatitis plus bilateral posterior cervical adenopathy and fatigue.

Diagnostic Considerations: EBV hepatitis is part of infectious mononucleosis and may be the presenting sign in adults. CMV hepatitis also may appear as a "mono-like" infection in normal hosts. In compromised hosts, hepatitis may be the primary manifestation of CMV infection. Diagnosis of EBV/ CMV hepatitis can be made by serology (positive mono spot test, high EBV VCA IgM titer, high CMV IgM titer, CMV early antigen detection (via shell vial cultures) or molecular amplification techniques.

Pitfalls: In normal and immunocompromised hosts with unexplained aminotransferase (ALT/AST) elevations, consider CMV hepatitis and order appropriate tests.

Treatment: None effective in EBV hepatitis; CMV hepatitis in normal hosts may be treated with Valganciclovir 900 mg (PO) q12h × 12 days.

Prognosis: In normal hosts EBV and CMV hepatitis are usually self-limited. In immunocompromised hosts, the prognosis of CMV hepatitis is related to the degree of Immunosuppression and the rapidity of onset of treatment.

Chronic Viral Hepatitis

Clinical Presentation: Often asymptomatic with persistently or intermittently elevated serum aminotransferases but in some aminotransferases are normal. Some present with signs and symptoms of chronic liver disease.

Diagnostic Considerations: Chronic hepatitis B is diagnosed by presence of HBsAg and HBV DNA. Chronic hepatitis C is diagnosed by positive tests for anti-HCV and HCV RNA. Chronic hepatitis D is diagnosed by positive tests for HBsAg and HDV RNA. Chronic hepatitis E is diagnosed by presence of anti-HEV and HEV RNA. Liver biopsy may be used to grade inflammation and stage fibrosis.

Pitfalls: Autoimmune hepatitis may present as an acute or chronic hepatitis but with elevated IgG levels, elevated ANAs, and anti-smooth muscle antibodies. For both HCV and HBV, rule out co-infection with HIV.

Therapeutic Considerations: In chronic hepatitis B use *either* tenofovir *or* entecavir until HBV DNA becomes undetectable, ALT normalizes, and for HBeAg-positive patients, HBeAg seroconversion occurs (then continue for 6–12 additional months). For chronic hepatitis C genotype 1, triple therapy with telaprevir *plus* pegylated interferon *and* ribavirin × 12 weeks *followed by continued treatment with just peginterferon and ribavirin* × 12 or 36 more weeks depending on virologic response and prior response to peginterferon plus ribavirin. Boceprevir *plus* peginterferon *and* ribavirin, following a 4-week lead-in without boceprevir is an alternate therapy. For chronic hepatitis C genotypes 4, 5, and 6, treat with peginterferon *plus* ribavirin as in genotype 1 (*without telaprevir or boceprevir*) × 48 weeks. For chronic hepatitis C genotypes 2 and 3, treat with peginterferon *plus lower doses of ribavirin* (800 mg daily in divided doses) × 24 weeks. For chronic hepatitis D prolonged treatment with peginterferon may be effective. For rare cases of chronic HEV, ribavirin, pegylated interferon or both have been suggested.

Prognosis: Sustained clearance of HCV RNA (measured 24 weeks after discontinuation of treatment) results in a cure in 99% of chronic hepatitis C patients. Sustained clearance of HBV DNA is linked with an improved prognosis in chronic hepatitis B.

Intraabdominal or Pelvic Peritonitis/Abscess

Subset	Usual Pathogens	Preferred IV Therapy	Alternate IV Therapy	PO Therapy or IV-to-PO Switch
Mild/ moderate peritonitis	Entero- bacteriaceae B. fragilis	Moxifloxacin 400 mg (IV) q24h[¥] **or** Cefoxitin 2 gm (IV) q6h[¥]	Ampicillin/ sulbactam 1.5 gm (IV) q6h[¥] **or combination therapy with** Clindamycin 600 mg (IV) q8h[¥] *plus* Aztreonam 2 gm (IV) q8h[¥]	Moxifloxacin 400 mg (PO) q24h[¥] **or** Amoxicillin/clavulanic acid 875/125 mg (PO) q12h[¥] **or combination therapy with** Clindamycin 300 mg (PO) q8h[¥] *plus* Levofloxacin 500 mg (PO) q24h[¥]
Severe peritonitis[‡]	Entero- bacteriaceae B. fragilis	Meropenem 1 gm (IV) q8h[¥] **or** Tigecycline 100 mg (IV) × 1 dose, then 50 mg (IV) q12h or 100 mg (IV) q24h[¥] **or** Piperacillin/ tazobactam 3.375 gm (IV) q6h[¥] **or** Ertapenem 1 gm (IV) q24h[¥]	Ampicillin/ sulbactam 3 gm (IV) q6h[¥] **or** Doripenem 1 gm (IV) q8h **or combination therapy with** Metronidazole 1 gm (IV) q24h[¥] **plus either** Ceftriaxone 1 gm (IV) q24h[¥] **or** Quinolone[¶] (IV)[¥]	Moxifloxacin 400 mg (PO) q24h[¥] **or** Amoxicillin/clavulanic acid 875/125 mg (PO) q12h[¥]
Fungal peritonitis/ abscess	C. albicans Non-albicans Candida	Treat as for Candidemia (see p. 153)		

Duration of therapy represents total time IV, PO, or IV + PO.
¥   Duration of therapy as clinically indicated or for 5–7 days following corrective surgery.

Intraabdominal or Pelvic Peritonitis/Abscess (cont'd)

Subset	Usual Pathogens	Preferred IV Therapy	Alternate IV Therapy	PO Therapy or IV-to-PO Switch
Spontaneous bacterial peritonitis (SBP)[‡]	Entero-bacteriaceae S. pneumoniae (children)	Ceftriaxone 1 gm (IV) q24h × 1–2 wks **or** Levofloxacin 500 mg (IV) × 1–2 weeks	Aztreonam 2 gm (IV) q8h × 1–2 weeks **or** Any aminoglycoside (IV) q24h × 1–2 wks	Quinolone[¶] (PO) × 1–2 weeks **or** Amoxicillin/clavulanic acid 875/125 mg (PO) q12h × 1–2 weeks
Chronic TB peritonitis	M. tuberculosis	Not applicable		Treat the same as pulmonary TB (p. 53)
CAPD-associated peritonitis[‡]	S. epidermidis (CoNS) S. aureus (MSSA) Entero-bacteriaceae Non-fermentative GNBs	_Before culture results_ Vancomycin 1 gm (IV) initial dose* **plus** Gentamicin 5 mg/kg or 240 mg (IV) initial dose*	_After culture results_ _MSSA/Enterobacteriaceae_ Meropenem 1 gm (IV) initial dose* _MRSA_ Vancomycin 1 gm (IV) initial dose* **or** Linezolid 600 mg (IV or PO)	

MSSA/MRSA = methicillin-sensitive/resistant S. aureus. Duration of therapy represents total time IV, PO, or IV + PO.

‡   Treat only IV or IV-to-PO switch.

*   Follow with maintenance dosing × 2 weeks after culture results are available. For maintenance dosing, use renal failure (CrCl < 10 mL/min) and post-peritoneal dialysis dosing (see Drug Summaries).

Intraabdominal or Pelvic Peritonitis/Abscess (Appendicitis/Diverticulitis/Septic Pelvic Thrombophlebitis)

Clinical Presentation: Spiking fevers with acute abdominal pain and peritoneal signs. In diverticulitis, the pain is localized over the involved segment of colon. Appendicitis ± perforation presents as RLQ pain/rebound tenderness or mass. Peri-diverticular abscess presents the same as intraabdominal/pelvic abscess, most commonly in the LLQ. Septic pelvic thrombophlebitis (SPT) presents as high spiking fevers unresponsive to antibiotic therapy following delivery/pelvic surgery.

Diagnostic Considerations: Diagnosis by CT/MRI scan of abdomen/pelvis.

Pitfalls: Tympany over liver suggests abdominal/visceral perforation. Pelvic peritonitis/abscess presents the same as intraabdominal abscess/peritonitis, but peritoneal signs are often absent.

Therapeutic Considerations: Patients with ischemic/inflammatory colitis should be treated the same as peritonitis, depending on severity. Obtain surgical consult for repair/lavage or abscess drainage. In SPT, fever rapidly falls when heparin is added to antibiotics.

Prognosis: Related to degree/duration of peritoneal spillage and rapidity/completeness of lavage. Prognosis for SPT is good if treated early and clots remain limited to pelvic veins.

Spontaneous Bacterial Peritonitis (SBP)

Clinical Presentation: Acute or subacute onset of fever ± abdominal pain.

Diagnostic Considerations: Diagnosis by positive blood cultures of SBP pathogens. For patients with abdominal pain, ascites, and a negative CT/MRI, paracentesis ascitic fluid with > 500 WBCs and > 100 PMNs predicts a positive ascitic fluid culture and is diagnostic of SBP. Some degree of splenic dysfunction usually exists, predisposing to infection with encapsulated organisms.

Pitfalls: Do not overlook GI source of peritonitis (e.g, appendicitis, diverticulitis); obtain CT/MRI.

Therapeutic Considerations: B. fragilis/anaerobes are not common pathogens in SBP, and B. fragilis coverage is unnecessary.

Prognosis: Related to degree of hepatitic/splenic dysfunction.

Chronic Tuberculous Peritonitis (Mycobacterium tuberculosis)

Clinical Presentation: Abdominal pain with fevers, weight loss, ascites over 1–3 months.

Diagnostic Considerations: "Doughy consistency" on abdominal palpation. Diagnosis by AFB on peritoneal biopsy/culture.

Pitfalls: Chest x-ray is normal in ~ 70%. Increased incidence in alcoholic cirrhosis.

Therapeutic Considerations: Treated the same as pulmonary TB.

Prognosis: Good if treated early.

CAPD-Associated Peritonitis

Clinical Presentation: Abdominal pain ± fever in a CAPD patient.

Diagnostic Considerations: Diagnosis by gram stain/culture and ↑ WBC count in peritoneal fluid. Lymphocytic predominance may suggest TB or fungi. Unlike SBP, there are not specific diagnostic criteria in peritoneal fluid.

Pitfalls: Fever is often absent.

Therapeutic Considerations: Treat with systemic antibiotics ± antibiotics in dialysate.

Prognosis: Good with early therapy and removal of peritoneal catheter.

Empiric Therapy of Genitourinary Tract Infections

Dysuria-Pyuria Syndrome (Acute Urethral Syndrome)

Subset	Usual Pathogens	IV Therapy	PO Therapy
Acute urethral syndrome	S. saprophyticus C. trachomatis E. coli (< 10^5 cfu/mL)	Not applicable	Doxycycline 100 mg (PO) q12h × 10 days **or** Quinolone (PO)* × 7 days

* Ciprofloxacin 500 mg q12h or Levofloxacin 500 mg q24h.

Clinical Presentation: Dysuria, frequency, urgency, lower abdominal discomfort, fevers < 102°F.
Diagnostic Considerations: Diagnosis by symptoms of cystitis with pyuria and no growth or low concentration of E. coli (≤ 10^3 colonies/mL) by urine culture. Clue to S. saprophyticus is alkaline urinary pH and RBCs in urine.
Pitfalls: Resembles "culture negative" cystitis.
Therapeutic Considerations: S. saprophyticus is susceptible to most antibiotics used to treat UTIs.
Prognosis: Excellent.

Cystitis (see Color Atlas for Urine Gram stains)

Subset	Usual Pathogens	Therapy
Bacterial	Enterobacteriaceae E. faecalis (VSE) S. agalactiae (group B streptococci) S. saprophyticus	Amoxicillin 500 mg (PO) × q12h × 3 days **or** TMP–SMX 1 SS tablet (PO) × q12h × 3 days **or** Levofloxacin 500 mg (PO) q24h × 3 days **or** Nitrofurantoin 100 mg (PO) q12h × 3 days
	MDR GNBs	Fosfomycin 3 gm (PO) q24h × 3 days
Fungal	C. albicans†	Fluconazole 200 mg (PO) × 1 dose, then 100 mg (PO) q24h × 4 days
	Fluconazole-resistant‡ Candida isolates or fluconazole-refractory disease	Amphotericin B 0.3 mg/kg (IV) × 1 dose

† C. albicans cystitis (see p. 104)
‡ Fluconazole-resistant (see p. 104)

Bacterial Cystitis

Clinical Presentation: Dysuria, frequency, urgency, lower abdominal discomfort, fevers < 102°F.

Diagnostic Considerations: Pyuria plus bacteriuria.

Pitfalls: Compromised hosts (chronic steroids, diabetes, SLE, cirrhosis, multiple myeloma) may require 3–5 days of therapy. A single dose of amoxicillin or TMP–SMX may be sufficient in acute uncomplicated cystitis in normal hosts.

Therapeutic Considerations: Pyridium 200 mg (PO) q8h after meals × 24–48h is useful to decrease dysuria (inform patients urine will turn orange).

Prognosis: Excellent in normal hosts.

Candida Cystitis

Diagnostic Considerations: Marked pyuria, urine nitrate negative ± RBCs. Speciate if not C. albicans.

Pitfalls: Lack of response suggests renal candidiasis or a "fungus ball" in the renal collecting system.

Therapeutic Considerations: If fluconazole fails, use amphotericin. For chronic renal failure/dialysis patients with candiduria, use amphotericin B deoxycholate bladder irrigation (as for catheter-associated candiduria, below). Removal of devices and correction of anatomic abnormalities are critical to success.

Prognosis: Patients with impaired host defenses, abnormal collecting systems, cysts, renal disease or stones are prone to recurrent UTIs/urosepsis.

Catheter-Associated Bacteriuria (CAB)/Candiduria (CAC)

Subset	Usual Pathogens	Therapy
Catheter-associated bacteriuria (CAB)[†][*]	E. coli E. faecalis (VSE)	Nitrofurantoin 100 mg (PO) q12h × 3 days **or** Amoxicillin 500 mg (PO) q12h × 3 days
	E. faecium (VRE)	Nitrofurantoin 100 mg (PO) q12h × 3 days
	MDR Klebsiella MDR Acinetobacter MDR P. aeruginosa	Doripenem 1 gm (IV) q8h × 3 days Fosomycin 3 gm (PO) q24h × 3 days Colistin 1.7 mg/kg (IV) q8h × 3 days Polymyxin B 1 mg/kg (IV) of q12h × 3 days

VSE/VRE = vancomycin-sensitive/resistant enterococci.

* **Remove/replace Foley catheter before initiating antibiotic therapy.**

† *Treat CAB/CAC in compromised hosts*, e.g., cirrhosis, SLE, DM, myeloma, steroids, immunosuppressives, and those with renal insufficiency.

Catheter-Associated Bacteriuria (CAB)/Candiduria (CAC) (cont'd)

Subset	Usual Pathogens	Therapy
Catheter-associated candiduria (CAC)†*	C. albicans	Fluconazole 200 mg (PO) × 1 dose, then 100 mg (PO) q24h × 2 weeks
	Fluconazole-resistant C. albicans/non-albicans Candida	Amphotericin B 0.3–0.6 mg/kg q24h × 1–7 days **or** Flucytosine 25 mg/kg QID (PO) × 7–10 days **or** Amphotericin B bladder irrigation (continuous: 50 mg in 1 liter sterile water over 24h × 1–2 days; intermittent: 50 mg in 200–300 ml sterile water q6-8h × 1–2 days)§

§   Limited efficacy.

Clinical Presentation: Indwelling urinary (Foley) catheter with bacteriuria and pyuria; no symptoms.

Diagnostic Considerations: Pyuria plus bacteriuria/candiduria. Usually afebrile or temperature < 101°F.

Pitfalls: Bacteriuria/candiduria often represent colonization, not infection. Persistent candiduria after amphotericin B deoxycholate bladder irrigation suggests renal candidiasis.

Therapeutic Considerations: Compromised hosts (diabetes, SLE, chronic steroids, multiple myeloma, cirrhosis) may require therapy for duration of catheterization. If bacteriuria/candiduria does not clear with appropriate therapy, change the catheter. For chronic renal failure/dialysis patients with candiduria, use amphotericin B deoxycholate bladder irrigation. Efficacy of therapy of catheter-associated candiduria is limited and relapse is frequent unless the catheter can be replaced or (preferably) removed. Avoid treating catheter-associated bacteriuria in normal hosts without GU tract abnormalities/disease.

Prognosis: Excellent in normal hosts. Untreated bacteriuria/candiduria in compromised hosts may result in ascending infection (e.g., pyelonephritis) or bacteremia/candidemia.

Epididymitis

Subset	Usual Pathogens	Preferred IV Therapy	Alternate IV Therapy	PO Therapy or IV-to-PO Switch
Acute *Young males*	C. trachomatis	Doxycycline 200 mg (IV) q12h × 3 days, then 100 mg (IV) q12h × 4 days	Levofloxacin 500 mg (IV) q24h × 7 days	Doxycycline 200 mg (PO) q12h × 3 days, then 100 mg (PO) q12h × 7 days* **or** Levofloxacin 500 mg (PO) q24h × 10 days **or** Ofloxacin 300 mg (PO) q12h × 10 days
Elderly males	P. aeruginosa	Cefepime 2 gm (IV) q8h × 10 days **or** Meropenem 1 gm (IV) q8h × 10 days	Ciprofloxacin 400 mg (IV) q8h × 10 days **or** Levofloxacin 750 mg (IV) q24h × 10 days	Ciprofloxacin 750 mg (PO) q12h × 10 days
Chronic	M. tuberculosis Blastomyces dermatiditis	Treat the same as pulmonary TB (see p. 53) or pulmonary blastomycosis (see p. 267)		

Duration of therapy represents total time IV, PO, or IV + PO. Most patients on IV therapy able to take PO meds should be switched to PO therapy soon after clinical improvement (usually < 72 hours).
* Loading dose is not needed PO if given IV with the same drug.

Acute Epididymitis (Chlamydia trachomatis/Pseudomonas aeruginosa)
Clinical Presentation: Acute unilateral testicular pain ± fever.
Diagnostic Considerations: Ultrasound to rule out torsion or tumor.
Pitfalls: Rule out torsion by absence of fever and ultrasound.
Therapeutic Considerations: Young males respond to treatment slowly over 1 week. Elderly males respond to anti-Pseudomonal therapy within 72 hours.
Prognosis: Excellent in young males. Related to health of host in elderly.

Chronic Epididymitis (Mycobacterium tuberculosis/ Blastomyces dermatiditis)
Clinical Presentation: Chronic epididymoorchitis with epididymal nodules.
Diagnostic Considerations: Diagnosis by AFB on biopsy/culture of epididymis. TB epididymitis is always associated with renal TB. Blastomyces epididymitis is a manifestation of systemic infection.
Pitfalls: Vasculitis (e.g., polyarteritis nodosum) and lymphomas may present the same way.
Therapeutic Considerations: Treated the same as pulmonary TB/blastomycosis.
Prognosis: Good.

Acute Pyelonephritis (see Color Atlas for Urine Gram stains)

Subset	Usual Pathogens	Preferred IV Therapy	Alternate IV Therapy	PO Therapy or IV-to-PO Switch
Acute pyelonephritis (Treat initially based on urine gram stain; see therapeutic considerations, below)	Entero-bacteriaceae	Ceftriaxone 1 gm (IV) q24h × 2 weeks **or** Levofloxacin 500 mg (IV) q24h × 2 weeks	Meropenem 1 gm (IV) q8h × 2 weeks **or** Aztreonam 2 gm (IV) q8h × 2 weeks **or** Gentamicin 240 mg (IV) q24h × 2 weeks	Levofloxacin 500 mg (PO) q24h × 2 weeks **or** Amoxicillin 1 gm (PO) q8h × 2 weeks
	Enterococcus faecalis (VSE)§	Ampicillin 1 gm (IV) q4h × 2 weeks **or** Linezolid 600 mg (IV) q12h × 2 weeks **or** Meropenem 1 gm (IV) q8h × 2 weeks	Quinolone† (IV) × 2 weeks	Amoxicillin 1 gm (PO) q8h × 2 weeks **or** Linezolid 600 mg (PO) q12h × 2 weeks **or** Levofloxacin 500 mg (PO) q24h × 2 weeks
	Enterococcus faecium (VRE)	Linezolid 600 mg (IV) q12h × 2 weeks	Quinupristin/ dalfopristin 7.5 mg/kg (IV) q8h × 2 weeks **or** Doxycycline 200 mg (IV) q12h × 3 days, then 100 mg q12h × 2 weeks	Linezolid 600 mg (PO) q12h × 2 weeks **or** Doxycycline 200 mg (PO) q12h × 3 days, then 100 mg (PO) q12h × 2 weeks*

VSE/VRE = vancomycin-sensitive/resistant enterococci. Duration of therapy represents total time IV, PO, or IV + PO. Most patients on IV therapy able to take PO meds should be switched to PO therapy after clinical improvement (usually < 72 hours).

*   Loading dose is not needed PO if given IV with the same drug.

§   Treat vancomycin resistant E. faecalis as VRE.

Chronic Pyelonephritis/Renal TB

Subset	Usual Pathogens	Preferred IV Therapy	Alternate IV Therapy	PO Therapy or IV-to-PO Switch
Chronic pyelonephritis	Entero-bacteriaceae	IV Therapy Not applicable	Quinolone[†] (PO) × 4–6 weeks **or** TMP–SMX 1 DS tab (PO) q12h × 4–6 weeks **or** Doxycycline 200 mg (PO) q12h × 3 days, then 100 mg (PO) q12h × 4–6 weeks total	
Renal TB	M. tuberculosis	IV Therapy Not applicable	Treated the same as pulmonary TB (p. 53)	

Duration of therapy represents total time IV, PO, or IV + PO. Most patients on IV therapy able to take PO meds should be switched to PO therapy after clinical improvement (usually < 72 hours).

†   Ciprofloxacin XR 1000 mg (PO) q24h or Ciprofloxacin 400 mg (IV) q12h or Levofloxacin 500 mg (IV or PO) q24h.

Acute Bacterial Pyelonephritis (Enterobacteriaceae, E. faecalis/faecium)

Clinical Presentation: Unilateral CVA tenderness with fevers ≥ 102°F.

Diagnostic Considerations: Bacteriuria plus pyuria with unilateral CVA tenderness and temperature ≥ 102°F. Bacteremia usually accompanies acute pyelonephritis; obtain blood and urine cultures.

Pitfalls: Temperature decreases in 72 hours with or without antibiotic treatment. If temperature does not fall after 72 hours of antibiotic therapy, suspect renal/perinephric abscess.

Therapeutic Considerations: Initial treatment is based on the urinary gram stain: If gram-negative bacilli, treat as Enterobacteriaceae. If gram-positive cocci in chains (enterococcus), treat as E. faecalis; if enterococcus is subsequently identified as E. faecium, treat accordingly. Acute pyelonephritis is usually treated initially for 1–3 days IV, then switched to PO to complete 4 weeks of antibiotics to minimize progression to chronic pyelonephritis. Obtain a CT/MRI in persistently febrile patients after 72 hours of antibiotics to rule out renal calculi, obstruction, abscess, or xanthomatous pyelonephritis.

Prognosis: Excellent if first episode is adequately treated with antibiotics for 4 weeks.

Chronic Bacterial Pyelonephritis (Enterobacteriaceae)

Clinical Presentation: Previous history of acute pyelonephritis with same symptoms as acute pyelonephritis but less CVA tenderness/fever.

Diagnostic Considerations: Diagnosis by CT/MRI showing changes of chronic pyelonephritis plus bacteriuria/pyuria. Urine cultures may be intermittently negative before treatment. Chronic pyelonephritis is bilateral pathologically, but unilateral clinically.

Pitfalls: Urine culture may be intermittently positive after treatment; repeat weekly × 4 to confirm urine remains culture-negative.

Therapeutic Considerations: Treat × 4–6 weeks. Impaired medullary vascular blood supply/renal anatomical distortion makes eradication of pathogen difficult.

Prognosis: Related to extent of renal damage.

Renal TB (Mycobacterium tuberculosis)

Clinical Presentation: Renal mass lesion with ureteral abnormalities (pipestem, corkscrew, or spiral ureters) microscopic hematuria/sterile pyuria. Painless unless complicated by ureteral obstruction.

Diagnostic Considerations: Combined upper/lower urinary tract abnormalities ± microscopic hematuria/urinary pH ≤ 5.5. Diagnosis by culture of TB from urine. Urine TB PCR is specific, but not very sensitive.

Pitfalls: Chest x-ray is normal in 50%, but most patients are PPD positive. Rule out other infectious/inflammatory causes of sterile pyuria (e.g., Trichomonas, interstitial nephritis).

Therapeutic Considerations: Treat the same as pulmonary TB.

Prognosis: Good if treated before renal parenchymal destruction/ureteral obstruction occur.

Renal Abscess (Intrarenal/Perinephric)

Subset	Usual Pathogens	Preferred IV Therapy	Alternate IV Therapy	PO Therapy or IV-to-PO Switch
Cortical (Treat initially for MSSA; if later identified as MRSA, treat accordingly)	S. aureus	<u>MSSA:</u> Nafcillin 2 gm (IV) q4h* **or** Ceftriaxone 1 gm (IV) q24h* **or** Clindamycin 600 mg (IV) q8h*	<u>MSSA</u> Meropenem 1 gm (IV) q8h* **or** Ertapenem 1 gm (IV) q24h*	<u>MSSA/MRSA</u> Linezolid 600 mg (PO) q12h* **or** Minocycline 100 mg (PO) q12h*
		<u>MRSA:</u> Linezolid 600 mg (IV) q12h* **or** Minocycline 100 mg (IV) q12h*	<u>MRSA</u> Vancomycin 1 gm (IV) q12h*	
Medullary	Entero-bacteriaceae	Quinolone (IV)†*	TMP–SMX 2.5 mg/kg (IV) q6h*	Quinolone (PO)†*

MSSA/MRSA = methicillin-sensitive/resistant S. aureus. Duration of therapy represents total time IV, PO, or IV + PO. Most patients on IV therapy able to take PO meds should be switched to PO therapy soon after clinical improvement.

*   Treat until renal abscess resolves completely or is no longer decreasing in size on CT/MRI.

†   Levofloxacin 500 mg (IV/PO) q24h.

Clinical Presentation: Similar to pyelonephritis but fever remains elevated after 72 hours of antibiotics.

Diagnostic Considerations: Obtain CT/MRI to diagnose perinephric/intra-renal abscess and rule out mass lesion. Cortical abscesses are usually secondary to hematogenous/contiguous spread. Medullary abscesses are usually due to extension of intrarenal infection.

Pitfalls: Urine cultures may be negative with cortical abscesses.
Therapeutic Considerations: Most large abscesses need to be drained. Multiple small abscesses are managed medically. Obtain urology consult.
Prognosis: Related to degree of baseline renal dysfunction.

Prostatitis/Prostatic Abscess

Subset	Usual Pathogens	Preferred IV Therapy	Alternate IV Therapy	PO Therapy or IV-to-PO Switch
Acute prostatitis/ acute prostatic abscess	Entero-bacteriaceae	Quinolone* (IV) × 2 weeks **or** Ceftriaxone 1 gm (IV) q24h × 2 weeks	TMP–SMX 2.5 mg/kg (IV) q6h × 2 weeks **or** Aztreonam 2 gm (IV) q8h × 2 weeks	Quinolone* (PO) × 2 weeks **or** Doxycycline 200 mg (PO) q12h × 3 days, then 100 mg (PO) q24h × 11 days **or** TMP–SMX 1 SS tablet (PO) q12h × 2 weeks
Chronic prostatitis	Entero-bacteriaceae	IV therapy not applicable	Quinolone* (PO) × 1–3 months **or** Doxycycline 100 mg (PO) q24h × 1–3 months **or** TMP–SMX 1 DS tablet (PO) q12h × 1–3 months	

Duration of therapy represents total time IV, PO, or IV + PO. Most patients on IV therapy able to take PO meds should be switched to PO therapy soon after clinical improvement (usually < 72 hours).
* Ciprofloxacin XR 1000 mg (PO) q24h or Ciprofloxacin 400 mg (IV) q12h or Levofloxacin 500 mg (IV or PO) q24h.

Acute Prostatitis/Acute Prostatic Abscess (Enterobacteriaceae)
Clinical Presentation: Acute prostatitis presents as an acute febrile illness in males with dysuria and no CVA tenderness. Prostatic abscess presents with hectic/septic fevers without localizing signs.
Diagnostic Considerations: Acute prostatitis is diagnosed by bacteriuria plus pyuria with exquisite prostate tenderness, and is seen primarily in young males. Positive urine culture is due to contamination of urine as it passes through infected prostate. Prostatic abscess is diagnosed by transrectal ultrasound or CT/MRI of prostate.

Pitfalls: Do not overlook acute prostatitis in males with bacteriuria without localizing signs, or prostatic abscess in patients with a history of prostatitis.

Therapeutic Considerations: Treat acute prostatitis for 2 full weeks to decrease progression to chronic prostatitis. Prostatic abscess is treated the same as acute prostatitis plus surgical drainage.

Prognosis: Excellent if treated early with full course of antibiotics (plus drainage for prostatic abscess).

Chronic Prostatitis (Enterobacteriaceae)

Clinical Presentation: Vague urinary symptoms (mild dysuria ± low back pain), history of acute prostatitis, and little or no fever.

Diagnostic Considerations: Diagnosis by bacteriuria plus pyuria with "boggy prostate" ± mild tenderness. Urine/prostate expressate is culture positive.

Pitfalls: Commonest cause of treatment failure is inadequate duration of therapy. Chronic prostatitis with prostatic calcifications (rectal ultrasound) will not clear with antibiotics; transurethral resection of prostate (TURP) with removal of *all* calcifications curative.

Therapeutic Considerations: In sulfa-allergic patients, TMP alone may be used in place of TMP–SMX.

Prognosis: Excellent if treated × 1–3 months. Prostatic abscess is a rare but serious complication (may cause urosepsis).

Urosepsis (see Color Atlas for Urine Gram stains)

Subset	Usual Pathogens	Preferred IV Therapy	Alternate IV Therapy	IV-to-PO Switch
Community-acquired (Treat initially based on urine gram stain)	Entero-bacteriaceae	Ceftriaxone 1 gm (IV) q24h × 7 days **or** Levofloxacin 500 mg (IV) q24h × 7 days	Amikacin 1 gm (IV) q24h × 7 days **or** Aztreonam 2 gm (IV) q8h × 7 days	Levofloxacin 500 mg (PO) q24h × 7 days **or** TMP–SMX 1 SS tablet (PO) q12h × 7 days
	E. faecalis (VSE) Group B streptococci	Ampicillin 2 gm (IV) q4h × 7 days	Meropenem 1 gm (IV) q8h × 7 days	Amoxicillin 1 gm (PO) q8h × 7 days **or** Levofloxacin 500 mg (PO) q24h × 7 days
(No urine gram stain)	Entero-bacteriaceae E. faecalis (VSE) Group B streptococci	Piperacillin/tazobactam 3.375 mg (IV) q6h × 7 days **or** Meropenem 1 gm (IV) q8h × 7 days	Doripenem 1 gm (IV) q8h × 7 days	Levofloxacin 500 mg (PO) q24h × 7 days

Duration of therapy represents total time IV or IV + PO. Most patients on IV therapy able to take PO meds should be switched to PO therapy after clinical improvement.

Urosepsis (cont'd) (see Color Atlas of Urine Gram stains)

Subset	Usual Pathogens	Preferred IV Therapy	Alternate IV Therapy	IV-to-PO Switch
Related to urological procedure (Treat intially for P. aeruginosa, etc; if later identified as non-aeruginosa Pseudomonas, treat accordingly)	P. aeruginosa Enterobacter Klebsiella Serratia	Ciprofloxacin 400 mg (IV) q8h × 7 days **or** Levofloxacin 750 mg (IV) q24h × 7 days **or** Cefepime 2 gm (IV) q8h × 7 days **or** Meropenem 1 gm (IV) q8h × 7 days	Piperacillin 4 gm (IV) q8h × 7 days **or** Aztreonam 2 gm (IV) q8h × 7 days **or** Amikacin 1 gm (IV) q24h × 7 days **or** Doripenem 1 gm (IV) q8h × 7 days	Ciprofloxacin 750 mg (PO) q12h × 7 days **or** Levofloxacin 750 mg (PO) q24h × 7 days
	Non-aeruginosa Pseudomonas (B. cepacia, S. maltophilia)	TMP–SMX 2.5 mg/kg (IV) q6h × 7 days **or** Minocycline 100 mg (IV) q12h	Doxycycline 200 mg (IV) q12h × 3 days, then 100 mg (IV) q12h × 7 days	TMP–SMX 1 SS tablet (PO) q12h × 7 days **or** Minocycline 100 mg (PO) q12h × 7 days **or** Doxycycline 100 mg (PO) q12h × 7 days

Duration of therapy represents total time IV or IV + PO. Most patients on IV therapy able to take PO meds should be switched to PO therapy after clinical improvement.

Community-Acquired Urosepsis

Clinical Presentation: Sepsis from urinary tract source.

Diagnostic Considerations: Blood and urine cultures positive for same uropathogen. If patient does not have diabetes, SLE, cirrhosis, myeloma, steroids, pre-existing renal disease or obstruction, obtain CT/MRI of GU tract to rule out abscess/obstruction. Prostatic abscess is rarely a cause of urosepsis.

Pitfalls: Mixed gram-positive/negative urine cultures suggest specimen contamination or enterovesicular fistula.

Therapeutic Considerations: Empiric treatment is based on urine gram stain. If urine gram stain shows pyuria and gram-positive cocci, treat as group D enterococci (E. faecalis-VSE). If gram-negative bacilli, treat as Enterobacteriaceae. S. aureus/S. pneumoniae are not uropathogens.

Prognosis: Related to severity of underlying condition causing urosepsis and health of host.

Urosepsis Following Urological Procedures

Clinical Presentation: Sepsis within 24 hours after GU procedure.

Diagnostic Considerations: Blood and urine cultures positive for same uropathogen. Use pre-procedural urine culture to identify uropathogen and guide therapy.

Pitfalls: If non-aeruginosa Pseudomonas in urine/blood, switch to TMP–SMX pending susceptibilities.

Therapeutic Considerations: Empiric P. aeruginosa monotherapy will cover most other uropathogens.

Prognosis: Related to severity of underlying condition causing urosepsis and health of host.

Pelvic Inflammatory Disease (PID), Salpingitis, Tuboovarian Abscess, Endometritis/Endomyometritis, Septic Abortion

Subset	Usual Pathogens	IV Therapy	PO Therapy or IV-to-PO Switch
Hospitalized patients[†]	B. fragilis Enterobacteriaceae N. gonorrhoeae C. trachomatis C. sordelli[§] (septic abortion)	**Monotherapy with** Moxifloxacin 400 mg (IV) q24h × 2 weeks **or combination therapy with** Doxycycline 200 mg (IV) q12h × 3 days, then 100 mg (IV) q12h × 11 days **plus either** Piperacillin 4 gm (IV) q6h × 2 weeks **or** Ertapenem 1 gm (IV) q24h × 3–10 days **or** Cefoxitin 2 gm (IV) q6h × 2 weeks **or** Cefotetan 2 gm (IV) q12h × 2 weeks **Alternate combination therapy** Doxycycline 200 mg (IV) q12h × 3 days, then 100 mg (IV) q12h × 11 days **plus** Ampicillin/sulbactam 3 gm (IV) q6h × 2 weeks **or** Quinolone[‡] (IV) q24h × 2 weeks **plus** Metronidazole 1 gm (IV) q24h × 2 weeks	**Monotherapy with** Moxifloxacin 400 mg (PO) q24h × 2 weeks
Outpatients (mild PID only)	N. gonorrhoeae C. trachomatis B. fragilis Enterobacteriaceae	Moxifloxacin 400 mg (PO) q24h × 2 weeks** **or** Doxycycline 100 mg (PO) q12h × 2 weeks	

Duration of therapy represents total time IV, PO, or IV + PO. Most patients on IV therapy able to take PO meds should be switched to PO therapy after clinical improvement.

† Treat only IV or IV-to-PO switch for salpingitis, tuboovarian abscess, endometritis, endomyometritis, septic abortion, or severe PID.

‡ Levofloxacin 500 mg (IV or PO) q24h or Ofloxacin 400 mg (IV or PO) q12h.

** Recent gonococcal resistance to quinolones requires careful follow-up during/after therapy.

§ Antibiotic therapy of septic abortion same as salpingitis/endometritis *plus* evacuation of uterine contents.

Clinical Presentation: PID/salpingitis presents with cervical motion/adnexal tenderness, lower quadrant abdominal pain, and fever. Endometritis/endomyometritis presents with uterine tenderness ± cervical discharge/fever. Endomyometritis is the most common post-partum infection.

Diagnostic Considerations: Unilateral lower abdominal pain in a female without a non-pelvic cause suggests PID/salpingitis.

Pitfalls: Obtain CT/MRI of abdomen/pelvis to confirm diagnosis and rule out other pathology or tuboovarian abscess.

Therapeutic Considerations: Tuboovarian abscess usually requires drainage/removal ± TAH/BSO, plus antibiotics (p. 113) × 1–2 weeks after drainage/removal. Septic abortion is treated the same as endometritis/endomyometritis plus uterine evacuation.

Prognosis: Related to promptness of treatment/adequacy of drainage if tuboovarian abscess. Late complications of PID/salpingitis include tubal scarring/infertility.

Empiric Therapy of Sexually Transmitted Diseases

Urethritis/Cervicitis

Subset	Usual Pathogens	IM Therapy	PO Therapy
Gonococcal (GC)	N. gonorrhoeae	Ceftriaxone 250 mg (IM) × 1 dose **plus** Azithromycin 1–2 gm (PO) × 1 dose	Cefixime† 400 mg (PO) × 1 dose† **or** Cefpodoxime† 400 mg (PO) × 1 dose† **or** Azithromycin† 2 gm (PO) × 1 dose†
Non-gonococcal (NGU)	C. trachomatis U. urealyticum M. genitalium	Not applicable	Azithromycin 1 gm (PO) × 1 dose **or** Doxycycline 100 mg (PO) q12h × 7 days **or** Quinolone*† (PO) × 7 days **or** Erythromycin 500 mg (PO) q6h × 7 days
	Trichomonas vaginalis	Not applicable	Tinidazole 2 gm (PO) × 1 dose **or** Metronidazole 2 gm (PO) × 1 dose

*   Levofloxacin 500 mg q24h or Moxifloxacin 400 mg q24h or Ofloxacin 300 mg q12h.
†   Increased resistance oral regimens should be considered alternate (second line) therapy and test of cure essential.

Gonococcal Urethritis/Cervicitis (Neisseria gonorrhoeae)
Clinical Presentation: Purulent penile/cervical discharge with burning/dysuria 3–5 days after contact.
Diagnostic Considerations: Rapid diagnosis in males by Gram stain of urethral discharge showing gram-negative diplococci; urethral cultures also positive. In females, diagnosis requires identification of organism by culture or DNA probe, not Gram stain. Rapid diagnosis in males/females by DNA probe. Obtain throat/rectal culture for N. gonorrhoeae. Co-infections are common; obtain syphilis and HIV serologies.
Pitfalls: Gram stain of cervical discharge showing gram-negative diplococci is not diagnostic of N. gonorrhoeae; must confirm by culture or nucleic acid amplification. N. gonorrhoeae infections are asymptomatic in 10% of men and 70% of women.

Therapeutic Considerations: Failure to respond suggests re-infection or relapse. Treat all GC with ceftriaxone. Because of frequent coinfection with agents of NGU, add oral azithromycin. Because of increasing resistance, consider using azithromycin 2 gm for dual therapy in patients with GC.
Prognosis: Good even with disseminated infection.

Non-Gonococcal Urethritis/Cervicitis (Chlamydia/Ureaplasma/Mycoplasma)

Clinical Presentation: Mucopurulent penile/cervical discharge ± dysuria ~ 1 week after contact.
Diagnostic Considerations: Diagnosis by positive chlamydial NAAT/Ureaplasma or Mycoplasma NAAT of urethral/cervical discharge. Evaluate urethral/cervical discharge to rule out N. gonorrhoeae. Co-infections are common; obtain syphilis and HIV serologies.
Pitfalls: C. trachomatis infections are asymptomatic in 25%.
Therapeutic Considerations: Failure to respond to doxycycline therapy suggests re-infection or Trichomonas/Ureaplasma/Mycoplasma infection. Failure to respond to azithromycin suggests trichomoniasis, or infection due to a resistant Mycoplasma (consider quinolone therapy).
Prognosis: Tubal scarring/infertility in chronic infection.

Trichomonas Urethritis/Cervicitis (Trichomonas vaginalis)

Clinical Presentation: Frothy, pruritic vaginal discharge.
Diagnostic Considerations: Trichomonas by wet mount/culture on special media.
Pitfalls: Classic "strawberry cervix" is infrequently seen.
Therapeutic Considerations: Use week-long regimen if single dose fails. Resistance now recognized as a cause of treatment failure.
Prognosis: Excellent if partner is also treated.

Vaginitis/Vaginosis

Subset	Usual Pathogens	PO Therapy
Bacterial vaginosis/ vaginitis	Polymicrobial (Gardnerella vaginalis, Mobiluncus, Prevotella, M. hominis, etc.)	Tinidazole 1 gm (PO) × 5 days **or** 2 gm (PO) × 2 days **or** Clindamycin 300 mg (PO) q12h × 7 days **or** Metronidazole 500 mg (PO) q12h × 7 days
Candida vaginitis/balanitis	Candida	Fluconazole 150 mg (PO) × 1 dose[†]

† Those failing to respond should be treated with Fluconazole 200 mg (PO) × 1 dose then 100 mg (PO) q24h × 1 week.

Bacterial Vaginosis/Vaginitis

Clinical Presentation: Non-pruritic vaginal discharge with "fishy" odor.
Diagnostic Considerations: Diagnosis by "clue cells" in vaginal fluid wet mount. Vaginal pH ≥ 4.5.
Pitfalls: "Fishy" odor from smear of vaginal secretions intensified when 10% KOH solution is added (positive "whiff test").
Therapeutic Considerations: As an alternative to oral therapy, clindamycin cream 2% intravaginally qHS × 7 days (avoid in pregnancy) or metronidazole gel 0.075% 1 application intravaginally q12h × 5 days can be used.
Prognosis: Complications include premature rupture of membranes, premature delivery, increased risk of PID. Recurrences very common.

Candida Vaginitis/Balanitis

Clinical Presentation: Pruritic white plaques in vagina/erythema of glans penis.

Diagnostic Considerations: Diagnosis by gram stain/culture of whitish plaques.

Pitfalls: Rule out Trichomonas, which also presents with pruritus in females.

Therapeutic Considerations: Uncomplicated vaginitis (mild sporadic infections in healthy individuals) responds readily to single-dose therapy. Complicated vaginitis (severe, recurrent, or in difficult-to-control diabetes) often requires ≥ 7 days of therapy (daily topical therapy or 2 doses of fluconazole 150 mg given 72h apart). Non-albicans infections respond poorly to azoles. Topical boric acid (600 mg/d in a gelatin capsule × 14 days) is often effective in this setting.

Prognosis: Good with systemic therapy. Diabetics/uncircumcised males may need prolonged therapy.

Genital Vesicles (Genital Herpes) (HSV-2/HSV-1)

Subset	PO Therapy
Initial therapy	Acyclovir 200 mg (PO) 5×/day × 10 days **or** Famciclovir 500 mg (PO) q12h × 7–10 days **or** Valacyclovir 1 gm (PO) q12h × 3 days
Recurrent/ intermittent therapy (< 6 episodes/year)	Acyclovir 200 mg (PO) 5×/day × 5 days **or** Valacyclovir (<u>normal host</u>: 500 mg [PO] q24h × 5 days; <u>HIV positive</u>: 1 gm [PO] q12h × 7–10 days)** **or** Famciclovir (<u>normal host</u>: 125 mg [PO] q12h × 5 days **or** 1 gm [PO] q12h × 1 day*; <u>HIV-positive</u>: 500 mg [PO] q12h × 7 days)
Chronic suppressive therapy (> 6 episodes/year)	Acyclovir 400 mg (PO) q12h × 1 year **or** Valacyclovir (<u>normal host</u>: 1 gm [PO] q24h × 1 year; <u>HIV-positive</u>: 500 mg [PO] q12h × 1 year) **or** Famciclovir 250 mg (PO) q12h × 1 year

*   Patient initiated therapy to be started immediately when recurrence begins.

**   Short-course therapy with Valaciclovir 500 mg (PO) q12h × 3 days or Acyclovir 800 mg (PO) q8h × 2 days also effective.

Clinical Presentation: Painful vesicles/ulcers on genitals with painful bilateral regional adenopathy ± low-grade fever.

Diagnostic Considerations: Diagnosis by clinical presentation may be misleading.

Pitfalls: 70% of newly acquired gential herpes is due to HSV-1. Elevated IgG HSV-2 titer indicates past exposure, not acute infection. HSV-2 IgM titers may be negative.

Therapeutic Considerations: If concomitant rectal herpes, increase acyclovir to 800 mg (PO) q8h × 7 days. For recurrent genital herpes, use acyclovir or valacyclovir (dose same as primary infection) for 7 days after each relapse. Recurrent episodes of HSV-2 are less painful than primary infection, and inguinal adenopathy is less prominent/painful.

Prognosis: HSV-2 tends to recur, especially during the first year. HSV-1 recurrences less frequent.

Genital Ulcers

Subset	Usual Pathogens	IM Therapy	PO Therapy
Primary syphilis	Treponema pallidum	Benzathine penicillin 2.4 mu (IM) × 1 dose	Doxycycline 100 mg (PO) q12h × 2 weeks **or** Azithromycin 2 gm (PO) × 1 dose**
Chancroid	Hemophilus ducreyi	Ceftriaxone 250 mg (IM) × 1 dose **or** Any 3rd generation cephalosporin 250–500 mg (IM) × 1 dose	Azithromycin 1 gm (PO) × 1 dose **or** Quinolone* (PO) × 3 days **or** Erythromycin base 500 mg (PO) q8h × 7 days

* Ciprofloxacin 500 mg q12h or Levofloxacin 500 mg or Moxifloxacin 400 mg q24h.

** Resistance increasing (careful followup essential).

Primary Syphilis (Treponema pallidum)
Clinical Presentation: Painless, indurated ulcers (chancres) with bilateral painless inguinal adenopathy. Syphilitic chancres are elevated, clean and indurated, but not undermined.
Diagnostic Considerations: Diagnosis by spirochetes on darkfield examination of ulcer exudate. Elevated non-treponemal (VDRL/RPR) titers after 1 week.
Pitfalls: Non-treponemal (VDRL/RPR) titers fall slowly within 1 year; failure to decline suggests treatment failure/HIV. Even after effective treatment some patients remain VDRL/RPR positive for life (serofast).
Therapeutic Considerations: Parenteral penicillin is the preferred antibiotic for all stages of syphilis. If treatment fails and VDRL/RPR titers do not decline, obtain HIV serology.
Prognosis: Good with early treatment.

Chancroid (Hemophilus ducreyi)
Clinical Presentation: Ragged, undermined, painful ulcer(s) + painful unilateral inguinal adenopathy.
Diagnostic Considerations: Diagnosis by streptobacilli in "school of fish" configuration on gram-stained smear of ulcer exudate/culture of H. ducreyi/NAAT.
Pitfalls: Co-infection is common; obtain Syphilis and HIV serologies.
Therapeutic Considerations: In HIV, multiple dose regimens or azithromycin is preferred. Resistance to erythromycin/ciprofloxacin has been reported.
Prognosis: Good with early treatment.

Suppurating Inguinal Adenopathy

Subset	Pathogens	IV Therapy	PO Therapy
Lympho-granuloma venereum (LGV)	Chlamydia trachomatis (L$_{1-3}$ serotypes)	Not applicable	Doxycycline 100 mg (PO) q12h × 3 wks **or** Erythromycin base 500 mg (PO) q6h × 3 weeks
Granuloma inguinale (Donovanosis)	Klebsiella (Calymmato-bacterium) granulomatis	Not applicable	Azithromycin 1 gm (PO) q week until cured. Doxycycline 100 mg (PO) q12h until cured **or** Erythromycin 500 mg (PO) q6h until cured **or** TMP–SMX 1 DS (PO) q12h until cured **or** Ciprofloxacin 750 mg (PO) q12h until cured

Lymphogranuloma Venereum (Chlamydia trachomatis) LGV
Clinical Presentation: Unilateral inguinal adenopathy ± discharge/sinus tract.
Diagnostic Consideration: Diagnosis by very high Chlamydia trachomatis L$_{1-3}$ titers. Do not biopsy site (often does not heal and may form a fistula). May present as FUO.
Pitfalls: Initial papule not visible at clinical presentation. Biopsy shows granulomas; may be confused with perianal Crohn's disease.
Therapeutic Considerations: Rectal LGV may require additional courses of treatment.
Prognosis: Fibrotic perirectal/pelvic damage does not reverse with therapy.

Granuloma Inguinale (Klebsiella [Calymmatobacterium] granulomatis) Donovanosis
Clinical Presentation: Pseudolymphadenopathy with painless inguinal ulcers.
Diagnostic Considerations: Donovan bodies ("puffed-wheat" appearance) in tissue biopsy.
Pitfalls: No true inguinal adenopathy, as opposed to LGV infection.
Therapeutic Considerations: Doxycycline or azithromycin preferred. Continue therapy until lesions are healed.
Prognosis: Good if treated early.

Genital/Perianal Warts (Condylomata acuminata)

Subset	Pathogens	Therapy
Genital/perianal warts	Human papilloma virus (HPV)	Podophyllin 10–25% in tincture of benzoin or podofilox or imiquimod (patient applies) **or** surgical/laser removal/cryotherapy with liquid nitrogen **or** cidofovir gel (1%) QHS × 5 days every other week for 6 cycles **or** trichloracetic acid (TCA)/bichloracetic acid (BCA) **or** intralesional interferon. Sinecatechins (15% ointment) q8h × 4 months

Clinical Presentation: Single/multiple verrucous genital lesions ± pigmentation, without inguinal adenopathy.

Diagnostic Considerations: Diagnosis by clinical appearance. Genital warts are usually caused by HPV types 6, 11. Anogenital warts caused by HPV types 16,18,31,33,35 and others are associated with cervical neoplasia. Females with anogenital warts need serial cervical PAP smears to detect cervical dysplasia/neoplasia.

Pitfalls: Most HPV infections are asymptomatic.

Therapeutic Considerations: Cidofovir cures/halts HPV progression in 50% of cases.

Prognosis: Related to HPV serotypes with malignant potential (HPV types 16,18,31,33,35). Preventative (not therapeutic) vaccines now available.

Syphilis

Subset	Pathogen	IV/IM Therapy	PO Therapy
Primary, secondary, or early latent (duration < 1 year) syphilis	Treponema pallidum	Benzathine penicillin 2.4 mu (IM) × 1 dose	Doxycycline 100 mg (PO) q12h × 2 weeks **or** Azithromycin 2 gm (PO) × 1 dose*
Late latent (duration > 1 year) or tertiary syphilis	Treponema pallidum	Benzathine penicillin 2.4 mu (IM) weekly × 3 weeks	Doxycycline 100 mg (PO) q12h × 4 weeks
Neurosyphilis	Treponema pallidum	Penicillin G 3–4 mu (IV) q4h or continuous infusion × 10–14 days **or** <u>Alternate:</u> Procaine penicillin 2.4 mu (IM) q24h × 10–14 days plus probenecid 500 mg (PO) q6h × 10–14 days **or** Ceftriaxone 2 gm (IV) q24h × 10–14 days	Doxycycline 100 mg (PO) q12h × 4 weeks **or** Minocycline 100 mg (PO) q12h × 4 weeks

*   Resistance increasing (careful follow up essential).

Duration of therapy represents total time IV, IM, or PO. All stages of syphilis in HIV patients usually respond to therapeutic regimens recommended for normal hosts. Syphilis in pregnancy should be treated according to the stage of syphilis; penicillin-allergic pregnant patients should be desensitized and treated with penicillin.

Primary Syphilis (Treponema pallidum)

Clinical Presentation: Painless, indurated ulcer(s) (chancre) with bilateral painless inguinal adenopathy.

Diagnostic Considerations: Diagnosis by spirochetes on darkfield or DFA examination of ulcer exudate. Reactive non-treponemal (VDRL/RPR) or treponemal (TPPA, others) test after 1 week. Patients with ↑ low titers of VDRL/RPR and – treponemal test may be BFP, e.g., SLE.

Pitfalls: VDRL/RPR titers fall slowly within 1 year; failure to decline suggests treatment failure.

Therapeutic Considerations: Parenteral penicillin is the preferred antibiotic for all stages of syphilis; if treatment fails and VDRL/RPR titers do not decline, obtain HIV serology. Some effectively treated patients remain VDRL/RPR positive in low titers eg 1:4 (serofast) for years.

Prognosis: Good with early treatment.

Secondary Syphilis (Treponema pallidum)

Clinical Presentation: Facial/truncal macular, papular, papulosquamous, non-pruritic, non-tender, symmetrical rash which may involve the palms/soles. Usually accompanied by generalized adenopathy. Typically appears 4–10 weeks after primary chancre, although stages may overlap. Alopecia, condyloma lata, mucous patches, iritis/uveitis may be present. Renal involvement ranges from mild proteinuria to nephrotic syndrome. Without treatment, spontaneous resolution occurs after 3–12 weeks.

Diagnostic Considerations: Diagnosis by clinical findings and VDRL/RPR in high titers (≥ 1:64). After treatment, RPR/VDRL titers usually ↓ × 4 < 6 months.

Pitfalls: If only undiluted serum is tested, prozone phenomenon may render VDRL/RPR falsely negative.

Therapeutic Considerations: Parenteral penicillin is the preferred antibiotic for all stages of syphilis.

Prognosis: Excellent with early treatment.

Latent Syphilis (Treponema pallidum)

Clinical Presentation: Patients are asymptomatic with elevated non-treponemal titers and reactive treponemal tests.

Diagnostic Considerations: Diagnosis by positive serology ± prior history, but no signs/symptoms of syphilis. Asymptomatic syphilis < 1 year in duration is termed "early" latent syphilis; asymptomatic syphilis > 1 year/unknown duration is termed "late" latent syphilis. Secondary syphilis may relapse in up to 25% of patients with early latent syphilis, but relapse is rare in late latent syphilis. Evaluate patients for neurosyphilis.

Pitfalls: Treponemal tests (FTA-ABS, MHA-TP, TPPA, others) usually remain positive for life, even after adequate treatment.

Therapeutic Considerations: Parenteral penicillin is the preferred antibiotic for all stages of syphilis. Repeat VDRL/RPR titers at 6, 12, and 24 months; therapeutic response is defined as a 4-fold reduction in RPR/VDRL titers (2 tube dilutions).

Prognosis: Excellent even if treated late.

Tertiary Syphilis (Treponema pallidum)

Clinical Presentation: May present with aortitis, neurosyphilis, iritis, or gummata 5–30 years after initial infection.

Diagnostic Considerations: Diagnosis by history of syphilis plus positive serological tests with signs/symptoms of late syphilis.

Pitfalls: Treat for signs of neurosyphilis on clinical exam or LP, even if VDRL/RPR are non-reactive.

Therapeutic Considerations: Parenteral penicillin is the preferred antibiotic for all stages of syphilis.

Prognosis: Related to extent of end-organ damage.

Neurosyphilis (Treponema pallidum)

Clinical Presentation: Patients are often asymptomatic, but may have ophthalmic/auditory symptoms, cranial nerve abnormalities, tabes dorsalis, paresis, psychosis, or signs of meningitis/dementia.

Diagnostic Considerations: Diagnosis by elevated CSF VDRL titers; no need to obtain CSF FTA-ABS titers. Diagnosis confirmed if CSF has pleocytosis (> 5 WBCs/hpf) or increased protein (> 50 mg/dL), and positive VDRL.

Pitfalls: Persistent CSF abnormalities suggest treatment failure. CSF VDRL (60% sensitive) may be negative in neurosyphilis.

Therapeutic Considerations: Parenteral penicillin is the preferred antibiotic for all stages of syphilis. CSF abnormalities should decrease in 6 months and return to normal after 2 years; repeat lumbar puncture 6 months after treatment. Failure rate with ceftriaxone is 20%.

Prognosis: Related to extent of end-organ damage.

Empiric Therapy of Bone and Joint Infections

Septic Arthritis/Bursitis

Subset	Usual Pathogens	Preferred IV Therapy	Alternate IV Therapy	PO Therapy or IV-to-PO Switch
Acute (Treat initially based on gram stain of synovial fluid. If gram-positive cocci in clusters, treat initially for MRSA; if later identified as MSSA, treat accordingly)	S. aureus (MSSA)	Ceftriaxone 1 gm (IV) q24h × 3 weeks **or** Cefazolin 1 gm (IV) q8h × 3 weeks **or** Clindamycin 600 mg (IV) q8h × 3 weeks	Nafcillin 2 gm (IV) q4h × 3 weeks **or** Meropenem 1 gm (IV) q8h × 3 weeks **or** Ertapenem 1 gm (IV) q24h × 3 weeks	Cephalexin 1 gm (PO) q6h × 3 weeks **or** Clindamycin 300 mg (PO) q8h× 3 weeks **or** Quinolone* (PO) q24h × 3 weeks
	S. aureus (MRSA)	Linezolid 600 mg (IV) q12h × 3 weeks **or** Quinupristin/dalfopristin 7.5 mg/kg (IV) q8h × 3 weeks **or** Minocycline 100 mg (IV) q12h × 3 weeks		Linezolid 600 mg (PO) q12h × 3 weeks **or** Minocycline 100 mg (PO) q12h × 3 weeks
	Group A,B,C,G streptococci	Ceftriaxone 1 gm (IV) q24h × 3 weeks **or** Clindamycin 600 mg (IV) q8h × 3 weeks	Cefazolin 1 gm (IV) q8h × 3 weeks **or** Quinolone* (IV) q24h × 3 weeks	Clindamycin 300 mg (PO) q8h × 3 weeks **or** Cephalexin 500 mg (PO) q6h × 3 weeks **or** Quinolone* (PO) q24h × 3 weeks

*   Moxifloxacin 400 mg or Levofloxacin 500 mg.

Septic Arthritis/Bursitis (cont'd)

Subset	Usual Pathogens	Preferred IV Therapy	Alternate IV Therapy	PO Therapy or IV-to-PO Switch
Acute (cont'd)	Entero-bacteriaceae	Ceftriaxone 1 gm (IV) q24h × 3 weeks **or** Cefepime 2 gm (IV) q12h × 3 weeks **or** Cefotaxime 2 gm (IV) q6h × 3 weeks **or** Ceftizoxime 2 gm (IV) q8h × 3 weeks	Aztreonam 2 gm (IV) q8h × 3 weeks **or** Quinolone‡ (IV) × 3 weeks	Quinolone‡ (PO) × 3 weeks
	P. aeruginosa	Meropenem 1 gm (IV) q8h × 3 weeks **or** Ciprofloxacin 400 mg (IV) q8h × 3 weeks	Aztreonam 2 gm (IV) q8h × 3 weeks **or** Cefepime 2 gm (IV) q8h × 3 weeks	Ciprofloxacin 750 mg (PO) q12h × 3 weeks **or** Levofloxacin 750 mg (PO) q24h x 3 weeks
	N. gonorrhoeae (PSNG/PPNG)	Ceftriaxone 1 gm (IV) q24h × 2 weeks **or** Ceftizoxime 2 gm (IV) q8h × 2 weeks	Levofloxacin 500 mg (IV) q24h × 2 weeks **or** Moxifloxacin 400 mg (IV) q24h × 2 weeks	Levofloxacin 500 mg (PO) q24h × 2 weeks **or** Moxifloxacin 400 mg (PO) q24h × 2 weeks
	Salmonella	Ceftriaxone 2 gm (IV) q24h × 2–3 weeks **or** Quinolone* (IV) × 2–3 weeks	Aztreonam 2 gm (IV) q8h × 2–3 weeks **or** TMP–SMX 2.5 mg/kg (IV) q6h × 2–3 weeks	Quinolone* (PO) × 2–3 weeks **or** TMP–SMX 1 DS tablet (PO) q12h × 2–3 weeks

‡   Moxifloxacin 400 mg (IV/PO) q24h or Levofloxacin 500 mg (IV/PO) q24h.

†   Loading dose is not needed PO if given IV with the same drug.

*   Ciprofloxacin 400 mg (IV) or 500 mg (PO) q12h or Levofloxacin 500 mg (IV or PO) q24h or Moxifloxacin 400 mg (IV or PO) q24h.

Septic Arthritis/Bursitis (cont'd)

Subset	Usual Pathogens	Preferred IV Therapy	Alternate IV Therapy	PO Therapy or IV-to-PO Switch
Secondary to animal bite wound	Pasteurella multocida Streptobacillus moniliformis Eikinella corrodens	Piperacillin/ tazobactam 3.375 gm (IV) q6h × 2 weeks **or** Ampicillin/ sulbactam 3 gm (IV) q6h × 2 weeks **or** Ticarcillin/ clavulanate 3.1 gm (IV) q6h × 2 weeks	Meropenem 1 gm (IV) q8h × 2 weeks **or** Ertapenem 1 gm (IV) q24h × 2 weeks **or** Doxycycline 200 mg (IV) q12h × 3 days, then 100 mg (IV) q12h × 11 days	Amoxicillin/ clavulanic acid 875/125 mg (PO) q12h × 2 weeks **or** Doxycycline 200 mg (PO) q12h × 3 days, then 100 mg (PO) q12h × 11 days[†] **or** Moxifloxacin 400 mg (PO) q24h × 2 weeks
Fungal arthritis	Coccidioides immitis	Not applicable	Itraconazole 200 mg (PO) solution q12h × 12 months or until cured* **or** Fluconazole 800 mg (PO) q24h until cured*	
	Sporothrix schenckii	Not applicable	Itraconazole 200 mg (PO) q12h until cured*	
TB arthritis	M. tuberculosis	Not applicable	Treat the same as for pulmonary TB (p. 53) except treat for 6–9 months	

MSSA/MRSA = methicillin-sensitive/resistant S. aureus. Duration of therapy represents total time IV, PO, or IV + PO. Most patients on IV therapy able to take PO meds should be switched to PO therapy after clinical improvement.

*   Itraconazole solution provides more reliable absorption than capsules.

Acute Septic Arthritis/Bursitis

Clinical Presentation: Acute joint pain with fever. Septic joint unable to bear weight. Septic bursitis presents with pain on joint motion, but patient is able to bear weight.

Diagnostic Considerations: Diagnosis by demonstrating organisms in synovial fluid by stain/culture. In septic bursitis (knee most common), there is pain on joint flexion (although the joint can bear weight), and synovial fluid findings are negative for septic arthritis. Except for N. gonorrhoeae, polyarthritis is not usually due to bacterial pathogens. Post-infectious polyarthritis is usually viral in origin, most commonly due to parvovirus B19, rubella, or HBV.

Pitfalls: Reactive arthritis may follow C. jejuni, Salmonella, Shigella, Yersinia, N. gonorrheae C. trachomatis, or C. difficile infections. Synovial fluid cultures are negative. Reactive arthritis is usually asymmetrical and is monoarticular/oligoarticular.

Therapeutic Considerations: See specific pathogen, below. Treat septic bursitis as septic arthritis.

Staphylococcus aureus (MSSA/MRSA)

Diagnostic Considerations: Painful hot joint; unable to bear weight. Diagnosis by synovial fluid pleocytosis and positive culture for joint pathogen. Examine synovial fluid to rule out gout (doubly birefringent crystals) and pseudogout (calcium pyrophosphate crystals). May occur in setting of endocarditis with septic emboli to joints; other manifestations of endocarditis are usually evident.

Pitfalls: Rule out causes of noninfectious arthritis (sarcoidosis, Whipple's disease, Ehlers-Danlos, etc.), which are less severe, but may mimic septic arthritis. In reactive arthritis following urethritis (C. trachomatis, Ureaplasma urealyticum, N. gonorrhoeae) or diarrhea (Shigella, Campylobacter, Yersinia, Salmonella), synovial fluid culture is negative, and synovial fluid WBCs counts are usually < 10,000/mm³ with normal synovial fluid lactic acid and glucose. Do not overlook infective endocarditis in mono/polyarticular MSSA/MRSA septic arthritis without apparent source.

Therapeutic Considerations: For MRSA septic arthritis, vancomycin penetration into synovial fluid is poor; use linezolid instead. Immobilization of infected joint during therapy is helpful. Local installation of antibiotics into synovial fluid has no advantage over IV/PO antibiotics.

Prognosis: Treat as early as possible to minimize joint damage. Repeated aspiration/open drainage may be needed to preserve joint function.

Group A, B, C, G Streptococci

Diagnostic Considerations: Usually monoarticular. Not usually due to septic emboli from endocarditis.

Prognosis: Related to extent of joint damage and rapidity of antibiotic treatment.

Enterobacteriaceae

Diagnostic Considerations: Diagnosis by isolation of gram-negative bacilli from synovial fluid.

Pitfalls: Septic arthritis involving an unusual joint (e.g., sternoclavicular, sacral) should suggest IV drug abuse until proven otherwise.

Therapeutic Considerations: Joint aspiration is essential in suspected septic arthritis of the hip and may be needed for other joints; obtain orthopedic surgery consult. Local installation of antibiotics into joint fluid is of no proven value.

Prognosis: Related to extent of joint damage and rapidity of antibiotic treatment.

Pseudomonas aeruginosa

Diagnostic Considerations P. aeruginosa septic arthritis/osteomyelitis may occur after water contaminated puncture wound (e.g., nail puncture of heel through shoes). Sternoclavicular/sacroiliac joint involvement is common in IV drug abusers (IVDAs).

Pitfalls: Suspect IVDA in P. aeruginosa septic arthritis without a history of trauma.

Therapeutic Considerations: If ciprofloxacin is used, treat with 750 mg (not 500 mg) dose for P. aeruginosa septic arthritis/osteomyelitis.

Prognosis: Related to extent of joint damage and rapidity of antibiotic treatment.

Neisseria gonorrhoeae

Diagnostic Considerations: Gonococcal arthritis may present as a monoarticular arthritis, or multiple joints may be affected as part of gonococcal arthritis-dermatitis syndrome (disseminated gonococcal infection). Bacteremia with positive blood cultures occurs early during rash stage while synovial fluid cultures are negative. Joint involvement follows with typical findings of septic arthritis and synovial fluid cultures positive for N. gonorrhoeae; blood cultures are negative at this stage. Acute tenosynovitis is often a clue to gonococcal septic arthritis.

Pitfalls: Spectinomycin is ineffective against pharyngeal gonorrhea.

Therapeutic Considerations: Gonococcal arthritis-dermatitis syndrome is caused by very susceptible strains of N. gonorrhoeae. Cephalosporins also eliminate incubating syphilis.

Prognosis: Excellent with arthritis-dermatitis syndrome; worse with only monoarticular arthritis.

Salmonella sp.

Diagnostic Considerations: Occurs in sickle cell disease and hemoglobinopathies. Diagnosis by blood/joint cultures.

Pitfalls: S. aureus, not Salmonella, is the most common cause of septic arthritis in sickle cell disease.

Prognosis: Related to severity of infection and underlying health of host.

Septic Arthritis Secondary to Animal Bite Wound

Clinical Presentation: Penetrating bite wound into joint space.

Diagnostic Considerations: Diagnosis by smear/culture of synovial fluid/blood cultures.

Pitfalls: May develop metastatic infection from bacteremia.

Therapeutic Considerations: Treat for at least 2 weeks of combined IV/PO therapy.

Prognosis: Related to severity of infection and underlying health of host.

Chronic Septic Arthritis

Clinical Presentation: Subacute/chronic joint pain with decreased range of motion and little or no fever. Able to bear weight on joint.

Diagnostic Considerations: Diagnosis by smear/culture of synovial fluid/synovial biopsy.

Coccidioides immitis

Diagnostic Considerations: Must grow organisms from synovium/synovial fluid for diagnosis.

Pitfalls: Synovial fluid the same as in TB (lymphocytic pleocytosis, low glucose, increased protein).

Therapeutic Considerations: Oral therapy is preferred; same cure rates as amphotericin regimens. HIV patients need life-long suppressive therapy.

Prognosis: Related to severity of infection and underlying health of host.

Sporothrix schenckii

Diagnostic Considerations: Usually a monoarticular infection secondary to direct inoculation/trauma.

Pitfalls: Polyarticular arthritis suggests disseminated infection.

Therapeutic Considerations: SSKI is useful for lymphocutaneous sporotrichosis, not bone/joint involvement.

Prognosis: Excellent for localized disease (e.g., lymphocutaneous sporotrichosis). In disseminated disease, prognosis is related to host factors.

Mycobacterium tuberculosis (TB)

Diagnostic Considerations: Clue is subacute/chronic tenosynovitis over involved joint. Unlike other forms of septic arthritis, which are usually due to hematogenous spread, TB arthritis may complicate adjacent TB osteomyelitis. Synovial fluid findings include lymphocytic pleocytosis, low glucose, and increased protein.

Pitfalls: Send synovial biopsy for AFB smear/culture in unexplained chronic monoarticular arthritis.

Therapeutic Considerations: TB arthritis is usually treated for 6–9 months.

Prognosis: Related to severity of infection and underlying health of host.

Lyme Disease*/Lyme Arthritis

Subset	Usual Pathogens	Preferred IV Therapy	Alternate IV Therapy	PO Therapy or IV-to-PO Switch
Lyme disease	Borrelia burgdorferi	Ceftriaxone 1 gm (IV) q24h × 2 weeks	Ceftizoxime 2 gm (IV) q8h × 2 weeks	Amoxicillin 1 gm (PO) q8h × 2 weeks **or** Doxycycline 200 mg (PO) q12h × 3 days, then 100 mg (PO) q12h × 11 days†
Lyme arthritis		Ceftriaxone 1 gm (IV) q24h × 4 weeks	Ceftizoxime 2 gm (IV) q8h × 4 weeks	Amoxicillin 1 gm (PO) q8h × 4 weeks **or** Doxycycline 200 mg (PO) q12h × 3 days, then 100 mg (PO) q12h × 4 weeks

Duration of therapy represents total time IV, PO, or IV + PO. Most patients on IV therapy able to take PO meds should be switched to PO therapy after clinical improvement.

*   See p. 21 for Lyme neuroborreliosis and p. 78 for Lyme myocarditis.

†   Doxycycline therapy × 10 days as effective as 2 weeks.

‡   For adult patients intolerant of Amoxicillin, Doxycycline, and Cefuroxime axetil, Azithromycin (500 mg orally per day for 7–10 days), Clarithromycin (500 mg orally twice per day for 14–21 days, if the patient is not pregnant), or Erythromycin (500 mg orally 4 times per day for 14–21 days) may be given. The recommended dosages of these agents for children are as follows: Azithromycin, 10 mg/kg per day (maximum of 500 mg per day); Clarithromycin, 7.5 mg/kg twice per day (maximum of 500 mg per dose); and Erythromycin, 12.5 mg/kg 4 times per day (maximum of 500 mg per dose).

Lyme Disease

Clinical Presentation: Can manifest acutely or chronically with local or disseminated disease following bite of tick infected with Borrelia spirochete. Erythema migrans (expanding, erythematous, annular lesion with central clearing) occurs in ~ 75% within 2 weeks of tick bite and may be associated with fever, headache, arthralgias/myalgias, meningismus. Other possible acute manifestations include meningitis, encephalitis, Bell's palsy, peripheral neuropathy, mild hepatitis, myocarditis with heart block, or arthritis. Chronic disease may present with arthritis, peripheral neuropathy, meningoencephalitis, or acrodermatitis chronica atrophicans (usually > 10 years after infection).

Diagnostic Considerations: Diagnosis by clinical presentation plus elevated IgM Lyme titers (IFA/ELISA). If Lyme titer is borderline or suspected to be a false-positive, obtain an IgM Western blot to confirm the diagnosis. IgM titers may take 4–6 weeks to increase after tick bite. Ixodes ticks are the principal vector; small rodents are the primary reservoir. In the United States, most cases occur in the coastal Northeast, upper Midwest, California, and western Nevada.

Pitfalls: Rash is not always seen, and tick bite is often painless and goes unnoticed (tick often spontaneously falls off after 1–2 days of feeding). Do not overlook Lyme disease in patients with unexplained heart block in areas where Ixodes ticks are endemic. Highest failure rater with macrolide therapy.

Therapeutic Considerations: B. burgdorferi is highly susceptible to all beta-lactams. For Bell's palsy or neuroborreliosis, minocycline (100 mg PO q12h × 2 weeks) may be preferred to doxycycline. Symptoms may persist for 1 year or more after adequate therapy. No rationale to re-treat persistent symptoms.

Prognosis: Excellent in normal hosts.

Lyme Arthritis

Clinical Presentation: Acute Lyme arthritis presents with joint pain, decreased range of motion, ability to bear weight on joint, and little or no fever. Chronic Lyme arthritis resembles rheumatoid arthritis.

Diagnostic Considerations: Usually affects children and large weight-bearing joints (e.g., knee). Acute Lyme arthritis is diagnosed by clinical presentation plus elevated IgM Lyme titer. Chronic Lyme arthritis is suggested by rheumatoid arthritis-like presentation with negative ANA and rheumatoid factor, and positive IgG Lyme titer and synovial fluid PCR.

Pitfalls: Acute Lyme arthritis joint is red but not hot, in contrast to septic arthritis. In chronic Lyme arthritis, a negative IgG Lyme titer essentially rules out chronic Lyme arthritis, but an elevated IgG Lyme titer indicates only past exposure to B. burgdorferi and is not diagnostic of Lyme arthritis. Joint fluid in chronic Lyme disease is usually negative by culture, but positive by PCR; synovial fluid PCR, however, does not differentiate active from prior infection.

Therapeutic Considerations: IgG Lyme titers remain elevated for life, and do not decrease with treatment. Joint symptoms often persist for months/years after effective antibiotic therapy due to autoimmune joint inflammation; treat with anti-inflammatory drugs, not repeat antibiotic courses. Oral therapy as effective as IV therapy.

Prognosis: Good in normal hosts. Chronic/refractory arthritis may develop in genetically predisposed patients with DRW 2/4 HLA types.

Infected Joint Prosthesis

Subset	Usual Pathogens	Preferred IV Therapy	Alternate IV Therapy	IV-to-PO Switch
Staphylococcal (Treat initially for MSSA; if later identified as MRSA/CoNS, treat accordingly)	S. epidermidis (CoNS)	Linezolid 600 mg (IV) q12h* **or** Vancomycin 1 gm (IV) q12h*	Cefotaxime 2 gm (IV) q6h*† **or** Ceftizoxime 2 gm (IV) q8h*†	Linezolid 600 mg (PO) q12h*
	S. aureus (MSSA)	Nafcillin 2 gm (IV) q4h* **or** Cefazolin 1 gm (IV) q8h* **or** Ceftriaxone 1 gm (IV) q24h*†	Meropenem 1 gm (IV) q8h* **or** Clindamycin 600 mg (IV) q8h*	Clindamycin 300 mg (PO) q8h* **or** Linezolid 600 mg (PO) q12h* **or** Cephalexin 1 gm (PO) q6h*
	S. aureus (MRSA)	Linezolid 600 mg (IV) q12h* **or** Vancomycin 1 gm (IV) q12h* **or** Minocycline 100 mg (IV) q12h* **or** Quinupristin/dalfopristin 7.5 mg/kg (IV) q8h*		Linezolid 600 mg (PO) q12h* **or** Minocycline 100 mg (PO) q12h*

MRSA/MSSA = methicillin-resistant/sensitive S. aureus; MSSE/MRSE = methicillin-sensitive/resistant S. epidermidis. Duration of therapy represents total time IV or IV + PO. Most patients on IV therapy able to take PO meds should be switched to PO therapy after clinical improvement.
*   Treat for 1 week after joint prosthesis is replaced.
†   Only if MSSE strain susceptible.

Clinical Presentation: Pain in area of prosthesis with joint loosening/instability ± low-grade fevers.

Diagnostic Considerations: Infected prosthesis is suggested by prosthetic loosening/lucent areas adjacent to prosthesis on plain films ± positive blood cultures. Diagnosis confirmed by bone scan. Use joint aspiration to identify organism.

Pitfalls: An elevated ESR with prosthetic loosening suggests prosthetic joint infection. Mechanical loosening without infection is comon many years after joint replacement, but ESR is normal.

Therapeutic Considerations: Infected prosthetic joints usually must be removed for cure. Replacement prosthesis may be inserted anytime after infected prosthesis is removed. To prevent infection of new joint prosthesis, extensive debridement of old infected material is important. *If replacement* *of infected joint prosthesis is not possible,* **chronic suppressive therapy** may be used with oral antibiotics e.g., minocycline 100 mg (PO) q12h. TMP–SMX 5 mg/kg (PO) q6h may be successful in long-term suppression/cure in total hip replacement (treat × 6 months) or total knee replacement (treat × 9 months) due to susceptible strains of MSSA/MSSE; adding rifampin 300 mg (PO) q12h may be helpful.

Prognosis: Related to adequate debridement of infected material when prosthetic joint is removed.

Osteomyelitis

Subset	Usual Pathogens	Preferred IV Therapy	Alternate IV Therapy	PO Therapy or IV-to-PO Switch
Acute (Treat initially for MSSA; if later identified as MRSA or Enterobacteriaceae, treat accordingly)	S. aureus (MSSA)	Cefazolin 1 gm (IV) q8h × 4–6 weeks **or** Ceftriaxone 1 gm (IV) q24h × 4–6 weeks **or** Meropenem 1 gm (IV) q8h × 4–6 weeks	Cefotaxime 2 gm (IV) q6h × 4–6 weeks **or** Ceftizoxime 2 gm (IV) q8h × 4–6 weeks	Clindamycin 300 mg (PO) q8h × 4–6 weeks **or** Cephalexin 1 gm (PO) q6h × 4–6 weeks **or** Respiratory quinolone‡ (PO) q24h × 4–6 weeks
	S. aureus (MRSA)	Linezolid 600 mg (IV) q12h × 4–6 weeks **or** Minocycline 100 mg (IV) q12h × 4–6 weeks **or** Vancomycin 2 gm (IV) q12h × 4–6 weeks **or** Quinupristin/dalfopristin 7.5 mg/kg (IV) q8h × 4–6 weeks		Linezolid 600 mg (PO) q12h × 4–6 weeks **or** Minocycline 100 mg (PO) q12h × 4–6 weeks
	Enterobacteriaceae	Ceftriaxone 1 gm (IV) q24h × 4–6 wks **or** Quinolone† (IV) × 4–6 weeks **or** Tigacycline 100 mg (IV) × 1 dose, then 50 mg (IV) q12h × 4–6 weeks	Cefotaxime 2 gm (IV) q6h × 4–6 wks **or** Ceftizoxime 2 gm (IV) q8h × 4–6 wks	Quinolone† (PO) × 4–6 weeks

Osteomyelitis (cont'd)

Subset	Usual Pathogens	Preferred IV Therapy	Alternate IV Therapy	PO Therapy or IV-to-PO Switch
Chronic *Diabetes mellitus/ Peripheral vascular disease*	Group A, B streptococci S. aureus (MSSA) E. coli P. mirabilis K. pneumoniae B. fragilis	Tigacycline 100 mg (IV) × 1 dose, then 50 mg (IV) q12h × 2–4 weeks **or** Meropenem 1 gm (IV) q8h* **or** Piperacillin/ tazobactam 3.375 gm (IV) q6h* **or** Ertapenem 1 gm (IV) q24h*	Moxifloxacin 400 mg (IV) q24h* **or** Ceftizoxime 2 gm (IV) q8h* **or** Ampicillin/ sulbactam 3 gm (IV) q6h* **or combination therapy with** Ceftriaxone 1 gm (IV) q24h* **plus** Metronidazole 1 gm (IV) q24h*	Clindamycin 300 mg (PO) q8h* **plus** Levofloxacin 500 mg (PO) q24h* **or** **monotherapy with** Moxifloxacin 400 mg (PO) q24h*
	Above pathogens/ S. aureus (MRSA)	Same as above **plus either** Minocycline 100 mg (IV) q12h × 2–4 weeks **or** Linezolid 600 mg (IV) q12h × 4–6 weeks **or monotheraphy with** Tigacycline 100 mg (IV) × 1 dose, then 50 mg (IV) q12h × 2–4 weeks	Minocycline 100 mg (IV) q12h × 2–4 weeks **plus either** Levofloxacin 500 mg (IV) q24h **or** Ceftriaxone 1 gm (IV) q24h × 2–4 weeks	Minocycline 100 mg (PO) q12h × 2–4 weeks **plus** Quinolone† (PO) q24h × 2–4 weeks
	Above pathogens/ B. fragilis (foul discharge)	Tigacycline 100 mg (IV) × 1 dose, then 50 mg (IV) q12h × 2–4 weeks	Moxifloxacin 400 mg (IV) q24h × 2–4 weeks **or** Ertapenem 1 gm (IV) q24h × 2–4 weeks	Moxifloxacin 400 mg (PO) q24h × 2–4 weeks

Osteomyelitis (cont'd)

Subset	Usual Pathogens	Preferred IV Therapy	Alternate IV Therapy	PO Therapy or IV-to-PO Switch
Chronic (cont'd)	Brucella	Streptomycin 1 gm (IM) q24h until cured **plus** Doxycycline 200 mg (IV) q12h × 3 days, then 100 mg (IV) q12h until cured	Gentamicin 5 mg/kg (IV) q24h until cured **plus** Doxycycline 200 mg (IV) q12h × 3 days, then 100 mg (IV) q12h until cured	Doxycycline 200 mg (PO) q12h × 3 days, then 100 mg (PO) q12h until cured† **plus** Rifampin 600 mg (PO) q24h until cured
TB osteomyelitis	M. tuberculosis	Treat the same as pulmonary TB (p. 53), but extend treatment to 6–9 months		

MSSA/MRSA = methicillin-sensitive/resistant S. aureus. Duration of therapy represents total time IV, PO, or IV + PO. Most patients on IV therapy able to take PO meds should be switched to PO therapy soon after clinical improvement.

*   Treat for 1 week after adequate debridement or amputation.

†   Moxifloxacin 400 mg or Levofloxacin 500 mg.

Acute Osteomyelitis

Clinical Presentation: Tenderness over infected bone. Fever and positive blood cultures common.

Diagnostic Considerations: Diagnosis by elevated ESR with positive bone scan. Bone biopsy is not needed for diagnosis. Bone scan is positive for acute osteomyelitis in first 24 hours.

Pitfalls: Earliest sign on plain films is soft tissue swelling; bony changes evident after 2 weeks.

Therapeutic Considerations: Treat 4–6 weeks with antibiotics. Debridement is not necessary for cure.

Prognosis: Related to adequacy/promptness of treatment.

Chronic Osteomyelitis
Diabetes Mellitus

Clinical Presentation: Afebrile or low-grade fever with normal WBC counts and deep penetrating ulcers ± draining sinus tracts.

Diagnostic Considerations: Diagnosis by elevated ESR and bone changes on plain films. Bone scan is not needed for diagnosis. Bone biopsy is preferred method of demonstrating organisms, since blood cultures are usually negative and cultures from ulcers/sinus tracts are unreliable.

Pitfalls: P. aeruginosa is a common colonizer and frequently cultured from deep ulcers/sinus tracts, but is not a pathogen in chronic osteomyelitis in diabetics.

Therapeutic Considerations: Surgical debridement is needed for cure; antibiotics alone are ineffective. Revascularization procedures usually do not help, since diabetes is a microvascular disease. Do not culture penetrating foot ulcers/draining sinus tracts; culture results reflect superficial flora. Bone biopsy during debridement is the best way to identify pathogen; if biopsy not possible, treat empirically.

Prognosis: Related to adequacy of blood supply/surgical debridement.

Non-Diabetics with Peripheral Vascular Disease (PVD)

Clinical Presentation: Absent or low-grade fever with normal WBC counts ± wet/dry digital gangrene.

Diagnostic Considerations: Diagnosis by clinical appearance of dusky/cold foot ± wet/dry gangrene. Chronic osteomyelitis secondary to PVD/open fracture is often polymicrobial.

Pitfalls: Wet gangrene usually requires surgical debridement/antibiotic therapy; dry gangrene may not.

Therapeutic Considerations: Surgical debridement needed for cure. Antibiotics alone are ineffective. Revascularization procedure may help treat infection by improving local blood supply.

Prognosis: Related to degree of vascular compromise.

Brucella Osteomyelitis (Brucella sp.)

Diagnostic Considerations: May be evidence of brucellosis elsewhere (epididymoorchitis). Suspect in patients with a history of animal/raw milk/cheese exposure. Serologic diagnosis by serum SAT, ELISA, or PCR.

Pitfalls: Brucella has predilection for vertebra, sacroiliac joints. Erosions of anterior vertebra adjacent to disc space typical vs. TB with diffuse vertebral destruction.

Therapeutic Considerations: May require 6 weeks of antibiotic therapy.

Prognosis: Joint destruction usually permanent.

TB Osteomyelitis (Mycobacterium tuberculosis)

Clinical Presentation: Presents similarly to chronic bacterial osteomyelitis. Vertebral TB (Pott's disease) affects disk spaces early and presents with chronic back/neck pain ± inguinal/paraspinal mass.

Diagnostic Considerations: Diagnosis by AFB on biopsy/culture of infected bone. T-spot PPD–positive.

Pitfalls: Chest x-ray is normal in 50%. May be confused with cancer, brucella osteomyelitis or chronic bacterial osteomyelitis.

Therapeutic Considerations: Treated the same as TB arthritis.

Prognosis: Good for non-vertebral TB/vertebral (if treated before paraparesis/paraplegia).

Empiric Therapy of Skin and Soft Tissue Infections

Cellulitis, Erysipelas, Impetigo, Lymphangitis (uSSSIs)

Subset	Usual Pathogens	Preferred IV Therapy	PO Therapy or IV-to-PO Switch
Above-the-waist (Treat initially for MSSA; if later identified as MRSA, treat accordingly)	S. aureus (MRSA)	Tigecycline 100 mg (IV) × 1 dose, then 50 mg (IV) q12h × 2 weeks **or** Linezolid 600 mg (IV) q12h × 2 weeks **or** Vancomycin 1 gm (IV) q12h × 2 weeks **or** Televancin 10 mg/kg (IV) q24h × 2 weeks **or** Daptomycin 4 mg/kg (IV) q24h × 2 weeks	Linezolid 600 mg (PO) q12h × 2 weeks **or** Minocycline 100 mg (PO) q12h × 2 weeks

Cellulitis, Erysipelas, Impetigo, Lymphangitis (uSSSIs) (cont'd)

Subset	Usual Pathogens	Preferred IV Therapy		PO Therapy or IV-to-PO Switch
Above-the-waist (cont'd)	Group A streptococci S. aureus (MSSA)	Ceftriaxone 1–2 gm (IV) q24h × 2 weeks **or** Cefazolin 1 gm (IV) q8h × 2 weeks	Nafcillin 2 gm (IV) q4h × 2 weeks **or** Clindamycin 600 mg (IV) q8h × 2 weeks	Cephalexin 500 mg (PO) q6h × 2 weeks **or** Clindamycin 300 mg (PO) q6h × 2 weeks
Below-the-waist	S. aureus (MRSA)	Treat the same as for MRSA above-the-waist cellulitis; see above		
(Treat initially for MSSA; if later identified as MRSA, treat accordingly)	Group A, B streptococci P. mirabilis K. pneumoniae E. coli S. aureus (MSSA)	Quinolone* (IV) q24h × 2 weeks **or** Ceftriaxone 1–2 gm (IV) q24h × 2 weeks **or** Cefazolin 1 gm (IV) q8h × 2 weeks	Piperacillin/ tazobactam 3.375 gm (IV) q6h × 2 weeks **or** Ampicillin/ sulbactam 3 gm (IV) q6h × 2 weeks **or** Ticarcillin/clavulanate 3.1 gm (IV) q6h × 2 weeks	Cephalexin 500 mg (PO) q6h × 2 weeks **or** Quinolone* (PO) q24h × 2 weeks

uSSSIs = uncomplicated skin skin structure infections.
MRSA/MSSA = methicillin-resistant/sensitive S. aureus. Duration of therapy represents total time IV, PO, or IV + PO. Most patients on IV therapy able to take PO meds should be switched to PO therapy soon after clinical improvement.
* Moxifloxacin 400 mg or Levofloxacin 750 mg.

Clinical Presentation: Cellulitis presents as warm, painful, non-pruritic skin erythema without discharge. Impetigo is characterized by vesiculopustular lesions, most commonly on the face/extremities. Erysipelas resembles cellulitis but is raised and sharply demarcated. Mastitis presents as cellulitis/abscess of the breast and is treated the same as cellulitis above the waist.

Diagnostic Considerations: Diagnosis by clinical appearance ± culture of pathogen from aspirated skin lesion(s). Group B streptococci are important pathogens in diabetics. Lower extremity cellulitis tends to recur. Chronic edema of an extremity predisposes to recurrent/persistent cellulitis.

Pitfalls: Streptococcal and staphylococcal cellulitis may be indistinguishable clinically, but regional adenopathy/lymphangitis favors Streptococci, and bullae favors S. aureus.

Therapeutic Considerations: Lower extremity cellulitis requires ~ 1 week of antibiotics to improve. Patients with peripheral vascular disease, chronic venous stasis, alcoholic cirrhosis, and diabetes take 1–2 weeks longer to improve and often require 3–4 weeks of treatment. Treat mastitis as cellulitis above-the-waist, and drain surgically if an abscess is present.

Prognosis: Related to degree of micro/macrovascular insufficiency.

Complicated Skin/Skin Structure Tissue Infections (cSSSIs)

Subset	Usual Pathogens	Preferred IV Therapy		IV-to-PO Switch
Mixed aerobic-anaerobic deep soft tissue infection	Entero-bacteriaceae Group A streptococci S. aureus (MSSA) Anaerobic streptococci Fusobacterium	Piperacillin/tazobactam 3.375 gm (IV) q6h × 2 weeks **or** Meropenem 1 gm (IV) q8h × 2 weeks	Ertapenem 1 gm (IV) q24h × 2 weeks **or** Doripenem 1 gm (IV) q8h **or** Moxifloxacin 400 mg (IV) q24h × 2 weeks	Moxifloxacin 400 mg (PO) q24h × 2 weeks **or combination therapy with** Clindamycin 300 mg (PO) q8h × 2 weeks **plus** Levofloxacin 750 mg (PO) q24h × 2 weeks
Clostridial myonecrosis (gas gangrene)	Clostridium sp.	<u>Preferred IV</u> Penicillin G 10 mu (IV) q4h × 2 weeks **or** Clindamycin 600 mg (IV) q8h × 2 weeks	<u>Alternate IV</u> Piperacillin 4 gm (IV) q8h × 2 weeks **or** Ertapenem 1 gm (IV) q24h × 2 weeks	Not applicable
Necrotizing fasciitis/synergistic gangrene/Fournier's gangrene	Group A streptococci Entero-bacteriaceae Anaerobic streptococci S. aureus (MSSA)	Piperacillin/tazobactam 3.375 gm (IV) q6h × 2 weeks **or** Ertapenem 1 gm (IV) q24h × 2 weeks	Clindamycin 600 mg (IV) q8h × 2 weeks **plus** Levofloxacin 500 mg (IV) q24h × 2 weeks	Clindamycin 300 mg (PO) q8h × 2 weeks **plus** Levofloxacin 750 mg (PO) q24h × 2 weeks
Severe cellulitis, fasciitis, phegmons, abscesses	MRSA/MSSA	Daptomycin 6 mg/kg (IV) q24h × 2 weeks **or** Linezolid 600 mg (IV) q12h × 2 weeks **or** Tigecycline† 200 mg (IV) × 1 dose, then 100 mg (IV) q24h × 2 weeks **or** Telavancin 10 mg/kg (IV) q24h × 2 weeks		Linezolid 600 mg (PO) q12h × 2 weeks **or** Minocycline 100 mg (PO) q12h × 2 weeks

cSSSIs = complicated skin skin structure infections.
CA-MRSA = community-acquired methicillin-resistant S. aureus (see p. 15), MSSA = methicillin-sensitive S. aureus. Duration of therapy represents total time IV or IV + PO. Most patients on IV therapy able to take PO meds should be switched to PO therapy after clinical improvement.
†   Tigecycline may be used if MRSA or VRE is suspected in addition to usual pathogens.

Complicated Skin/Skin Structure Tissue Infections (cSSSIs) (cont'd)

Subset	Usual Pathogens	Preferred IV Therapy	IV-to-PO Switch
Pyomyositis/ necrotizing abscesses	Community-acquired MRSA (CA-MRSA)§	Daptomycin 6 mg/kg (IV) q24h × 2 weeks **or** Linezolid 600 mg (IV) q12h × 2 weeks	Linezolid 600 mg (PO) q12h × 2 weeks **or** Minocycline 100 mg (PO) q12h × 2 weeks

CA-MRSA = community-acquired methicillin-resistant S. aureus (see p. 15), MSSA = methicillin-sensitive S. aureus.
§   CA-MRSA PVL-positive strains (see p. 15).

Mixed Aerobic/Anaerobic Deep Soft Tissue Infection

Clinical Presentation: Local pain/tenderness ± gross gas deep in soft tissues and usually high fevers. More common in diabetics.

Diagnostic Considerations: Diagnosed clinically. Bacteriologic diagnosis by gram stain/culture of aspirated fluid. Patients usually have high fevers. Wound discharge is foul when present.

Pitfalls: Gross crepitance/prominent gas in soft tissues on x-ray suggests a mixed aerobic/anaerobic necrotizing infection, not gas gangrene. Gas gangrene extremely rare in diabetics.

Therapeutic Considerations: Prompt empiric therapy and surgical debridement may be lifesaving.

Prognosis: Related to severity of infection, adequacy of debridement, and underlying health of host.

Gas Gangrene (Clostridial Myonecrosis)

Clinical Presentation: Fulminant infection of muscle with little or n fever. Infected area is extremely painful, indurated, and discolored with or without bullae.

Diagnostic Considerations: Diagnosis is clinical. Aspiration of infected muscle shows few PMNs and gram-positive bacilli without spores (C. perfringens only). Gas gangrene is not accompanied by high fever. Patients are often apprehensive with relative bradycardia ± diarrhea. Wound discharge, if present, is sweetish and not foul. Rapidly progressive hemolytic anemia is characteristic.

Pitfalls: Gas gangrene (clostridial myonecrosis) has little visible gas on plain film x-rays; abundant gas should suggest a mixed aerobic/anaerobic infection, not gas gangrene. Gas gangrene extremely rare in diabetics.

Therapeutic Considerations: Surgical debridement is life saving and the only way to control infection.

Prognosis: Related to speed/extent of surgical debridement. Progression/death may occur in hours.

Necrotizing Fasciitis/Synergistic Gangrene

Clinical Presentation: Acutely ill patient with high fevers and extreme local pain without gas in tissues. If scrotum involved (± abdominal wall involvement), the diagnosis is Fournier's gangrene.

Diagnostic Considerations: Diagnosis by CT/MRI of involved extremity showing infection confined to one or more muscle compartments/fascial planes. Patients are febrile and ill. Gas is not present on exam or x-rays. May be polymicrobial or due to a single organism. Foul smelling exudate from infected soft tissues indicates anaerobes are present.

Pitfalls: Extreme pain in patients with deep soft tissue infections should suggest a compartment syndrome/necrotizing fasciitis. No hemolytic anemia, diarrhea, or bullae as with gas gangrene.

Therapeutic Considerations: Control/cure of infection requires surgical, debridement of dead tissue, and antimicrobial therapy. Clindamycin may be added for its anti-exotoxin effects if pathogen group A streptococci.

Prognosis: Related to rapidity/extent of surgical debridement.

Severe Cellulitis (Fascitis, Phegmons, Abscesses)

Clinical Presentation: MSSA/MRSA cellulitis often accompanied by bullae. Fascitis presents with pain out of proportion to clinical findings in the distribution of fascial planes, a phegmon (pre-abscess before abscess wall forms) presents with pain ± overlying cellulitis. MSSA/MRSA abscesses are clinically indistinguishable from other abscesses, but remain the most common pathogens in cSSSI abscesses.

Diagnostic Considerations: Diagnosis of cellulitis and abscesses is clinical. Demonstration of fascitis, phegmons, of abscesses are by imaging studies by CT/MRI.

Pitfalls: Bullae with cellulitis should suggest MSSA/MRSA (not group A streptococci). Bullae in DM/bullous diseases are not accompanied by fever/cellulitis.

Therapeutic Considerations: Cellulitis and phegmons may be treated with antibiotic therapy alone. Fasciitis and abscesses usually require debridement (fascitis) or drainage (abscesses).

Prognosis: Good if treated appropriately/early.

Pyomyositis/Necrotizing Abscesses (CA-MRSA)

Clinical Presentation: Abrupt onset of severe/deep muscle infection ± large abscesses should suggest community-acquired MRSA (CA-MRSA).

Diagnostic Considerations: The diagnosis of CA-MRSA is made on the basis of the distinctively fulminant/severe clinical presentation and by culturing MRSA from muscle/abscess. If available, test isolate for SCC *mec* IV ± Panton-Valentine leukocidin (PVL) gene.

Pitfalls: CA-MRSA susceptible to clindamycin, TMP–SMX, and doxycycline.

Therapeutic Considerations: Prompt/complete incision and drainage of abscesses and early use of anti-CA-MRSA drugs may be life-saving. Antibiotics effective against CA-MRSA (TMP–SMX, clindamycin, doxycycline) are ineffective against CO-MRSA/HA-MRSA; antibiotics effective against CO-MRSA/HA-MRSA are also effective against CA-MRSA (see p. 15). Use minocycline instead of doxycycline for CA-MRSA/CO-MRSA. Doxycycline resistance with CA-MRSA of concern. Minocycline more effective than doxycycline, TMP-SMX or clindamycin for CA-MRSA.

Prognosis: Related to presence of PVL gene CA-MRSA. CA-MRSA PVL negative infections are similar in severity to MSSA infections.

Skin Ulcers

Subset	Usual Pathogens	Preferred IV Therapy	Alternate IV Therapy	PO Therapy or IV-to-PO Switch
Decubitus ulcers (*above the waist*)	Group A streptococci E. coli, P. mirabilis K. pneumoniae S. aureus (MSSA)	Cefazolin 1 gm (IV) q8h* **or** Ceftriaxone 1 gm (IV) q24h*	Cefotaxime 2 gm (IV) q6h* **or** Ceftizoxime 2 gm (IV) q8h*	Cephalexin 500 mg (PO) q6h*
(*sacral ulcers/ ulcers below the waist*) *stage III/ IV ulcers* = ***chronic osteomyelitis***	B. fragilis Group A streptococci E. coli P. mirabilis K. pneumoniae S. aureus (MSSA) S. aureus (MRSA)[†] (*not P. aeruginosa*[§])	Tigecycline 100 mg (IV) × 1 dose, then 50 mg (IV) q12h* **or** Ertapenem 1 gm (IV) q24h* **or** Piperacillin/ tazobactam 3.375 gm (IV) q6h* **or** Meropenem 1 gm (IV) q8h*	Moxifloxacin 400 mg (IV) q24h* **or** **combination therapy with** Clindamycin 600 mg (IV) q6h* **plus** Levofloxacin 500 mg (IV) q24h*	Moxifloxacin 400 mg (PO) q24h* **or** **combination therapy with** Clindamycin 300 mg (PO) q8h* **plus** Levofloxacin 500 mg (PO) q24h*

Duration of therapy represents total time IV, PO, or IV + PO. Most patients on IV therapy able to take PO meds should be switched to PO therapy soon after clinical improvement.

*   Treat Stages I/II (superficial) decubitus ulcers with local care. If no underlying chronic osteomyelitis, treat Stages III/IV (deep) decubitus ulcers with antibiotics and adequate *bone* debridement.

†   MRSA: Tigecycline 100 mg (IV) × 1 dose then 50 mg (IV) q12h* alone or one of above non-MRSA antibiotics *plus* [Daptomycin 4 mg/kg (IV) q24h* or Linezolid 600 mg (IV) q12h*] or Vancomycin 1 gm (IV) q12h* or Minocycline 100 mg (IV) q12h*. PO therapy or IV-to-PO switch if MRSA: Linezolid 600 mg (PO) q12h* or Minocycline 100 mg (PO) q12h* *plus* one of above antibiotics.

§   Deep penetrating ulcers (stage III/IV) in diabetics represent underlying *chronic osteomyelitis* and are *not due to P. aeruginosa*. However, P. aeruginosa (a water associated organism) can be cultured from > 90% of deep diabetic foot ulcers and represents superficial colonization (from moist socks, moist dressings, whirlpool baths, etc.)

Skin Ulcers (cont'd)

Subset	Usual Pathogens	Preferred IV Therapy	Alternate IV Therapy	PO Therapy or IV-to-PO Switch
Diabetic foot ulcers (deep/ complicated) (Treat initially for MSSA; if later identified as Group A streptococci, MRSA, etc., treat accordingly)	S. aureus (MRSA)	Tigacycline 100 mg (IV) × 1 dose, then 50 mg (IV) q12h **or** Telavancin 10 mg/kg (IV) q24h[†]	Vancomycin 1 gm (IV) q12h[†] **or** Daptomycin 4 mg/kg (IV) q24h[†] **or** Linezolid 600 mg (IV) q12h[†]	Linezolid 600 mg (PO) q12h[†] **or** Minocycline 100 mg (PO) q12h[†]
	Group A, B streptococci S. aureus (MSSA) E. coli P. mirabilis K. pneumoniae B. fragilis	Ertapenem 1 gm (IV) q24h[†] **or** Piperacillin/ tazobactam 3.375 gm (IV) q6h[†] **or** Moxifloxacin 400 mg (IV) q24h[†]	Cefoperazone 2 gm (IV) q12h **or** Doripenem 1 gm (IV) q8h **or** Ampicillin/ sulbactam 3 gm (IV) q6h[†] **or combination therapy with** Ceftriaxone 1 gm (IV) q24h[†] **plus** Metronidazole 1 gm (IV) q24h[†] **or** Clindamycin 600 mg (IV) q8h[†] **plus either** Ciprofloxacin 400 mg (IV) q12h[†] **or** Levofloxacin 750 mg (IV) q24h[†]	Moxifloxacin 400 mg (PO) q24h[†] **or** **combination therapy with** Minocycline 100 mg (PO) q12h[†] **or** Clindamycin 300 mg (PO) q8h[†] **plus** Levofloxacin 500 mg (PO) q24h[†]
	Any pathogen(s) above **plus** S. aureus (MRSA)	<u>IV Therapy:</u> MRSA drug **plus** a non-MRSA drug (see above) <u>PO Therapy or IV-to-PO Switch:</u> MRSA drug (PO) **plus** a non-MRSA drug (PO) (see above)		

†   Treat × 1 week after adequate debridement/amputation.

Skin Ulcers (cont'd)

Subset	Usual Pathogens	Preferred IV Therapy	Alternate IV Therapy	PO Therapy or IV-to-PO Switch
Ischemic foot ulcers (Treat initially for MSSA; if later identified as Gp. A strep, MRSA, etc., treat accordingly)	S. aureus (MRSA)	Treat the same as for deep/complicated diabetic foot ulcers, above		
	Group A streptococci E. coli S. aureus (MSSA)	Cefazolin 1 gm (IV) q8h × 2 weeks **or** Ceftriaxone 1 gm (IV) q24h × 2 weeks	Quinolone* (IV) q24h × 2 weeks	Quinolone* (PO) q24h × 2 weeks
	Any pathogen(s) above **plus** S. aureus (MRSA)	<u>IV Therapy:</u> MRSA drug **plus** a non-MRSA drug (see diabetic foot ulcers) <u>PO Therapy or IV-to-PO Switch:</u> MRSA drug **plus** a non-MRSA drug (see diabetic foot ulcers)		

MSSA = methicillin-sensitive S. aureus. Duration of therapy represents total time IV, PO, or IV + PO. Most patients on IV therapy able to take PO meds should be switched to PO therapy soon after clinical improvement.
*   Levofloxacin 750 mg or Moxifloxacin 400 mg.

Decubitus Ulcers
Clinical Presentation: Painless ulcers with variable depth and infectious exudate ± fevers ≤ 102°F.
Diagnostic Considerations: Diagnosis by clinical appearance. Obtain ESR/bone scan to rule out underlying osteomyelitis with deep (Stage III/IV) decubitus ulcers.
Pitfalls: Superficial decubitus ulcers do not require systemic antibiotics.
Therapeutic Considerations: Deep decubitus ulcers require antibiotics and debridement, superficial ulcers do not. Coverage for B. fragilis is needed for deep perianal decubitus ulcers. Good nursing care is important in preventing/limiting extension of decubitus ulcers.
Prognosis: Related to fecal contamination of ulcer and bone involvement (e.g., osteomyelitis).

Diabetic Foot Ulcers/Chronic Osteomyelitis
Clinical Presentation: Ulcers/sinus tracts on bottom of foot/between toes; usually painless. Fevers ≤ 102°F and a foul smelling exudate are common.
Diagnostic Considerations: In diabetics, deep, penetrating, chronic foot ulcers/draining sinus tracts are diagnostic of chronic osteomyelitis. ESR ≥ 100 mm/hr in a diabetic with a foot ulcer/sinus tract is diagnostic of chronic osteomyelitis. Foot films confirm chronic osteomyelitis. Bone scan is needed only in acute osteomyelitis.
Pitfalls: Do not rely on culture results of deep ulcers/sinus tracts to choose antibiotic coverage, since cultures reflect skin colonization, not bone pathogens. Treat empirically.
Therapeutic Considerations: B. fragilis coverage is required in deep penetrating diabetic foot ulcers/ fetid foot infection. P. aeruginosa is often cultured from diabetic foot ulcers/sinus tracts, but represents colonization, not infection. P. aeruginosa is a "water" organism that colonizes feet from moist socks/ dressings, irrigant solutions, or whirlpool baths. Surgical debridement is essential for cure of chronic osteomyelitis in diabetics. Treat superficial diabetic foot ulcers the same as cellulitis in non-diabetics (p. 132).
Prognosis: Related to adequacy of debridement of infected bone.

Ischemic Foot Ulcers

Clinical Presentation: Ulcers often clean/dry ± digital gangrene. No fevers/exudate.

Diagnostic Considerations: Diagnosis by clinical appearance/location in a patient with peripheral vascular disease. Ischemic foot ulcers most commonly affect the toes, medial malleoli, dorsum of foot, or lower leg.

Pitfalls: In contrast to ulcers in diabetics, ischemic ulcers due to peripheral vascular disease usually do not involve the plantar surface of the ulcer.

Therapeutic Considerations: Dry gangrene should not be treated with antibiotics unless accompanied by signs of systemic infection. Wet gangrene should be treated as a mixed aerobic/anaerobic infection. Both dry/wet gangrene may require debridement for cure/control. Do not rely on ulcer cultures to guide treatment; treat empirically if necessary. Evaluate for revascularization.

Prognosis: Related to degree of vascular insufficiency.

Skin Abscesses/Infected Cysts (Skin Pustules, Skin Boils, Furunculosis) (uSSSIs/cSSSIs)

Subset	Usual Pathogens	Preferred IV Therapy	Alternate IV Therapy	PO Therapy or IV-to-PO Switch
cSSSIs (Deep/multiple skin abscesses) (Treat initially for MSSA; if later identified as MRSA, treat accordingly)	S. aureus (MRSA)	Tigecycline 100 mg (IV) × 1 dose, then 50 mg (IV) q12h × 2 weeks **or** Linezolid 600 mg (IV) q12h × 2 weeks **or** Daptomycin 4 mg/kg (IV) q24h × 2 weeks **or** Telavancin 10 mg/kg (IV) q24h × 2 weeks **or** Minocycline 100 mg (IV) q12h × 2 weeks **or** Vancomycin 1 mg (IV) q12h × 2 weeks		Linezolid 600 mg (PO) q12h × 2 weeks **or** Minocycline 100 mg (PO) q12h × 2 weeks
	S. aureus (MSSA)	Cefazolin 1 gm (IV) q8h × 2 weeks **or** Nafcillin 2 gm (IV) q4h × 2 weeks	Clindamycin 600 mg (IV) q8h × 2 weeks **or** Ceftriaxone 1 gm (IV) q24h × 2 weeks	Cephalexin 500 mg (PO) q6h × 2 weeks **or** Clindamycin 300 mg (PO) q8h × 2 weeks

uSSSIs = uncomplicated skin skin structure infections; cSSSs = complicated skin skin structure infections. *MRSA/MSSA = methicillin-resistant/sensitive S. aureus.* Duration of therapy represents total time IV, PO, or IV + PO. Most patients on IV therapy able to take PO meds should be switched to PO therapy soon after clinical improvement.

Skin Abscesses/Infected Cysts (Skin Pustules, Skin Boils, Furunculosis) (cSSSIs/uSSSIs) (cont'd)

Subset	Usual Pathogens	Preferred IV Therapy	Alternate IV Therapy	PO Therapy or IV-to-PO Switch
uSSSIs *Infected pilonidal cysts*	Group A streptococci E. coli P. mirabilis K. pneumoniae S. aureus (MSSA)	Ceftriaxone 1 gm (IV) q24h × 2 weeks **or** Ceftizoxime 2 gm (IV) q8h × 2 weeks **or** Cefoxitin 2 gm (IV) q6h × 2 weeks	Levofloxacin 500 mg (IV) q24h × 2 weeks **or** Moxifloxacin 400 mg (IV) q24h × 2 weeks	Levofloxacin 500 mg (PO) q24h × 2 weeks **or** Moxifloxacin 400 mg (PO) q24h × 2 weeks
Hydradenitis suppurativa	S. aureus (MSSA)	Not applicable	TMP–SMX 1 SS tablet (PO) q12h × 2–4 weeks **or** Clindamycin 300 mg (PO) q8h × 2–4 weeks **or** Minocycline 100 mg (PO) q12h × 2–4 weeks	
	S. aureus (MRSA)	Not applicable	Minocycline 100 mg (PO) q12h × 2–4 weeks	

uSSSIs = uncomplicated SSSIs.
cSSSIs = complicated SSSIs.
MRSA/MSSA = methicillin-resistant/sensitive S. aureus. Duration of therapy represents total time IV, PO, or IV + PO. Most patients on IV therapy able to take PO meds should be switched to PO therapy soon after clinical improvement.

Skin Abscesses

Clinical Presentation: Warm painful nodules ± bullae, low-grade fever ± systemic symptoms, no lymphangitis. Skin boils/furunculosis present as acute, chronic, or recurrent skin pustules, and remain localized without lymphangitis.

Diagnostic Considerations: Specific pathogen diagnosed by gram stain of abscess. Recurring S. aureus abscesses are not uncommon and should be drained. Blood cultures are rarely positive. Suspect Job's syndrome if recurring abscesses with peripheral eosinophilia. Skin boils/furunculosis are diagnosed by clinical appearance (skin pustules).

Pitfalls: Recurring S. aureus skin infections may occur on immune basis but immunologic studies are usually negative.

Therapeutic Considerations: Repeated aspiration of abscesses may be necessary. Surgical drainage is required if antibiotics fail. Treat boils/furunculosis as in hydradenitis suppurativa.

Prognosis: Excellent if treated early.

Infected Pilonidal Cysts

Clinical Presentation: Chronic drainage from pilonidal cysts.
Diagnostic Considerations: Diagnosis by clinical appearance. Deep/systemic infection is rare.
Pitfalls: Culture of exudate is usually unhelpful.
Therapeutic Considerations: Surgical debridement is often necessary.
Prognosis: Good with adequate excision.

Hydradenitis Suppurativa

Clinical Presentation: Chronic, indurated, painful, raised axillary/groin lesions ± drainage/sinus tracts.
Diagnostic Considerations: Diagnosis by clinical appearance/location of lesions. Infections are often bilateral and tend to recur.
Pitfalls: Surgical debridement is usually not necessary unless deep/extensive infection.
Therapeutic Considerations: Most anti-S. aureus antibiotics have poor penetration and usually fail.
Prognosis: Good with recommended antibiotics. Surgery, if necessary, is curative.

Skin Vesicles (Non-Genital)

Subset	Pathogen	Therapy
Herpes simplex	Herpes simplex virus (HSV)	Acyclovir 400 mg (PO) q8h × 10 days **or** Valacyclovir 1 gm (PO) q12h × 7–10 days **or** Famciclovir 250 mg (PO) q8h × 10 days
Chickenpox	Varicella zoster virus (VZV)	Acyclovir 800 mg (PO) q6h × 5 days **or** Valacyclovir 1 gm (PO) q8h × 5 days **or** Famciclovir 500 mg (PO) q8h × 5 days
Herpes zoster *Dermatomal zoster (shingles)*	Varicella zoster virus (VZV)	Acyclovir 800 mg (PO) 5x/day × 7–10 days **or** Valacyclovir 1 gm (PO) q8h × 7–10 days **or** Famciclovir 500 mg (PO) q8h × 7–10 days
Disseminated zoster		<u>IV therapy:</u> Acyclovir 10 mg/kg (IV) q8h × 7–10 days <u>PO therapy:</u> Valacyclovir 1 gm (PO) q8h × 7–10 days **or** Famciclovir 500 mg (PO) q8h × 7–10 days
Herpes whitlow	HSV-1	Acyclovir 400 mg (PO) q8h × 7–10 days **or** Valacyclovir 1 gm (PO) q12h × 7–10 days **or** Famciclovir 250 mg (PO) q8h × 7–10 days

Herpes Simplex (HSV)

Clinical Presentation: Painful, sometimes pruritic vesicles that form pustules or painful erythematous ulcers. Associated with fever, myalgias.
Diagnostic Considerations: Diagnosis by clinical appearance and demonstration of HSV by culture of vesicle fluid/vesicle base. May be severe in HIV.

Pitfalls: Painful vesicular lesions surrounded by prominent induration distinguishes HSV from insect bites (pruritic) and cellulitis (no induration).

Therapeutic Considerations: Topical acyclovir ointment may be useful early when vesicles erupt, but is ineffective after vesicles stop erupting. For severe/refractory cases, use acyclovir 5 mg/kg (IV) q8h × 2–7 days, then if improvement, switch to acyclovir 400 mg (PO) q8h to complete 10-day course.

Prognosis: Related to extent of tissue involvement/degree of cellular immunity dysfunction.

Chickenpox (VZV)

Clinical Presentation: Abrupt appearance of discrete/diffuse pruritic vesicles. Appear in successive crops over 3 days, then no more new lesions. Patients do not appear toxic.

Diagnostic Considerations: Chickenpox lesions are central and typically concentrated on the trunk, although vesicles may also occur in the mouth, GI or GU tract. Vesicles are seen at different stages of development, and are superficial with the classic "dew drop on a rose petal" appearance. Tzanck test is positive in chickenpox (negative in smallpox).

Pitfalls: Vesicles are not deep/umbilicated like smallpox. Smallpox patients are sick/toxic, and vesicles are at the same stage of development in each anatomical area. Vesicles begin and are concentrated on the face with smallpox.

Therapeutic Considerations: Begin therapy as early as possible before appearance of successive crops of vesicles appear. Treat VZV pneumonia early with acyclovir.

Prognosis: Children do better than adults. Worst prognosis in smokers/pregnancy (may develop chickenpox/VZV pneumonia).

Herpes Zoster (VZV)

Clinical Presentation: Painful, vesicular eruption in dermatomal distribution. Pain may be difficult to diagnose.

Diagnostic Considerations: Diagnosis by appearance/positive Tzanck test of vesicle base scrapings.

Pitfalls: Begin therapy within 2 days of vesicle eruption.

Therapeutic Considerations: Higher doses of acyclovir are required for VZV than HSV. See p. 343 for disseminated VZV, ophthalmic nerve/visceral involvement, or acyclovir-resistant strains.

Prognosis: Good if treated early. Some develop painful post-herpetic neuralgia of involved dermatomes.

Herpes Whitlow

Clinical Presentation: Multiple vesicopustular lesions on fingers and hands. Lymphangitis, adenopathy, fever/chills are usually present, suggesting a bacterial infection.

Diagnostic Considerations: Common in healthcare workers giving patients oral care/suctioning.

Pitfalls: No need for antibiotics even though lesions appear infected with "pus."

Therapeutic Considerations: Never incise/drain herpes whitlow; surgical incision will flare/prolong the infection.

Prognosis: Excellent, unless incision/drainage has been performed.

Wound Infections (for rabies, see pp. 362, 374–375)

Subset	Usual Pathogens	Preferred IV Therapy	Alternate IV Therapy	PO Therapy or IV-to-PO Switch
Animal bite wounds[†]	Group A streptococci P. multocida Capnocytophaga canimorsus (DF2) S. aureus (MSSA)	Piperacillin/ tazobactam 3.375 gm (IV) q6h × 2 weeks **or** Tigecycline 200 mg (IV) × 1 dose, then 100 mg (IV) q24h × 2 weeks	Ertapenem 1 gm (IV) q24h × 2 weeks **or** Ampicillin/ sulbactam 3 gm (IV) q6h × 2 weeks	Amoxicillin/ clavulanic acid 500/125 mg (PO) q8h or 875/125 mg (PO) q12h × 2 weeks **or** Doxycycline 200 mg (PO) q12h × 3 days, then 100 mg (PO) q12h × 11 days
Human bite wounds	Oral anaerobes Group A streptococci E. corrodens S. aureus (MSSA)	Same as for animal bite wounds, above	Same as for animal bite wounds, above	Same as for animal bite wounds, above
Cat scratch disease (CSD)	Bartonella henselae (invasive disease)	Doxycycline 200 mg (IV) q12h × 3 days, then 100 mg (IV) q12h × 4–8 weeks **or** Azithromycin 500 mg (IV) q24h × 4–8 weeks	Chloramphenicol 500 mg (IV) q6h × 4–8 weeks **or** Erythromycin 500 mg (IV) q6h × 4–8 weeks	Doxycycline 200 mg (PO) q12h × 3 days, then 100 mg (PO) q12h × 4–8 weeks* **or** Azithromycin 250 mg (PO) q24h × 4–8 weeks **or** Quinolone[‡] (PO) × 4–8 weeks
	B. henselae (lymphaden-opathy only)	PO therapy: Azithromycin 500 mg (PO) × 1 dose, then 250 mg (PO) × 4 days		

MSSA = methicillin-sensitive S. aureus. Duration of therapy represents total time IV, PO, or IV + PO.

*   Loading dose is not needed PO if given IV with the same drug.

‡   Ciprofloxacin 400 mg (IV) or 500 mg (PO) q12h or Levofloxacin 500 mg (IV or PO) q24h or Moxifloxacin 400 mg (IV or PO) q24h.

†   Rabies (see p. 362)

Wound Infections (cont'd) (for rabies, see pp. 362, 374–375)

Subset	Usual Pathogens	Preferred IV Therapy	Alternate IV Therapy	PO Therapy or IV-to-PO Switch
Burn wounds (severe)†	Group A streptococci S. aureus (MSSA) Enterobacter P. aeruginosa	Doripenem 1 gm (IV) q8h × 2 weeks **or** Meropenem 1 gm (IV) q8h × 2 weeks	Cefepime 2 gm (IV) q8h × 2 weeks **or** Cefoperazone 2 gm (IV) q12h × 2 weeks	Not applicable
Freshwater-exposed wounds	Aeromonas hydrophilia	Quinolone‡ (IV) × 2 weeks **or** TMP–SMX 2.5 mg/kg (IV) q6h × 2 weeks	Ceftriaxone 1 gm (IV) q24h × 2 weeks **or** Aztreonam 2 gm (IV) q8h × 2 weeks **or** Gentamicin 240 mg (IV) q24h × 2 weeks	Quinolone‡ (PO) × 2 weeks **or** TMP–SMX 1 SS tablet (PO) q12h × 2 weeks
Saltwater-exposed wounds	Vibrio vulnificus Vibrio sp.	Doxycycline 200 mg (IV) q12h × 3 days, then 100 mg (IV) q12h × 11 days **or** Quinolone‡ (IV) × 2 weeks	Ceftriaxone 2 gm (IV) q12h × 2 weeks **or** Chloramphenicol 500 mg (IV) q6h × 2 weeks	Doxycycline 200 mg (PO) q12h × 3 days, then 100 mg (PO) q12h × 11 days* **or** Quinolone‡ (PO) × 2 weeks

MSSA = methicillin-sensitive S. aureus. Duration of therapy represents total time IV, PO, or IV + PO. Most patients on IV therapy able to take PO meds should be switched to PO therapy soon after clinical improvement.

† Treat only IV or IV-to-PO switch.
* Loading dose is not needed PO if given IV with the same drug.
‡ Ciprofloxacin 400 mg (IV) or 500 mg (PO) q12h or Levofloxacin 500 mg (IV or PO) q24h or Moxifloxacin 400 mg (IV or PO) q24h.

Animal Bite Wounds (for rabies, see p. 362)
Clinical Presentation: Cellulitis surrounding bite wound.
Diagnostic Considerations: Diagnosis by culture of bite wound exudate. Deep bites may also cause tendinitis/osteomyelitis, and severe bites may result in systemic infection with bacteremia.
Pitfalls: Avoid erythromycin in penicillin-allergic patients (ineffective against P. multocida).
Therapeutic Considerations: For facial/hand bites, consult a plastic surgeon.
Prognosis: Related to adequacy of debridement and early antibiotic therapy.

Human Bite Wounds

Clinical Presentation: Cellulitis surrounding bite wound.

Diagnostic Considerations: Diagnosis by culture of bite wound exudate. Infection often extends to involve tendon/bone.

Pitfalls: Compared to animal bites, human bites are more likely to contain anaerobes, S. aureus, and Group A streptococci.

Therapeutic Considerations: Avoid primary closure of human bite wounds.

Prognosis: Related to adequacy of debridement and early antibiotic therapy.

Cat Scratch Disease (Bartonella henselae)

Clinical Presentation: Subacute presentation of obscure febrile illness associated with cat bite/contact. Usually accompanied by adenopathy.

Diagnostic Considerations: Diagnosis by wound culture/serology for Bartonella. Cat scratch fever/disease may follow a cat scratch, but a lick from a kitten contaminating an inapparent micro-laceration is more common. May present as an FUO. Culture of exudate/node is unlikely to be positive, but silver stain of biopsy material shows organisms.

Pitfalls: Rule out lymphoma, which may present in similar fashion. Titers may cross react with C. burnetii (Q fever).

Therapeutic Considerations: For invasive disease, treat until symptoms/signs resolve. For lymph-adenopathy, oral azithromycin decreases the size of nodes but may not reduce fever/systemic symptoms. Bartonella are sensitive in vitro to cephalosporins and TMP–SMX, but these antibiotics are ineffective in vivo.

Prognosis: Related to health of host.

Burn Wounds

Clinical Presentation: Severe (3rd/4th degree) burns ± drainage.

Diagnostic Considerations: Semi-quantitative bacterial counts help differentiate colonization (low counts) from infection (high counts). Burn wounds quickly become colonized.

Pitfalls: Treat only infected 3rd/4th degree burn wounds with systemic antibiotics.

Therapeutic Considerations: Meticulous local care/eschar removal/surgical debridement is key in preventing and controlling infection.

Prognosis: Related to severity of burns and adequacy of eschar debridement.

Freshwater-Exposed Wounds (Aeromonas hydrophilia)

Clinical Presentation: Fulminant wound infection with fever and diarrhea.

Diagnostic Considerations: Diagnosis by stool/wound/blood culture.

Pitfalls: Suspect A. hydrophilia in wound infection with fresh water exposure followed by diarrhea.

Therapeutic Considerations: Surgical debridement of devitalized tissue may be necessary.

Prognosis: Related to severity of infection and health of host.

Saltwater-Exposed Wounds (Vibrio vulnificus/Vibrio sp.)

Clinical Presentation: Fulminant wound infection with fever, painful hemorrhagic bullae, diarrhea.

Diagnostic Considerations: Diagnosis by stool/wound/blood culture. Vibrio vulnificus is a fulmi-nant, life-threatening infection that may be accompanied by hypotension.

Pitfalls: Suspect V. vulnificus in acutely ill patients with fever, diarrhea, and bullous lesions after salt-water exposure.

Therapeutic Considerations: Surgical debridement of devitalized tissue may be necessary.
Prognosis: Related to extent of infection and health of host.

Superficial Fungal Infections of Skin and Nails

Subset	Usual Pathogens	Topical Therapy	PO Therapy
Mucocutaneous (local/non-disseminated) candidiasis	C. albicans	Clotrimazole 1% cream twice daily × 2 weeks	Fluconazole 400 mg (PO) × 1 dose, then 200 mg (PO) q24h × 2 weeks
Tinea corporis (body ringworm)	Trichophyton rubrum Epidermophyton floccosum Microsporum canis Trichophyton mentagrophytes	Clotrimazole 1% cream twice daily × 4–8 weeks **or** Miconazole 2% cream twice daily × 2 weeks **or** Econazole 1% cream twice daily × 2 weeks	Terbinafine 250 mg (PO) q24h × 4 weeks **or** Ketoconazole 200 mg (PO) q24h × 4 weeks **or** Fluconazole 200 mg (PO) weekly × 4 weeks
Tinea capitis (scalp ringworm)	Same as Tinea corporis, above	Selenium sulfide shampoo daily × 2–4 weeks	Same as Tinea corporis (see above)
Tinea cruris (jock itch)	T. cruris	Same as Tinea corporis, above	Same as Tinea corporis (see above)
Tinea pedis (athlete's foot)	Same as Tinea corporis, above	Same as Tinea corporis, above	Terbinafine 250 mg (PO) q24h × 2 weeks **or** Ketoconazole 200 mg (PO) q24h × 4 weeks **or** Itraconazole 200 mg (PO)* q24h × 4 weeks

* Itraconazole solution provides more reliable absorption than Itraconazole capsules.

Superficial Fungal Infections of Skin and Nails (cont'd)

Subset	Usual Pathogens	Topical Therapy	PO Therapy
Tinea versicolor (pityriasis)	Malasezzia furfur (Pityrosporum orbiculare)	Clotrimazole cream (1%) or miconazole cream (2%) or ketoconazole cream (2%) daily × 7 days	Ketoconazole 200 mg (PO) q24h × 7 days **or** Itraconazole 200 mg (PO)* q24h × 7 days **or** Fluconazole 400 mg (PO) × 1 dose
Onychomycosis (nail infection)	Epidermophyton floccosum Trichophyton mentagrophytes Trichophyton rubrum C. albicans	Not applicable	Fluconazole 200 mg (PO) q24h *pulse dosed*, i.e., 1 week per month × 3 months (fingernail infection) or 6 months (toenail infection) **or** Itraconazole 200 mg (PO)* q24h *pulse dosed, i.e.,* 1 week per month × 2 months (fingernail infection) or 3 months (toenail infection) **or** Terbinafine 250 mg (PO) q24h × 6 weeks (fingernail infection) or 12 weeks (toenail infection)

*   Itraconazole solution provides more reliable absorption than itraconazole capsules.

Mucocutaneous (Local/Non-disseminated) Candidiasis

Clinical Presentation: Primary cutaneous findings include an erythematous rash with satellite lesions, which may be papular, pustular, or ulcerated. Lesions can be limited or widespread over parts of body. Chronic mucocutaneous candidiasis manifests as recurrent candidal infections of skin, nails, or mucous mebranes.

Diagnostic Considerations: Diagnosis by demonstrating organism by stain/culture in tissue specimen. In HIV, Candida is very common on skin/mucous membranes.

Pitfalls: Do not confuse with the isolated, multinodular lesions of disseminated disease, which may resemble ecthyma gangrenosa or purpura fulminans.

Therapeutic Considerations: Diabetics and other compromised hosts may require prolonged therapy. In contrast to local disease, nodular cutaneous candidiasis represents disseminated disease (p. 290).

Prognosis: Related to extent of disease/host defense status.

Tinea Corporis (Body Ringworm)

Clinical Presentation: Annular pruritic lesions on trunk/face with central clearing.

Diagnostic Considerations: Diagnosis by clinical appearance/skin scraping.

Pitfalls: Do not confuse with erythema migrans, which is not pruritic.

Therapeutic Considerations: If topical therapy fails, treat with oral antifungals.

Prognosis: Excellent.

Tinea Capitis (Scalp Ringworm)

Clinical Presentation: Itchy, annular scalp lesions.

Diagnostic Considerations: Scalp lesions fluoresce with ultraviolet light. Culture hair shafts.

Pitfalls: T. capitis is associated with localized areas of alopecia.

Therapeutic Considerations: Selenium sulfide shampoo may be used first for 2–4 weeks. Treat shampoo Failures with oral ketoconazole, terbinafine, or fluconazole.

Prognosis: Excellent.

Tinea Cruris (Jock Itch)

Clinical Presentation: Groin, inguinal, perineal, or buttock lesions that are pruritic and serpiginous with scaling borders/central clearing.

Diagnostic Considerations: Diagnosis by clinical appearance/culture.

Pitfalls: Usually spares penis/scrotum, unlike Candida.

Therapeutic Considerations: In addition to therapy, it is important to keep area dry.

Prognosis: Excellent.

Tinea Pedis (Athlete's Foot)

Clinical Presentation: Painful cracks/fissures between toes.

Diagnostic Considerations: Diagnosis by clinical appearance/skin scraping.

Pitfalls: Must keep feet dry or relapse/reinfection may occur.

Therapeutic Considerations: In addition to therapy, it is important to keep area dry.

Prognosis: Excellent.

Tinea Versicolor (Pityriasis)

Clinical Presentation: Oval hypo- or hyperpigmented scaly lesions that coalesce into large confluent areas typically on upper trunk; chronic/relapsing.

Diagnostic Considerations: Diagnosis by clinical appearance and culture of affected skin lesions.

Pitfalls: M. furfur also causes seborrheic dermatitis, but seborrheic lesions are typically on the face/scalp.

Therapeutic Considerations: If topical therapy fails, treat with oral antifungals. Treat non-scalp seborrheic dermatitis with ketoconazole cream (2%) daily until cured.

Prognosis: Excellent.

Dermatophyte Nail Infections

Clinical Presentation: Chronically thickened, discolored nails.

Diagnostic Considerations: Diagnosis by culture of nail clippings.

Pitfalls: Nail clipping cultures often contaminated by bacterial/fungal colonizers. Green nail discoloration suggests P. aeruginosa, not a fungal nail infection; treat with ciprofloxacin 500 mg (PO) q12h × 2–3 weeks.

Therapeutic Considerations: Lengthy therapy is required. However, terbinafine and itraconazole remain bound to nail tissue for months following dosing and thus therapy with these compounds is not continued until clearance of the nail bed.

Prognosis: Excellent if infection is totally eradicated from nail bed. New nail growth takes months.

Skin Infestations

Subset	Usual Pathogens	Therapy
Scabies	Sarcoptes scabiei	Treat whole body with Permethrin cream 5% (Elimite); leave on for 8–10 hours **or** Ivermectin 18 mg (three 6-mg pills) (PO) × 1 dose
Head lice	Pediculus humanus var. capitis	Shampoo with Permethrin 5% (Elimite) or 1% (NIX) cream × 10 minutes
Body lice	Pediculus humanus var. corporis	Body lice removed by shower. Removed clothes should be washed in hot water or sealed in bags for 1 month, or treated with DDT powder 10% or malathion powder 1%
Pubic lice (crabs)	Phthirus pubis	Permethrin 5% (Elimite) or 1% (NIX) cream × 10 minutes to affected areas

Scabies (Sarcoptes scabiei)
Clinical Presentation: Punctate, serpiginous, intensely pruritic black spots in webbed spaces of hands/feet and creases of elbows/knees.
Diagnostic Considerations: Diagnosis by visualization of skin tracts/burrows. Incubation period up to 6 weeks after contact. Spread by scratching from one part of body to another.
Pitfalls: Mites are not visible, only their skin tracks, but mites may be scraped out of tracts for diagnosis.
Therapeutic Considerations: Permethrin cream is usually effective. If itching persists after treatment, do not retreat (itching is secondary to hypersensitivity reaction of eggs in skin burrows). Treat close contacts. Vacuum bedding/furniture.
Prognosis: Norwegian scabies is very difficult to eradicate.

Head Lice (Pediculus humanus var. capitis)
Clinical Presentation: White spots may be seen on hair shafts of head/neck, but not eyebrows.
Diagnostic Considerations: Nits on hair are unhatched lice eggs, seen as white dots attached to hair shaft. May survive away from body × 2 days.
Pitfalls: May need to retreat in 7 days to kill any lice that hatched from surviving nits.
Therapeutic Considerations: Shampoo with Permethrin 5% (Elimite) or 1% (NIX) cream kills lice/nits. Clothes and non-washables should be tied off in plastic bags × 2 weeks to kill lice. Alternately, wash and dry clothes/bed linens; heat from dryer/iron kills lice.
Prognosis: Related to thoroughness of therapy.

Body Lice (Pediculus humanus var. corporis)
Clinical Presentation: Intense generalized pruritus.
Diagnostic Considerations: Smaller than head lice and more difficult to see. May survive away from body × 1 week.
Pitfalls: Body lice live in clothes; leave only for a blood meal, then return to clothing.
Therapeutic Considerations: Can survive in seams of clothing × 1 week.
Prognosis: Good if clothes are also treated.

Pubic Lice (Phthirus pubis) Crabs

Clinical Presentation: Genital pruritus.

Diagnostic Considerations: Seen on groin, eyelashes, axilla. May survive away from body × 1 day.

Pitfalls: Smaller than head lice, but easily seen.

Therapeutic Considerations: Treat partners. Wash, dry, and iron clothes; heat from dryer/iron kills lice. Non-washables may be placed in a sealed bag × 7 days.

Prognosis: Good if clothes are also treated.

Ischiorectal/Perirectal Abscess

Subset	Pathogens	Preferred Therapy
Ischiorectal/ perirectal abscess	Enterobacteriaceae B. fragilis	Treat the same as mild/severe peritonitis (p. 100) ± surgical drainage depending on abscess size/severity

Clinical Presentation: Presents in normal hosts with perirectal pain, pain on defecation, leukocytosis, erythema/tenderness over abscess ± fever/chills. In febrile neutropenia, there is only tenderness.

Diagnostic Considerations: Diagnosis by erythema/tenderness over abscess or by CT/MRI.

Pitfalls: Do not confuse with perirectal regional enteritis (Crohn's disease) in normal hosts, or with ecthyma gangrenosum in febrile neutropenics.

Therapeutic Considerations: Antibiotic therapy may be adequate for mild cases. Large abscesses require drainage plus antibiotics × 1–2 weeks post-drainage. With febrile neutropenia, use an antibiotic that is active against both P. aeruginosa and B. fragilis e.g., meropenem.

Prognosis: Good with early drainage/therapy.

Sepsis/Septic Shock

Sepsis/Septic Shock

Subset	Usual Pathogens	Preferred IV Therapy	Alternate IV Therapy	IV-to-PO Switch
Unknown source	Entero- bacteriaceae B. fragilis E. faecalis (VSE)†	Meropenem 1 gm (IV) q8h × 2 weeks **or** Piperacillin/ tazobactam 3.375 gm (IV) q6h × 2 weeks	Quinolone* (IV) × 2 weeks **plus either** Metronidazole 1 gm (IV) q24h × 2 weeks **or** Clindamycin 600 mg (IV) q8h × 2 weeks	Moxifloxacin 400 mg (PO) q24h × 2 weeks

VSE/VRE = vancomycin-sensitive/resistant enterococci. Duration of therapy represents total time IV or IV + PO.

* Ciprofloxacin 400 mg (IV) q12h or Levofloxacin 500 mg (IV or PO) q24h.

† Treat initially for E. faecalis (VSE); if later identified as E. faecium (VRE), treat accordingly (urosepsis see pp. 154–155).

Sepsis/Septic Shock (cont'd)

Subset	Usual Pathogens	Preferred IV Therapy	Alternate IV Therapy	IV-to-PO Switch
Lung source *Community-acquired pneumonia*§	S. pneumoniae H. influenzae K. pneumoniae	Quinolone‡ (IV) q24h × 2 weeks **or** Ceftriaxone 1 gm (IV) q24h × 2 weeks	Any 2nd generation cephalosporin (IV) × 2 weeks	Quinolone‡ (PO) q24h × 2 weeks **or** Doxycycline 200 mg (PO) q12h × 3 days, then 100 mg (PO) q12h × 11 days
	Influenza A (ILI **with** rapidly cavitating <72 hours multiple pulmonary infiltrates)	MSSA/MRSA	(see pp. 62–63)	(see p. 52)
Nosocomial pneumonia	P. aeruginosa K. pneumoniae E. coli S. marcescens (*not* MSSA/ MRSA)	Same as ventilator-associated pneumonia (see p. 68)		
CVC source** *Bacteremia* (Treat initially for MSSA; if later identified as MRSA, etc., treat accordingly)	S. epidermidis (CoNS) S. aureus (MSSA) Klebsiella Enterobacter Serratia	Meropenem 1 gm (IV) q8h × 2 weeks **or** Cefepime 2 gm (IV) q12h × 2 wks	Ceftriaxone 1 gm (IV) q24h × 2 wks **or** Quinolone* (IV) q24h × 2 wks	Quinolone* (PO) q24h × 2 weeks **or** Cephalexin 500 mg (PO) q6h × 2 weeks
	S. aureus (MRSA)	Daptomycin 6 mg/kg (IV) q24h × 2 weeks **or** Linezolid 600 mg (IV) q12h × 2 weeks		Linezolid 600 mg (PO) q12h × 2 weeks

ILI = Influenza like illness.

MRSA/MSSA = methicillin resistant/sensitive S. aureus. Duration of therapy represents total time IV or IV + PO.

*   Moxifloxacin 400 mg or Levofloxacin 500 mg.

**   If clinically possible, remove CVC as soon as possible.

†   Patients with ILI/influenza A (human/swine) presenting with *simultaneous* MSSA/MRSA CAP often present in shock.

‡   Levofloxacin 750 mg (IV) q24h or Moxifloxacin 400 mg (IV) q24h.

§   *Uncomplicated by cardiopulmonary decompensation/failure, CAP does not present with hypotension/shock in normal hosts. Hyposplenia/asplenia should be suspected if CAP presents with hypotension/shock in patients with good cardiopulmonary function.*

Sepsis/Septic Shock (cont'd)

Subset	Usual Pathogens	Preferred IV Therapy	Alternate IV Therapy	IV-to-PO Switch
			Quinupristin/dalfopristin 7.5 mg/kg (IV) q8h × 2 weeks **or** Vancomycin 1 gm (IV) q12h × 2 weeks	Minocycline 100 mg (PO) q12h × 2 weeks
Candidemia (disseminated/ invasive) Unless species is known, empiric therapy as for non-albicans/ possibly fluconazole-resistant Candida is preferred if recent prior azole therapy, severe illness, neutropenia or high risk for infection with C. glabrata or C. krusei	Candida albicans (or other fluconazole-susceptible species)¶	If less critically ill, not neutropenic, and no recent azole exposure: fluconazole is usual first choice alternates an echinocandin may be used. In critically ill, neutropenia or recent azole exposure: an echinocandin is preferred. **or** Micafungin 100 mg (IV) q24h × 2 weeks† **or** Caspofungin 70 mg (IV) × 1 dose, then 50 mg (IV) q24h × 2 weeks† Fluconazole 800 mg (IV) × 1, then 400 mg (IV) q24h × 2 weeks† **or** Lipid-associated formulation of amphotericin B (p. 525) (IV) q24h × 2 weeks† **or** Amphotericin B deoxycholate 0.7 mg/kg (IV) q24h × 2 weeks† **or** Voriconazole (see "usual dose," p. 714) **or** Anidulafungin 200 mg (IV) × 1 dose, then 100 mg (IV) q24h × 2 weeks†	Fluconazole 400 mg (PO) q24h × 2 weeks† **or** Voriconazole (see "usual dose," p. 714)
	Non-albicans Candida¶ (possibly fluconazole-resistant)	Choices are as for C. albicans (see above), but Fluconazole should *not* be used and an echinocandin is preferred. Micafungin 100 mg (IV) q24h × 2 weeks† **or** Caspofungin (see C. albicans, above) Use an Amphotericin or Voriconazole if additional mould coverage is desired **or** Lipid amphotericin B (p. 525) (IV) q24h† **or** Amphotericin B deoxycholate (see C. albicans, above) × 2 weeks† **or** Voriconazole (see "usual dose," p. 714) × 2 weeks¶† **or** Itraconazole (see C. albicans, above) **or** Anidulafungin 200 mg (IV) × 1 dose, then 100 mg (IV) q24h × 2 weeks†	Voriconazole (see "usual dose," p. 714) × 2 weeks¶†

¶   Best agent depends on infecting species. Fluconazole-susceptibility varies predictably by species. (See Fluconazole Drug Summary) also, see Amphotericin B (deoxycholate and lipid-associated formulations) Drug Summaries.
†   Treat candidemia for 2 weeks after negative blood cultures.

Sepsis/Septic Shock (cont'd)

Subset	Usual Pathogens	Preferred IV Therapy	Alternate IV Therapy	IV-to-PO Switch
Intra-abdominal/ pelvic source	Entero-bacteriaceae B. fragilis	Ertapenem 1 gm (IV) q24h × 2 weeks **or** Tigacycline 200 mg (IV) × 1 dose, then 100 mg (IV) q24h × 2 weeks **or** Meropenem 1 gm (IV) q8h × 2 weeks **or** Piperacillin/ tazobactam 3.375 gm (IV) q6h × 2 weeks	**Combination therapy with either** Ceftriaxone 1 gm (IV) q24h × 2 weeks **or** Levofloxacin 500 mg (IV) q24h × 2 weeks **plus** Metronidazole 1 gm (IV) q24h × 2 weeks	Moxifloxacin 400 mg (PO) q24h × 2 weeks **or** **combination therapy with** Clindamycin 300 mg (PO) q8h × 2 weeks **plus** Levofloxacin 500 mg (PO) q24h × 2 weeks
Urosepsis (*community-acquired*)	Entero-bacteriaceae E. faecalis (VSE)	Levofloxacin 500 mg (IV) q24h × 1–2 weeks **or** Piperacillin/ tazobactam 3.375 gm (IV) q6h × 1–2 weeks	Meropenem 1 gm (IV) q8h × 1–2 weeks **or** Levofloxacin 500 mg (IV) q24h	Levofloxacin 500 mg (PO) q24h × 1–2 weeks
	E. faecium (VRE)	Linezolid 600 mg (IV) q12h × 1–2 weeks	Quinupristin/ dalfopristin 7.5 mg/kg (IV) q8h × 1–2 weeks	Linezolid 600 mg (PO) q12h × 1–2 weeks **or** Minocycline 100 mg (PO) q12h × 1–2 weeks
(*nosocomial*)	P. aeruginosa Entero-bacteriaceae	Meropenem 1 gm (IV) q8h × 1–2 weeks **or** Ciprofloxacin 400 mg (IV) q8h × 1–2 weeks **or** Levofloxacin 750 mg (IV) q24h × 1–2 weeks	Aztreonam 2 gm (IV) q8h × 1–2 weeks **or** Cefepime 2 gm (IV) q12h × 1–2 weeks **or** Colistin 1.7 mg/kg (IV) q8h × 1–2 weeks Doripenem 1 gm (IV) q8h × 1–2 weeks	Levofloxacin 500 mg (PO) q24h × 1–2 weeks

Sepsis/Septic Shock

Subset	Usual Pathogens	Preferred IV Therapy	Alternate IV Therapy	IV-to-PO Switch
Urosepsis (*group D enterococci*)	E. faecalis (VSE)	Ampicillin 2 gm (IV) q4h × 1–2 weeks **or** Linezolid 600 mg (IV) q12h × 1–2 weeks **or combination therapy with** Vancomycin 1 gm (IV) q12h × 1–2 weeks **plus** Gentamicin 240 mg (IV) q24h × 1 week		Amoxicillin 1 gm (PO) q8h × 1–2 weeks **or** Levofloxacin 500 mg (PO) q24h × 1–2 weeks
	E. faecium (VRE)	Linezolid 600 mg (IV) q12h × 1–2 weeks **or** Quinupristin/dalfopristin 7.5 mg/kg (IV) q8h × 1–2 weeks		Linezolid 600 mg (PO) q12h × 1–2 weeks **or** Minocycline 100 mg (PO) q12h × 3 days, then 100 mg (PO) q12h × 4–11 days
Overwhelming sepsis with purpura (asplenia or hyposplenia)	S. pneumoniae H. influenzae N. meningitidis	Ceftriaxone 2 gm (IV) q24h × 2 weeks **or** Levofloxacin 500 mg (IV) q24h × 2 weeks	Cefepime 2 gm (IV) q12h × 2 weeks **or** Cefotaxime 2 gm (IV) q6h × 2 weeks	Levofloxacin 500 mg (PO) q24h × 2 weeks **or** Amoxicillin 1 gm (PO) q8h × 2 weeks
Steroids (high chronic dose)	Aspergillus	Treat as Aspergillus pneumonia (see p. 55)		
Miliary TB	M. tuberculosis	Treat as pulmonary TB (see p. 53) plus steroids × 1–2 wks		
Miliary BCG (disseminated BCG)	Bacille Calmette-Guérin (BCG)	Treat with INH plus RIF × 9 months; EMB, until susceptibilities known; may add steroids e.g., prednisolone 40 mg q24h × 1–2 weeks		
Septic shock	Gram-negative or gram-positive bacteria	Empiric site appropriate antimicrobial therapy plus surgical decompression/drainage if needed		

Duration of therapy represents total time IV or IV + PO.

Sepsis (Unknown Source)

Clinical Presentation: Abrupt onset of high spiking fevers, rigors ± hypotension.

Diagnostic Considerations: Diagnosis suggested by high-grade bacteremia (2/4–4/4 positive blood cultures) with unexplained hypotension. Rule out pseudosepsis (GI bleed, myocardial infarction, pulmonary embolism, acute pancreatitis, adrenal insufficiency, etc.). Sepsis usually occurs from a GI, GU, or IV source, so coverage is directed against GI and GU pathogens if IV line infection is unlikely.

Pitfalls: Most cases of fever/hypotension are *not* due to sepsis. Before the label of "sepsis" is applied to febrile/hypotensive patients, first consider treatable/reversible mimics (see p. 151).

Therapeutic Considerations: Resuscitate shock patients initially with rapid adequate volume replacement, followed by pressors, if needed. Do not give pressors before volume replacement or hypotension may continue/worsen. Use normal saline, plasma expanders, or blood for volume replacement, not D_5W. If patient is persistently hypotensive despite volume replacement, consider relative adrenal insufficiency: Obtain a serum cortisol level, then give cortisone 100 mg (IV) q6h × 24–72h; blood pressure will rise promptly if relative adrenal insufficiency is the cause of volume-unresponsive hypotension. Do not add/change antibiotics if patient is persistently hypotensive/febrile; look for GI bleed, myocardial infarction, pulmonary embolism, pancreatitis, undrained abscess, adrenal insufficiency, or IV line infection. Drain abscesses as soon as possible. Remove IV lines if the entry site is red or a central line has been in place for ≥ 7 days and there is no other explanation for fever/hypotension. Early antibiotic therapy/surgical drainage of abscesses, debridement of necrotic tissue eg. necrotizing fasciitis or relief of obstruction is critical.

Prognosis: Related to severity of septic process and underlying cardiopulmonary/immune status.

Sepsis (Lung Source)

Clinical Presentation: Normal hosts with community-acquired pneumonia (CAP) do not present with sepsis. CAP with sepsis suggests the presence of impaired immunity/hyposplenic function (see "sepsis in hyposplenia/asplenia," p. 157). Nosocomial pneumonia uncommonly presents as (or is complicated by) sepsis with otherwise unexplained hypotension.

Diagnostic Considerations: Impaired splenic function may be inferred by finding Howell-Jolly bodies (small, round, pinkish or bluish inclusion bodies in red blood cells) in the peripheral blood smear. The number of Howell-Jolly bodies is proportional to the degree of splenic dysfunction.

Pitfalls: CAP with hypotension/sepsis should suggest hyposplenic function, impaired immunity, or an alternate diagnosis that can mimic CAP/shock. Be sure to exclude acute MI, acute heart failure/COPD, PE/infarction, overzealous diuretic therapy, concomitant GI bleed, and acute pancreatitis.

Therapeutic Considerations: Patients with malignancies, myeloma, or SLE are predisposed to CAP, which is not usually severe or associated with shock. Be sure patients with CAP receiving steroids at less than "stress doses" do not have hypotension/shock from relative adrenal insufficiency. In patients with SLE, try to distinguish between lupus pneumonitis and CAP; SLE pneumonitis usually occurs as part of a SLE flare, CAP usually does not.

Prognosis: Related to underlying cardiopulmonary/immune status. Early treatment is important.

Sepsis (Central Venous Catheter [CVC] Source)

Clinical Presentation: Temperature ≥ 102°F ± IV site erythema.

Diagnostic Considerations: Diagnosis by semi-quantitative catheter tip culture with ≥ 15 colonies plus blood cultures with same pathogen. If no other explanation for fever and line has been in place ≥ 7 days, remove CVC and obtain semi-quantitative catheter tip culture. Suppurative thrombophlebitis presents with hectic/septic fevers and pus at IV site ± palpable venous cord.

Pitfalls: Temperature ≥ 102°F with CVC infection, in contrast to phlebitis (temperature ≤ 102°F). Acute bacterial endocarditis (ABE) may complicate intracardiac or CVC (not peripheral) infection.

Therapeutic Considerations: Line removal is usually curative, but antibiotic therapy is usually given for 1 week after CVC removal for gram-negative bacilli or 2 weeks after CVC removal for S. aureus (MSSA/MRSA). Antifungal therapy is also usually given for 2 weeks after CVC removal for candidemia. Dilated ophthalmoscopy by an ophthalmologist is important to exclude candidal endophthalmitis following candidemia.

Prognosis: Good if CVC is removed before endocarditis/metastatic spread.

Sepsis (Intra-abdominal/Pelvic Source)

Clinical Presentation: Fever, peritonitis ± hypotension. Usually a history of an intra-abdominal disorder that predisposes to sepsis (e.g., diverticulosis, gallbladder disease, recent intra-abdominal/pelvic surgery). Signs and symptoms are referable to the abdomen/pelvis.

Diagnostic Considerations: Clinical presentation plus imaging studies (e.g., abdominal/pelvic CT or MRI to demonstrate pathology) are diagnostic.

Pitfalls: Elderly patients may have little/no fever and may not have rebound tenderness. Be sure to exclude intra-abdominal mimics of sepsis (e.g., GI bleed, pancreatitis).

Therapeutic Considerations: Empiric coverage should be directed against aerobic gram-negative bacilli plus B. fragilis. Anti-enterococcal coverage is not essential. Antibiotic therapy is ineffective unless ruptured viscus is repaired, obstruction is relieved, abscesses are drained.

Prognosis: Related to rapidity/adequacy of abscess drainage and repair/lavage of ruptured organs. The preoperative health of the host is also important.

Sepsis (Urinary Source)

Clinical Presentation: Fever/hypotension in a patient with diabetes mellitus, SLE, myeloma, pre-existing renal disease, stone disease, or partial/total urinary tract obstruction.

Diagnostic Considerations: Urine gram stain determines initial empiric coverage. Pyuria is also present. Diagnosis confirmed by culturing the same isolate from urine and blood.

Pitfalls: Pyuria without bacteriuria and bacteremia due to same pathogens is not diagnostic of urosepsis. Urosepsis does not occur in normal hosts; look for host defect (e.g., diabetes, renal disease).

Therapeutic Considerations: If stones/obstruction are not present, urosepsis resolves rapidly with appropriate therapy. Delayed/no response suggests infected/obstructed stent, stone, partial/total urinary tract obstruction, or renal abscess.

Prognosis: Good if stone/stent removed, obstruction relieved, abscess drained. Fatalities rare with urosepsis.

Sepsis (Hyposplenia/Asplenia)

Clinical Presentation: Presents as overwhelming septicemia/shock with petechiae.

Diagnostic Considerations: Diagnosis by gram stain of buffy coat of blood or by blood cultures. Organism may be stained/cultured from aspirated petechiae. Howell-Jolly bodies in the peripheral smear are a clue to decreased splenic function. Conditions associated with hyposplenism include sickle cell trait/disease, cirrhosis, rheumatoid arthritis, SLE, systemic necrotizing vasculitis, amyloidosis, celiac disease, chronic active hepatitis, Fanconi's syndrome, IgA deficiency, intestinal lymphangiectasia, intravenous gamma-globulin therapy, myeloproliferative disorders, non-Hodgkin's lymphoma, regional enteritis, ulcerative colitis, Sezary syndrome, splenic infarcts/malignancies, steroid therapy, systemic mastocytosis, thyroiditis, infiltrative diseases of spleen, mechanical compression of splenic artery/spleen, Waldenstrom's macroglobulinemia, hyposplenism of old age, congenital absence of spleen.

Pitfalls: Suspect hyposplenia/asplenia in unexplained overwhelming infection.

Therapeutic Considerations: In spite of early aggressive antibiotic therapy and supportive care, patients often die within hours from overwhelming infection, especially due to S. pneumoniae.
Prognosis: Related to degree of splenic dysfunction.

Sepsis (Chronic High Dose Steroids)

Clinical Presentation: Subacute onset of fever with disseminated infection (Candida, Aspergillus) in multiple organs.
Diagnostic Considerations: Diagnosis by positive blood cultures for fungi or demonstration of invasive fungal infection from tissue biopsy specimens. Sepsis is most commonly due to fungemia.
Pitfalls: Obtain blood cultures to diagnose fungemias and rule out bacteremias (uncommon).
Therapeutic Considerations: Empirical approach is the same as for invasive candidiasis (p. 153) or invasive *aspergillosis* (p. 159 and p. 164). Therapy focused solely on candidiasis (e.g., fluconazole alone) should be used only if *aspergillosis* seems unlikely following careful review of the epidemiologic and clinical presentation.
Prognosis: Related to degree of immunosuppression.

Miliary (Disseminated) TB (Mycobacterium tuberculosis)

Clinical Presentation: Unexplained, prolonged fevers without localizing signs.
Diagnostic Considerations: Diagnosis by AFB on biopsy/culture of liver or bone marrow.
Pitfalls: Chest x-ray is negative early in 1/3. Subtle miliary (2 mm) infiltrates on chest x-ray 1–4 weeks).
Therapeutic Considerations: Treated the same as pulmonary TB ± steroids initially.
Prognosis: Death within weeks without treatment.

Miliary (Disseminated) BCG (Bacille Calmette-Guérin)

Clinical Presentation: Fever, circulatory collapse, DIC days to weeks after intravesicular BCG.
Diagnostic Considerations: Usually occurs in compromised hosts (e.g., transplants, active TB, congenital/acquired immunodeficiencies [e.g., HIV], leukemias/lymphomas). Rare in normal hosts.
Pitfalls: Avoid intravesicular BCG immediately after traumatic catheterization, bladder biopsy, TURP.
Therapeutic Considerations: Treat with 4 anti-TB drugs plus steroids. Do not repeat BCG therapy.
Prognosis: Good with early treatment.

Febrile Neutropenia

Febrile Neutropenia

Subset	Usual Pathogens	Preferred IV Therapy	Alternate IV Therapy	IV-to-PO Switch
Febrile leukopenia **< 7 days**	P. aeruginosa Entero-bacteriaceae (*not* MSSA/MRSA)¶	Meropenem 1 gm (IV) q8h* **or** Levofloxacin 750 mg (IV) q24h*	Cefepime 2 gm (IV) q8h* **or** Doripenem 1 gm (IV) q8h*	Levofloxacin 750 mg (PO) q24h*

Febrile Neutropenia (cont'd)

> 7 days	C. albicans Non-albicans Candida Aspergillus	Micafungin 100 mg (IV) q24h* **or** Voriconazole (see "usual dose," p. 714)* **or** Caspofungin 70 mg (IV) × 1 dose, then 50 mg (IV) q24h* **or** Lipid- associated formulation of amphotericin B (IV) (p. 525) q24h*	Amphotericin B deoxycholate 1.5 mg/kg (IV) q24h until 1–2 gm given	Itraconazole 200 mg (PO) q12h* **or** Voriconazole (see "usual dose," p. 714)*
	MSSA (2° to CVC)†	Same as above (have good GNB and MSSA activity)	Same as above (have good GNB and MSSA activity)	Linezolid 600 mg (PO) q12h **or** Minocycline§ 100 mg (PO) q12h
	MRSA (2° to CVC)†	Meropenem 1 gm (IV) q8h* **or** Levofloxacin 750 mg (IV) q24h* **plus** Daptomycin§ 6 mg/kg (IV) q24h **or** Vancomycin§ 1 gm (IV) q12h	Cefepime 2 gm (IV) q8h* **or** Doripenem 1 gm (IV) q8h* **plus either** Linezolid 600 mg (IV) q12h **or** Quinupristin/ dalfopristin§ 7.5 mg/kg (IV) q8h	Linezolid 600 mg (PO) q12h **or** Minocycline§ 100 mg (PO) q12h

MSSA = methicillin-sensitive S. aureus. Duration of therapy represents total time IV or IV + PO.
* Treat until neutropenia resolves.
† If clinically possible, remove CVC.
§ Treat for 2 weeks post–CVC removal.
¶ Neutropenia, per se, does not predispose to MSSA/MRSA bacteremias. MSSA/MRSA bacteremias in febrile neutropenia are 2° to CVC associated infection, *not* neutropenia.

Clinical Presentation: Incidence of infection rises as PMN counts fall below 1000/mm³.
Diagnostic Considerations: Febrile neutropenia < 7 days ± positive blood cultures. After blood cultures are drawn, anti-P. aeruginosa coverage should be initiated. Do not overlook ischiorectal or perirectal abscess as sources of fever.
Pitfalls: Suspect fungemia if abrupt rise in temperature occurs after 7 days of appropriate anti-P. aeruginosa antibiotic therapy. Fungemias usually do not occur in first 7 days of neutropenia. Viridans streptococci (S. mitis) may present with bacteremia, shock, ARDs, and rash in febrile neutropenia.

Therapeutic Considerations: If a patient is neutropenic for > 2 weeks and develops RUQ/LUQ pain/increased alkaline phosphatase, suspect hepatosplenic candidiasis; confirm diagnosis with abdominal CT/MRI showing mass lesions in liver/spleen and treat as systemic/invasive candidiasis (p. 79). S. aureus is not a common pathogen in neutropenic compromised hosts without central IV lines, and B. fragilis/anaerobes are not usual pathogens in febrile neutropenia. If IV line infection/perirectal abscess are ruled out, consider tumor fever or drug fever before changing antibiotic therapy.

Prognosis: Related to degree and duration of neutropenia.

Transplant Infections

Transplant Infections

Subset	Usual Pathogens	Preferred IV Therapy	Alternate IV Therapy	PO Therapy or IV-to-PO Switch
BACTEREMIA OR CANDIDEMIA				
Bacteremia Post-**BMT** (*leukopenic pre-engraftment*) **< 7 days**	P. aeruginosa Entero-bacteriaceae S. aureus (MSSA) Viridans streptococci E. faecalis (VSE)	Meropenem 1 gm (IV) q8h* **or** Piperacillin 4 gm (IV) q6h*	Quinolone† (IV) q24h* **plus either** Aztreonam 2 gm (IV) q8h* **or** Amikacin 1 gm (IV) q24h*	Quinolone† (PO) q24h* **or** Ciprofloxacin 750 mg (PO) q12h*
	S. aureus (Co-MRSA/HA-MRSA)	Daptomycin 6 mg/kg (IV) q24h × 2 weeks **or** Linezolid 600 mg (IV) q12h × 2 weeks **or** Quinupristin/dalfopristin 7.5 mg/kg (IV) q8h × 2 weeks **or** Vancomycin 1 gm (IV) q12h × 2 weeks		Linezolid 600 mg (PO) q12h × 2 weeks **or** Minocycline 100 mg (PO) q12h × 2 weeks
	E. faecium (VRE)	Linezolid 600 mg (IV) q12h × 1–2 weeks	Daptomycin 6 mg/kg (IV) q24h × 1–2 weeks	Linezolid 600 mg (PO) q12h × 1–2 weeks **or** Minocycline 100 mg (PO) q12h × 1–2 weeks

BMT/SOT = bone marrow/solid organ transplant, CO/HA-MRSA = community-onset/hospital-acquired methicillin-resistant S. aureus (see p. 14), MSSA = Methicillin-sensitive S. aureus.
† Levofloxacin 750 mg or Moxifloxacin 400 mg.
* Treat until neutropenia resolves.

Transplant Infections (cont'd)

Subset	Usual Pathogens	Preferred IV Therapy	Alternate IV Therapy	PO Therapy or IV-to-PO Switch
Candidemia Post-**BMT** (leukopenic pre-engraftment) **> 7 days**	C. albicans Non-albicans Candida	Micafungin 100 mg (IV) q24h Ambisome (L-Amb) 3–5 mg/kg (IV) q24h* **or** Caspofungin 70 mg (IV) × 1 dose, then 50 mg (IV) q24h* **or** Voriconazole (see "usual dose," p. 714)¶ **or** Anidulafungin 200 mg (IV) × 1 dose, then 100 mg (IV) q24h	Itraconazole 200 mg (IV) q12h × 2 days, then 200 mg (IV) q24h*¶ **or** Amphotericin B deoxycholate 0.6–1.5 mg/kg (IV) q24h until 1–2 gm given (significant toxicity likely—alternate therapy preferred)	Itraconazole 200 mg (PO) q12h*¶ **or** Voriconazole (see "usual dose," p. 714)*¶ **or** Fluconazole 800 mg (PO) × 1, then 400 mg (PO) q24h*‡
Bacteremia Post-**SOT** (Treat initially for MSSA; if later identified as MRSA, treat accordingly)	S. aureus (MSSA) Entero-bacteriaceae	Meropenem 1 gm (IV) q8h × 2 weeks **or** Ceftriaxone 1 gm (IV) q24h × 2 weeks	Quinolone† (IV) q24h × 2 weeks **or** Cefepime 2 gm (IV) q12h × 2 weeks	Quinolone† (PO) q24h × 2 weeks **or** Cephalexin 500 mg (PO) q6h × 2 weeks
	S. aureus (CO-MRSA/HA-MRSA)	Linezolid 600 mg (IV) q12h × 2 weeks **or** Daptomycin 6 mg/kg (IV) q24h × 2 weeks **or** Vancomycin 1 gm (IV) q12h × 2 weeks **or** Quinupristin/dalfopristin 7.5 mg/kg (IV) q8h × 2 weeks		Linezolid 600 mg (PO) q12h × 2 weeks **or** Minocycline 100 mg (PO) q12h × 2 weeks

BMT/SOT = bone marrow/solid organ transplant, CO/HA-MRSA = community-onset/hospital-acquired methicillin-resistant S. aureus (see p. 14), MSSA = methicillin-sensitive S. aureus.

†   Levofloxacin 750 mg or Moxifloxacin 400 mg.
*   Treat until neutropenia resolves.
‡   Loading dose is not needed PO if given IV with the same drug.
¶   Significant drug interactions are possible with usual immunosuppressive agents (e.g., sirolinus, cyclosporine, tacrolimus).
    Review all concomitant medications for potential interactions. *Voriconazole contraindicated in patients with sirolinus.*

Transplant Infections (cont'd)

	Viremia	
CMV	Ganciclovir 5 mg/kg (IV) q12h until clinical/ virologic response (not < 2 weeks) **or** Valganciclovir 900 mg (PO) q12h until clinical/virologic response (not < 2 weeks)	Follow therapy with 1-3 months of CMV prophylaxis (see p. 368) or frequent clinical/virologic followup. Risk of CMV disease greatest 3-6 months post-organ transplant in D+/R- patients during the period of maximum immuno-suppression. Coinfection with HHV-6/7 may increase risk of CMV disease. Risk also high where ALG is used for induction therapy to treat organ rejection. Also, CMV disease risk higher in lung, pancreas and intestine transplants (kidney, liver have lower risk). Lowest risk of CMV disease in D-/R- transplants (should be given leukodepleted blood products and CMV negative blood). Consider IVIG† in patients with CMV pneumonia or consider CMVIG†† in patients with CMV pneumonia or severe CMV infection.
HHV-6	Ganciclovir: 5 mg/ kg (IV) q12h until viremia/infection clears. **or** Foscarnet 90 mg/ kg (IV) q12h until viremia/infection clears. **or** Cidofovir 5 mg/kg (IV) q week × 2, then q other week* until viremia/infection clears.	*Reduction of immunosuppression remains the mainstay of treatment.* HHV-6-A may be gangcyclovir resistant. HHV-6-B variants susceptible to Ganciclovir and Foscarnet Treatment recommended for HHV-6 CNS disease with Ganciclovir, Foscarnet or a combination of both.
BK virus	Cidofovir 0.25 –1 mg/kg (IV) q2 weeks* **or**	*Reduction of immunosuppression remains the mainstay of treatment.* Treatment indicated for BKV viremia/BKV nephropathy. *No treatment necessary for asymptomatic BKV infection.* BV viremia predicts presence of BK nephropathy which precedes viruria. "Decoy cells" in urine indicate BK viruria. BK viruria is common and preceeds viremia and invasive infection. ALG: antilymphoayte globulin (thymoglobulin).

*   IVIG: 500 mg/kg (IV) q48h.
†† CMVIG:
   Renal Transplants: 150 mg/kg (IV) within 72 hours post-transplant, then 100 mg/kg (IV) at weeks 2, 4, 6, 8, then 50 mg/kg (IV) at weeks 12 and 16.
   Non-Renal Transplants: 150 mg/kg (IV) given within 72 hours post-transplant, then 150 mg/kg (IV) at weeks 2, 4, 6, 8, then 100 mg/kg (IV) at weeks 12 and 16 after transplant.

Transplant Infections (cont'd)

	Viremia (cont'd)	
	Leflunomide (given as mycophenolate replacement) **Loading Dose:** 100 mg (PO) q24h × 5 days, then **Maintenance Dose:** 40 mg (PO) q24h until viremia/ infection clears.	Measure leflunomide trough levels to ensure therapeutic concentrations (50–100 mcg/ml).
EBV/PTLD	Rituximab **or** Chemotherapy/ surgery	*Reduction or discontinuation of immunosuppression remains the mainstay of treatment of PTLD (spontaneous regression in ¼ – ½ of cases).*
RSV	Ribavirin 20 mg/ mL (aerosol) for 12–18 hours q24h × 3–7 days.	*Reduction of immunosuppression remains the mainstay of treatment. Palivizumab may prevent progression from upper to lower RTI. IVIG may be added in severe cases.*
Adenovirus	Ribavirin **Loading Dose:** 30 mg/ kg (IV), then **Maintenance Dose:** 16 mg/kg (IV) q6h × 4 days, then 8 mg/kg (IV) q8h until viremia/ infection clears. **or** Cidofovir 5 mg/kg (IV) q 1–2 weeks (with saline hydration and probenecid) until viremia/infection clears.§	*Reduction of immunosuppression remains the mainstay of treatment.* Oral ribavirin may be effective, but outcomes are variable and may be adenovirus-serotype specific.

§   Probenecid 2 gm (PO) 3 hours prior to cidofovir, 1 gm at 2 hours and 8 hours after completion of infusion. Patient should receive 1 liter normal saline (IV) prior to each infusion of cidofovir; a second liter may be administered over 1-3 hours at the start of cidofovir infusion or immediately following infusion.

*   With hydration/probenecid (see Cidofovir Drug Summary).

Transplant Infections (cont'd)

		CNS INFECTIONS		
Encephalitis/ meningitis	CMV HHV-6	Ganciclovir 5 mg/kg (IV) q12h × 2–4 weeks or until resolution of symptoms and viremia IVIG or CMVIG may be beneficial in severe cases Valganciclovir 900 mg (PO) q24h × 3 months. After successful treatment, a course of 2° prophylaxis is recommended		
	CMV (ganciclovir-resistant CMV: MIC ≥ 3 mcg/mL) or UL 54 or UL 97 mutations	Cidofovir 5 mg/kg (IV) of 1–2 weeks with saline plus probenecid (see p. 163) **or** Foscarnet 60 mg/kg (IV) q8h × 2 weeks **or** Foscarnet plus Ganciclovir (see above) **or** Cidofovir (see above) may be used in severe cases		
	Listeria, HSV, C. neoformans, M. tuberculosis treated the same as in normal/other compromised hosts (see pp. 25–26)			
Brain abscess/ mass lesions	Aspergillus	Voriconazole (see "usual dose," p. 714) until cured¶	Ambisome (L-Amb) 5 mg/kg (IV) q24h until cured **or** Amphotericin B 1.5 mg/kg (IV) q24h until cured	Voriconazole (see "usual dose," p. 714) until cured¶
	Nocardia	TMP–SMX 5 mg/kg (IV) q6h **or** Minocycline 200 mg (IV) q12h until clinical improvement, then (PO) therapy for at least 9–12 months or until cured	Linezolid 600 mg (IV) q12h until clinical improvement, then (PO) therapy for at least 9–12 months or until cured **or** Meropenem 2 gm (IV) q8h for at least 9–12 months or until cured	TMP–SMX 2 DS (PO) q8h **or** Minocycline 200 mg (PO) q12h **or** Linezolid 600 mg (PO) q12h for at least 9–12 months or until cured
	T. gondii	<u>Preferred Therapy</u> Sulfadiazine 1–1.5 gm (PO) q6h + Pyrimethamine 200 mg (PO) × 1 dose then 50 mg (PO) q6h + folinic acid 10 mg (PO) q24h × 6–8 weeks until CT/MRI clinical response.		

¶ Significant drug interactions are possible with usual immunosuppressive agents (e.g., sirolimus, cyclosporine tacrolimus). Review all concomitant medications for potential interactions. *Voriconazole contraindicated in patients on sirolimus.*

Transplant Infections (cont'd)

		CNS INFECTIONS (cont'd)
		Follow with sulfadiazine 1 gm (PO) q12h + Pyrimethamine 50 mg (PO) q24h + folinic acid 10 mg (PO) q24h until cured <u>Alternate Therapy</u> Clindamycin 600 mg (IV or PO) q6h + Pyrimethamine 200 mg (PO) × 1 dose then 50 mg (PO) q6h + folinic acid 10 mg (PO) q24h × 6–8 weeks until CT/MRI clinical response. Follow with Sulfadiazine 1 gm (PO) q12h + Pyrimethamine 50 mg (PO) q24h + folinic acid 10 mg (PO) q24h until cured
	C. neoformans	Treat the same as in chronic meningitis (see p. 21)
		PNEUMONIAS
Focal/ segmental/ nodular infiltrates *Acute*	Legionella	Treat the same as in normal hosts (see pp. 49–55)
Subacute	Aspergillus	<u>Preferred Therapy</u> Voriconazole (see "usual dose," p. 714) until cured*¶ **or** Lipid amphotericin (p. 525) (IV) q24h until cured **or** Amphotericin B 1–1.5 mg/kg (IV) q24h until 2–3 gm given <u>Alternate Therapy</u> Itraconazole 200 mg (IV) q12h × 2 days, then 200 mg (IV) q24h × 1–2 weeks, then 200 mg (PO) solution q12h until cured¶
	M. tuberculosis C. neoformans Nocardia	For TB (see p. 53). For C. neoformans (see p. 269). For Nocardia (see p. 268).
Diffuse infiltrates	S. stercoralis (hyperinfection syndrome)	<u>Preferred Therapy</u> Ivermectin 200 mcg/kg (PO) q24h until cured <u>Alternate Therapy</u> Thiabendazole 25–50 mg/kg (PO) q12h (max. 3 gm/day) until cured

Duration of therapy represents total time PO, IV, or IV + PO. Most patients on IV therapy able to take PO medications should be switched to PO therapy after clinical improvement.

*   If < 40 kg, use 100 mg (PO) maintenance dose.

¶   Significant drug interactions are possible with usual immunosuppressive agents (e.g., sirolimus, cyclosporine, tacrolimus). Review all concomitant medications for potential interactions. *Voriconazole contraindicated in patients on sirolimus.*

Transplant Infections (cont'd)

PNEUMONIAS (cont'd)		
	PCP/RSV	Treat the same as in other compromised hosts (see p. 325)
	CMV, HHV-6	Treat the same as CMV (see p. 55), HHV-6 (see p. 164)
HEPATITIS		
Viral hepatitis	CMV	Treat the same as for CMV pneumonia (see p. 55)
	HBV, HCV	Treat the same as in normal hosts (see pp. 97–98)

Bacteremia/Candidemia (Bacteremia)

Clinical Presentation: Fever and shaking chills ± localizing signs. If localizing signs are present, the organ involved indicates the origin of the bacteremia (e.g., urinary tract findings suggest urosepsis).

Diagnostic Considerations: Diagnosis is clinical and is confirmed by positive blood cultures.

Pitfalls: 3/4 or 4/4 positive blood cultures indicates bacteremia. Even 1/4 positive blood cultures of an unusual pathogen may be clinically significant in BMT/SOT. The significance of 1/4 blood cultures with coagulase-negative staphylococci is less clear. S. epidermidis bacteremia is usually IV-line related, but in some compromised hosts, it may be pathogenic without an IV line focus.

Therapeutic Considerations: In SOT, coverage should be directed against S. aureus and Enterobacteriaceae. Anti-P. aeruginosa coverage is usually not needed since these patients are not neutropenic. If the source of infection is a central IV line, the line should be removed. In pre-engraftment BMT, coverage should be directed against P. aeruginosa until leukopenia resolves. Continued fever after 1 week of appropriate antibiotic therapy suggests the presence of candidemia, or another invasive fungal infection.

Prognosis: Good with early antibiotic therapy and, if appropriate, IV line removal.

Bacteremia/Candidemia (Candidemia)

Clinical Presentation: Fever and shaking chills ± localizing signs. If localizing signs are present, the organ involved indicates the origin of the fungemia (e.g., reddened central IV line site suggests IV line-related fungemia).

Diagnostic Considerations: Candida and Fusarium are the most common fungi associated with fungemia in BMT/SOT.

Pitfalls: Do not assume that all Candida are C. albicans. Non-albicans Candida are more common in SOT patients. Empiric therapy should be directed against non-albicans Candida pending speciation, which will also cover C. albicans (including fluconazole-resistant strains). Because mortality/morbidity associated with candidemia exceeds that of bacteremia, empiric therapy should be started as soon as candidemia is suspected. Aspergillus, common after BMT/SOT, rarely grows in blood cultures.

Prognosis: Related to underlying immune status and promptness of empiric antifungal therapy, and if appropriate, CVC removal.

CNS Infections (Encephalitis/Meningitis)

Clinical Presentation: Typical encephalitis/meningitis presentation (fever, headache, ± stiff neck, change in mental status).

Diagnostic Considerations: CSF usually reveals a lymphocytic predominance with a normal or normal CSF lactic acid and low glucose. The diagnosis of HSV, CMV, HHV-6 encephalitis can be made by CSF PCR.

Pitfalls: Patients with Listeria encephalitis often have a negative CSF Gram stain, but Listeria nearly always grows on CSF culture. HSV and listeria encephalitis typically have RBCs in the CSF. Head CT/MRI rules out CNS mass lesions. Nuchal rigidity may be absent in meningitis.

Therapeutic Considerations: CMV encephalitis is rare but treatable, resulting in clinical/radiological improvement. However, neurological deficits usually remain. CMV retinitis, common in HIV (p. 327), is unusual in BMT/SOT.

Prognosis: Related to underlying immune status and promptness of therapy.

CNS Infections (Brain Abscess/Mass Lesions)

Clinical Presentation: BMT/SOT patients with brain abscesses/mass lesions present with seizures/cranial nerve abnormalities. Mental status is clear, in contrast to patients with encephalitis, and nuchal rigidity is absent, in contrast to most patients with meningitis.

Diagnostic Considerations: Head CT/MRI is the preferred diagnostic modality, and brain biopsy is the definitive diagnostic method. CSF analysis is not usually helpful in mass lesions, with the exception of infection due to M. tuberculosis or C. neoformans. With C. neoformans, the CSF cryptococcal antigen test is positive, and the CSF India ink preparation may be positive. With M. tuberculosis, acid fast smear of the CSF is sometimes positive, but culture has a higher yield and PCR is the preferred diagnostic modality.

Pitfalls: Patients with brain abscesses/mass lesions should have a head CT/MRI before lumbar puncture. To avoid herniation during lumbar puncture when a mass lesion is present, lumbar puncture should be performed by an experienced operator, and a minimal amount of CSF should be withdrawn.

Therapeutic Considerations: M. tuberculosis and C. neoformans are readily treatable. Be sure to use antimicrobial therapy that penetrates into CSF/brain. If TMP, TMP–SMX, or minocycline cannot be used for CNS Nocardia, linezolid or meropenem (meningeal doses) may be useful.

Prognosis: Related to underlying immune status and promptness of therapy.

Pneumonias (Focal, Segmental, or Nodular Pulmonary Infiltrates)

Clinical Presentation: Acute or subacute community-acquired pneumonia (CAP) with respiratory symptoms and fever.

Diagnostic Considerations: BMT/SOT patients with focal/segmental infiltrates are most commonly infected with the usual CAP pathogens affecting normal hosts (e.g., S. pneumoniae, H. influenzae, Legionella). The clinical presentation of CAP in organ transplants is indistinguishable from that in normal hosts. However, BMT/SOT patients presenting subacutely with focal/segmental infiltrates are usually infected with pulmonary pathogens with a slower clinical onset (e.g., Nocardia, Aspergillus). Empiric therapy will not cover all possible pathogens; tissue biopsy is necessary for definitive diagnosis and specific therapy. Preferred diagnostic modalities include transbronchial lung biopsy, percutaneous thin needle biopsy, or open lung biopsy, not BAL which may be negative in tissue invasive infections, e.g., Aspergillus.

Pitfalls: Patients presenting with subacute onset of CAP have a different pathogen distribution than those presenting with acute CAP. PCP/CMV does not present with focal/segmental infiltrates.

Therapeutic Considerations: BMT/SOT patients with acute onset of CAP are treated with the same antibiotics used to treat CAP in normal hosts. Empiric coverage is directed against both typical and atypical bacterial pathogens. If no improvement in clinical status after 72 hours, proceed to transbronchial biopsy or lung biopsy to identify nonbacterial pathogens (e.g., Nocardia, Aspergillus). Nocardia reinfection may require 6–12 months of therapy.

Prognosis: Best with acute focal/segmental infiltrates. Not as good with subacute or chronic focal/segmental infiltrates.

Pneumonias (Diffuse Pulmonary Infiltrates)

Clinical Presentation: Insidious onset of interstitial pneumonia usually accompanied by low-grade fevers. Focal/segmental infiltrates are absent.

Diagnostic Considerations: Bilateral diffuse infiltrates, which can be minimal or extensive, fall into two clinical categories: those with and without hypoxemia/↑ A-a gradient. Diffuse pulmonary infiltrates without hypoxemia suggest a noninfectious etiology (e.g., CHF, pulmonary drug reaction, pulmonary hemorrhage). The differential diagnosis of diffuse pulmonary infiltrates with hypoxemia includes PCP, CMV, HSV, RSV, HHV-6, VZV. Quantitative PCR testing of BAL fluid for CMV, VZV, RSV, HHV-6 may be diagnostically helpful. For interstitial infiltrates with hypoxemia, the chest x-ray may be only minimally abnormal, but chest CT scans are more revealing. CMV/PCP may require tissue biopsy for definitive diagnosis. A very highly elevated LDH suggests PCP. Transbronchial biopsy is preferable, but BAL may be used. The incidence of CMV pneumonia is highest in lung transplants and BMTs.

Pitfalls: Because infections in BMT/SOT are sequential, many patients with PCP pneumonia may have underlying CMV or HHV-6. In BMT, CMV found alone on lung biopsy suggests it is the primary pathogen. Serological tests are unhelpful for CMV; quantitative CMV PCR is preferred. Candida pneumonia does not exist as a separate entity but only as part of disseminated/invasive candidiasis.

Therapeutic Considerations: Among the subacute diffuse pneumonias, PCP is readily treatable. Initiate treatment for CMV pneumonia with ganciclovir IV; after clinical improvement, complete therapy with valganciclovir (PO) until cured. If after treatment, there is an ↑ in CMV antigen levels or quantitative PCR, treat pre-emptively to prevent CMV pneumonia with valganciclovir 900 mg (PO) q24h until CMV antigen levels return to previous levels or quantitative PCR becomes undetectable.

Prognosis: Related to underlying immune status, promptness of therapy, and general health of host.

Hepatitis (Viral)

Clinical Presentation: Fever with ↑ SGOT/SGPT ± RUQ pain.

Diagnostic Considerations: Because CMV is of such critical importance in BMT/SOT, CMV testing should always be done in organ transplants with ↑ SGOT/SGPT. Liver biopsy with immunohisto chemical staining is diagnostic; quantitative PCR may be helpful. Prior to SOT, HIV, HBV, HCV testing should be performed on donor and recipient. Other viruses causing acute viral hepatitis post-transplant include EBV, HHV-6, VZV, adenovirus, and influenza. Viral hepatitis is usually accompanied by some degree of leukopenia. A few atypical lymphocytes may be present, and serum transaminases may be mildly or markedly elevated. CMV viremia is the commonest manifestation of CMV infection in BMT/SOT patients. CMV has a predilection for infecting the organ transplanted, and CMV hepatitis is particularly common in liver transplants. Anicteric hepatitis is more common than icteric hepatitis.

Pitfalls: The diagnosis of active CMV hepatitis in organ transplant patients is critical because it is an immunomodulating virus, adding to the net immunosuppressive effect of immunosuppressive therapy. Do not rely on CMV IgM/IgG titers for diagnosis.

Therapeutic Considerations: CMV should be treated aggressively to minimize its potentiating immunoregulatory defects, which may predispose to non-viral opportunistic pathogens and ↑ risk of chronic rejection in SOT. CMV antigen levels or quantitative PCR increase before CMV infection. Therefore, when CMV antigen levels or quantitative PCR increase, begin early pre-emptive therapy with valganciclovir 900 mg (PO) q12h until CMV antigen levels or quantitative PCR return to previous levels. There is no treatment for EBV.

Prognosis: Treated early, CMV responds well to therapy. CMV is associated with chronic allograft rejection in SOT recipient so that prevention or early diagnosis/therapy are critical.

Toxin-Mediated Infectious Diseases

Toxin-Mediated Infectious Diseases

Subset	Usual Pathogens	IV Therapy	PO Therapy or IV-to-PO Switch
Toxic shock syndrome (TSS)* (Treat initially for MRSA; if later identified as MSSA, treat accordingly)	S. aureus (MRSA)	<u>Preferred IV Therapy</u> Vancomycin 1 gm (IV) q12h × 2 weeks **or** Linezolid 600 mg (IV) q12h × 2 weeks <u>Alternate IV Therapy</u> Minocycline 100 mg (IV) q12h × 2 weeks **or** Daptomycin 6 mg/kg (IV) q24h × 2 weeks	Linezolid 600 mg (PO) q12h × 2 weeks **or** Minocycline 100 mg (PO) q12h × 2 weeks
	S. aureus (MSSA)	<u>Preferred IV Therapy</u> Cefazolin 1 gm (IV) q8h × 2 weeks <u>Alternate IV Therapy</u> Nafcillin 2 gm (IV) q4h × 2 weeks **or** Clindamycin 600 mg (IV) q8h × 2 weeks	Cephalexin 500 mg (PO) q6h × 2 weeks **or** Clindamycin 300 mg (PO) q6h × 2 weeks
	Clostridium sordelli	<u>Preferred IV Therapy</u> Penicillin G 10 mu (IV) q4h × 2 weeks **or** Clindamycin 600 mg (IV) q8h × 2 weeks **or** Piperacillin 4 gm (IV) q8h × 2 weeks <u>Alternate IV Therapy</u> Meropenem 1 gm (IV) q8h × 2 weeks **or** Ertapenem 1 gm (IV) q24h × 2 weeks	Not applicable

MRSA/MSSA = methicillin-resistant/sensitive S. aureus. Duration of therapy represents total time IV, PO, or IV + PO. Most patients on IV therapy able to take PO meds should be switched to PO therapy after clinical improvement.
*   Treat only IV or IV-to-PO switch.

Toxin-Mediated Infectious Diseases (cont'd)

Subset	Usual Pathogens	IV Therapy	PO Therapy or IV-to-PO Switch
Botulism (food, infant, wound)	Clostridium botulinum	<u>Preferred Therapy</u> 2 vials of type-specific trivalent (types A,B,E) or polyvalent (types A,B,C,D,E) antitoxin (IV)	<u>Alternate Therapy</u> Amoxicillin 1 gm (PO) q8h × 7 days (wound botulism only)
Tetanus	Clostridium tetani	<u>Preferred Therapy</u> Tetanus immune globulin (TIG) 3,000–6,000 units (IM) (50% into deltoid, 50% into wound site) **plus either** Penicillin G 4 mu (IV) q4h × 10 days **or** Doxycycline 200 mg (IV or PO) q12h × 3 days, then 100 mg (IV or PO) × 7 days	<u>Alternate Therapy</u> Tetanus antitoxin 1,500–3,000 units (IM/IV) **plus** Metronidazole 1 gm (IV) q12h × 10 days
Diphtheria (pharyngeal, nasal, wound, myocarditis)	Coryne-bacterium diphtheriae C. ulcerans	Diphtheria antitoxin (IV) over 1 hour (pharyngeal diphtheria = 40,000 units; nasopharyngeal diphtheria = 60,000 units; systemic diphtheria or diphtheria > 3 days duration = 100,000 units) **plus either** Penicillin G 1 mu (IV) q4h × 14 days **or** Erythromycin 500 mg (IV) q6h × 14 days	Diphtheria antitoxin (IV) over 1 hour (pharyngeal diphtheria = 40,000 units; nasopharyngeal diphtheria = 60,000 units; systemic diphtheria or diphtheria > 3 days duration = 100,000 units) **plus** Procaine penicillin 600,000 units (IM) q24h × 14 days

Duration of therapy represents total time IV, PO, or IV + PO. Most patients on IV therapy able to take PO meds should be switched to PO therapy after clinical improvement.

Toxic Shock Syndrome (S. aureus)

Clinical Presentation: Scarlatiniform rash ± hypotension. Spectrum ranges from minimal infection to multiorgan system failure/shock. ↑ CPK common.

Diagnostic Considerations: Diagnosis by clinical presentation with mucous membrane, renal, liver, and skin involvement/culture of TSS-1 toxin-producing strain of S. aureus from mouth, nares, vagina, or wound.

Pitfalls: Toxic shock syndrome wound discharge is clear, not purulent.

Therapeutic Considerations: Remove source of toxin production if possible (e.g., remove tampon, drain collections). Clindamycin may be added for its anti-toxin effect.

Prognosis: Good in early/mild form. Poor in late/multisystem disease form.

Toxic Shock Syndrome (C. sordelli)

Clinical Presentation: Resembles clostridial myonecrosis (gas gangrene) with soft tissue necrotizing infection are local edema. Hypotension with acute onset of nausea/vomiting and weakness characteristic. Associated with IVDA (black tar heroin), trauma, parturition, abortion, cadaver graft surgery. Hemoconcentration with leukocytosis typical; leukemoid reactions common with WBC counts > 50k/mm^3.

Diagnostic Considerations: Clinical diagnosis. Culture of C. sordelli from necrotic soft tissue.

Pitfalls: Gas gangrene like clinical presentation but with hemoconcentration not hemolytic anemia. Nausea/vomiting instead of diarrhea as with gas gangrene. Shock with no/low fever and ↑ WBC should suggest the diagnosis. Muscle involvement (clostridial myonecrosis) and bullae typical of gas gangrene not a feature of C. sordelli TSS.

Therapeutic Considerations: Early/adequate debridement critical. Anti-anerobic antibiotics and supportive measures important.

Prognosis: Like gas gangrene, prognosis related to early diagnosis and early/adequate surgical debridement.

Botulism (Clostridium botulinum)

Clinical Presentation: Descending symmetrical paralysis beginning with cranial nerve involvement, induced by botulinum toxin. Onset begins with blurry vision, followed rapidly by ocular muscle paralysis, difficulty speaking, and inability to swallow. Respiratory paralysis may occur in severe cases. Mental status is unaffected. Usual incubation period is 10–12 hours. Incubation is shortest for Type E strain (hours), longest for Type A strain (up to 10 days), and is inversely proportional to the quantity of toxin consumed (food botulism). Wound botulism (Types A or B) may follow C. botulinum entry into IV drug abuser injection site, surgical or traumatic wounds. Infant (< 1 year) botulism (most commonly Type A or B) is acquired from C. botulinum containing honey. Patients with botulism are afebrile, and have profuse vomiting without diarrhea.

Diagnostic Considerations: Detection of botulinum toxin from stool, serum, or food (especially home canned foods with neutral or near neutral pH [~ 7] or smoked fish [Type E]) is diagnostic of food botulism. Wound botulism is diagnosed by culturing C. botulinum from the wound or by detecting botulinum toxin in the serum.

Pitfalls: Clinical diagnosis based on descending paralysis with cranial nerve involvement in an afebrile patient must be differentiated from Guillain-Barre (fever, ascending paralysis, sensory component) and polio (fever, pure ascending motor paralysis). Do not diagnose botulism in the absence of ocular/pharyngeal paralysis.

Therapeutic Considerations: Antitoxin neutralizes only unbound toxin, and does not reverse toxin-induced paralysis. Botulism is a toxin-mediated infection and antibiotic therapy (wound botulism) is adjunctive. Guanidine has been used with variable effect. Ventilator support is needed for respiratory paralysis. Bioterrorist botulism presents clinically and is treated the same as naturally-acquired botulism.

Prognosis: Good if treated early, before respiratory paralysis.

Tetanus (Clostridium tetani)

Clinical Presentation: Begins with jaw stiffness/difficulty chewing induced by C. tetani toxin (tetanospasmin). Trismus rapidly follows with masseter muscle spasm, followed by spasm of the abdominal/back muscles. Rigidity and convulsions may occur. Patients are afebrile unless there is hypothalamic involvement (central fever), in which case fevers may exceed 106°F. Usual incubation period is 3–21 days.

Diagnostic Considerations: Diagnosis suggested by muscle spasms/rigidity in a patient with trismus.

Pitfalls: In rabies, muscle spasms are localized and usually involve the face/neck, rather than primary involvement of the extremities, as in tetanus.

Therapeutic Considerations: Tetanus is self-limited with intensive supportive care. Sedation is important, and avoidance of all stimuli is mandatory to reduce the risk of convulsions. Avoid unnecessary handling/movement of patient. Antitoxin is effective only in neutralizing unbound toxin. Tracheostomy/respiratory support can be lifesaving in severe cases.

Prognosis: Good if not complicated by spinal fractures, aspiration pneumonia, or CNS involvement (hyperpyrexia, hyper/hypotension).

Diphtheria (Corynebacterium diphtheriae/Corynebacterium ulcerans)

Clinical Presentation: Within 1 week following insidious onset of sore throat without fever, pharyngeal patches coalesce to form a gray diphtheric membrane (surrounded by a red border), which is adherent/bleeds easily when removed. Membrane begins unilaterally; may extend to the soft palate, uvula and contralateral posterior pharynx; are accompanied by prominent bilateral anterior adenopathy; become necrotic (green/black); and have a foul odor (fetor oris). Submandibular edema ("bull neck") and hoarseness (laryngeal stridor) precede respiratory obstruction/death. Cutaneous diphtheria may follow C. diphtheriae contaminated wounds (traumatic, surgical) or insect/human bites, and is characterized by a leathery eschar (cutaneous membrane) covering a deep punched out ulcer. Serosanguineous discharge is typical of nasal diphtheria (membrane in nares). Diphtheric myocarditis may complicate any form of diphtheria (most commonly follows pharyngeal form), and usually occurs in the second week, but may occur up to 8 weeks after infection begins. Diphtheric polyneuritis is a common complication. Cardiac/neurologic complications are due to elaboration of a potent toxin.

Diagnostic Considerations: Diagnosis is suggested by unilateral membranous pharyngitis/palatal paralysis, absence of fever, and relative tachycardia. Diagnosis is confirmed by culture of C. diphtheriae from nares, membrane, or wound.

Pitfalls: Differentiated from Arcanobacterium (Corynebacterium) haemolyticum (which also forms a pharyngeal membrane) by culture and absence of scarlatiniform rash with C. diphtheriae. C.ulcerans has the same clinical features as C. diphtheriae.

Therapeutic Considerations: Antibiotic therapy treats the infection and stops additional toxin production. Antitoxin is effective against unbound toxin, but will not reverse toxin-mediated myocarditis/neuropathy. Serum sickness is common 2 weeks after antitoxin. Respiratory/cardiac support may be lifesaving. C.ulcerans is treated the same as C. diptheriae.

Prognosis: Poor with airway obstruction or myocarditis. Myocarditis may occur despite early treatment.

Bioterrorist Agents

Bioterrorist Agents in Adults[¶]

Subset	Pathogen	IV/IM Therapy	IV-to-PO Switch
Anthrax *Inhalation, oropharyngeal, gastrointestinal*	Bacillus anthracis	Quinolone* (IV) × 2 weeks **or** Doxycycline 200 mg (IV) q12h × 3 days, then 100 mg (IV) q12h × 11 days[‡] **or** Penicillin G 4 MU (IV) q4h ± clindamycin 600 mg (IV) q8h × 2 weeks	Quinolone* (PO) × 2 weeks **or** Doxycycline 200 mg (PO) q12h × 3 days, then 100 mg (PO) q12h × 11 days (loading dose not needed PO if given IV). Duration of IV + PO therapy = 60 days
Cutaneous		Treat severe cases with same (PO) antibiotics as for inhalation anthrax	
Meningitis		If penicillin susceptible, treat with Penicillin G4 MU (IV) q24h **or** Meropenem 2 gm (IV) q8h for at least 2 weeks or markedly improved and complete 60–100 days of therapy as described in the inhalation, oropharyngeal or gastrointestinal forms, in addition to quinolones or doxycycline. Consider adjunctive steroid therapy. Penicillin should NOT be used as a single agent. Not susceptible to cephalosporins or TMP–SMX.	
Tularemia pneumonia	Francisella tularensis	Streptomycin 1 gm (IM) q12h × 10 days **or** Gentamicin 5 mg/kg (IM or IV) q24h × 10 days **or** Doxycycline 200 mg (IV) q12h × 3 days, then 100 mg (IV) q12h × 11–18 days[‡] **or** Chloramphenicol 500 mg (IV) q6h × 14 days **or** Quinolone* (IV) × 10 days <u>If meningitis:</u> add chloramphenicol	Doxycycline 200 mg (PO) q12h × 3 days, then 100 mg (PO) q12h × 11–18 days (loading dose not needed PO if given IV) **or** Quinolone* (PO) × 10 days <u>If meningitis:</u> add chloramphenicol

Duration of therapy represents total treatment time.

[‡] Patients who remain critically ill after Doxycycline 200 mg (IV) q12h × 3 days should continue receiving 200 mg (IV) q12h for the full course of therapy. For patients who have improved after 3 days, the dose may be decreased to 100 mg (IV or PO) q12h to complete the course of therapy. Total duration of IV + PO therapy = 60 days.

* Ciprofloxacin 400 mg (IV) q12h or 500 mg (PO) q12h or Levofloxacin 500 mg (IV or PO) q24h.

[¶] Additional information can be obtained at www.bt.cdc.gov. For post-exposure prophylaxis, see p. 358.

Bioterrorist Agents in Adults¶ (cont'd)

Subset	Pathogen	IV/IM Therapy	IV-to-PO Switch
Pneumonic plague	Yersinia pestis	Treat the same as tularemic pneumonia (see p. 176)	
Botulism	Clostridium botulinum	Contrary to the package insert, administer 50 mg/kg up to 1 vial of type-specific trivalent (types A,B,E) or polyvalent (types A,B,C,D,E) antitoxin (IV) after skin testing. Antitoxin administration is not repeated (circulating antitoxin's half-life = 5–8 days). Treatment with 1 vial resulted in adverse effects in < 1%; treatment with 2–4 times present dose resulted in hypersensitivity reactions in 9%. Antibiotics do not neutralize toxin	
Smallpox	Variola virus	Smallpox vaccine ≤ 4 days after exposure. Cidofovir 5 mg/kg (IV) × 1 dose may be protective for up to 6 days post-exposure.	
Ebola	Ebola virus	No specific therapy. Supportive therapy can be life saving	

Duration of therapy represents total treatment time.

* Ciprofloxacin 400 mg (IV) q12h or 500 mg (PO) q12h or Levofloxacin 500 mg (IV or PO) q24h.

¶ Additional information can be obtained at www.bt.cdc.gov. For post-exposure prophylaxis, see p. 358.

‡ Patients who remain critically ill after Doxycycline 200 mg (IV) q12h × 3 days should continue receiving 200 mg (IV) q12h for the full course of therapy. For patients who have improved after 3 days, the dose may be decreased to 100 mg (IV or PO) q12h to complete the course of therapy. Total duration of IV + PO therapy = 60 days.

Anthrax (B. anthracis)

Clinical Presentation: Bioterrorist anthrax usually presents as cutaneous or inhalational anthrax. Cutaneous anthrax has the same clinical presentation as naturally-acquired anthrax: Lesions begin as painless, sometimes mildly pruritic papules, usually on the upper extremities, neck, or face, and evolve into a vesicular lesion which may be surrounded by satellite lesions. A "gelatinous halo" surrounds the vesicle as it evolves into an ulcer, and a black eschar eventually develops over the ulcer. Inhalational anthrax is a biphasic illness. Initially, there is a viral illness-like prodrome with fever, chills, and myalgias with chest discomfort 3–5 days after inhaling anthrax spores. Bacteremia is common. Patients often improve somewhat over the next 1–2 days, only to rapidly deteriorate and become critically ill with high fevers, dyspnea, cyanosis, crushing substernal chest pain, and shock. Oropharyngeal anthrax presents with fever, soft tissue edema, painful cervical adenopathy. Lesions in oropharynx ulcerate in ~ 2 weeks. GI anthrax presents with fever, malaise ± syncope, followed in 24 hours by mild nausea/vomiting, severe abdominal pain, and then ascites, ↑ abdominal pain, flushed face, and shock.

Diagnostic Considerations: Cutaneous anthrax is a clinical diagnosis suggested by the lack of pain relative to the size of the lesion. A presumptive microbiologic diagnosis is made by finding gram-positive bacilli in the fluid from the gelatinous halo surrounding the ulcer or from under the eschar. Blood cultures may reveal B. anthracis. Definitive diagnosis depends on identifying B. anthracis from culture of the skin lesions or blood cultures. Inhalation anthrax is suspected in patients with fevers, chest pain, and mediastinal widening accompanied by bilateral pleural effusions on chest x-ray. If chest x-ray findings are equivocal, then a chest CT/MRI is recommended to demonstrate mediastinal lymph node enlargement. Inhalational anthrax presents as a hemorrhagic mediastinitis, not community-acquired pneumonia. The diagnosis is clinical but supported by Gram stain of hemorrhagic pleural fluid demonstrating gram-positive bacilli. Patients with inhalational anthrax often have positive blood cultures and may have associated anthrax meningitis. If meningitis is present, the CSF is hemorrhagic and CSF Gram stain shows gram-positive bacilli, which, when cultured, is B. anthracis.

Pitfalls: Cutaneous anthrax is most often initially confused with ringworm or a brown recluse spider bite. Subacute/chronic lesions may initially resemble ringworm, but the skin lesion in ringworm has an annular configuration, is painless, and is accompanied by prominent pruritus, particularly at the edges of the lesion. Patients with ringworm have no fever or systemic symptoms. Brown recluse spider bites produce extremely painful lesions with irregular edges, which eventually develop a necrotic center followed by eschar formation. The lesions of the brown recluse spider bite are irregular, not accompanied by fever, and intensely painful. In contrast, cutaneous anthrax lesions are painless, round, and are not primarily pruritic in nature. Be alert to the possibility of smallpox following outbreaks of other bioterrorist agents such as anthrax, as the genome of smallpox is easily modified and can be incorporated into bacteria.

Therapeutic Considerations: B. anthracis is highly susceptible to nearly all antibiotics; in the U.S. bioterrorist experience, no strains were resistant to antibiotics. Traditionally, penicillin has been used to treat natural anthrax, but because of concern for resistant bioterrorist strains, doxycycline or quinolones are preferred. Because meningitis is frequently associated with inhalational anthrax, penicillin in (IV) meningeal doses may be added as a second or third antibiotic to quinolones or doxycycline. For meningeal anthrax use penicillin G or meropenem in meningeal doses. Clindamycin is active against B. anthracis and has been used in combination therapy because of its potential anti-exotoxin activity. Some patients seemed to respond somewhat better when clindamycin 600 mg (IV) q8h or 300 mg (PO) q8h plus rifampin 300 mg (PO) q12h is added to either a quinolone or doxycycline. Corticosteroids should be considered for severe mediastinal edema or meningitis. Depending upon antimicrobial susceptibility testing, rifampin, vancomycin, penicillin, ampicillin, chloramphenicol, imipenem, clindamycin or clarithromycin may be added if the need arises. Prolonged therapy of 100 days with or without anthrax vaccine has been recommended by some authors. Three doses of anthrax vaccine (BioThraxT, formerly AVA - anthrax vaccine absorbed) have been recommended by the ACIP and the John Hopkins Working Group on Civilian Bio-Defense with antimicrobials for prophylaxis after aerosolized exposure, but as it is not licensed, it must be administered under an IND application. Some B. anthracis strains produce cephalosporinase and inducible beta-lactamase that make penicillins drugs less suitable for initial therapy. In general, the organism is resistant to trimethoprim-sulfamethoxazole.

Prognosis: Prognosis of cutaneous anthrax is uniformly good. With inhalational anthrax, prognosis is related to the inhaled dose of the organism, underlying host status, and rapidity of initiating antimicrobial therapy. Inhalational anthrax remains a highly lethal infectious disease, but with early intervention/supportive care, some patients survive. Patients with associated anthrax meningitis have a poor prognosis.

Tularemic Pneumonia (F. tularensis)

Clinical Presentation: Fever, chills, myalgias, headache, dyspnea and a nonproductive cough may occur, but encephalopathy is absent. Chest x-ray resembles other causes of community-acquired pneumonia, but tularemic pneumonia is usually accompanied by hilar adenopathy and pleural effusion, which is serosanguineous or frankly bloody. Cavitation sometimes occurs. Relative bradycardia is not present and serum transaminases are not elevated.

Diagnostic Considerations: Tularemic pneumonia can resemble other atypical pneumonias, but in a patient presenting with community-acquired pneumonia, the presence of hilar adenopathy with pleural effusions should suggest the diagnosis. F. tularensis may be seen in the Gram stain of the sputum or bloody pleural effusion fluid as a small, bipolar staining, gram-negative bacillus. Diagnosis is confirmed serologically or by culture of the organism from respiratory fluid/blood.

Pitfalls: Gram-negative bacilli in the sputum may resemble Y. pestis but are not bipolar staining. Chest x-ray may resemble inhalational anthrax (hilar adenopathy/mediastinal widening). Both tularemic pneumonia and inhalational anthrax may be accompanied by bloody pleural effusions. In contrast to inhalational anthrax (which may be accompanied by anthrax meningitis), CNS involvement is not a feature of tularemic pneumonia.

Therapeutic Considerations: Streptomycin is the antibiotic traditionally used to treat tularemia. Gentamicin may be substituted for streptomycin if it is not available. Doxycycline, chloramphenicol, or a quinolone are also effective.

Prognosis: Depends on inoculum size and health of host. Mortality rates for severe untreated infection can be as high as 30%, although early treatment is associated with mortality rates < 1%.

Pneumonic Plague (Y. pestis)

Clinical Presentation: Bioterrorist plague presents as pneumonic plague and has the potential for person-to-person spread. After an incubation period of 1–4 days, the patient presents with acute onset of fever, chills, headache, myalgias and dizziness, followed by pulmonary manifestations including cough, chest pain, dyspnea. Hemoptysis may occur, and increasing respiratory distress and circulatory collapse are common. Compared to community-acquired pneumonia, patients presenting with plague pneumonia are critically ill. Sputum is pink and frothy and contains abundant bipolar staining gram-negative bacilli. Chest x-ray is not diagnostic.

Diagnostic Considerations: Yersinia pestis may be demonstrated in sputum Gram stain (bipolar staining gram-negative bacilli) and may be recovered from blood cultures. Laboratory confirmation requires isolation of Y. pestis from body fluid or tissue culture. Consider the diagnosis in any critically ill patient with pneumonia and bipolar staining gram-negative bacilli in the sputum.

Pitfalls: Plague pneumonia can resemble tularemic pneumonia, but there are several distinguishing features. Unlike plague, tularemic pneumonia is usually associated with hilar enlargement and pleural effusion. Although gram-negative bacilli may be present in the sputum of patients with tularemia, the organisms are not bipolar staining.

Therapeutic Considerations: Streptomycin is the preferred drug for pneumonic plague. Doxycycline or a quinolone is also effective.

Prognosis: Depends on inoculum size, health of the host, and the rapidity of treatment. Left untreated, mortality rates exceed 50%. ARDS, DIC, and other manifestations of gram-negative sepsis are more common when treatment is delayed.

Botulism (C. botulinum) (see p. 171)

Smallpox
Clinical Presentation: After an incubation period of 1–12 days, typical smallpox is heralded by high fever, headache, and gastrointestinal complaints (vomiting, colicky pain). No rash is present at this time. After 1–2 days, the fever decreases to near normal level, and macules begin to appear on the head, usually at the hairline. Macules progress to papules, then vesicles, then finally pustules. The rash begins on the face/head and rapidly spreads to the extremities with relative sparing of the trunk. The mucous membranes of the oropharynx and upper/lower airways are also affected early. Lesions initially are umbilicated, then later lose their umbilication. The fully formed smallpox pustule is located deep in the dermis. The appearance of the pustules is accompanied by recrudescence of fever. Hemorrhagic smallpox is a fulminant form of smallpox that begins with petechial lesions in a "swimming trunk" distribution and results in widespread hemorrhage into the skin and mucous membranes. Patients look toxemic and have high fevers with no other signs of smallpox; death from toxemia often occurs before the typical rash appears.

Diagnostic Considerations: Smallpox is most likely to be confused with chickenpox or drug eruptions. Patients with chickenpox are less toxemic and the lesion distribution is different from smallpox. Chickenpox lesions occur in crops for the first 72 hours, then stop. The lesions of chickenpox are superficial, not deep in the dermis like smallpox, and chickenpox vesicles are predominantly centripetal rather than centrifugal. The chickenpox vesicle has been described as a "dewdrop on a rose petal" because of its fragility and superficial location on the skin. If there is any doubt, a Tzanck test should be performed by unroofing the vesicle, scraping cells from the base of the vesicle, and staining the cells. A positive Tzanck test indicates chickenpox, not smallpox. Alternatively, a monoclonal VZV test can be performed on vesicle base cells. Drug eruptions are not accompanied by toxemia and are usually accompanied by relative bradycardia if fever is present.

Pitfalls: Smallpox is easily missed before the rash and is difficult to diagnose. Look for the combination of high fever/headache with gastrointestinal symptoms (e.g., abdominal pain) that precedes the rash. GI complaints may be confused with appendicitis. A petechial rash in a swimming trunk distribution does not occur with any other infectious disease and should immediately suggest smallpox. Recently human monkeypox has occurred in the Western Hemisphere after transmission via imported African rodent pets. After an incubation period of 7–19 days, patients develop fever, headache, and malaise. Skin lesions appear on head, trunk, and extremities (including palms/soles). Rash begins like smallpox as macules, then papules, and finally umbilicated vesicles. Some exudative pharyngitis/tonsillitis with cervical adenopathy may be present. Encephalitis is very rare. Laboratory results are nonspecific. Unlike smallpox, human monkeypox patients are not toxic, have pharyngitis/tonsillitis with cervical adenopathy, and have focal hemorrhage into some lesions (in hemorrhagic smallpox, hemorrhages are extensive/widespread). Patients immunized against smallpox are unlikely to acquire human monkeypox.

Therapeutic Considerations: Smallpox vaccination should be initiated as soon as the diagnosis is suspected. Smallpox vaccine may be given at full strength or in a 1:5 dilution, which is also protective. Cidofovir may prove useful but dose for smallpox is not established.

Prognosis: Variable in typical smallpox, with deep, permanent scarring, especially on the face. Hemorrhagic smallpox is highly lethal.

Ebola/Lassa Fever

Clinical Presentation: After an incubation period of 3–9 days, abrupt onset of high fevers, severe headache/myalgias followed by diarrhea, extreme malaise. Hemorrhagic phenomenon–GI, renal, vaginal, conjunctival bleeding-occur at 5–7 days. Patients rapidly become critically ill. Fever is biphasic. Patients usually have leukopenia, thrombocytopenia, and hepatic/renal dysfunction. Conjunctival suffusion is also an early finding in half the cases. If a patient is not a traveler from an endemic area (e.g., Africa), suspect bioterrorist Ebola/Lassa fever. Lassa fever differs from Ebola in having prominent head/neck edema. CNS finding (oculogyric crisis, seizures, deafness) are characteristic of Lassa fever.

Diagnostic Considerations: Ebola is a hemorrhagic fever clinically indistinguishable from Yellow fever and other African hemorrhagic fevers (e.g., Lassa fever, Marburg virus disease). Presumptive diagnosis is clinical; definitive diagnosis is confirmed by specific virologic/serologic studies.

Pitfalls: Patients with Ebola may complain initially of a sore throat and dry cough, with or without chest pain. Diarrhea/abdominal pain is not uncommon. The rash is maculopapular before it becomes hemorrhagic. Failure to consider the diagnosis may occur early when sore throat/GI symptoms are prominent (i.e., before hemorrhagic manifestations appear).

Therapeutic Considerations: There is no effective therapy available for Ebola infection. Supportive therapy can be life saving.

Prognosis: Varies with severity of infection and health of the host.

REFERENCES AND SUGGESTED READINGS

Azad AF. Pathogenic rickettsiae as bioterrorism agents. Clin Infec Dis 45 Suppl 1:S52–S55, 2007.

Alvarez-Lerma F, Grau S, Alvarez-Beltran. Levofloxacin in the treatment of ventilator-associated pneumonia. Clin Microbiol Infect 12:81–92, 2006.

Baddour LM, Bettmann MA, Bolger AF, et al. Nonvascular cardiovascular device-related infections. Circulation 108:2015–2031, 2003.

Bartlett JG, Inglesby TV, JR, Bono L. Management of anthrax. Clin Infect Dis 35:851–858, 2002.

Bouza E, Burillo A, Munoz P. Antimicrobial Therapy of Clostridium difficile-associated diarrhea. Med Clin N Am 90:1141–63, 2006.

Boyce JM. Methicillin-resistant Staphylococcus aureus. Lancet Infect Dis 5:653–663, 2005.

Bradley SF. Infections in long-term-care residents. Infect Med 22:168–172, 2005.

Bratu S. Therapeutic approach to complicated skin and soft tissue infections: methicillin-susceptible and methicillin-resistant Staphylococcus aureus. Antibiotics for Clinicians 10:S35–28, 2006.

Breman JG, Henderson DA. Diagnosis and management of smallpox. N Engl J Med 346:1300–1308, 2002.

Carratala J, Martin-Herrero JE, Mykietiuk A, et al. Clinical experience in the management of community-acquired pneumonia: lessons from the use of fluoroquinolones. Clin Microbiol Infect 12:2–11, 2006.

Castro P, Soriano A, Escrich C, et al. Linezolid treatment of ventriculoperitoneal shunt infection without implant removal. Eur J Clin Microbiol Infect Dis 24:603–06, 2005.

Celebi G, Baruonu F, Ayoglu F, et al. Tularemia, a reemerging disease in northwest Turkey: epidemiological investigation and evaluation of treatment responses. Jpn J Infect Dis 59:229–234, 2006.

Centers for Disease Control. Anthrax: preventive therapy. Downloaded from http://www/bt.cdc.gov/ agent/anthrax/ faq/preventive.asp, 2006.

Centers for Disease Control. Consensus statement: tularemia as a biological weapon: medical and public health management http://www.bt.cec.gov/agent/ tularemia/tularemia-biological-weapon-abstract.asp, 2006.

Chastre J, Wolff M, Fagon JY, et al. Comparison of 8 vs 15 days of antibiotic therapy for ventilator-associated pneumonia in adults. JAMA 290:2588–2598, 2003.

Chen XM, Leithly JS, Paya CV, et al. Cryptosporidiosis. N Engl J Med 346:1723–1731, 2002.

Chiou CC, Does penicillin remain the drug of choice for pneumococcal pneumonia in view of emerging in vitro resistance? Clin Infect Dis 42:234–7, 2006.

Collins J, Ali-Ibrahim A, Smoot DT. Antibiotic therapy for Helicobacter pylori. Med Clin N Am 90:1125–40, 2006.

Cono J, Craga JD, Jamieson DJ, et al. Prophylaxis and treatment of pregnant women for emerging infections and bioterrorism emergencies. Emerg Infect Dis 12:1631–1637, 2006.

Cunha BA. Antibiotic selection in the penicillin-allergic patient. Med Clin North Am 90:1257–64, 2006.

Cunha BA. Antimicrobial therapy of multidrug-resistant Streptococcus pneumoniae, vancomycin-resistant enterococci, and methicillin-resistant Staphylococcus aureus. Med Clin North Am 90:1165–82, 2006.

Cunha BA. The atypical pneumonias: clinical diagnosis and importance. Clin Microbiol Infect 12:12–4, 2006.

Cunha BA. Oral antibiotic therapy of serious systemic infections. Med Clin North Am 90:1197–222, 2006.

Cunha BA. Persistent S. aureus bacteremia: Clinical Pathway for diagnosis and treatment. Antibiotics for Clinicians 10:S39–46, 2006.

Cunha BA. Staphylococcal aureus acute bacterial endocarditis (ABE): clinical pathway for diagnosis and treatment. Antibiotics for Clinicians 10:S29–33, 2006.

Cunha BA. Ventilator-associated pneumonia: monotherapy is optimal if chosen wisely. Crit Care 10:141, 2006.

Cunha BA. Herpes Simplex-1 (HSV-1) pneumonia. Infect Dis Practice 29:375–78, 2005.

Cunha BA. Malaria vs. Typhoid fever: a diagnostic dilemma? Am J of Med 118:1442–43, 2005.

Cunha BA. Methicillin-resistant Staphylococcus aureus: clinical manifestations and antimicrobial therapy. Clin Microbiol Infect 11:33–42, 2005.

Cunha BA. Pseudomonas aeruginosa: resistance and therapy. Semin Respir Infect 17:231–9, 2002.

Cunha BA. Clinical relevance of penicillin-resistant Streptococcus pneumoniae. Semin Respir Infect 17:204–14, 2002.

Cunha BA. Smallpox: An Oslerian primer. Infectious Disease Practice 26:141–148, 2002.

Cunha BA. Osteomyelitis in the elderly. Clin Infect Dis 35:287–273, 2002.

Cunha BA. Bioterrorism in the emergency room: Anthrax, tularemia, plague, ebola and smallpox. Clinical Microbiology & Infection 8:489–503, 2002.

Cunha BA. Central nervous system infections in the compromised host. A diagnostic approach. Infect Dis Clin 15:67–590, 2001.

Cunha BA. Effective antibiotic resistance and control strategies. Lancet 357:1307–1308, 2001.

Cunha BA. Nosocomial pneumonia: Diagnostic and therapeutic considerations. Medical Clinics of North America 85:79–114, 2001.

Cunha BA. Community acquired pneumonia: diagnostic and therapeutic considerations. Medical Clinics of North America 85:43–77, 2001.

Cunha BA. Pneumonias in the compromised host. Infect Dis Clin 15:591–612, 2001.

Cunha BA. Community-acquired pneumonias re-revisited. Am J Med 108:436–437, 2000.

Daver NG, Shelburne SA, Atmar RL, et al. Oral step-down therapy is comparable to intravenous therapy for Staphylococcus aureus osteomyelitis. Journal of Infection 54:539–544, 2007.

Demirturk N, Usluer G, Ozgunes I, et al. Comparison of different treatment combinations for chronic hepatitis B infection. J Chemother 14:285–9, 2002.

DiBisceglie AM. Combination therapy for hepatitis B. Gut 50:443–5, 2002.

Eckburg PB, Schneider JJ, Renault CA. Avian influenza in humans: A practical review for clinicians. Infect Med 22:535–542, 2005.

Ferrer M, Liapikou A, Valencia M, et al. Validation of the American Thoracic Society-Infectious Diseases Society of America Guidelines for hospital-acquired pneumonia in the intensive care unit. Clin Infect. Dis. 50:945–952, 2010.

Fihn SD. Acute uncomplicated urinary tract infection in women. N Engl J Med 349:259–66, 2003.

File TM Jr. Community-acquired pneumonia. Lancet 362:1991–2001, 2003.

Fishbain J, Peleg AY. Treatment of Acinetobacter Infections. Clin Infect. Dis. 51:79–84, 2010.

Fishman, JA. Infection in solid-organ transplant recipients. N Engl J Med 357:2601–2614, 2007.

Frieden TR, Sterling TR, Munsiff SS, et al. Tuberculosis. Lancet 362:887–99, 2003.

Furin J, Nardell EA. Multidrug-resistant tuberculosis: An update on the best regimens. J Respir Dis 27:172–82, 2006.

Gagliotti C, Nobilio L, Milandri M, et al. Macrolide prescriptions and erythromycin resistance for Streptococcus pyogenes. Clin Infect Dis 42:1153–6, 2006.

Giamarellou H, Treatment options for multidrug-resistant bacteria. Anti Infect Ther 4:601–18, 2006.

Gomes CC, Vormittag E, Santos CR, Levin AS. Nosocomial infection with cefalosporin-resistant Klebsiella pneumoniae Is not associated with increased mortality. Infect Control and Hosp Epidemiol 27:907–12, 2006.

Gould IM. The clinical significance of methicillin-resistant Staphylococcus aureus. J Hosp Infect 61:277–282, 2005.

Grabenstein JD. Vaccines: Countering anthrax: vaccines and immunoglobulins. Clin Infect Dis 46:129–136, 2008.

Gupta R, Warren T, Wald A. Genital herpes. Lancet 370:2127–2137, 2007.

Haque NZ, Zervos MJ. Vancomycin-Resistant Enterococcal Infections: clinical manifestations and Management. Infections in Medicine 23:14–19, 2006.

Hayakawa K, Nakagawa K. Treatment of infected total knee arthroplasty. Infect Diseases in Clin Practice 14:211–215, 2006.

Heldman AW, Hartert TV, Ray SC, et al. Oral antibiotic treatment of right-sided staphylococcal endocarditis in injection drug users: prospective randomized comparison with parenteral therapy. Am J Med 101: 68–76, 1996.

Hotchkiss RS, Karl IE. The pathophysiology and treatment of sepsis. N Engl J Med 348:138–50, 2003.

Huang H, Flynn NM, King JH, et al. Comparisons of community-associated methicillin-resistant Staphylococcus aureus (MRSA) and hospital-associated MSRA infections in Sacramento, California. Journal of Clinical Microbiology. 44:2423–28, 2006.

Johnson DH, Cunha BA. Infections in alcoholic cirrhosis. Infectious Disease Clinics 16:363–372, 2001.

Johnson LB, Saravolatz LD. Community-acquired MRSA: current epidemiology and management issues. Infections in Medicine 23:6–10, 2006.

Joseph SM, Peiris MD, D. Phil et al. The severe acute respiratory syndrome. N Engl J Med 349:2431–41, 2003.

Kallen AJ, Mu Y, Bulens S, et al. Health care-associated invasive MRSA infections, 2005–2008. JAMA 304: 641–648, 2010.

Kanafani ZA, Khalife N, Kanj SS, Araj GF, Khalifeh M, Sharara AI. Antibiotic use in acute cholecystitis: practice patterns in the absence of evidence-based guidelines. J Infect 51:128–134, 2005.

Kauffman CA. Endemic mycoses in patients with hematologic malignancies. Semin Respir Infect 17:106–12, 2002.

Kauffman CA. Managing fungal pneumonias: a review of the new therapies. J Crit Illness 20:30–35, 2005.

Kawai N, Idematsu H, Iwaki N, et al. Comparisons of the effectiveness of zanamivir and oseltamivir against influenza A/H₁N₁, A/H3N2, and B. Clin Infect Dis 48:996–99, 2009.

Khardori N, Kanchanapoom T. Overview of biological terrorism: Potential agents and preparedness. Clin Microbiol News 27:1, 2005.

Kim AI, Saab S. Treatment of hepatitis C. Am J Med 118:808–815, 2005.

Kimberlin DW, Rouse DJ. Genital herpes. N Engl J Med 350:1970–7, 2004.

Lai CL, Ratziu V, Yuen MF, et al. Viral hepatitis B. Lancet 362:2089–94, 2003.

Lamas C. Diagnostic strategy for blood culture-negative endocarditis. Clin Infect. Dis. 51:141–142, 2010.

Leather HL, Wingard JR. Infections following hematopoietic stem cell transplantation. Infect Dis Clin North Am 15:483–520, 2001.

Linden PK. Treatment options for vancomycin-resistant enterococcal infections. Drugs 62: 425–41, 2002.

Lipsky BA, Berendt AR, Deery HG, et al. Diagnosis and Treatment of Diabetic Foot Infections. Clin Infect Dis 39:885–910, 2004.

Lipsky BA, Byren I, Hoey CT. Treatment of bacterial prostatitis. Clin Infect Dis. 50:1641–1652, 2010.

Loddenkemper R, Sagebiel D, Brendel A. Strategies against multidrug-resistant tuberculosis. Eur Respir J Suppl 36:66s-77s, 2002.

Lok AS. Chronic hepatitis B. N Engl J Med 346:1682–3, 2002.

Lok AS, MacMahon BJ. Chronic hepatitis B. Hepatology 45:507–539, 2007.

Maartens G, Wilinson RJ. Tuberculosis. Lancet 370:2030–2043, 2007.

Martin SS, Hollingsworth CL, Norfolk SG, et al. Reversible cardiac dysfunction associated with pandemic 2009 influenza A (H1N1). Chest. 137:1195–1997, 2010.

McLaughlin SP, Carson CC. Urinary tract infections in women. Med Clin North Am 88:417–29, 2004.

Meddings J, Rogers MAM, Macy M, et al. Systematic review and meta-analysis: reminder systems to reduced catheter-associated urinary tract infections and urinary catheter use in hospitalized patients. Clin Infect Dis. 51:550–560, 2010.

Mermel LA. What is the Predominant Source of Intravascular Catheter Infections? Clin Infect Dis 52:211–212, 2011.

Metlay JP, Fishman NO, Joffe MM, et al. Macrolide resistance in adults with bacteremic pneumococcal pneumonia. Emerging Infect Dis 12:1223–30, 2006.

Michalopoulos A, Falagas ME. Treatment of Acinetobacter infections. Expert Opin Pharmacotherapy. 11:779–788, 2010.

Minnaganti V, Cunha BA. Infections associated with uremia and dialysis. Infect Dis Clin 16:385–406, 2001.

Musher DM, Musher BJ. Contagious acute gastrointestinal infections. N Engl J Med 351:2417–27, 2004.

Musher DM, Aslam S, Logan N, et al. Relatively poor outcome after treatment of Clostridium difficile colitis with metronidazole. Clin Infect Dis 40:1586–1590, 2005.

Mylonakis E, Calderwood SB. Infective endocarditis in adults. N Engl J Med 345:1318, 2001.

Nicholson KG, Wood JM, Zambon M. Influenza. Lancet 362:1733–45, 2003.

Nucci M, Anaissie E, Betts RF, et al. Early removal of central venous catheter in patients with candidemia does not improve outcome: analysis of 842 patients from 2 randomized clinical trials. Clin Infect. Dis. 51:295–303, 2010.

Parry CM, Hien TT, Dougan G, et al. Typhoid fever. N Engl J Med 347:1770–82, 2002.

Peipert JF. Genital Chlamydial Infections. N Engl J Med 349:2424–30, 2003.

Perea S, Patterson TF. Invasive Aspergillus infections in hematologic malignancy patients. Semin Respir Infect 17:99–105, 2002.

Perencevich EN, Diekema DJ. Decline in invasive MRSA infection. where to go from here? JAMA 304: 687–689, 2010.

Peterson LR. Penicillin for treatment of pneumococcal pneumonia: does In vitro resistance really matter? Clin Infect Dis 42:224–33, 2006.

Piccirillo JF. Acute bacterial sinusitis. N Engl J Med 351:902–10, 2004.

Razonable RR. Management of cytomegalovirus infection after renal transplantation. Infect Dis in Clinical Practice 17:220–230, 2009.

Relman DA. Bioterrorism preparedness: what practitioners need to know. Infect Med 18:497–515, 2001.

Rex JH. Approach to the treatment of systemic fungal infectious. In: Kelley WN (ed), Kelley's Textbook of Internal Medicine, 4th ed., 2279–2281, 2000.

Rodriguez-Bano J. Selection of empiric therapy in patients with catheter-related infections. Clin Microbiol Infect 8:275–81, 2002.

Ross AGP, Bartley PB, Sleigh AC, et al. Schistosomiasis. N Engl J Med 346:1212–1220, 2002.

Rovers MM, Schilder AGM, Zielhuis GA, et al. Otitis media. Lancet 363:465–73, 2004.

Ruhe JJ, Monson T, Bradsher RW, Menon A. Use of long-acting tetracyclines for methicillin-resistant Staphylococcus aureus infections: case series and review of the literature. Clin Infect Dis 40:1429–1434, 2005.

Safdar A, Bryan CS, Stinfon S, et al. Prosthetic valve endocarditis due to vancomycin-resistant Enterococcus faecium: treatment with chloramphenicol plus minocycline. Clin Infect Dis 34:61–3, 2002.

Schlossberg D. Treatment of multi-drug resistant turberculosis. Antibiotics for Clinicians 9:317–321, 2005.

Slenczka W, Klenk HD. Fort years of Marburg virus. J Infect Dis 196:S131–S135, 2007.

Small PM, Fujiwara PI. Management of tuberculosis in the United States. N Engl J Med 345:189–200, 2001.

Sobel J. Botulism. Clin Infect Dis 41:1167–1173, 2005.

Sobel JD, Wiesenfeld HC, Martens M, et al. Maintenance fluconazole therapy for recurrent vulvovaginal candidiasis. N Engl J Med 351:876–83, 2004.

Spellberg BJ, Filler SG, Edwards JE. Current treatment strategies for disseminated candidiasis. Clin Infect Dis 42:244–251, 2006.

Stanek G, Strle F. Lyme borreliosis. Lancet 362:1639–47, 2003.

Strader DB, Wright T, Thomas DL, et al. Diagnosis, management, and treatment of hepatitis C. Hepatology 39:1147–1171, 2004.

Tegnell A, Wahren B, Elgh G. Smallpox - eradicated, but a growing terror threat. Clin Microbiol Infect 8:504–509, 2002.

Teshae EH, Hu DJ, Holmberg SD. The two faces of hepatitis E virus. Clin Infect Dis. 51:328–334, 2010.

Thielman NM, Guerrant RL. Acute infectious diarrhea. N Engl J Med 350:38–47, 2004.

Tolkoff-Rubin NE, Rubin RH. Recent advances in the diagnosis and management of infection in the organ transplant recipient. Semin Nephrol 20:148–163, 2000.

Tunkel AR, Hartman BJ, Kaplan SL, et al. Practical guidelines for the management of bacterial meningitis. Clin Infect Dis 39:1267–84, 2004.

van de Beek D, de Gans J, Spanjaard L, et al. Clinical features and prognostic factors in adults with bacterial meningitis. N Engl J Med 351:1849–59, 2004.

van de Beek D, de Gans J, Tunkel AR, Wijdicks EFM. Community-acquired bacterial meningitis in adults. N Engl J Med 354:44–53, 2006.

Viale P, STefani S. Vascular catheter-associated infections: a microbiological and therapeutic update. Journal of Chemotherapy 18:235–49, 2006.

Walsh TJ, Rex JH. All catheter-related candidemia is not the same: assessment of the balance between the risks and benefits of removal of vascular catheters. Clin Infect Dis 34:600–602, 2002.

Wormser, GP. Discovery of new infections diseases Bartonella species. N Engl J of Med 356:2346–2347, 2007.

Wormser, GP. Early Lyme Disease. N Engl J Med 354:2794–801, 2006.

Yeh E, Luo RF, Dyner L, et al. Preferential lower respiratory tract infection in swine-origin 2009 A (H1N1) influenza. Clin Infect. Dis. 50:391–394, 2010.

GUIDELINES

Bhattacharya D, This CL. Review of Hepatitis B Therapeutics. Clin Infect Dis 51:1201–1208, 2010.

Bisno AL, Gerber MA, Gwaltney JM Jr, Kaplan EL, Schwartz RH. Practice guidelines for the diagnosis and management of group A streptococcal pharyngitis. Infectious Diseases Society of America. Clin Infect Dis 35:113–25, 2002.

CDC MMWR Sexually transmitted diseases treatment guidelines, 2010. (RR-12) 59:1–110, 2010.

Chapman SW, Bradsher RW Jr, Cambell CD Jr, et al. Practice guidelines for the management of patients with blastomycosis. Infectious Diseases Society of America. Clin Infect Dis 30:679–83, 2000.

Cordonnier C, Pautas C, Maury S, Vekhoff A, et al. Empirical versus preemptive antifungal therapy for high-risk, febrile, neutropenic patients: A randomized, controlled trial. Clin Infect Dis 48:1042–1051, 2009.

Dworkin RH, Johnson RW, Breuer J. Recommendations for the management of Herpes zoster. Clin Infect Dis 44:S1–26, 2007.

Dykewicz CA. Summary of the guidelines for preventing opportunistic infectious among hematopoietic stem cell transplant recipients. Clin Infect Dis 33:139–44, 2001.

File TM. Recommendations for treatment of hospital-acquired and ventilator-associated pneumonia: review of recent international guidelines. Clin Infect. Dis. 51:S42–S47, 2010.

Freifeld A, Bow E, Sepkowitz K, et al. Clinical Practice Guideline for the Use of Antimicrobial Agents in Neutropenic Patients with Cancer: 2010 Update by the Infectious Diseases Society of America. Clin Infect Dis 52:e56–e93, 2011.

Galgiani JN, Ampel NM, Blair JE, et al. Coccidioidomycosis. Clin Infect Dis 41:1217–23, 2005.

Goodman EL. Practice guidelines for evaluating new fever in critically ill adult patients. Clin Infect Dis 30:234, 2000.

Guerrant RL, Van Gilder T, Sterner TS, et al. Practice guidelines for the management of infectious diarrhea. Clin Infect Dis 15:321–4, 2001.

Gupta K, Hooton T, Naber K, et al. International Clinical Practice Guidelines for the Treatment of Acute Uncomplicated Cystitis and Pyelonephritis in Women: A 2010 Update by the Infectious Diseases Society of America and the European Society for Microbiology and infectious Diseases. Clinical infectious Diseases. 52:e103–e120, 2011.

Horsburgh CR Jr, Feldman S, Ridzon R. Practice guidelines for the treatment of tuberculosis. Clin Infect Dis 31:633–9, 2000.

Hughes WT, Armstrong D, Bodey GP, et at guidelines for the use of antimicrobial agents in neutropenic patients with cancer. Clin Infect Dis 34:730–51, 2002.

Kauffman CA, Hajjeh R, Chapman SW. Practice guidelines for the management of patients with sporotrichosis. For the mycoses study group, Infectious Diseases Society of America. Clin Infect Dis 30:684–7, 2000.

Krol V, Hamid NS, Cunha BA. Neurosurgically related nosocomial Acinetobacter baumannii meningitis: report of two cases and literature review. J Hospital Infection. 71:176–180, 2009.

Lipsky BA, Berendt AR, Deery HG, et al. Diagnosis and treatment of diabetic foot infections. Infect Dis 39:885–910, 2004.

Liu C, Bayer A, Cosgrove S, et al. Clinical Practice Guidelines by the Infectious Diseases Society of America for the Treatment of Methicillin-Resistant Staphylococcus Aureus Infections in Adults and Children. Clinical Infectious Diseases. 52:1–38, 2011.

Mandell LA, Wunderink RG, Anzueto A, et al. Infectious diseases society of america/american thoracic society consensus guidelines on the management of community-acquired pneumonia in adults. Clin Infect Dis 44(S2):S27–S72, 2007.

Marr K, Boeckh M. Practice guidelines for fungal infections: a risk-guided approach. Clin Infect Dis 32:331–51, 2001.

Mermel LA, Allon M, Bouza E, Craven DE, et al. Clinical practice guidelines for the diagnosis and management of intravascular catheter-related infection: 2009 update by the Infectious Diseases Society of America. Clin Infect Dis 49:1–45, 2009.

Nicolle LE, Bradley S, Colgan R, et al. Infectious Diseases Society of America guidelines for the diagnosis and treatment of asymptomatic bacteriuria in adults. Clin Infect Dis 40:643–54, 2005.

O'Grady NP, Barie PS, Bartlett JG, et al. Practice guidelines for evaluating new fever in critically ill adult patients. Clin Infect Dis 26:1042–1059, 1998.

Pappas PG, Rex JH, Sobel JD, et al. Guidelines for treatment of candidiasis. Clin Infect Dis 38:161–89, 2004.

Pappas PG, Kauffman CA, Andes D, et al. Clinical practice guidelines for the management of candidiasis: 2009 update by the Infectious Diseases Society of America. Clin Infect Dis 48:503–535, 2009.

Rolston KV. The Infectious Diseases Society of America 2002 guidelines for the use of antimicrobial agents in patients with cancer and neutropenia: salient features and comments. Clin Infect Dis 39 Suppl 1:S44-8, 2004.

Saag MS, Graybill RJ, Larsen RA, Pappas PG, et al. Practice guidelines for the management of cryptococcal disease. Infectious Diseases Society of America. Clin Infect Dis 30:710-8, 2000.

Sobel JD. Practice guidelines for the treatment of fungal infections. For the mycoses study group. Infectious diseases society of america. Clin Infect Dis 30:652, 2000.

Solomkin JS, Mazuski JE, Bradley JS, et al. Diagnosis and management of complicated intra-abdominal infection in adults and children: guidelines by the surgical infection society and the infectious diseases society of america. Clin Infect. Dis 50:133-164, 2010.

Solomon JS, Mazuski JE, Baron EJ, et al. Guidelines for the selection of anti-infective agents for complicated intra-abdominal infections. Clin Infect Dis 37:997-1005, 2003.

Stevens DA, Dan VL, Judson MA, Morrison VA, et al. Practice guidelines for diseases caused by Aspergillus. infectious diseases society of america. Clin Infect Dis 30:696-709, 2000.

Stevens DL, Bisno AL, Chambers HF, et al. Practice guidelines for the diagnosis and management of skin and soft-tissue infections. Clin Infect Dis 41:1373-1406, 2005.

Talmor M, Li P, Barie PS. Acute paranasal sinusitis in critically ill patients: guidelines for prevention, diagnosis, and treatment. Clin Infect Dis 25:1441-6, 1997.

Tice AD, Rehm SJ, Dalovisio JR, et al. Practice guidelines for outpatient parenteral antimicrobial therapy. IDSA guidelines. Clin Infect Dis 38:1651-72, 2004.

Tunkel AR, Hartman BJ, Kaplan SL, et al. Practice guidelines for the management of bacterial meningitis. Clin Infect Dis 39:1267-1284, 2004.

U.S. Preventive Services Task Force. Screening for Syphilis Infection in Pregnancy: U.S. Preventive Services Task Force Reaffirmation Recommendation Statement. Ann Intern Med 150:705-709, 2009.

Van Bambeke F, Michot J-M, Van Eldere J, Tulkens PM. Quinolones in 2005: an update. Clin Microbiol Infect 11:256-280, 2005.

Walker M, Kublin JG, Zunt JR. Parasitic central nervous system infections in immunocompromised hosts: Malaria, microsporidiosis, Leishmaniasis, and African trypanosomiasis. Clin Infect Dis 42:115-125, 2006.

Warren JW, Abrutyn E, Hebel JR, et al. Guidelines for antimicrobial treatment of uncomplicated acute bacterial cystitis and acute pyelonephritis in women. Infectious Diseases Society of America. Clin Infect Dis 29:745-58, 1999.

Wheat LJ, Freifeld AG, Kleiman MB, et al. Clinical practice guidelines for the management of patients with histoplasmosis: 2007 update by the Infectious Diseases Society of America. Clin Infect Dis 45:807-25, 2007.

Wheat LJ, Musial CE, Jenny-Avital E. Diagnosis and management of central nervous system histoplasmosis. Clin Infect Dis 40:844-852, 2005.

Workowski KA. Sexually transmitted diseases treatment guidelines. Clin Infect Dis 44:S73-174, 2007.

Wormser GP, Nadelman RB, Battwyler RJ, et al. Practice guidelines for the treatment of Lyme disease. Infectious Disease Society of America. Clin infect Dis 31 (Suppl 1):1-14, 2000.

Yu VL, Ramirez J, Roig J, et al. Legionnaires disease and the updated IDSA guidelines for community-acquired pneumonia. Clin Infect Dis 39:1734-7, 2004.

TEXTBOOKS

Arikan S Rex JH (eds). Antifungal Drugs in Manual of Clinical Microbiology, 8th Edition, 2003.

Baddour L, Gorbach SL (eds). Therapy of Infectious Diseases. Saunders, Philadelphia, Pennsylvania, 2003.

Bodey GP, Feinstein V (eds). Candidiasis. New York, Raven Press, 1985.

Bowden RA, Ljungman P, Snydman DR (eds). Transplant Infections 3rd Edition, Lippincott Williams & Wilkins, Philadelphia, PA, 2010.

Brandstetter R, Cunha BA, Karetsky M (eds). The Pneumonias. Mosby, Philadelphia, 1999.

Brook I (ed). Sinusitis. Taylor & Francis Group, New York, New York, 2006.

Brusch JL Endocarditis Essentials. Jones & Bartlett, Sudbury, MA, 2010.

Brusch, JL. Infective Endocarditis: Management in the Era of Intravascular Devices. Informa Healthcare, New York 2007.

Bryskier A (ed). Antimicrobial Agents. ASM Press, Washington, D.C., 2005.

Calderone RA (ed). Candida and Candidiasis. ASM Press, Washington DC, 2002.

Cimolai N (ed). Laboratory Diagnosis of Bacterial Infections. New York, Marcel Dekker, 2001.

Cook GC. (eds). Manson's Tropical Diseases, 21st Edition. W.B. Saunders Company Ltd., London, 2003.

Cunha BA (ed). Infectious Disease in Critical Care Medicine, 3rd Edition, Informa Healthcare, New York, 2010.

Cunha BA (ed). Tick-Borne Infectious Diseases. Marcel Dekker, New York, 2005.

Cunha BA (ed). Infectious Disease in the Elderly. John Wright & Co., London, 1988.

Despommier DD, Gwadz RW Hotez PJ, Knirsh CA (eds). Parasitic Diseases, 5th Edition, Apple Tree Productions, LLC, New York, New York, 2005.

Faro S, Soper DE (eds). Infectious Diseases in Women. WB Saunders Company, Philadelphia, 2001.

Glauser MP, Pizzo PA (eds). Management of Infection in Immunocompromised Patients. W.B. Saunders, London, 2000.

Gorbach SL, Bartlett JG, Blacklow NR (eds). Infectious Diseases, ed 3. Philadelphia, Lippincott, Williams & Wilkins, 2004.

Grayson ML (ed). Kucers' The Use of Antibiotics, 6th Edition, ASM Press, Washington, DC, 2010.

Guerrant RL, Walker DH, Weller PF (eds). Tropical Infectious Disease: Principles, Pathogens & Practice, 3rd Edition, Elsevier, Philadelphia, 2011.

Halperin JJ. Encephalitis: Diagnosis and Treatment. Informa Healthcare, New York, 2008.

Hauser AR, Rello J (eds). Severe Infections Caused by Pseudomonas Aeruginosa. Kluwer Academic Publishers, Boston, Massachusetts, 2003.

Koff RS Hepatitis Essentials, Jones & Bartlett, Sudbury, MA, 2011.

Madkour MM (ed). Tuberculosis. Springer-Verlag, Berlin Germany, 2004.

Maertens JA, Marr KA. Diagnosis of Fungal Infections. Informa Healthcare, New York, 2007.

Mandell GL, Bennett JE, Dolin R (eds). Mandell, Douglas, and Bennett's Principles and Practice of infectious Diseases, 7th Edition, Philadelphia, Elsevier Churchill Livingstone, 2010.

McMillan A, Young H, Ogilvie MM, Scott GR (eds). Clinical practice in Sexually Transmissible Infections, Saunders, London, England, 2002.

Pilch RF, Ziliinskas RA (eds). Encyclopedia of Bioterrorism Defense. Wiley-Liss, Hoboken, New Jersey, 2005.

Raoult D, Parola P. Rickettsial Diseases. Informa Healthcare, New York, 2007.

Rom WN, Garay SM (eds). Tuberculosis. Lippincott Williams & Wilkins, Philadelphia, Pennsylvania, 2004.

Scheld W, Whitley R, Marra C (eds). Infections of the Central Nervous System, 3rd Edition, Lippincott Williams & Wilkins, Philadelphia, 2005.

Schlossberg D (ed). Tuberculosis & Nontuberculous Mycobacterial Infections, 6th Edition, New York, McGraw-Hill, 2011.

Schlossberg D (ed). Clinical Infections Diseases. Cambridge University Press, London, 2008.

Schlossberg D (ed). Current Therapy of Infectious Disease, 3rd Edition, Mosby-Yearbook, St. Louis, 2008.

Schlossberg D (ed). Medical Interventions for Bioterrorism and Emerging Infections. Handbooks in Healthcare Co., Newtown, Pennsylvania, 2004.

Singh N, Aguado JM (eds). Infectious Complications in Transplant Patients. Kluwer Academic Publishers, Boston, 2000.

Studahl M, Cinque P, Bergstrom T (eds). Herpes Simplex Viruses. Taylor & Francis Group, New York, New York, 2006.

Wingard JR, Anaissie EL (eds). Fungal Infections in the Immunocompromised Patient. Taylor & Francis Group, Boca Raton, Florida, 2005.

Woods JB (ed). USAMRIID's Medical management of biological casualties handbook, 6th Edition, US Army Medical Research Institute of Infections Disease, Fort Detrick, Frederick, Maryland, 2005.

Yoshikawa TT, Rajagopalan S (eds). Antibiotic Therapy for Geriatric Patients. Taylor & Francis Group, New York, New York, 2006.

Yu, V, Edwards G, McKinnon PS, Peloquin C, Morse G (eds). Antimicrobial Therapy and Vaccines, Volume II: Antimicrobial Agents, 2nd Edition, ESun Technologies, Pittsburgh, Pennsylvania, 2005.

Chapter 3

Antibiotic Susceptibility Profiles and Initial Therapy of Isolates Pending Susceptibility Results

Burke A. Cunha, MD, Paul E. Schoch, PhD, Edward J. Bottone, PhD, John H. Rex, MD, Stephanie Strollo, MD, Uzma Syed, DO

*****Color Atlas for CSF, Sputum, and Urine Gram stains** (see center of book).

To determine if an isolate is likely to be susceptible to an antibiotic, see **Antibiotic Susceptibility Profiles** (Tables 3.1–3.3).

When bacteria are isolated from a body site and reported, the clinical significance of the organism should be determined before deciding on potential antibiotic treatment.

The tables in this chapter serve as a guide to the clinical significance of isolates recovered from various body sites. In general, isolates listed as pathogens (P) should be treated with antibiotics, while those listed as non-pathogens (NP), colonizers (C), or skin contaminants (C*) ordinarily should not. **To determine the clinical significance of an isolate in selecting appropriate initial antibiotic therapy pending susceptibility testing** (Tables 3.5–3.8).

Table 3.1. Antibiotic Susceptibility Profiles (Penicillins, Macrolides, Tetracyclines, and Others)

ORGANISMS	Penicillins							Anti-Pseudomonal Penicillins				Macrolides				Tetra-Cyclines			Miscellaneous				
	Penicillin G (IV)	Penicillin V (PO)	Ampicillin (IV/PO)	Ampicillin/Sulbactam (IV)	Amoxicillin (PO)	Amoxicillin/Clavulanate (PO)	Nafcillin (IV)	Ticarcillin (IV)	Ticarcillin/Clavulanate (IV)	Piperacillin (IV)	Piperacillin/Tazobactam (IV)	Erythromycin (IV/PO)	Clarithromycin (PO)	Azithromycin (IV/PO)	Telithromycin (PO)	Tetracycline (IV/PO)	Doxycycline (IV/PO)	Minocycline (IV/PO)	Clindamycin (IV/PO)	Metronidazole (IV/PO)	Rifampin (PO)	TMP-SMX (IV/PO)	Chloramphenicol (IV/PO)
Aerobic Gram Positive Cocci (Clusters)																							
Staphylococcus aureus (MSSA)	0	0	1	2	0	2	3	0	0	0	3	3	0	0	0	0	2	1	1	0	2	1	2
Staphylococcus aureus (HA/CO-MRSA)	0	0	0	0	0	0	0	0	0	0	0	0	0	0	0	0	2†	1	2†	0	2	3†	0
S. aureus (CA-MRSA)	0	0	0	0	0	0	0	0	0	0	0	0	0	0	0	0	2	1	2	0	0	2	0
S. epidermidis (CoNS)	0	0	0	0	0	0	0	0	0	0	0	0	0	0	0	0	2	2	2	0	2	2	0
Aerobic Gram Positive Cocci (Chains)																							
Enterococcus faecalis (VSE)	0	0	1	2	1	1	0	2	2	2	2	3	0	0	0	0	0	0	0	0	0	3	3
Enterococcus faecium (VRE)††	0	0	0	0	0	0	0	0	0	0	0	0	0	0	0	0	3	2	0	0	0	0	3
Group A, B, C, F, G	1	1	2	2	1	2	0	2	2	2	2	3	3	3	0	0	0	0	1	0	0	0	3

Organism																									
Streptococcus (bovis) gallolyticus	1	1	2	2	1	2	0	2	2	2	3	3	0	0	0	0	2	0	0	0	0	0	3	0	0
Viridans streptococci (S. mitior, milleri, mitis, mutans, oralis, sanguis, parasanguis, salivarius)	1	1	2	2	1	2	0	2	2	3	3	3	3	0	0	1	2	1	1	2	0	3*	3*	0	3
Aerobic Gram Positive Cocci (Pairs)																									
Streptococcus pneumoniae (PSSP)	1	1	3*	2	1	2	0	2	2	2	3*	3*	3*	2	0	3*	1	2	3*	0	1	3*	3*	0	3
Streptococcus pneumoniae (PRSP)	1	0	0*	2	1	2	0	2	3	3	0	0	0	2	0	0	1	1	2	0	2	2	0	0	3
Streptococcus pneumoniae (MDRSP)	0	0	0	0	0	0	0	0	0	0	0	0	0	2	0	0	2	3	3	0	3	3	0	0	3
Aerobic Gram Negative Cocci (Pairs)																									
Neisseria gonorrhoeae	0	0	2	2	0	2	0	2	2	2	3	2	0	3*	2	2	0	2	0	0	1	2	0	0	3
Neisseria meningitidis	1	2	2	2	2	2	0	3	0	0	0	0	0	0	0	3	0	3	0	0	2	2	0	0	2
Aerobic Gram Positive Bacilli																									
Bacillus anthracis	2	2	2	3	2	3	0	0	0	0	3	3	2	2	0	3	0	3	0	0	2	2	0	0	2
Corynebacterium diphtheriae	2	0	0	0	0	0	0	0	0	0	0	0	0	0	0	0	0	0	0	0	0	0	0	0	0

1 = Preferred antibiotic—High degree of activity against the isolate and likely to be clinically effective, most strains susceptible, has a favorable PK/PD characteristics, has a good safety profile, and has a "low resistance" potential (see Chapter 11 Drug Summaries for antibiotic dosing details). 2 = Alternate choice—With many attributes of a preferred antibiotic. 3 = Acceptable, but preferably select an alternate antibiotic. 0 = No activity or no data or limited experience. * = May be effective initially but as a "high resistance" antibiotic potential, resistance may develop during/after therapy. † = Preferably use another CA-MRSA antibiotic, e.g., minocycline. †† = Same for vancomycin resistant E. faecalis. PSSP = Penicillin sensitive S. pneumoniae; PRSP = Penicillin resistant S. pneumoniae; MDRSP = Multidrug resistant S. pneumoniae.

Table 3.1. Antibiotic Susceptibility Profiles (Penicillins, Macrolides, Tetracylines, and Others) (cont'd)

ORGANISMS	Penicillin G (IV)	Penicillin V (PO)	Ampicillin (IV/PO)	Ampicillin/Sulbactam (IV)	Amoxicillin (PO)	Amoxicillin/Clavulanate (PO)	Nafcillin (IV)	Ticarcillin (IV)	Ticarcillin/Clavulanate (IV)	Piperacillin (IV)	Piperacillin/Tazobactam (IV)	Erythromycin (IV/PO)	Clarithromycin (PO)	Azithromycin (IV/PO)	Telithromycin (PO)	Tetracycline (IV/PO)	Doxycycline (IV/PO)	Minocycline (IV/PO)	Clindamycin (IV/PO)	Metronidazole (IV/PO)	Rifampin (PO)§	TMP-SMX (IV/PO)	Chloramphenicol (IV/PO)
Corynebacterium jeikeium (JK)	0	0	0	0	0	0	0	0	0	0	0	0	0	0	0	0	0	0	0	0	2	0	0
Listeria monocytogenes	2	2	1	2	1	2	0	2	2	2	2	3	0	0	0	3	3	3	0	0	2	1	1
Nocardia	0	0	0	0	0	0	0	0	0	0	0	0	0	0	0	3	1	2	0	0	0	1	0
Aerobic Gram-Negative Bacilli																							
Acinetobacter sp.	0	0	0	1	0	0	0	0	3	0	3	0	0	0	0	0	3	2	0	0	3	3	0
Aeromonas hydrophila	0	0	0	3	0	3	0	3	3	3	3	0	0	0	0	0	2	3	0	0	0	2	2
Bordetella sp.	0	0	0	0	0	0	0	0	0	0	0	1	1	1	3	3	3	3	0	0	3	2	3
Brucella sp.	0	0	0	0	0	0	0	0	0	0	0	0	0	0	0	3	2	3	0	0	3	3	3
Burkholderia (Pseudomonas) cepacia	0	0	0	0	0	0	0	3	3	0	0	0	0	0	0	0	3	2	0	0	0	3	3
Citrobacter sp.	0	0	0	0	0	0	0	3	3	3	3	0	0	0	0	0	0	0	0	0	0	3	3
Enterobacter sp.	0	0	0	0	0	0	0	3	3	3	3	0	0	0	0	0	0	0	0	0	0	3	0

Organism	1	2	3	4	5	6	7	8	9	10	11	12	13	14	15	16	17	18	19	20	21	22	23	24	25	26
Escherichia coli	0	0	3*	2	2	0	2	2	2	0	0	0	0	0	0	0	2	0	0	0	2	3	0	0	3	2
Francisella tularensis	0	0	0	0	2	0	0	2	2	0	0	0	0	0	0	0	2	0	0	0	2	0	0	3	3	3
Haemophilus sp.	0	0	3*	2	2	0	3	3	3	3	3	3	0	0	3*	1	3	0	0	3*	1	3	0	3	3	2
Klebsiella sp.	0	0	0	2	3	0	0	3	3	3	0	0	2	0	0	0	0	0	0	0	0	0	0	0	0	3
Moraxella catarrhalis	0	0	0	0	3	0	3	2	3	3	0	3	0	0	0	1	3	0	3	0	1	3	0	0	3*	3
Morganella sp.	0	0	3	0	0	0	3	2	3	3	0	3	2	0	0	0	0	0	0	0	0	0	0	0	3*	3
P. aeruginosa	0	0	0	0	0	0	3	3	3	3	0	0	0	0	0	0	0	0	0	0	0	0	0	0	0	0
Proteus sp.	0	0	3	0	0	0	3	3	3	3	0	0	0	0	0	0	0	0	0	0	0	0	0	0	3*	3
Providencia sp.	0	0	3	0	0	0	3	3	3	3	0	0	0	0	0	0	0	0	0	0	0	0	0	0	3*	3
Salmonella sp.	0	0	3	0	0	0	3	3	3	3	0	0	0	0	3*	0	3	0	0	3*	2	0	0	0	3	2
Serratia marcescens	0	0	0	0	0	0	3	0	3	3	0	0	0	0	0	0	0	0	0	0	0	0	0	0	3	0
Shigella sp.	0	0	3	0	0	0	3	3	3	3	0	0	0	0	0	0	3	0	0	0	3	3	0	0	3*	2
Stenotrophomonas (Pseudomonas) maltophilia	0	0	0	0	0	0	3	3	3	3	0	0	0	0	0	0	0	0	0	0	2	2	0	0	2	3
Vibrio vulnificus	0	0	0	0	0	0	0	2	3	3	0	0	0	0	3	1	3	0	0	3	1	3	0	0	0	3
Yersinia enterocolitica	0	2	1	0	0	0	2	2	3	3	0	0	0	0	0	0	0	0	0	3	0	0	0	0	1	2
Anaerobic Gram Positive Cocci (chains)																										
Peptostreptococcus	1	1	2	2	2	0	2	2	2	2	0	3	3	3	3	3	3	2	2	3	2	2	2	0	0	2

1 = Preferred antibiotic–High degree of activity against the isolate and likely to be clinically effective, most strains susceptible, has a favorable PK/PD characteristics, has a good safety profile, and has a "low resistance" potential (see Chapter 11 Drug Summaries for antibiotic dosing details). 2 = Alternate choice–With many attributes of a preferred antibiotic. 3 = Acceptable, but preferably select an alternate antibiotic. 0 = No activity or no data or limited experience. * = May be effective initially but as a "high resistance" antibiotic potential, resistance may develop during/after therapy.
§ = Always use in combination with another antibiotic.

Table 3.1. Antibiotic Susceptibility Profiles (Penicillins, Macrolides, Tetracyclines, and Others) (cont'd)

ORGANISMS	Penicillins							Anti-Pseudomonal Penicillins					Macrolides				Tetra-Cyclines			Miscellaneous				
	Penicillin G (IV)	Penicillin V (PO)	Ampicillin (IV/PO)	Ampicillin/Sulbactam (IV)	Amoxicillin (PO)	Amoxicillin/Clavulanate (PO)	Nafcillin (IV)	Ticarcillin (IV)	Ticarcillin/Clavulanate (IV)	Piperacillin (IV)	Piperacillin/Tazobactam (IV)	Erythromycin (IV/PO)	Clarithromycin (PO)	Azithromycin (IV/PO)	Telithromycin (PO)	Tetracycline (IV/PO)	Doxycycline (IV/PO)	Minocycline (IV/PO)	Clindamycin (IV/PO)	Metronidazole (IV/PO)	Rifampin (PO)§	TMP-SMX (IV/PO)	Chloramphenicol (IV/PO)
Anaerobic Gram Positive Bacilli																							
Actinomyces sp.	1	1	1	2	1	2	0	0	0	0	0	2	2	2	0	2	2	2	2	0	0	0	0
Anaerobic Gram Negative Bacilli																							
Bacteroides fragilis group (B. distasonis, ovatus, thetaiotaomicron, vulgatus)	0	0	0	2	0	2	0	2	2	2	2	3	3	3	0	3	2	2	1	1	0	0	2
Prevotella sp.	1	1	1	1	1	2	0	2	2	2	2	2	2	2	2	2	2	2	1	1	0	0	2

1 = Preferred antibiotic—High degree of activity against the isolate and likely to be clinically effective, most strains susceptible, has a favorable PK/PD characteristics, has a good safety profile, and has a "low resistance" profile, and has a "low resistance" potential (see Chapter 11 Drug Summaries for antibiotic dosing details). 2 = Alternate choice—With many attributes of a preferred antibiotic. 3 = Acceptable, but preferably select an alternate antibiotic. 0 = No activity or no data or limited experience. § = Always use in combination with another antibiotic.

Table 3.2. Antibiotic Susceptibility Profiles (Cephalosporins)

ORGANISMS	CEPHALOSPORINS																					
	1st GC (IV)	1st GCs (PO)		2nd GCs (IV)			2nd GCs (PO)				3rd GCs (IV)			3rd GCs (PO)					Anti-Pseudomonal 3rd GC (IV)		4th GC (IV)	Anti-MRSA* (IV)
	Cefazolin (IV)	Cefadroxil (PO)	Cephalexin (PO)	Cefoxitin (IV)	Cefuroxime (IV)	Cefotetan (IV)	Cefaclor (PO)	Loracarbef (PO)	Cefprozil (PO)	Cefuroxime axetil (PO)	Cefotaxime (IV)	Ceftizoxime (IV)	Ceftriaxone (IV)	Cefixime (PO)	Ceftibuten (PO)	Cefpodoxime (PO)	Cefdinir (PO)	Cefditoren (PO)	Cefoperazone (IV)	Ceftazidime (IV)	Cefepime (IV)	Ceftaroline fosamil (IV)
Aerobic Gram Positive Cocci (Clusters)																						
Staphylococcus aureus (MSSA)	1	2	1	2	2	3	3	0	3	2	2	2	2	0	0	2	2	0	2	3	2	2
Staphylococcus aureus (HA/CO-MRSA)	0	0	0	0	0	0	0	0	0	0	0	0	0	0	0	0	0	0	0	0	0	1
S. aureus (CA-MRSA)	0	0	0	0	0	0	0	0	0	0	0	0	0	0	0	0	0	0	0	0	0	2
S. epidermidis (CoNS)	3	0	0	3	3	3	0	0	0	0	3	3	3	0	0	0	0	0	3	0	3	0

1 = Preferred antibiotic—High degree of activity against the isolate and likely to be clinically effective, most strains susceptible, has a favorable PK/PD characteristics, has a good safety profile, and has a "low resistance potential" (see Chapter 11 Drug Summaries for antibiotic dosing details); 2 = Alternate choice—With many attributes of a preferred antibiotic. 3 = Acceptable, but preferably select an alternate antibiotic. 0 = No activity or no data or limited experience. * = Ceftaroline fosamil is approved for MRSA in ABSSSI and has not been evaluated in clinical trials for any other MRSA infections.

Table 3.2. Antibiotic Susceptibility Profiles (Cephalosporins) (cont'd)

ORGANISMS	1st GC (IV)	1st GCs (PO)		2nd GCs (IV)			2nd GCs (PO)				3rd GCs (IV)			3rd GCs (PO)					Anti-Pseudomonal 3rd GC (IV)		4th GC (IV)	Anti-MRSA* (IV)
	Cefazolin (IV)	Cefadroxil (PO)	Cephalexin (PO)	Cefoxitin (IV)	Cefuroxime (IV)	Cefotetan (IV)	Cefaclor (PO)	Loracarbef (PO)	Cefprozil (PO)	Cefuroxime axetil (PO)	Cefotaxime (IV)	Ceftizoxime (IV)	Ceftriaxone (IV)	Cefixime (PO)	Ceftibuten (PO)	Cefpodoxime (PO)	Cefdinir (PO)	Cefditoren (PO)	Cefoperazone (IV)	Ceftazidime (IV)	Cefepime (IV)	Ceftaroline fosamil (IV)
Aerobic Gram Positive Cocci (Chains)																						
Enterococcus faecalis (VSE)	0	0	0	0	0	0	0	0	0	0	0	0	0	0	0	0	0	0	3	0	0	0
Enterococcus faecium (VRE)	0	0	0	0	0	0	0	0	0	0	0	0	0	0	0	0	0	0	0	0	0	0
Group A, B, C, F, G	1		1	2	2	2	2		1	2	1	1	1	2	3	2	2	2	1	3	2	2†
Streptococcus (bovis) gallolyticus	1		1	2	2	2	2		2	2	1	1	1	2	3	2	2	2	1	3	2	0

Organism																					
Viridans streptococci (S. mitior, milleri, mitis, mutans, oralis, sanguis, par sanguis, salivarius)	1	1	2	2	2	2	3	2	2	2	1	1	1	2	2	2	2	1	2	2	0
Aerobic Gram Positive Cocci (Pairs)																					
Streptococcus pneumoniae (PSSP)	1	1	2	2	2	2	1	2	2	1	2	2	3	0	3	2	2	2	3	3	2
Streptococcus pneumoniae (PRSP)	1	1	2	2	2	2	1	2	2	1	2	2	2	0	2	2	2	2	3	3	2
Streptococcus pneumoniae (MDRSP)	1	1	2	2	2	2	1	2	2	1	2	2	2	0	2	2	2	2	3	3	2
Aerobic Gram Negative Cocci (Pairs)																					
Neisseria gonorrhoeae	2	0	2	2	3	2	3	3	2	1	2	1	1	3	2	2	2	2	3	2	0
Neisseria meningitidis	3	0	3	2	3	3	3	3	2	1	3	3	3	3	2	2	2	3	3	2	0

1 = Preferred antibiotic—High degree of activity against the isolate and likely to be clinically effective, most strains susceptible, has a favorable PK/PD characteristics, has a good safety profile, and has a "low resistance potential" (see Chapter 11 Drug Summaries for antibiotic dosing details). 2 = Alternate choice—With many attributes of a preferred antibiotic. 3 = Acceptable, but preferably select an alternate antibiotic. 0 = No activity or no data or limited experience. * = Ceftaroline fosamil is approved for MRSA in ABSSSI and has not been evaluated in clinical trials for any other MRSA infections.
† Group A & B only.

Table 3.2. Antibiotic Susceptibility Profiles (Cephalosporins) (cont'd)

CEPHALOSPORINS

ORGANISMS	1st GC (IV)	1st GCs (PO)		2nd GCs (IV)			2nd GCs (PO)				3rd GCs (IV)			3rd GCs (PO)					Anti-Pseudomonal 3rd GC (IV)		4th GC (IV)	Anti-MRSA* (IV)
	Cefazolin (IV)	Cefadroxil (PO)	Cephalexin (PO)	Cefoxitin (IV)	Cefuroxime (IV)	Cefotetan (IV)	Cefaclor (PO)	Loracarbef (PO)	Cefprozil (PO)	Cefuroxime axetil (PO)	Cefotaxime (IV)	Ceftizoxime (IV)	Ceftriaxone (IV)	Cefixime (PO)	Ceftibuten (PO)	Cefpodoxime (PO)	Cefdinir (PO)	Cefditoren (PO)	Cefoperazone (IV)	Ceftazidime (IV)	Cefepime (IV)	Ceftaroline fosamil (IV)
Aerobic Gram Positive Bacilli																						
Bacillus anthracis	0	0	0	0	0	0	0	0	0	0	0	0	0	0	0	0	0	0	0	0	0	0
Corynebacterium diphtheriae	0	0	0	0	0	0	0	0	0	0	0	0	0	0	0	0	0	0	0	0	0	0
Corynebacterium jeikeium (JK)	0	0	0	0	0	0	0	0	0	0	0	0	0	0	0	0	0	0	0	0	0	0
Listeria monocytogenes	0	0	0	0	0	0	0	0	0	0	0	0	0	0	0	0	0	0	0	0	0	0
Nocardia sp.	0	0	0	0	3	0	0	0	0	0	3	0	3	0	0	0	0	0	0	0	0	0
Aerobic Gram-Negative Bacilli																						
Acinetobacter sp.	0	0	0	0	0	0	0	0	0	0	0	0	0	0	0	0	0	0	0	3	2	0

Organism																			
Aeromonas hydrophila	0	0	3	2	0	0	3	3	2	2	3	0	3	3	0	3	3	3	0
Bordetella pertussis	0	0	0	0	0	0	0	0	0	0	0	0	0	0	0	0	0	0	0
Brucella sp.	0	0	3	0	0	0	0	0	2	2	2	3	2	0	0	2	2	2	0
Burkholderia (Pseudomonas) cepacia	0	0	2	0	0	0	0	0	3	3	0	0	2	2	0	0	0	0	0
Campylobacter sp.	0	0	0	0	0	0	0	0	0	0	0	0	3	2	0	0	0	0	0
Citrobacter sp.	0	1	2	0	0	0	0	0	2	2	3	0	2	0	0	2	3	0	0
Enterobacter sp.	0	1	3	0	0	0	3	0	3	3	0	0	2	0	0	2	3	3	0
Escherichia coli	3	2	2	1	2	2	2	2	1	1	2	2	2	2	2	1	2	2	2
Francisella tularensis	0	0	0	0	0	0	0	0	0	0	0	2	0	0	0	0	0	0	0
Haemophilus sp.	2†	1	2	1	2	2	2	1	1	1	1	2	1	3	2	2	2	1	1
Klebsiella sp.	0	2	2	2	2	2	2	1	1	1	2	2	1	0	2	2	2	2	2
Moraxella catarrhalis	0	2	2	2	2	2	2	2	2	2	2	2	2	0	2	2	2	2	2
Morganella sp.	0	2	3	2	0	0	0	3	2	2	3	0	2	0	2	2	3	3	2
P. aeruginosa	0	2	3	2	0	0	0	0	0	0	0	0	0	0	0	0	3	3	2
Providencie sp.	0	2	3	2	0	0	3	0	2	2	3	0	2	0	2	2	3	3	2
Proteus sp.	0	2	3	2	0	0	3	0	2	2	3	0	2	0	2	2	3	3	2
Salmonella sp.	0	0	3	2	0	0	0	0	1	1	0	0	1	0	0	2	3	3	0

1 = Preferred antibiotic—High degree of activity against the isolate and likely to be clinically effective, most strains susceptible, has a favorable PK/PD characteristics, has a good safety profile, and has a "low resistance potential" (see Chapter 11 Drug Summaries for antibiotic dosing details). 2 = Alternate choice—With many attributes of a preferred antibiotic. 3 = Acceptable, but preferably select an alternate antibiotic. 0 = No activity or no data or limited experience. * = Ceftaroline fosamil is approved for MRSA in ABSSSI and has not been evaluated in clinical trials for any other MRSA infections.
† H. influenzae only.

Table 3.2. Antibiotic Susceptibility Profiles (Cephalosporins) (cont'd)

ORGANISMS	1st GC (IV)	1st GCs (PO)		2nd GCs (IV)			2nd GCs (PO)				3rd GCs (IV)			3rd GCs (PO)					Anti-Pseudomonal 3rd GC (IV)		4th GC (IV)	Anti-MRSA* (IV)
	Cefazolin (IV)	Cefadroxil (PO)	Cephalexin (PO)	Cefoxitin (IV)	Cefuroxime (IV)	Cefotetan (IV)	Cefaclor (PO)	Loracarbef (PO)	Cefprozil (PO)	Cefuroxime axetil (PO)	Cefotaxime (IV)	Ceftizoxime (IV)	Ceftriaxone (IV)	Cefixime (PO)	Ceftibuten (PO)	Cefpodoxime (PO)	Cefdinir (PO)	Cefditoren (PO)	Cefoperazone (IV)	Ceftazidime (IV)	Cefepime (IV)	Ceftaroline fosamil (IV)
Serratia marcescens	0	0	0	3	0	2	0	0	0	0	1	1	1	0	0	3	0	3	1	2	1	0
Shigella sp.	0	0	0	3	0	3	0	0	0	0	2	2	2	0	0	0	0	0	2	3	2	0
Stenotrophomonas (Pseudomonas) maltophilia	0	0	0	0	0	0	0	0	0	0	0	0	0	0	0	3	0	0	0	0	0	0
Vibrio vulnificus	0	0	0	0	0	0	0	0	0	0	2	0	0	0	0	0	0	0	0	2	0	0
Yersinia enterocolitica	0	0	0	3	3	3	0	0	0	0	2	2	2	2	2	0	2	0	2	3	2	0
Anaerobic Gram Positive Cocci (chains)																						

Peptostreptococcus	2		2	2	2	2	3	2	2	2	2	0	0	0	2	2	2	3	3	2	0
Anaerobic Gram Positive Bacilli																					
Actinomyces sp.	0		0	0	0	0	0	2	3	3	2	0	0	0	0	3	0	3	0	0	0
Anaerobic Gram Negative Bacilli																					
Bacteroides fragilis group (B distasonis, ovatus, thetaiotaomicron, vulgatus)	0		0	0	2	0	0	2	0	3	2	0	0	0	0	2	2	2	0	0	0
Prevotella sp.	2		2	2	2	2	2	2	2	2	2	2	2	2	2	2	2	2	0	2	0

1 = Preferred antibiotic—High degree of activity against the isolate and likely to be clinically effective, most strains susceptible, has a favorable PK/PD characteristics, has a good safety profile, and has a "low resistance potential" (see Chapter 11 Drug Summaries for antibiotic dosing details).

2 = Alternate choice—With many attributes of a preferred antibiotic.

3 = Acceptable, but preferably select an alternate antibiotic.

0 = No activity or no data or limited experience.

* Ceftaroline fosamil is approved for MRSA in ABSSSI and has not been evaluated in clinical trials for any other MRSA infections.

Table 3.3. Antibiotic Susceptibility Profiles (Aminoglycosides, Fluoroquinolones, Carbapenems, and Others)

ORGANISMS	Gentamicin (IV)	Tobramycin (IV)	Amikacin (IV)	Ciprofloxacin (IV/PO)	Levofloxacin (IV/PO)	Moxifloxacin (IV/PO)	Colistimethate/Polymyxin B (IV)	Aztreonam (IV)	Tigecycline (IV)	Vancomycin (IV)	Quinupristin/dalfopristin (IV)	Linezolid (IV/PO)	Daptomycin (IV)	Telavancin (IV)	Nitrofurantoin↑ (PO)	Fosfomycin↑ (PO)	Imipenem (IV)	Meropenem (IV)	Ertapenem (IV)	Doripenem (IV)
Aerobic Gram Positive Cocci (Clusters)																				
Staphylococcus aureus (MSSA)	2	3	3	3*	2	2	0	0	1	3	1	1	1	1	0	0	2	2	2	2
Staphylococcus aureus (HA/CO-MRSA)	0	0	0	0	0	0	0	0	1	2	1	1	1	1	0	3	0	0	0	0
S. aureus (CA-MRSA)	0	0	0	0	0	0	0	0	1	1	1	1	1	1	0	0	0	0	0	0
S. epidermidis (CoNS)	0	0	0	0	3	3	0	0	1	1	1	1	1	1	0	0	3	3	3	3
Aerobic Gram Positive Cocci (Chains)																				
Enterococcus faecalis (VSE)	0	0	0	0	3	2	0	0	1	2	0	1	2	3	1	3	2	2	0	3
Enterococcus faecium (VRE)	0	0	0	0	0	0	0	0	1	0	1	1	2	3	1	3	0	0	0	3
Group A, B, C, F, G	0	0	0	0	3	2	0	0	2	2	3	2	2	2	2	0	2	2	2	3
Streptococcus (bovis) galloyticus	0	0	0	0	3	2	0	0	2	2	2	2	2	2	0	0	2	2	0	2

Organism																			
Viridans streptococci (S. mitior, milleri, mitis, mutans, oralis, sanguis, parasanguis, salivarius)	0	0	0	0	0	0	0	0	2	2	0	2	2	0	2	2	2	0	2
Aerobic Gram Positive Cocci (Pairs)																			
Streptococcus pneumoniae (PSSP)	0	0	3*	1	2	0	0	1	2	2	0	3	2	0	2	2	2	2	2
Streptococcus pneumoniae (PRSP)	0	0	3*	1	2	0	0	1	2	2	0	3	2	0	2	2	2	2	2
Streptococcus pneumoniae (MDRSP)	0	0	3*	1	2	0	0	1	2	2	0	3	2	0	2	2	2	2	2
Aerobic Gram Negative Cocci (Pairs)																			
Neisseria gonorrhoeae	0	0	1	1	2	0	2	0	0	0	0	0	0	0	0	2	0	3	3
Neisseria meningitidis	0	0	2	2	2	0	2	0	0	0	0	0	0	0	0	2	0	2	2
Aerobic Gram Positive Bacilli																			
Bacillus anthracis	0	0	1	1	1	0	0	0	0	0	0	0	0	0	0	0	0	0	0
Corynebacterium diphtheriae	0	0	0	0	0	0	0	0	0	3	0	0	0	0	0	0	0	0	0
Corynebacterium jeikeium (JK)	0	0	0	0	0	0	0	2	0	1	3	2	0	0	0	0	0	0	0

1 = Preferred antibiotic—High degree of activity against the isolate and likely to be clinically effective, most strains susceptible, has a favorable PK/PD characteristics, has a good safety profile, and has a "low resistance" potential (see Chapter 11 Drug Summaries for antibiotic dosing details). 2 = Alternate drug choice—With many attributes of a preferred antibiotic. 3 = Acceptable, but preferably select an alternate antibiotic. 0 = No activity or no data or limited experience. * = May be effective initially but as a "high resistance" antibiotic potential, resistance may develop during/after therapy.

Table 3.3. Antibiotic Susceptibility Profiles (Aminoglycosides, Fluoroquinolones, Carbapenems, and Others) (cont'd)

ORGANISMS	Amino-Glycosides			Fluoro-Quinolones			Miscellaneous										Carbapenems			
	Gentamicin (IV)	Tobramycin (IV)	Amikacin (IV)	Ciprofloxacin (IV/PO)	Levofloxacin (IV/PO)	Moxifloxacin (IV/PO)	Colistimethate/ Polymyxin B (IV)	Aztreonam (IV)	Tigecycline (IV)	Vancomycin (IV)	Quinupristin/ dalfopristin (IV)	Linezolid (IV/PO)	Daptomycin (IV)	Telavancin (IV)	Nitrofurantoin † (PO)	Fosfomycin † (PO)	Imipenem (IV)	Meropenem (IV)	Ertapenem (IV)	Doripenem (IV)
Listeria monocytogenes	3	3	3	0	0	0	0	0	3	0	3	3	0	0	0	0	3	2	0	0
Nocardia	0	0	2	0	0	0	0	0	0	0	0	3	0	0	0	0	3	2	0	0
Aerobic Gram-Negative Bacilli																				
Acinetobacter sp.	1	2		3*	2	3	2	1	2*	0	0	0	0	0	0	0	2*	1	0	1
Aeromonas hydrophila	2	2	2	1	1	1	0	3	2	0	0	0	0	0	0	0	3	2	3	0
Bordetella sp.	0	0	0	3	3	3	0	0	0	0	0	0	0	0	0	0	3	3	3	0
Brucella sp.	2	0	0	3	3	0	0	0	0	0	0	0	0	0	0	0	0	0	0	0
Burkholderia (Pseudomonas) cepacia	0	0	0	3*	3	3	3	0	0	0	0	0	0	0	0	0	3	2	3	0
Campylobacter sp.	3	0	0	1	1	1	0	0	0	0	0	0	0	0	0	0	3	3	3	3
Citrobacter sp.	1	1	2	3	2	3	3	0	2	0	0	0	0	0	2	3	3	3	3	1
Enterobacter sp.	1	1	1	2*	2	2	3	2	2	0	0	0	0	0	3	2	1	1	1	1
Escherichia coli	2	2	1	2	2	2	3	2	1	0	0	0	0	0	2	2	2	2	2	2
Francisella tularensis	1	3	0	2	2	2	0	0	0	0	0	0	0	0	0	2	0	1	0	0

Organism																										
Haemophilus sp.	3	3	3	2	2	2	2	3	3	2	0	2	0	0	0	0	0	2	3	0	2	2	2	2	2	2
Moraxella catarrhalis	3	3	3	2	2	2	0	2	2	2	0	2	0	0	0	0	0	2	2	0	2	2	2	2	2	2
Morganella sp.	2	2	1	3	3	2	0	2	2	2	0	0	0	0	0	2	2	2	2	1	2	2	2	2	2	—
P. aeruginosa	3	3	1	1*	1*	1	1	1*	2	2	1	1*	0	0	0	0	0	1	2*	1	2*	1	1	0	1	—
Proteus sp.	2	2	3	3	3	2	0	2	1	2	0	2	0	0	0	0	0	2	2	2	2	2	2	2	2	—
Providencia sp.	2	2	3	3	3	1	0	2	1	2	0	2	0	0	0	0	0	2	2	2	2	2	2	2	2	—
Salmonella sp.	0	0	1	1	1	1	0	2	1	1	0	0	0	0	0	0	0	0	0	0	2	2	2	2	2	—
Serratia marcescens	3	2	1*	1*	3	1	2	2	1	2	0	3	0	0	0	0	0	2	2	3	2	2	2	2	2	2
Shigella sp.	3	3	1	1	3	3	2	2	1	2	0	3	0	0	0	0	0	2	2	0	2	2	2	2	2	2
Stenotrophomonas (Pseudomonas) maltophilia	0	0	3	3	0	2	2	0	2	2	3	0	0	0	0	0	0	0	0	0	0	0	0			
Vibrio vulnificus	0	0	3	3	0	3	3	0	3	3	0	0	0	0	0	0	0	2	3							
Yersinia enterocolitica	2	2	2	2	2	2	0	2	3	3	3	2	0	0	0	0	0	3	3	0	2	2	2	2	2	0
Anaerobic Gram Positive Cocci (chains)																										
Peptostreptococcus	0	0	0	0	0	0	2	2	0	0	3	2	2	0	0	0	0	0	2	2		2	2	2		2
Anaerobic Gram Positive Bacilli																										
Actinomyces sp.	0	0	0	0	0	0	3	3	0	3	0	0	0	0	0	0	2	2	2	0		2	2	2		0

1 = Preferred antibiotic—High degree of activity against the isolate and likely to be clinically effective, most strains susceptible, has a favorable PK/PD characteristics, has a good safety profile, and has a "low resistance" potential (see Chapter 11 Drug Summaries for antibiotic dosing details). 2 = Alternate choice—With many attributes of a preferred antibiotic. 3 = Acceptable, but preferably select an alternate antibiotic. 0 = No activity or no data or limited experience. * = May be effective initially but as a "high resistance" antibiotic potential, resistance may develop during/after therapy.

Table 3.3. Antibiotic Susceptibility Profiles (Aminoglycosides, Fluoroquinolones, Carbapenems, and Others) (cont'd)

ORGANISMS	Amino-Glycosides			Fluoro-Quinolones			Miscellaneous										Carbapenems			
	Gentamicin (IV)	Tobramycin (IV)	Amikacin (IV)	Ciprofloxacin (IV/PO)	Levofloxacin (IV/PO)	Moxifloxacin (IV/PO)	Colistimethate/Polymyxin B (IV)	Aztreonam (IV)	Tigecycline (IV)	Vancomycin (IV)	Quinupristin/dalfopristin (IV)	Linezolid (IV/PO)	Daptomycin (IV)	Telavancin (IV)	Nitrofurantoin † (PO)	Fosfomycin † (PO)	Imipenem (IV)	Meropenem (IV)	Ertapenem (IV)	Doripenem (IV)
Anaerobic Gram Negative Bacilli																				
Bacteroides fragilis group (*B distasonis, ovatus, thetaiotaomicron, vulgatus*)	0	0	0	0	0	2	0	0	1	0	3	0	0	0	0	0	1	1	1	1
Prevotella sp.	0	0	0	2	2	2	0	0	2	0	0	0	0	0	0	0	2	2	2	2

1 = Preferred antibiotic—High degree of activity against the isolate and likely to be clinically effective, most strains susceptible, has a favorable PK/PD characteristics, has a good safety profile, and has a "low resistance" potential (see Chapter 11 Drug Summaries for antibiotic dosing details).

2 = Alternate choice—With many attributes of a preferred antibiotic.

3 = Acceptable, but preferably select an alternate antibiotic.

0 = No activity or no data or limited experience.

* = May be effective initially but as a "high resistance" antibiotic potential, resistance may develop during/after therapy.

† = For lower tract infections (UTIs)/catheter associated bacteriuria (CAB).

Isolates by Gram Stain Characteristics, Morphologic Arrangement, Oxygen Requirement

AEROBIC ISOLATES

* Oxidase negative.   (α) = α (alpha) hemolysis on BAP.   (m) = motile.
† Catalase positive.   (β) = β (beta) hemolysis on BAP.   (v) = Gram variable bacilli.
§ Non-lactose fermenter.   (γ) = γ (gamma) hemolysis on BAP.

CAPNOPHILIC ISOLATES[+]

GRAM-NEGATIVE BACILLI

+ Capnophilic organisms grow best under increased CO² tension.   (m) = motile.

ANAEROBIC ISOLATES

GRAM-POSITIVE COCCI (CHAINS)

GRAM-POSITIVE BACILLI

++ **Microaerophilic organisms. Grow best under decreased O$_2$ concentration.**
* **Oxidase negative.** (m) = **motile.**
† **Catalase positive.** (v) = **Gram variable bacilli.**

YEASTS/FUNGI

Alphabetical Index of Isolates

Table 3.4. Key Factors in Antibiotic Selection When the Isolate is Known

- **Select an antibiotic with a high degree of activity against the presumed pathogen** (*not colonizer*).

- **Dose appropriate for the target tissue to assure therapeutic/effective concentrations at site of infection**. If necessary, adjust dose ↑ for tissue targets that require higher doses, e.g., bacterial meningitis, endocarditis, etc., or ↓ dose for sites with antibiotic concentrations that are above serum concentrations, e.g., skin, urine, etc.

- **Select an empiric antibiotic with a "low resistance" potential** avoid, if possible, antibiotics with a "high resistance" potential (also with a high degree of activity against the presumed pathogen). Select a "low resistance" potential antibiotic for the same/different class with a high degree of activity.

- **Select antibiotic with a good safety profile** and minimal potential for drug-drug interactions.

- **Select antibiotic that is relatively cost effective** (that first takes into account the above principles).

- **Preferentially use PO antibiotics** unless patient critically ill, unable to take oral medications, or if no oral equivalent antibiotic available.

Table 3.5. Clinical Significance of AEROBIC Isolates Pending Susceptibility Testing

	GRAM-POSITIVE COCCI (CLUSTERS)		
Isolate	Isolate Significance	Therapy	Comments
Staphylococcus aureus (MSSA/MRSA) (also see p. 14)	• CSF = C*, P (CNS shunts) • Blood = C*, P (from soft tissue/bone infection, abscess, IV line infection, ABE, PVE) • Sputum = C, P (S. aureus pneumonia is rare; usually only after viral influenza) • Urine = C, P (S. aureus in urine is usually due to skin contamination or rarely overwhelming S. aureus bacteremia) • Stool = C, P (enterocolitis) • Wound = C, P (cellulitis, abscess)	MSSA: Nafcillin (IV), Cefazolin (IV), Clindamycin (IV/PO), a "respiratory quinolone" (IV/PO), Minocycline (IV/PO), Daptomycin (IV), any carbapenem (IV), Linezolid (IV/PO), Tigecycline (IV), Telavancin (IV) Hospital-acquired MRSA (HA-MRSA)/Community-onset MRSA (CO-MRSA): Daptomycin (IV), Linezolid (IV/PO), Tigecycline (IV/PO), Vancomycin (IV), Minocycline (IV/PO), Quinupristin/dalfopristin (IV), Telavancin (IV) Community acquired MRSA (CA-MRSA): Doxycycline*, TMP-SMX, Clindamycin VISA/VRSA: Linezolid (IV/PO), Daptomycin (IV), Telavancin (IV)	MSSA: For oral treatment, 1st generation cephalosporins are better than oral anti-staphylococcal penicillins (e.g., dicloxacillin) MRSA: in-vitro susceptibility testing is unreliable; treat MRSA infections empirically. Most effective drugs for MRSA are vancomycin, linezolid, ceftaroline fosamil (ABSSSI only), quinupristin/dalfopristin, minocycline, daptomycin, tigecycline. **Preferentially use minocycline** **instead of doxycycline for MSSA/MRSA.** Community-acquired MRSA (CA-MRSA) SCC mec IV, V CA-MRSA has different susceptibilities than HA-MRSA/CO-MRSA (see p. 14). CA-MRSA strains with Panton-Valentin Leukocidin PVL+ gene cause two distinct clinical syndromes: severe necrotizing pneumonia (with viral influenza) and severe necrotizing fasciitis/pyomyositis. **CA-MRSA is usually susceptible to doxycycline** **in vitro, but minocycline more effective in** **vivo than doxycycline,** TMP-SMX, clindamycin. Drugs effective against HA-MRSA/CO-MRSA are also effective against CA-MRSA. However, drugs effective against CA-MRSA are may not be effective against HA-MRSA/CO-MRSA MSSA/MRSA: Noncontinuous low-grade blood culture positivity indicates skin contamination during venipuncture. Continuous high-grade blood culture positivity (3/4 or 4/4) indicates intravascular infection or abscess

Staphylococcus epidermidis (MSSE/MRSE) or coagulase-negative staphylococci (CoNS) Staphylococcus lugdunensis	• CSF = C*, P (CNS shunts) • Blood = C*, P (from IV lines, infected implants, prosthetic valve endocarditis [PVE], rarely from native valve subacute bacterial endocarditis [SBE]) • Sputum = C • Urine = C (may be reported as S. saprophyticus; request novobiocin sensitivity to differentiate S. epidermidis from other coagulase-negative staphylococci) • Stool = NP • Wound = C, P (infected foreign body drainage)	**MSSE:** Linezolid (IV/PO), Daptomycin (IV), Vancomycin (IV), Telavancin (IV), any carbapenem (IV), a "respiratory quinolone" (IV/PO), Minocycline (IV/PO) **MRSE:** Linezolid (IV/PO), Daptomycin (IV), Vancomycin (IV), Quinupristin/dalfopristin (IV), Minocycline (IV/PO)	<u>VISA/VRSA:</u> MICs for vancomycin sensitive (VSSA), heteroresistant vancomycin intermediate (hVISA), intermediate (VISA), and resistant (VRSA) S. aureus are < 4 mcg/mL, < 4 mcg/mL (with subpopulations > 4 mcg/mL), 8–16 mcg/mL, and ≥ 32 mcg/mL, respectively. Usually non-pathogenic in absence of prosthetic/implant materials. Common cause of PVE; rare cause of native valve SBE. Treat foreign body-related infection until foreign body is removed. S. lugdunensis is a CoNS but is often misidentified as S. aureus since it produces "clumping factor" which gives a + rapid short tube coagulase test (long tube test −) although a CoNS resembles S. aureus in terms of invasiveness/virulence. Unlike S. aureus, S. lugdunensis is pan-sensitive to antibiotics which is another clue the isolate is not S. aureus. S. lugdunensis bacteremia associated with community acquired (not nosocomial) SBE.

C = colonizer; C* = skin contaminant; NP = non-pathogen at site; P = pathogen at site; (IV/PO) = IV or PO. See p. xi for all other abbreviations.

* Minocycline (IV/PO) preferred.

Table 3.5. Usual Clinical Significance of AEROBIC Isolates Pending Susceptibility Testing (cont'd)

Isolate	Isolate Significance	Preferred Therapy	Alternate Therapy	Comments
GRAM-POSITIVE COCCI (CLUSTERS)				
Staphylococcus saprophyticus (coagulase-negative staphylococci)	• CSF = NP • Blood = NP • Sputum = NP • Urine = P (cystitis, pyelo) • Stool = NP • Wound = NP	Preferred therapy Amoxicillin (PO) TMP-SMX (PO) Nitrofurantoin (PO) Alternate therapy Any quinolone (PO) Any 1st generation cephalosporin (PO)		S. saprophyticus UTI is associated with a urinary "fishy odor," alkaline urine pH, and microscopic hematuria. Novobiocin sensitivity differentiates coagulase-negative staphylococci (sensitive) from S. saprophyticus (resistant).
GRAM-POSITIVE COCCI (CHAINS)				
Enterococcus faecalis (VSE)	• CSF = NP (except from S. stercoralis hyperinfection or V-P shunt infection) • Blood = C*, P (from GI/GU source, SBE) • Sputum = NP • Urine = C, P (cystitis, pyelonephritis) • Stool = C, P • Wound = C, P (cellulitis)	Non-SBE Ampicillin (IV) Amoxicillin (PO) Meropenem (IV) Piperacillin (IV) Linezolid (IV/PO) Tigecycline (IV) Daptomycin (IV) SBE Gentamicin + ampicillin (IV) or vancomycin (IV) Meropenem (IV) Piperacillin (IV) Linezolid (IV/PO)	Non-SBE Cefoperazone (IV) Chloramphenicol (IV) Levofloxacin (IV/PO) Moxifloxacin (IV/PO) Nitrofurantoin (PO) (UTIs only) SBE Any quinolone (IV/PO) Cefoperazone (IV)	Sensitive to ampicillin, not penicillin. Cause of intermediate (severity between ABE and SBE) endocarditis, hepatobiliary infections, and UTIs. Enterococci (E. faecalis, E. faecium) are the only cause of SBE (below the waist) from GI/GU sources. Permissive pathogen (i.e., usually does not cause infection alone) in the abdomen/pelvis (except in gallbladder or urinary bladder/kidneys). Cefoperazone is the only cephalosporin with anti-E. faecalis (VSE) activity (MIC ~ 32 mcg/mL). Quinupristin/dalfopristin is not active against E. faecalis (VSE). Treat vancomycin resistant E. faecalis as VRE (see E. faecium VRE p. 211).

Enterococcus faecium (VRE)	• CSF = NP (except from S. stercoralis hyperinfection or V-P shunt infection) • Blood = C*, P (from GI/GU source, SBE) • Sputum = C • Urine = C, P (cystitis, pyelo) • Stool = NP • Wound = C, P (cellulitis)	**Non-SBE** Linezolid (IV/PO), quinupristin/dalfopristin (IV), doxycycline (IV/PO), tigecycline (IV), chloramphenicol (IV/PO), nitrofurantoin (PO) (UTIs only) **SBE** Linezolid (IV/PO) Quinupristin/dalfopristin (IV)	Same spectrum of infection as E. faecalis. Colonization common; infection uncommon. Fecal carriage is intermittent but prolonged. In vitro sensitivity = in vivo efficacy. Increased prevalence of E. faecalis (VRE) related to vancomycin IV (not PO) use. Nitrofurantoin preferred for VRE lower UTIs/catheter-associated bacteriuria.
Group A streptococci	• CSF = C*, P (rare cause of ABM) • Blood = P (from skin/soft tissue infection) • Sputum = P (rare cause of CAP) • Urine = NP • Stool = NP • Wound = C, P (cellulitis) • Throat = C, P (pharynx is colonized with Group A streptococci in ~ 30% of patients with EBV mono)	Amoxicillin (PO) Any β-lactam (IV/PO) Penicillin (PO) Clindamycin (IV/PO)	For Group A streptococcal pharyngitis, amoxicillin is preferred over penicillin. Clindamycin is best for elimination of carrier states, and for penicillin-allergic patients with streptococcal pharyngitis. Any β-lactam is equally effective against Group A streptococci. Nafcillin is the most active anti-staphylococcal penicillin against Group A streptococci. Erythromycin is no longer reliable against Group A streptococci due to increasing resistance. Doxycycline has little/no activity against Group A streptococci.
Group B streptococci (S. agalactiae)	• CSF = P • Blood = P (from IV line/urine source, SBE)	**Non-SBE, non-CNS** Clindamycin (IV/PO) **Non-SBE, non-CNS** Vancomycin (IV) Amoxicillin (PO)	Cause of UTIs and IV line infections in diabetics and the elderly. Cause of neonatal meningitis. Infection is uncommon in the general population. Rarely a cause of SBE in

C = colonizer; C* = skin contaminant; NP = non-pathogen at site; P = pathogen at site; (IV/PO) = IV or PO. See p. xi for all other abbreviations.

Table 3.5. Usual Clinical Significance of AEROBIC Isolates Pending Susceptibility Testing (cont'd)

		GRAM-POSITIVE COCCI (CHAINS)	
Isolate	Isolate Significance	Preferred Therapy	Alternate Therapy	Comments
	• Sputum = NP • Urine = P (CAB, UTIs, especially in diabetics, elderly) • Stool = NP • Wound = C, P (diabetic foot infections)	Any 1st, 2nd, 3rd generation cephalosporin (IV/PO) <u>SBE</u> Ceftriaxone (IV) Penicillin (IV) Vancomycin (IV) <u>CNS</u> Ceftriaxone (IV) Penicillin (IV)	<u>SBE</u> Meropenem (IV) Ertapenem (IV) Linezolid (IV/PO) <u>CNS</u> Chloramphenicol (IV) Linezolid (IV/PO)	Non-pregnant adults. On gram stain, GBS appear larger/rounder than S. pneumoniae. Colonies of GBS on BAP have a "sheen" (vs. S. pneumoniae). Aminoglycosides and tetracyclines are ineffective.
Group C, F, G streptococci	• CSF = P (meningitis) • Blood = P (from skin/soft tissue infection, SBE) • Sputum = P (rare cause of CAP) • Throat = C (especially with viral pharyngitis), P (pharyngitis in medical personnel) • Urine = NP • Stool = NP • Wound = P (cellulitis)	Ceftriaxone (IV) Penicillin (IV) Ampicillin (IV) Clindamycin (IV/PO)	Vancomycin (IV) Amoxicillin (PO) Any 1st, 2nd, 3rd generation cephalosporin (IV) Meropenem (IV) Ertapenem (IV)	Group C, G streptococci may cause pharyngitis, wound infections, and rarely SBE. Group G streptococci associated with malignancies. Common pharyngeal colonizers in medical personnel.

GRAM-NEGATIVE COCCI (CHAINS)

Streptococcus (bovis) gallolyticus	• CSF = NP • Blood = P (SBE from GI source) • Sputum = NP • Urine = NP • Stool = NP • Wound = NP	Ceftriaxone (IV) Ampicillin (IV) Clindamycin (IV/PO)	Vancomycin (IV) Amoxicillin (PO) Any 1st, 2nd, 3rd generation cephalosporin (IV)	Associated with GI malignancies. Non-enterococcal Group D streptococci (e.g., S. bovis) are sensitive to penicillin.
Viridans streptococci (S. mitior, milleri, mitis, mutans, oralis, sanguis, parasanguis, salivarius)	• CSF = NP (aseptic meningitis with SBE) • Blood = C*, P (1° bacteremia, SBE) • Sputum = NP • Urine = NP • Stool = NP • Wound = NP	Ceftriaxone (IV) Penicillin (IV)	Amoxicillin (PO) Any 1st, 2nd, 3rd generation cephalosporin (IV/PO) Meropenem (IV) Ertapenem (IV) Vancomycin (IV)	Viridans streptococci are commonly isolated from blood cultures. Low-grade blood culture positivity (1/4) indicates contamination during venipuncture. Continuous/high-grade blood culture positivity (3/4 or 4/4) indicates SBE until proven otherwise. S. milleri is associated with metastatic abscesses.

GRAM-POSITIVE COCCI (PAIRS)

Leuconostoc	• CSF = NP • Blood = P (PVE) • Sputum = NP • Urine = P (UTIs) • Stool = NP • Wound = NP	Penicillin (IV) Ampicillin (IV) Clindamycin (IV/PO)	Amoxicillin (PO) Erythromycin (IV) Minocycline (IV/PO) Clarithromycin XL (PO)	Coccobacillary forms resemble streptococci/ enterococci. Cause of infection in compromised hosts. Rare cause of IV line infection. Usually vancomycin-resistant.
Streptococcus pneumoniae	• CSF = P (ABM) • Blood = P (from respiratory tract source) • Sputum = C, P • Urine = NP • Stool = NP	Multidrug Resistant S. pneumoniae (MDRSP) A "respiratory quinolone" (IV/PO); telithromycin (PO); ertapenem (IV); meropenem (IV); cefepime (IV); linezolid (IV/PO); vancomycin (IV)	Penicillin (IV) Ampicillin (IV) Clindamycin (IV/PO)	Amoxicillin (PO) Erythromycin (IV) Minocycline (IV/PO) Clarithromycin XL (PO)	Penicillin-resistant S. pneumoniae (PRSP) are still sensitive to full-dose/high-dose β-lactams. If possible, avoid macrolides, as > 30% of S. pneumoniae are macrolide resistant (MRSP). (~ 20–25% are naturally resistant and 10–15% acquire macrolide resistance).

C = colonizer; C* = skin contaminant; NP = non-pathogen at site; P = pathogen at site; (IV/PO) = IV or PO. See p. xi for all other abbreviations.

Table 3.5. Usual Clinical Significance of AEROBIC Isolates Pending Susceptibility Testing (cont'd)

Isolate	Isolate Significance	GRAM-POSITIVE COCCI (PARIS)		Comments
		Preferred Therapy	Alternate Therapy	
	• Wound = P (cellulitis only in SLE)		Sensitive or relatively PCN-resistant Doxycycline (IV/PO); any cephalosporin (IV/PO); clindamycin (IV/PO); amoxicillin/clavulanic acid (PO)	
		GRAM-NEGATIVE COCCI (PARIS)		
Neisseria gonorrhoeae (GC)	• CSF = NP • Blood = P (from pharyngitis, proctitis, ABE) • Sputum = NP • Urine = P (urethritis) • Stool = NP • Wound = NP • Rectal discharge = P (GC proctitis)	Penicillin-sensitive N. gonorrhoeae (PSNG) Ceftriaxone (IV/IM) Any quinolone (IV/PO) PRNG Ceftriaxone (IV/IM)	Penicillin-sensitive N. gonorrhoeae (PSNG) Penicillin (IV/IM) Amoxicillin (PO) Doxycycline (IV/PO) PPNG Spectinomycin (IM) Any quinolone (PO) Any 1st, 2nd, 3rd gen. cephalosporin (IV/IM)	Cause of "culture negative" right-sided ABE. May be cultured from synovial fluid/blood in disseminated GC infection (arthritis-dermatitis syndrome). Spectinomycin is ineffective against pharyngeal GC/incubating syphilis. PRNG are tetracycline-resistant (TRNG). GC strains from Hawaii/California have increased quinolone resistance; use cefixime or ceftriaxone for such strains. Treat possible Chlamydia trachomatis co-infection and sexual partners.
Neisseria meningitidis	• CSF = P (ABM) • Blood = P (acute/chronic meningococcemia) • Sputum = C, P (only in closed populations, e.g., military recruits)	Penicillin (IV) Ampicillin (IV) Any 3rd generation cephalosporin (IV)	Chloramphenicol (IV) Cefepime (IV) Meropenem (IV)	In ABM, do not decrease meningeal dose of β-lactam antibiotics as patient improves, since CSF penetration/concentration decreases as meningeal inflammation decreases. Chloramphenicol is an excellent choice for penicillin-allergic patients. Preferred meningococcal prophylaxis is an oral quinolone (single dose).

		GRAM-POSITIVE BACILLI		
• Urine C, P (urethritis rarely) • Stool = NP • Wound = NP				
Arcanobacterium (Corynebacterium) haemolyticum	• CSF = NP • Blood = NP • Sputum = P (oropharyngeal secretions) • Urine = NP • Stool/Wound = NP	Doxycycline (PO)	Erythromycin (PO) Azithromycin (PO) Any 1st, 2nd, 3rd generation cephalosporin (PO) Clarithromycin XL (PO)	Causes membranous pharyngitis with scarlet fever-like rash. Differentiate from C. diphtheriae by culture. Penicillin and ampicillin are less effective than erythromycin or doxycycline.
Bacillus anthracis (naturally acquired) (For potential bioterrorist anthrax, see p. 173)	• CSF = P (ABM) • Blood = P (septicemia; isolation required; dangerous) • Sputum = P (mediastinitis; anthrax pneumonia rare) • Urine = NP • Stool = NP • Wound = P (ulcer; isolation required; dangerous)	Penicillin (IV) Doxycycline (IV/PO) Any quinolone (IV/PO)	Amoxicillin (PO) Ampicillin (IV)	Doxycycline may be used for therapy/outbreak prophylaxis. Streptobacillary configuration in blood. Causes hemorrhagic meningitis, wound infections, and bacteremia. Quinolones are effective. Alert microbiology laboratory of potentially biohazardous specimens.
Bacillus cereus, subtilis, megaterium	• CSF = NP • Blood = C*, P (leukopenic compromised hosts)	Vancomycin (IV) Clindamycin (IV/PO)	Meropenem (IV) Any quinolone (IV/PO)	Soil organisms not commonly pathogenic for humans. Suspect pseudoinfection if isolated from clinical specimens. Look for soil/dust contamination of blood culture tube top/

C = colonizer; C* = skin contaminant; NP = non-pathogen at site; P = pathogen at site; (IV/PO) = IV or PO. See p. xi for all other abbreviations.

Table 3.5. Usual Clinical Significance of AEROBIC Isolates Pending Susceptibility Testing (cont'd)

Isolate	Isolate Significance	Preferred Therapy	Alternate Therapy	Comments
	• Sputum = NP • Urine = NP • Stool = NP • Wound = NP			apparatus. Rare pathogen in leukopenic compromised hosts.
Corynebacterium diphtheriae	• CSF = NP • Blood = NP • Sputum = P (oropharyngeal secretions) • Urine = NP • Stool = NP • Wound = P (wound diphtheria)	Penicillin (IV) Erythromycin (IV) Clindamycin (IV/PO)	Doxycycline (IV/PO) Clarithromycin XL (PO) Rifampin (PO)	Administer diphtheria antitoxin as soon as possible (p. 170). Antibiotic therapy is adjunctive, since diphtheria is a toxin-mediated disease. Patients may die unexpectedly from toxin-induced myocarditis during recovery.
Corynebacterium jeikeium (JK)	• CSF = C*, P (CSF shunts) • Blood = C*, P (from IV lines) • Sputum = NP • Urine/Stool = NP • Wound = C	Vancomycin (IV) Linezolid (IV/PO)	Quinupristin/ dalfopristin (IV)	Cause of IV line/foreign body infections. In-vitro testing is not always reliable. Highly resistant to most anti-gram positive antibiotics.
Erysipelothrix rhusiopathiae	• CSF = NP • Blood = P (from SBE) • Sputum = NP • Urine = NP • Stool = NP • Wound = P (chronic erysipelas-like skin lesions)	Penicillin (IV) Ampicillin (IV)	Any 3rd generation cephalosporin (IV) Any quinolone (IV/PO)	Cause of "culture-negative" SBE. Susceptible to clindamycin but resistant to vancomycin.

Listeria monocytogenes	• CSF = P (ABM) • Blood = P (1° bacteremia, SBE) • Sputum = NP • Urine = NP • Stool = NP • Wound = NP	Ampicillin (IV) Amoxicillin (PO) Chloramphenicol (IV) <u>CNS</u> Ampicillin (IV) TMP–SMX (IV/PO) Chloramphenicol (IV/PO) <u>SBE</u> Ampicillin (IV)	Doxycycline (IV/PO) Erythromycin (IV) Meropenem (IV) <u>CNS</u> Meropenem (IV) (Meningeal dosed) Linezolied (IV/PO) <u>SBE</u> Meropenem (IV) Linezolied (IV/PO)	Listeria ABM is common in T-cell deficiencies (e.g., lymphoma, steroids, HIV). Causes SBE in normal hosts, and is the commonest cause of bacteremia in non-neutropenic cancer patients. 3rd generation cephalosporins are ineffective against Listeria.
Nocardia asteroides, brasiliensis	• CSF = P (brain abscess) • Blood = P (from lung/ soft tissue source) • Sputum = P (pneumonia, lung abscess) • Urine/Stool = NP • Wound = P (skin lesions from direct inoculation or dissemination)	TMP–SMX (IV/PO) Minocycline (IV/PO)	Imipenem (IV) plus either amikacin (IV) or any 3rd generation cephalosporin (IV)	Branched, filamentous, beady hyphae are typical, but coccobacillary and bacillary forms are also common. Nocardia are gram-positive, aerobic, and acid fast. Linezolid is active against Nocardia and may be effective if other agents cannot be used. Quinolones and macrolides are usually ineffective.
Rhodococcus equi	• CSF = NP • Blood = P (from pneumonia, lung abscess) • Sputum = P (pneumonia with abscess/cavitation)	Any quinolone (IV/PO) Vancomycin (IV)	Erythromycin (IV) Imipenem (IV) Meropenem (IV) Doxycycline (IV/PO) TMP–SMX (IV/PO)	Causes TB-like community-acquired pneumonia in AIDS patients. Filamentous bacteria break into bacilli/cocci. Aminoglycosides and β-lactams are relatively ineffective.

C = colonizer; C* = skin contaminant; NP = non-pathogen at site; P = pathogen at site; (IV/PO) = IV or PO. See p. xi for all other abbreviations.

Table 3.5. Usual Clinical Significance of AEROBIC Isolates Pending Susceptibility Testing (cont'd)

Isolate	Isolate Significance	Preferred Therapy	Alternate Therapy	Comments
		GRAM-POSITIVE BACILLI		
	• Urine = NP • Stool = NP • Wound = NP			
		GRAM-NEGATIVE BACILLI		
Acinetobacter baumannii, lwoffi, calcoaceticus, haemolyticus	• CSF = C* P (ABM) • Blood = P (from IV line, lung, or urine source) • Sputum = C, P (VAP) • Urine = C, P (CAB) • Stool = NP • Wound = C (common), P (rare)	Any carbapenem (IV) Ampicillin/ sulbactam (IV)	Colistin Polymyxin B Any 3rd generation cephalosporin (IV) (except ceftazidime) Cefepime (IV)	Colonization common; infection uncommon. Occurs in outbreaks of ventilator-associated pneumonia. Usually associated with respiratory support equipment. Test susceptibility to each carbapenem (may be susceptible to one but not others). Use meropenem for MDR susceptible isolates. For meropenem resistant MDR isolates, use colistin, polymyxin B, tigacycline or doripenem.
Aeromonas hydrophila	• CSF = NP • Blood = P (from wound, urine, or GI source) • Sputum = NP • Urine = C, P (CAB) • Stool = P (diarrhea) • Wound = P (cellulitis)	Gentamicin (IV) TMP-SMX (IV/PO) Any quinolone (IV/PO)	Doxycycline (IV/PO) Any 3rd generation cephalosporin (IV/PO) Any carbapenem (IV) Aztreonam (IV)	Cause of wound infection, septic arthritis, diarrhea, and necrotizing soft tissue infection resembling gas gangrene.
Aggregatibacter (Actinobacillus) actinomycetem-comitans	• CSF = NP • Blood = P (from abscess, SBE) • Sputum = NP • Urine/Stool = NP	Any quinolone (IV/PO) Any 3rd generation cephalosporin (IV/PO)	Penicillin (IV) + gentamicin (IV) TMP-SMX (IV/PO)	Cause of "culture-negative" SBE. One of the HACEK organisms. Found with Actinomyces in abscesses. Resistant to erythromycin and clindamycin.

Organism	Site/Pathogen	Preferred Therapy	Alternate Therapy	Comments
	• Wound = P (from abscess, draining fistulous tract)			
Alcaligenes (Achromobacter) xylosoxidans	• CSF = P (rarely ABM) • Blood = P (from urine) • Sputum = NP • Urine = P (CAB) • Stool = NP • Wound = P (cellulitis rare)	Imipenem (IV) Meropenem (IV) Any 3rd generation cephalosporin (IV/PO)	Any quinolone (IV/PO) Cefepime (IV) Aztreonam (IV)	Water-borne pathogen resembling Acinetobacter microbiologically. Resistant to aminoglycosides and 1st, 2nd generation cephalosporins.
Bartonella henselae, quintana, bacilliformis	• CSF = NP • Blood = P (from skin source, SBE) • Sputum = NP • Urine = NP • Stool = NP • Wound = P (skin lesions)	Doxycycline (IV/PO) Azithromycin (PO)	Clarithromycin XL (PO) Any quinolone (IV/PO) Any aminoglycoside (IV)	B. henselae (bacteremia, endocarditis, peliosis hepatis, bacillary angiomatosis); B. quintana (relapsing, trench fever, bacillary angiomatosis); B. baciliformis (Oroyo fever, Carrion's disease). May present as FUO. Titers may cross react with C. burnetii (Q fever). TMP–SMX and cephalosporins are ineffective.
Bordetella pertussis, parapertussis	• CSF = NP • Blood = P (from respiratory tract source) • Sputum = C, P (pertussis) • Urine = NP • Stool = NP • Wound = NP	Erythromycin (IV) Clarithromycin XL (PO) Azithromycin (IV/PO)	Any quinolone (IV/PO) TMP–SMX (IV/PO) Doxycycline (IV/PO)	Causes pertussis in children and incompletely/ non-immunized adults. Macrolides remain the preferred therapy. Resistant to penicillins, cephalosporins, and aminoglycosides.
Brucella abortus, canis, suis, melitensis	• CSF = P (meningitis) • Blood = P (from abscess, SBE)	Doxycycline (IV/PO) + gentamicin (IV)	TMP–SMX (IV/PO) + gentamicin (IV)	Causes prolonged relapsing infection. Zoonotic cause of brucellosis/Malta fever. Resistant to penicillins.

C = colonizer; C* = skin contaminant; NP = non-pathogen at site; P = pathogen at site; (IV/PO) = IV or PO. See p. xi for all other abbreviations.

Table 3.5. Usual Clinical Significance of AEROBIC Isolates Pending Susceptibility Testing (cont'd)

		GRAM-NEGATIVE BACILLI		
Isolate	Isolate Significance	Preferred Therapy	Alternate Therapy	Comments
	• Sputum = NP • Urine = P (pyelonephritis) • Stool/Wound = NP	Doxycycline + streptomycin (IM)	Doxycycline (IV/PO) + rifampin (PO) Any quinolone (IV/PO) + rifampin (PO)	
Burkholderia (Pseudomonas) cepacia	• CSF = NP • Blood = P (usually from IV line/urinary tract infection) • Sputum = C (not a cause of VAP) • Urine = C • Stool = NP • Wound = NP	TMP-SMX (IV/PO) Minocycline (IV/PO)	A "respiratory quinolone" (IV/PO) Chloramphenicol (IV/PO)	Rare cause of urosepsis following urologic instrumentation. Common water-borne colonizer in intensive care units. Opportunistic pathogen in cystic fibrosis/bronchiectasis. Resistant to aminoglycosides, colistin, and polymyxin B.
Burkholderia (Pseudomonas) pseudomallei	• CSF = NP • Blood = P (from septicemic melioidosis) • Sputum = P (chronic cavitary pneumonia) • Urine = NP • Stool = NP • Wound = NP	Imipenem (IV) Meropenem (IV) Ceftazidime (IV) Doxycycline (IV/PO)	Chloramphenicol (IV) TMP-SMX (IV/PO) Amoxicillin/clavulanic acid (PO)	Acute (septicemia)/chronic (cavitary CAP/abscesses) melioidosis endemic in S.E. Asia. Chronic melioidosis resembles reactivation TB, but has lower lobe distribution. Prolonged latency until reactivation years later. Slow response to effective therapy (1–2 weeks). Prolonged therapy needed to prevent relapse (≥ 3 months). Oxidase positive. Resistant to penicillin, aminoglycosides, colistin.
Campylobacter fetus	• CSF = P (ABM) • Blood = P (from vascular source)	Gentamicin (IV) Imipenem (IV) Meropenem (IV)	Chloramphenicol (IV) Ampicillin (IV)	Causes invasive infection with spread to CNS. CNS infection may be treated with meningeal doses of chloramphenicol, ampicillin,

	• Sputum = NP • Urine = NP • Stool = NP • Wound = NP	Any 3rd generation cephalosporin (IV)	or a 3rd generation cephalosporin. Resistant to erythromycin.
Campylobacter jejuni	• CSF = NP • Blood = P (from GI source) • Sputum = NP • Urine = NP • Stool = P (diarrhea) • Wound = NP	Any quinolone (IV/PO) Erythromycin (PO) Doxycycline (IV/PO)	Azithromycin (PO) Clarithromycin XL (PO)	Commonest cause of acute bacterial diarrhea. Resistant to TMP–SMX.
Cardiobacterium hominis	• CSF = NP • Blood = P (from SBE) • Sputum = NP • Urine = NP • Stool = NP • Wound = NP	Penicillin (IV) + gentamicin (IV) Ampicillin (IV) + gentamicin (IV)	Any 3rd generation cephalosporin (IV) + gentamicin (IV)	Pleomorphic bacillus with bulbous ends. Often appears in clusters resembling rosettes. Indole positive. Cause of "culture-negative" SBE (one of the HACEK organisms). Rare cause of abdominal abscess. Grows best with CO_2 enhancement. Resistant to macrolides and clindamycin.
Chromobacterium violaceum	• CSF = NP • Blood = P (from wound infection) • Sputum = NP • Urine = NP • Stool = NP • Wound = P (drainage from deep soft tissue infection)	Gentamicin (IV) Doxycycline (IV/PO)	Chloramphenicol (IV)	Cause of cutaneous lesions primarily in tropical/subtropical climates. Often mistaken for Vibrio or Alcaligenes. Resistant to β-lactams.
Chryseobacterium (Flavobacterium) meningosepticum	• CSF = P (ABM) • Blood = P (from IV line infection, PVE) • Sputum = NP	<u>CNS</u> TMP–SMX (IV/PO)	<u>CNS</u> Chloramphenicol (IV)	Rare cause of ABM in newborns and PVE in adults. Only unencapsulated Flavobacterium species. Clindamycin, clarithromycin, and vancomycin are useful only in non-CNS

C = colonizer; C* = skin contaminant; NP = non-pathogen at site; P = pathogen at site; (IV/PO) = IV or PO. See p. xi for all other abbreviations.

Table 3.5. Usual Clinical Significance of AEROBIC Isolates Pending Susceptibility Testing (cont'd)

Isolate	Isolate Significance	GRAM-NEGATIVE BACILLI Preferred Therapy	Alternate Therapy	Comments
	• Urine = C, P (from urologic instrumentation) • Stool = NP • Wound = C, P (cellulitis)	<u>Non-CNS</u> Vancomycin (IV) + rifampin (PO) Any quinolone (IV/PO)	<u>Non-CNS</u> Clarithromycin XL (PO) + rifampin (PO) Clindamycin (IV/PO)	infections. Resistant to aztreonam and carbapenems.
Citrobacter diversus, freundii, koseri	• CSF = C*, P (from NS procedure) • Blood = C*, P (from IV line/urinary tract infection) • Sputum = C (not pneumonia) • Urine = C, P (from urologic instrumentation) • Stool = NP • Wound = C, P (rarely in compromised hosts)	Any carbapenem (IV) Cefepime (IV) Any quinolone (IV/PO)	Aztreonam (IV) Piperacillin (IV) Any 3rd generation cephalosporin (IV)	Common wound/urine colonizer. Rare pathogen in normal hosts. Often aminoglycoside resistant. (C. freundii is usually more resistant than C. koseri).
Edwardsiella tarda	• CSF = NP • Blood = P (from liver abscess) • Sputum/Urine = NP • Stool = P • Wound C, P (wound infection)	Ampicillin (IV) Amoxicillin (PO) Any quinolone (IV/PO)	Doxycycline (IV/PO) Any 3rd generation cephalosporin (IV/PO)	Cause of bacteremia, usually from liver abscess or wound source.

Organism	Sites/Pathogen Status	First-line	Alternatives	Comments
Enterobacter agglomerans, aerogenes, cloacae	• CSF = C*, P (from NS procedure) • Blood = C*, P (from IV line/urinary tract infection) • Sputum = C (not a cause of pneumonia) • Urine = C, P (post-urologic instrumentation) • Stool = NP • Wound = C, P (rarely in compromised hosts)	Any carbapenem (IV)	Any quinolone (IV/PO) Aztreonam (IV) Piperacillin (IV) Cefepime (IV)	Not a cause of community-acquired or nosocomial pneumonia. Common colonizer of respiratory secretions and wound/urine specimens. Antibiotic resistance to E. cloacae > E. aerogenes > E. agglomerans. Treatment of Enterobacter colonizers with ceftazidime or ciprofloxacin may result in MDR/ESBL Enterobacter sp. NDM-1 metallo β-lactamase strains are carbapenem resistant and usually susceptible only to colistin, tigacycline.
Escherichia coli	• CSF = P (ABM) • Blood = P (from GI/GU source) • Sputum = P (rarely CAP from urinary source, VAP) • Urine = C, P (CAB, cystitis, pyelonephritis) • Stool = C, P (diarrhea) • Wound = P (cellulitis)	Any 1st, 2nd, 3rd generation cephalosporin (IV/PO) Amoxicillin (PO) Any quinolone (IV/PO) Ceftriaxone (IV) Nitrofurantoin (PO) (UTIs only)	Aztreonam (IV) Gentamicin (IV) TMP-SMX (IV/PO)	Common pathogen, usually from GI/GU source. Many strains are resistant to ampicillin and some to 1st generation cephalosporins. ESBL-producing E. coli may be treated with a carbapenem. NDM-1 metallo β-lactamase strains are carbapenem resistant and usually susceptible only to colistin, tigacycline.
Francisella tularensis	• CSF = NP • Blood = P (isolation dangerous) • Sputum = P (tularemic pneumonia; isolation dangerous)	Doxycycline (IV/PO) Gentamicin (IV/IM) Streptomycin (IM)	Chloramphenicol (IV/PO) Any quinolone (IV/PO)	Six clinical tularemia syndromes. Alert microbiology laboratory of potentially biohazardous specimens. Do not culture. Resistant to penicillins and cephalosporins. Bioterrorist tularemia is treated the same as naturally-acquired tularemia.

C = colonizer; C* = skin contaminant; NP = non-pathogen at site; P = pathogen at site; (IV/PO) = IV or PO. See p. xi for all other abbreviations.

Table 3.5. Usual Clinical Significance of AEROBIC Isolates Pending Susceptibility Testing (cont'd)

		GRAM-NEGATIVE BACILLI		
Isolate	Isolate Significance	Preferred Therapy	Alternate Therapy	Comments
Hafnia alvei	• Urine/Stool = NP • Wound = P (isolation dangerous)			
	• CSF = C, P (from NS procedure) • Blood = C*, P (from IV line/urinary tract infection) • Sputum = C (not pneumonia) • Urine = C, P (post-urologic instrumentation) • Stool = NP • Wound = C, P (rarely in compromised hosts)	Cefepime (IV) Any quinolone (IV/PO) Aztreonam (IV)	Piperacillin (IV) Imipenem (IV) Meropenem (IV)	Formerly Enterobacter hafniae. Uncommon nosocomial pathogen. Rarely pathogenic in normal hosts. Cause of UTIs in compromised hosts.
Helicobacter (Campylobacter) pylori	• CSF = NP • Blood = NP • Sputum = NP • Urine = NP • Stool = P (from upper GI tract biopsy specimens, not stool) • Wound = NP	Omeprazole (PO) + clarithromycin XL (PO) Omeprazole (PO) + amoxicillin (PO) Metronidazole (PO) + amoxicillin (PO) + bismuth subsalicylate (PO)	Doxycycline (PO) + metronidazole (PO) + bismuth subsalicylate (PO)	Optimal therapy awaits definition. Treat until cured. Some strains of resistant H. pylori may respond to treatment with a quinolone. TMP–SMX is ineffective.

Organism	Site	For all Hemophilus species	For all Hemophilus species	Comments
Hemophilus influenzae, parainfluenzae, aphrophilus, paraphrophilus	• CSF = P (ABM) • Blood = P (from respiratory tract or cardiac source) • Sputum = C, P (CAP) • Urine = NP • Stool = NP • Wound = P	For all Hemophilus species Any 2nd, 3rd generation cephalosporin (IV/PO) Any quinolone (IV/PO) Doxycycline (IV/PO)	For all Hemophilus species Chloramphenicol (IV) TMP-SMX (IV/PO) Azithromycin (PO) Aztreonam (IV) Ampicillin-resistant H. influenzae Meropenem (IV) Imipenem (IV) Ertapenem (IV) Cefepime (IV) Aztreonam (IV)	1st generation cephalosporins, erythromycin, and clarithromycin have limited anti-H. influenzae activity; doxycycline and azithromycin are better. Hemophilus species are common colonizers of the respiratory tract. Rarely a cause of "culture-negative" SBE (H. parainfluenzae/aphrophilus are HACEK organisms). H. influenzae and H. parainfluenzae (pathogens) may be differentiated from the throat commensals H. hemolyticus and H. parahemolyticus (non-pathogens) by hemolysis on sheep agar.
Kingella (Moraxella) kingae	• CSF = NP • Blood = P (from skeletal or cardiac source) • Sputum = C • Urine = NP • Stool/wound = NP	Ampicillin (IV) + any aminoglycoside (IV)	Any 3rd generation cephalosporin + any aminoglycoside (IV) Imipenem (IV) Meropenem (IV) Any quinolone (IV/PO)	Common colonizer of respiratory tract, but rarely a respiratory pathogen. Causes septic arthritis/osteomyelitis in children and endocarditis in adults (one of HACEK organisms). Oxidase positive. Growth enhanced with CO_2.
Klebsiella pneumoniae, oxytoca	• CSF = P (ABM) • Blood = P (from respiratory, GI, GU source)	Tigecycline (IV) Any carbapenem (IV)	Any 3rd generation cephalosporin (IV, PO) except ceftazidime Any quinolone (IV/PO)	TMP-SMX may be ineffective in systemic infection. Anti-pseudomonal penicillins have limited anti-Klebsiella activity. Klebsiella usually susceptible to carbapenems. Carbapenem resistant MDR Klebsiella usually susceptible to tigecycline, colistin, polymyxin B.

C = colonizer; C* = skin contaminant; NP = non-pathogen at site; P = pathogen at site; (IV/PO) = IV or PO. See p. xi for all other abbreviations.

Table 3.5. Usual Clinical Significance of AEROBIC Isolates Pending Susceptibility Testing (cont'd)

		GRAM-NEGATIVE BACILLI		
Isolate	Isolate Significance	Preferred Therapy	Alternate Therapy	Comments
Klebsiella ozaenae, rhinoscleromatis	• Sputum = C, P (CAP/ VAP) • Urine = C (CAB), P • Stool = NP • Wound = C, P		Aztreonam (IV) Cefepime (IV)	NDM-1 metallo β-lactamase strains are carbapenem resistant and usually susceptible only to colistin, tigacycline.
	• CSF = NP • Blood = NP • Sputum = NP • Urine = NP • Stool = NP • Wound = P (rhinoscleromatis lesions)	Any quinolone (PO)	TMP–SMX (PO) + rifampin (PO)	Skin infection usually requires prolonged treatment for cure (weeks-to-months).
Legionella sp.	• CSF = NP • Blood = NP • Sputum = P (CAP or VAP) • Urine = NP • Stool = NP • Wound = NP	Any quinolone (IV/PO) Doxycycline (IV/PO) Tigacycline (IV) Azithromycin (IV/PO)	Clarithromycin XL (PO) Erythromycin (IV) Telithromycin (PO)	Anti-Legionella activity: quinolones > doxycycline > erythromycin. Erythromycin failures are not uncommon. Rarely a cause of culture-negative SBE/PVE.
Leptospira interrogans	• CSF = P (ABM) • Blood = P (1° bacteremia) • Sputum = NP • Urine = P (excreted in urine) • Stool = NP • Wound = NP	Doxycycline (IV/PO) Penicillin G (IV) Any 3rd generation cephalosporin (IV/PO)	Amoxicillin (PO)	Blood/urine cultures may be positive during initial/bacteremic phase, but are negative during immune phase. Relapse is common. Resistant to chloramphenicol.

Organism	Site			Comments
Moraxella (Branhamella) catarrhalis	• CSF = NP • Blood = P (rarely from CAP) • Sputum = C, P (CAP) • Urine = NP • Stool = NP • Wound = NP	Any 2nd, 3rd generation cephalosporin (IV/PO) Any quinolone (IV/PO) Telithromycin (PO) Doxycycline (IV/PO)	Azithromycin (PO) Clarithromycin XL (PO) TMP–SMX (IV/PO) Amoxicillin/clavulanic acid (PO)	Almost all strains are β-lactamase positive and resistant to penicillin/ampicillin. β-lactamase-resistant β-lactams are effective. Resembles Acinetobacter on sputum gram stain.
Morganella morganii	• CSF = NP • Blood = P (from GU source) • Sputum = NP • Urine = P (CAB, cystitis, pyelonephritis) • Stool = NP • Wound = P (cellulitis rare)	Any quinolone (IV/PO) Any 3rd generation cephalosporin (IV) Any carbapenem (IV)	Any aminoglycoside (IV) Aztreonam (IV) Cefepime (IV)	Common uropathogen. Causes bacteremia with urosepsis. Rare cause of wound infections.
Ochrobactrum anthropi (CDC group Vd)	• CSF = NP • Blood = P (from IV line infections) • Sputum = C • Urine = C • Stool/Wound = C	Any quinolone (IV/PO) TMP–SMX (IV/PO)	Any aminoglycoside (IV) Imipenem (IV) Meropenem (IV)	Pathogen in compromised hosts. Oxidase and catalase positive. Resistant to β-lactams.
Pasteurella multocida	• CSF = P (ABM) • Blood = P (from respiratory source, bite wound/abscess) • Sputum = C, P (CAP, bronchiectasis)	Amoxicillin (PO) Doxycycline (IV/PO) Penicillin G (IV)	Ampicillin/sulbactam (IV) Piperacillin (IV) Any quinolone (IV/PO)	Common cause of infection following dog/cat bites. Many antibiotics are effective, but erythromycin is ineffective. Resembles Hemophilus sp. on sputum gram stain.

C = colonizer; C* = skin contaminant; NP = non-pathogen at site; P = pathogen at site; (IV/PO) = IV or PO. See p. xi for all other abbreviations.

Table 3.5. Usual Clinical Significance of AEROBIC Isolates Pending Susceptibility Testing (cont'd)

		GRAM-NEGATIVE BACILLI		
Isolate	Isolate Significance	Preferred Therapy	Alternate Therapy	Comments
	• Urine = C, P (pyelonephritis) • Stool = NP • Wound = P (human/animal bites)			Infrequent cause of diarrhea, less commonly dysentery. Oxidase positive. β-lactamase strains are increasing. Resistant to penicillins.
Plesiomonas shigelloides	• CSF = NP • Blood = P (from GU source) • Sputum = NP • Urine = NP • Stool = P (diarrhea) • Wound = NP	Any quinolone (PO) TMP-SMX (PO)	Doxycycline (PO) Aztreonam (PO)	
Proteus mirabilis, vulgaris	• CSF = NP • Blood = P (from urinary source) • Sputum = C • Urine = C, P (from urologic instrumentation) • Stool = NP • Wound = C, P (wound infection)	P. mirabilis, indole (−) Ampicillin (IV) Any 1st, 2nd, 3rd gen. cephalosporin (IV/PO) P. vulgaris, indole (+) Any 3rd generation cephalosporin (IV/PO) Cefepime (IV) Any quinolone (IV/PO)	P. mirabilis, indole (−) TMP-SMX (IV/PO) Amoxicillin (PO) P. vulgaris, indole (+) Any carbapenem (IV) Any aminoglycoside (IV)	Usually a uropathogen. Most antibiotics are effective against P. mirabilis (indole-negative); P. penneri (indole-negative P. vulgaris is resistant to ceftriaxone. Indole-positive Proteus sp. require potent antibiotics to treat non-UTIs. P. penneri (indole-negative P. vulgaris) resistant to 3rd gen. cephalosporins; use cefepime, carbapenem, or quinolone.

Providencia alcalifaciens, rettgeri, stuartii	• CSF = NP • Blood = C*, P (from GU source) • Sputum/Stool = NP • Urine = C, P • Wound = C, P (rare)	Any quinolone (IV/PO) Any 3rd generation cephalosporin (IV/PO) Cefepime (IV) Meropenem (IV) Ertapenem (IV)	Any aminoglycoside (IV) Aztreonam (IV) Piperacillin (IV) Imipenem (IV)	Almost always a uropathogen. Formerly classified as indole-positive Proteus.
Pseudomonas aeruginosa	• CSF = NP • Blood = P (from respiratory, GU source) • Sputum = C (usually), P (rarely indicates VAP) • Urine = C, P (from urologic instrumentation) • Stool = NP • Wound = C (almost always)	Monotherapy Meropenem (IV) Cefepime (IV) Combination therapy either meropenem (IV) or cefepime (IV) plus amikacin	Doripenem (IV) Colistin (IV) Polymyxin B (IV) Amikacin (IV) Aztreonam (IV)	For serious systemic P. aeruginosa infection, double-drug therapy preferred. All double anti-P. aeruginosa regimens are equally effective. Individual differences in activity (MICs) are unimportant if combination therapy is used. If MDR P. aeruginosa meropenem susceptible, treat with meropenem. If MDR P. aeruginosa meropenem resistant, treat with colistin, polymyxin B, or doripenem.
Pseudomonas (Chryseomonas) luteola (CDC group Ve-1)	• CSF = NP • Blood = P (from IV line infection) • Sputum = NP • Urine = NP • Stool = NP • Wound = NP	Imipenem (IV) Meropenem (IV) Cefepime (IV)	Piperacillin/ tazobactam (IV) Aztreonam (IV)	Opportunistic pathogen primarily in compromised hosts.

C = colonizer; C* = skin contaminant; NP = non-pathogen; P = pathogen at site; (IV/PO) = IV or PO. See p. xi for all other abbreviations.

Table 3.5. Usual Clinical Significance of AEROBIC Isolates Pending Susceptibility Testing (cont'd)

		GRAM-NEGATIVE BACILLI		
Isolate	**Isolate Significance**	**Preferred Therapy**	**Alternate Therapy**	**Comments**
Pseudomonas (Flavimonas) oryzihabitans (CDC group Ve-2)	• CSF = P (NS procedures) • Blood = P (from IV line infection) • Sputum = NP • Urine = NP • Stool = NP • Wound = P (rare)	Imipenem (IV) Meropenem (IV) Cefepime (IV)	Any 3rd generation cephalosporin (IV) Piperacillin (IV) Aztreonam (IV)	Rare cause of central IV line infections in compromised hosts (usually in febrile neutropenics). Rare cause of peritonitis in CAPD patients. Oxidase negative, unlike other Pseudomonas species.
Salmonella typhi, non-typhi	• CSF = NP • Blood = P (from GI source) • Sputum = NP • Urine = P (only with enteric fever) • Stool = C (carrier), P (gastroenteritis, enteric fever) • Wound = NP	Any quinolone (IV/PO) Any 3rd generation cephalosporin (IV)	Chloramphenicol (IV) TMP–SMX (IV/PO) Doxycycline (IV/PO)	Carrier state is best eliminated by a quinolone or TMP–SMX. If drug therapy fails to eliminate carrier state, look for hepatic/bladder calculi for persistent focus. Many strains are resistant to ampicillin/amoxicillin.
Serratia marcescens	• CSF = P (from NS procedures) • Blood = P (from IV line or urinary source) • Sputum = C, P (rarely in VAP) • Urine = C, P (post-urologic instrumentation) • Stool = NP • Wound = C, P (rare)	Any 3rd generation cephalosporin (IV/PO) (except ceftazidime) Any quinolone (IV/PO) Cefepime (IV)	Any carbapenem (IV) Gentamicin (IV) Aztreonam (IV) Piperacillin (IV)	Enterobacteriaceae. Associated with water sources. Common colonizer of respiratory secretions/urine in ICU. Serratia nosocomial pneumonia and PVE are rare. Cause of septic arthritis, osteomyelitis, and SBE (IV drug abusers). Among the aminoglycosides, gentamicin has the greatest anti-Serratia activity.

Shigella boydii, sonnei, flexneri, dysenteriae	• CSF = NP • Blood = P (from GI source) • Sputum = NP • Urine = NP • Stool = P (Shigella dysentery) • Wound = NP	Any quinolone (IV/PO)	TMP–SMX (IV/PO) Azithromycin (IV/PO)	No carrier state. Severity of dysentery varies with the species: S. dysenteriae (most severe) > S. flexneri > S. sonnei/boydii (least severe).
Steno-trophomonas (Pseudomonas, Xanthomonas) maltophilia	• CSF = C, P (from NS procedures) • Blood = C*, P (from IV line infection, GU source) • Sputum = C (not VAP) • Urine = C, P (from urologic instrumentation) • Stool = NP • Wound = C, P (rarely in compromised hosts)	TMP–SMX (IV/PO) Minocycline (IV/PO)	Cefepime (IV) Any respiratory quinolone (IV/PO)	Potential pulmonary pathogen only in bronchiectasis/cystic fibrosis. Resistant to aminoglycosides and carbapenems. Although usually carbapenem resistant, ~60% of strains demonstrate synergy with meropenem + levofloxacin. Susceptible to chloramphenicol, rifampin, colistin, polymyxin B.
Streptobacillus moniliformis	• CSF = P (brain abscess) • Blood = P (from wound) • Sputum = P (lung abscess) • Urine = NP • Stool = NP • Wound = P (from rat bite)	Penicillin (IV) Ampicillin (IV) Amoxicillin (PO)	Oxycycline (IV/PO) Erythromycin (IV) DClindamycin (IV/PO)	Cause of Haverhill fever and rat-bite fever, with abrupt onset of severe headache/arthralgias after bite wound has healed. No regional adenopathy. Morbilliform/petechial rash. Arthritis in 50%. May cause SBE.

C = colonizer; C* = skin contaminant; NP = non-pathogen at site; P = pathogen at site; (IV/PO) = IV or PO. See p. xi for all other abbreviations.

Table 3.5. Usual Clinical Significance of AEROBIC Isolates Pending Susceptibility Testing (cont'd)

		GRAM-NEGATIVE BACILLI		
Isolate	Isolate Significance	Preferred Therapy	Alternate Therapy	Comments
Vibrio cholerae	• CSF = NP • Blood = P (from GI source) • Sputum = NP • Urine = NP • Stool = P (cholera) • Wound = NP	Doxycycline (IV/PO) Any quinolone (IV/PO)	TMP–SMX (IV/PO)	No carrier state. Treat for 3 days. Single-dose therapy is often effective. Resistant to ampicillin.
Vibrio parahaemolyticus	• CSF = NP • Blood = P (from GI source) • Sputum = NP • Urine = NP • Stool = P (diarrhea) • Wound = P	Doxycycline (IV/PO) Any quinolone (IV/PO)	Any quinolone (IV/PO)	Most cases of gastroenteritis caused by V. parahaemolyticus are self-limited and require no treatment.
Vibrio vulnificus, alginolyticus	• CSF = NP • Blood = P (from GI/wound source) • Sputum = NP • Urine = NP • Stool = P (diarrhea) • Wound = P (water-contaminated wound raw oysters, other shell fish ingestion)	Doxycycline (IV/PO) Any quinolone (IV/PO)	Piperacillin (IV) Ampicillin/sulbactam (IV)	Causes necrotizing soft tissue infection resembling gas gangrene. Patients are critically ill with fever, bullous lesions, diarrhea, and hypotension. Treat wound infection, bacteremia. Aminoglycoside susceptibilities are unpredictable.
Yersinia enterocolitica	• CSF = NP • Blood = P (from GI source)	Any quinolone (IV/PO)	TMP–SMX (IV/PO) Any 3rd generation cephalosporin (IV/PO)	Cause of diarrhea with abdominal pain. If pain in is right lower quadrant, may be mistaken for acute appendicitis.

	• Sputum = NP • Urine = NP • Stool = P (diarrhea) • Wound = NP	Gentamicin (IV) Doxycycline (IV/PO)	
Yersinia pestis	• CSF = NP • Blood = P (septicemic plague; isolation required; dangerous) • Sputum = P (pneumonic plague; isolation required; dangerous) • Urine = NP • Stool = NP • Wound = P (lymph nodes, lymph node drainage; bubonic plague; isolation required; dangerous)	Doxycycline (IV/PO) Streptomycin (IM) Gentamicin (IV/IM) Any quinolone (IV/PO)	Chloramphenicol (IV/PO)	Cause of bubonic, septicemic, and pneumonic plague. Doxycycline or any quinolone may be used for prophylaxis. Alert microbiology laboratory of potentially biohazardous specimens. Do not culture. Bioterrorist plague is treated the same as naturally-acquired plague.

SPIROCHETES			
Borrelia burgdorferi	• CSF = P (neuroborreliosis) • Blood = P (rarely isolated; requires special media) • Sputum = NP • Urine = NP • Stool = NP • Wound = P (rarely isolated from erythema migrans lesions)	Doxycycline (PO) Amoxicillin (PO)	Any cephalosporin (PO) Azithromycin (PO) Erythromycin (PO)	Cause of Lyme disease. β-lactams and doxycycline are effective. Erythromycin least effective for erythema migrans. Minocycline may be preferred to doxycycline for neuroborreliosis.

C = colonizer; C* = skin contaminant; NP = non-pathogen at site; P = pathogen at site; (IV/PO) = IV or PO. See p. xi for all other abbreviations.

Table 3.5. Usual Clinical Significance of AEROBIC Isolates Pending Susceptibility Testing (cont'd)

		SPIROCHETES		
Isolate	Isolate Significance	Preferred Therapy	Alternate Therapy	Comments
Borrelia recurrentis	• CSF = P (ABM) • Blood = P (1° bacteremia) • Sputum = NP • Urine = NP • Stool = NP • Wound = NP	Doxycycline (IV/PO) Azithromycin (IV/PO)	Erythromycin (IV) Penicillin (IV) Ampicillin (IV) Any 1st, 2nd, 3rd generation cephalosporin (IV/PO)	Cause of relapsing fever. May be recovered from septic metastatic foci. Septic emboli may cause sacroiliitis, SBE, myositis, orchitis, or osteomyelitis.
Spirillum minus	• CSF = NP • Blood = P (from wound source, SBE) • Sputum = NP • Urine = NP • Stool = NP • Wound = P (from rat bite)	Penicillin (IV) Amoxicillin (PO)	Doxycycline (IV/PO) Any quinolone (IV/PO)	Cause of rat-bite fever. Bite wound heals promptly, but 1–4 weeks later becomes painful, purple and swollen, and progresses to ulceration and eschar formation. Painful regional adenopathy. Central maculopapular rash is common (rarely urticarial). Arthralgias/arthritis is rare compared to rat-bite fever from Streptobacillus moniliformis. Rarely causes SBE.

C = colonizer; C* = skin contaminant; NP = non-pathogen at site; P = pathogen at site; (IV/PO) = IV or PO. See p. xi for all other abbreviations.

Table 3.6. Clinical Significance of CAPNOPHILIC Isolates Pending Susceptibility Testing

		GRAM-NEGATIVE BACILLI		
Isolate	Isolate Significance	Preferred Therapy	Alternate Therapy	Comments
Capnocytophaga canimorsus/ cynodegni (DF-2 like)	• CSF = NP • Blood = P (from GI source, bite wound) • Sputum = NP • Urine = NP • Stool = NP • Wound = P (from dog/cat bite)	Ampicillin/ sulbactam (IV) Piperacillin/ tazobactam (IV) Imipenem (IV) Meropenem (IV) Ertapenem (IV)	Clindamycin (IV/PO) Any quinolone (IV/PO) Doxycycline (IV/PO)	Associated with animal bites or cancer. May cause fatal septicemia in cirrhotics/asplenics. Resistant to aminoglycosides, metronidazole, TMP–SMX, and aztreonam.
Capnocytophaga ochraceus (DF-1)	• CSF = NP • Blood = P (from GI, wound, abscess source) • Sputum = NP • Urine = NP • Stool = NP • Wound = P	Ampicillin/ sulbactam (IV) Piperacillin/ tazobactam (IV) Imipenem (IV) Meropenem (IV) Ertapenem (IV)	Clindamycin (IV/PO) Any quinolone (IV/PO) Doxycycline (IV/PO)	Thin, spindle-shaped bacilli resemble Fusobacteria morphologically. "Gliding motility" seen in hanging drop preparations. Cause of septicemia, abscesses, and wound infections. Resistant to aminoglycosides, metronidazole, TMP–SMX, and aztreonam.
Eikenella corrodens	• CSF = NP • Blood = P (SBE in IV drug abusers) • Sputum = NP • Urine = NP • Stool = NP • Wound = P (IV drug abusers)	Penicillin (IV) Ampicillin (IV) Imipenem (IV) Meropenem (IV) Ertapenem (IV)	Piperacillin (IV) Ampicillin/ sulbactam (IV) Doxycycline (IV/PO) Amoxicillin (PO)	Cause of "culture-negative" SBE (one of the HACEK organisms). Resistant to clindamycin and metronidazole.

C = colonizer; C* = skin contaminant; NP = non-pathogen at site; P = pathogen at site; (IV/PO) = IV or PO. See p. xi for all other abbreviations.

Table 3.7. Usual Clinical Significance of ANAEROBIC Isolates Pending Susceptibility Testing

Isolate	Isolate Significance	Preferred Therapy	Alternate Therapy	Comments
GRAM-POSITIVE BACILLI				
Peptococcus	• CSF = P (brain abscess) • Blood = P (from GI/pelvic source) • Sputum = C, P (aspiration pneumonia, lung abscess) • Urine/Stool = NP • Wound = P (rarely a sole pathogen)	Penicillin (IV) Ampicillin (IV) Amoxicillin (PO) Clindamycin (IV/PO)	Chloramphenicol (IV) Erythromycin (IV) Any carbapenem (IV) Moxifloxacin (IV/PO)	Normal flora of mouth, GI tract, and pelvis. Associated with mixed aerobic/anaerobic dental, abdominal, and pelvic infections, especially abscesses.
Peptostreptococcus	• CSF = P (brain abscess) • Blood = P (GI/pelvic source) • Sputum = C, P (aspiration pneumonia, lung abscess) • Urine/Stool = NP • Wound = P (rarely a sole pathogen)	Penicillin (IV) Ampicillin (IV) Amoxicillin (PO) Clindamycin (IV/PO)	Chloramphenicol (IV) Erythromycin (IV) Any carbapenem (IV) Moxifloxacin (IV/PO)	Normal flora of mouth, GI tract, and pelvis. Associated with mixed aerobic/anaerobic dental, abdominal, and pelvic infections, especially abscesses.
GRAM-POSITIVE BACILLI				
Actinomyces israelii, odontolyticus	• CSF = P (brain abscess) • Blood = NP	Amoxicillin (PO) Doxycycline (PO)	Erythromycin (PO) Clindamycin (PO)	Anaerobic and non-acid fast. Usually presents as cervical, facial, thoracic, or abdominal masses/fistulas. Prolonged

Organism	Site	Preferred Therapy	Alternative Therapy	Comments
	• Sputum = C, P (lung abscess) • Urine = NP • Stool = NP • Wound = P (fistulas/underlying abscess)			(6–12 month) treatment is needed for cure. Unlike Nocardia, Actinomyces rarely causes CNS infections. May be cultured from polymicrobial brain abscess of pulmonary origin. Quinolones, aminoglycosides, metronidazole, and TMP–SMX have little activity.
Arachnia propionica	• CSF = P (brain abscess) • Blood = P (from dental, GI, lung source) • Sputum = C, P (lung abscess) • Urine = NP • Stool = NP • Wound = NP	Clindamycin (IV/PO) Ampicillin (IV) + gentamicin (IV)	Erythromycin (IV)	Polymicrobial pathogen in dental, lung, and brain abscesses.
Bifidobacterium sp.	• CSF = P (brain abscess) • Blood = NP • Sputum = C, P (lung abscess) • Urine/Stool = NP • Wound = NP	Clindamycin (IV/PO) Ampicillin (IV) + gentamicin (IV)	Erythromycin (IV)	Usually part of polymicrobial infection.
Clostridium botulinum	• CSF = NP • Blood = NP • Sputum = NP • Urine/Stool = NP • Wound = P (wound botulism)	Penicillin (IV)	Clindamycin (IV/PO) Imipenem (IV) Meropenem (IV)	Give trivalent equine antitoxin (p. 170) as soon as possible. Antibiotic therapy is adjunctive.

C = colonizer; C* = skin contaminant; NP = non-pathogen at site; P = pathogen at site; (IV/PO) = IV or PO. See p. xi for all other abbreviations.

Table 3.7. Usual Clinical Significance of ANAEROBIC Isolates Pending Susceptibility Testing

		GRAM-POSITIVE BACILLI		
Isolate	**Isolate Significance**	**Preferred Therapy**	**Alternate Therapy**	**Comments**
Clostridium difficile	• CSF = NP • Blood = P (rarely from GI source) • Sputum = NP • Urine = NP • Stool = C (normal fecal flora), P (antibiotic-associated diarrhea/colitis) • Wound = NP	_C. difficile diarrhea_ Vancomycin (PO) Nitazoxanide (PO) _C. difficile colitis_ Metronidazole (IV/PO) Nitazoxanide (PO)	_C. difficile diarrhea_ Metronidazole (PO) _C. difficile colitis_ Tigacycline (IV)	**C. difficile diarrhea** PO vancomycin preferred. _PO vancomycin more reliably effective than PO metronidazole._ Nitazoxanide also highly effective. PO metronidazole, not PO vancomycin, increases prevalence of VRE. **C. difficile colitis,** use IV or PO metronidazole (IV vancomycin ineffective). Nitazoxanide (PO) or tigacycline (IV) also highly effective. Diagnose C. difficile diarrhea by stool C. difficile toxin assay/PCR. Diagnose C. difficile colitis by C. difficile + toxin assay/PCR plus colitis on abdominal CT scan/colonoscopy.
Clostridium perfringens, septicum, novyi	• CSF = NP • Blood = P (from GI source/malignancy) • Sputum = NP • Urine = NP • Stool = NP • Wound = P (gas gangrene)	Penicillin (IV) Piperacillin/ tazobactam (IV) Meropenem (IV) Ertapenem (IV)	Clindamycin (IV) Chloramphenicol (IV) Imipenem (IV)	Usual cause of myonecrosis (gas gangrene). Surgical debridement is crucial; antibiotic therapy is adjunctive. Also causes emphysematous cholecystitis/cystitis. Does not form spores in blood cultures as does C. sordelli.
Clostridium tetani	• CSF = NP • Blood = NP	Penicillin (IV) Clindamycin (IV)	Imipenem (IV) Meropenem (IV)	Prompt administration of tetanus immune globulin is crucial (p. 170). Antibiotic therapy is adjunctive.

	• Sputum = NP • Urine/Stool = NP • Wound = P (wound tetanus)			
Eubacterium sp.	• CSF = P (brain abscess) • Blood = P (from dental, GI, GU, lung source) • Sputum = P (lung abscess) • Urine/Stool = NP • Wound = NP	Clindamycin (IV/PO) Ampicillin (IV) + gentamicin (IV)	Erythromycin (IV)	Pathogen in lung/pelvic/brain abscesses, and chronic periodontal disease. Eubacterium bacteremias are associated with malignancies.
Lactobacillus sp.	• CSF = P (ABM) • Blood = P (1° bacteremia, SBE, or from endometritis) • Sputum = NP • Urine = P (rare) • Stool = NP • Wound = NP	Ampicillin (IV) + gentamicin (IV) Clindamycin (IV/PO)	Erythromycin (IV)	Uncommon pathogen in normal/ compromised hosts. Rare cause of SBE. Variably resistant to cephalosporins and quinolones. Some clindamycin-resistant strains. Resistant to metronidazole and vancomycin.
Propionibacterium acnes	• CSF = C*, P (meningitis from NS shunts) • Blood = C*, P (from IV line infection, SBE) • Sputum = NP • Urine = NP • Stool = NP • Wound = C	Penicillin (IV) Clindamycin (IV/PO)	Doxycycline (IV/PO)	Common skin colonizer/blood culture contaminant. Rarely causes prosthetic joint infection, endocarditis, or CNS shunt infection. Resistant to metronidazole.

C = colonizer; C* = skin contaminant; NP = non-pathogen at site; P = pathogen at site; (IV/PO) = IV or PO. See p. xi for all other abbreviations.

Table 3.7. Usual Clinical Significance of ANAEROBIC Isolates Pending Susceptibility Testing (cont'd)

Isolate	Isolate Significance	GRAM-NEGATIVE BACILLI Preferred Therapy	Alternate Therapy	Comments
Bacteroides fragilis group (B. distasonis, ovatus, thetaiotao-micron, vulgatus)	• CSF = P (meningitis from Strongyloides hyperinfection) • Blood = P (from GI/pelvic source) • Sputum = NP • Urine = NP, P (only from colonic fistula) • Stool = NP • Wound = NP	Tigecycline (IV) Piperacillin/tazobactam (IV) Any carbapenem (IV)	Moxifloxacin (IV/PO) Ampicillin/sulbactam (IV) Clindamycin (IV/PO) or combination of Metronidazole (IV/PO) plus either ceftriaxone (IV) or levofloxacin (IV/PO)	Major anaerobe below the diaphragm. Usually part of polymicrobial lower intra-abdominal and pelvic infections. Cefotetan is less effective against B. fragilis DOT strains (B. distasonis, B. ovatus, B. thetaiotaomicron). Resistant to penicillin.
Fusobacterium nucleatum	• CSF = P (brain abscess) • Blood = P (from lung, GI source) • Sputum = P (aspiration pneumonia, lung abscess) • Urine = NP • Stool = NP • Wound = P (rarely)	Clindamycin (IV/PO) Piperacillin/tazobactam (IV) Ampicillin/sulbactam (IV)	Chloramphenicol (IV) Metronidazole (IV/PO)	Mouth flora associated with dental infections and anaerobic lung infections. F. nucleatum is associated with jugular vein septic phlebitis and GI cancer. Resembles Capnophagia sp. on sputum gram stain.
Prevotella (Bacteroides) bivia	• CSF = NP • Blood = P (from dental, lung, pelvic source) • Sputum = P (lung abscess)	Penicillin (IV/PO) Any β-lactam (IV/PO)	Any quinolone (IV/PO) Doxycycline (IV/PO) Clindamycin (IV/PO)	Cause of dental, oropharyngeal, and female genital tract infections.

Prevotella (Bacteroides) melaninogenicus, intermedius	• Urine = NP • Stool = NP • Wound = NP • CSF = P (brain abscess) • Blood = P (from oral/pulmonary source) • Sputum = P (from aspiration pneumonia, lung abscess) • Urine = NP • Stool = NP • Wound = NP	Aspiration pneumonia/lung abscess Any β-lactam (IV/PO) Any quinolone (IV/PO) Brain abscess Penicillin (IV)	Aspiration pneumonia/lung abscess Doxycycline (IV/PO) Brain abscess Chloramphenicol (IV)	Predominant anaerobic flora of mouth. Known as "oral pigmented" Bacteroides (e.g., B. melanogenicus). Antibiotics used to treat community-acquired pneumonia are effective against oral anaerobes (e.g., Prevotella) in aspiration pneumonia; does not require anti-B. fragilis coverage with clindamycin, metronidazole, or moxifloxacin.

C = colonizer; C* = skin contaminant; NP = non-pathogen at site; P = pathogen at site; (IV/PO) = IV or PO. See p. xi for all other abbreviations.

Table 3.8. Clinical Significance of YEAST/FUNGI Pending Susceptibility Testing

		YEAST/FUNGI		
Isolate	**Usual Isolate Significance	Preferred Therapy	Alternate Therapy	Comments
Aspergillus species	• CSF = P (only from disseminated infection) • Blood = C, P (1° fungemia or from pulmonary source) • Sputum = C, P (pneumonia) • Urine = NP • Stool = NP • Wound = NP, P (rarely, but possible with extensive wounds, e.g., burns)	See p. 55: Voriconazole (IV/PO) Amphotericin B lipid formulation (IV)	See p. 55: Posaconazole (PO) Amphotericin B deoxycholate (IV)	A. fumigatus is the usual cause of invasive aspergillosis. Growth of Aspergillus sp. from a specimen can represent airborne contamination, but repeated growth or growth from a significantly immunocompromised patient with a consistent syndrome should be considered as evidence of possible infection. Aspergillus pneumonia and disseminated aspergillosis are common in patients receiving chronic steroids or immuno-suppressive therapy (esp. organ transplants). Recovery of Aspergillus from Sputum or BAL is not diagnostic of Aspergillus pneumonia and/or (increasingly available) detection of circulating galactomannan are used to confirm the diagnosis.
Candida albicans	• CSF = P (only from disseminated infection) • Blood = P (1° candidemia or from IV line infection) • Sputum = C, P (only from disseminated infection)	Fluconazole (IV/PO) Micafungin (IV) Caspofungin (IV) Anidulafungin (IV) Posaconazole (PO)	Amphotericin B deoxycholate (IV/PO) Amphotericin B lipid formulation (IV) Itraconazole (IV/PO) Voriconazole (IV/PO)	Common colonizer of GI/GU tracts. Colonization common in diabetics, alcoholics, patients receiving steroids/antibiotics. Commonest cause of fungemia in hospitalized patients. Candidemia secondary to central IV lines should always be treated as possible disseminated disease even though this is not invariably the case. Repeated blood cultures and careful follow-up (including

	• Urine = C, P (from cystitis, pyelonephritis) • Stool = C (source of candiduria) • Wound = NP		ophthalmoscopy) should be undertaken to exclude possible occult dissemination following even a single positive blood culture. Primary candidal pneumonia is rare.
Candida non-albicans	• CSF = P (only from disseminated infection) • Blood = P (1° candidemia or from IV line infection) • Sputum = NP • Urine = C (indwelling catheters), P (from cystitis, pyelonephritis) • Stool = C (source of candiduria) • Wound = NP	Micafungin (IV) Caspofungin (IV) Anidulafungin (IV) Posaconazole (PO) Voriconazole (IV/PO)	Fluconazole (IV/PO) Amphotericin B deoxycholate (IV/PO) Amphotericin B lipid formulation (IV) Itraconazole (IV/PO)	Non-albicans Candida cause the same spectrum of invasive disease as C. albicans. Fluconazole-susceptibility varies predictably by species. C. glabrata (usually) and C. krusei (almost always) are resistant to fluconazole. C. lusitaniae is often resistant to amphotericin B (deoxycholate and lipid-associated formulations). Other species are generally susceptible to all agents.
Cryptococcus neoformans	• CSF = P (meningitis, brain abscess) • Blood = P (from pulmonary source) • Sputum = P (pneumonia) • Urine = NP • Stool = NP • Wound = NP*	<u>CNS</u> Amphotericin B deoxycholate (IV) ± flucytosine (PO) <u>Non-CNS</u> Amphotericin B deoxycholate (IV)	<u>CNS</u> Fluconazole (IV/PO) <u>Non-CNS</u> Itraconazole (IV/PO) Fluconazole (IV/PO)	C. neoformans meningitis may occur with or without dissemination. Cryptococcal pneumonia frequently disseminates to CNS. C. neoformans in blood cultures occurs in compromised hosts (e.g., HIV) and indicates disseminated infection.

C = colonizer; C* = skin contaminant; NP = non-pathogen at site; P = pathogen at site; (IV/PO) = IV or PO. See p. xi for all other abbreviations. Isolation of a fungus from any normal sterile site should be cause for a careful review of the patient's epidemiology, risk factors, and clinical presentation.

* Cutaneous cryptococcus represents disseminated infection. ** Fungi can produce disseminated infections that involve essentially any organ.

Table 3.8. Usual Clinical Significance of YEAST/FUNGI Pending Susceptibility Testing (cont'd)

| | | YEAST/FUNGI | | |
Isolate	**Usual Isolate Significance	Preferred Therapy	Alternate Therapy	Comments
Histoplasma capsulatum	• CSF = P (from disseminated infection, pneumonia) • Blood = P (1° fungemia, rarely SBE) • Sputum = P (pneumonia, mediastinitis) • Urine = P • Stool = P • Wound = P	Itraconazole (IV/PO) Amphotericin B deoxycholate (IV) Amphotericin B lipid formulation (IV)	Fluconazole (IV/PO) Amphotericin B lipid formulation (IV)	Histoplasma recovered from CSF/blood cultures indicates dissemination. Disseminated (reactivated latent) histoplasmosis is most common in compromised hosts (e.g., HIV). Itraconazole is ineffective for meningeal histoplasmosis, but is preferred for chronic suppressive therapy.
Malassezia furfur	• CSF = NP • Blood = P (from IV line infection) • Sputum = NP • Urine = NP • Stool = NP • Wound = P (eosinophilic folliculitis)	Itraconazole (IV/PO) Ketoconazole (PO)	Fluconazole (IV/PO)	M. furfur IV line infections are associated with IV lipid hyperalimentation emulsions. Fungemia usually resolves with IV line removal. Morphology in blood is blunt buds on a broad base yeast. M. furfur requires long chain fatty acids for growth (overlay agar with thin layer of olive oil, Tween 80, or oleic acid).

| Penicillium marneffei | • CSF = NP
• Blood = P (usually from dissemination)
• Sputum = P (pneumonia)
• Urine = NP
• Stool = NP
• Wound = NP* | Amphotericin B deoxycholate (IV)
Itraconazole (IV/PO) | Amphotericin B lipid formulation (IV) | Histoplasma-like yeast forms seen in lymph nodes, liver, skin, bone marrow, blood. Characteristic red pigment diffuses into agar. Closely resembles histoplasmosis yeast forms (H. capsulatum has narrow based budding yeast forms, but P. marneffei has transverse septa). Skin lesions indicate dissemination. May resemble molluscum contagiosum. Hepatosplenomegaly is common. |

C = colonizer; C* = skin contaminant; NP = non-pathogen at site; P = pathogen at site; (IV/PO) = IV or PO. See p. xi for all other abbreviations.

*   Cutaneous lesions represents disseminated infection.

** Fungi can produce disseminated infections that involve essentially any organ. Isolation of a fungus from any normal sterile site should be cause for a careful review of the patient's epidemiology, risk factors, and clinical presentation.

Table 3.9. Technique for Gram Stain and Giemsa Stain

GRAM STAIN

Clinical applications: CSF, sputum, urine

Technique:

1. Place specimen on slide.
2. Heat fix smear on slide by passing it quickly over a flame.
3. Place crystal violet solution on slide for 20 seconds.
4. Wash gently with water.
5. Apply Gram iodine solution to slide for 20 seconds.
6. Decolorize the slide quickly in solution of acetone/ethanol.
7. Wash slide gently with water.
8. Counterstain slide with safranin for 10 seconds.
9. Wash gently with water; air dry or blot dry with bibulous paper.

Interpretation: Gram-negative organisms stain red; gram-positive organisms stain blue. B fragilis stains weakly pink. Fungi stain deep blue. See Tables 3.10–3.12 for interpretation of Gram stain findings in CSF, urine, sputum, and feces, respectively.

GIEMSA STAIN

Clinical applications: Blood buffy coat, bone marrow

Technique:

1. Place specimen on slide.
2. Fix smear by placing slide in 100% methanol for 1 minute.
3. Drain methanol off slide.
4. Flood slide with Giemsa stain (freshly diluted 1:10 with distilled water) for 5 minutes.
5. Wash slide gently with water; air dry.

Interpretation: Fungi/parasites stain light/dark blue.

Table 3.10. Clinical Use of CSF Gram Stain, WBC Type, Glucose (see Color Atlas of CSF Gram stains)

Gram Stain	Organism/Condition	
Gram-positive bacilli	Pseudomeningitis (Bacillus, Corynebacteria)	Listeria
Gram-negative bacilli	H. influenzae (small, encapsulated, pleomorphic)	Non-enteric/enteric aerobic bacilli (larger, unencapsulated)
Gram-positive cocci	Gp A, B, D, streptococci (pairs/chains) S. pneumoniae (pairs)	S. aureus (pairs/clusters) S. epidermidis (pairs/clusters)
Gram-negative diplococci	Neisseria meningitidis	

Table 3.10. Clinical Use of CSF Gram Stain, WBC Type, Glucose (cont'd)

Gram Stain	Organism/Condition	
Mixed organisms (polymicrobial)	Pseudomeningitis Anaerobic organisms (brain abscess with meningeal leak)	Neonatal meningitis Meningitis 2° to penetrating head trauma

WBC Type/Glucose	Organism/Condition	
Purulent CSF, no organisms	Neisseria meningitidis	Listeria
Clear CSF, no organisms	Viral meningitis Viral encephalitis TB/fungal meningitis Sarcoidosis meningitis Meningeal carcinomatosis Brain abscess Parameningeal infection Septic emboli 2° to SBE SLE cerebritis Lyme's disease	Lymphocytic choriomeningitis (LCM) Drug induced aseptic meningitis Listeria HIV Syphilis Leptospirosis Bacterial meningitis (very early/partially-treated) Meningitis (leukopenic host) Rocky Mountain Spotted Fever
Cloudy CSF, no WBCs	S. pneumoniae	
Predominantly PMNs, decreased glucose	Bacterial meningitis (partially-treated) Listeria HSV-1/2 encephalitis TB (early/beginning therapy) Sarcoidosis	Parameningeal infection Septic emboli 2° to SBE Amebic meningoencephalitis Syphilis (early) Posterior-fossa syndrome
Predominantly lymphocytes, normal glucose	Bacterial meningitis (partially-treated) Sarcoidosis Lyme's disease HIV Leptospirosis Rocky Mountain Spotted Fever	Viral meningitis Viral encephalitis Parameningeal infection TB/fungal meningitis Parasitic meningitis Meningeal carcinomatosis
Predominantly lymphocytes, decreased glucose	Bacterial meningitis (partially-treated) TB/fungal meningitis Sarcoidosis Lymphocytic choriomeningitis (LCM) Mumps	Enteroviral meningitis Listeria Leptospirosis Syphilis Meningeal carcinomatosis
Red blood cells	Traumatic tap CNS bleed/tumor Listeria Leptospirosis Herpes (HSV-1) encephalitis	TB meningitis Amebic (Naegeleria) meningoencephalitis Anthrax

Table 3.11. Clinical Use of the Sputum Gram Stain (see Color Atlas of Sputum Gram stains)

Gram Stain	Organism	Comments
Gram-positive diplococci	S. pneumoniae	Lancet-shaped encapsulated diplococci (not streptococci)
Gram-positive cocci (grape-like clusters)	S. aureus	Clusters predominant. Short chains or pairs may also be present
Gram-positive cocci (short chains or pairs)	Group A streptococci	Virulence inversely proportional to length of streptococci. Clusters not present
Gram-positive beaded/ filamentous branching organisms	Nocardia	Coccobacillary forms common
Gram-negative cocco-bacillary organisms	H. influenzae	Pleomorphic may be encapsulated. Gram negative cocci/bacilli. Lightly stained
Gram-negative bacilli	Klebsiella P. aeruginosa	Plump and encapsulated Thin and often arranged in end-to-end pairs
Gram-negative diplococci	Moraxella (Branhamella) catarrhalis Neisseria meningitidis	Kidney bean-shaped diplococci

Table 3.12. Clinical Use of the Urine Gram Stain (see Color Atlas of Urine Gram stains)

Gram Stain	Organism	Comments
Gram-positive cocci (clusters)*	S. aureus S. epidermidis S. saprophyticus	Skin flora contaminant Skin flora contaminant Uropathogen

Gram-positive cocci (chains)	Group B streptococci
	Group D streptococci
	  E. faecalis
	  E. faecium
		Uropathogen
		Uropathogen
		May represent colonization or infection
		May represent colonization or infection

Gram-negative bacilli*	Coliform bacilli	Uropathogen; may represent colonization or infection
Gram-negative diplococci*	N. gonorrhoeae N. meningitidis	Gonococcal urethritis Rare cause of urethritis

*   Staphylococci (except S. saprophyticus), S. pneumoniae, and B. fragilis are *not* uropathogens.

Table 3.13. Clinical Use of the Fecal Gram Stain

Gram Stain	Possible Organisms	
Fecal leukocytes present	Enteropathogenic E. coli (EPEC) Enteroinvasive E. coil (EIEC) Shigella Yersinia Campylobacter Salmonella Vibrio parahaemolyticus Vibrio vulnificus	Aeromonas hydrophila Chlamydia trachomatis Plesiomonas shigelloides Neisseria gonorrhoeae (proctitis) Herpes simplex virus (HSV-1) *Noninfectious:* Ulcerative colitis
No fecal leukocytes	Enterovirus Rotavirus Coronavirus Enterotoxigenic E. coli (ETEC) S. aureus Clostridium perfringens Adenovirus	Norwalk virus Vibrio cholerae Bacillus cereus (food poisoning) Giardia lamblia Isospora belli Cryptosporidia Strongyloides stercoralis
Fecal leukocytes variable	Clostridium difficile Enterohemorrhagic E. coli (EHEC)	Cytomegalovirus (CMV) Herpes simplex virus (HSV-1)
Red blood cells present	Shigella Salmonella Campylobacter EPEC EHEC Enteroinvasive E. coli (EIEC) Enterohemorrhagic E. coli (EHEC)	Clostridium difficile Cytomegalovirus (CMV) Yersinia Plesiomonas shigelloides *Noninfectious:* Ulcerative colitis

REFERENCES AND SUGGESTED READINGS

Aridan S, Paetznick V, Rex JH. Comparative evaluation of disk diffusion with microdilution assay in susceptibility of caspofungin against Aspergillus and fusarium isolates. Antimicrob Agents Chemother 46:3084–7, 2002.

Baldis MM, Keidich SD, Mukhejee PK, et al. Mechanisms of fungal resistance: an overview. Drugs 62:1025–40, 2002.

Bartlett JG. Antibiotic-associated diarrhea. N Engl J Med 346:334–9, 2002.

Bingen E, Leclercq R, Fitoussi F, et al. Emergence of group A streptococcus strains with different mechanisms of macrolide resistance. Antimicrob Agents Chemother 46:1199–203, 2002.

Bouza E, Cercenado E. Klebsiella and enterobacter: antibiotic resistance and treatment implications. Semin Respir Infect 17:215–30, 2002.

Boyce JM. Methicillin-resistant Staphylococcus aureus. Lancet Infect Dis 5:653–63, 2005.

Brueggemann AB, Coffmen SL, Rhomberg P, et al. Fluoroquinolone resistance in Streptococcus pneumoniae in United States. Antimicrob Agents Chemother 46:680–8, 2002.

Courvalin P. Vancomycin resistance in gram-positive cocci. Clin Infect Dis 42:S25–S34, 2006.

Cunha BA. Clinical relevance of penicillin-resistant Streptococcus pneumoniae. Semin Respir Infect 17:204–14, 2002.

Cunha BA. Pseudomonas aeruginosa: resistance and therapy. Semin Respir Infect 17:231–9, 2002.

Cunha BA. MRSA & VRE: In vitro susceptibility versus in vivo efficacy. Antibiotics for Clinicians 4:31–32, 2000.

Cunha BA. The significance of antibiotic false sensitivity testing with in vitro testing. J Chemother 9:25–35, 1997.

Daneman N, McGeer, Green K, Low DE. Macrolide Resistance in Bacteremic Pneumococcal Disease: Implications for Patient Management. Clin Infect Dis 43:432–8, 2006.

Doern GV. Macrolide and Ketolide Resistance with Streptococcus pneumoniae. Med Clin N Am 90:1109–24, 2006.

Espinel-Ingroff A, Chaturvedi V, Fothergill A, et al. Optimal testing conditions for determining MICs and minimum fungicidal concentrations of new and established antifungal agents for uncommon molds: NCCLS collaborative study. J Clin Microbiol 40:3776–81, 2002.

Falagas ME, Kasiakou SK. Colistin: the revival of polymyxins for the management of multidrug-resistant gram-negative bacterial infections. Clin Infect Dis 40:1333–41, 2005.

Fuchs PC, Barry AL, Brown SD. In vitro activity of telithromycin against Streptococcus pneumoniae resistant to other antibiotics, including cefotaxime. J Antimicrob Chemother 49:399–401, 2002.

Gould IM. The clinical significance of methicillin-resistant Staphylococcus aureus. J Hosp Infect 61:277–282, 2005.

Halstead DC, Abid J, Dowzicky MJ. Antimicrobial susceptibility among Acinetobacter calcoaceticus-baumannii complex and enterobacteriacae collected as part of the tigecycline evaluation and surveillance trial. Journal of Infection 55:49–57, 2007.

Holmes A, Ganner M, McGuane S, et al. Staphylococcus aureus isolates carrying Panton-Valentine leucocidin genes in England and Wales: frequency, characterization, and association with clinical disease. J Clin Microbiol 43:2384–90, 2005.

Jain R, Danziger LH. Multidrug-resistant Acinetobacter infections: an emerging challenge to clinicians. Ann Pharmacother 38:1449–59, 2004.

Jevitt LA, Thorne GM, Traczewski MM, et al. Multicenter evaluation of the Etest and disk diffusion methods for differentiating Daptomycin-susceptible from non-Daptomycin-susceptible Staphylococcus aureus isolates. J Clin Microbiol 44:3098–3104, 2006.

Jiang X, Zhang Z, Li M, et al. Detection of Extended-Spectrum B-Lactamases in Clinical Isolates of Pseudomonas aeruginosa. Antimicrobial Agents and Chemotherapy 50:2990–95, 2006.

King A, Bathgate T, Phillips I. Erythromycin susceptibility of viridans streptococci from the normal throat flora of patients treated with azithromycin or clarithromycin. Clin Microbiol Infect 8:85–92, 2002.

Kocazeybek B, Arabaci U, Erenturk S. Investigation of various antibiotic combinations using the E-Test method in multiresistant Pseudomonas aeruginosa strains. Chemotherapy 48:31–5, 2002.

Kontoyiannis DP, Lewis RE. Antifungal drug resistance of pathogenic fungi. Lancet 359:1135–44, 2002.

Kralovic SM, Danko LH, Roselle GA. Laboratory reporting of Staphylococcus aureus with reduced susceptibility to vancomycin in United States Department of Veterans Affairs facilities. Emerg Infect Dis 8:402–7, 2002.

Kremery V, Barnes AJ. Non-albicans Candida spp. causing fungaemia: pathogenicity and antifungal resistance. J Hosp Infect 50:243–60, 2002.

Laverdiere M, Hoban D, Restieri C, et al. In vitro activity of three new triazoles and one echinocandin against Candida bloodstream isolates from cancer patients. J Antimicrob Chemother 50:119–23, 2002.

Linden PK. Treatment options for vancomycin-resistant enterococcal infections. Drugs 62:425–41, 2002.

Linder JA, Stafford RS. Erythromycin-resistant group A streptococci. N Engl J Med 347:614–5, 2002.

Lonks JR, Garau J, Gomez L, et al. Failure of macrolide antibiotic treatment in patients with bacteremia due to erythromycin-resistant Streptococcus pneumoniae. Clin Infect Dis 35:556–64, 2002.

Metlay JP, Fishman NO, Joffe MM, et al. Macrolide Resistance in Adults with Bacteremic Pneumococcal Pneumonia. Emerging Infect Dis 12, 1223–30, 2006.

Midolo PD, Matthews D, Fernandez CD, et al. Detection of extended spectrum beta-lactamases in the routine clinical microbiology laboratory. Pathology 34:362–4, 2002.

Mollering RC Jr. Problems with antimicrobial resistance in gram-positive cocci. Clin Infect Dis 26:1177–8, 1998.

Naas T, Fortineau N, Spicq C, et al. Three-year survey of community-acquired methicillin-resistant Staphylococcus aureus producing Panton-Valentine leukocidin in a French university hospital. J Hosp Infect 61:321–9, 2005.

Paterson DL, Bonomo RA. Extended-spectrum β-lactamases: a clinical update. Clin Microbiol Rev 18:657–86, 2005.

Pelaez T, Alcala L, Alonso R, et al. Reassessment of Clostridium difficile susceptibility to metronidazole and vancomycin. Antimicrob Agents Chemother 46:1647–50, 2002.

Perri MB, Hershberger E, Ionescu M, et al. In vitro susceptibility of vancomycin-resistant enterococci (VRE) to fosfomycin. Diagn Microbiol Infect Dis 42:269–71, 2002.

Poole K. Aminoglycoside resistance in Pseudomonas aeruginosa. Antimicrob Agents Chemother 49:479–87, 2005.

Rex JH, Pfaller MA, Walsh TJ, et al. Antifungal susceptibility testing: practical aspects and current challenges. Clin Microbiol Rev 14:643–658, 2002.

Rex JH, Rinaldi MG, Pfaller MA. Resistance of Candida species to fluconazole. Antimicrob Agents Chemother 39:1–8, 1995.

Robinson DA, Sutcliffe JA, Tweodros W, et al. Evolution and global dissemination of macrolide-resistant group A streptococci. Antimicrobial Agents and Chemotherapy 50:2903–11, 2006.

Ruhe JJ, Monson T, Bradsher RW, et al. Use of long-acting tetracyclines for methicillin-resistant Staphylococcus aureus infections: case series and review of the literature. Clin Infect Dis 40:142–934, 2005.

Stratton CW. In vitro susceptibility testing versus in vivo effectiveness. Med Clin N Am 90:1077–88, 2006.

Suzuki S, Yamazaki T, Narita M, et al. Clinical evaluation of macrolide-resistant Mycoplasma pneumoniae. Antimicrobial Agents and Chemotherapy 50:709–12, 2006.

Swenson JM, Killgore GE, Tenover FC. Antimicrobial susceptibility testing of Acinetobacter spp. by NCCLS broth microdilution and disk diffusion methods. J Clin Microbiol 42:5102–8, 2004.

Syndman DR, Jacobut NV, McDermott LA, et al. National survey on the susceptibility of Bacteroides fragilis: report and analysis of trends for 1997–2000. Clin Infect Dis 35(Suppl 1):S126–34, 2002.

Taccone FS, Rodriguez-Villalobos H, DeBacker D, et al. Successful treatment of septic shock due to pan-resistant Acinetobacter baumannii using combined antimicrobial therapy including tigecycline. Eur J Clin Microbiol Infect Dis 25:257–60, 2006.

Tenover FC, Moellering RC. The rationale for revising the clinical and laboratory standards institute vancomycin minimal inhibitory concentration interpretive criteria for Staphylococcus aureus. Clin Infect Dis 44:1208–1215, 2007.

Tomioka H, Sato K, Shimizu T, et al. Anti-Mycobacterium tuberculosis activities of new fluoroquinolones in combination with other antituberculous drugs. J Infect 44:160–5, 2002.

Turner PJ. Trends in antimicrobial susceptibilities among bacterial pathogens isolated from patients hospitalized in European medical centers: 6-year report of the MYSTIC Surveillance Study (1997–2002). Diagn Microbiol Infect Dis 51:281–9, 2005.

Wagenvoort JHT, Ciraci VE, Penders RJR, et al. Superior discriminative performance of ceftizoxime disk diffusion test for detecting methicillin-resistant Staphylococcus aureus. Eur J Clin Microbiol Infect Dis 25:405–6, 2006.

Walsh FM, Amyes SG. Microbiology and drug resistance mechanisms of fully resistant pathogens. Curr Opin Microbiol 7:439–44, 2004.

Yong D, Lee K, Yum JH, et al. Imipenem-EDTA disk method for differentiation of metallo-beta-lactamase-producing clinical isolates of Pseudomonas spp. and Acinetobacter spp. J Clin Microbiol 40:3798–801, 2002.

Yuan S, Astion ML, Shapiro J, et al. Clinical impact associated with corrected results in clinical microbiology testing. J Clin Microbiol 43:2188–93, 2005.

TEXTBOOKS

Anaissie EJ, McGinnis MR, Pfaller MA (eds). Clinical Mycology. Churchill Livingstone, New York, 2003.

Bottone EJ (ed). An Atlas of the Clinical Microbiology of Infectious Diseases, Volume 1. Bacterial Agents. The Parthenon Publishing Group, Boca Raton, 2004.

Bottone EJ (ed). An Atlas of the Clinical Microbiology of Infectious Diseases, Volume 2. Viral, fungal, and parasitic agents. Taylor and Francis, 2006.

Bowden RA, Ljungman P, Snydman DR (eds). Transplant Infections 3rd Edition, Lippincott Williams & Wilkins, Philadelphia, PA, 2010.

Bryskier A (ed). Antimicrobial Agents. ASM Press, Washington, D.C., 2005.

de la Maza LM, Pezzlo MT, Shigei JT, et al. (eds). Color Atlas of Medical Bacteriology. ASM Press, Washington, D.C., 2004.

Forbes BA, Sahm DF, Weissfeld AS, et al. (eds). Bailey & Scott's Diagnostic Microbiology, 12th Edition, St. Louis, Mosby, 2007.

Gorbach SL, Bartlett JG, Blacklow NR (eds). Infectious Diseases, 3rd Edition, Philadelphia, Lippincott, Williams & Wilkins, 2004.

Grayson ML (ed). Kucers' The Use of Antibiotics, 6th Edition, ASM Press, Washington, DC, 2010.

Janda JM, Abbott SL (eds). The Enterobacteria, 2nd Edition, ASM Press, Washington, D.C., 2006.

Koneman EW, Allen SD, Janda WM, et al. (eds). Color Atlas and Textbook of Diagnostic Microbiology, 5th Edition, Lippincott-Raven Publishers, Philadelphia, 1997.

Lorian V (ed). Antibiotics in Laboratory Medicine. 5th Edition, Lippincott Williams & Wilkins, Philadelphia, 2005.

Madigan MT, Martinko JM, Parker J (eds). Brock Biology of Microorganisms. 10th Edition, Prentice Hall, Upper Saddle River, NJ, 2003.

Mandell GL, Bennett JE, Dolin R (eds). Mandell, Douglas, and Bennett's Principles and Practice of infectious Diseases, 7th Edition, Philadelphia, Elsevier Churchill Livingstone, 2010.

Scholar EM Pratt WB (eds). The Antimicrobial Drugs, 2nd Edition, Oxford University Press, New York, 2000.

Versalovic J, Carroll KC, Funke G, et al. (eds). Manual of Clinical Microbiology, 10th Edition, Washington, DC, ASM Press, 2011.

Chapter 4

Parasites, Fungi, Unusual Organisms*

Kenneth F. Wagner, DO, James H. McGuire, MD
Burke A. Cunha, MD, Jean E. Hage, MD
John H. Rex, MD, Edward J. Bottone, PhD

Color Atlas of Fungal stains (see center of book).

Parasites, Fungi, Unusual Organisms in Blood

Microfilaria in Blood

Subset	Pathogen	Preferred Therapy	Alternate Therapy
Filariasis	Brugia malayi	Diethylcarbamazine: day 1: 50 mg (PO) day 2: 50 mg (PO) q8h day 3: 100 mg (PO) q8h days 4–14: 2 mg/kg (PO) q8h	Ivermectin 200 mcg/kg (PO) × 1 dose ± albendazole 400 mg (PO) × 1 dose
	Wuchereria bancrofti	Albendazole 400 mg (PO) × 1 dose plus diethylcarbamazine: day 1: 50 mg (PO) day 2: 50 mg (PO) q8h day 3: 100 mg (PO) q8h days 4–14: 2 mg/kg (PO) q8h ± doxycycline 100 mg (PO) q12h × 6 weeks	Ivermectin 400 mcg/kg (PO) × 1 dose.

Brugia malayi
Clinical Presentation: May present as an obscure febrile illness, chronic lymphedema, lymphangitis, or cutaneous abscess. "Filarial fevers" usually last 1 week and spontaneously remit.

Diagnostic Considerations: Diagnosis by demonstrating microfilaria on Giemsa's stained thick blood smear or by using the concentration method; yield is increased by passing blood through a Millipore filter before staining. Several smears should be taken over 24 hours. Adult worms may be detected in scrotal lymphatics by ultrasound. Common infection in Southeast Asia (primarily China, Korea, India, Indonesia, Malaysia, Philippines, Sri Lanka). Most species have nocturnal periodicity (microfilaria in blood at night). Eosinophilia is most common during periods of acute inflammation.

Pitfalls: Genital manifestations—scrotal edema, epididymitis, orchitis, hydrocele—are frequent with W. bancrofti, but rare with B. malayi.

Prognosis: Related to state of health and extent of lymphatic obstruction. No satisfactory treatment is available. Single-dose ivermectin is effective treatment for microfilaremia, but does not kill the adult worm (although diethylcarbamazine kills some). If no microfilaria in blood, full-dose diethylcarbamazine (2 mg/kg q8h) can be started on day one. Antihistamines or corticosteroids may decrease allergic reactions from disintegration of microfilaria.

Wuchereria bancrofti
Clinical Presentation: May present as an obscure febrile illness, chronic lymphedema, lymphangitis, or cutaneous abscess. Genital (scrotal) lymphatic edema, groin lesions, epididymitis, orchitis, hydroceles are characteristic. Chyluria may occur. "Filarial fevers" usually last 1 week and spontaneously remit. Lymphedema worsened by cellulitis associated with Tinea pedis infections.

Diagnostic Considerations: Diagnosis by demonstrating microfilaria on Giemsa's stained thick blood smear or by using the concentration method; yield is increased by passing blood through a Millipore filter before staining. Several smears should to be taken over 24 hours. W. bancrofti is the most common human filarial infection, particularly in Asia (China, India, Indonesia, Japan, Malaysia, Philippines), Southeast Asia, Sri Lanka, Tropical Africa, Central/South America, and Pacific Islands. Most species have nocturnal periodicity (microfilaria in blood at night). Eosinophilia is common.

Pitfalls: Differentiate from "hanging groins" of Loa Loa, which usually do not involve the scrotum.

Prognosis: Related to state of health and extent of lymphatic obstruction. No satisfactory treatment is available. Single-dose ivermectin is effective treatment for microfilaremia, but does not kill the adult worm (although diethylcarbamazine kills some). If no microfilaria in blood, full-dose diethylcarbamazine (2 mg/kg q8h) can be started on day one. Antihistamines or corticosteroids decrease allergic reactions from disintegration of microfilaria. Wolbachia bacteria are endosymbionts in W. bancrofti filariasis. Treatment with doxycycline effective against Wolbachia which are important in microfilarial reproduction.

Trypanosomes in Blood

Subset	Pathogen	Preferred Therapy	Alternate Therapy
Chagas' disease (American trypanosomiasis)	Trypanosoma brucei cruzi	Nifurtimox 2–3 mg/kg/day (PO) q6h × 30–90 days	Benznidazole 2.5–3.5 mg/kg (PO) q12h × 60 days
Loa Loa (Loiasis)	L. loa	Diethylcarbamazine 2–3 mg/kg (PO) q8h × 3 weeks	Albendazole 200 mg (PO) q12h × 3 weeks
Sleeping sickness *West African (Gambian) trypanosomiasis*	Trypanosoma brucei gambiense	<u>Early disease</u> Pentamidine 4 mg/kg (IM) q24h × 7 days	
		<u>Late disease</u> Melarsoprol 2.2 mg/kg (IV) q24h × 10 days **plus** Nifurtimox 15 mg/kg (PO) q8h × 10 days **or** Eflornithine 100 mg/kg (PO) q6h × 10 days	
East African (Rhodesian) trypanosomiasis	Trypanosoma brucei rhodesiense	<u>Early disease</u> Suramin test dose of 4–5 mg/kg (IV) day 1, then five injections of 20 mg/kg (IV) q 7 days (max. dose 1 gm/injection day 3, 10, 17, 24, 31) max .dose 1 gm/injection	
		<u>Late disease</u> Melarsoprol 3 series of 1.8, 2.16, 2.52 mg/kg (IV) q24h; 3 series of 2.52, 2.88, 3.25 mg/kg (IV) q24h; 3 series of 3.6, 3.6, 3.6 mg/kg (IV) q24h; the series given at intervals of 7 days	

Chagas' Disease (Trypanosoma brucei cruzi) American Trypanosomiasis

Clinical Presentation: Presents acutely after bite of infected reduviid bug with unilateral painless edema of the palpebrae/periocular tissues (Romaña's sign), or as an indurated area of erythema and swelling with local lymph node involvement (chagoma). Fever, malaise, and edema of the face and lower extremities may follow. Generalized lymphadenopathy and hepatosplenomegaly occur. Patients with chronic disease may develop cardiac involvement (cardiomyopathy with arrhythmias, heart block, heart failure, thromboembolism), GI involvement (megaesophagus, megaduodenum, megacolon) or CNS involvment in HIV/immunosuppressed.

Diagnostic Considerations: Common in Central and South America. Acquired from infected reduviid bug, which infests mud/clay parts of primitive dwellings. Transmitted by blood transfusion (~10%), organ transplants, and congenitally. Diagnosis in acute disease by detecting trypanosomes in wet prep of anticoagulated blood or stained buffy coat smears. Amastigote forms present intracellularly in monocytes/histiocytes in Giemsa-stained smears, bone marrow or lymph node aspirates, or by xenodiagnosis. Screening test ELISA IFA; confirmatory test RIPA (radioimmuno precipitation assay).

Pitfalls: Do not overlook the diagnosis in patients from endemic areas with unexplained heart block ± apical ventricular aneurysms. May be transmitted by blood transfusion/organ transplantation.

Prognosis: Related to extent of cardiac GI, or CNS involvement.

Sleeping Sickness (T. brucei gambiense/rhodesiense) West African/East African Trypanosomiasis

Clinical Presentation: Sleeping sickness from T. brucei gambiense is milder than sleeping sickness from T. brucei rhodesiense, which is usually a fulminant infection. A few days to weeks after bite of tsetse fly, patients progress through several clinical stages:

- *Chancre stage:* Trypanosomal chancre occurs at bite site and lasts several weeks.
- *Blood/lymphatic stage:* Blood parasitemia is associated with intermittent high fevers, headaches and insomnia, followed by generalized adenopathy. Posterior cervical lymph node enlargement (Winterbottom's sign) is particularly prominent with T. brucei gambiense. Hepatosplenomegaly and transient edema/pruritus/irregular circinate rash are common. Myocarditis (tachycardia unrelated to fevers) occurs early (before CNS involvement) and is responsible for acute deaths from T. brucei rhodesiense.
- *CNS stage:* Occurs after a few months of non-specific symptoms, and is characterized by increasing lethargy, somnolence (sleeping sickness), and many subtle CNS findings. Coma and death ensue without treatment. With melarsoprol, use prednisolone 1 mg/kg (PO) q24h (start steroid 1 day prior to first dose and continue to last dose)**.**

Diagnostic Considerations: Diagnosis by demonstrating trypanosomes in blood, chancre, or lymph nodes aspirates by Giemsa-stained thin and thick preparations, light microscopy, or buffy coat concentrates with acridine orange. CSF determines early vs. late stage disease (> 20 WBCs/mm^3).

Pitfalls: Do not miss other causes of prominent bilateral posterior cervical lymph node enlargement, e.g., lymphoma, EBV.

Prognosis: Related to extent of cardiac/CNS involvement. Relapse may occur.

Loa Loa (Loiasis)

Clinical Presentation: Cutaneous swellings (Calabar swellings) with pruritus. Adults may be visible when migrations under the conjuctiva or under the skin. Disappear in 10 minutes. Calabar swellings are painless and appear on the extremities. Eosinophilia prominent.

Diagnostic Considerations: Demonstrates of microfilariae in blood (at noon) or by demonstration of L. loa in skin/eye. Immunodiagnosis unhelpful.

Pitfalls: Calabar swellings occur one at time and may last for hours/days; may persist for years.

Prognosis: Poorest with CNS involvement.

Spirochetes in Blood

Subset	Pathogen	Preferred Therapy	Alternate Therapy
Relapsing fever *Louse-borne* *(LBRF)* *Tick-borne* *(TBRF)*	Borrelia recurrentis > 15 Borrelia species (U.S. B. hermsi; Africa: B. duttonii; Africa/Middle East: B. crocidurae)	LBRF Erythromycin 500 mg (IV or PO) q6h × 7 days TBRF Doxycycline 200 mg (PO) × 3 days, then 100 mg (PO) q12h × 7 days	TBRF with CNS involvement Penicillin G 2 mu (IV) q4h × 2 weeks **or** Ceftriaxone 1 gm (IV) q12h × 2 weeks **or** Cefotaxime 3 gm (IV) q6h × 2 weeks
Rat bite fever	Spirillum minus	Penicillin G 4 mu (IV) q4h × 2 weeks **or** Ceftriaxone 1 g (IV) q24h × 2 weeks **or** Doxycycline 200 mg (IV or PO) q12h × 3 days, then 100 mg (IV or PO) q12h × 11 days	Amoxicillin 1 gm (PO) q8h × 2 weeks **or** Erythromycin 500 mg (IV or PO) q6h × 2 weeks **or** Chloramphenicol 500 mg (IV) q6h × 2 weeks

Relapsing Fever, Louse-Borne (LBRF) / Tick-Borne (TBRF)

Clinical Presentation: Abrupt onset of "flu-like" illness with high fever, rigors, headache, myalgias, arthralgias, tachycardia, dry cough, abdominal pain after exposure to infected louse or tick. Truncal petechial rash and conjunctival suffusion are common. Hepatosplenomegaly/DIC may occur. Bleeding or rash at bite site. Complications more common in LBRF. Fevers last ~ 1 week, remit for a week, and usually relapse only once in LBRF, but several times in TBRF. Relapses usually last 2–3 days. Fevers are often higher in TBRF.

Diagnostic Considerations: Borreliae seen in Wright/Giemsa-stained blood smears. LBRF is endemic in South American Andes, Central and East Africa, and is associated with crowded, unhygienic conditions. Soft ticks (Ornithodoros) TBRF main vector. Bite at night, patients do not recall tick bite. TBRF is seen throughout the world, and is endemic in Western U.S., British Columbia, Mexico, Central/South America, Mediterranean, Central Asia, and Africa. With TBRF, meningismus ± facial nerve palsy common with B. duttoni rare with B. hermsii.

Pitfalls: Spirochetes are most likely to be seen during febrile periods. Blood smears may be negative if not obtained during fever.

Prognosis: Good if treated early. Usually no permanent sequelae.

Rat Bite Fever (Spirillum minus)

Clinical Presentation: Infection develops 1–4 weeks following bite of a rat. Healed rat bite becomes red, painful, swollen and ulcerated, with regional lymphangitis/adenopathy. Recurrent fevers occurs in 2–4 day fever cycles. Fevers are usually accompanied by chills, headache, photophobia, nausea, vomiting. Rash on palms/soles develops in > 50%. Arthritis, myalgias, and SBE are rare.

Diagnostic Considerations: Spirochetes are seen in Wright/Giemsa-stained blood smears. Differential diagnosis includes Borrelia, malaria, and lymphoma. VDRL is positive.

Pitfalls: May be confused with syphilis, due to rash on palms/soles and false-positive syphilis serology in 50%. SBE occurs with Streptobacillus moniliformis, not S. minus (unless there is preexisting valvular disease). Bite wound ulcerates in S. minus, not Streptobacillus moniliformis.

Prognosis: Patients with arthritis have a protracted course.

Intracellular Inclusion Bodies in Blood

Subset	Pathogen	Preferred Therapy	Alternate Therapy
Babesiosis	Babesia microti	Azithromycin 500 mg (PO) × 1, then 250 mg (PO) q24h × 7 days **plus** Atovaquone (suspension) 750 mg (PO) q12h × 7 days	Clindamycin 600 mg (PO) q8h × 7 days **plus** Quinine 650 mg (PO) q8h × 7 days
Ehrlichiosis/ anaplasmosis *Human monocytic ehrlichiosis (HME)* *Human granulocytic anaplasmosis (HGA)*	Ehrlichia chaffeensis, ewubguum Anaplasma (Ehrlichia) phagocytophilium	Doxycycline 200 mg (IV or PO) q12h × 3 days, then 100 mg (IV or PO) q12h × 1–2 weeks total	Any once-daily quinolone (IV or PO) × 1–2 weeks **or** Rifampin 300 mg (PO) q12h × 1–2 weeks* **or** Chloramphenicol 500 mg (IV or PO) q6h × 1–2 weeks*
Severe Malaria (Usually P. falciparum)	**Quinidine gluconate *plus* either doxycycline or clindamycin** 6.25 mg base/ kg (= 10 mg salt/kg) loading dose (IV) over 1–2 h, then 0.0125 mg base/kg/ min (= 0.02 mg salt/kg/min) continuous infusion for at least 24h. An alternative regimen is 15 mg base/kg (= 24 mg salt/kg) loading dose infused over 4 hours, followed by 7.5 mg base/kg (= 12 mg salt/kg) infused over 4 hours every 8 hours, starting 8 hours after the loading dose. Once parasitemia <1%; and patient can take oral medications, complete therapy with oral quinine or an oral regimen. (see below chloroquine-sensitive or resistant). **Quinidine/quinine course = 7 days in Southeast Asia; = 3 days in Africa or south America.**		

*   May be used in pregnancy.

Intracellular Inclusion Bodies in Blood (cont'd)

Subset	Therapy
	or
	Quinine 20 mg (salt)/kg (IV) over 4 hours (in D_5W), then 10 mg (salt)/kg (IV) over 2 hours q8h until able to take oral meds; complete 7 days total therapy with **doxycycline** or **oral regimen** (*see below* chloroquine-sensitive or resistant).
	or
	Artemether-lumefantrine 3.2 mg/kg (IM) × 1 dose, then 1.6 mg/kg (IM) q24h until able to take oral meds; complete 7 days total therapy with **doxycycline** or **oral regimen** (*see below* chloroquine-sensitive or resistant).
	or
	Artesunate 2.4 mg/kg (IV) initially and at 12, 24, and 48 hours, then q24h until able to take oral meds; complete 7 days total therapy with **doxycycline** or **oral regimen** (*see below* chloroquine-sensitive or resistant).
Uncomplicated Malaria (P. falciparum, P. malariae, P. knowlesi or unidentified species) P. vivax and P. ovale	*Chloroquine-sensitive* **Chloroquine phosphate** 600 mg base (= 1000 mg salt) (PO) immediately, followed by 300 mg base (= 500 mg salt) (PO) at 6,24, and 48 hours. Total dose = 1500 mg base (= 2500 mg salt).
	or
	Hydroxychloroquine 620 mg base (= 800 mg salt) (PO) loading dose, then 310 mg base (= 400 mg salt) (PO) at 6, 24, and 48 hours.
	Plus **primaquine phosphate** 30 mg base (PO) q24h × 2 weeks.
	Chloroquine-resistant **Quinine sulfate** 625 mg base (= 625 mg salt) (PO) q8h × 7 days *plus* **doxycycline** 200 mg (PO) q12h × 3 days, then 100 mg (PO) q12h × 4 days.
	or
	Atovaquone/proguanil (250/100 gm PO tab) 4 tablets as single dose or 4 tablets (PO) q12h × 3 days.
	or
	Artesunate 4 mg/kg (PO) × 3 days *plus* **Mefloquine** 684 mg base (= 750 mg salt) (PO) as initial dose followed by 456 mg base (= 500 mg salt) (PO) given 6–12 hours after initial dose. Total dose = 1250 mg salt.
	or
	Artemether/lumefantrine 4 tabs = 1 dose (20/120 mg tablets) give initial dose, followed by second dose 8h later, then 1 dose (PO) q12h for the following 2 days.
	or
	Dihydroartemisinin 40 mg plus piperaquine 320 mg (PO) q24h × 3 days.

For CDC guidelines for malaria in US (see p. 721).

Babesiosis (Babesia microti)

Clinical Presentation: "Malarial-like illness" with malaise, fever, relative bradycardia, shaking chills, myalgias, arthralgias, headache, abdominal pain, and splenomegaly. Laboratory abnormalities include anemia, atypical lymphocytes, relative lymphopenia, thrombocytopenia, mildly elevated LFTs, highly elevated ↑ ESR, ↑ ferritin, and ↓ LDH. Transmitted by infected Ixodes ticks.

Diagnostic and Considerations: Characteristic four merozoites (often pear shaped) arranged in "Maltese cross" formation (tetrads). Serology diagnostic of acute infection. Hyposplenic patients may have profound hemolytic anemia and life-threatening infection.

Pitfalls: Co-infection with Lyme disease may occur. No serological cross-reactivity between Babesia and Borrelia (Lyme disease). Merozoites only may be confused with P. falciparum malaria. Extra-RBC forms and vacuolated RBCs distinguish babesiosis from malaria. Travel history is important. Doxycycline ineffective.

Prognosis: May be more severe with Lyme disease co-infection. Severe/fatal if ↓/absent splenic function. Exchange transfusions may be life saving.

Ehrlichiosis (HME/HGA)

Clinical Presentation: Acute febrile illness with chills, headache, malaise, myalgias, leukopenia, relative lymphopenia, atypical lymphocytes, thrombocytopenia, ↑ LFTs, ↓ ESR, ↑ ferritin. No vasculitis. Resembles Rocky Mountain spotted fever (RMSF), but without rash.

Diagnostic Considerations: Characteristic "morula" (spherical, basophilic, mulberry-shaped, cytoplasmic inclusion bodies) may be seen in peripheral blood neutrophils in HGA. PCR from blood is 86% sensitive and highly specific for early diagnosis. Obtain acute and convalescent IFA serology. HGA vector is Ixodes ticks clinical co-infection with B. burgdorferi (Lyme Disease) is rare, but may occur. Main HME vector Ambylomma americanum (lone star tick).

Pitfalls: No morula with HME. Rash uncommon in HME and rare in HGA. E. chaffeensis (HME) titers will not be elevated with A. phagocytophilium (HGA) and vice versa.

Prognosis: Good if treated early. Delayed response or may be more severe with in co-infection with Lyme disease.

Malaria (Plasmodium ovale/vivax/falciparum/malariae/knowlesi)

Clinical Presentation: Presents acutely with fever/chills, severe headaches, cough, nausea/vomiting, diarrhea, abdominal/back pain. Typical "malarial paroxysm" consists of chills, fever and profuse sweating, followed by extreme prostration. There are a paucity of physical findings, but most have tender hepatomegaly/splenomegaly and relative bradycardia. ↑ T.bilirubin, thrombocytopenia, atypical lymphocytes, and ↑ LFTs are common.

Diagnostic Considerations: Diagnosis by visualizing Plasmodium on thick/thin Giemsa or Wright-stained smears.

Pitfalls: Be wary of diagnosing malaria without headache. Dengue most closely resembles malaria. On abdominal US, dengue patients have gallbladder wall thickening/splenomegaly but not hepatomegaly vs.malaria patients which have a normal gallbladder, splenomegaly/heptomegaly. If no atypical lymphocytes on smear (auto cell counters are insensitive to atypical lymphocytes), question the diagnosis of malaria. P. knowlesi (monkey malaria emerging cause of human malaria. Resembles P. malariae (microscopically) but may be severe resembing P. falciparum (clinically). Treat P. knowlesi as chloroquine sensitive (P. vivax, P. ovale, P. malariae) malaria.

Prognosis: Related to species degree of parasitemia P. falciparum with high-grade parasitemia is most severe, and may be complicated by coma, hypoglycemia, renal failure, or non-cardiogenic pulmonary edema. If parasitemia exceeds 15%, consider exchange transfusions.

Fungi/Mycobacterium in Blood

See histoplasmosis (p. 341), Mycobacterium tuberculosis (treat as pulmonary TB, p. 326), Mycobacterium avium-intracellulare (p. 321, 342).

Parasites, Fungi, Unusual Organisms in CSF/Brain

Cysts/Mass Lesions in CSF/Brain

Subset	Pathogens	Preferred Therapy	Alternate Therapy
Cerebral nocardiosis	Nocardia sp.	<u>Preferred IV Therapy:</u> TMP–SMX (TMP 5 mg/kg, SMX 15 mg/kg) (IV) q6h until clinical improvement, then (PO) therapy <u>Alternate IV PO Therapy:</u> Minocycline or Doxycycline 100 mg (IV) q12h until clinical improvement, then (PO) therapy	<u>Preferred PO Therapy</u> TMP–SMX 1 DS tablet (PO) q12h × 6 months <u>Alternate PO Therapy</u> Minocycline 100 mg (PO) q12h × 6 months **or** Doxycycline 100 mg (PO) q12h × 6 months
Cryptococcal meningitis/ cryptococcomas	Cryptococcus neoformans	See p. 22	
Cerebral amebiasis	Entamoeba histolytica	Metronidazole 750 mg (PO) q8h × 10 days **or** Tinidazole 800 mg (PO) q8h × 5 days	
Primary amebic meningo-encephalitis	Naegleria fowleri	See p. 21	
Granulomatous amebic encephalitis	Acanthamoeba	See p. 22	
Cerebral echinococcosis (hydatid cyst disease)	Echinococcus granulosus or multilocularis	Surgical resection plus Albendazole 400 mg* (PO) q12h until cured	Surgical resection plus Mebendazole 50 mg/kg (PO) q24h until cured
Cerebral gnathostomiasis	Gnathostoma spinigerum	Surgical resection	Albendazole 400 mg (PO) q12h × 3 weeks **or** Ivermectin 200 mcg/kg/d × 2 days
Cerebral coenurosis	Taenia multiceps	Surgical resection	

Cysts/Mass Lesions in CSF/Brain (cont'd)

Subset	Pathogens	Preferred Therapy	Alternate Therapy
Neurocysticercosis	Taenia solium	Albendazole 400 mg* (PO) q12h × 2 weeks	Praziquantel 33 mg/kg (PO) q8h × 1day, then 15 mg/kg (PO) q8h × 2–4 weeks ± cimetidine 400 mg (PO) q8h (to ↑ praziquantel levels)
Cerebral paragonimiasis (lung fluke)	Paragonimus westermani	Praziquantel 25 mg/kg (PO) q8h × 2 days	Bithionol 50 mg/kg (PO) q48h × 2 weeks **or** Tridabendazole 10 mg/kg (PO) q24h × 2 days
Cerebral toxoplasmosis	Toxoplasma gondii	See pp. 331–332	
Chagas' disease (American trypanosomiasis)	Trypanosoma brucei cruzi	Nifurtimox 2 mg/kg (PO) q6h × 4 months	Benznidazole 3.5 mg/kg (PO) q12h × 2 months

*   If < 60 kg, give albendazole 7.5 mg/kg.

Cerebral Nocardiosis

Clinical Presentation: CNS mass lesion resembling brain tumor/abscess. Symptoms are highly variable, and result from local effects of granulomas/abscesses in CNS. Up to 40% of patients with systemic nocardiosis have associated mass lesions in CNS.

Diagnostic Considerations: Diagnosis by demonstrating Nocardia (gram positive, delicate, beaded, branching filaments) in brain biopsy specimens. Notify laboratory for modified acid fast specimen staining/aerobic cultures if suspect Nocardia. Nocardia are weakly acid-fast and aerobic.

Pitfalls: Usually not limited to brain. Look for Nocardia in skin, lungs or liver. Use in-vitro susceptibility data to guide therapy for refractory cases. IV regimens are recommended for critically ill patients. HIV patients require life-long suppression with TMP–SMX.

Prognosis: Related to health of host, degree of immunosuppression, and extent of lesions.

Cerebral Amebiasis (Entamoeba histolytica)

Clinical Presentation: Rare cause of brain abscess. Onset is frequently abrupt with rapid progression. Suspect in patients with a history of amebiasis and altered mental status/focal neurologic signs. If present, meningeal involvement resembles acute bacterial meningitis. CT/MRI shows focal lesions.

Diagnostic Considerations: Diagnosis by demonstrating E. histolytica trophozoites in wet preps or by trichrome stain from aspirated brain lesions under CT guidance. Worldwide distribution. Mass lesions may be single or multiple, and more commonly involve the left hemisphere. Most patients have concomitant liver ± lung abscesses.

Pitfalls: Trophozoites/cysts in stool are not diagnostic of CNS disease. E. histolytica serology is often positive, but is nonspecific. E. histolytica trophozoites are not present in CSF.

Prognosis: Related to size/location of CNS lesions.

Primary Amebic Meningoencephalitis (Naegleria fowleri) (see p. 23)

Granulomatous Amebic Encephalitis (Acanthamoeba) (see p. 23)

Cerebral Echinococcosis (Echinococcus granulosus) Hydatid Cyst Disease

Clinical Presentation: Most cysts are asymptomatic. Mass lesions may cause seizures, cranial nerve abnormalities, other focal neurologic symptoms.

Diagnostic Considerations: CT/MRI typically shows a single large cyst without edema or enhancement. Multiple cysts are rare. Diagnosis by demonstrating protoscolices in "hydatid sand" in cysts. Usually associated with liver/lung hydatid cysts.

Pitfalls: E. granulosus serology lacks specificity.

Prognosis: Related to size/location of CNS cysts. CSF eosinophilia is not a feature of CNS involvement. Treatment consists of surgical removal of total cyst after instilling cysticidal agent (hypertonic saline, iodophor, ethanol) into cyst plus albendazole.

Cerebral Echinococcosis (Echinococcus multilocularis) Hydatid Cyst Disease

Clinical Presentation: Frequently associated with hydatid bone cysts (may cause spinal cord compression), liver/lung cysts. Peripheral eosinophilia occurs in 50%, but eosinophils are not seen in the CSF.

Diagnostic Considerations: E. multilocularis ELISA is sensitive and specific.

Pitfalls: Praziquantel is ineffective for CNS hydatid cyst disease. Imaging studies suggest carcinoma/sarcoma. Diagnosis is frequently not made until brain biopsy.

Prognosis: If treatment is effective, improvement of CNS lesions is evident in 8 weeks. Brain/bone cysts are difficult to cure.

Cerebral Gnathostomiasis (Gnathostoma spinigerum)

Clinical Presentation: Nausea, vomiting, increased salivation, skin flushing, pruritus, urticaria, and upper abdominal pain 1–6 days after exposure. Cerebral form presents as eosinophilic meningitis with radiculomyeloencephalitis, with headache and severe sharp/shooting pains in extremities often followed by paraplegia and coma. Any cranial nerve may be involved. The most characteristic feature is changing/migratory neurological findings. Intense peripheral eosinophilia occurs in 90% of patients. CSF has eosinophilic pleocytosis and may have RBCs.

Diagnostic Considerations: In cases with ocular involvement, the worm may be seen in the anterior chamber of eye. Specific Gnathostoma serology of CSF is helpful in establishing the diagnosis. Acquired from infected cat/dog feces. Most cases occur in Southeast Asia also Central/South America (Mexico, Peru) and most recently in Africa (Botswana). Few other CNS infections have both RBCs and eosinophils in the CSF.

Pitfalls: Do not miss associated eye involvement or characteristic episodic non-pitting subcutaneous edema.

Prognosis: Related to invasion of medulla/brainstem.

Cerebral Coenurosis (Taenia multiceps)

Clinical Presentation: CNS mass lesion with seizures/cranial nerve abnormalities, often presenting as a posterior-fossa syndrome. Common sites of CNS involvement include paraventricular and basal subarachnoid spaces. Eosinophils not in CSF.

Diagnostic Considerations: Diagnosis by demonstrating protoscolices in brain cyst specimens. Worldwide distribution. Transmitted via dog feces.
Pitfalls: Do not miss associated ocular lesions, which mimic intraocular neoplasms/granulomas.
Prognosis: Related to size/extent of CNS lesions.

Neurocysticercosis (Taenia solium)

Clinical Presentation: Chronic eosinophilic meningitis/mass lesions with seizures. Hydrocephalus is common. Spinal involvement may result in paraplegia. Cerebral cysts are usually multiple.
Diagnostic Considerations: CT/MRI shows multiple enhancing and non-enhancing unilocular cysts. Diagnosis by specific T. solium serology of serum/CSF or excision of cyst. Neurocysticercosis is the most common CNS parasite. Worldwide in distribution; most common in Eastern Europe, Asia, Latin America.
Pitfalls: Cranial nerve abnormalities are uncommon.
Prognosis: Related to extent/location of CNS lesions. Adjunctive therapy includes corticosteroids, anti-epileptics, and shunt for hydrocephalus.

Cerebral Paragonimiasis (Paragonimus westermani) Lung Fluke

Clinical Presentation: Can resemble epilepsy, cerebral tumors, or brain embolism. Primary focus of infection is pulmonary, with pleuritic chest pain, cough, and night sweats. CNS findings are a manifestation of extrapulmonary (ectopic) organ involvement.
Diagnostic Considerations: Diagnosis by demonstrating operculated eggs in sputum, pleural fluid, or feces. Multiple sputum samples are needed to demonstrate P. westermani eggs. Charcot-Leyden crystals are seen in sputum. Endemic in Far East, India, Africa, and Central/South America.
Pitfalls: Extrapulmonary (ectopic) organ involvement (cerebral, subcutaneous, abdominal) is common. Up to 20% of patients have normal chest x-rays.
Prognosis: Related to size/location of CNS cysts and extent of lung involvement.

Cerebral Toxoplasmosis (T. gondii) (see pp. 331–332)

Cerebral Cryptococcosis (C. neoformans) (see pp. 329–330)

Chagas' Disease (Trypanosoma brucei cruzi) American Trypanosomiasis

Clinical Presentation: Acute unilateral periorbital cellulitis (Romaña's sign) or regional adenopathy and edema of extremity at site of infected reduviid bug (Chagoma). Chronic disease manifests as myocarditis/heart block or megaesophagus, megaduodenum, megacolon. Hepatosplenomegaly is common. Overt CNS signs are frequently absent. CNS Chagas' disease typically have hypodense ring enhancing lesions with surrounding edema on head CT/MRI scans. If meningoencephalitis develops, the prognosis is very poor. In immunosuppressed patients (especially AIDS), recrudescence of disease occurs with development of T. brucei cruzi brain abscesses.
Diagnostic Considerations: Diagnosis in acute disease by demonstrating trypanosomes in wet prep of anticoagulated blood or stained buffy coat smears. Amastigote forms present intracellularly in monocytes/histiocytes in Giemsa-stained smear of bone marrow/lymph node aspirate, or by xenodiagnosis. Serology (mostly used for chronic disease) has limited value in endemic areas due to lack of specificity, but is useful in non-endemic areas. Common in Central/South America. Acquired from infected reduviid bugs, which infest mud/clay/stone parts of primitive dwellings. Infection in humans occurs in areas containing reduviids that defecate during or immediately after a blood meal.

Diagnostic Considerations: Screening test ELISA IFA; confirmatory test RIPA (radioimmuno precipitation assay).

Pitfalls: Do not overlook diagnosis in persons from endemic areas with unexplained heart block. For children ages 11–16 years, use nifurtimox 3.5 mg/kg (PO) q6h × 3 months. For children < 11 years, use nifurtimox 5 mg/kg (PO) q6h × 3 months.

Prognosis: Related to extent of GI cardiac or CNS involvement. The addition of gamma interferon to nifurtimox × 20 days may shorten the acute phase of the disease.

Parasites, Fungi, Unusual Organisms in Lungs

Pulmonary Cystic Lesions/Masses

Subset	Pathogens	Preferred Therapy	Alternate Therapy
Alveolar echinococcosis	Echinococcus multilocularis	<u>Operable cases</u> Wide surgical resection plus Albendazole 400 mg* (PO) q12h or Mebendazole 50 mg/kg (PO) q24h until cured	<u>Inoperable cases:</u> Albendazole 400 mg* (PO) q12h × 1 month, then repeat therapy after 2 weeks × 3 cycles (i.e., 4 total months of albendazole)
Pulmonary amebiasis	Entamoeba histolytica	Metronidazole 750 mg (PO) q8h × 10 days	Tinidazole 800 mg (PO) q8h × 5 days
Pulmonary paragonimiasis (lung fluke)	Paragonimus westermani	Praziquantel 25 mg/kg (PO) q8h × 2 days	Bithionol 50 mg/kg (PO) q48h × 4 weeks **or** Tridabendazole 10 mg/kg (PO) q24h × 2 days

* If < 60 kg, give albendazole 7.5 mg/kg.

Alveolar Echinococcosis (Echinococcus multilocularis)

Clinical Presentation: Slowly growing cysts remain asymptomatic for 5–20 years, until space-occupying effect elicits symptoms. Rupture/leak into bronchial tree can cause cough, chest pain, and hemoptysis.

Diagnostic Considerations: Diagnosis is suggested by typical "Swiss cheese calcification" findings on chest x-ray, and confirmed by specific E. multilocularis serology (which does not cross react with E. granulosus). Most common in Northern forest areas of Europe, Asia, North America, and Arctic. Acquired by ingestion of viable parasite eggs in food. Tapeworm-infected canines/cats or wild rodents are common vectors. Less common than infection with E. granulosus.

Pitfalls: Do not confuse central cavitary lesions with squamous cell carcinoma.

Prognosis: Related to size/location of cysts.

Pulmonary Amebiasis (Entamoeba histolytica)

Clinical Presentation: Cough, pelvic pain, fever, and right lung/pleural mass mimicking pneumonia or lung abscess. Bronchopleural fistulas may occur. Sputum has "liver-like" taste if cyst ruptures into bronchus. Bacterial co-infection is rare. Amebic lung lesions are associated with hepatic liver abscesses, and invariably involve the right lobe of lung/diaphragm.

Diagnostic Considerations: Diagnosis by aspiration of lungs cysts, which may be massive. Amebic serology is sensitive and specific. Worldwide distribution. Acquired by ingesting amebic cysts. Key to diagnosis is concomitant liver involvement; liver abscess presents years after initial diarrheal episode.

Pitfalls: Lung involvement is rarely the sole manifestation of amebic infection, and is usually due to direct extension of amebic liver abscess (10–20% of amebic liver abscesses penetrate through the diaphragm and into the lungs). Follow metronidazole with paromomycin 500 mg (PO) q8h × 7 days to eliminate intestinal focus.

Prognosis: Related to severity/extent of cysts.

Pulmonary Paragonimiasis (Paragonimus westermani) Lung Fluke

Clinical Presentation: Mild infection; may be asymptomatic. Acute phase of infection is accompanied by abdominal pain, diarrhea and urticaria, followed by pleuritic chest pain/eosinophilic pleural effusion. Chronic symptoms occur within 6 months after exposure, with dyspnea/dry cough leading to productive cough ± hemoptysis. Complications include lung abscess, bronchiectasis, cough, and night sweats. Eosinophilia may be present acutely.

Diagnostic Considerations: Oriental lung fluke acquired by ingestion of freshwater crayfish/crabs. After penetration of the gut/peritoneal cavity, the fluke migrates through the diaphragm/pleural space and invades lung parenchyma. Incubation period is 2–20 days. Diagnosis by demonstrating operculated eggs in sputum, pleural fluid, or feces. Multiple sputum samples are needed to demonstrate P. westermani eggs. Charcot-Leyden crystals are seen in sputum, and characteristic chest x-ray findings of ring-shaped/crescent infiltrates with "thin-walled" cavities are evident in ~ 60%. Endemic in Asia, Africa, and Latin America. Chest x-ray findings take months to resolve.

Pitfalls: May have extrapulmonary (ectopic) organ involvement, e.g., cerebral, subcutaneous, abdominal. Up to 20% have normal chest x-rays. Commonest cause of eosinophilic pleural effusions in endemic areas. Diagnosis should be questioned if pleural effusion fluid does not have eosinophils.

Prognosis: Related to degree of lung damage, e.g., bronchiectasis and extrapulmonary organ involvement, especially CNS.

Pulmonary Coin Lesions

Subset	Pathogens	Preferred Therapy	Alternate Therapy
Dog heartworm	Dirofilaria immitis	No therapy necessary	
Aspergilloma	Aspergillus	No therapy if asymptomatic. Surgery for massive hemoptysis	Itraconazole 200 mg (PO) solution q24h × 3–6 months **or** Voriconazole (see "usual dose," p. 714) × 3–6 months

Dog Heartworm (Dirofilaria immitis)

Clinical Presentation: Asymptomatic "coin lesion" after bite of infected mosquito transmits parasite from dogs to humans. Differential diagnosis includes granulomas and malignancy.

Diagnostic Considerations: Diagnosis by specific serology or pathological demonstration of organism in granuloma, usually when a coin lesion is biopsied to rule out malignancy. Worldwide distribution. Acquired from pet dogs. Dirofilariasis causes dog heartworm in carrier, but presents as a solitary lung nodule in humans.

Pitfalls: Often confused with malignancy.

Prognosis: Excellent.

Pulmonary Aspergilloma

Clinical Presentation: Coin lesion(s) ± productive cough, hemoptysis, wheezing. May be asymptomatic. Usually occurs in pre-existing cavitary lung lesions, especially TB with cavity > 2 cm.

Diagnostic Considerations: Diagnosis by chest x-ray appearance of fungus ball in cavity and Aspergillus precipitins/biopsy or by demonstrating Aspergillus hyphae and "fruiting bodies" (conidiophores) in respiratory specimens. May present with "crescent sign" on chest x-ray (white fungus ball silhouetted against black crescent of the cavity).

Pitfalls: Role of itraconazole or voriconazole as therapy is unclear.

Prognosis: Related to degree of hemoptysis.

Pulmonary Infiltrates/Mass Lesions¶

Subset	Pathogens	Preferred Therapy	Alternate Therapy
Pulmonary blastomycosis	Blastomyces dermatitidis	Mild illness: Itraconazole 200 mg (PO) TID × 3 days and then QD or BID for a total of 6–12 months (adequate serum levels should be confirmed). Moderately severe or severe illness: lipid amphotericin for 1–2 weeks followed by itraconazole as for mild illness.	Fluconazole has been disappointing; its use is limited to specialized settings such as CNS blastomycosis. Amphotericin B 0.7–1 mg/kg may be used as initial therapy instead of lipid amphotericin.
Pulmonary histoplasmosis	Histoplasma capsulatum	Mild illness: Therapy is not always needed, but symptoms lasting more than a month may be treated with Itraconazole 200 mg (PO) TID × 3 days and then QD or BID for a total of 6–12 weeks. Moderately severe or severe illness: lipid amphotericin for 1–2 weeks followed by Itraconazole as for mild illness. Chronic cavity histoplasmosis requires at least a year of therapy & confirmation of adequate blood levels.	Strategies are complex (See Wheat LJ et al. Clin Infect Dis 45:807–825, 2007).
Pulmonary paracoccidioidomycosis (South American blastomycosis)	Paracoccidioides brasiliensis	Itraconazole 200 mg (PO) q24h × 6 months **or** Ketoconazole 400 mg (PO) q24h × 18 months	Amphotericin B 0.5 mg/kg (IV) q24h until 1.5–2.5 grams given

¶ **See Color Atlas** (center of book).

Pulmonary Infiltrates/Mass Lesions (cont'd)

Subset	Pathogens	Preferred Therapy	Alternate Therapy
Pulmonary actinomycosis	Actinomyces israelii	Amoxicillin 1 gm (PO) q8h × 6 months **or** Doxycycline 100 mg (PO) q12h × 6 months	Clindamycin 300 mg (PO) q8h × 6 months **or** Chloramphenicol 500 mg (PO) q6h × 6 months
Pulmonary aspergillosis *BPA*	Aspergillus	Systemic oral steroids	Itraconazole 200 mg (PO) q12h × 8 months
	Aspergillus	See p. 323	
Acute invasive pneumonia/ aspergillus *Chronic pneumonia aspergillus*	Aspergillus	Treat the same as on p. 165	Treat the same as on p. 165
Pulmonary sporotrichosis	Sporothrix schenckii	Lipid amphotericin (p. 525) (IV) q24h × 3 weeks **or** Amphotericin B 0.5 mg/kg (IV) q24h until 1–2 grams given	Itraconazole 200 mg (PO)* q12h until cured **or** Lipid amphotericin (p. 525) (IV) q24h until cured
Pulmonary coccidioido-mycosis	Coccidioides immitis	Itraconazole 200 mg (PO)* q12h until cured **or** Fluconazole 800 mg (IV or PO) × 1 dose, then 400 mg (PO) q24h until cured	Amphotericin B 1 mg/kg (IV) q24h × 7 days† **or** Lipid amphotericin (p. 525) (IV) q24h × 7 days
Pulmonary nocardiosis	Nocardia asteroides	TMP–SMX 5–10 mg/kg/d (TMP) in 2–4 doses (IV) × 3–6 weeks, then 1 DS tablet (PO) q12h until cured	Minocycline 100 mg (PO) q12h until cured

*　Initiate therapy with Itraconazole 200 mg (IV) q12h × 7–14 days.
†　Follow with Itraconazole 200 mg (PO) solution q12h until cured.

Pulmonary Infiltrates/Mass Lesions (cont'd)

Subset	Pathogens	Preferred Therapy	Alternate Therapy
Pulmonary cryptococcosis	Cryptococcus neoformans	Fluconazole 800 mg (IV or PO) × 1 dose, then 400 mg (PO) q24h until cured	Amphotericin B 0.5 mg/kg (IV) q24h until 1–2 grams given **or** Lipid amphotericin (p. 525) (IV) q24h × 3 weeks
Pulmonary zygomycosis (mucormycosis)	Rhizopus/ Mucor/Absidia	Lipid amphotericin (p. 525) (IV) q24h × 1–2 weeks† or × 3 wks **or** Amphotericin B 1–1.5 mg/kg (IV) q24h × 1–2 wks† or until 2–3 grams given	Itraconazole 200 mg (PO)* q12h until cured
Pulmonary pseudall-escheriasis	Pseudallescheria boydii/ Scedosporium apiospermum	Voriconazole (see "usual dose," p. 714) until cured	Itraconazole 200 mg (PO)* q12h until cured

BPA = bronchopulmonary aspergillosis.

* Initiate therapy with itraconazole 200 mg (IV) q12h × 7–14 days.

† Follow with itraconazole 200 mg (PO) solution q12h until cured.

Pulmonary Blastomycosis (Blastomyces dermatitidis)

Clinical Presentation: Highly variable. May present as a chronic/non-resolving pneumonia with fever/cough and characteristic "right-sided perihilar infiltrate" ± small pleural effusion.

Diagnostic Considerations: Usual sites of dissemination include skin, bones and prostate, not CNS or adrenals. Blastomyces serology may XR (false +) with Aspergillus, Coccidiodides, Histoplasma, or paracoccidiomycosis.

Pitfalls: Dissemination to extra-pulmonary sites may occur years after pneumonia.

Prognosis: Related to severity/extent of infection. One-third of cases are self-limited and do not require treatment.

Pulmonary Histoplasmosis (Histoplasma capsulatum)

Clinical Presentation: Acute primary infection presents as self-limiting flu-like illness with fever, headache, nonproductive cough, chills, and chest pain. Minority of patients become overtly ill with complicated respiratory or progressive pulmonary infection. Can cause arthralgias, E. nodosum, E. multiforme, or pericarditis. May occur in outbreaks. Chronic infection presents as chronic pneumonia resembling TB or chronic disseminated infection. Eosinophilia common.

Diagnostic Considerations: May be recovered from sputum or demonstrated in lung tissue specimens. Worldwide distribution, but most common in Central/South Central United States. Acute disseminated histoplasmosis suggests HIV. Intracellular (PMNs/monocytes) organisms may be seen in Wright/Giema stained peripheral blood smears/buffy coat smears in disseminated infection. Acute histoplasmosis with immunodiffusion (ID) assay M band precipitins; chronic histoplasmosis with ID assay M band precipitins or CF ≥ 1:32. Histoplasma urinary antigen useful in diagnosis of acute/disseminated histoplasmosis. Histoplasma serology may XR (false +) with coccidiomycosis, blastomycosis, TB or sarcoidosis. Histoplasma urinary antigen may XR with acute/chronic coccidiomycosis (false + histoplasma urinary antigen may provide a clue to the presence of coccidiomycosis.)

Pitfalls: Pleural effusion is uncommon. Do not treat old/inactive/minimal histoplasmosis, histoplasmosis pulmonary calcification, or histoplasmosis fibrosing mediastinitis. Differentiate from TB and kala-azar. Resembles kala-azar histologically, but rod-shaped kinetoplasts (kala-azar) are absent extracellularly.

Prognosis: Related to severity/extent of infection. No treatment is needed for self-limiting acutehistoplasmosis presenting as flu-like illness. HIV patients should receive life-long suppressive therapy with itraconazole 200 mg (PO) solution q24h.

Pulmonary Paracoccidioidomycosis (South American Blastomycosis)

Clinical Presentation: Typically presents as a chronic pneumonia syndrome with productive cough, blood-tinged sputum, dyspnea, and chest pain. May also develop fever, malaise, weight loss, mucosal ulcerations in/around mouth and nose, dysphagia, changes in voice, cutaneous lesions on face/limbs, or cervical adenopathy. Can disseminate to prostate, epididymis, kidneys, or adrenals.

Diagnostic Considerations: Characteristic "pilot wheel" shaped yeast in sputum. Diagnosis by culture and stain (Gomori) of organism from clinical specimen. Found only in Latin American. One-third of cases have only pulmonary involvement. Skin test is non-specific/non-diagnostic.

Pitfalls: No distinguishing radiologic features. No clinical adrenal insufficiency, in contrast to TB or histoplasmosis. Hilar adenopathy/pleural effusions are uncommon.

Prognosis: Related to severity/extent of infection. HIV require life-long suppression with TMP–SMX 1 DS tablet (PO) q24h or itraconazole 200 mg (PO) solution q24h.

Pulmonary Actinomycosis (Actinomyces israelii)

Clinical Presentation: Indolent, slowly progressive infiltrates involving the pulmonary parenchyma ± pleural space. Presents with fever, chest pain, weight loss. Cough/hemoptysis are less common. Chest wall sinuses frequently develop. Chest x-ray shows adjacent dense infiltrate. "Sulfur granules" are common in sinus drainage fluid.

Diagnostic Considerations: Diagnosis by stain/culture of drainage from sinuses or lung/bone biopsy specimens. Actinomyces are non-acid fast and anaerobic to microaerophilic.

Pitfalls: No CNS lesions, but bone erosion is common with chest lesions. Prior antibiotic therapy may interfere with isolation of organism.

Prognosis: Excellent when treated until lesions resolve. Use IV regimen in critically ill patients, then switch to oral regimen.

Bronchopulmonary Aspergillosis (BPA / ABPA)

Clinical Presentation: Migratory pulmonary infiltrates in chronic asthmatics. Eosinophilia is common, and sputum shows Charcot-Leyden crystals/brown flecks containing Aspergillus.

Diagnostic Considerations: Diagnosis by Aspergillus in sputum and high-titers of Aspergillus precipitins in serum. BPA is an allergic reaction in chronic asthmatics, *not* an infectious disease. Pulmonary infiltrates with peripheral eosinophilia in chronic asthmatics suggests the diagnosis.

Pitfalls: Correct diagnosis is important since therapy is steroids, not antifungals.

Prognosis: Related to severity/duration of asthma and promptness of steroid therapy.

Acute Invasive Aspergillus Pneumonia (see p. 67)

Chronic Aspergillus Pneumonia

Clinical Presentation: Occurs in patients with AIDS, chronic granulomatous disease, alcoholism, diabetes, and those receiving steroids for chronic pulmonary disease. Usual features include chronic productive cough ± hemoptysis, low-grade fever, weight loss, and malaise. Chronic Aspergillus pneumonia resembles TB, histoplasmosis, melioidosis.

Diagnostic Considerations: Diagnosis by lung biopsy demonstrating septate hyphae invading lung parenchyma. Aspergillus may be in sputum, but is not diagnostic of Aspergillus pneumonia.

Pitfalls: May extend into chest wall, vertebral column, or brachial plexus.

Prognosis: Related to severity/extent of infection. Cavitation is a favorable prognostic sign.

Pulmonary Sporotrichosis (Sporothrix schenckii)

Clinical Presentation: Usually presents as productive cough, low-grade fever, and weight loss. Chest x-ray shows cavitary thin-walled lesions with associated infiltrate. Hemoptysis is unusual. Differential diagnosis includes other thin-walled cavitary lung lesions (e.g., coccidioidomycosis, atypical TB, paragonimiasis).

Diagnostic Considerations: Diagnosis by lung biopsy demonstrating invasive lung disease, not broncho-alveolar lavage. Usually a history of puncture/traumatic wound involving an extremity. May be associated with septic arthritis/osteomyelitis.

Pitfalls: Sporotrichosis in lungs implies disseminated disease. May need repeated attempts at culture.

Prognosis: Related to extent of infection/degree of immunosuppression.

Pulmonary Coccidioidomycosis (Coccidioides immitis)

Clinical Presentation: Usually presents as a solitary, peripheral, thin-walled cavitary lesion in early or later stage of primary infection. May present as a solitary pulmonary nodule. E. nodosum and bilateral hilar adenopathy are common (in contrast to sporotrichosis). Hemoptysis is unusual.

Diagnostic Considerations: Diagnosis by demonstration of spherules with endospores in sputum/BAL or biopsy specimens/Coccidioides serology. Increased incidence of dissemination in Filipinos, Blacks, and American Indians. Eosinophils in CSF in disseminated infection with CNS involvement. May be associated with chronic meningitis/osteomyelitis. CF IgG titer ≥ 1:32 diagnostic of active disease. Coccidioides CF may XR (false +) with Blastomyces, Histoplasma, Cryptococci, Torulopsis, or TB (XR minimal with EIA). (False + histoplasma urinary antigen may provide a clue to the presence of coccidiomycosis.)

Pitfalls: Dissemination is preceded by ↓ Coccidioides titers/disappearance of Erythema nodosum.

Prognosis: Related to extent of infection/degree of immunosuppression.

Pulmonary Nocardiosis (Nocardia asteroides)

Clinical Presentation: Usually presents as a dense lower lobe lung mass ± cavitation. May have associated mass lesions in CNS. Chest wall sinuses are more common with Actinomycosis.

Diagnostic Considerations: Diagnosis by demonstrating organisms by stain/culture of lung specimens. Nocardia are weakly acid-fast and aerobic.

Pitfalls: Use IV regimens in critically ill patients. HIV patients require life-long suppressive therapy with TMP–SMX or minocycline.

Prognosis: Related to extent of infection/degree of immunosuppression.

Pulmonary Cryptococcosis (Cryptococcus neoformans)

Clinical Presentation: Individual focus of infection is usually inapparent/minimal when patient presents with disseminated cryptococcal infection. Pneumonia is typically a minor part of disseminated disease; CNS manifestations usually predominate (e.g., headache, subtle cognitive changes, occasional meningeal signs, focal neurological deficits).

Diagnostic Considerations: Diagnosis by serum cryptococcal antigen, by demonstrating encapsulated yeasts in sputum/lung specimens, or by culture of pulmonary specimens.

Pitfalls: Clinical presentation of isolated cryptococcal pneumonia is rare. In HIV, false + cryptococcal antigen may occur with BBL Port-A-Cul transport vials. Patients require life-long suppressive therapy with fluconazole.

Prognosis: Related to extent of dissemination/degree of immunosuppression.

Pulmonary Zygomycosis (Mucormycosis) (Rhizopus/Mucor/Absidia/Cunninghamella)

Clinical Presentation: Progressive pneumonia with fever, dyspnea, hemoptysis and cough unresponsive to antibiotic therapy. Usually seen only in compromised hosts. Chest x-ray is not characteristic, but shows infiltrate with consolidation in > 50% of patients. Cavitation occurs in 40% as neutropenia resolves.

Diagnostic Considerations: Diagnosis by demonstrating branched non-septate "ribbon-like" hyphae with right angle branching in biopsy specimens in lung biopsy. Pleural effusion is not a feature of pulmonary mucormycosis.

Pitfalls: Causes rhinocerebral mucormycosis in diabetics, pneumonia in leukopenic compromised hosts.

Prognosis: Related to degree of immunosuppression and underlying disease. Angioinvasive with a propensity for dissemination.

Pulmonary Pseudallescheriasis (P. boydii/S. apiospermum)

Clinical Presentation: Progressive pulmonary infiltrates indistinguishable from Aspergillosis or Mucor. Usually seen only in compromised hosts (e.g., prolonged neutropenia, high-dose steroids, bone marrow or solid organ transplants, AIDS). Manifests as cough, fever, pleuritic pain, and often hemoptysis. No characteristic chest x-ray appearance.

Diagnostic Considerations: Diagnosis by culture of organisms in lung biopsy. Hemoptysis is common in patients with cavitary lesions. CNS involvement is rare.

Pitfalls: One of few invasive fungi unresponsive to amphotericin B deoxycholate. Cause of sinusitis in diabetics, and pneumonia in leukopenic compromised hosts.

Prognosis: Related to severity/extent of infection and degree of immunosuppression. Cavitary lesions causing hemoptysis often require surgical excision. Disseminated infection is often fatal.

Parasites, Fungi, Unusual Organisms in Heart

Chagas' Disease (Trypanosoma brucei cruzi) American Trypanosomiasis

Subset	Pathogens	Preferred Therapy	Alternate Therapy
Chagas' disease (American trypanosomiasis)	Trypanosoma brucei cruzi	Benznidazole 2.5–3.5 mg/kg (PO) q12h × 60 days	Nifurtimox 2–3 mg/kg/day (PO) q6–8h × 90 days

Parasites, Fungi, Unusual Organisms in the Liver

Liver Flukes

Subset	Pathogens	Preferred Therapy	Alternate Therapy
Fascioliasis	Fasciola hepatica Fasciola gigantica	Tridabendazole 10 mg/kg (PO) × 1 or 2 doses	Bithionol 30–50 mg/kg (PO) q48h × 20–30 days **or** Nitazoxanide 500 mg (PO) q12h × 7 days
Clonorchiasis/ Opisthorchiasis	Clonorchis sinensis Opisthorchis viverrini	Praziquantel 25 mg/kg (PO) q8h × 2 days	C. sinensis/O. viverrini Albendazole 10 mg/kg (PO) q24h × 7 days O. viverrini: Tribendimidine 400 mg (PO) × 1 dose

Hepatic Fascioliasis (F. hepatica/F. gigantica)

Clinical Presentation: Frequently asymptomatic, but may present acutely with fever, right upper quadrant pain, nausea, diarrhea, wheezing, urticaria, hepatomegaly, eosinophilia, anemia. ELISA, IHA, CF, CIE serology helpful with acute diagnosis. Aspiration of biliary fluid may show flukes/eggs. Chronic disease is associated with gallstones, cholecystitis, cholangitis, liver abscess, generalized adenopathy. Subacute nodules, hydrocele, lung/brain abscess can be seen in ectopic forms.

Diagnostic Consideration: Diagnosis by F. hepatica/F. gigantica eggs in stool. Endemic in sheep-raising areas (sheep liver flukes). Acquired from freshwater plants (watercress). Not associated with cholangiocarcinoma.

Pitfalls: May present as Katayama syndrome resembling schistosomiasis, with high fever, eosinophilia, and hepatosplenomegaly. Unlike other trematodes, praziquantel is ineffective. Chronic F. hepatica often asymptomatic, but may present with intermittent biliary colic. No eosinophilia. Abdominal ultrasound/CT shows crescentic/leaf shaped defects in gallbladder/hepatic ducts.

Prognosis: Related to extent/location of liver damage.

Hepatic Clonorchiasis (C. sinensis) / Opisthorchiasis (O. viverrini)

Clinical Presentation: Frequently asymptomatic, but may present 2–4 weeks after ingestion of fluke with fever, tender hepatomegaly, rash, and eosinophilia. Chronically presents as recurrent cholangitis, chronic cholecystitis, or pancreatitis. Associated with cholangiocarcinoma (unlike fascioliasis).

Diagnostic Considerations: Diagnosis by visualizing C. sinensis/O. viverrini (operculated lemon-shaped) eggs in stool. Clonorchiasis is acquired from ingesting raw/inadequately cooked infected freshwater (Cyprinoid) fish in Southeast Asia. Opisthorchiasis is acquired from ingesting raw/inadequately cooked infected freshwater fish/crayfish from Laos, Cambodia, or Thailand.

Pitfalls: Cholecystitis with eosinophilia should suggest clonorchiasis.

Prognosis: Related to extent/location of hepatic damage. Associated with cholangiocarcinoma.

Cystic Masses in Liver

Subset	Pathogens	Preferred Therapy	Alternate Therapy
Hepatic amebiasis	Entamoeba histolytica	Metronidazole 750 mg (PO) q8h × 7–10 days	Tinidazole 2 gm/day (PO) in 3 divided doses × 3 days
Hepatic echinococcosis (hydatid cyst disease)	Echinococcus granulosus	<u>Operable</u> Surgical resection **plus** Albendazole 400 mg* (PO) q12h × 1–6 months	<u>Inoperable</u> Albendazole 400 mg* (PO) q12h × 1–6 months

*   If < 60 kg, give albendazole 7.5 mg/kg.

Hepatic Amebiasis (Entamoeba histolytica)

Clinical Presentation: Presents insidiously with weight loss and night sweats or acutely ill with fever, nausea, vomiting, right upper quadrant pain. Typically, amebic liver abscesses are single, affect the right posterior lobe of liver, and do not show air/fluid levels. (In contrast, bacterial liver abscesses are usually multiple, and in all lobes of liver, and often show air/fluid levels.) Amebic liver abscesses do not calcify like hydatid cysts.

Diagnostic Considerations: Diagnosis by E. histolytica serology/E. histolytica in abscess wall. Worldwide distribution. Acquired by ingesting amebic cysts. Amebic liver abscess usually presents years after initial mild amebic dysenteric episode.

Pitfalls: Amebic abscess fluid ("anchovy paste") contains no PMNs or amebas; amebas are found only in abscess wall. Eosinophilia is not a feature of amebiasis.

Prognosis: Related to health of host/extrapulmonary spread.

Hepatic Echinococcosis (Echinococcus granulosus) Hydatid Cyst Disease

Clinical Presentation: Right upper quadrant pain/mass when cysts enlarge enough to cause symptoms. Hepatic cysts are unilocular in 70%, multilocular in 30%.

Diagnostic Considerations: Diagnosis by demonstrating E. granulosus scolices/hooklets in cyst/hydatid sand. Serology is unreliable. Worldwide distribution in sheep/cattle raising areas. Acquired by ingestion of eggs from dogs.

Pitfalls: Eosinophilia not a feature of hydatid cyst disease. Hydatid cysts are multifaceted, loculated, and calcified.

Prognosis: Related to location/extent of extrahepatic cysts. Large cysts are best treated by surgical removal after injection with hypertonic saline, alcohol, or iodophor to kill germinal layer/daughter cysts. Percutaneous drainage under ultrasound guidance plus albendazole may be effective.

Hepatomegaly

Subset	Pathogens	Preferred Therapy	Alternate Therapy
Visceral leishmaniasis (Kala-azar)	Leishmania donovani	Antimony stibogluconate 20 mg/kg (IV/IM) q24h × 28 days **or** Lipid amphotericin (Immunocompetent adults: 3 mg/kg (IV) q24h on days 1–5, 14, and 21; Immunocompromised adults: 4 mg/kg (IV) q24h on days 1–5, 10, 17, 24, 31, and 38)*	Miltefosine 2.5 mg/kg* (PO) q24h × 28 days **or** Paromomycin 15 mg/kg (IM) q24h × 21 days
Indian (Bihar state) visceral leishmaniasis (Kala-azar)	L. donovani	AmBisome (L-Amb)† 5 mg/kg (IV) × 1 dose, then Miltefosine 50 mg (PO with food) q12h × 7–14 days	
Schistosomiasis	Schistosoma mansoni	Praziquantel 20 mg/kg (PO) q12h × 2 doses	Oxamniquine 15 mg/kg (PO) × 1 dose¶
	Schistosoma japonicum	Praziquantel 20 mg/kg (PO) q8h × 3 doses	None

* Maximum 150 mg (PO)/day.

† Ultra short course therapy with AmBisome is 10 mg/kg (IV) × 2 days.

¶ In Africa, give 20 mg/kg (PO) q24h × 3 days.

Visceral Leishmaniasis (Leishmania donovani) Kala-azar

Clinical Presentation: Subacute or chronic systemic cases manifest months to years after initial exposure to Leishmania, most often with fever, weight loss, anemia, hepatosplenomegaly ± generalized adenopathy. Long eyelashes in some. Laboratory abnormalities include leukopenia, anemia, and polyclonal gammopathy on SPEP. Incubation period is usually 3–8 months. May have atypical presentation in HIV (e.g., no splenomegaly). Acutely can mimic malaria with chills/temperature spikes. Post–kala-azar dermatitis may resemble leprosy, and is persistent/common on face.

Diagnostic Considerations: Double quotidian fever (double daily temperature spike) in persons from endemic areas with hepatosplenomegaly suggests the diagnosis. Kala-azar in children may have ↑ triglycerides/↓ HDL. Diagnosis by liver/bone marrow or buffy coat smear. Histologically, Kala-azar resembles histoplasmosis. Key diagnostic finding in tissue biopsy specimens is intracellular amastigotes with adjacent rod-shaped kinetoplasts. L. donovani serology is specific; immunochromatographic Anti-K39 strip test is also useful. Most common in Southern Europe, Middle East, Asia, Africa, South America. Facial lesion is a clue to the diagnosis.

Pitfalls: In acute cases, can mimic malaria with chills and temperature spikes, but no thrombocytopenia or atypical lymphocytes. Antimony resistance is common in India (Bihar state).

Prognosis: Related to degree of liver/spleen involvement.

Hepatic Schistosomiasis (Schistosoma mansoni/japonicum)

Clinical Presentation: May present acutely with Katayama fever (serum sickness-like illness with wheezing and eosinophilia) 4–8 weeks after exposure. May be accompanied or followed by fever/chills, headache, cough, abdominal pain, diarrhea, generalized lymphadenopathy, or hepatosplenomegaly. Laboratory abnormalities include leukocytosis, eosinophilia, and polyclonal gammopathy on SPEP. Resolves spontaneously after 2–4 weeks. After 10–15 years, may present chronically as hepatosplenic schistosomiasis, with pre-sinusoidal portal hypertension, hepatomegaly (L > R lobe enlargement), no jaundice, and intact liver function.

Diagnostic Considerations: Diagnosis by S. mansoni/S. japonicum eggs in stool/liver biopsy. Serology is good for acute (not chronic) schistosomiasis. CT/MRI of liver shows "turtle back" septal calcifications. Rare complications include cor pulmonale and protein-losing enteropathy. Increased incidence of hepatitis B/C and chronic Salmonella infections. Renal complications include glomerulonephritis and nephrotic syndrome.

Pitfalls: Chronic schistosomiasis is not associated with eosinophilia. S. hematobium does not infect the liver/spleen. Oxamniquine is contraindicated in pregnancy.

Prognosis: Related to egg burden.

Parasites, Fungi, Unusual Organisms in Stool/Intestines

Intestinal Protozoa

Subset	Pathogens	Preferred Therapy	Alternate Therapy
Amebiasis	E. histolytica	See p. 88	
Giardiasis	Giardia lamblia	Tinidazole 2 gm (PO) × 1 dose **or** Metronidazole 250 mg (PO) q8h × 5–7 days	
Isospora	Isospora belli	TMP–SMX 1 DS tablet (PO) q12h × 10 days **or** Nitazoxanide 500 mg (PO) × 3 days (for HIV, see p. 334)	Ciprofloxacin 500 mg (PO) q12h × 7 days **or** Pyrimethamine 75 mg (PO) q24h + folinic acid 10 mg (PO) q24h × 2 weeks then q12h × 3 weeks
Dientamoebiasis	Dientamoeba fragilis	Iodoquinol 650 mg (PO) q8h × 20 days	Doxycycline 100 mg (PO) q12h × 10 days **or** Metronidazole 500–750 mg (PO) q8h × 10 days
Blastocystis	Blastocystis hominis	Nitazoxanide 500 mg (PO) q12h × 3 days	Iodoquinol 650 mg (PO) q8h × 20 days **or** TMP–SMX 1 DS tablet (PO) q12h × 7 days

Intestinal Protozoa (cont'd)

Subset	Pathogens	Preferred Therapy	Alternate Therapy
Cyclospora	Cyclospora	TMP–SMX 1 DS (PO) q12h × 10 days **or** Nitazoxanide 500 mg (PO) q12h × 3 days (for HIV, see p. 335)	
Cryptosporidiosis	Cryptosporidia	Nitazoxanide 500 mg (PO) q12h × 3 days (for HIV, see p. 334)	
Balantidiasis	Balantidium coli	Doxycycline 100 mg (PO) q12h × 10 days	Iodoquinol 650 mg (PO) q8h × 20 days **or** Metronidazole 750 mg (PO) q8h × 5 days

Amebiasis (Entamoeba histolytica) (see p. 91)

Giardiasis (Giardia lamblia) (see p. 90)

Isosporiasis (Isospora belli)
Clinical Presentation: Acute/subacute onset of diarrhea. Isospora belli is the only protozoa to cause diarrhea with eosinophils in stool.
Diagnostic Considerations: Diagnosis by demonstrating cysts in stool and organisms in intestinal biopsy specimen. Associated with HIV, immigration from Latin America, daycare centers, and mental institutions. If stool exam is negative, "string test"/duodenal aspirate and biopsy may be helpful.
Pitfalls: Difficult to eradicate; may last months. Multiple stool samples may be needed for diagnosis. Add folinic acid 10 mg (PO) q24 if pyrimethamine is used. In HIV, may need life-long suppressive therapy with TMP–SMX 1–2 DS tablet (PO) q24h (pp. 331–332, 335).
Prognosis: Related to adequacy of treatment/degree of immunosuppression.

Dientamoebiasis (Dientamoeba fragilis)
Clinical Presentation: Acute/subacute onset of diarrhea. No cyst stage. Lives only as trophozoite.
Diagnostic Considerations: Diagnosis by demonstrating trophozoites in stool/intestinal by trichrome stain. Mucus in diarrheal stools, not blood. May have abdominal pain. Diarrhea may last for months/years.
Pitfalls: Frequently associated with pinworm (Enterobius vermicularis) infection.
Prognosis: Related to adequacy of fluid replacement/underlying health of host.

Blastocystis (Blastocystis hominis)
Clinical Presentation: Acute/subacute onset of diarrhea.
Diagnostic Considerations: Diagnosis by demonstrating cysts and trophozoites in stool by trichrome stain. Trichrome stain reveals characteristic "halo" (slime capsule) in stool specimens.
Pitfalls: Uncommon GI pathogen. Consider as cause of diarrhea only after other pathogens excluded.
Prognosis: Related to adequacy of fluid replacement/underlying health of host.

Cyclospora (see p. 90; for HIV, see p. 335)

Cryptosporidiosis (see p. 90; for HIV, see p. 334)

Balantidiasis (Balantidium coli)

Clinical Presentation: Acute/subacute onset of diarrhea. Fecal WBCs only with mucosal invasion. Largest intestinal protozoa and only ciliated protozoa to infect humans.

Diagnostic Considerations: Diagnosis by demonstrating organism in stool/intestinal biopsy specimen. Identifying features include darkly staining "kidney shaped" nucleus and large size. Fulminant dysentery seen only in debilitated/compromised hosts.

Pitfalls: Stools not bloody. Diarrhea may be intermittent.

Prognosis: Related to adequacy of fluid replacement/underlying health of host.

Intestinal Nematodes (Roundworms)

Subset	Pathogens	Preferred Therapy	Alternate Therapy
Capillariasis	Capillaria (Aonchotheca) philippinensis	Mebendazole 200 mg (PO) q12h × 20 days	Albendazole 400 mg (PO) q24h × 10 days
Angiostrongyliasis (rodent lung/ intestinal worm)	Angiostrongylus cantonensis	Albendazole 400 mg (PO) q12h × 2–3 weeks **plus** corticosteroids	Mebendazole 200–400 mg (PO) q8h × 10 days
Hookworm	Necator americanus/ Ancylostoma duodenale	Albendazole 400 mg (PO) × 1 dose **or** Mebendazole 100 mg (PO) q12h × 3 days or 500 mg (PO) × 1 dose	Pyrantel pamoate 11 mg/kg (PO) q24h × 3 days (max. 1 gm/ day)
Strongyloidiasis	Strongyloides stercoralis	Ivermectin 200 mcg/kg (PO) q24h × 2 days **or** Thiabendazole 25 mg/kg (PO) q12h × 2 days (max. 3 gm/day)	Albendazole 400 mg (PO) q24h × 3 days
Ascariasis	Ascaris lumbricoides	Albendazole 400 mg (PO) × 1 dose **plus** Pyrantel pamoate 11 mg/kg (PO) q24h × 3 days (max. 1gm/ day) **or** Mebendazole 100 mg (PO) q12h × 3 days or 500 mg (PO) × 1 dose	Ivermectin 200 mcg/kg (PO) × 1 dose*
Trichostrongyliasis	Trichostrongylus orientalis	Pyrantel pamoate 11 mg/kg (PO) × 1 dose (max. 1 gm)	Albendazole 400 mg (PO) × 1 dose **or** Mebendazole 100 mg (PO) q12h × 3 days

*   Avoid in young children and pregnant adults.

Intestinal Nematodes (Roundworms) (cont'd)

Subset	Pathogens	Preferred Therapy	Alternate Therapy
Pinworm	Enterobius vermicularis	Pyrantel pamoate 11 mg/kg (PO) × 1 dose (max. 1 gm); repeat in 2 weeks **or** Albendazole 400 mg (PO) × 1 dose; repeat in 2 weeks	Ivermectin 200 mcg/kg (PO) × 1 dose **or** Mebendazole 100 mg (PO) × 1 dose; repeat in 2 weeks
Whipworm	Trichuris trichiura	Mebendazole 100 mg (PO) q12h × 3–7 days	Albendazole 400 mg (PO) q24h × 3 days **or** Ivermectin 200 mcg/kg (PO) q24h × 3 days

Capillariasis (Capillaria philippinensis)

Clinical Presentation: Intermittent voluminous watery diarrhea ± malabsorption. Fever is uncommon.

Diagnostic Considerations: Diagnosis by demonstrating ova or parasite in stools. Resembles Trichuris, but C. philippinensis ova are larger and have a "pitted shell" with prominent polar plugs. Peripheral eosinophilia is uncommon until after therapy.

Pitfalls: Serology is positive in 85%, but cross-reacts with other parasites.

Prognosis: Related to severity of malabsorption/extra-intestinal disease.

Angiostrongyliasis (A. cantonensis) Rodent Lung/Intestinal Worm

Clinical Presentation: Presents as appendicitis (worm resides and deposits eggs in arteries/arterioles around ileocecum/appendix).

Diagnostic Considerations: Diagnosis by demonstrating organism in biopsied/excised tissue. May involve proximal small bowel, liver, CNS. When in CNS, a cause of eosinophilic meningitis.

Pitfalls: Can present as RLQ mass/fever resembling regional enteritis (Crohn's disease), but with eosinophilia and leukocytosis.

Prognosis: Related to severity of malabsorption and extra-intestinal disease.

Hookworm (Necator americanus/Ancylostoma duodenale)

Clinical Presentation: Pruritic, vesicular eruptions at site of filariform larval entry ("ground itch"). Pulmonary symptoms and transient eosinophilia may occur during migratory phase to intestines. Later, abdominal pain, diarrhea, weight loss, hypoalbuminemia, and anemia develop.

Diagnostic Considerations: Diagnosis by demonstrating eggs in stools. Larvae rare in fresh stool specimens (eggs may hatch if stools allowed to stand too long prior to examination). N. americanus can ingest 0.3 ml of blood/worm/day, much greater than A. duodenale. Anemia may be severe with heavy infestation (up to 100 mL/day).

Pitfalls: Eggs in fresh stool, not rhabditiform larvae. Eggs in hyperinfection syndrome.

Prognosis: Related to severity of anemia/malabsorption.

Strongyloidiasis (Strongyloides stercoralis)

Clinical Presentation: Pruritic, papular, erythematous rash. Pulmonary symptoms (cough, asthma) may occur during lung migration phase. May develop Loeffler's syndrome (pulmonary infiltrates with eosinophilia) or ARDS in heavy infections. Intestinal phase associated with colicky abdominal pain, diarrhea, and malabsorption.

Diagnostic Considerations: Diagnosis by demonstrating larvae in stool specimens/duodenal fluid. Usually asymptomatic in normal hosts, but causes "hyperinfection syndrome" in compromised hosts. CNS strongyloides (part of hyperinfection syndrome) should suggest diagnosis of HIV in non-immunosuppressed patients. Diarrhea/abdominal pain mimics regional enteritis (Crohn's disease) or ulcerative colitis. Malabsorption is common and mimics tropical sprue. Anemia is usually mild.
Pitfalls: Usually rhabditiform larvae (not eggs) in stools.
Prognosis: Related to severity of malabsorption.

Ascariasis (Ascaris lumbricoides)

Clinical Presentation: Pulmonary symptoms (cough, asthma) may occur during larval lung migration phase. May develop Loeffler's syndrome (pulmonary infiltrates with eosinophilia), as with hookworm/Strongyloides. Intestinal symptoms develop late. Usually asymptomatic until intestinal/biliary obstruction occurs. Can obstruct the appendix/pancreatic duct.
Diagnostic Considerations: Diagnosis by demonstrating eggs in stool specimens. Abdominal ultrasound can detect obstruction from adult worms. Most infections are asymptomatic; symptoms are related to "worm burden"/ectopic migration. Each female worm may produce up to 250,000 eggs/day.
Pitfalls: Lung involvement (bronchospasm, bronchopneumonia, lung abscess) is prominent in HIV.
Prognosis: Related to worm burden/extra-intestinal organ invasion.

Trichostrongyliasis (Trichostrongylus orientalis)

Clinical Presentation: Mild intestinal symptoms with persistent eosinophilia.
Diagnostic Considerations: Diagnosis by demonstrating eggs in stool specimens. Most prevalent in the Middle East and Asia. Mild anemia. Eosinophilia is usually > 10%.
Pitfalls: Must differentiate eggs from hookworm, and rhabditiform larvae from Strongyloides. T. orientalis eggs have "pointed ends."
Prognosis: Related to extent of disease/underlying health of host.

Pinworm (Enterobius vermicularis)

Clinical Presentation: Primarily affects children. Perianal pruritus (ectopic migration) is the main symptom. Worm lives in the cecum, but patients do not have intestinal symptoms.
Diagnostic Considerations: Scotch tape of anus at night can be used to detect eggs left by migrating female worms (Scotch tape test).
Pitfalls: Abdominal pain and diarrhea should prompt search for Dientamoeba fragilis, since co-infection is common.
Prognosis: Excellent.

Whipworm (Trichuris trichiura)

Clinical Presentation: May present as "chronic appendicitis." Severe infestation may cause bloody diarrhea/abdominal pain ("Trichuris dysentery syndrome"), rectal prolapse.
Diagnostic Considerations: Diagnosis by demonstrating large eggs with bile-stained, triple-layered eggshell walls and doubly operculated transparent plugs. Most patients are asymptomatic or mildly anemic.
Pitfalls: Commonly co-exists with Ascaris, hookworm, or E. histolytica.
Prognosis: Related to severity/extent of dysentery. May need retreatment if heavy infection.

Intestinal Cestodes (Tapeworms)

Subset	Pathogens	Preferred Therapy	Alternate Therapy
Beef tapeworm	Taenia saginata	Praziquantel 5–10 mg/kg (PO) × 1 dose	Niclosamide 2 gm (PO) × 1 dose **or** Nitazoxanide 500 mg (PO) q12h × 3 days
Pork tapeworm	Taenia solium	Praziquantel 5–10 mg/kg (PO) × 1 dose	Niclosamide 2 gm (PO) × 1 dose **or** Nitazoxanide 500 mg (PO) q12h × 3 days
Dwarf tapeworm	Hymenolepis nana	Praziquantel 25 mg/kg (PO) × 1 dose	Nitazoxanide 500 mg (PO) q12h × 3 days **or** Niclosamide 2 gm (PO) × 1 dose, then 1.5 gm q24h × 6 days
Fish tapeworm	Diphyllobothrium latum	Praziquantel 10 mg/kg (PO) × 1 dose	Niclosamide 2 gm (PO) × 1 dose **or** Nitazoxanide 500 mg (PO) q12h × 3 days

Beef Tapeworm (Taenia saginata)/Pork Tapeworm (Taenia solium)

Clinical Presentation: Usually mild symptoms (weight loss, anemia), since most infections are caused by a single tapeworm.

Diagnostic Considerations: Diagnosis by demonstrating proglottids in stool. Taenia eggs in stool cannot be speciated; all are brown and spherical with a radially-striated inner shell. T. saginata may survive for 10 years, T. solium for 25 years.

Pitfalls: Severe cases may cause appendicitis, intestinal obstruction/perforation.

Prognosis: Related to severity of malabsorption/intestinal obstruction.

Dwarf Tapeworm (Hymenolepis nana)

Clinical Presentation: Usually asymptomatic.

Diagnostic Considerations: Diagnosis by demonstrating typical eggs in stool, with two shells enclosing inner oncosphere with hooklets. ELISA is positive in 85%, but cross-reacts with Taenia/Cysticercosis. GI symptoms develop with stool egg counts > 15,000/gm.

Pitfalls: Abdominal pain and diarrhea in heavy infestations.

Prognosis: Related to severity of malabsorption/underlying health of host.

Fish Tapeworm (Diphyllobothrium latum)

Clinical Presentation: Symptoms secondary to macrocytic anemia from vitamin B_{12} deficiency. Most infestations are asymptomatic.

Diagnostic Considerations: Diagnosis by demonstrating operculated eggs and proglottids in stool.

Pitfalls: Vitamin B$_{12}$ deficiency anemia requires prolonged infection (> 3 years).
Prognosis: Related to severity of B$_{12}$ deficiency anemia/underlying health of host.

Intestinal Trematodes (Flukes/Flatworms)

Subset	Pathogens	Preferred Therapy
Fasciolopsiasis	Fasciolopsis buski	Praziquantel 25 mg/kg (PO) q8h × 3 doses
Heterophyiasis	Heterophyes heterophyes Metagonimus yokogawai	Praziquantel 25 mg/kg (PO) q8h × 3 doses

Fasciolopsiasis (Fasciolopsis buski)
Clinical Presentation: Diarrhea with copious mucus in stool. Most cases are asymptomatic.
Diagnostic Considerations: Diagnosis by demonstrating eggs in stool. May have eosinophilia, low-grade fever ± malabsorption. Intestinal obstruction is the most serious complication.
Pitfalls: Mimics peptic ulcer disease with upper abdominal pain relieved by food.
Prognosis: Related to severity/extent of malabsorption/intestinal obstruction.

Heterophyiasis (Heterophyes heterophyes/Metagonimus yokogawai)
Clinical Presentation: Usually asymptomatic or mild intestinal symptoms. Embolization of eggs may result in myocarditis, myocardial fibrosis, or cerebral hemorrhage. Eosinophilia may be present.
Diagnostic Considerations: Diagnosis by demonstrating large operculated eggs in stool. Small intestine fluke.
Pitfalls: Difficult to differentiate from clonorchis sinensis.
Prognosis: Related to extent/severity of extra-intestinal dissemination to heart, lungs, CNS.

Other Intestinal Infections

Subset	Pathogen	Preferred Therapy
Whipple's disease	Tropheryma whippelii	Ceftriaxone 2 gm (IV) q24h × 2 weeks*
		or
		Penicillin G 6 mu (IV) q6h × 2 weeks **plus** Streptomycin 1 gm (IM) q24h × 2 weeks*
		or
		Ceftriaxone 1 gm (IV) q24h × 2 weeks **plus** Streptomycin 1 gm (IM) q24h × 2 weeks*

*   Follow with TMP–SMX 1 DS tablet (PO) q12h × 1 year or Doxycycline 100 mg (PO) q12h × 1 year.

Whipple's Disease (Tropheryma whippelii)
Clinical Presentation: Diarrhea, fever, encephalopathy/dementia, weight loss, polyarthritis, myocarditis, pericarditis, general lymphadenopathy ± malabsorption.
Diagnostic Considerations: Diagnosis by demonstrating organism by PAS staining macrophages in small bowel biopsy specimens.
Pitfalls: May present with dementia mimicking Alzheimer's disease, or FUO mimicking celiac disease or lymphoma. Optimum length of treatment is unknown. Relapses occur.
Prognosis: Related to severity/extent of extra-intestinal disease.

Parasites, Fungi, Unusual Organisms in Skin/Muscle

Infiltrative Skin/Subcutaneous Lesions

Subset	Pathogens	Preferred Therapy
Cutaneous leishmaniasis *Old World*	Leishmania major Leishmania tropica	Sodium stibogluconate 20 mg/kg (IV or IM) q24h × 20 days **or** Pentamidine 2–3 mg/kg (IM) q48h × 4–7 days **or**
New World	Leishmania mexicana Leishmania braziliensis	Lipid amphotericin 3 mg/kg (IV) q24h on days 1–5, 14, and 21 **or** Miltefosine 2.5 mg/kg (PO) q24h × 28 days (max. 150 mg/day)
Leprosy *Lepromatous*	Mycobacterium leprae	Dapsone 100 mg (PO) q24h × 1–2 years **plus** Clofazimine 50 mg (PO) q24h × 1–2 years **plus** Rifampin 600 mg (PO) monthly × 1–2 years
Non-lepromatous (tuberculoid)	Mycobacterium leprae	Dapsone 100 mg (PO) q24h × 6 months **plus** Rifampin 600 mg (PO) monthly × 6 months
Loa Loa (Loiasis)	L. loa	Diethylcarbamazine 2–3 mg/kg (PO) q8h × 2–3 weeks **or** Albendazole 200 mg (PO) q12h × 3 weeks
Erythrasma	Corynebacterium minutissimum	Erythromycin 250 mg (PO) q6h × 2 weeks

Cutaneous Leishmaniasis (Old World/New World)

Clinical Presentation: Variable presentation. Typically, a nodule develops then ulcerates, with a raised/erythematous outer border and a central area of granulation tissue. May be single or multiple. Usually non-pruritic/non-painful. Occurs weeks after travel to endemic areas (New World leishmaniasis: Latin America; Old World leishmaniasis: Central Asia).

Diagnostic Considerations: Diagnosis by demonstrating Leishmania amastigotes in biopsy specimen.

Pitfalls: Most skin lesions undergo spontaneous resolution. However, treatment is advisable for lesions caused by L. braziliensis or related species causing mucosal leishmaniasis.

Prognosis: Excellent.

Lepromatous Leprosy (Mycobacterium leprae)

Clinical Presentation: Diffuse, symmetrical, red or brown skin lesions presenting as macules, papules, plaques, or nodules. May also present as diffuse thickening of skin, especially involving ear lobes, face, and extremities. Loss of eyebrows/body hair may occur.

Diagnostic Considerations: Diagnosis by demonstrating organism in acid fast stain of tissue specimens. Afebrile bacteremia is frequent, and buffy coat smears positive for M. leprae. Erythema nodosum and polyclonal gammopathy on SPEP are common, and lepromin skin test/PPD are negative (anergic). When present, peripheral neuropathy is often symmetrical and acral in distribution.
Pitfalls: Differential diagnosis is large. Consider leprosy in patients with unexplained skin diseases.
Prognosis: Good if treated early.

Non-Lepromatous (Tuberculoid) Leprosy (Mycobacterium leprae)
Clinical Presentation: Small number of asymmetrical, hypopigmented skin lesions, which are often scaly with sharp borders and associated anesthesia. Asymmetric peripheral nerve trunk involvement is common.
Diagnostic Considerations: Diagnosis by demonstrating granulomas with few acid-fast bacilli. Differentiate from cutaneous leishmaniasis by skin biopsy. Lepromin skin test/PPD are positive and SPEP is normal (in contrast to lepromatous leprosy).
Pitfalls: Wide spectrum of presentations depending on immune status and duration of disease. Differential diagnosis is large. Consider leprosy in patients with unexplained skin diseases.
Prognosis: Good if treated early.

Erythrasma (Corynebacterium minutissimum)
Clinical Presentation: Reddened/raised skin lesions on face/trunk. Not hot or pruritic.
Diagnostic Considerations: Differentiated from Tinea versicolor by culture. C. minutissimum skin lesions fluoresce red under UV light.
Pitfalls: Resembles Tinea versicolor, but lesions primarily involve the face, not trunk.
Prognosis: Excellent.

Infiltrative Skin Lesions ± Ulcers/Sinus Tracts/Abscesses

Subset	Pathogens	Preferred Therapy
Cutaneous histoplasmosis	Histoplasma capsulatum	Treat as for disseminated histoplasmosis (p. 267) if part of systematic syndrome. If solely involves the skin, Itraconazole 200 mg (PO) q12h until resolution.
Cutaneous blastomycosis	Blastomyces dermatitidis	Treat the same as pulmonary infection (p. 267)
Cutaneous coccidioidomycosis	Coccidioides immitis	Treat the same as pulmonary infection (p. 268)
Cutaneous actinomycosis	Actinomyces israelii	Treat the same as pulmonary infection (p. 268)
Cutaneous nocardiosis	Nocardia sp.	Treat the same as pulmonary infection (p. 268)
Cutaneous amebiasis	Entamoeba histolytica	Treat the same as pulmonary infection (p. 265)

Infiltrative Skin Lesions ± Ulcers/Sinus Tracts/Abscesses (cont'd)

Subset	Pathogens	Preferred Therapy
Cutaneous mycobacteria *Scrofula*	Mycobacterium tuberculosis	Treat same as pulmonary TB. See p. 53
	M. scrofulaceum	Surgical excision is curative
M. haemophilum	M. haemophilum	Surgical excision/TMP–SMX 1 DS tablet (PO) q12h **or** Minocycline 100 mg (PO) q12h **or** quinolone (PO) until cured
M. chelonae	M. chelonae	Clarithromycin 500 mg (PO) q12h × 6 months
M. fortuitum	M. fortuitum	Minocycline 100 mg (PO) q12h × 6–12 months **or** Doxycycline 100 mg (PO) q12h × 6–12 months **plus** TMP–SMX 1 DS tablet (PO) q12h × 6–12 months
Swimming pool granuloma	M. marinum	Clarithromycin XL 1 gm (PO) q24h × 3 months **plus** Rifampin 600 mg (PO) q24h × 3 months **or** TMP–SMX 1 DS tablet (PO) q12h × 3 months **plus** Ethambutol 15 mg/kg (PO) q24h × 3 months **or** Doxycycline 100 mg (PO) q12h × 3 months
Buruli ulcer	M. ulcerans	TMP–SMX 1 DS tablet (PO) q12h **plus** Ethambutol 15 mg/kg (PO) q24h × 6 weeks
Cutaneous MAI	Mycobacterium avium-intracellulare	Ethambutol 15 mg/kg (PO) q24h **plus** Azithromycin 1200 mg (PO) weekly × 6 months

Cutaneous Histoplasmosis (Histoplasma capsulatum)
Clinical Presentation: Chronic, raised, verrucous lesions.
Diagnostic Considerations: Diagnosis by demonstrating organism by culture/tissue staining.
Pitfalls: Skin nodules represent disseminated histoplasmosis, not isolated skin infection. Look for histoplasmosis elsewhere (e.g., lung, liver, bone marrow). Skin nodules (± chronic pneumonia) with osteolytic bone lesions suggests. African histoplasmosis due to H. capsulation var. duboisii.
Prognosis: Related to extent of infection/degree of immunosuppression.

Cutaneous Blastomyces (Blastomyces dermatitidis)
Clinical Presentation: Painless, erythematous, well-circumscribed, hyperkeratotic, crusted nodules or plaques that enlarge over time. Some may ulcerate and leave an undermined edge.
Diagnostic Considerations: Diagnosis by demonstrating organism by culture/tissue staining. Blastomyces dermatitidis affects many organs.

Pitfalls: When found in skin, look for Blastomyces elsewhere (e.g., lungs, prostate).
Prognosis: Related to extent of infection/degree of immunosuppression.

Cutaneous Coccidioidomycosis (Coccidioides immitis)
Clinical Presentation: Skin lesions take many forms, including raised verrucous lesions, cold subcutaneous abscesses, indolent ulcers, or small papules.
Diagnostic Considerations: Diagnosis by demonstrating organism by culture/tissue staining.
Pitfalls: Skin nodules represent disseminated coccidioidomycosis, not isolated skin infection. Look for Coccidioides elsewhere (e.g., CNS, bone, lungs).
Prognosis: Related to extent of infection/degree of immunosuppression.

Cutaneous Actinomycosis (Actinomyces israelii)
Clinical Presentation: Erythematous, uneven, indurated, woody, hard, cervicofacial tumor. Localized single/multiple sinus tracts in chest wall, abdominal wall, or inguinal/pelvic area may be present.
Diagnostic Considerations: Diagnosis by demonstrating organism by culture/tissue staining.
Pitfalls: Look for underlying bone involvement.
Prognosis: Good with early/prolonged treatment.

Cutaneous Nocardia (Nocardia brasiliensis)
Clinical Presentation: Subcutaneous abscesses may rupture to form chronically draining fistulas.
Diagnostic Considerations: Diagnosis by demonstrating organism by culture/tissue staining. May present as "Madura foot."
Pitfalls: Look for underlying immunosuppressive disorder.
Prognosis: Related to extent of infection/degree of immunosuppression.

Cutaneous Amebiasis (Entamoeba histolytica)
Clinical Presentation: Ulcers with ragged edges, sinus tracts, amebomas, and strictures may develop around the anus/rectum or abdominal wall.
Diagnostic Considerations: Diagnosis by demonstrating organism by tissue staining.
Pitfalls: If abdominal sinus tract is present, look for underlying ameboma and evidence of infection in other organs (e.g., CNS, lung, liver).
Prognosis: Related to extent of infection/degree of organ damage.

Scrofula (Mycobacterium tuberculosis)
Clinical Presentation: Cold, chronic, anterior cervical adenopathy ± sinus tracts. Usually in children.
Diagnostic Considerations: Diagnosis by acid-fast stain and culture of node/drainage.
Pitfalls: Cured by antibiotic therapy alone. No need for surgical excision.
Prognosis: Excellent with treatment.

Scrofula (Mycobacterium scrofulaceum)
Clinical Presentation: Cold, chronic, anterior cervical adenopathy ± sinus tracts. Usually in adults.
Diagnostic Considerations: Diagnosis by acid-fast stain and culture of node/drainage.
Pitfalls: Highly resistant to anti-TB therapy.
Prognosis: Excellent with surgical excision.

Cutaneous Mycobacterium haemophilum

Clinical presentation: Particularly common in immunosuppressed/HIV patients, presents as multiple, painful cutaneous ulcers/abscesses ± draining fistulas.

Diagnostic Considerations: Diagnose by PCR, RT-PCR assay.

Pitfalls: Suspect M. haemophilum if drainage from ulcer/abscess is AFB smear + but fails to grow on AFB media. M. haemophilus grows only on AFB media supplemented with ferric containing compounds i.e., hemin, hemoglobin, or ferric ammonium citrate. Susceptible to minocycline, TMP–SMX, or quinolones, but most strains resistant to INH, EMB, RIF, PZA.

Prognosis: Good with surgical excision/prolonged treatment.

Cutaneous Mycobacterium chelonae

Clinical presentation: Present as cold abscesses with draining fistulas.

Diagnostic Considerations: AF culture of wound drainage.

Pitfalls: Some strains clarithromycin resistant. May be susceptible to quinolones, doxycycline, or minocycline.

Prognosis: Good with effective therapy.

Cutaneous Mycobacterium fortuitum

Clinical Presentation: Usually associated with chronic foreign body infection, especially infected breast implants. Associated with nail salon footbaths. Present as cold abscesses with draining fistulas.

Diagnostic Considerations: Diagnosis by demonstrating organism by acid fast smear are culture of drainage/infected prosthetic material.

Pitfalls: Highly resistant to anti-TB therapy, may be susceptible to quinolones or linezolid.

Prognosis: Good with surgical excision/prolonged treatment.

Swimming Pool Granuloma (Mycobacterium marinum)

Clinical Presentation: Begins as erythema with tenderness at inoculation site, followed by a papule or violaceous nodule that ulcerates and drains pus. May have sporotrichoid spread. Presents as a skin lesion unresponsive to antibiotics after abrasive water exposure (e.g., fish tank, swimming pool/lake).

Diagnostic Considerations: Diagnosis by demonstrating organism by acid-fast smear/culture.

Pitfalls: Resistant to INH/pyrazinamide. Surgical excision of isolated lesions may be needed.

Prognosis: Good with prolonged therapy.

Buruli Ulcer (Mycobacterium ulcerans)

Clinical Presentation: Begin as a firm, painless, movable, subcutaneous nodule. In 1–2 months, nodule becomes fluctuant, ulcerates, and develops an undermined edge. May have edema around lesion and in extremity (if involved).

Diagnostic Considerations: Diagnosis by acid-fast stain and culture of punch biopsy of ulcer rim. Patient is usually from Africa, but M. ulcerans also exists in Asia, Australia, and Central/South America.

Pitfalls: Steroids/skin grafting sometimes needed.

Prognosis: Good with surgical excision.

Cutaneous MAI (Mycobacterium avium-intracellulare)

Clinical Presentation: Nodules, abscesses, ulcers, plaques, ecthyma and draining sinuses can occur, but are uncommon in normal hosts and usually only seen in immunosuppressed patients.

Diagnostic Considerations: Diagnosis by demonstrating organism by acid-fast staining and culture (for species identification) of tissue biopsy specimens.
Pitfalls: Usually represents disseminated infection. Look for non-cutaneous evidence of infection (e.g., lungs, bone marrow, liver/spleen).
Prognosis: Related to extent of organ damage/degree of immunosuppression.

Skin Vesicles/Bullae

Subset	Pathogens	Preferred Therapy
Herpes simplex	Herpes simplex virus (HSV)	See p. 142 (for HIV, see p. 340)
Herpes zoster	Varicella zoster virus (VZV)	See p. 142 (for HIV, see p. 319, 343)

Subcutaneous Serpiginous Lesions

Subset	Pathogens	Preferred Therapy
Cutaneous larva migrans (creeping eruption)	Ancylostoma braziliense	Ivermectin 200 mcg/kg (PO) × 1 dose **or** Albendazole 400 mg (PO) q24h × 3–7 days. Children may be treated topically with albendazole ointment (10%) q8h × 10 days
Guinea worm	Dracunculus medinensis	Surgical removal of worm near skin surface. Metronidazole 250 mg (PO) q8h × 10 days facilitates worm removal
Cutaneous gnathostomiasis	Gnathostoma spinigerum	Surgical removal **or** Albendazole 400 mg (PO) q12h × 3 weeks **or** Ivermectin 200 mcg/kg (PO) q24h × 2 days

Cutaneous Larva Migrans (Ancylostoma braziliense) Creeping Eruption
Clinical Presentation: Intensely pruritic, migratory, subcutaneous, raised serpiginous lesions.
Diagnostic Considerations: Diagnosis by clinical appearance.
Pitfalls: Must be differentiated from "swimmer's itch" caused by schistosomal cercariae.
Prognosis: Excellent with treatment.

Guinea Worm (Dracunculus medinensis)
Clinical Presentation: Serpiginous, raised, subcutaneous tract overlying worm.
Diagnostic Considerations: Diagnosis by demonstrating Dracunculus worm when surgically removed.
Pitfalls: Resembles cutaneous larva migrans, but worm is visible below the skin and lesions are serpiginous with Dracunculus. May be complicated by painful arthritis.
Prognosis: Excellent with treatment. Soaking extremity in warm water promotes emergence/removal of worm. Metronidazole can also be used to decrease inflammation and facilitate worm removal. Mebendazole 200–400 mg (PO) q12h × 6 days may kill worms directly.

Cutaneous Gnathostomiasis (Gnathostoma spinigerum)

Clinical Presentation: Painful, intermittent, subcutaneous swelling with local edema, intense pruritus, and leukocytosis with eosinophilia. Acquired by eating undercooked fish, frogs, and other intermediate larvae-containing hosts. May be complicated by eosinophilic meningitis.

Diagnostic Considerations: Diagnosis by demonstrating Gnathostoma in tissue specimens. Relatively common infection in Thailand and parts of Japan, South America, and Southeast Asia.

Prognosis: Good if limited to the skin and surgically removed. Poor with CNS involvement. Albendazole is preferred.

Skin Papules/Nodules/Abscesses

Subset	Pathogens	Preferred Therapy
Bacillary angiomatosis	Bartonella henselae Bartonella quintana	Doxycycline 100 mg (PO) q12h **or** azithromycin 250 mg (PO) q24h **or** any quinolone (PO) × 8 weeks
Cutaneous Alternaria	Alternaria alternata	Amphotericin B 0.7–1.0 mg/kg (IV) q24h × 2–3 grams‡ <u>Alternate therapy:</u> Voriconazole, itraconazole, posaconazole, caspofungin. (See Drug Summaries Chapter 11 for dosage.) Treat until cured.
Entomophthoromycosis	E. basidiobolus E. conidiobolus	Amphotericin B 0.7–1.0 mg/kg (IV) q24h × 1–2 grams‡ **or** TMP–SMX 1 DS tablet (PO) q24h until cured
Chromomycosis	Fonsecaea pedrosoi, compactum Phialophora verrucosa, others	<u>Few small lesions:</u> Wide/deep surgical excision or cryosurgery with liquid nitrogen <u>Larger lesions:</u> Itraconazole 200 mg (PO) solution q24h until lesions regress ± cryosurgery
Cutaneous Fusarium	Fusarium solani	Amphotericin B 0.7–1.0 mg/kg (IV) q24h × 2–3 grams‡ **or** Voriconazole (see "usual dose," p. 714)
Cutaneous Penicillium	Penicillium marneffei	Amphotericin B 0.6 mg/kg (IV) q24h × 14 days,‡ then Itraconazole 200 mg (IV) q12 × 2 days followed by 200 mg (PO) q12h × 10 weeks. For HIV, continue with Itraconazole 200 mg (PO) q24h indefinitely
Cutaneous Prototheca	Prototheca wikermanii	Surgical excision. If excision is incomplete, add either Amphotericin B 0.7–1.0 mg/kg (IV) q24h × 2–3 grams‡ **or** Itraconazole 200 mg (PO)† q12h until cured
Trichosporon	Trichosporon beigelii	Amphotericin B 0.7–1.0 mg/kg (IV) q24h × 2–3 grams‡

‡ Liposomal amphotericin (p. 525) may be a suitable alternative.

† Initiate therapy with Itraconazole 200 mg (IV) q12h × 7–14 days.

Skin Papules/Nodules/Abscesses (cont'd)

Subset	Pathogens	Preferred Therapy
Cutaneous aspergillosis	Aspergillus sp.	Voriconazole (see "usual dose," p. 714) **or** Itraconazole 200 mg (IV) q12h × 7–14 days, then 200 mg (PO) solution q12h until cured
Cutaneous zygomycosis (mucormycosis)	Mucor/Rhizopus/Absidia	Treat as for pulmonary zygomycosis (see p. 269)
Cutaneous coccidioido-mycosis	Coccidioides immitis	Fluconazole 800 mg (PO) × 1 dose, then 400 mg (PO) q24h until cured **or** Itraconazole 200 mg (PO)† q12h until cured <u>Alternate therapy</u> Amphotericin B 1 mg/kg (IV) q24h × 7 days, then 0.8 mg/kg (IV) q48h × 2–3 grams total dose‡
Cutaneous histoplasmosis	Histoplasma capsulatum	See p. 284
Cutaneous cryptococcosis	Cryptococcus neoformans	Amphotericin B 0.5 mg/kg (IV) q24h × 1–2 grams‡ **or** Lipid amphotericin (p. 525) (IV) q24h × 3 weeks, **then** Fluconazole 800 mg (PO) × 1 dose, then 400 mg (PO) q24h × 8–10 weeks
Cutaneous sporotrichosis	Sporothrix schenckii	Itraconazole 200 mg (PO). If HIV, chronic suppressive therapy may be needed q24h until 2–4 weeks after all lesions have resolved (typically 3–6 months in total).
Nodular/pustular candidiasis	Candida sp.	If occurs in moist skin areas (under breasts, groin, etc.), therapy is for mucocutaneous candidiasis (see p. 147). Nodular candidiasis occuring in non-moist skin areas in compromised hosts is a manifestation of disseminated disease and should be treated as such (see p. 148–149)
Cutaneous onchocerciasis	Onchocerca volvulus	Ivermectin 150 mcg/kg (PO) × 1 dose, repeated q12 months until asymptomatic **plus** Doxycycline 100 mg (PO) q12h × 6 weeks

† Initiate therapy with Itraconazole 200 mg (IV) q12h × 7–14 days.
‡ Lipid amphotericin (p. 525) may be a suitable alternative.

Bacillary Angiomatosis (Bartonella henselae/quintana) Peliosis Hepatis

Clinical Presentation: Skin lesions resemble Kaposi's sarcoma. Liver lesions resemble CMV hepatitis in HIV patients.

Diagnostic Considerations: Diagnosis by demonstrating organism by stain/culture of skin lesions or by blood culture after lysis-centrifugation.

Pitfalls: Requires life-long suppressive therapy.

Prognosis: Related to extent of infection/degree of immunosuppression.

Cutaneous Alternaria (Alternaria alternata)

Clinical Presentation: Bluish/purple papules that are often painful and non-pruritic. Usually seen only in leukopenic compromised hosts.

Diagnostic Considerations: Diagnosis by demonstrating organism by stain/culture in tissue specimen.

Pitfalls: Skin lesions usually represent disseminated disease in compromised hosts, not local infection. Fluconazole and micafungin ineffective.

Prognosis: Poor and related to degree of immunosuppression.

Cutaneous Entomophthoromycosis (E. basidiobolus / E. conidiobolus)

Clinical Presentation: E. conidiobolus infection presents as swelling of nose, paranasal tissues and mouth, accompanied by nasal stuffiness, drainage, and sinus pain. Begins as swelling of inferior nasal turbinates and extends until generalized facial swelling occurs. Subcutaneous nodules can be palpated in tissue. E. basidiobolus infection presents as a non-painful, firm, slowly progressive, subcutaneous nodule of the trunk, arms, legs, or buttocks.

Diagnostic Considerations: Diagnosis by demonstrating organism by stain/culture in tissue specimen. Skin lesions usually represent disseminated disease in compromised hosts, not localized infection.

Pitfalls: Unlike Mucor, E. basidiobolus does not usually invade blood vessels, although tissue infarction/necrosis is occasionally seen in diabetics and immunocompromised patients.

Prognosis: May spontaneously resolve. Surgical removal of accessible nodules and reconstructive surgery may be helpful for disfigurement.

Cutaneous Chromomycosis (F. pedrosoi/compactum, P. verrucosa, others)

Clinical Presentation: Warty papule/nodule that enlarges slowly to form a scarred, verrucous plaque. May also begin as a pustule, plaque, or ulcer. Over time, typical papule/nodule ulcerates, and the center becomes dry/crusted with raised margins. Lesions can be pedunculated/cauliflower-like.

Diagnostic Considerations: Diagnosis by demonstrating organism by stain/culture in tissue specimen. Chromomycosis remains localized within cutaneous/subcutaneous tissues.

Pitfalls: May resemble other fungal diseases. Sclerotic bodies in tissue and exudate distinguish chromomycosis from other related fugal diseases.

Prognosis: Related to degree of organ damage.

Cutaneous Fusarium (Fusarium solani)

Clinical Presentation: Presents in compromised hosts as multiple papules or painful nodules, initially macular with central pallor, which then become raised, erythematous, and necrotic. Seen mostly in leukopenic compromised hosts (especially acute leukemia and bone marrow transplants). Also a cause of mycetoma/onychomycosis.

Diagnostic Considerations: Diagnosis by demonstrating organism by stain/culture from blood/tissue.

Pitfalls: Skin lesions usually represent disseminated disease, not localized infection.

Prognosis: Poor/fair. Related to degree of immunosuppression. Amphotericin B lipid formulation (p. 525), colony-stimulating granulocyte factor, and granulocyte transfusions may be useful.

Cutaneous Penicillium (Penicillium marneffei)

Clinical Presentation: Papules, pustules, nodules, ulcers, or abscesses. Mostly seen in HIV (requires life-long suppressive therapy with itraconazole).

Diagnostic Considerations: Diagnosis by demonstrating organism by stain/culture in tissue specimen. Affects residents/visitors of Southeast Asia/Southern China.

Pitfalls: Lesions commonly become umbilicated and resemble molluscum contagiosum. May present as disseminated infection.

Prognosis: Poor and related to degree of immunosuppression.

Cutaneous Prototheca (Prototheca wickermanii)

Clinical Presentation: Most common presentation is a single plaque or papulonodular lesion of the skin or subcutaneous tissue. Lesions are usually painless, slowly progressive (enlarge over weeks to months without healing), well-circumscribed, and may become eczematoid/ulcerated.

Diagnostic Considerations: Diagnosis by demonstrating organism by stain/culture in tissue specimen. Skin lesions in HIV are not different from normal hosts.

Pitfalls: Lesions are usually painless and may resemble eczema.

Prognosis: Poor/fair. Related to degree of immunosuppression. Surgical excision has been successful.

Cutaneous Trichosporon (Trichosporon beigelii)

Clinical Presentation: Seen mostly in leukopenic compromised hosts (especially in acute leukemia, but also in HIV, burn wounds, and organ transplants). Usually presents as multiple red-bluish/purple papules, which are often painful and non-pruritic.

Diagnostic Considerations: Diagnosis by demonstrating organism by stain/culture in tissue specimen.

Pitfalls: Skin lesions usually represent disseminated disease, not localized infection.

Prognosis: Related to extent of infection/degree of immunosuppression.

Cutaneous Aspergillosis (Aspergillus fumigatus)

Clinical Presentation: Seen at site of IV catheter insertion or adhesive dressing applied to skin in leukopenic, compromised hosts. Lesion is similar to pyoderma gangrenosum. May also invade burn wounds and cause rapidly progressive necrotic lesions.

Diagnostic Considerations: Diagnosis by demonstrating organism by stain/culture in tissue specimen.

Pitfalls: Infiltrative/ulcerative skin lesions usually represent disseminated disease in compromised hosts, not localized infection. May cause invasive dermatitis/skin lesions in HIV.

Prognosis: Related to extent of infection/degree of immunosuppression.

Cutaneous Mucormycosis/Rhizopus/Absidia

Clinical Presentation: Necrotic skin lesion secondary to vascular invasion. Involves epidermis and dermis. Black eschars are evident.

Diagnostic Considerations: Diagnosis by demonstrating broad, non-septate hyphae with branches at right angles by stain/culture in tissue specimen.
Pitfalls: Skin lesions usually represent disseminated disease in compromised hosts, not localized infection. Contaminated elastic bandages have been associated with cutaneous Mucor.
Prognosis: Related to extent of infection/degree of immunosuppression.

Cutaneous Coccidioidomycosis (Coccidioides immitis)
Clinical Presentation: Skin lesions may take many forms, including verrucous granulomas, cold subcutaneous abscesses, indolent ulcers, or small papules.
Diagnostic Considerations: Diagnosis by demonstrating organism by stain/culture in tissue specimen.
Pitfalls: Skin lesions usually represent disseminated disease in compromised hosts, not local infection.
Prognosis: Related to extent of infection/degree of immunosuppression.

Cutaneous Histoplasmosis (Histoplasma capsulatum)
Clinical Presentation: Common cutaneous findings include maculopapular eruption, petechiae, and ecchymosis. Histopathology reveals necrosis around superficial dermal vessels.
Diagnostic Considerations: Diagnosis by demonstrating organism by stain/culture in tissue specimen.
Pitfalls: Skin lesions usually represent disseminated disease in compromised hosts, not local infection.
Prognosis: Related to extent of infection/degree of immunosuppression.

Cutaneous Cryptococcosis (Cryptococcus neoformans)
Clinical Presentation: May present as single or multiple papules, pustules, erythematous indurated plaques, soft subcutaneous masses, draining sinus tracts, or ulcers with undermined edges.
Diagnostic Considerations: Diagnosis by demonstrating spherules with endospores by stain/culture in tissue specimen.
Pitfalls: Skin lesions usually represent disseminated disease in compromised hosts, not localized infection. In AIDS patients, umbilicated papules resemble molluscum contagiosum. In organ transplants, cellulitis with necrotizing vasculitis may occur.
Prognosis: Related to extent of infection/degree of immunosuppression.

Cutaneous Sporotrichosis (Sporothrix schenckii)
Clinical Presentation: Primary cutaneous lymphatic sporotrichosis starts as a small, firm, movable, subcutaneous nodule, which then becomes soft and breaks down to form a persistent, friable ulcer. Secondary lesions usually develop proximally along lymphatic channels, but do not involve lymph nodes. Plaque form does not spread locally.
Diagnostic Considerations: Diagnosis by demonstrating organism by stain/culture in tissue specimen. Cutaneous disease arises at sites of minor trauma with inoculation of fungus into skin. Skin lesions usually represent disseminated disease in compromised hosts, not localized infection.
Pitfalls: HIV patients with $CD_4 < 200$ may have widespread lymphocutaneous disease that ulcerates and is associated with arthritis. Unusual in axilla due to increased temperature.
Prognosis: Related to extent of infection/degree of immunosuppression.

Nodular/Pustular Candidiasis (sepsis in chronic steroids, see p. 158)

Cutaneous Onchocerciasis (Onchocerca volvulus)

Clinical Presentation: Early manifestation is pruritic, papular rash with altered pigmentation. Later, papules, scaling, edema, and depigmentation may develop. Nodules develop in deep dermis/subcutaneous tissue (especially over bony prominences) or in deeper sites near joints, muscles, bones. Endemic in Middle East, Central Africa, Central America.

Diagnostic Considerations: Diagnosis by serology/demonstration of microfilaria in thin snips of involved skin or in anterior chamber (by slit lamp) if eye involvement. Intradermal edema produces "peau d'orange" effect with pitting around hair follicles/sebaceous glands.

Pitfalls: Ivermectin is effective against microfilaria, not adult worms. Adults live ~ 18 years.

Prognosis: Related to location/extent of organ damage.

Rickettsia (Fever/Petechial Skin Rash)

Subset	Pathogens	Preferred Therapy	Alternate Therapy
Rocky Mountain spotted fever (RMSF)	Rickettsia rickettsii (tick borne)	Doxycycline 200 mg (IV or PO) q12h × 3 days, then 100 mg (IV or PO) × 4 days	Any quinolone (IV or PO) × 7 days **or** Chloramphenicol 500 mg (IV or PO) q6h × 7 days
Epidemic (louse-borne) typhus, flying squirrel typhus	Rickettsia prowazekii	Same as RMSF	Same as RMSF
Murine (flea-borne) typhus	Rickettsia typhi	Same as RMSF	Same as RMSF
Scrub (chigger/mite-borne) typhus (Tsutsugamushi fever)	Rickettsia tsutsugamushi	Same as RMSF, **or** in mild cases Azithromycin 500 mg (PO) × 1 dose	Rifampin 600–900 mg (PO) q24h × 7 days
Rickettsialpox	Rickettsia akari	Same as RMSF	Same as RMSF
Tick typhus fevers (Mediterranean spotted fever, Boutonneuse fever, Israeli spotted fever)	Rickettsia conorii Rickettsia parkeri	Same as RMSF	Same as RMSF
African tick bite fever	Rickettsia africae	Same as RMSF	Same as RMSF

Rocky Mountain Spotted Fever (Rickettsia rickettsia) RMSF

Clinical Presentation: Fever with relative bradycardia, severe frontal headache, severe myalgias of abdomen/back/legs 3–12 days after tick bite. Rash begins as erythematous macules on wrists and ankles 3–5 days after tick bite, and progresses to petechiae/palpable purpura with confluent areas of ecchymosis. Periorbital edema, conjunctival suffusion, acute deafness, and edema of the dorsum of the hands/feet are important early signs. Abdominal pain can mimic acute abdomen, and meningismus and headache can mimic meningitis. Hepatosplenomegaly, cough, and coma may develop late. Laboratory findings include normal leukocyte count, thrombocytopenia, ↑ LFTs, and pre-renal azotemia. Hypotension/shock may occur secondary to myocarditis, which is the most common causes of death. Primary vector in United States is the Dermacentor tick; primary animal reservoir is small wild animals.

Diagnosis: Primarily a clinical diagnosis requiring a high index of suspicion and early empiric therapy. Early/rapid diagnosis can be made by DFA of biopsy specimen of rash (Weil-Felix reactions: OX-19: + + +, OX-2: +, OX-K: −). Specific R. rickettsii IFA, complement fixation, ELISA antibody titers are confirmatory. Include RMSF in differential diagnosis of any patient with fever and potential tick exposure, especially during the summer months.

Pitfalls: Most cases occur in eastern and southeastern United States, not Rocky Mountain area. Many cases go unrecognized due to nonspecific early findings. Early antibiotic therapy may blunt/ eliminate serologic response. Patients with signs/symptoms of RMSF but without a rash should be considered as having ehrlichiosis ("spotless RMSF") until proven otherwise. Early therapy is essential; begin empiric therapy as soon as RMSF is suspected. Other adjunctive measures may be required.

Prognosis: Late (after day 5) initiation of treatment increases the risk of death by 5-fold. Adverse prognostic factors include myocarditis and severe encephalitis.

Epidemic (Louse-Borne) Typhus (Rickettsia prowazekii)

Clinical Presentation: High fever with relative bradycardia, chills, headache, conjunctival suffusion, and myalgias. A macular, rubella-like, truncal rash develops in most on the fifth febrile day, which may become petechial and involve the extremities, but spares the palms/soles. Facial swelling/flushing occurs at end of first week, along with CNS symptoms (e.g., tinnitus, vertigo, delirium) and GI complaints (diarrhea, constipation, nausea, vomiting, abdominal pain). Hypotension, pneumonia, renal failure, gangrene, cerebral infarction may develop late. Laboratory findings include normal leukocyte count, thrombocytopenia, and ↑ serum creatinine/LFTs. Primary vector is the human body louse; primary reservoir is humans.

Diagnosis: Primarily a clinical diagnosis requiring a high index of suspicion and early empiric therapy (Weil-Felix reactions: OX-19: + + +, OX-2: +, OX-K: −). Specific R. prowazekii antibody titers are confirmatory. Consider epidemic (louse-borne) typhus in febrile impoverished persons infested with lice, especially in Africa and parts of Latin America. Rarely seen in the United States. Milder recrudescent form (Brill-Zinsser disease) is also rare.

Pitfalls: Many cases go unrecognized due to nonspecific early findings. Early therapy is essential.

Prognosis: Gangrene of nose, ear lobes, genitalia, toes, and fingers may develop in severe cases. Death occurs in 10–50% of untreated patients.

Murine (Flea-Borne) Typhus (Rickettsia typhi)

Clinical Presentation: Similar to epidemic typhus but less severe, with fever in most, and head-ache, myalgias, and a macular rash in half. Laboratory findings include a normal leukocyte count, mild thrombocytopenia, and mildly ↑ LFTs. Primary vector is the Asian rat flea (Xenopsylla cheopis); primary reservoir is the commensal rat (Rattus genus). Uncommon in United States; most cases from Texas, California, Florida, Hawaii.

Diagnosis: Primarily a clinical diagnosis requiring a high index of suspicion. More common during summer and fall (Weil-Felix reactions: OX-19: + + +, OX-2: +, OX-K: −). Specific R. typhi antibody titers are confirmatory.

Pitfalls: Many cases go unrecognized due to nonspecific findings. Rash becomes maculopapular, compared to epidemic typhus, which remains macular. A similar illness is caused by R. felis.

Prognosis: Good if treated early. Death occurs in < 1%.

Scrub Typhus (Rickettsia tsutsugamushi) Tsutsugamushi Fever

Clinical Presentation: Fever, chills, headache, myalgias, arthralgias, GI symptoms, other nonspecific complaints. Eschar at mite bite site (tache noire) ± regional adenopathy. A macular, truncal rash develops in most, usually in the first week, and may progress to involve the extremities and face, but spares the palms/soles. Vasculitis may lead to cardiopulmonary, CNS, hematologic abnormalities during the second week. Hepatosplenomegaly is common. Primary vector/reservoir is the larval (chigger) trombiculid mite. Endemic areas include northern Australia, southeastern Asia, Indian subcontinent.

Diagnosis: Presumptive diagnosis is clinical (Weil-Felix reactions: OX-19: −, OX-2: −, OX-K: + + +). Specific R. tsutsugamushi serology is confirmatory.

Pitfalls: Incomplete therapy frequently results in relapse.

Prognosis: Excellent if treated early.

Rickettsialpox (Rickettsia akari)

Clinical Presentation: Milder illness than other rickettsioses, with initial eschar at bite site, high fever, and generalized rash (usually erythematous papules which become vesicular and spares the palms/soles). Fever peak is usually < 104°F, occurs 1–3 weeks after mite bite, and lasts ~ 1 week without therapy. Headache, photophobia, marked diaphoresis, sore throat, GI complaints (nausea/vomiting following initial headache) may occur. Most labs are normal, although leukopenia may be present. Primary vector is the mouse mite; primary animal reservoir is the house mouse. Rare in the United States.

Diagnosis: Presumptive diagnosis by clinical presentation (Weil-Felix reactions: OX-19: −, OX-2: −, OX-K: ±). Specific R. akari serology is confirmatory.

Pitfalls: Do not confuse with African tick-bite fever, which may also have a vesicular rash.

Prognosis: Excellent even without therapy.

Tick Typhus Fevers (Rickettsia conorii, Rickettsia parkeri) Mediterranean Spotted Fever, Boutonneuse Fever, Israeli Fever

Clinical Presentation: Similar to RMSF with fever, chills, myalgias, but less severe. Unlike RMSF, an eschar is usually present at the site of the tick bite ± regional adenopathy. Leukocyte count is normal and thrombocytopenia is common. Transmitted by the brown dog tick, Rhipicephalus sanguineus.

Diagnosis: Presumptive diagnosis by clinical presentation (Weil-Felix reactions: OX-19: +, OX-2: +, OX-K: +). Specific R. conorii serology is confirmatory.

Pitfalls: Suspect in travelers from endemic areas with a RMSF-like illness. Consider different diagnosis in absence of an eschar.

Prognosis: Good with early treatment. Prostration may be prolonged even with proper therapy.

African Tick Bite Fever (Rickettsia africae)

Clinical Presentation: Similar to murine typhus with fever, chills, myalgias, but regional adenopathy and multiple eschars are common. Incubation period ~ 6 days. Amblyomma hebreum/variegatum tick vectors frequently bite humans multiple times.

Diagnosis: Presumptive diagnosis by clinical presentation (Weil-Felix reactions: OX-19: +, OX-2: +, OX-K: +). Specific R. africae serology is confirmatory.

Pitfalls: Rash is transient, and may be vesicular or absent.

Prognosis: Good even without therapy; excellent with therapy.

Other Skin Lesions

Subset	Pathogens	Topical Therapy	PO Therapy
Tinea versicolor (pityriasis)	Malassezia furfur (Pityrosporum orbiculare)	Clotrimazole cream (1%) or miconazole cream (2%) **or** Ketoconazole cream (2%) daily × 7 days	Ketoconazole 200 mg (PO) q24h × 7 days **or** Itraconazole 200 mg (PO) q24h × 7 days **or** Fluconazole 400 mg (PO) × 1 dose
Eosinophilic folliculitis	Malassezia furfur (Pityrosporum orbiculare)	<u>Preferred Therapy</u> Ketoconazole cream (2%) topically × 2–3 weeks ± Ketoconazole 200 mg (PO) q24h × 2–3 weeks	

Tinea Versicolor/Pityriasis (Malassezia furfur)

Clinical Presentation: Hyper- or hypopigmented scaling papules (0.5–1 cm), which may coalesce into larger plaques. Most commonly affects the upper trunk and arms. May be asymptomatic or pruritic.

Diagnostic Considerations: M. furfur also causes eosinophilic folliculitis in HIV, and catheter-acquired sepsis mostly in neonates or immunosuppressed patients. Diagnosis is clinical.

Pitfalls: Skin pigmentation may take months to return to normal after adequate therapy.

Prognosis: Excellent.

Eosinophilic Folliculitis (Malassezia furfur)

Clinical Presentation: Intensely pruritic folliculitis, usually on lower extremities.

Diagnostic Considerations: Tissue biopsy shows eosinophilic folliculitis. Diagnosis by demonstrating organism by culture on Sabouraud's agar overlaid with olive oil.

Pitfalls: Resembles folliculitis, but lesions are concentrated on lower extremities (not on trunk as with cutaneous candidiasis).

Prognosis: Related to degree of immunosuppression. Use oral therapy if topical therapy fails.

Myositis

Subset	Pathogens	Preferred Therapy
Chromomycosis	Cladosporium/Fonsecaea	Itraconazole 200 mg (PO) q24h until cured **or** Terbinafine 250 mg (PO) q24h until cured
Trichinosis	Trichinella spiralis	Albendazole 400 mg (PO) q12h × 8–14 days **or** Mebendazole 200–400 mg (PO) q8h × 3 days, then 400–500 mg q8h × 10 days

Chromomycosis (Cladosporium/Fonsecaea)

Clinical Presentation: Subcutaneous/soft tissue nodules or verrucous lesions.

Diagnostic Considerations: Diagnosis by demonstrating organism by culture/tissue biopsy specimen.

Pitfalls: May resemble Madura foot or cause ulcerative lesions in muscle.

Prognosis: Related to degree of immunosuppression.

Trichinosis (Trichinella spiralis)

Clinical Presentation: Muscle tenderness, low-grade fevers, peripheral eosinophilia, conjunctival suffusion.

Diagnostic Considerations: Diagnosis by Trichinella serology or by demonstrating larvae in muscle biopsy.

Pitfalls: ESR is very low (near zero), unlike other causes of myositis, which have elevated ESRs.

Prognosis: Excellent with early treatment. Short-term steroids may be useful during acute phase. Therapy is ineffective against calcified larvae in muscle.

REFERENCES AND SUGGESTED READINGS

Adjei GO, Goka BQ, Kurtzhals AL. Neurotoxicity of Artemisinin Derivatives. Clin Infect Dis 43:1616–17, 2006.

Alexander BD, Pfaller MA. Contemporary Tools for the Diagnosis and Management of Invasive Mycoses. Clin Infect Dis 43:S15–S27, 2006.

Ansart S, Perez L, Vergely O, et al. Illnesses in travelers returning from the tropics: a prospective study of 622 patients. J Travel Med 12:312–18, 2005.

Avulunov A, Klaus S, Vardy D. Fluconazole for the treatment of cutaneous leishmaniasis. N Engl J Med 347:370–1, 2002.

Ayeh-Kumi PF, Petri Jr. WA. Amebiasis: An Update on Diagnosis and Treatment. Infections in Medicine 23:301–10, 2006.

Bisser S, N'Siesi FX, Lejon V, et al. Equivalence trial of melarsoprol and nifurtimox monotherapy and combination

therapy for the treatment of second-stage Trypanosoma brucei gambiense sleeping sickness J Infect Dis 195:322–9, 2007.

Chayakulkeeree M, Ghannoum MA, Perfect JR. Zygomycosis: the re-emerging fungal infection. Clin Infect Dis 25:215–229, 2006.

Chen XM, Keithly JS, Paya CV, et al. Cryptosporidiosis. N Engl J Med 346:1723–1731, 2002.

Cheng AC, Currie BJ. Melioidosis: epidemiology, pathophysiology, and management. Clin Microbiol Rev 18:383–16, 2005.

Cisneros Herreros JM, Cordero Matia E. Therapeutic armamentarium against systemic fungal infections. Clin Microbiol and Infection 12:S53–64, 2006.

Croft SL, Yardley V. Chemotherapy of leishmaniasis. Curr Pharm Des 8:319–42, 2002.

Cunha BA. Malaria vs. Typhoid Fever: A Diagnostic Dilemma? Am J Med 118:1442–43, 2005.

DeGroote MA, Huitt G. Infections Due to Rapidly Growing Mycobacteria. Clin Infect Dis 42:1756–63, 2006.

Galgiani JN, Ampel NM, Blair JE, Catanzaro A, et al. Coccidioidomycosis. Clin Infect Dis 41: 1217–23, 2005.

Griffith, KS; Lewis, LS; Mali, S; Parise, ME. Treatment of Malaria in the United States. JAMA 297:2264–2277, 2007.

Haque R, Huston CD, Hughes M et al. Amebiasis. N Engl J Med 348:1565–73, 2003.

Herbrecht R, Natarajan A, Letscher-Bru V, et al. Invasive pulmonary aspergillosis. Semin Respir Crit Care Med 25:191–202, 2004.

International Artemisinin Study Group. Artesunate combinations for treatment of malaria: meta-analysis. Lancet 363:9–17, 2004.

Kremsner PG, Krishna S. Antimalarial combinations. Lancet 364:285–94, 2004.

Montoya JG, Liesenfeld O. Toxoplasmosis. Lancet 363: 1965–76, 2004.

Munoz P, Guinea J, Bouza E. Update on invasive aspergillosis: clinical and diagnostic aspects. Clin Microbiol and Infection 12:S24–39, 2006.

Murray HW. Treatment of visceral leishmaniasis in 2004. Am J Trop Med Hyg 71:787–94, 2004.

Mushatt DM, Mihm LB, Dreisbach AW, et al. Antibiotic Dosing in Slow Extended Daily Dialysis. Clin Infect Dis 49:433–437, 2009.

Olliaro PL, Guerin PJ, Gerstl S, et al. Treatment options for visceral leishmaniasis: a systematic review of clinical studies done in India, 1980–2004. Lancet Infect Dis 5:763–4, 2005.

Ouellette M, Drummelsmith J, Papadopoulou B. Leishmaniasis: drugs in the clinic, resistance and new developments. Drug Resist Updat 7:257–66, 2004.

Perea S, Patterson TF. Invasive Aspergillus infections in hematologic malignancy patients. Semin Respir Infect 17:99–105, 2002.

Pirisi M, Salvador E, Bisoffi Z, et al. Unsuspected strongyloidiasis in hospitalized elderly patients with and without eosinophilia. Clin Microbiol Infect 12:787–92, 2006.

Priotto G, Kasparian S, Mutombo W, et al. Nifurtimox-eflornithine combination therapy for second-stage African Trypanosoma brucei gambiense trypanosomiasis: a multicentre, randomized, phase III, noninferiority trial. Lancet 374:56–64, 2009.

Ross AGP, Bartley PB, Sleigh AC, et al. Schistosomiasis. N Engl J Med 346:1212–1220, 2002.

Segal BH, WalshTJ.Current Approaches to Diagnosis and Treatment of Invasive Aspergillosis.Am J Respir Crit Care Med 173:707–17, 2006.

Sinha PK, Ranjan A, Singh VP, Das VNR, et al. Visceral leishmaniasis (kala-azar)—the Bihar (India) perspective. Journal of Infection 53:60–64, 2006.

Sobel JD.Combination therapy for invasive mycosis: evaluation of past clinical trial designs. Clin Infect Dis 15; 39 Suppl 4:S224–7, 2004.

Soto J. Miltefosine for new world cutaneous leishmaniasis. Clin Infect Dis 38:1266–72, 2004.

Tortoli E. Clinical Manifestations of nontuberculous mycobacteria infections. Clin Microbiol Infect 15:906–910, 2009.

Udall DN.Recent Updates on Onchocerciasis: Diagnosis and Treatment. Clin Infect Dis 44:53–60, 2007.

Vardakas KZ, Michalopoulos A, Kiriakidou KG, et al. Candidaemia: Incidence, risk factors, characteristics and outcomes in immunocompetent critically ill patients. Clinical Microbiology and Infectious Diseases 15:286–295, 2009.

White AC. New Developments in the Management of Neurocysticercosis. J of Infectious Diseases 199: 1261–1262, 2009.

GUIDELINES

Chapman SW, Bradsher RW Jr, Campbell GD Jr, et al. Practice guidelines for the management of patients with blastomycosis. Infectious Diseases Society of America. Clin Infect Dis 30:679–83, 2000.

Galgiani JN, Ampel NM, Catanzaro A. et al. Practice guidelines for the treatment of coccidiomycosis. Infectious Diseases Society of America. Clin Infect Dis 30:658–61, 2000.

Hill DR, Ericsson CD, Pearson RD, Keystone JS, et al. The Practice of Travel Medicine: Guidelines by the Infectious Diseases Society of America. Clin Infect Dis 43: 1499–539, 2006.

Kauffman CA, Hajjeh R, Chapman SW.Practice guidelines for the management of patients with sporotrichosis. For the Mycoses Study Group.Infectious Diseases Society of America. Clin Infect Dis 30:684–7, 2000.

Pappas PG, Rex JH, Sobel JD, Filler SG, et al. Guidelines for the Treatment of Candidiasis. Clin Infect Dis 38: 161–89, 2004.

Perfect JR, Dismukes WE, Dromer F, et al. Clinical Practice Guidelines for the Management of Cryptococcal Disease: 2010 Update by the Infectious Disease Society of America. Clin Infect Disease 50:291–322, 2010.

Sobel JD. Practice guidelines for the treatment of fungal infections. For the Mycoses Study Group. Infectious Diseases Society of America. Clin Infect Dis 30:652, 2000.

Walsh TH, Anaissie EJ, Denning DW, et al. Treatment of Aspergillosis: Clinical Practice Guidelines of the Infectious Diseases Society of America. Clin Infect Dis 46: 327–60, 2008.

Wheat J, Sarosi G, McKinsey D, Hamill R, et al. Practice guidelines for the management of patients with histoplasmosis. Infectious Diseases Society of America. Clin Infect Dis 30:688–95, 2000.

Wormser GP, Dattwyler RJ, Shapiro ED, Halperin JJ, et al. The Clinical Assessment, Treatment, and Prevention of Lyme Disease, Human Granulocytic Anaplasmosis, and Babesiosis: Clinical Practice Guidelines by the Infectious Diseases Society of America. Clin Infect Dis 43:1089–134, 2006.

TEXTBOOKS

Anaissie EJ, McGinnis MR. Pfaller MA (eds). Clinical Mycology, 2nd Edition, Churchill Livingston, New York, 2009.

Arikan S Rex JH. Antifungal Drugs. In: Manual of Clinical Microbiology, 8th Edition, ASM Press, Washington, D.C., 2003.

Bottone EJ (ed). An Atlas of the Clinical Microbiology of Infectious Diseases, Volume 1. Bacterial Agents. The Parthenon Publishing Group, Boca Raton, 2004.

Bottone EJ (ed). An Atlas of the Clinical Microbiology of Infectious Diseases, Volume 2. Viral, fungal, and parasitic agents. Taylor and Francis, 2006.

Bryskier A (ed). Antimicrobial Agents. ASM Press, Washington, D.C., 2005.

Calderone RA (ed). Candida and Candidiasis. ASM Press, Washington D.C., 2002.

Cook GC (ed). Manson's Tropical Diseases, 23rd Edition, WB Saunders Company, Ltd., London, 2009.

Cunha BA (ed). Tick-Borne Infectious Diseases. Marcel Dekker, New York, 2000.

Despommier DD, Gwadz RW, Hotez PJ, Knirsch CA (eds). Parasitic Diseases, 4th Edition, Apple Trees Productions, LLC, New York, 2000.

Garcia LS (ed). Practical guide to Diagnostic Parasitology. ASM Press, Washington, DC, 2009.

Gorbach SL, Bartlett JG, Blacklow NR (eds). Infectious Diseases, 3rd Edition, Philadelphia, Lippincott, Williams & Wilkins, 2004.

Guerrant RL, Walker DH, Weller PF (eds). Tropical Infectious Disease: Principles, Pathogens & Practice, 3rd Edition, Elsevier, Philadelphia, 2011.

Gutierrez Y (ed). Diagnostic Pathology of Parasitic Infections with Clinical Correlations, 2nd Edition, Oxford University Press, New York, 2000.

Howard DH (ed). Pathogenic Fungi in Humans and Animals. 2nd Edition, New York, Marcel Dekker, 2003.

Jong E, Sanford C (eds). The Travel and Tropical Medicine Manual. 4th Edition, Philadelphia: Saunders Elsevier, 2008.

Keystone JS, Kozarsky PE, Freedman DO, Nothdurft HO, Connor B. Travel Medicine 2nd Edition, Philadelphia: Mosby Elsevier, 2008.

Knipe DM, Howley PM (eds). Fields, Virology, 5th Edition, Lippincott Williams & Wilkins, Philadelphia, 2008.

Krauss H, Weber A, Appel M (eds). Zoonoses. Infectious Diseases Transmissible from Animals to Humans, 3rd Edition, ASM Press, Washington, D.C. 2003.

Maertens JA, Marr KA (eds). Diagnosis of Fungal Infections. Informa Healthcare, New York, 2007.

Mandell GL, Bennett JE, Dolin R (eds). Mandell, Douglas, and Bennett's Principles and Practice of infectious Diseases, 7th Edition, Philadelphia, Elsevier, 2010.

Porterfield JS (ed). Exotic Viral Infections. Chapman & Hall Medical, London, 1995.

Raoult D, Parola P. Rickettsial Diseases. Informa Healthcare, New York, 2007.

Richman DD, Whitley RJ, Hayden FG (eds). Clinical Virology, 2nd Edition, ASM Press, Washington, DC, 2002.

Schlossberg DM (ed). Current Therapy of Infectious Diseases, 3rd Edition, Mosby St. Louis, 2008.

Strickland GT (ed). Hunter's Tropical Medicine and Emerging Infectious Diseases, 8th Edition, W.B. Saunders Company, Philadelphia, 2000.

Sun T (ed). Parasitic Disorders: Pathology, Diagnosis, and Management, 2nd Edition, Williams & Wilkins, Baltimore, 1999.

Walker DH (ed). Biology of Rickettsial Diseases. CRC Press, Boca Raton, 2000.

Warrell DA, Gilles HM. Essential Malariology, 4th Edition, Oxford University Press, New York, 2002.

Yu VL, Jr., Merigan TC, Jr., and Barriere SL (eds.). Antimicrobial Therapy & Vaccines, 2nd Edition, Williams & Wilkins, Baltimore, MD, 2005.

Chapter 5

HIV Infection

Paul E. Sax, MD
Jean E. Hage, MD
Arthur Gran, MD

HIV INFECTION OVERVIEW

Paul E. Sax, M.D.

Infection with Human Immunodeficiency Virus (HIV-1) leads to a chronic and without treatment usually fatal infection characterized by progressive immunodeficiency, a long clinical latency period, and opportunistic infections. The hallmark of HIV disease is infection and viral replication within T-lymphocytes expressing the CD_4 antigen (helper-inducer lymphocytes), a critical component of normal cell-mediated immunity. Qualitative defects in CD_4 responsiveness and progressive depletion in CD_4 cell counts increase the risk for opportunistic infections such as Pneumocystis (carinii) jiroveci pneumonia, and neoplasms such as lymphoma and Kaposi's sarcoma. HIV infection can also disrupt blood monocyte, tissue macrophage, and B-lymphocyte (humoral immunity) function, predisposing to infection with encapsulated bacteria. Direct attack of CD_4-positive cells in the central and peripheral nervous system can cause HIV meningitis, peripheral neuropathy, and dementia. More than 1 million people in the United States and 30 million people worldwide are infected with HIV. Without treatment, the average time from acquisition of HIV to an AIDS-defining opportunistic infection is about 10 years; survival then averages 1–2 years. There is tremendous individual variability in these time intervals, with some patients progressing from acute HIV infection to death within 1–2 years, and others not manifesting HIV-related immunosuppression for > 20 years after HIV acquisition. Antiretroviral therapy and prophylaxis against opportunistic infections have markedly improved the overall prognosis of HIV disease. The approach to HIV infection is shown in Figure 5.1.

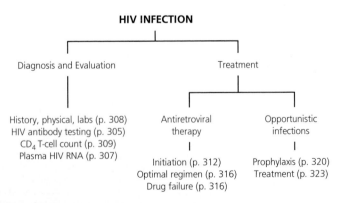

Figure 5.1. Diagnosis, Evaluation, and Treatment of HIV Infection

STAGES OF HIV INFECTION

A. **Viral Transmission.** HIV infection is acquired primarily by sexual intercourse (anal, vaginal, infrequently oral), exposure to contaminated blood (primarily needle transmission), or maternal-fetus (perinatal) transmission. Sexual practices with the highest risk of transmission include unprotected receptive anal intercourse (especially with mucosal tearing), unprotected receptive vaginal intercourse (especially during menses), and unprotected rectal/vaginal intercourse in the presence of genital ulcers (e.g., primary syphilis, genital herpes, chancroid). Lower risk sexual practices include insertive anal/vaginal intercourse and oral-genital contact. The risk of transmission after a single encounter with an HIV source has been estimated to be 1 in 150 with needle sharing, 1 in 300 with occupational percutaneous exposure, 1 in 300–1000 with receptive anal intercourse, 1 in 500–1250 with receptive vaginal intercourse, 1 in 1000–3000 with insertive vaginal intercourse, and 1 in 3000 with insertive anal intercourse. Transmission risk increases with the number of encounters and with higher HIV RNA plasma levels. The mode of transmission does not affect the natural history of HIV disease.

B. **Acute (Primary) HIV Infection (p. 304).** Acute HIV occurs 1–4 weeks after transmission, and is accompanied by a burst of viral replication with a decline in CD_4 cell count. Most patients manifest a symptomatic mononucleosis-like syndrome, which is often overlooked. Acute HIV infection is confirmed by a high HIV RNA in the absence of HIV antibody.

C. **Seroconversion.** Development of a positive HIV antibody test usually occurs within 4 weeks of acute infection, and invariably (with few exceptions) by 6 months.

D. **Asymptomatic HIV Infection** lasts a variable amount of time (average 8–10 years), and is accompanied by a gradual decline in CD_4 cell counts and a relatively stable HIV RNA level (sometimes referred to as the viral "set point").

E. **Symptomatic HIV Infection.** Previously referred to as "AIDS Related Complex (ARC)," findings include thrush or vaginal candidiasis (persistent, frequent, or poorly responsive to treatment), cervical dysplasia/carcinoma in-situ, herpes zoster (recurrent episodes or involving multiple dermatomes), oral hairy leukoplakia, peripheral neuropathy, diarrhea, or constitutional symptoms (e.g., low-grade fevers, weight loss).

F. **AIDS** is defined by a CD_4 cell count < 200/mm^3, a CD_4 cell percentage of total lymphocytes <14%, or one of several AIDS-related opportunistic infections. Common opportunistic infections include Pneumocystis (carinii) jiroveci pneumonia, cryptococcal meningitis, recurrent bacterial pneumonia, Candida esophagitis, CNS toxoplasmosis, tuberculosis, and non-Hodgkin's lymphoma. Other AIDS indicators in HIV-infected patients include candidiasis of the bronchi, trachea, or lungs; disseminated/extrapulmonary coccidiomycosis, cryptococcosis, or histoplasmosis; chronic (>1 month) intestinal cryptosporidiosis or isosporiasis; Kaposi's sarcoma; lymphoid interstitial pneumonia/pulmonary lymphoid hyperplasia; disseminated/extrapulmonary Mycobacterium (avium-intracellulare, kansasii, other species) infection; progressive multifocal leukoencephalopathy (PML); recurrent Salmonella septicemia; or HIV wasting syndrome.

G. Advanced HIV Disease is diagnosed when the CD_4 cell count is < 50/mm³. Most AIDS-related deaths occur at this point. Common late stage opportunistic infections are caused by CMV disease (retinitis, colitis) or disseminated Mycobacterium avium-intracellulare (MAI).

ACUTE (PRIMARY) HIV INFECTION

A. Description. Acute clinical illness associated with primary acquisition of HIV, occurring 1–4 weeks after viral transmission (range: 6 days to 6 weeks). Symptoms develop in 50–90%, but are often mistaken for the flu, mononucleosis, or other nonspecific viral syndrome. More severe symptoms may correlate with a higher viral set point and more rapid HIV disease progression. Even without therapy, most patients recover, reflecting development of a partially effective immune response and depletion of susceptible CD_4 cells.

B. Differential Diagnosis includes **EBV, CMV**, viral hepatitis, enteroviral infection, 2° syphilis, toxoplasmosis, HSV with erythema multiforme, drug reaction, Behcet's disease, acute lupus.

C. Signs and Symptoms usually reflect hematogenous dissemination of virus to lymphoreticular and neurologic sites:
- Fever (97%).
- Pharyngitis (73%). Typically non-exudative (unlike EBV, which is usually exudative).
- Rash (77%). Maculopapular viral exanthem of the face and trunk is most common, but can involve the extremities, palms and soles.
- Arthralgia/myalgia (58%).
- Neurologic symptoms (12%). Headache is most common. Neuropathy, Bell's palsy, and meningoencephalitis are rare, but may predict worse outcome.
- Oral/genital ulcerations, thrush, nausea, vomiting, diarrhea, weight loss.

D. Laboratory Findings
1. **CBC.** Lymphopenia followed by lymphocytosis (common). Atypical lymphocytosis is variable, but usually low level (unlike EBV, where atypical lymphocytosis may be 20–30% or higher). Thrombocytopenia occurs in some.
2. **Elevated transaminases** in some but not all patients.
3. **Depressed CD_4 cell count.** Can rarely be low enough to induce opportunistic infections.
4. **HIV antibody.** Usually negative, although persons with prolonged symptoms of acute HIV may have positive antibody tests if diagnosed late during the course of illness.

E. Confirming the Diagnosis of Acute HIV Infection

1. **Obtain HIV antibody** after informed consent (if required by state law) to exclude prior disease.

2. **Order viral load test (HIV RNA PCR),** preferably RT-PCR. HIV RNA confirms acute HIV infection prior to seroconversion. Most individuals will have very high HIV RNA (>100,000 copies/mL). Be suspicious of a false-positive test if the HIV RNA is low (< 20,000 copies/mL). For any positive test, it is important to repeat HIV RNA and HIV antibody testing. p24 antigen can also be used to establish the diagnosis, but is less sensitive than HIV RNA PCR.

3. **Order other tests/serologies if HIV RNA test is negative.** Order throat cultures for bacterial/viral respiratory pathogens, EBV VCA IgM/IgG, CMV IgM/IgG, HHV-6 IgM/IgG, and hepatitis serologies as appropriate to establish a diagnosis for patient's symptoms.

F. Management of Acute HIV Infection

1. **Initiate antiretroviral therapy.** The rationale behind this change is to treat a greater proportion of people with HIV, regardless of disease stage, is based on accumulating evidence of the benefits of earlier initiation of HIV treatment and, conversely, the potential for uncontrolled viral replication and CD_4 depletion.

2. **Obtain HIV resistance genotype** (see p. 317) because of a rising background prevalence of transmission of antiretroviral therapy-resistant virus. A genotype resistance test is preferred; therapy can be st arted pending results of the test.

3. **Possible benefits for treatment of acute HIV infection.** Possible (but unproven) benefits include hastening symptom resolution, reducing viral transmission, lowering virologic "set point," and preserving virus-specific CD_4 responses.

APPROACH TO HIV TESTING (Figure 5.2)

A. Standard HIV Antibody Tests. Most patients produce antibody to HIV within 6–8 weeks of exposure; half will have a positive antibody test in 3–4 weeks, and nearly 100% will have detectable antibody by 6 months.

1. **ELISA.** Usual screening test. All positives must be confirmed with Western blot or other more specific tests.

2. **Western blot.** CDC criteria for interpretation: **positive:** at least two of the following bands: p24, gp41, gp160/120; **negative:** no bands; **indeterminate:** any HIV band, but does not meet criteria for positivity.

3. **Test performance.** Standard method is ELISA screen with Western blot confirmation.

   a. **ELISA negative:** Western blot is not required (ELISA sensitivity 99.7%, specificity 98.5%). Obtain HIV RNA if acute HIV infection is suspected.

   b. **ELISA positive:** Confirm with Western blot. Probability that ELISA and Western blot are both false-positives is extremely low (< 1 per 140,000). Absence of p31 band could be a clue to a false positive Western blot.

   c. **Unexpected ELISA/Western blot:** Repeat test to exclude clerical/computer error.

4. **Indeterminate Western Blot.** Common clinical problem, affecting 4–20% of reactive ELISAs. Usually due to a single p24 band or weak other bands. Causes include seroconversion in progress, advanced HIV disease with loss of antibody response,

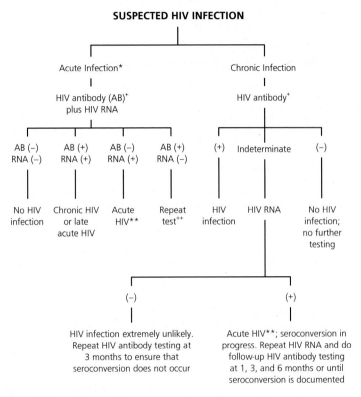

SUSPECTED HIV INFECTION

Acute Infection*

HIV antibody (AB)+
plus HIV RNA

| AB (–) | AB (+) | AB (–) | AB (+) |
| RNA (–) | RNA (+) | RNA (+) | RNA (–) |

No HIV infection

Chronic HIV or late acute HIV

Acute HIV**

Repeat test++

Chronic Infection

HIV antibody+

(+)   Indeterminate   (–)

HIV infection

HIV RNA

No HIV infection; no further testing

(–)   (+)

HIV infection extremely unlikely. Repeat HIV antibody testing at 3 months to ensure that seroconversion does not occur

Acute HIV**; seroconversion in progress. Repeat HIV RNA and do follow-up HIV antibody testing at 1, 3, and 6 months or until seroconversion is documented

Figure 5.2. Approach to HIV Testing

(–) = negative test; (+) = positive test.

* Occurs 1–4 weeks after viral transmission. Most patients manifest a viral syndrome (fever, pharyngitis ± rash/arthralgias), which is often mistaken for the flu and therefore overlooked.

** HIV RNA in acute HIV infection should be very high (usually > 100,000 copies/mL).

+ All positive ELISA tests must be confirmed by Western Blot; usually this is done automatically in clinical laboratories.

++ May be long-term non-progressor or laboratory error.

cross-reacting antibody from pregnancy, blood transfusions, organ transplantation, autoantibodies from collagen vascular disease, infection with HIV-2, influenza vaccination, or recipient of HIV vaccine. In low-risk patients, an indeterminate result almost never represents true HIV infection. Since seroconversion in progress is generally associated with high HIV RNA levels, the recommended approach is to order an HIV RNA test.

B. Quantitative Plasma HIV RNA (HIV Viral Load Assays)

1. **Description.** Measures amount of HIV RNA in plasma. High sensitivity of assays allows detection of virus in most patients not on antiviral therapy. Used to diagnose acute HIV infection and more commonly to monitor the response to antiretroviral therapy.

2. **Uses of HIV RNA Assay**

   a. **Confirms diagnosis of acute HIV infection.** A high HIV RNA with a negative HIV antibody test confirms acute HIV infection prior to seroconversion.

   b. **Helpful in initial evaluation of HIV infection.** Establishes baseline HIV RNA and helps (along with CD_4 cell count) determine whether to initiate or defer therapy, as HIV RNA correlates with rate of CD_4 decline.

   c. **Monitors response to antiviral therapy.** HIV RNA changes rapidly decline 2–4 weeks after starting or changing effective antiretroviral therapy, with slower decline thereafter. Patients with the greatest HIV RNA response have the best clinical outcome. No change in HIV RNA suggests therapy will be ineffective.

   d. **Estimates risk for opportunistic infection.** For patients with similar CD_4 cell counts, the risk of opportunistic infections is higher with higher HIV RNAs.

3. **Assays and Interpretation**

   a. **Tests, sensitivities, and dynamic range.** Three main assays, each with advantages and disadvantages, are widely used. Any assay can be used to diagnose acute HIV infection and guide/monitor therapy, but the same test should be used to follow patients longitudinally.

      1. **RT-PCR Amplicor** (Roche): Sensitivity = 400 copies/mL; dynamic range = 400–750,000 copies/mL.

      2. **RT-PCR Ultrasensitive 1.5** (Roche): Sensitivity = 50 copies/mL; dynamic range = 50–75,000 copies/mL.

      3. **bDNA Versant 3.0** (Bayer): Sensitivity = 75 copies/mL; dynamic range = 50–500,000 copies/mL.

   b. **Correlation between HIV RNA and CD_4.** HIV RNA assays correlate inversely with CD_4 cell counts, but do so imperfectly (e.g., some patients with high CD_4 counts have relatively high HIV RNA levels, and vice versa.) For any given CD_4, higher HIV RNA levels correlate with more rapid CD_4 decline. In response to antiretroviral therapy, changes in HIV RNA generally precede changes in CD_4 cell count.

c. **Significant change in HIV RNA assay** is defined by at least a 2-fold (0.3 log) change in viral RNA (accounts for normal variation in clinically stable patients), or a 3-fold (0.5 log) change in response to new antiretroviral therapy (accounts for intra-laboratory and patient variability). For example, if a HIV RNA result = 50,000 copies/mL, then the range of possible actual values = 25,000–100,000 copies/mL, and the value needed to demonstrate antiretroviral activity is ≤ 17,000 copies/mL.

4. **Indications for HIV RNA Testing.** Usually performed in conjunction with CD_4 cell counts. Indicated for the diagnosis of acute HIV infection, and for initial evaluation of newly diagnosed HIV. Also recommended 2–8 weeks after initiation of antiretroviral therapy and every 3–4 months in all HIV patients.

5. **When to Avoid HIV RNA Testing**
   a. **During acute illnesses and immunizations.** Patients with acute infections (opportunistic infection, bacterial pneumonia, even HSV recurrences) may experience significant (> 5-fold) rises in HIV RNA, which return to baseline 1–2 months after recovery. Although data are conflicting, many studies show at least a transient increase in HIV RNA levels following influenza and other immunizations, which return to baseline after 1–2 months.
   b. **When results of test would not influence therapy.** Frequent scenario in patients with advanced disease who have no antiretroviral options or cannot tolerate therapy.
   c. **As a screening test for HIV infection,** except if acute (primary) HIV disease is suspected during the HIV antibody window (i.e., first 3–6 weeks after viral transmission).

INITIAL ASSESSMENT OF HIV INFECTION

A. **Clinical Evaluation.** History and physical exam should focus on diagnoses associated with HIV infection. Compared to patients without HIV, the severity, frequency, and duration of these conditions are usually increased in HIV disease.

1. **Dermatologic:** Severe herpes simplex (oral/anogenital); herpes zoster (especially recurrent, cranial nerve, or disseminated); molluscum contagiosum; staphylococcal abscesses; tinea nail infections; Kaposi's sarcoma (from HHV-8 infection); petechiae (from ITP); seborrheic dermatitis; new or worsening psoriasis; eosinophilic pustular folliculitis; severe cutaneous drug eruptions (especially sulfonamides).

2. **Oropharyngeal:** Oral candidiasis; oral hairy leukoplakia (from EBV); Kaposi's sarcoma (most commonly on palate or gums); gingivitis/periodontitis; warts; aphthous ulcers (especially esophageal/perianal).

3. **Constitutional symptoms:** Fatigue, fevers, chronic diarrhea, weight loss.

4. **Lymphatic:** Persistent, generalized lymphadenopathy.

5. **Others:** Active TB (especially extrapulmonary); non-Hodgkin's lymphoma (especially CNS); unexplained leukopenia, anemia, thrombocytopenia (especially ITP); myopathy; miscellaneous neurologic conditions (cranial/peripheral neuropathies, Guillain-Barre syndrome, mononeuritis multiplex, aseptic meningitis, cognitive impairment).

B. **Baseline Laboratory Testing (Table 5.1)**

C. **CD$_4$ Cell Count (lymphocyte subset analysis)**
   1. **Overview.** Acute HIV infection is characterized by a decline in CD$_4$ cell count, followed by a gradual rise associated with clinical recovery. Chronic HIV infection shows progressive declines (~ 50–80 cells/year) in CD$_4$ cell count without treatment, followed by more rapid decline 1–2 years prior to opportunistic infection (AIDS-defining diagnosis). Cell counts remain stable over 5–10 years in 5% of patients, while others may show rapid declines (> 300 cells/year). Since variability exists within individual patients and between laboratories, it is useful to *repeat any value before making management decisions.*

   2. **Uses of CD$_4$ Cell Count**
      a. **Gives context of degree of immunosuppression** for interpretation of symptoms/signs (Table 5.2).
      b. **Used to guide therapy.** Guidelines support CD$_4$ < 500/mm^3 as the threshold for initiating treatment, regardless of HIV RNA or symptoms. For prophylaxis against PCP, toxoplasmosis, and MAI/CMV infection, CD$_4$ cell counts of 200/mm^3, < 100/mm^3, and < 50/mm^3 are used as threshold levels, respectively.
      c. **Provides estimate of risk of opportunistic infection or death.** CD$_4$ cell counts < 50/mm^3 are associated with a markedly increased risk of death (median survival 1 year), although some patients with low counts survive > 3 years even without antiretroviral therapy. Prognosis is heavily influenced by HIV RNA, presence/history of opportunistic infections or neoplasms, performance status, and the immune reconstitution response to antiretroviral therapy.

D. **HIV RNA Assay (HIV RNA PCR) (p. 307)**

Table 5.1. Baseline Laboratory Testing for HIV-Infected Patients

Test	Rationale
Repeat HIV serology (ELISA/confirmatory Western blot)	Indicated for patients unable to document a prior positive test, and for "low risk" individuals with a positive test (to detect computer/clerical error). Repeat serology is now less important since HIV RNA testing provides an additional means of confirming HIV infection.

Table 5.1. Baseline Laboratory Testing for HIV-Infected Patients (cont'd)

Test	Rationale
CBC with differential, platelets	Detects cytopenias (e.g., ITP) seen in HIV. Needed to calculate CD_4 cell count.
Chemistry panel ("SMA 20") and fasting lipid panel	Detects renal dysfunction and electrolyte/LFT abnormalities, which may accompany HIV and associated infections (e.g., HIV nephropathy, HCV). Provides baseline lipid profile (many antiretroviral drugs can affect lipids).
CD_4 cell count	Determines the need for antiretroviral therapy and opportunistic infection (OI) prophylaxis. Best test for defining risk of OIs and prognosis.
HIV RNA assay ("viral load")	Provides a marker for the pace of HIV disease progression. Determines indication for and response to antiretroviral therapy.
Tuberculin skin test (standard 5 TU of PPD)	Detects latent TB infection and targets patients for preventive therapy. Anergy skin tests are no longer indicated due to poor predictive value. HIV is the most powerful co-factor for the development of active TB.
PAP smear	Risk of cervical cancer is nearly twice as high in HIV-positive women compared to uninfected controls.
HLA-B*5701	Needed if abacavir therapy is planned, to assess risk for severe abacavir hypersensitivity reactions.
Toxoplasmosis serology (IgG)	Identifies patients at risk for subsequent cerebral/systemic toxoplasmosis and the need for prophylaxis. Those with negative tests should be counseled on how to avoid infection.
Syphilis serology (VDRL or RPR)	Identifies co-infection with syphilis, which is epidemiologically-linked to HIV. Disease may have accelerated course in HIV patients.
Hepatitis C serology (anti-HCV)	Identifies HCV infection and usually chronic carriage. If positive, follow with HCV genotype and HCV viral load assay. If the patient is antibody-negative and at high-risk for hepatitis, order HCV RNA to exclude a false-negative result.
Hepatitis B serologies (HBsAb, HBcAb, HBsAg)	Identifies patients who are immune to hepatitis B (HBsAb) or chronic carriers (HBsAg). If all three are negative, hepatitis B vaccine is indicated.

Table 5.1. Baseline Laboratory Testing for HIV-Infected Patients (cont'd)

Test	Rationale
G6PD screen	Identifies patients at risk for dapsone or primaquine-associated hemolysis.
CMV serology (IgG)	Identifies patients who should receive CMV-negative or leukocyte-depleted blood if transfused.
VZV serology (IgG)	Identifies patients at risk for varicella (chickenpox), and those who should avoid contact with active varicella or herpes zoster patients. Serology-negative patients exposed to chickenpox should receive varicella-zoster immune globulin (VZIG).
Chest x-ray	Sometimes ordered as a baseline test for future comparisons. May detect healed granulomatous diseases/other processes. Indicated in all tuberculin skin test positive patients.

Table 5.2. Use of CD$_4$ Cell Count for Interpretation of Patient Signs/Symptoms

CD$_4$ Cell Count (cells/mm³)	Associated Conditions
> 500	Most illnesses are similar to those in HIV-negative patients. Some increased risk of bacterial infections (pneumococcal pneumonia, sinusitis), herpes zoster, tuberculosis, skin conditions.
200–500*	Bacterial infections (especially pneumococcal pneumonia, sinusitis), cutaneous Kaposi's sarcoma, vaginal candidiasis, ITP.
50–200*	Thrush, oral hairy leukoplakia, classic HIV-associated opportunistic infections (e.g., P. [carinii] jiroveci pneumonia, cryptococcal meningitis, toxoplasmosis). For patients receiving prophylaxis, most opportunistic infection do not occur until CD$_4$ cell counts fall significantly below 100/mm³.
< 50*	"Final common pathway" opportunistic infections (disseminated M. avium-intracellulare, CMV retinitis), HIV-associated wasting, neurologic disease (neuropathy, encephalopathy).

*   Patients remain at risk for all processes noted in earlier stages.

INDICATIONS FOR TREATMENT OF HIV INFECTION

Table 5.3. Initiation of Antiretroviral Therapy in HIV-1 Infected Patients

Clinical Condition and/or CD$_4$ count	Recommendation
Symptomatic HIV disease	ART strongly recommended regardless of CD$_4$ cell count
Pregnant women	
HIV-1 RNA > 100,000 copies/mm^3	
Rapid decline in CD$_4$ cell count, >100 cells/mm^3 per year	
Acute hepatitis B coinfection	
Acute hepatitis C coinfection	
Active or high risk for cardiovascular disease	
HIV associated neuropathy	
Symptomatic primary HIV infection	
High risk for secondary HIV transmission (e.g., serodiscordant couples)	
Asymptomatic (any CD$_4$ cell count)	ART is recommended

ART = antiretroviral therapy.

Adapted from: Panel on Antiretroviral Guidelines for Adults and Adolescents. Department of Health and Human Services. Guidelines for the use of antiretroviral agents in HIV-infected adults and adolescents. http://aidsinfo.nih.gov/ConsentFiles/AdultandAdolescentGL.pdf, 2012.

ANTIRETROVIRAL TREATMENT

Table 5.4. ART Therapy for Treatment-Naive Patients from DHHS Guidelines 2012

Regimen	Preferred Regimen	Alternate Regimen	Acceptable Regimen
NNRTI-based (1 NNRTI + 2 NRTIs)	Efavirenz (EFV) + Tenofovir (TDF) + Emtricitabine (FTC)	Efavirenz (EFV) + Abacavir (ABC) + Lamivudine (3TC) Rilpivirine (RPV) **plus** Tenofovir (TDF) + Emtricitabine (FTC) **or** Abacavir (ABC) + Lamivudine (3TC)	Efavirenz (EFV) + Zidovudine (ZDV) + Lamivudine (3TC) Nevirapine (NVP) **plus** Tenofovir (TDF) + Emtricitabine (FTC) **or** Zidovudine (ZDV) + Lamivudine (3TC)
PI-based (1 PI + 2 NRTIs)	Atazanavir (ATV)/r + Tenofovir (TDF) + Emtricitabine (FTC) Darunavir (DRV)/r + Tenofovir (TDF) + Emtricitabine (FTC)	Atazanavir (ATV)/r + Abacavir (ABC) + Lamivudine (3TC) Darunavir (DRV)/r + Abacavir (ABC) + Lamivudine (3TC) Fosamprenavir (FPV)/r **plus** Abacavir (ABC) + Lamivudine (3TC) **or** Tenofovir (TDF) + Emtricitabine (FTC) Lopinavir (LPV)/r **plus** Abacavir (ABC) + Lamivudine (3TC) **or** Tenofovir (TDF) + Emtricitabine (FTC)	Atazanavir (ATV) + [Abacavir (ABC) or Zidovudine (ZDV)] + Lamivudine (3TC) Atazanavir (ATV)/r **or** Darunavir DRV/r **or** Fosamprenavir (FPV)/r **or** Lopinavir (LPV)/r **plus** Zidovudine (ZDV) + Lamivudine (3TC)

Table 5.4. ART Therapy for Treatment-Naive Patients from DHHS Guidelines 2012 (cont'd)

Regimen	Preferred Regimen	Alternate Regimen	Acceptable Regimen
INSTI-based (1 INSTI + 2 NRTIs)	Raltegravir (RAL) + Tenofovir (TDF) + Emtricitabine (FTC)	Raltegravir (RAL) + Abacavir (ABC) + Lamivudine (3TC) Elvitegravir (EVG) + Combicistat (COBI) + Emtricitabine (FTC) + Tenofovir (TDF)	Raltegravir (RAL) + Zidovudine (ZDV) + Lamivudine (3TC)
CCR5 Antagonist-based (1 CCR5 + 2 NRTIs)	N/A	N/A	Maraviroc (MVC) **plus** Zidovudine (ZDV) + Lamivudine (3TC) **or** Tenofovir (TDF) + Emtricitabine (FTC) **or** Abacavir (ABC) + Lamivudine (3TC)

Adapted from: Panel on Antiretroviral Guidelines for Adults and Adolescents. Department of Health and Human Services. Guidelines for the use of antiretroviral agents in HIV-infected adults and adolescents. http://aidsinfo.nih.gov/ConsentFiles/AdultandAdolescentGL.pdf, 2012.

Regimens for Pregnant Women LPV/r (bid) ZDV/3TC Recommendations for use of antiretroviral drugs in pregnant HIV-infected women for maternal health and interventions to reduce perinatal HIV transmission in the United States at http://aidsinfo.nih.gov/guidelines.

- Efavirenz should not be used during the first trimester of pregnancy or in women trying to conceive or in those not using effective and consistent contraception.
- Lamivudine may substitute for emtricitabine or vice versa.
- Abacavir should not be used in patients who test positive for HLA-B*5701 and should be used with caution in patients at high risk for cardiovascular disease or with pretreatment HIV-RNA > 100,000 copies/ml.
- Nevirapine should not be used in patients with moderate to severe hepatic impairment. It should not be used in women with pre-ARV CD_4+ > 250 cells/mm^3 or men with pre-ARV CD_4+ > 400 cells/mm^3.
- Atazanavir/r should not be used in patients who requires > 20 mg omeprazole per day.
- Atazanavir/r is generally preferred over atazanavir. Unboosted atazanavir may be used when ritonavir boosting is not possible.
- Abacavir should not be used in patients who test positive for HLA-B*5701 and should be used with caution in patients at high risk for cardiovascular disease or with pretreatment HIV-RNA > 100,000 copies/ml.
- Lopinavir/r qd is not recommended for pregnant women.

Table 5.5. Recommended initial Antiretroviral Therapy from IAS-USA Guidelines

	Recommended regimen	Alternate regimen	Comments
NNRTI-based	Efavirenz + Tenofovir + Emtricitabine Efavirenz + Abacavir + Lamivudine	Nevirapine + Tenofovir + Emtricitabine Nevirapine + Abacavir + Lamivudine Rilpivirine + Tenofovir + Emtricitabine Rilpivirine + Abacavir + Lamivudine	Abacavir only in HLA-B*5701-negative patients with HIV-1 RNA < 100000 copies/mL. Severe hepatotoxicity and rash with nevirapine are more common in initial therapy when CD4 cell count > 250/μL in women and > 400/μL in men
PI-based	Darunavir/r + Tenofovir + Emtricitabine Atazanavir/r + Tenofovir + Emtricitabine Atazanavir/r + Abacavir +Lamivudine	Darunavir/r + Abacavir + Lamivudine Lopinavir/r + Tenofovir + Emtricitabine Lopinavir/r + Abacavir + Lamivudine	Other alternative PIs include fosamprenavir/r and saquinavir/r but indications to use these options for initial treatment are rare
InSTI-based	Raltegravir + Tenofovir + Emtricitabine	Ralegravir + Abacavir + Lamivudine Elvitegravir + Combicistat + Tenofovir + Emtricitabine	Raltegravir is given twice daily. Experience with elvitegravir/combicistat/ tenofovir/emtricitabine is limited to 48-week data

Adapted from: Thompson MA, Aberg JA, Hoy JF, et al. Antiretroviral treatment of adult HIV infection: 2012 recommendations of the International Antiviral Society-USA Panel. JAMA 308:387–402, 2012.

Selection of Optimal Antiretroviral Therapy. Selection of the optimal initial antiretroviral regimen must take into consideration antiviral potency, tolerability, and safety. In the DHHS and IAS-USA Guidelines (Tables 5.4 and 5.5).

ANTIRETROVIRAL TREATMENT FAILURE (Table 5.6)

Antiretroviral treatment failure can be defined in various ways, as described below. Causes of treatment failure include inadequate adherence, preexisting drug resistance, regimen complexity, side effects, and suboptimal pharmacokinetics. All of these factors can lead to persistent viral replication and evolution of drug resistance. Poor medication adherence is the most common cause of treatment failure.

A. Types of Treatment Failure

1. **Virologic Failure** is most strictly defined as the inability to achieve or maintain virologic suppression. In a treatment-naïve patient, the HIV RNA level should be < 400 copies/mL after 24 weeks or < 50 copies/mL by 48 weeks after starting therapy. Virologic rebound is seen when there is repeated detection of HIV RNA after virologic suppression in either treatment-naïve or treatment-experienced patients.

2. **Immunologic Failure** can occur in the presence or absence of virologic failure and is defined as a failure to increase the CD_4 cell count by 25–50 cells/mm³ above baseline during the first year of therapy, or as a decrease in CD_4 cell count to below baseline count while on therapy.

3. **Clinical Failure** is the occurrence or recurrence of HIV-related events after at least 3 months on potent antiretroviral therapy, excluding events related to an immune reconstitution syndrome.

4. **Usual Sequence of Treatment Failure.** Virologic failure usually occurs first, followed by immunologic failure, and finally by clinical progression. These events may be separated by months or years and may not occur in this order in all patients.

B. Goals After Virologic Failure.
When patients have detectable HIV RNA on treatment, clinicians should attempt to identify the cause of their lack of response and set a treatment goal of achieving full virologic suppression (HIV RNA < 50 copies/mL). In addition to improving clinical and immunologic outcomes, this strategy will also prevent the selection of additional resistance mutations. Provided that medication adherence issues and regimen tolerability have been addressed, the regimen should be changed sooner than later. On the other hand, achieving an undetectable HIV RNA level in patients with an extensive prior treatment history may not be possible. The main goals in these patients should be partial suppression of HIV RNA below the pretreatment level to preserve immune function and prevent clinical progression.

C. Resistance Testing and Selection of New Antiretroviral Therapy.
Genotypic assays characterize nucleotide sequences of the reverse transcriptase/protease portions of the virus, and identify resistance mutations associated with various drugs.

Phenotypic assays attempt to grow the virus in the presence of drugs, providing a more intuitively applicable measurement of resistance (similar to that done with bacteria). Compared to phenotypic assays, genotypic assays are faster (1–2 weeks vs. 2–4 weeks for results), less expensive ($400 vs. $1000), and have less inter-laboratory variability; however, mutations do not always correlate with resistance and results are difficult to interpret.

Table 5.6. Management of Antiretroviral Treatment Failure

Type of Failure	Recommended Approach	Comments
Virologic failure Limited or intermediate prior treatment	Assess for adherence and regimen tolerability. Obtain genotype resistance test. Select new regimen based on resistance test results and tolerability.	Usually associated with limited or no detectable resistance. If no resistance is found, consider re-testing for resistance 2–4 weeks after resuming antivirals. Stop NNRTI's if resistance is detected. Virologic suppression is likely if adherence is good.
Extensive prior treatment	Assess for adherence and regimen tolerability. Obtain resistance test – consider phenotype, "virtual phenotype," or phenotype-genotype combination if level of resistance is likely to be high. Obtain viral tropism assay to assess possible use of CCR5 antagonist. Select new regimen using at least 2 new active agents; if 2 new active agents not available, continue a "holding" regimen.	In patients with resistance to NRTI's, NNRTI's and PI's, the new regimen should generally contain at least: (1) at least one drug from a new drug class (integrase inhibitor, CCR5 antagonist, or fusion inhibitor); (2) a boosted PI with activity against resistant viruses (tipranavir or darunavir); and (3) one or two NRTI's, one of them 3TC or FTC. A holding regimen should always contain 3TC or FTC plus a boosted PI; NNRTI's should never be used.
Low-level HIV RNA (50–1000 copies)	Assess for adherence, drug-drug interactions, intercurrent illness, recent immunizations. Repeat test in 3–4 weeks.	For low-level viremia followed by undetectable HIV RNA ("blip"), no treatment change is necessary. If HIV RNA is persistently detectable at > 500 copies/mL, obtain resistance test as described above, and treat accordingly. If HIV RNA is persistently detectable at 50–500 copies/mL, consider regimen "intensification" with use of an additional agent.

Table 5.6. Management of Antiretroviral Treatment Failure (cont'd)

Type of Failure	Recommended Approach	Comments
Immunologic failure *Detectable HIV RNA*	Assess for adherence and tolerability. If non-adherent, resume treatment after barriers to adherence are addressed. If adherent, obtain resistance testing and alter therapy as described above.	If HIV RNA is back to pre-treatment baseline, non-adherence is the most likely explanation.
Suppressed HIV RNA	Investigate for modifiable conditions that may be associated with impaired CD$_4$ response (chronic HCV, treatment with ZDV, TDF + ddI). If no modifiable conditions found, continue current regimen.	Prognosis for patients with suppressed HIV RNA and immunologic failure better than for those with comparable CD$_4$ cell counts and detectable viremia.
Clinical failure *Detectable HIV RNA*	Treat OI with appropriate anti-infective therapy. Assess for antiretroviral adherence and tolerability. Send resistance test and choose new regimen based on results of test and other treatment options.	OI's (IRIS excluded) most commonly occur in those not on antiretroviral therapy due to poor compliance and/or regimen tolerability.
Suppressed HIV RNA	Continue current antiretrovirals. Treat OI with appropriate anti-infective therapy. If symptoms persist and IRIS is likely, use adjunctive corticosteroids.	IRIS most likely when baseline CD$_4$ cell count is low (< 200/mm^3); onset usually weeks-to-months after starting a potent regimen. IRIS been reported with virtually all OI's. True clinical progression with suppressed HIV RNA is unusual; IRIS should not be considered a sign of treatment failure.

IRIS = immune reconstitution inflammatory syndrome, OI = opportunistic infection.

PROPHYLAXIS OF OPPORTUNISTIC INFECTIONS IN HIV (Tables 5.7, 5.8)

Patients with HIV disease are at risk for infectious complications not otherwise seen in immunocompetent patients. Such opportunistic infections occur in proportion to the severity of immune system dysfunction (reflected by CD_4 cell count depletion). While community acquired infections (e.g., pneumococcal pneumonia) can occur at any CD_4 cell count, "classic" HIV-related opportunistic infections (PCP, toxoplasmosis, cryptococcus, disseminated M. avium-intracellulare, CMV) do not occur until CD_4 cell counts are dramatically reduced. Specifically, it is rare to encounter PCP in HIV patients with $CD_4 > 200/mm^3$, and CMV and disseminated MAI occur at median CD_4 cell counts $< 50/mm^3$.

Table 5.7. Overview of Prophylaxis (See Table 5.8 for details)

Infection	Indication	Intervention
PCP	$CD_4 < 200/mm^3$	TMP–SMX
TB (M. tuberculosis)	PPD > 5 mm (current or past) or contact with active case	INH
Toxoplasma	IgG Ab (+) and $CD_4 < 100/mm^3$	TMP–SMX
MAI	$CD_4 < 50/mm^3$	Azithromycin or Clarithromycin
S. pneumoniae	$CD_4 > 200/mm^3$	Pneumococcal vaccine
Hepatitis B (HBV)	Susceptible patients	Hepatitis B vaccine
Hepatitis A (HAV)	HCV (+) and HA Ab (–); HCV (–) and HA Ab (–) gay men and travelers to endemic areas, chronic liver disease	Hepatitis A vaccine
Influenza	All patients	Annual flu vaccine Swine influenza (H_1N_1) vaccine
VZV	Exposure to chickenpox or shingles; no prior history	VZIG

Abbreviations: Ab = antibody; HAV = Hepatitis A virus; HCV = Hepatitis C virus; VZIG = varicella-zoster immune globulin; VZV = varicella- zoster virus; other abbreviations (p. xi).

Table 5.8. Prophylaxis of Opportunistic Infections in HIV

Infection	Indications and Prophylaxis	Comments
P. (carinii) jiroveci pneumonia (PCP)	<u>Indications:</u> CD$_4$ < 200/mm^3, oral thrush, constitutional symptoms, or previous history of PCP <u>Preferred prophylaxis:</u> TMP–SMX 1 DS tablet (PO) q24h or 1 SS tablet (PO) q24h. 1 DS tablet (PO) 3×/week is also effective, but daily dosing may be slightly more effective <u>Alternate prophylaxis:</u> Dapsone 100 mg (PO) q24h (preferred as second-line by most; more effective than aerosolized pentamidine when CD$_4$ cell count < 100) **or** Atovaquone 1500 mg (PO) q24h (comparably effective to dapsone and aerosolized pentamidine; more GI toxicity vs. dapsone, but less rash) **or** Aerosolized pentamidine 300 mg via Respirgard II nebulizer once monthly (exclude active pulmonary TB first to avoid nosocomial transmission)	Without prophylaxis, 80% of AIDS patients develop PCP, and 60–70% relapse within one year after the first episode. Prophylaxis with TMP–SMX also reduces the risk for toxoplasmosis and possibly bacterial infections. Among patients with prior non-life-threatening reactions to TMP–SMX, 55% can be successfully rechallenged with 1 SS tablet daily, and 80% can be rechallenged with gradual dose escalation using TMP–SMX elixir (8 mg TMP + 40 mg SMX/mL) given as 1 mL × 3 days, then 2 mL × 3 days, then 5 mL × 3 days, then 1 SS tablet (PO) q24h. Macrolide-regimens for MAI (azithromycin, clarithromycin) add to efficacy of PCP prophylaxis. Primary and secondary prophylaxis may be discontinued if CD$_4$ cell counts increase to > 200 cells/mm^3 for 3 months or longer in response to antiretroviral therapy (i.e., immune reconstitution). Prophylaxis should be resumed if the CD$_4$ cell count decreases to < 200/mm^3.
Toxoplasmosis	<u>Indications:</u> CD$_4$ < 100/mm^3 with positive toxoplasmosis serology (IgG) <u>Preferred prophylaxis:</u> TMP–SMX 1 DS tablet (PO) q24h <u>Alternate prophylaxis:</u> Dapsone 50 mg (PO) q24h + pyrimethamine 50 mg (PO) weekly + folinic acid 25 mg (PO) weekly **or**	Incidence of toxoplasmosis in seronegative patients is too low to warrant chemoprophylaxis. Primary prophylaxis can be discontinued if CD$_4$ cell counts increase to > 200/mm^3 for at least 3 months in response to antiretroviral therapy. Secondary prophylaxis (chronic maintenance therapy) may be discontinued in patients who responded to initial therapy, remain asymptomatic, and whose CD$_4$ counts increase to > 200/mm^3 for 6 months or longer in response to

Table 5.8. Prophylaxis of Opportunistic Infections in HIV (cont'd)

Infection	Indications and Prophylaxis	Comments
	Dapsone 100 mg/pyrimethamine 50 mg twice weekly (no folinic acid) **or** Atovaquone 1500 mg (PO) q24h	antiretroviral therapy. Prophylaxis should be restarted if the CD_4 count decreases to < 200/mm³. Some experts would obtain an MRI of the brain as part of the evaluation prior to stopping secondary prophylaxis.
M. tuberculosis (TB)	<u>Indications:</u> PPD induration ≥ 5 mm or history of positive PPD without prior treatment, or close contact with active case of TB. Must exclude active disease (chest x-ray mandatory). Indicated at any CD_4 cell count <u>Preferred prophylaxis:</u> INH 300 mg (PO) q24h × 9 months + pyridoxine 50 mg (PO) q24h × 9 months <u>Alternate prophylaxis:</u> Rifampin 600 mg (PO) q24h × 2 months + pyrazinamide 20 mg/kg (PO) q24h × 2 months. Rifampin should not be given to patients receiving PI's	Consider prophylaxis for skin test negative patients when the probability of prior TB exposure is > 10% (e.g., patients from developing countries, IV drug abusers in some cities, prisoners). However, a trial testing this strategy in the U.S. did not find a benefit for empiric prophylaxis. INH prophylaxis delayed progression to AIDS and prolonged life in Haitian cohort with positive PPD treated × 6 months. Rifampin plus pyrazinamide × 2 months was effective in a multinational clinical trial (but the combination may ↑ hepatotoxicity). Rifabutin may be substituted for rifampin in rifampin-containing regimens.
M. avium-intracellulare (MAI)	<u>Indications:</u> CD_4 < 50/mm³ <u>Preferred prophylaxis:</u> Azithromycin 1200 mg (PO) once a week (fewest number of pills; fewest drug interactions; may add to efficacy of PCP prophylaxis) **or** Clarithromycin 500 mg (PO) q12h (more effective than rifabutin; associated with survival advantage; resistance detected in some breakthrough cases) <u>Alternate prophylaxis:</u> Rifabutin (less effective). See TB (p. 326) for dosing	Macrolide options (azithromycin, clarithromycin) preferable to rifabutin. Azithromycin is preferred for patients on protease inhibitors (fewer drug interactions). Primary prophylaxis may be discontinued if CD_4 cell counts increase to > 100/mm³ and HIV RNA suppresses for 3–6 months or longer in response to antiretroviral therapy. Secondary prophylaxis may be discontinued for CD_4 cell counts that increase to > 100/mm³ × 6 months or longer in response to antiretroviral therapy if patients have completed 12 months of MAI therapy and have no evidence of disease. Resume MAI prophylaxis for CD_4 < 100/mm³.

Table 5.8. Prophylaxis of Opportunistic Infections in HIV (cont'd)

Infection	Indications and Prophylaxis	Comments
Pneumococcus (S. pneumoniae)	<u>Indications:</u> $CD_4 > 200/mm^3$ <u>Preferred prophylaxis:</u> Pneumococcal polysaccharide (23 valent) vaccine.* Re-vaccinate × 1 at 5 years	Incidence of invasive pneumococcal disease is > 100-fold higher in HIV patients. Efficacy of vaccine is variable in clinical studies.
Influenza (human seasonal)	<u>Indications:</u> Generally recommended for all patients <u>Preferred prophylaxis:</u> Influenza vaccine (inactivated whole virus and split virus vaccine)*	Give annually (optimally October–January). Some experts do not give vaccine if CD_4 is < $100/mm^3$ (antibody response is poor). New intranasal live virus vaccine is contraindicated in immunosuppressed patients.
Hepatitis B (HBV)	<u>Indications:</u> All susceptible (anti-HBcAb negative and anti-HBsAg negative) patients <u>Preferred prophylaxis:</u> Hepatitis B recombinant DNA vaccine*	Response rate is lower than in HIV-negative controls. Repeat series if no response, especially if CD_4 was low during initial series and is now increased.
Hepatitis A (HAV)	<u>Indications:</u> All susceptible patients who are also infected with hepatitis C; HAV-susceptible seronegative gay men or travelers to endemic areas; chronic liver disease; illegal drug users <u>Preferred prophylaxis:</u> Hepatitis A vaccine*	Response rate is lower than in HIV-negative controls.
Measles, mumps, rubella	<u>Indications:</u> Patients born after 1957 and never vaccinated; patients vaccinated between 1963–1967 <u>Preferred prophylaxis:</u> MMR (measles, mumps, rubella) vaccine*	Single case of vaccine-strain measles pneumonia in severely immuno-compromised adult who received MMR; vaccine is therefore contraindicated in patients with severe immunodeficiency (CD_4 < 200).

*   Same dose as for normal hosts (see pp. 372–375). If possible, give vaccines early in course of HIV infection, while immune system may still respond. Alternatively, to increase the likelihood of response in patients with advanced HIV disease, vaccines may be administered after 6–12 months of effective antiretroviral therapy. Vaccines should be given when patients are clinically stable, not acutely ill (e.g., give during a routine office visit, rather than during hospitalization for an opportunistic infection). Live vaccines (e.g., oral polio, oral typhoid, Yellow fever) are generally contraindicated, but measles vaccine is well-tolerated in children, and MMR vaccine is recommended for adults as described above.

Table 5.8. Prophylaxis of Opportunistic Infections in HIV (cont'd)

Infection	Indications and Prophylaxis	Comments
H. influenzae	<u>Indications:</u> Not generally recommended for adults <u>Preferred prophylaxis:</u> H. influenzae type B polysaccharide vaccine*	Incidence of H. influenzae disease is increased in HIV patients, but 65% are caused by non-type B strains. Unclear whether vaccine offers protection.
Travel vaccines*	<u>Indications:</u> Travel to endemic areas	All considered safe except oral polio, yellow fever, and live oral typhoid—each a live virus vaccine.

* Same dose as for normal hosts (see pp. 372–375). If possible, give vaccines early in course of HIV infection, while immune system may still respond. Alternatively, to increase the likelihood of response in patients with advanced HIV disease, vaccines may be administered after 6–12 months of effective antiretroviral therapy. Vaccines should be given when patients are clinically stable, not acutely ill (e.g., give during a routine office visit, rather than during hospitalization for an opportunistic infection). Live vaccines (e.g., oral polio, oral typhoid, Yellow fever) are generally contraindicated, but measles vaccine is well-tolerated in children, and MMR vaccine is recommended for adults as described above.

TREATMENT OF OPPORTUNISTIC INFECTIONS IN HIV

Antiretroviral therapy (ART) and specific antimicrobial prophylaxis regimens have led to a dramatic decline in HIV-related opportunistic infections. Today, opportunistic infections occur predominantly in patients not receiving ART (due to undiagnosed HIV infection or nonacceptance of therapy), or in the period after starting ART (due to lack of immune reconstitution or from eliciting a previously absent inflammatory host response). Despite high rates of virologic failure in clinical practice, the rate of opportunistic infections in patients compliant with ART remains low, presumably due to continued immunologic response despite virologic failure, a phenomenon that may be linked to impaired "fitness" (virulence) of resistant HIV strains. For patients on or off ART, the absolute CD_4 cell count provides the best marker of risk for opportunistic infections.

Respiratory Tract Opportunistic Infections

Aspergillosis, Invasive Pulmonary

Pathogen	Preferred Therapy	Alternate Therapy
Aspergillus fumigatus (rarely other species)	Voriconazole 400 mg (IV or PO) q12h × 2 days, then 200 mg (IV or PO) q12h until cured (typically 6–18 months)	Amphotericin B 1 mg/kg (IV) q24h until 2–3 gm total dose given (optimal duration of therapy poorly defined) **or** Lipid amphotericin (Abelcet or Ambisome) 5 mg/kg/day (IV) until cured

Clinical Presentation: Pleuritic chest pain, hemoptysis, cough in a patient with advanced HIV disease. Additional risk factors include neutropenia and use of corticosteroids.

Diagnostic Considerations: Diagnosis by bronchoscopy with biopsy/culture. Open lung biopsy (usually video-assisted thorascopic surgery) is sometimes required. Radiographic appearance includes cavitation, nodules, sometimes focal consolidation. Dissemination to CNS may occur, and manifests as focal neurological deficits.

Pitfalls: Positive sputum culture for Aspergillus in advanced HIV disease should heighten awareness of possible infection.

Therapeutic Considerations: Decrease/discontinue corticosteroids, if possible. If present, treat neutropenia with granulocyte-colony stimulating factor (G-CSF) to achieve absolute neutrophil count > 1000/mm³. There are insufficient data to recommend chronic suppressive or maintenance therapy.

Prognosis: Poor unless immune deficits can be corrected.

Bacterial Pneumonia

Usual Pathogens	Preferred Therapy	Comments
Streptococcus pneumoniae (most common) Haemophilus influenzae Pseudomonas aeruginosa	**Monotherapy with** Levofloxacin 750 mg (PO/IV) q24h or Moxifloxacin 400 mg (PO/IV) q24h × 7–14 days, depending on severity **or combination therapy with** Ceftriaxone 1–2 gm (IV) q24h (or Cefotaxime 1 gm [IV] q8h) **plus** Azithromycin 500 gm q24h × 7–14 days	For severe immunodeficiency (CD₄ < 100/mm³), neutropenia, or a prior history of pseudomonas infection, broaden coverage to include *P. aeruginosa* and other gram-negative bacilli by adding **either** Ceftazidime 1 gm (IV) q8h **or** Cefepime 1 gm (IV) q12h **or** Ciprofloxacin 750 mg (PO) q12h or 400 mg (IV) q8h.

Clinical Presentation: HIV-infected patients with bacterial pneumonia present similar to those without HIV, with a relatively acute illness (over days) that is often associated with chills, rigors, pleuritic chest pain, and purulent sputum. Patients who have been ill over weeks to months are more likely have PCP, tuberculosis, or a fungal infection. Since bacterial pneumonia can occur at any CD₄ cell count, this infection is frequently the presenting symptom of HIV disease, prompting initial HIV testing and diagnosis.

Diagnostic Considerations: The most common pathogens are Streptococcus pneumoniae, followed by Haemophilus influenzae. The pathogens of atypical pneumonia (Legionella pneumophila, Mycoplasma pneumoniae, and Chlamydia pneumoniae) are rarely encountered, even with extensive laboratory investigation. A lobar infiltrate on chest radiography is a further predictor of bacterial pneumonia. Blood cultures should be obtained, as HIV patients have an increased rate of bacteremia compared to those without HIV.

Pitfalls: Sputum gram stain and culture are generally only helpful if collected prior to starting antibiotics, and only if a single organism predominates. HIV patients with bacterial pneumonia may rarely have a more subacute opportunistic infection concurrently, such as PCP or TB.

Therapeutic Considerations: Once improvement has occurred, a switch to oral therapy is generally safe. Patients with advanced HIV disease are at greater risk of bacteremic pneumonia due to gram-negative bacilli, and should be covered empirically for this condition.

Prognosis: Response to therapy is generally prompt and overall prognosis is good.

Pneumocystis (carinii) jiroveci Pneumonia (PCP)

Subset	Preferred Therapy	Alternate Therapy
Severe disease (pO₂< 70 mmHg, A-a gradient > 35)	TMP–SMX (5 mg/kg TMP) (IV) q6h × 21 days **plus** Prednisone 40 mg (PO) q12h on days 1–5, then 40 mg (PO) q24h on days 6–10, then 20 mg (PO) q24h on days 11–21. Methylprednisolone (IV) can be substituted at 75% of prednisone dose	Pentamidine 4 mg/kg (IV) q24h (infused over ≥ 60 minutes) × 21 days *plus* prednisone × 21 days. (Dose reduction of pentamidine to 3 mg/kg [IV] q24h may reduce toxicity) **or** Primaquine 30 mg (PO) q24h × 21 days plus clindamycin 600 mg (PO) q8h × 21 days
Mild or moderate disease (pO₂ > 70 mmHg, A-a gradient < 35)	TMP–SMX 2 DS tablets (PO) q6h × 21 days	Dapsone 100 mg (PO) q24h × 21 days plus TMP 5 mg/kg (PO) q8h × 21 days **or** Primaquine 30 mg (PO) q24h × 21 days *plus* clindamycin 600 mg (PO) q8h × 21 days **or** Atovaquone 750 mg (PO) q12h (with food) × 21 days

Clinical Presentation: Fever, cough, dyspnea; often indolent presentation. Physical exam is usually normal. Chest x-ray is variable, but commonly shows a diffuse interstitial pattern. Elevated LDH/↑ β-glucan levels and exercise desaturation are highly suggestive of PCP.

Diagnostic Considerations: Diagnosis by immunofluorescent stain of induced sputum or bronchoscopy specimen. Check ABG if O_2 saturation is abnormal or respiratory rate is increased.

Pitfalls: Slight worsening of symptoms is common after starting therapy, especially if not treated with steroids. Do not overlook superimposed bacterial pneumonia or other secondary infections, especially while on pentamidine. Patients receiving second-line agents for PCP prophylaxis—in particular aerosolized pentamidine–may present with atypical radiographic findings, including apical infiltrates, multiple small-walled cysts, pleural effusions, pneumothorax, or single/multiple nodules.

Therapeutic Considerations: Outpatient therapy is possible for mild disease, but only when close follow-up is assured. Adverse reactions to TMP–SMX (rash, fever, GI symptoms, hepatitis, hyperkalemia, leukopenia, hemolytic anemia) occur in 25–50% of patients, many of whom will need a second-line regimen to complete therapy (e.g., trimethoprim-dapsone or atovaquone). Unless an adverse reaction to TMP–SMX is particularly severe (e.g., Stevens-Johnson syndrome or other life-threatening problem), TMP–SMX may be considered for PCP prophylaxis, since prophylaxis requires a much lower dose (only 10–15% of treatment dose). Patients being treated for severe PCP with TMP–SMX who do not improve after one week may be switched to pentamidine, although there are no prospective data to confirm this approach. In general, patients receiving antiretroviral therapy when PCP develops should have their treatment continued, since intermittent antiretroviral therapy can lead to drug resistance. For newly-diagnosed or antiretroviral-naive HIV patients, treatment of PCP may be completed before starting antiretroviral therapy. Steroids should be tapered, not discontinued abruptly. Adjunctive steroids increase the risk of thrush/herpes simplex infection, but probably not CMV, TB, or disseminated fungal infection.

Prognosis: Usually responds to treatment. Adverse prognostic factors include ↑ A-a gradient, hypoxemia, ↑ LDH.

Pulmonary Tuberculosis (for isolates sensitive to INH and rifampin)

Pathogen	Patients NOT Receiving PI's or NNRTI's	Patients Receiving PI's or NNRTI's*
Mycobacterium tuberculosis (TB)	Initial phase (8 weeks) INH 300 mg (PO) q24h **plus** Rifampin† 600 mg (PO) q24h **plus** Pyrazinamide (PZA) 25 mg/kg (PO) q24h **plus** Ethambutol (EMB) 15–20 mg/kg (PO) q24h Continuation phase (18 weeks) INH 300 mg (PO) q24h **plus** Rifampin† 600 mg (PO) q24h	Initial phase (8 weeks) INH 300 mg (PO) q24h **plus** Rifabutin* **plus** PZA 25 mg/kg (PO) q24h **plus** EMB 15 mg/kg (PO) q24h × 8 weeks. Continuation phase (18 weeks) INH 300 mg (PO) q24h **plus** Rifabutin*

* Rifabutin dose: If PI is nelfinavir, indinavir, amprenavir or fosamprenavir, then rifabutin dose is 150 mg (PO) q24h. If PI is ritonavir, lopinavir/ritonavir or atazanavir, then rifabutin dose is 150 mg (PO) 2–3 times weekly. If NNRTI is efavirenz, then rifabutin dose is 450 mg (PO) q24h or 600 mg (PO) 2–3 times weekly. If NNRTI is nevirapine, then rifabutin dose is 300 mg (PO) q24h. Rifabutin is **contraindicated** in patients receiving delavirdine rilpivirine, etravirine + ritonavir boosted PI or hard-gel saquinavir. Patients receiving PI's AND NNRTI's: as above, except adjust rifabutin to 300 mg (PO) q24h.

† For patients receiving triple NRTI regimens, substitute rifabutin 300 mg (PO) q24h for rifampin.

Clinical Presentation: May present atypically. HIV patients with high (> 500/mm³) CD$_4$ cell counts are more likely to have a typical pulmonary presentation, but patients with advanced HIV disease may have a diffuse interstitial pattern, hilar adenopathy, or a normal chest x-ray. Tuberculin skin testing (TST) is helpful if positive, but unreliable if negative due to anergy.

Diagnostic Considerations: In many urban areas, TB is one of the most common HIV-related respiratory illnesses. In other areas, HIV-related TB occurs infrequently except in immigrants or patients arriving from highly TB endemic areas. Maintain a high Index of suspicion for TB in HIV patients with unexplained fevers/pulmonary infiltrates.

Pitfalls: Extrapulmonary and pulmonary TB often coexist, especially in advanced HIV disease.

Therapeutic Considerations: Treatment by directly observed therapy (DOT) is strongly recommended for all HIV patients. If patients have cavitary disease or either positive sputum cultures or lack of clinical response at 2 months, total duration of therapy should be increased up to 9 months. If hepatic transaminases are elevated (AST > 3 times normal) before treatment initiation, treatment options include: (1) standard therapy with frequent monitoring; (2) rifamycin (rifampin or rifabutin) + EMB + PZA for 6 months; or (3) INH + rifamycin + EMB for 2 months, then INH + rifamycin for 7 months. Once-weekly rifapentine is not recommended for HIV patients. Non-severe immune reconstitution inflammatory syndrome (IRIS) may be treated with nonsteroidal anti-inflammatory drugs (NSAIDs); severe cases should be treated with corticosteroids. In all cases of IRIS, antiretroviral therapy should be continued if possible. Monitor carefully for signs of rifabutin drug toxicity (arthralgias, uveitis, leukopenia).

Prognosis: Usually responds to treatment. Relapse rates are related to the degree of immunosuppression and local risk of re-exposure to TB.

CNS Opportunistic Infections

CMV Retinitis

Preferred Therapy, Duration of Therapy, Chronic Maintenance	Alternate Therapy	Other Options/Issues
Preferred therapy for CMV retinitis *For immediate sight-threatening lesions* Ganciclovir intraocular implant + valganciclovir 900 mg (PO) q12h for 14–21 days, then q24h daily) One dose of intravitreal ganciclovir may be administered immediately after diagnosis until ganciclovir implant can be placed *For small peripheral lesions* Valganciclovir 900 mg (PO) q12h × 14–21 days, then 900 mg (PO) q24h	Alternative therapy for CMV retinitis Ganciclovir 5 mg/kg (IV) q12h × 14–21 days, then 5 mg/kg (IV) q24h; **or** Ganciclovir 5 mg/kg (IV) q12h × 14–21 days, then valganciclovir 900 mg (PO) q24h **or** Foscarnet 60 mg/kg (IV) q8h or 90 mg/kg (IV) q12h × 14–21 days, then 90–120 mg/kg (IV) q24h; **or** Cidofovir 5 mg/kg (IV) q week × 2 weeks, then 5 mg/kg (IV) every other week with saline hydration before and after therapy plus probenecid 2 g (PO) 3 hours before the dose followed by 1 g (PO) 2 hours after the dose, and 1 g (PO) 8 hours after the dose (total of 4 g) **Note:** This regimen should be avoided in patients with sulfa allergy because of cross hypersensitivity with probenecid	The choice of initial therapy for CMV retinitis should be individualized, based on location and severity of the lesion(s), level of immunosuppression, and other factors such as concomitant medications and ability to adhere to treatment Initial therapy in patients with CMV retinitis, esophagitis, colitis, and pneumonitis should include initiation or optimization of ART In patients with CMV neurological disease, localized morbidity might occur because of IRIS, a brief delay in initiation of ART until clinical improvement might be prudent Maintenance therapy for CMV retinitis can be safely discontinued in patients with inactive disease and sustained CD_4+ count

CMV Retinitis (cont'd)

Preferred Therapy, Duration of Therapy, Chronic Maintenance	Alternate Therapy	Other Options/Issues
Preferred chronic maintenance therapy (secondary prophylaxis) for CMV retinitis Valganciclovir 900 mg (PO) daily **or** Ganciclovir implant (may be replaced every 6–8 months if CD₄+ count remains < 100 cells/μL) + Valganciclovir 900 mg (PO) q24h until immune recovery	Alternative chronic maintenance (secondary prophylaxis) for CMV retinitis Ganciclovir 5 mg/kg IV 5–7 times weekly **or** Foscarnet 90–120 mg/kg (IV) q24h **or** Cidofovir 5 mg/kg (IV) of other week with saline hydration and probenecid (as above)	(> 100 cells/mm^3 for ≥ 3–6 months); consultation with ophthalmologist is advised Patients with CMV retinitis who discontinued maintenance therapy should undergo regular eye examination, optimally every 3 months, for early detection of relapse or immune recovery uveitis (IRU) IRU might develop in the setting of immune reconstitution. Treatment of IRU: periocular corticosteroid or short courses of systemic steroid

CMV Encephalitis

Pathogen	Preferred Therapy	Alternate Therapy
Cytomegalovirus (CMV)	Acute therapy Ganciclovir (GCV) 5 mg/kg (IV) q12h until symptomatic improvement (typically > 3 weeks). *For severe cases*, consider acute therapy with Ganciclovir 5 mg/kg (IV) q12h plus Foscarnet 90 mg/kg (IV) q24h until improvement Follow with lifelong suppressive therapy Valganciclovir 900 mg (PO) q24h	Acute therapy Foscarnet 60 mg/kg (IV) q8h or 90 mg/kg (IV) q12h × 3 weeks Follow with lifelong suppressive therapy Valganciclovir 900 mg (PO) q24h

CMV Retinitis
Clinical Presentation: Blurred vision, scotomata, field cuts common. Often bilateral, even when initial symptoms are unilateral.

Diagnostic Considerations: Diagnosis by characteristic hemorrhagic ("tomato soup and milk") retinitis on funduscopic exam. Consult ophthalmology in suspected cases.

Pitfalls: May develop immune reconstitution vitreitis after starting antiretroviral therapy.

Therapeutic Considerations: Oral valganciclovir is the preferred option for initial and maintenance therapy. Lifelong maintenance therapy for CMV retinitis is required for CD_4 counts < 100/mm³, but may be discontinued if CD_4 counts increase to > 100–150/mm³ for 6 or more months in response to antiretroviral therapy (in consultation with ophthalmologist). Patients with CMV retinitis who discontinue therapy should undergo regular eye exams to monitor for relapse. Ganciclovir intraocular implants might need to be replaced every 6–8 months for patients who remain immunosuppressed with CD_4 < 100–150/mm³. Immune recovery uveitis (IRU) may develop in the setting of immune reconstitution due to ART and be treated by ophthalmologist with periocular corticosteroid, sometimes systemic corticosteroid.

Prognosis: Good initial response to therapy. High relapse rate unless CD_4 improves with antiretroviral therapy.

CMV Encephalitis

Clinical Presentation: Encephalitis presents as fever, mental status changes, and headache evolving over 1–2 weeks. True meningismus is rare. CMV encephalitis occurs in advanced HIV disease (CD_4 < 50/mm³), often in patients with prior CMV retinitis. Polyradiculitis presents as rapidly evolving weakness/sensory disturbances in the lower extremities, often with bladder/bowel incontinence. Anesthesia in "saddle distribution" with ↓ sphincter tone possible.

Diagnostic Considerations: CSF may show lymphocytic or neutrophilic pleocytosis; glucose is often decreased. For CMV encephalitis, characteristic findings on brain MRI include confluent periventricular abnormalities with variable degrees of enhancement. Diagnosis is confirmed by CSF CMV PCR (preferred), CMV culture, or brain biopsy.

Pitfalls: For CMV encephalitis, a wide spectrum of radiographic findings are possible, including mass lesions (rare). Obtain ophthalmologic evaluation to exclude active retinitis. For polyradiculitis, obtain sagittal MRI of the spinal cord to exclude mass lesions, and CSF cytology to exclude lymphomatous involvement (can cause similar symptoms).

Therapeutic Considerations: For any established CMV disease, optimization of antiretroviral therapy is important along with initiating anti-CMV therapy. Ganciclovir plus foscarnet may be beneficial as initial therapy for severe cases. Consider discontinuation of valganciclovir maintenance therapy if CD_4 increases to > 100–150/mm³ × 6 months or longer in response to antiretroviral therapy.

Prognosis: Unless CD_4 cell count increases in response to antiretroviral therapy, response to anti-CMV treatment is usually transient, followed by progression of symptoms.

Cryptococcal Meningitis

Pathogen	Preferred Therapy	Alternate Therapy
Cryptococcus neoformans	Acute infection (induction therapy) Amphotericin B 0.7 mg/kg (IV) q24h × 2 weeks ± flucytosine (5-FC) 25 mg/kg (PO) q6h × 2 weeks **or**	Acute infection (induction therapy) Amphotericin B 0.7 mg/kg/day (IV) × 2 weeks **or** Fluconazole 400–800 mg (IV or PO) q24h × 6 weeks (less severe disease) **or**

Cryptococcal Meningitis (cont'd)

Pathogen	Preferred Therapy	Alternate Therapy
	Lipid amphotericin 4 mg/kg (IV) q24h × 2 weeks ± flucytosine (5-FC) 25 mg/kg (PO) q6h × 2 weeks	Fluconazole 400–800 mg (IV or PO) q24h *plus* flucytosine (5-FC) 25 mg/kg (PO) q6h × 4–6 weeks
	Consolidation therapy Fluconazole 400 mg (PO) q24h × 8 weeks or until CSF cultures are sterile	Consolidation therapy Itraconazole 200 mg (PO) q12h × 8 weeks or until CSF cultures are sterile
	Chronic maintenance therapy (secondary prophylaxis) Fluconazole 200 mg (PO) q24h	Chronic maintenance therapy Itraconazole 200 mg (PO) q24h for intolerance to fluconazole or failed fluconazole therapy

Clinical Presentation: Often indolent onset of fever, headache, subtle cognitive deficits. Occasional meningeal signs and focal neurologic findings, though non-specific presentation is most common.

Diagnostic Considerations: Diagnosis usually by cryptococcal antigen; India ink stain of CSF is less sensitive. Diagnosis is essentially excluded with a negative serum cryptococcal antigen (sensitivity of test in AIDS patients approaches 100%). If serum cryptococcal antigen is positive, CSF antigen may be negative in disseminated disease without spread to CNS/meninges. Brain imaging is often normal, but CSF analysis is usually abnormal with a markedly elevated opening pressure.

Pitfalls: Be sure to obtain a CSF opening pressure, since reduction of increased intracranial pressure is critical for successful treatment. Remove sufficient CSF during the initial lumbar puncture (LP) to reduce closing pressure to < 200 mm H_2O or 50% of opening pressure. Increased intracranial pressure requires repeat daily lumbar punctures until CSF pressure stabilizes; persistently elevated pressure should prompt placement of a lumbar drain or ventriculo-peritoneal shunting. Adjunctive corticosteroids are not recommended.

Therapeutic Considerations: Optimal total dose/duration of amphotericin B prior to fluconazole switch is unknown (2–3 weeks is reasonable if patient is doing well). Treatment with 5-FC is optional; however, since 5-FC is associated with more rapid sterilization of CSF, it is reasonable to start 5-FC and then discontinue it for toxicity (neutropenia, nausea). Fluconazole is preferred over itraconazole for life-long maintenance therapy. Consider discontinuation of chronic maintenance therapy in patients who remain asymptomatic with CD_4 >100–200/mm^3 for > 6 months due to ART.

Prognosis: Variable. Mortality up to 40%. Adverse prognostic factors include increased intracranial pressure, abnormal mental status.

Progressive Multifocal Encephalopathy (PML)

Pathogen	Therapy
Reactivation of latent papovavirus (JC strain most common)	Effective antiretroviral therapy with immune reconstitution

Clinical Presentation: Hemiparesis, ataxia, aphasia, other focal neurologic defects, which may progress over weeks to months. Usually alert without headache or seizures on presentation.

Diagnostic Considerations: Demyelinating disease caused by reactivation of latent papovavirus (JC strain most common). Diagnosis by clinical presentation and MRI showing patchy demyelination of white matter ± cerebellum/brainstem. JC virus PCR of CSF is useful for noninvasive diagnosis. In confusing or atypical presentation, biopsy may be needed to distinguish PML from other opportunistic infections, CNS lymphoma, or HIV encephalitis/encephalopathy.

Pitfalls: Primary HIV-related encephalopathy has a similar appearance on MRI.

Therapeutic Considerations: Most effective therapy is antiretroviral therapy with immune reconstitution. Some patients experience worsening neurologic symptoms once ART is initiated due to immune reconstitution induced inflammation. ART should be continued, with consideration of adjunctive steroids. Randomized controlled trials have evaluated cidofovir and vidarabine—neither is effective nor recommended.

Prognosis: Rapid progression of neurologic deficits over weeks to months is common. Best chance for survival is immune reconstitution in response to antiretroviral therapy, although some patients will have progressive disease despite immune recovery.

Toxoplasma Encephalitis

Pathogen	Preferred Therapy	Alternate Therapy
Toxoplasma gondii	<u>Acute therapy (× 6–8 weeks until good clinical response)</u> Pyrimethamine 200 mg (PO) × 1 dose, then 50 mg (< 60 kg body weight) or 75 mg (> 60 kg) (PO) q24h **plus** Sulfadiazine 1000 mg (< 60 kg) or 1500 mg (> 60 kg) (PO) q6h **plus** Leucovorin 10–25 mg (PO) q24h *For severely ill patients who cannot take oral medications*, treat with TMP–SMX (5 mg/kg TMP and 25 mg/kg SMX) (IV) q12h	<u>Acute therapy (× 6–8 weeks until good clinical response)</u> Pyrimethamine 200 mg (PO) × 1 dose, then 50 mg (< 60 kg body weight) or 75 mg (> 60 kg) (PO) q24h *plus* clindamycin 600 mg (IV or PO) q6h plus leucovorin 10 mg (PO) q24h **or** TMP–SMX (5 mg/kg TMP (IV or PO) q12h **or** Atovaquone 1500 mg (PO) q12h (with meals or nutritional supplement) plus pyrimethamine (as above) **or** Atovaquone 1500 mg (PO) q12h (with meals or nutritional supplement) *plus* sulfadiazine 1000–1500 mg (PO) q6h **or** Atovaquone 1500 mg (PO) q12h (with meals) **or** Pyrimethamine (see above) *plus* leucovorin 10 mg (PO) q24h *plus* azithromycin 900–1200 mg (PO) q24h

Toxoplasma Encephalitis (cont'd)

Pathogen	Preferred Therapy	Alternate Therapy
	<u>Follow with lifelong suppressive therapy</u> Sulfadiazine 500–1000 mg (PO) q6h **plus** Pyrimethamine 50 mg (PO) q24h **plus** Leucovorin 10–25 mg (PO) q24h	<u>Lifelong suppressive therapy</u> Clindamycin 600 mg (PO) q8h plus pyrimethamine 50 mg (PO) q24h *plus* leucovorin 10–25 mg (PO) q24h (2nd choice regimen) **or** Atovaquone 750 mg (PO) q12h ± pyrimethamine 25 mg (PO) q24h *plus* leucovorin 10 mg (PO) q24h (3rd choice regimen)

Clinical Presentation: Wide spectrum of neurologic symptoms, including sensorimotor deficits, seizures, confusion, ataxia. Fever/headache are common.

Diagnostic Considerations: Diagnosis by characteristic radiographic appearance and response to empiric therapy in a for T. gondii seropositive patient.

Pitfalls: Use leucovorin (folinic acid) 10 mg (PO) daily with pyrimethamine-containing regimens, not folate/folic acid. Radiographic improvement may lag behind clinical response.

Therapeutic Considerations: Alternate agents include atovaquone, azithromycin, clarithromycin, minocycline (all with pyrimethamine if possible). Decadron 4 mg (PO or IV) q6h is useful for edema/mass effect. Chronic suppressive therapy can be discontinued if patients are free from signs and symptoms of disease and have a CD_4 cell count > 200/mm³ for > 6 months due to ART.

Prognosis: Usually responds to treatment if able to tolerate drugs. Clinical response is evident by 1 week in 70%, by 2 weeks in 90%. Radiographic improvement is usually apparent by 2 weeks. Neurologic recovery is variable.

Gastrointestinal Tract Opportunistic Infections

Campylobacter (C. jejuni) Enteritis

Subset	Preferred Therapy
Mild disease	Might withhold therapy unless symptoms persist for several days
Moderate disease	Ciprofloxacin 500 mg (PO) q12h × 1 week **or** Azithromycin 500 mg (PO) q24h × 1 week
Bacteremia	Ciprofloxacin 500 mg (PO) q12h × 2 weeks* **or** Azithromycin 500 mg (PO) q24h × 2 weeks*

*   Consider addition of aminoglycoside in bacteremic patients.

Clinical Presentation: Acute onset of diarrhea, sometimes bloody; constitutional symptoms may be prominent.

Diagnostic Considerations: Diagnosis by stool culture; bacteremia may rarely occur, so blood cultures also indicated. Suspect campylobacter in AIDS patient with diarrhea and curved gram-negative rods in blood culture. Non-jejuni species may be more strongly correlated with bacteremia.

Therapeutic Considerations: Optimal therapy not well defined. Treat with quinolone or azithromycin; modify therapy based on susceptibility testing. Quinolone resistance can occur and correlates with treatment failure. Role of aminoglycoside is unclear.

Prognosis: Depends on underlying immune status; prognosis is generally good.

Clostridium difficile Diarrhea/Colitis

Pathogen	Preferred Therapy	Alternate Therapy
C. difficile	Metronidazole 500 mg (PO) q8h × 10–14 days. Avoid use of other C. difficile associated antibiotics if possible.	Vancomycin 125 mg (PO) q6h × 10–14 days. Avoid use of C. difficile associated antibiotics if possible.

Clinical Presentation: Diarrhea and abdominal pain following antibiotic therapy. Diarrhea may be watery or bloody. Proton pump inhibitors increase the risk. Among antibiotics, clindamycin and beta-lactams are most frequent. Rarely due to aminoglycosides, linezolid, doxycycline, TMP–SMX, carbapenems, daptomycin, vancomycin.

Diagnostic Considerations: Most common cause of bacterial diarrhea in U.S. among HIV patients. Watery diarrhea with positive C. difficile toxin in stool specimen. C. difficile stool toxin test is sufficiently sensitive/specific. If positive, no need to retest until negative (endpoint is end of diarrhea); if negative, no need to retest (repeat tests will be negative). C. difficile colitis may be distinguished clinically from C. difficile diarrhea by temperature > 102°F, ↑ WBC, ↑ ESR, and/or abdominal pain. C. difficile virulent epidemic strain is type B1 (toxinotype III), which produces 20-times the amount of toxin A/B compared to less virulent strains.

Pitfalls: In a patient with C. difficile diarrhea, C. difficile colitis is suggested by the presence of ↑ WBC, ↑ ESR, abdominal pain and temperature > 102°F; confirm diagnosis with CT of abdomen, which will show colonic wall thickening. New virulent strain of C. difficile may present with colitis with temperature ≤ 102°F, little/no ↑ WBC, and little/no abdominal pain; confirm diagnosis with CT/MRI of abdomen. C. difficile toxin may remain positive in stools for weeks following treatment; do not treat positive stool toxin unless patient has symptoms.

Therapeutic Considerations: Initiate therapy for mild disease with metronidazole; symptoms usually begin to improve within 2–3 days. For moderate or severe disease, or with evidence of colitis clinically (leukocytosis, fever, colonic thickening on CT scan), vancomycin has become the preferred agent in many centers due to concern for the more virulent strain, and based on the results of some observational studies suggesting vancomycin is more effective. The duration of therapy should be extended beyond 14 days if other systemic antibiotics must be continued. Relapse occurs in 10–25% of patients, and rates may be higher in patients with HIV due to the frequent need for other antimicrobial therapy. First relapses can be treated with a repeat of the initial regimen of metronidazole or vancomycin. For multiple relapses, a long-term taper is appropriate: week 1–125 mg 4x/day; week 2–125 mg 2x/day; week 3–125 mg once daily; week 4–125 mg every other day; weeks 5 and 6–125 mg every three days. Every effort should be made to resume a normal diet and to avoid other antibacterial therapies. Probiotic treatments (such as lactobacillus or Saccharomyces boulardii) have not yet been shown to reduce the risk of relapse in controlled clinical trials.

Prognosis: Prognosis with C. difficile colitis is related to severity of the colitis.

CMV Esophagitis/Colitis

Infection	Preferred Therapy	Alternate Therapy
Initial infection	Ganciclovir 5 mg/kg (IV) q12h × 3–4 weeks or until signs and symptoms have resolved. **or** Valganciclovir 900 mg (PO) q12h can be used if able to tolerate oral intake. Maintenance therapy is generally not necessary but should be considered after relapses	Foscarnet 90 mg/kg (IV) q12h × 3–4 weeks or until signs and symptoms have resolved **or** Cidofovir 5 mg/kg (IV) q every other week with saline hydration and probenecid (see CMV retinitis)
Relapses	Valganciclovir 900 mg (PO) q24h indefinitely; consider discontinuation if $CD_4 > 200/mm^3$ for ≥ 6 months on ART	

Clinical Presentation: Localizing symptoms, including odynophagia, abdominal pain, diarrhea, sometimes bloody stools.

Diagnostic Considerations: Diagnosis by finding CMV inclusions on biopsy. CMV can affect the entire GI tract, resulting in oral/esophageal ulcers, gastritis, and colitis (most common). CMV colitis varies greatly in severity, but typically causes fever, abdominal cramping, and sometimes bloody stools.

Pitfalls: CMV colitis may cause colonic perforation and should be considered in any AIDS patient presenting with an acute abdomen, especially if radiography demonstrates free intraperitoneal air.

Therapeutic Considerations: Duration of therapy is dependent on clinical response, typically 3–4 weeks. Consider chronic suppressive therapy for recurrent disease. Screen for CMV retinitis.

Prognosis: Relapse rate is greatly reduced with immune reconstitution due to antiretroviral therapy.

Cryptosporidia Enteritis

Pathogen	Preferred Therapy	Alternate Therapy
Cryptosporidium sp.	Effective ART with immune reconstitution to $CD_4 > 100/mm^3$ can result in complete resolution of symptoms and clearance of infection	Nitazoxanide 500 mg (PO) q12h × 4–6 weeks **or** Paromomycin 1 gm (PO) q12h × 2–4 weeks

Clinical Presentation: High-volume watery diarrhea with weight loss and electrolyte disturbances, especially in advanced HIV disease.

Diagnostic Considerations: Spore-forming protozoa. Diagnosis by AFB smear of stool demonstrating characteristic oocyte. Malabsorption may occur.

Pitfalls: No fecal leukocytes; organisms are not visualized on standard ova and parasite exams (need to request special stains).

Therapeutic Considerations: Anecdotal reports of antimicrobial success. Newest agent nitazoxanide may be effective in some settings, but no increase in cure rate for nitazoxanide if $CD_4 < 50/mm^3$. Immune reconstitution in response to antiretroviral therapy is the most effective therapy, and may induce prolonged remissions and cure. Anti-diarrheal agents (Lomotil, Pepto-Bismol) are useful to control symptoms. Hyperalimentation may be required for severe cases.

Prognosis: Related to degree of immunosuppression/response to antiretroviral therapy.

Isospora (Isospora belli) Enteritis

Subset	Preferred Therapy	Alternate Therapy
Acute infection	TMP 160 mg and SMX 800 mg (IV or PO) q6h × 10 days **or** TMP 320 mg and SMX 1600 mg (IV or PO) q12h × 10–14 days	Pyrimethamine 50–75 mg (PO) q24h *plus* leucovorin 5–10 mg (PO) q24h **or** Ciprofloxacin 500 mg (PO) q12h or other fluoroquinolones
Chronic maintenance therapy for CD$_4$ < 200 (secondary prophylaxis)	TMP 320 mg *plus* SMX 1600 mg (PO) q24h*	Pyrimethamine 25 mg (PO) q24h *plus* leucovorin 5–10 mg (PO) q24h*

* Discontinuation of secondary prophylaxis may be considered if CD$_4$ > 200/mm³ for > 3 months.

Clinical Presentation: Severe chronic diarrhea without fever/fecal leukocytes.
Diagnostic Considerations: Spore-forming protozoa (Isospora belli). Oocyst on AFB smear of stool larger that cryptosporidium (20–30 microns vs. 4–6 microns). More common in HIV patients from the tropics (e.g., Haiti). Less common than cryptosporidium or microsporidia. Malabsorption may occur.
Pitfalls: Multiple relapses are possible.
Therapeutic Considerations: Chronic suppressive therapy may be required if CD$_4$ does not increase.
Prognosis: Related to degree of immunosuppression/response to antiretroviral therapy.
Comments: Immune reconstitution with ART results in fewer relapses.

Microsporidia Enteritis

Pathogen	Therapy*
Microsporidia other than Enterocytozoon bienuesi	Albendazole 400 mg (PO) q12h (continue until CD$_4$ > 200/mm³)
Enterocytozoon bienuesi	Nitazoxanide 1 gm (PO) q12h × 60 days **or** Fumagillin 60 mg (PO) q24h (not available in the U.S.)
Trachipleistophora or Brachiola	Itraconazole 400 mg (PO) q24h plus albendazole 400 mg (PO) q12h

* Regardless of species, ART with immune reconstitution is a critical component of treatment.

Clinical Presentation: Intermittent chronic diarrhea without fever/fecal leukocytes.
Diagnostic Considerations: Spore-forming protozoa (S. intestinalis, E. bieneusi). Diagnosis by modified trichrome or fluorescent antibody stain of stool. Microsporidia can rarely disseminate to sinuses/cornea. Severe malabsorption may occur.
Pitfalls: Microsporidia is too small for detection by routine microscopic examination of stool.
Therapeutic Considerations: Albendazole is less effective for E. bieneusi than S. intestinalis, but speciation is usually not possible. May consider treatment discontinuation for CD$_4$ < 200/mm³ if patient remains asymptomatic (no signs or symptoms of microsporidiosis). If ocular infection is present, continue treatment indefinitely.
Prognosis: Related to degree of immunosuppression/response to antiretroviral therapy.

Oropharyngeal/Esophageal Candidiasis

Infection	Therapy	Fluconazole-Resistance
Oropharyngeal candidiasis (thrush)	<u>Preferred therapy</u> Fluconazole 100 mg (PO) q24h × 1–2 weeks <u>Alternate therapy</u> Itraconazole oral solution 200 mg (PO) q24h × 1–2 weeks **or** Clotrimazole troches 10 mg (PO) 5x/day × 1–2 weeks **or** nystatin suspension 4–6 mL q6h or 1–2 flavored pastilles 4–5x/day × 1–2 weeks	Fluconazole at doses up to 800 mg (PO) q24h × 1–2 weeks <div align="center">**or**</div>Caspofungin 70 mg (IV) on day 1, then 50 mg (IV) q24h × 1–2 weeks <div align="center">**or**</div>Micafugin 150 mg (IV) q24h × 1–2 weeks
Esophageal candidiasis	<u>Preferred therapy</u> Fluconazole 100 mg (up to 400 mg) (IV or PO) q24h × 1–2 weeks <u>Alternate therapy</u> Itraconazole oral solution 200 mg (PO) q24h × 2–3 weeks **or** Voriconazole 200 mg (PO) q24h × 2–3 weeks **or** Caspofungin 50 mg (IV) q24h × 2–3 weeks	Amphotericin B 0.3 mg/kg (IV) q24h × 1–2 weeks <div align="center">**or**</div>Lipid amphotericin 3–5 mg/kg (IV) q24h × 1–2 weeks

Oral Thrush (Candida)

Clinical Presentation: Dysphagia/odynophagia. More common/severe in advanced HIV disease.

Diagnostic Considerations: Pseudomembranous (most common), erythematous, and hyperplastic (leukoplakia) forms. Pseudomembranes (white plaques on inflamed base) on buccal muscosa/ tongue/gingiva/palate scrape off easily, hyperplastic lesions do not. Diagnosis by clinical appearance ± KOH/gram stain of scraping showing yeast/pseudomycelia. Other oral lesions in AIDS patients include herpes simplex, aphthous ulcers, Kaposi's sarcoma, oral hairy leukoplakia.

Pitfalls: Patients may be asymptomatic.

Therapeutic Considerations: Fluconazole is superior to topical therapy in preventing relapses of thrush and treating Candida esophagitis. Continuous treatment with fluconazole may lead to fluconazole-resistance, which is best treated initially with itraconazole suspension and, if no response, with IV caspofungin or amphotericin. Chronic suppressive therapy is usually only considered for severely immunosuppressed patients.

Prognosis: Improvement in symptoms are often seen within 24–48 hours.

Candida Esophagitis

Clinical Presentation: Dysphagia/odynophagia, almost always in the setting of oropharyngeal thrush. Fever is uncommon.

Diagnostic Considerations: Most common cause of esophagitis in HIV disease. For persistent symptoms despite therapy, endoscopy with biopsy/culture is recommended to confirm diagnosis and assess azole-resistance.

Pitfalls: May extend into stomach. Other common causes of esophagitis include CMV, herpes simplex, and aphthous ulcers. Rarely, Kaposi's sarcoma, non-Hodgkin's lymphoma, zidovudine, dideoxycytidine, and other infections may cause esophageal symptoms.

Therapeutic Considerations: Systemic therapy is preferred over topical therapy. Failure to improve on empiric therapy mandates endoscopy to look for other causes, especially herpes viruses/aphthous ulcers. Consider maintenance therapy with fluconazole for frequent relapses, although the risk of fluconazole resistance is increased. Fluconazole-resistance is best treated initially with itraconazole suspension and, if no response, with IV caspofungin, micafungin, or amphotericin.

Prognosis: Relapse rate related to degree of immunosuppression.

Salmonella Gastroenteritis (non-typhi)

Subset	Preferred Therapy	Alternate Therapy
Mild disease	Ciprofloxacin 750 mg (PO) q12h × 1–2 weeks	TMP–SMX 1 DS (PO) q12h × 2 weeks **or**
CD$_4$ < 200	Ciprofloxacin 750 mg (PO) q12h × 4–6 weeks	Ceftriaxone 2 gm (IV) q24h × 2 weeks **or**
Bacteremia	Ciprofloxacin 750 mg (PO) q12h × 4–6 weeks, then 500 mg (PO) q12h indefinitely	Cefotaxime 1 gm (IV) q8h × 2 weeks

Clinical Presentation: Patients with HIV are at markedly increased risk of developing salmonellosis. Three different presentations may be seen: (1) self-limited gastroenteritis, as typically seen in immunocompetent hosts; (2) a more severe and prolonged diarrheal disease, associated with fever, bloody diarrhea, and weight loss; or (3) Salmonella septicemia, which may present with or without gastrointestinal symptoms.

Diagnostic Considerations: The diagnosis is established through cultures of stool and blood. Given the high rate of bacteremia associated with Salmonella gastroenteritis—especially in advanced HIV disease—blood cultures should be obtained in any HIV patient presenting with diarrhea and fever.

Pitfalls: A distinctive feature of salmonella bacteremia in patients with AIDS is its propensity for relapse (rate > 20%).

Therapeutic Considerations: The mainstay of treatment is a fluoroquinolone; greatest experience is with ciprofloxacin, but newer quinolones (moxifloxacin, levofloxacin) may also be effective. For uncomplicated salmonellosis in an HIV patient with CD$_4$ > 200/mm^3, 1–2 weeks of treatment is reasonable to reduce the risk of extraintestinal spread. For patients with advanced HIV disease (CD$_4$ < 200/mm^3) or who have salmonella bacteremia, at least 4–6 weeks of treatment is required. Chronic suppressive therapy, given for several months or until antiretroviral therapy-induced immune reconstitution ensues, is indicated for patients who relapse after cessation of therapy. Consider using ZDV as part of the antiretroviral regimen (ZDV is active against Salmonella).

Prognosis: Usually responds well to treatment. Relapse rate in AIDS patients with bacteremia is > 20%.

Shigella (Shigella sp.) Enteritis

Subset	Preferred Therapy	Alternate Therapy
No bacteremia	Fluoroquinolone (IV or PO) × 3–7 days	TMP–SMX 1 DS tablet (PO) q12h × 3–7 days **or** Azithromycin 500 mg (PO) on day 1, then 250 mg (PO) q24h × 4 days
Bacteremia	Extend treatment duration to 14 days	Extend treatment duration to 14 days

Clinical Presentation: Acute onset of bloody diarrhea/mucus.

Diagnostic Considerations: Diagnosis by demonstrating organism in stool specimens. Shigella ulcers in colon are linear, serpiginous, and rarely lead to perforation. More common in gay men.

Therapeutic Considerations: Shigella dysentery is more acute/fulminating than amebic dysentery. Shigella has no carrier state, unlike Entamoeba. Shigella infections acquired outside of United States have high rates of TMP–SMX resistance. Therapy is indicated to shorten the duration of illness and to prevent spread of infection. Shigella has no carrier state.

Prognosis: Good if treated early. Severity of illness related to Shigella species: S. dysenteriae (most severe) > S. flexneri > S. boydii/S. sonnei (mildest).

TREATMENT OF OTHER OPPORTUNISTIC INFECTIONS IN HIV

Candida Vaginitis

Pathogen	Therapy
Candida albicans	Intravaginal miconazole suppository 200 mg q24h × 3 days or miconazole 3% × 7 days **or** Nystatin vaginal tablet 100,000U q24h × 14 days **or** Itraconazole 200 mg (PO) q12h × 1 day (or 200 mg q24h × 3 days) **or** Fluconazole 150 mg (PO) × 1 dose

Clinical Presentation: White, cheesy, vaginal discharge or vulvar rash ± itching/pain. Local infection not a sign of disseminated disease.

Diagnostic Considerations: Local infection. Not a manifestation of disseminated disease.

Pitfalls: Women with advanced AIDS receiving fluconazole may develop fluconazole-resistant Candida.

Therapeutic Considerations: For recurrence, consider maintenance with fluconazole 100–200 mg (PO) weekly.

Prognosis: Good response to therapy. Relapses are common.

Coccidioidomycosis (C. immitis) Infection

Infection	Therapy*
Non-meningeal infection	Acute therapy (diffuse pulmonary or disseminated disease) Amphotericin B 0.5–1.0 mg/kg (IV) q24h until clinical improvement (usually 500–1000 mg total dose). Some specialists add an azole to amphotericin B therapy Acute therapy (milder disease) Fluconazole 400–800 mg (PO) q24h or Itraconazole 200 mg (PO) q12h Chronic maintenance therapy (secondary prophylaxis) Preferred: Fluconazole 400 mg (PO) q24h indefinitely; alternative: or Itraconazole 200 mg capsule (PO) q12h indefinitely
Meningeal infection*	Acute therapy Fluconazole 400–800 mg (IV) or (PO) q24h. Intrathecal amphotericin B if no response to azole therapy Chronic maintenance therapy (secondary prophylaxis) Fluconazole 400 mg (PO) q24h or itraconazole 200 mg capsule (PO) q12h indefinitely

* Therapy for meningeal infection should be lifelong with fluconazole 400–800 mg q24h. There are insufficient data to recommend discontinuation of chronic maintenance therapy in other settings.

Clinical Presentation: Typically a complication of advanced HIV infection (CD$_4$ cell count < 200/mm³). Most patients present with disseminated disease, which can manifest as fever, diffuse pulmonary infiltrates, adenopathy, skin lesions (multiple forms – verrucous, cold abscesses, ulcers, nodules), and/or bone lesions. Approximately 10% will have spread to the CNS in the form of meningitis (fever, headache, altered mental status).

Diagnostic Considerations: Consider the diagnosis in any patient with advanced HIV-related immunosuppression who has been in a C. immitis endemic area (Southwestern US, northern Mexico) and presents with a systemic febrile syndrome. Diagnosis can be made by culture of the organism, visualization of characteristic spherules on histopathology, or a positive complement-fixation antibody (≥ 1:16). In meningeal cases, CSF profile shows low glucose, high protein, and lymphocytic pleocytosis.

Pitfalls: Antibody titers often negative on presentation. CSF profile of meningitis can be similar to TB.

Prognosis: Related to extent of infection and degree of immunosuppression. Clinical response tends to be slow, especially with a high disease burden and advanced HIV disease. Meningeal disease is treated life-long regardless of CD$_4$ recovery.

Extrapulmonary Tuberculosis

Pathogen	Therapy
Mycobacterium tuberculosis	Treat the same as pulmonary TB (see p. 326). May require longer duration of therapy based on clinical response

Clinical Presentation: Multiple presentations possible (e.g., lymphadenitis, osteomyelitis, meningitis, hepatitis). Dissemination is more common in patients with low CD$_4$ cell counts (< 100/mm³).

Diagnostic Considerations: Diagnosis by isolator blood cultures or tissue biopsy.
Pitfalls: Patients with disseminated disease frequently have pulmonary disease, which has implications for infection control.
Therapeutic Considerations: Response to therapy may be slower than in normal hosts.
Prognosis: Usually responsive to therapy.

Herpes Simplex Virus (HSV) Disease

Infection	Preferred Therapy	Alternate Therapy
Orolabial lesions or initial/recurrent genital HSV	Famciclovir 500 mg (PO) q12h × 1–2 weeks **or** valacyclovir 1 gm (PO) q12h × 1–2 weeks **or** acyclovir 400 mg (PO) q8h × 1–2 weeks	<u>Acyclovir-resistant HSV</u> Foscarnet 60–100 mg/kg (IV) q12h until clinical response **or** Cidofovir 5 mg/kg (IV) weekly until clinical response
Moderate-to-severe mucocutaneous HSV	Initial therapy: Acyclovir 5 mg/kg (IV) q8h × 2–7 days. If improvement, switch to famciclovir 500 mg (PO) q12h **or** valacyclovir 1 gm (PO) q12h **or** acyclovir 400 mg (PO) q8h to complete 7–10 days	<u>Acyclovir-resistant HSV</u> Foscarnet 60–100 mg/kg (IV) q12h until clinical response **or** Cidofovir 5 mg/kg (IV) weekly until clinical response
HSV keratitis	Trifluridine 1% ophthalmic solution, one drop onto cornea q2h, not to exceed 9 drops per day and no longer than 21 days. Treatment in conjunction with ophthalmology consultation	<u>Acyclovir-resistant HSV</u> Foscarnet 60–100 mg/kg (IV) q12h until clinical response **or** Cidofovir 5 mg/kg (IV) weekly until clinical response
HSV encephalitis	Acyclovir 10 mg/kg (IV) q8h × 2–3 weeks **or** Valacyclovir 1 gm (PO) q6h × 2–3 weeks	<u>Acyclovir-resistant HSV</u> Foscarnet 60–100 mg/kg (IV) q12h until clinical response **or** Cidofovir 5 mg/kg (IV) weekly until response
Multiple mucocutaneous (oral or anogenital) relapses (chronic suppressive therapy)	Acyclovir 400 mg (PO) q12h **or** Famciclovir 250 mg (PO) q12h **or** Valacyclovir 500 mg (PO) q12h	Patients may be able to titrate dose downward to maintain response

Herpes Simplex (genital/oral)

Clinical Presentation: Painful, grouped vesicles on an erythematous base that rupture, crust, and heal within 2 weeks. Lesions may be chronic, severe, ulcerative with advanced immunosuppression.
Diagnostic Considerations: Diagnosis by viral culture of swab from lesion base/roof of blister; alternative diagnostic techniques include Tzanck prep or immunofluorescence staining.

Pitfalls: Acyclovir prophylaxis is not required in patients receiving ganciclovir or foscarnet.

Therapeutic Considerations: In refractory cases, consider acyclovir resistance and treat with foscarnet. Topical trifluridine ophthalmic solution (Viroptic 1%) may be considered for direct application to small, localized areas of refractory disease; clean with hydrogen peroxide, then debride lightly with gauze, apply trifluridine, and cover with bacitracin/polymyxin ointment and nonadsorbent gauze; topical cidofovir (requires compounding) also may be tried. Chronic suppressive therapy with oral acyclovir, famciclovir, or valacyclovir may be indicated for patients with frequent recurrences, dosing similar to HIV-negative patients.

Prognosis: Responds well to treatment except in severely immunocompromised patients, in whom acyclovir resistance may develop. Prognosis for HSV meningitis is excellent.

Herpes Encephalitis (HSV-1)

Clinical Presentation: Acute onset of fever and change in mental status.

Diagnostic Considerations: EEG is abnormal early (< 72 hours), showing unilateral temporal lobe abnormalities. Brain MRI is abnormal before CT scan, which may require several days before a temporal lobe focus is seen. Definitive diagnosis is by CSF PCR for HSV-1 DNA. Profound decrease in sensorium is characteristic of HSV meningoencephalitis. CSF may have PMN predominance and low glucose levels, unlike other viral causes of meningitis. A different clinical entity is HSV meningitis, which is usually associated with HSV-2 and can recur with lymphocytic meningitis.

Pitfalls: Rule out noninfectious causes of encephalopathy. Surprisingly, HIV encephalitis is a relatively rare cause of encephalitis in patients with HIV.

Therapeutic Considerations: Treat as soon as possible since neurological deficits may be mild and reversible early on, but severe and irreversible later.

Prognosis: Related to extent of brain injury and early antiviral therapy. Prognosis for HSV meningitis is excellent.

Histoplasmosis (H. capsulatum), Disseminated

Subset	Preferred Therapy	Alternate Therapy
Acute phase (3–10 days or until clinically improved)	Liposomal amphotericin B 3 mg/kg × 1–2 weeks or other lipid associated formulations at 5 mg/kg	Amphotericin B doxychloate 0.7–1 mg/kg **or** Intravenous itraconazole (200 mg q12 × 4 doses then 200 mg q24)
Continuation phase	Itraconazole 200 (PO) TID × 3 days and then QD or BID for atleast 12 months (adequate serum levels should be confirmed). Immunosuppressed patients may require lifelong suppressive therapy.	Itraconazole oral solution 200 mg (PO) q12h × 12 weeks **or** Fluconazole 800 mg (PO) q24h × 12 weeks
Meningitis	Amphotericin B deoxycholate 0.7 mg/kg (IV) q24h × 12–16 weeks **or** Liposomal amphotericin B 4 mg/kg (IV) q24h × 12–16 weeks	Fluconazole 800 mg (PO) q24h × 12 weeks

*   Duration of therapy dependent on response to therapy.

Clinical Presentation: Two general forms: Mild disease with fever/lymph node enlargement (e.g., cervical adenitis), or severe disease with fever, wasting ± diarrhea/meningitis/GI ulcerations.

Diagnostic Considerations: Diagnosis by urine/serum histoplasmosis antigen, sometimes by culture of bone marrow/liver or isolator blood cultures. May occur in patients months to years after having lived/moved from an endemic area.

Pitfalls: Relapse is common after discontinuation of therapy. Cultures may take 7–21 days to turn positive.

Therapeutic Considerations: Initial therapy depends on severity of illness on presentation. Extremely sick patients should be started on amphotericin B deoxycholate, with duration of IV therapy dependent on response to treatment. Mildly ill patients can be started on itraconazole. All patients require chronic suppressive therapy, with possible discontinuation for immune reconstitution with CD_4 counts > 100/mm^3 for at least 6 months. HIV patients with CD_4 > 500/mm^3 and acute pulmonary histoplasmosis might not require therapy, but a short course of itraconazole (4–8 weeks) is reasonable to prevent systemic spread.

Prognosis: Usually responds to treatment, except in fulminant cases.

Mycobacterium avium-intracellulare (MAI)

Pathogen	Preferred Therapy	Alternate Therapy
Mycobacterium avium-intracellulare (MAI)	<u>At least 2 drugs as initial therapy</u> Clarithromycin 500 mg (PO) q12h plus ethambutol 15 mg/kg (PO) q24h (usually 800 mg or 1200 mg daily). Consider adding third drug, rifabutin 300 mg (PO) q24h, for patients with CD_4 < 50/mm^3, high mycobacterial loads and severely symptomatic disease. Duration of therapy is **lifelong**, although consider discontinuation in asymptomatic patients with > 12 months therapy and CD_4 > 100/mm^3 for > 6 months in response to ART	<u>Alternative to clarithromycin</u> Azithromycin 500–600 mg (PO) q24h <u>Alternative 3rd or 4th drug for severe symptoms or disseminated disease</u> Ciprofloxacin 500–750 mg (PO) q12h **or** Levofloxacin 500 mg (PO) q24h **or** Amikacin 10–15 mg/kg (IV) q24h

Clinical Presentation: Typically presents as a febrile wasting illness in advanced HIV disease (CD_4 < 50/mm^3). Focal invasive disease is possible, especially in patients with advanced immunosuppression after starting antiretroviral therapy. Focal disease likely reflects restoration of pathogen-specific immune response to subclinical infection ("immune reconstitution inflammatory syndrome" [IRIS]), and typically manifests as lymphadenitis (mesenteric, cervical, thoracic) or rarely disease in the spine mimicking Pott's disease. Immune reconstitution syndrome usually occurs within weeks to months after starting antiretroviral therapy for the first time, but may occur a year or more later.

Diagnostic Considerations: Diagnosis by isolation of organism from a normally sterile body site (blood, lymph node, bone marrow, liver biopsy). Lysis centrifugation (DuPont Isolator) is the preferred blood culture method. Anemia/↑ alkaline phosphatase are occasionally seen.

Pitfalls: Isolator blood cultures may be negative, especially in immune reconstitution inflammatory syndrome initially.

Therapeutic Considerations: Some studies suggest benefit for addition of rifabutin 300 mg (PO) q24h, others do not. Rifabutin may require dosage adjustment with NNRTI's and PI's. For concurrent use with nelfinavir, indinavir, or amprenavir, decrease rifabutin to 150 mg (PO) q24h. For concurrent use with ritonavir, decrease rifabutin to 150 mg (PO) 2–3x/week. For concurrent use with efavirenz, increase rifabutin to 450–600 mg (PO) q24h. The dose of PI's or NNRTI's may need to be increased by 20–25%. Monitor carefully for rifabutin drug toxicity (arthralgias, uveitis, leukopenia). Treat IRIS initially with NSAIDs; if symptoms persist, systemic corticosteroids (prednisone 20–40 mg daily) for 4–8 weeks can be used. Some patients will require a more prolonged course of corticosteroids with a slow taper over months. Azithromycin is often better tolerated than clarithromycin and has fewer drug-drug interactions. Optimal long-term management is unknown, though most studies suggest that treatment can be discontinued in asymptomatic patients with > 12 months of therapy and CD_4 > 100/mm³ for > 6 months.

Prognosis: Depends on immune reconstitution in response to antiretroviral therapy. Adverse prognostic factors include high-grade bacteremia or severe wasting.

Varicella Zoster Virus (VZV)

Infection	Preferred Therapy
Primary VZV infection (chickenpox)	Acyclovir 10 mg/kg (IV) q8h × 7–10 days. Can start with or change to oral therapy with Valacyclovir 1 gm (PO) q8h or Famciclovir 500 mg (PO) q8h after defervescence if no evidence of visceral involvement exists
Local dermatomal herpes zoster	Famciclovir 500 mg (PO) q8h × 7–10 days **or** Valacyclovir 1 gm (PO) q8h × 7–10 days
Extensive cutaneous or visceral involvement	Acyclovir 10 mg/kg (IV) q8h until cutaneous and visceral disease has clearly resolved and the patient is clinically improved
Acute retinal necrosis	Acyclovir 10 mg/kg (IV) q8h until progression stops, then Valacyclovir 1 gm (PO) q8h × 6 weeks. Treat in conjunction with close ophthalmologic consultation

Clinical Presentation: Primary varicella (chickenpox) presents as clear vesicles on an erythematous base that heal with crusting and sometimes scarring. Zoster usually presents as painful tense vesicles on an erythematous base in a dermatomal distribution. In patients with HIV, primary varicella is more severe/prolonged, and zoster is more likely to involve multiple dermatomes/disseminate. VZV can rarely cause acute retinal necrosis, which requires close consultation with ophthalmology.

Diagnostic Considerations: Diagnosis is usually clinical. In atypical cases, immunofluorescence can be used to distinguish herpes zoster from herpes simplex.

Pitfalls: Extend treatment beyond 7–10 days if new vesicles are still forming after initial treatment period. Corticosteroids for dermatomal zoster are not recommended in HIV-positive patients.

Therapeutic Considerations: IV therapy is generally indicated for severe disease/cranial nerve zoster.

Prognosis: Usually responds slowly to treatment.

HIV COINFECTIONS (HBV/HCV)

Hepatitis B Virus (HBV)

Preferred Therapy, Duration of Therapy, Chronic Maintenance	Alternate Therapy	Other Options/Issues
Therapy for patients who require ART Patients should be treated with agents active against both HIV and HBV or with agents with independent activity against each virus	Treatment for patients who do not require ART Use agents with sole activity against HBV and with the least potential of selecting HIV resistance mutations	Emtricitabine, entecavir, lamivudine, or tenofovir should not be used for the treatment of HBV infection in patients who are not receiving combination ART
Consider tenofovir + emtricitabine as part of HIV and HBV regimen	Consider early initiation of ART, especially for patients with high HBV DNA *For patients with CD$_4$+ count > 350 cells/μL, HBeAg (-), HBV DNA > 2,000 IU/mL (> 20,000 copies/mL)* Adefovir 10 mg PO daily	Among patients coinfected with HIV, HBV, and HCV, consideration of starting ART should be the first priority. If ART is not required, an interferon-based regimen, which suppresses both HCV & HBV, should be considered
Lamivudine or emtricitabine-naïve patients [Lamivudine 150 mg PO BID (or 300 mg PO daily) or emtricitabine 200 mg PO daily] + tenofovir (TDF) 300 mg PO daily (+ additional agent[s] active against HIV)		If IFN-based treatment for HCV has failed, treatment of chronic HBV with nucleoside or nucleotide analogs is recommended
Lamivudine or emtricitabine-experienced patients with detectable HBV DNA (assume lamivudine-resistance)		Cross-resistance to emtricitabine or telbivudine should be assumed in patients with suspected or proven 3TC resistance
If not on TDF: Add TDF 300 mg PO daily as part of an ART regimen + lamivudine or emtricitabine; **or** Adefovir 10 mg PO daily + lamivudine or emtricitabine + other combination ART; **or**	*For patients with CD$_4$+ count > 350 cells/μL, HBeAg (+), HBV DNA > 20,000 IU/mL (> 200,000 copies/mL), and elevated ALT*	When changing ART regimens, continue agents with anti-HBV activity because of the risk of IRIS

Hepatitis B Virus (HBV) (cont'd)

Preferred Therapy, Duration of Therapy, Chronic Maintenance	Alternate Therapy	Other Options/Issues
Entecavir 1 mg PO daily can be considered in patients with complete HIV suppression (while on ART) who do not demonstrate YMDD (M204V/I) motif mutations in HBV DNA Duration of therapy: Because of the high rates of relapse, certain specialists recommend continuing therapy indefinitely	Peginterferon alfa-2a 180 µg SQ weekly x 48 weeks—with careful follow-up of HBeAg conversion	If anti-HBV therapy is discontinued and a flare occurs, therapy should be reinstituted, as it can be potentially life saving

Adapted from: Sax PE, Cohen CJ, Kuritzkes DR. HIV Essentials, 4th edition. Jones & Bartlett, Sudbury, MA, 2011.

Epidemiology: Hepatitis B virus (HBV) infection is relatively common in patients with HIV, with approximately 60% showing some evidence of prior exposure. Chronic hepatitis B infection interacts with HIV infection in several important ways:

- HBV increases the risk of liver-related death and hepatotoxicity from antiretroviral therapy
- 3TC, FTC, and tenofovir each have anti-HBV activity. Thus selection of antiretroviral therapy for patients with HBV can have clinical and resistance implications for HBV as well as HIV. This is most notable with 3TC and FTC, as a high proportion of coinfected patients will develop HBV-associated resistance to these drugs after several years of therapy. This resistance reduces response to subsequent non-3TC or FTC anti-HBV therapy.
- Cessation of anti-HBV therapy may lead to exacerbations of underlying liver disease; in some cases, these flares have been fatal.
- Immune reconstitution may lead to worsening of liver status, presumably because HBV disease is immune mediated. This is sometimes associated with loss of HBEAg.
- Entecavir can no longer be recommended for HIV/HBV coinfected patients, as it has anti-HIV activity and may select for HIV resistance mutation M184V. If needed, it should be used only with a fully suppressive HIV regimen.

Diagnostic Consideration: Obtain HBSAb, HBSAg, and HBCAb at baseline in all patients. If negative, hepatitis B vaccination is indicated. If chronic HBV infection (positive HBSAg) is identified, obtain HBEAg, HBEAb, and HBV DNA levels. As with HCV infection, vaccination with hepatitis A vaccine and counseling to avoid alcohol are important components of preventive care. Isolated Hepatitis B Core Antibody: Many patients with HIV have antibody to hepatitis B core (anti-HBc) but are negative for both HBSAg and HBSAb. This phenomenon appears to be more common in those with HCV coinfection (Clin Infec Dis 2003 36:1602–6). In this scenario, diagnostic considerations include: (1) recently acquired HBV, before development of HBSAb; (2) chronic HBV, with HBSAg below the levels of detection; (3) immunity to HBV, with HBSAb below the levels of detection; (4) false-positive anti-HBV core. As the incidence of HBV is relatively low in most populations and anti-HBc alone is usually a stable phenomenon over years, recent acquisition of HBV is rarely the explanation. We recommend checking HBV DNA in this situation: If positive, this indicates chronic HBV; if negative, then low-level immunity or false-positive anti-HBV core remain as possible explanations; since distinguishing between these possibilities cannot be done, we recommend immunization with the hepatitis B vaccine series. It is useful to measure HBV serologic markers periodically in this population, as improvement in immune status due to ART may lead to increasing titers of HBSAb and subsequently confirm immunity.

Therapeutic Considerations: The optimal treatment for HBV infection is in evolution. Current guidelines suggest treatment of HBV in all patients with active HBV replication, defined as a detectable HBEAg or HBV DNA. Pending long-term studies defining optimal management, the recommendations set forth in the grid above are reasonable. Patients being treated with regimens for HBV should be monitored for ALT every 3–4 months. HBV DNA levels provide a good marker for efficacy of therapy and should be added to regular laboratory monitoring. The goal of therapy is to reduce HBV DNA to as low a level as possible, preferably below the limits of detection. The duration of HBV therapy is not well established; with development of HBEAb, while some individuals without HIV can stop therapy after reversion of HBEAg to negative, there are no clear stopping rules for HIV-coinfected patients.

Hepatitis C Virus (HCV)

Preferred Therapy, Duration of Therapy, Chronic Maintenance	Alternate Therapy	Other Options/Issues
<u>Genotype 1, 4, 5 or 6</u> Peginterferon alfa-2a 180 μg SQ weekly, **or** Peginterferon alfa-2b 1.5 mg/kg SQ weekly **plus** Ribavirin PO (wt-based dosing) < 75 kg: 600 mg qAM and 400 mg qPM; ≥ 75 kg: 600 mg qAM and 600 mg qPM	<u>In patients for whom ribavirin is contraindicated (e.g. unstable cardiopulmonary disease, pre-existing anemia unresponsive to erythropoietin, renal failure, or hemoglobinopathy)</u> Peginterferon alfa-2a 180 μg SQ weekly, **or** Peginterferon alfa-2b 1.5 μg/kg SQ weekly	For patients with CD$_4$+ count < 200 cells/μL, initiation of ART may be considered before HCV treatment Didanosine + Ribavirin may lead to increased mitochondrial toxicities; concomitant use is contraindicated

Hepatitis C Virus (HCV) (cont'd)

Preferred Therapy, Duration of Therapy, Chronic Maintenance	Alternate Therapy	Other Options/Issues
<u>Genotype 2 or 3</u> Peginterferon alfa-2a 180 μg SQ weekly, **or** Peginterferon alfa-2b 1.5 mg/kg SQ weekly **plus** Ribavirin (fixed dose) PO 400 mg qAM and 400 mg qPM Duration of therapy: 48 weeks-genotypes 1 or 4, 5 or 6 and genotypes 2 and 3 At least 24 weeks–treatment of acute HCV infection (< 6 months from HCV exposure)	<u>In patients with decompensated liver disease</u> Liver transplantation if feasible	HCV therapy is not recommended in patients with hepatic decompensation. Liver transplantation, if feasible, should be the primary treatment option Interferon is abortifacient in high doses and ribavirin is teratogenic. HCV treatment is not recommended in pregnant women or women who are not willing to use birth control

Adapted from: Sax PE, Cohen CJ, Kuritzkes DR. HIV Essentials, 5th edition. Jones & Bartlett, Sudbury, MA, 2012 (see also p. 97–100).

Epidemiology: Hepatitis C virus (HCV) infection is transmitted primarily through blood exposure; sexual and perinatal transmission are also possible but less efficient. A notable exception is sexually transmitted HCV among gay men. Since modes of transmission of HIV and HCV are similar, there are high rates of HCV coinfection in HIV—an estimated 16% of HIV patients overall, including 80% or more of IDUs and 5–10% of gay men. Genotype 1 accounts for 75% of HCV in the United States. HIV accelerates the progression of chronic HCV infection to cirrhosis, liver failure, and hepatocellular carcinoma. Data are conflicting regarding the independent effect of HCV on HIV disease progression, but several studies have shown a markedly higher rate of antiretroviral therapy-induced hepatotoxicity in those with chronic HCV. In some series, liver failure from HCV is one of the leading causes of death in HIV/HCV coinfected individuals.

Clinical Presentation: Persistently elevated liver transaminases; usually asymptomatic.

Diagnostic Considerations: All HIV-positive patients should be tested for HCV antibody. If the antibody test is negative but the likelihood of HCV infection is high (IDU, unexplained increase in LFTs), obtain an HCV RNA since false-negative antibody tests may occur, especially in advanced HIV disease. Since LFT elevation does not correlate well with underlying HCV activity, a liver biopsy is the best way to assess the degree of fibrosis and inflammation.

Therapeutic Considerations:

<u>Once Diagnosis is Established</u>. Advise patients to abstain from alcohol and administer vaccinations for hepatitis A and B (if non-immune). Also obtain HCV RNA levels with genotype assessment. HCV RNA levels do not have prognostic significance for underlying degree of liver disease, but higher levels make treatment for cure less likely. Genotype results also correlate with cure rates (reported

cure rates: 60–75% for genotypes 2 and 3; 15–25% for genotype 1). Some clinicians elect to treat HCV without a liver biopsy due to: the risks, costs, and discomfort of the test; the potential to underestimate the degree of HCV activity due to sampling error; and the high rate of treatment success for genotypes 2 and 3.

Optimal Patient Characteristics for HCV Treatment in HIV include no active psychiatric disease or substance abuse; stable HIV disease with undetectable HIV RNA and higher CD$_4$ cell count; receiving an antiretroviral regimen that does not contain ddI (in particular), d4T, or ZDV; and adherent to medications, follow-up visits, and blood test monitoring. Only a small proportion of patients will meet all these criteria; therefore, to maximize treatment effect, it is important to optimize clinical status prior to starting HCV therapy. Patients should be fully educated regarding the goals and risks of treatment, with provision of written information about side effects, local support groups, and whom to contact with questions. It is useful to administer the first dose of treatment in the office in order to provide instructions on injection techniques.

Choice of Drug Therapy. The treatment of choice for HCV infection is pegylated interferon plus ribavirin. All patients should also receive hepatitis A vaccine and counseling to avoid alcohol use.

- **Pegylated Interferon**. Two different formulations of pegylated interferon are available for treatment of HCV infection: (1) peginterferon alfa-2a (Pegasys), supplied as a pre-mixed solution and administered subcutaneously as a fixed dose of 180 mcg once a week; and (2) peginterferon alfa-2b (Peg-Intron), supplied as a powder that is reconstituted in saline and administered subcutaneously as a weight-based dose once a week. Efficacy and toxity of these two peginterferon preparations appear to be similar. Three clinical trials have shown that pegylated interferon plus ribavirin is more effective than standard interferon plus ribavirin (N Engl J Med 2004;351:451–9; N Engl J Med 2004;351:438–50; JAMA 2004;292:2839–48). Interferon has numerous side effects, the most important of which are listed in Table 5.9.

- **Ribavirin**. Ribavirin is available in 200-mg capsules. Although the dose used in clinical trials was 800 mg daily (400 mg BID), it appears that a higher initial dose is associated with greater efficacy. Standard dose is now 400 mg qAM and 600 mg qPM for weight < 75 kg, and 600 mg qAM and 600 mg qPM for weight > 75 kg. Ribavirin causes hemolytic anemia that predictably leads to a measurable decline in hemoglobin; this stabilizes by week 4–8 of treatment. Hemolytic anemia may be exacerbated in patients receiving ZDV; if possible an alternative NRTI should be chosen, with preference for tenofovir or abacavir. For symptomatic anemia or patients with coexisting conditions exacerbated by anemia, erythropoietin is used to maintain hemoglobin levels > 10 gm/dL or higher as needed. The typical starting dose of erythropoietin is 40,000 units SQ once a week. ddI is contraindicated during ribavirin administration due to an increased risk of mitochondrial toxicity and hepatic decompensation (Clin Infect Dis 2004;38:e79–e80). d4T should also be avoided because of its potential for inducing mitochondrial toxicity itself. Finally, some data suggest that ABC may interact with ribavirin, reducing efficacy of HCV therapy. Another common side effect of ribavirin is GI distress, which can overlap with a similar effect of interferon. Ribavirin is pregnancy category × (potent teratogen), and can only be used in sexually active women of childbearing potential if they are using 2 forms of birth control. Pregnancy should be avoided until at least 6 months after stopping ribavirin.

Monitoring. The monitoring plan for HIV/HCV coinfected patients consists of both safety and efficacy evaluations (Table 5.10). Results of HCV RNA testing are used to decide between completing 48 weeks of HCV therapy vs. discontinuing treatment at 12 or 24 weeks due to low probability of cure (Figure 5.3).

Figure 5.3. Management of HCV Infection Based on HCV RNA Testing

HCV RNA should be assessed at week 12. If the HCV viral load has not dropped by more than 2 logs (100–fold), then the likelihood of achieving a cure is extremely low. Many patients and providers will elect to discontinue therapy at this point, although theoretically low-dose peg-interferon may help improve liver fibrosis independent of its antiviral effect. (This strategy is being tested in clinical trials.) HCV RNA should be measured at weeks 24 and 48. If undetectable at week 48, additional measurements should be obtained at weeks 4, 12, and 24 after stopping treatment. An undetectable HCV RNA at week 24 post-treatment is the current standard for assessing a "sustained virologic response" (SVR), which can be equated with cure. Importantly, patients cured of HCV are susceptible to re-acquisition and should be cautioned about resuming high-risk behavior.

Table 5.9. Adverse Effects Associated with Interferon

Side Effect	Comments
Fatigue and flu-like symptoms (fever, chills, muscle aches, headache)	Dose at night so that some initial symptoms can be slept through. Symptoms may not peak until 48–78 hours after weekly dose and can be managed with acetaminophen (maximum 1300 mg/day) or ibuprofen plus good hydration. Fatigue is sometimes a manifestation of thyroid dysregulation or anemia; monitor thyroid function tests and CBC

Table 5.9. Adverse Effects Associated with Interferon (cont'd)

Side Effect	Comments
Depression	Interferon can aggravate life-threatening psychiatric conditions. Low threshold for initiating anti-depressant therapy. Patients with a pre-existing history of depression or other psychiatric disease should be followed closely by mental health professionals during HCV treatment
Leukopenia, thrombocytopenia, anemia	Cytopenias are more common in HIV/HCV co-infection. Can treat with G-CSF 300 mcg 3x/week if absolute neutrophil count is < 500/mm^3. If neutropenia persists, decrease dose of interferon. If platelet count falls to < 80,000/mm^3, also consider decreasing interferon dose (some clinicians tolerate counts down to 50,000/mm^3). Low threshold for use of erythropoietin (EPO) 40,000 U/week for anemia (see section on ribavirin)
Mouth ulcers	Topical viscous lidocaine or sucralfate is helpful in some
Gastrointestinal symptoms	Nausea and anorexia are the most common, often leading to weight loss. Advise patients to eat several small meals daily rather than a few large meals
Hair loss	Reversible after completion of therapy

Table 5.10. Monitoring Plan During Treatment for HCV Infection

	Weeks of Treatment								
	Baseline	2	4	8	12	16	20	24	24–28
CBC	X	X	X	X	X	X	X	X	q4 weeks
LFTs + metabolic panel	X		X	X	X	X	X	X	q4 weeks
HCV RNA	X		X¶		X*			X**	q12 weeks
HIV RNA + CD$_4$ profile	X				X†			X	q12 weeks

* Patients who have not dropped ≥ 2 logs from baseline HCV RNA at 12 weeks (early virologic response) have < 3% chance of obtaining a sustained viral response (undetectable HCV RNA 6 months post-treatment). Optimally, the HCV RNA will be undetectable by week 12 ("complete" early virologic response). One proposed strategy for patients with low-level detectable HCV RNA at week 12 ("partial" early virologic response) is to lengthen the course of therapy to 72 weeks or longer to reduce the risk of relapse; this is currently under investigation.

** If undetectable HCV RNA at 24 weeks, continue therapy for an additional 24 weeks (if known genotype 2 or 3 discuss option to stop, but some experts agree co-infected patients should continue treatment for 48 weeks to decrease risk of relapse). If HCV RNA is positive at 24 weeks, consider discontinuing HCV therapy. Even in patients without viral response, treatment may improve liver histology. Also see Figure 5.1.

† *Anticipate decrease in absolute cell count but stable CD$_4$%.*

¶ Check HCV RNA at week 4; if no decline in HIV RNA is seen, response is extremely unlikely. In contrast, ≥ 1 log decline can be very motivating and treatment should be continued. Best chance at cure is with an undetectable HIV RNA at 4 weeks, sometimes called a "rapid virologic response."

Table 5.10. Monitoring Plan During Treatment for HCV Infection (cont'd)

	Weeks of Treatment								
	Baseline	2	4	8	12	16	20	24	24–28
TSH	X				X			X	q12 weeks
Depression	X	X	X	X	X	X	X	X	ongoing
Ophthalmologic exam	X‡				X			X	q12 weeks
PT	X					X			q12 weeks
Pregnancy test	Perform at regular intervals if appropriate								

‡   Necessary for patients with a history of retinopathy; IFN package insert recommends screening for all patients prior to treatment. Many clinicians choose to defer the initial exam and monitor for disturbances in vision and loss of color perception.

Adapted from: Sax PE, Cohen CJ, Kuritzkes DR. HIV Essentials, 4th Edition, Jones & Bartlett, Sudbury, MA, 2011.

REFERENCES AND SUGGESTED READINGS

GUIDELINES

Antiretroviral Postexposure Prophylaxis After Sexual, Injection-Drug Use, or Other Nonoccupational Exposure to HIV in the United States. MMWR 54(RR02): 1–20, 2005.

Guidelines for Treating Opportunistic Infections Among HIV-Infected Adults and Adolescents. www.hivatis.org. January 29, 2008.

Management of Possible Sexual, Infection-Drug-Use, or Other Nonoccupational Exposure to HIV, Including Considerations Related to Antiretroviral Therapy 2005. www.hivatis.org.

Panel on Antiretroviral Guidelines for Adults and Adolescents. Department of Health and Human Services. Guidelines for the use of antiretroviral agents in HIV-infected adults and adolescents. http://aidsinfo.nih.gov/ConsenFiles/AdultandAdolescentGL.pdf, 2012.

Public Health Service Task Force Recommendations for Use of Antiretroviral Drugs in Pregnant HIV-1–Infected Women for Maternal Health and Interventions to Reduce Perinatal HIV-1 Transmission in the United States www.hivatis.org. November 2, 2007.

Thompson MA, Aberg JA, Cahn P. et al. Antiretroviral treatment of adult HIV infection: 2012 recommendations of the International Antiviral Society—USA panel. JAMA 308:387–402, 2012.

Updated Public Health Service Guidelines for the management of occupational exposures to HIV and recommendations for post-exposure prophylaxis. MMWR 54(RR-9):1–17, Sept. 30, 2005.

Updated U.S. Public Health Service Guidelines for the management of occupational exposures to HBV, HCV, and HIV and recommendations for postexposure prophylaxis. MMWR 50(RR-11); 1–42, June 29, 2001.

TEXTBOOKS

Dolin R, Masur H, Saag MS (eds). AIDS Therapy, 2nd Edition, Churchill Livingstone, New York, 2003.

Gorbach SL, Bartlett JG, Blacklow NR (eds). Infectious Diseases, 3rd Edition, Philadelphia, Lippincott, Williams & Wilkins, 2004.

Mandell GL, Bennett JE, Dolin R (eds). Mandell, Douglas, and Bennett's Principles and Practice of Infectious Diseases, 7th Edition, Philadelphia, Elsevier, 2010.

Sax PE, Cohen CJ, Kuritzkes DR (eds). HIV Essentials. 5th Edition, Jones & Bartlett, Sudbury, MA, 2012.

Wormser GP (ed). AIDS, 4th Edition, Elsevier, Philadelphia, 2004.

Chapter 6

Prophylaxis and Immunizations

Pierce Gardner, MD
John L. Brusch, MD
Jean E. Hage, MD
Ronald L. Nichols, MD
Staci A. Fischer, MD
Arthur Gran, MD
Burke A. Cunha, MD

*   For additional information on the prophylaxis of opportunistic infections in HIV see Chapter 5, pp. 320–323.

SURGICAL PROPHYLAXIS

Antibiotic prophylaxis is designed to prevent infection for a defined period of time. **Prophylaxis is most likely to be effective when given for a short duration against a single pathogen with a known sensitivity pattern,** and least likely to be effective when given for a long duration against multiple organisms with varying/unpredictable sensitivity patterns (Table 6.1). It is a common misconception that antibiotics used for prophylaxis should not be used for therapy and vice versa. **The only difference between prophylaxis and therapy is the inoculum size and the duration of antibiotic administration:** In prophylaxis, there is no infection, so the inoculum is minimal/none and antibiotics are administered only for the duration of exposure/surgical procedure. With therapy, the inoculum is large (infection already exists), and antibiotics are continued until the infection is eradicated.

Table 6.1. Factors Affecting the Efficacy of Surgical Antibiotic Prophylaxis

Number of Organisms	Susceptibility Pattern	Duration of Protection	Efficacy of Prophylaxis
Single organism	Predictable	Short	Excellent
Multiple organisms	Predictable	Short	Excellent
Single organism	Unpredictable	Short	Good
Single organism	Predictable	Long	Good
Multiple organisms	Unpredictable	Long	Poor/none

Antibiotic prophylaxis is designed to achieve effective antibiotic serum/tissue concentrations at the time of initial surgical incision, and is maintained throughout the "vulnerable period" of the procedure (i.e., time between skin incision and skin closure) (Table 6.2). If prophylaxis is given too early, antibiotic levels will be suboptimal/nonexistent when protection is needed. Properly timed pre-operative antibiotic prophylaxis is desirable for optimal effectiveness since **antibiotics given after skin closure are unlikely to be effective.** When no infection exists prior to surgery (clean/clean contaminated surgery), single-dose prophylaxis is preferred. When infection is present/likely prior to surgery ("dirty" surgery, e.g., perforated colon, TURP in the presence of positive urine cultures, repair of open fracture), antibiotics are given for > 1 day and represent early therapy, not true prophylaxis. Parenteral cephalosporins are commonly used for surgical prophylaxis, and ordinarily given as a bolus injection/rapid IV infusion 15–60 minutes prior to the procedure. Prophylaxis with vancomycin or gentamicin is given by slow IV infusion over 1–2 hours, starting ~1–2 hours prior to the procedure.

Table 6.2. Surgical Prophylaxis

Procedure	Usual Organisms	Preferred Prophylaxis	Alternate Prophylaxis	Comments
CNS shunt (VP/VA) placement, craniotomy, open CNS trauma	S. epidermidis (CoNS) S. aureus (MSSA)	MRSA/MRSE unlikely Ceftriaxone 1 gm (IV) × 1 dose MRSA/MRSE likely Linezolid 600 mg (IV) × 1 dose	MRSA/MRSE unlikely Cefotaxime 2 gm (IV) × 1 dose **or** Ceftizoxime 2 gm (IV) × 1 dose MRSA/MRSE likely Linezolid 600 mg (PO) × 1 dose **or** Vancomycin 1 gm (IV) × 1 dose **or** Minocycline 200 mg (IV) × 1 dose	Administer immediately prior to procedure. Vancomycin protects against wound infections, but may not prevent CNS infections. Give vancomycin slowly IV over 1 hour prior to procedure.
Thoracic (non-cardiac) surgery	S. aureus (MSSA)	Cefazolin 1 gm (IV) × 1 dose **or** Ceftriaxone 1 gm (IV) × 1 dose	Cefotaxime 2 gm (IV) × 1 dose **or** Ceftizoxime 2 gm (IV) × 1 dose	Administer immediately prior to procedure.
Cardiac valve replacement surgery	S. epidermidis (MSSE/MRSE) S. aureus (MSSA/ MRSA) Enterobacter	Vancomycin 1 gm (IV) × 1 dose **plus** Gentamicin 120 mg (IV) × 1 dose	Linezolid 600 mg (IV) × 1 dose **plus** Gentamicin 120 mg (IV) × 1 dose	Administer vancomycin and gentamicin slowly IV over 1 hour prior to procedure.
Coronary artery bypass graft (CABG) surgery	S. aureus (MSSA)	Cefazolin 2 gm (IV) × 1 dose **or** Ceftriaxone 1 gm (IV) × 1 dose	Cefotaxime 2 gm (IV) × 1 dose **or** Ceftizoxime 2 gm (IV) × 1 dose	Administer immediately prior to procedure. Except for ceftriaxone, repeat dose intraoperatively for procedures lasting > 3 hours.
Biliary tract surgery	E. coli Klebsiella E. faecalis (VSE)	Meropenem 1 gm (IV) × 1 dose **or** Piperacillin 4 gm (IV) × 1 dose	Ampicillin/ sulbactam 3 gm (IV) × 1 dose	Administer immediately prior to procedure (anaerobic coverage unnecessary).

Table 6.2. Surgical Prophylaxis (cont'd)

Procedure	Usual Organisms	Preferred Prophylaxis	Alternate Prophylaxis	Comments
Hepatic surgery	E. coli Klebsiella E. faecalis (VSE) B. fragilis	Ampicillin/ sulbactam 3 gm (IV) × 1 dose **or** Piperacillin 4 gm (IV) × 1 dose	Meropenem 1 gm (IV) × 1 dose **or** Moxifloxacin 400 mg (IV) × 1 dose	Administer immediately prior to procedure.
Stomach, upper small bowel surgery	S. aureus (MSSA) Group A streptococci	Ceftriaxone 1 gm (IV) × 1 dose **or** Cefazolin 1 gm (IV) × 1 dose	Cefotaxime 2 gm (IV) × 1 dose **or** Ceftizoxime 2 gm (IV) × 1 dose	Administer immediately prior to procedure (anaerobic coverage unnecessary).
Distal small bowel, colon surgery	E. coli Klebsiella B. fragilis	<u>Oral</u> Neomycin* **plus either** Erythromycin base* **or** Metronidazole* <u>Parenteral</u> Ertapenem 1 gm (IV) × 1 dose	Piperacillin 3 gm (IV) × 1 dose **or** Cefoxitin 2 gm (IV) × 1 dose **or combination therapy with** Metronidazole 1 gm (IV) × 1 dose **plus either** Ceftriaxone 1 gm (IV) × 1 dose **or** Levofloxacin 500 mg (IV) × 1 dose **or** Gentamicin 240 mg (IV) × 1 dose	Administer immediately prior to procedure. Give gentamicin slowly IV over 1 hour.
Pelvic (OB/GYN) surgery	Aerobic GNBs Anaerobic streptococci B. fragilis	Ceftriaxone 1 gm (IV) × 1 dose **plus** Metronidazole 1 gm (IV) × 1 dose	Cefotetan 2 gm (IV) × 1 dose **or** Cefoxitin 2 gm (IV) × 1 dose **or** Ceftizoxime 2 gm (IV) × 1 dose	Administer immediately prior to procedure.

* After appropriate diet and catharsis give either neomycin 1 gm (PO) plus erythromycin base 1 gm (PO) at 1 pm, 2 pm, and 11 pm, or give neomycin 2 gm (PO) plus metronidazole 2 gm (PO) at 7 pm and 11 pm the day before an 8 am operation.

Table 6.2. Surgical Prophylaxis (cont'd)

Procedure	Usual Organisms	Preferred Prophylaxis	Alternate Prophylaxis	Comments
Orthopedic prosthetic implant surgery (total hip/knee replacement)	S. epidermidis (CoNS) S. aureus (MSSA)	<u>MRSA/MRSE unlikely</u> Cefazolin 2 gm (IV) × 1 dose <u>MRSA/MRSE likely</u> Vancomycin 1 gm (IV) × 1 dose	<u>MRSA/MRSE unlikely</u> Ceftriaxone 1 gm (IV) × 1 dose <u>MRSA/MRSE likely</u> Linezolid 600 mg (IV) × 1 dose	Administer immediately prior to procedure. Postoperative doses are ineffective and unnecessary.
Arthroscopy	S. aureus (MSSA)	Cefazolin 1 gm (IV) × 1 dose **or** Ceftriaxone 1 gm (IV) × 1 dose	Cefotaxime 2 gm (IV) × 1 dose **or** Ceftizoxime 2 gm (IV) × 1 dose	Pre-procedure prophylaxis is usually unnecessary in clean surgical procedures.
Orthopedic surgery (open fracture)	S. aureus (MSSA) Aerobic GNBs	Ceftriaxone 1 gm (IV) × 1 week	Clindamycin 600 mg (IV) q8h × 1 week **plus** Gentamicin 240 mg (IV) q24h × 1 week	Represents early therapy, not true prophylaxis. Duration of post-op antibiotics depends on severity of infection.
Urological implant surgery	S. aureus (MSSA) Aerobic GNBs bacilli	Ceftriaxone 1 gm (IV) × 1 dose	Cefotaxime 2 gm (IV) × 1 dose **or** Ceftizoxime 2 gm (IV) × 1 dose	Administer immediately prior to procedure.
TURP, cystoscopy	P. aeruginosa P. cepacia P. maltophilia E. faecalis (VRE) Aerobic GNBs	Ciprofloxacin 400 mg (IV) × 1 dose **or** Piperacillin 4 gm (IV) × 1 dose	Levofloxacin 500 mg (IV) × 1 dose **or** Gatifloxacin 400 mg (IV) × 1 dose	Prophylaxis given to TURP patients with positive pre-op urine cultures. Represents early therapy, not true prophylaxis.
	E. faecium (VRE)	Linezolid 600 mg (IV) × 1 dose	Quinupristin/ dalfopristin 7.5 mg/kg (IV) × 1 dose	No prophylaxis required for TURP if pre-op urine culture is negative.

MSSA/MRSA = methicillin-sensitive/resistant S. aureus; MSSE/MRSE = methicillin-sensitive/resistant S. epidermidis.

POST-EXPOSURE PROPHYLAXIS

Some infectious diseases can be prevented by post-exposure prophylaxis (PEP). To be maximally effective, PEP should be administered within 24 hours of the exposure, since the effectiveness of prophylaxis > 24 hours after exposure decreases. PEP is usually reserved for persons with close/intimate contact with an infected individual. Casual contact does not warrant PEP.

Table 6.3. Post-Exposure Prophylaxis

Exposure	Usual Organisms	Preferred Prophylaxis	Alternate Prophylaxis	Comments
Meningitis	N. meningitidis	Any quinolone (PO) × 1 dose	Minocycline 100 mg (PO) q12h × 2 days **or** Rifampin 600 mg (PO) q12h × 2 days	Must be administered within 24 hours of close face-to-face exposure to be effective. Otherwise, observe and treat if infection develops. Avoid tetracyclines in children ≤ 8 years.
	H. influenzae	Rifampin 600 mg (PO) q24h × 3 days	Any quinolone (PO) × 3 days	Must be administered within 24 hours of close face-to-face exposure to be effective. H. influenzae requires 3 days of prophylaxis.
Viral influenza (human seasonal)	Influenza virus, type A or B	Oseltamivir (Tamiflu) 75 mg (PO) q24h for duration of outbreak (or at least 7 days after close contact to an infected person). For CrCl 10–30 cc/min, give 75 mg (PO) q48h‡	Rimantadine 100 mg (PO) q12h* for duration of outbreak (or at least 7–10 days after close contact to infected person) **or** Amantidine 200 mg (PO) q24h† for duration of outbreak (or at least 7–10 days after close contact to infected person)	Give to non-immunized contacts and high-risk contacts even if immunized. Begin at onset of outbreak or within 3 days of close contact to an infected person. Oseltamivir is active against both influenza A and B; rimantadine and amantadine are only active against influenza A. Oseltamivir may be ineffective due to resistance.

Table 6.3. Post-Exposure Prophylaxis (cont'd)

Exposure	Usual Organisms	Preferred Prophylaxis	Alternate Prophylaxis	Comments
Avian influenza	Influenza A (H_5N_1)	Oseltamivir (as for viral influenza, above)	Rimantadine **or** Amantadine[†] (as for viral influenza, above)	Oseltamivir may be ineffective due to resistance.
Swine influenza	Influenza A (H_1N_1)	Oseltamivir above (as for viral influenza, above)	None	Amantadine/rimantadine ineffective Continue PEP for swine influenza (H_1N_1) × 10 days post-close exposure.[‡]
Pertussis	B. pertussis	Erythromycin 500 mg (PO) q6h × 2 weeks	TMP–SMX 1 SS tablet (PO) q12h × 2 weeks **or** Levofloxacin 500 mg (PO) q24h × 2 weeks	Administer as soon as possible after exposure. Effectiveness is greatly reduced after 24 hours.
Diphtheria	C. diphtheriae	Erythromycin 500 mg (PO) q6h × 1 week **or** Benzathine penicillin 1.2 mu (IM) × 1 dose	Azithromycin 500 mg (PO) q24h × 3 days	Administer as soon as possible after exposure. Effectiveness is greatly reduced after 24 hours.
TB	M. tuberculosis	Rifampin 600 mg (PO) q24h × 4 months[§] **or** INH 300 mg (PO) q24h × 9 months	Rifapentine 900 mg (PO) q week **plus** INH 900 mg (PO) q week × 3 months (D.O.T.)	For INH, monitor SGOT/SGPT weekly × 4, then monthly. Mild elevations are common and resolve spontaneously. D/C INH if SGOT/SGPT levels ≥ 5 × normal.

* For elderly, severe liver dysfunction, or CrCl < 10 cc/min, give 100 mg (PO) q24h.

† For age ≥ 65 years, give 100 mg (PO) q24h. For renal dysfunction, give 200 mg (PO) load followed by 100 mg q24h (CrCl 30–50 ml/min), 100 mg q48h (CrCl 15–29 ml/min), or 200 mg weekly (CrCl < 15 ml/min).

‡ *Pediatric prophylaxis:* < 15 kg: 30 mg PO qd for 10 days, > 15-24 kg: 45 mg PO qd for 10 days, 24-40 kg: 60 mg PO qd for 10 days, > 40 kg: same as adults.

§ INH preferred if patient uses contact lens, has HIV, or is taking medications that may interact with rifampin.

Table 6.3. Post-Exposure Prophylaxis (cont'd)

Exposure	Usual Organisms	Preferred Prophylaxis	Alternate Prophylaxis	Comments
Gonorrhea (GC)	N. gonorrhoeae	Ceftriaxone 125 mg (IM) × 1 dose	Spectinomycin 2 gm (IM) × 1 dose **or** Any oral quinolone × 1 dose	Administer as soon as possible after sexual exposure (≤ 72 hours). Ceftriaxone also treats incubating syphilis.
Syphilis	T. pallidum	Benzathine penicillin 2.4 mu (IM) × 1 dose	Doxycycline 100 mg (PO) q12h × 1 week	Administer as soon as possible after sexual exposure. Obtain HIV serology.
Chancroid	H. ducreyi	Ceftriaxone 250 mg (IM) × 1 dose	Azithromycin 1 gm (PO) × 1 dose **or** Any oral quinolone × 3 days	Administer as soon as possible after sexual exposure. Obtain HIV and syphilis serologies.
Non-gonococcal urethritis (NGU)	C. trachomatis U. urealyticum M. genitalium	Azithromycin 1 gm (PO) × 1 dose **or** Doxycycline 100 mg (PO) q12h × 1 week	Any oral quinolone × 1 week	Administer as soon as possible after sexual exposure. Also test for gonorrhea/Ureaplasma.
Varicella (chicken-pox)	VZV	<u>Preferred:</u> For exposure < 72 hours, give varicella-zoster immune globulin (VZIG) 625 mcg (IM) × 1 dose to immuno-compromised hosts and pregnant women (esp. with respiratory conditions). For others or exposure > 72 hours, consider acyclovir 800 mg (PO) 5x/day × 5–10 days <u>Alternate:</u> Varicella vaccine 0.5 mL (SC) × 1 dose. Repeat in 4 weeks		Administer as soon as possible after exposure (≤ 72 hours). Varicella vaccine is a live attenuated vaccine and should not be given to immunocompromised or pregnant patients. If varicella develops, start acyclovir treatment immediately.

Table 6.3. Post-Exposure Prophylaxis (cont'd)

Exposure	Usual Organisms	Preferred Prophylaxis	Alternate Prophylaxis	Comments
Hepatitis A (HAV)	Hepatitis A virus	HAV vaccine 1 mL (IM) × 1 dose	Immune serum globulin (IG) 0.02 mL/kg (IM) × 1 dose	Give HAV vaccine alone if within 14 days after exposure.
Hepatitis B (HBV)	Hepatitis B virus	<u>Unvaccinated</u> Hepatitis B immune globulin (HBIG) 0.06 mL/kg (IM) × 1 dose **plus** HBV vaccine (40 mcg HBsAg/mL) deep deltoid (IM) at 0, 1, 6 months (can use 10-mcg dose in healthy adults < 40 years)	<u>Previously vaccinated</u> *Known responder* (anti-HBsAg antibody levels ≥ 10 IU/mL): No treatment. *Known non-responder* (anti-HBsAg antibody levels < 10 IU/mL): Treat as if unvaccinated. *Antibody status unknown:* Obtain HBsAg antibody levels to determine immunity status. If testing is not possible or results are not available within 24 hours of exposure, give HBIG plus 1 dose of HBV vaccine (booster).	
Hepatitis C (HCV)	Hepatitis C virus	None		
Rocky Mountain spotted fever	R. rickettsia	Doxycycline 100 mg (PO) q12h × 1 week	Any oral quinolone × 1 week	Administer prophylaxis after removal of Dermacentor tick.
Lyme disease	B. burgdorferi	Doxycycline 200 mg (PO) × 1 dose	Amoxicillin* 1 gm (PO) q8h × 3 days **or** Any oral 1st gen. cephalosporin* × 3 days **or** Azithromycin* 500 mg (PO) q24h × 3 days	If tick is in place ≥ 72 hours or is grossly engorged, prophylaxis may be given after tick is removed. Otherwise, prophylaxis is usually not recommended.

HDCV = human diploid cell vaccine, HRIG = human rabies immune globulin, PCEC = purified chick embryo cells, RVA = rabies vaccine absorbed.

* All or as much of the full dose of HRIG should be injected into the wound, and the remaining vaccine should be injected IM into the deltoid. Do not give HRIG at the same site or through the same syringe with PCEC, RVA, or HDCV.

Table 6.3. Post-Exposure Prophylaxis (cont'd)

Exposure	Usual Organisms	Preferred Prophylaxis	Alternate Prophylaxis	Comments
		* Although experience is limited, single-dose prophylaxis with these agents is probably also effective.		
Zoonotic diseases (plague, anthrax)	B. anthracis Y. pestis	Doxycycline 100 mg (PO) q12h for duration of exposure	Any oral quinolone for duration of exposure	Continued for the duration of a naturally-acquired exposure/outbreak. See p. 363 for bioterrorist plague/anthrax recommendations.
Rabies	Rabies virus	<u>No Previous Immunization</u> HRIG 20 IU/kg/* **plus either** PCEC 1 mL (IM) in deltoid **or** RVA 1 mL (IM) in deltoid **or** HDCV 1 mL (IM) in deltoid PCEC, RVA, HDCV given on days 0, 3, 7, 14, and 28 post-exposure	<u>Previous Immunization</u> PCEC 1 mL (IM) in deltoid on days 0 and 3 **or** RVA 1 mL (IM) in deltoid on days 0 and 3 **or** HDCV 1 mL (IM) in deltoid on days 0 and 3	Following unprovoked or suspicious dog or cat bite, immediately begin prophylaxis if animal develops rabies during a 10-day observation period. If dog or cat is suspected of being rabid, begin vaccination sequence immediately. Raccoon, skunk, bat, fox, and most wild carnivore bites should be regarded as rabid, and bite victims should be vaccinated against rabies immediately (contact local health department regarding rabies potential of animals in your area). All potential rabies wounds should immediately be thoroughly cleaned with soap and water. Do not inject rabies vaccine IV (may cause hypotension/shock). Serum sickness may occur with HDCV.

HDCV = human diploid cell vaccine, HRIG = human rabies immune globulin, PCEC = purified chick embryo cells, RVA = rabies vaccine absorbed.

* All or as much of the full dose of HRIG should be injected into the wound, and the remaining vaccine should be injected IM into the deltoid. Do not give HRIG at the same site or through the same syringe with PCEC, RVA, or HDCV.

Table 6.3. Post-Exposure Prophylaxis (cont'd)

Exposure	Usual Organisms	Preferred Prophylaxis	Alternate Prophylaxis	Comments
BIOTERRORIST AGENTS				
Anthrax *Inhalation/ cutaneous*	B. anthracis	Doxycycline 100 mg (PO) q12h × 60 days **or** Ciprofloxacin 500 mg (PO) q12h × 60 days **or** Levofloxacin 500 mg (PO) q24h × 60 days	Amoxicillin 1 gm (PO) q8h × 60 days	Duration of anthrax PEP based on longest incubation period of inhaled spores in nares.
Tularemia pneumonia	F. tularensis	Doxycycline 100 mg (PO) q12h × 2 weeks	Ciprofloxacin 500 mg (PO) q12h × 2 weeks **or** Levofloxacin 500 mg (PO) q24h × 2 weeks	Duration of PEP for tularemia is 2 weeks, not 1 week as for plague.
Pneumonic plague	Y. pestis	Doxycycline 100 mg (PO) q12h × 7 days **or** Ciprofloxacin 500 mg (PO) q12h × 7 days **or** Levofloxacin 500 mg (PO) q24h × 7 days	Chloramphenicol 500 mg (PO) q6h × 7 days	Pneumonic plague should be considered bioterrorism since most natural cases of plague are bubonic plague.
Smallpox	Variola virus	Smallpox vaccine ≤ 4 days after exposure	None	Smallpox vaccine is protective when diluted 1:5.
Viral hemorrhagic fever	Lassa fever	Ribavarin loading dose: 35mg/kg (PO) (not to exceed 2.5 g), then 15 mg/kg (PO) (not to exceed 1g) q8h × 10 days	None	Decrease maintenance dose to 7.5 mg/kg (PO) q8h if CrCl < 50/ml/min.

CHRONIC MEDICAL PROPHYLAXIS

Some infectious diseases are prone to recurrence/relapse and may benefit from intermittent or chronic suppressive therapy. The goal of suppressive therapy is to minimize the frequency/severity of recurrent infectious episodes.

Table 6.4. Chronic Medical Prophylaxis

Disorder	Usual Organisms	Preferred Prophylaxis	Alternate Prophylaxis	Comments
Asplenia/ impaired splenic function	S. pneumoniae H. influenzae N. meningitidis	Amoxicillin 1 gm (PO) q24h indefinitely	Respiratory quinolone* (PO) q24h indefinitely	Long-term prophylaxis effective. Vaccines may be given but are not always protective. Use amoxicillin in children.
UTIs (recurrent)	Gram-negative bacilli Enterococci	Nitrofurantoin 100 mg (PO) q24h × 6 months	Amoxicillin 500 mg (PO) q24h × 6 mos **or** TMP–SMX 1 SS tablet (PO) q24h × 6 months	Prophylaxis for reinfection UTIs (≥ 3 per year). Relapse UTIs should be investigated for stones, abscesses, or structural problems.
Asymptomatic bacteriuria in pregnancy	Gram-negative bacilli	Nitrofurantoin 100 mg (PO) q24h × 1 week	Amoxicillin 1 gm (PO) q24h × 1 week	Prophylaxis prevents symptomatic infections.
Prophylaxis of fungal infections in neutropenic patients†	Candida albicans Non-albicans Candida Aspergillus	Posaconazole 200 mg (PO) q8h **or** Itraconazole 200 mg (PO) q12h		Prophylaxis given until neutropenia resolves (absolute neutrophil count ≥ 500 cells/mm³).
Recurrent genital herpes (< 6 episodes/ year)	H. simplex (HSV-2)	Famciclovir 125 mg (PO) q12h × 5 days **or** Valacyclovir 500 mg (PO) q24h × 5 days	Acyclovir 200 mg (PO) 5x/day × 5 days	Begin therapy as soon as lesions appear. (For HIV disease, see Ch. 5.) Famciclovir 1 gm (PO) q12h × 1 day ↓ lesion progression by 2 days.
Recurrent genital herpes (> 6 episodes/ year)	H. simplex (HSV-2)	Famciclovir 250 mg (PO) q12h × 1 year **or** Valacyclovir 1 gm (PO) q24h × 1 year	Acyclovir 400 mg (PO) q12h × 1 year	Suppressive therapy is indicated for frequent recurrences. (For HIV disease, see Ch. 5.)

Table 6.4. Chronic Medical Prophylaxis (cont'd)

Disorder	Usual Organisms	Preferred Prophylaxis	Alternate Prophylaxis	Comments
Acute exacerbation of chronic bronchitis (AECB)	S. pneumoniae H. influenzae M. catarrhalis	Moxifloxacin 400 mg or levofloxacin 500 mg or gatifloxacin 400 mg or gemifloxacin 320 mg (PO) q24h × 5 days **or** Amoxicillin/clavulanic acid XR 2 tablets (PO) q12h × 5 days **or** Clarithromycin XL 1 gm (PO) q24h × 5 days **or** Doxycycline 100 mg (PO) q12h × 5 days **or** Azithromycin 500 mg (PO) × 3 days		Treat each episode individually.
Acute rheumatic fever (ARF)	Group A streptococci	Benzathine penicillin 1.2 mu (IM) monthly until age 30	Amoxicillin 500 mg (PO) q24h **or** Azithromycin 500 mg (PO) q72h until age 30	Group A streptococcal pharyngitis and acute rheumatic fever are uncommon after age 30.
Neonatal Group B streptococcal (GBS) infection (primary prevention)	Group B streptococci	Ampicillin 2 gm (IV) q4h at onset of labor until delivery	Clindamycin 600 mg (IV) q8h at onset of labor until delivery **or** Vancomycin 1 gm (IV) q12h at onset of labor until delivery	Indications: previous infant with GBS infection, maternal GBS colonization/infection during pregnancy, vaginal/rectal culture of GBS after week 35 of gestation, delivery ≤ week 37 of gestation without labor/ruptured membranes, ruptured membranes ≥ 12 hrs, or intrapartum temp ≥ 100.4°F.

*   Levofloxacin 500 mg (PO) or gatifloxacin 400 mg (PO) q24h or moxifloxacin 400 mg (PO).
†   During induction chemotherapy for acute myelogenous leukemia (AML) or myelodysplastic syndrome (MDS).

Table 6.5. Pre-Exposure Prophylaxis (PrEP)

Disorder	Usual Organisms	Preferred Prophylaxis	Alternate Prophylaxis	Comments
Repeated potential HIV exposures	HIV	Truvada 1 tablet (PO) q24h × 90 days (recheck HIV status)		Avoid if CrCl < 60 ml/min. Avoid if breast feeding.

Table 6.6. HIV Post-Exposure Prophylaxis (PEP)

Exposure	Preferred regimen	Recommended regimen	Alternate recommended regimen	Comments
HIV	**Truvada 1** tablet (PO) q24h [tenofovir 300 mg (PO) q24h + emtricitabine 200 mg (PO) q24h] × 4 weeks **plus** Raltegravir 400 mg (PO) q12h × 4 weeks	**Truvada 1** tablet (PO) q24h [tenofovir 300 mg (PO) q24h + emtricitabine 200 mg (PO) q24h] × 4 weeks **plus** (*one of the following*) Darunavir 800 mg (PO) q24h × 4 weeks **or** Atazanavir 300 mg (PO) q24h × 4 weeks **or** Fosamprenavir 1400 mg (PO) q24h × 4 weeks **plus** Ritonavir 100 mg (PO) q24h × 4 weeks	**Truvada 1** tablet (PO) q24h [tenofovir 300 mg (PO) q24h + emtricitabine 200 mg (PO) q24h] × 4 weeks **plus** Zidovudine 300 mg (PO) q12h × 4 weeks **or** **Truvada 1** tablet (PO) q24h [tenofovir 300 mg (PO) q24h + emtricitabine 200 mg (PO) q24h] × 4 weeks **plus** **Kaletra** 2 tablets (PO) q12h [lopinavir 200 mg (PO) q12h + ritonavir 50 mg (PO) q12h] × 4 weeks	...

Table 6.7. HIV: Prophylaxis of Opportunistic Infections

Disorder	Usual organism	Indication for Prophylaxis	Intervention
HIV	PCP	$CD_4 < 200/mm^3$	TMP-SMX: 1 SS tablet or 1 DS tablet (PO) q24h **or** Atovaquone 1500 mg (PO) q24h
	TB	PPD > 5 mm (current or past) or contact with active case	INH: 300 mg (PO) q24h × 9 months Rifabutin: Dose based on concomitant ART × 4 months
	Toxoplasmosis	IgG (+) and $CD_4 < 100/mm^3$	TMP-SMX: 1 DS tablet (PO) q24h
	MAI	$CD_4 < 50/mm^3$	Azithromycin: 1200 mg (PO) q week
	S.pneumoniae	$CD_4 > 200/mm^3$	Pneumococcal vaccine
	Hepatitis B (HBV)	Susceptible patients	Hepatitis B vaccine
	Hepatitis A (HAV)	Susceptible patients	Hepatitis A vaccine
	Influenza	All patients	Annual influenza vaccine
	VZV	$CD_4 > 200/mm^3$, VZV antibody negative	VZV vaccine

Table 6.8. Transplant Prophylaxis (BMT/SOT)

Exposure	Usual organism	Preferred prophylaxis	Alternate prophylaxis	Comments
Herpes simplex (HSV)	Herpes simplex	<u>HSV → < 6 recurrences/year</u> Valacyclovir 500 mg (PO) q24h × 30 days **or** Famciclovir 1 g (PO) q12 × 30 days	Acyclovir 400 mg (PO) q8h × 30 days post-BMT	<u>Acute prophylaxis</u> Nearly all post-tranplant HSV infections occur < 1 month. Transplants receiving CMV prophylaxis with ganciclovir, or valganciclovir are protected against HSV (see CMV prophylaxis).
		<u>HSV → > 6 recurrences/year</u> Valacyclovir 1 gm (PO) q24h × 90 days **or** Famciclovir 250 mg (PO) q12 × 30 days	Acyclovir 400 mg (PO) q8h × 90 days post-BMT	<u>Chronic prophylaxis</u> Valacyclovir 500 mg (PO) q12h **or** Famciclovir 500 mg (PO) q12h **or** Acyclovir 400 mg (PO) q8h
Varicella zoster virus (VZV)	Varicella zoster virus	<u>VZV seropositive recipient</u> Valacyclovir 500 mg (PO) q12h post-transplant x 4–24 months	Acyclovir 400 mg (PO) q8h post-transplant x 4–24 months	Post-transplant VZV infections occur later than HSV. > 95% of adults are VZV seropositive. In transplants, most VZV infections are due to reactivation rather than primary infection. Patients may develop shingles after prophylaxis is discontinued.
		<u>VZV seronegative recipient (VZV seropositive graft)</u> Valacyclovir 1 g (PO) q8h post-transplant x 4–24 months	Acyclovir 800mg (PO) 5x/day post-transplant x 4–24 months	Transplant recipients on CMV prophylaxis with gangciclovir or valganciclovir do not require VZV prophylaxis.

Table 6.8. Transplant Prophylaxis (BMT/SOT) (cont'd)

Exposure	Usual organism	Preferred prophylaxis	Alternate prophylaxis	Comments
Cytomegalovirus (CMV)	Transplants (SOT) D+/R-, D+/ R+, D-/R+	Valganciclovir 900 mg (PO) q24h × 3–6 months	Ganciclovir 5 mg/kg (IV) q24h × 3–6 months	Alternately, preemptive therapy may be used. When quantitative CMV PCR/pp 65 antigenemia levels become +/↑. D-/R- patients should receive CMV negative blood and leukocyte depleted RBCs but do not require antiviral prophylaxis.
PCP	SOT/ BMT (with GVHD)	TMP-SMX 1 DS tablet (PO) q week × 12 months	TMP-SMX 1 SS tablet (PO) q24h × 12 months *or* Atovaquone 1500 mg (PO) q24h × 12 months (with a meal)	See Drug Summaries for drug-drug interactions.
Toxoplasmosis	Heart transplants	TMP-SMX 1 DS tablet (PO) q24h	Atovaquone 1500 mg (PO) q24h (take with a meal)	See Drug Summaries for drug-drug interactions.
Candida sp.	Liver/ pancreas transplants	Fluconazole 400 mg (IV/PO) q24h × 4 weeks	Posacona-zole 200 mg (PO) q8h × 4 weeks	See Drug Summaries for drug-drug interactions.
Aspergillus sp.	Allogeneic BMT/lung transplants	Voriconazole 200 mg (PO) q12h	Posacona-zole 200 mg (PO) q8h	Until engrafted (BMT); duration in lung transplants unclear. See Drug Summaries for drug-drug interactions.

GVHD = graft vs. host disease.

ENDOCARDITIS PROPHYLAXIS

Endocarditis prophylaxis is now recommended only for previous endocarditis, prosthetic cardiac valve or prosthetic cardiac valve material, congenital heart disease (CHD), unrepaired cyanotic CHD, including palliative shunts and conduits, completely repaired congenital heart defects with prosthetic material/devices (placed by surgery or by catheter intervention during the first 6 months post-procedure), repaired CHD with residual defects adjacent to the site of prosthetic patch/device, and cardiac transplantation with cardiac valvupathy.

Table 6.9. Previous Indications for Infective Endocarditis (IE) Prophylaxis*

Subset	Prophylaxis Recommended (Column A)	Prophylaxis Not Recommended (Column B)
Cardiac conditions	• Ostium primum ASD • Prosthetic heart valves, including bioprosthetic and homograft valves • Previous infective endocarditis • Most congenital cardiac malformations • Rheumatic valve disease • Hypertrophic cardiomyopathy • MVP with significant valvular regurgitation • Calcific aortic stenosis	• Isolated ostium secundum ASD • Surgical repair without residue beyond 6 months of ostium secundum ASD or PDA • Previous coronary artery bypass surgery • MVP without valvular regurgitation • Physiologic, functional, or innocent murmurs • Previous Kawasaki's cardiac disease or rheumatic fever without valve disease
Procedures	• Dental procedures known to induce gingival/mucosal bleeding, including dental cleaning • Tonsillectomy or adenoidectomy • Surgical operations involving intestinal or respiratory mucosa • Cystoscopy or urethral dilation • Urethral catheterization or urinary tract surgery if UTI is present • Prostate surgery • I & D of infected tissue	• Dental procedures not likely to induce gingival bleeding • Tympanostomy tube insertion • Flexible bronchoscopy ± biopsy • Endotracheal intubation • Endoscopy ± gastrointestinal biopsy • Cesarean section • D & C, IUD insertion/removal, or therapeutic abortion in the absence of infection • Cardiac pacemaker/defibrillator insertion

* Wilson W, et al. Prevention of Infective Endocarditis. Circulation 116:1736–1754, 2007.

Table 6.9. Previous Indications for Infective Endocarditis (IE) Prophylaxis* (cont'd)

Subset	Prophylaxis Recommended (Column A)	Prophylaxis Not Recommended (Column B)
	• Biopsies of infected respiratory mucosa or infected skin/soft tissues • Any surgical procedure involving an infected field	• Coronary stent implantation • Percutaneous transluminal coronary angioplasty (PTCA) • Cardiac catheterization

ASD = atrial septal defect, D & C = dilatation and curettage, I & D = incision and drain, IUD = intrauterine device, MVP = mitral valve prolapse, PDA = patent ductus arteriosus, UTI = urinary tract infection.

*   Prophylaxis is indicated for patients with cardiac conditions in Column A undergoing procedures in Column A. Prophylaxis is not recommended for patients or procedures in Column B. See Tables 6.9 and 6.10 for prophylaxis regimens for above-the-waist and below-the-waist procedures, respectively.

Table 6.10. Endocarditis Prophylaxis for Above-the-Waist (Dental, Oral, Esophageal, Respiratory Tract) Procedures*

Prophylaxis	Reaction to Penicillin	Antibiotic Regimen
Oral prophylaxis	None	Amoxicillin 2 gm (PO) 1 hour pre-procedure†
	Non-anaphylactoid	Cephalexin 1 gm (PO) 1 hour pre-procedure
	Anaphylactoid	Clindamycin 300 mg (PO) 1 hour pre-procedure††
IV prophylaxis	None	Ampicillin 2 gm (IV) 30 minutes pre-procedure
	Non-anaphylactoid	Cefazolin 1 gm (IV) 15 minutes pre-procedure
	Anaphylactoid	Clindamycin 600 mg (IV) 30 minutes pre-procedure

*   Endocarditis prophylaxis is directed against viridans streptococci, the usual SBE pathogen above the waist. Macrolide regimens are less effective than other regimens; clarithromycin/azithromycin regimens (500 mg PO 1 hour pre-procedure) are of unproven efficacy.
†   Some recommend a 3 gm dose of amoxicillin, which is excessive given the sensitivity of viridans streptococci to amoxicillin.
††   Some recommend a 600 mg dose of clindamycin, but a 300 mg dose gives adequate blood levels and is better tolerated (less diarrhea).

Table 6.11. Endocarditis Prophylaxis for Below-the-Waist (Genitourinary, Gastrointestinal) Procedures Involving an Infected Field*†

Prophylaxis	Reaction to Penicillin	Antibiotic Regimen
Oral prophylaxis	None	Amoxicillin 2 gm (PO) 1 hour pre-procedure
	Non-anaphylactoid, anaphylactoid	Linezolid 600 mg (PO) 1 hour pre-procedure

COLOR ATLAS

CSF, Sputum, and Urine Gram Stains

Paul E. Schoch, PhD
Edward J. Bottone, PhD
Daniel Caplivski, MD

Staphylococcus aureus

Listeria monocytogenes

H. influenzae

Neisseria meningitidis

Klebsiella pneumoniae

Streptococcus pneumoniae

Streptococcus pneumoniae

Klebsiella pneumoniae

Hemophilus influenzae

Staphylococcus aureus

Moraxella catarrhalis

Pseudomonas aeruginosa

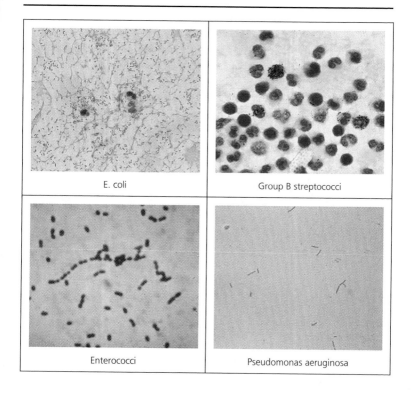

E. coli

Group B streptococci

Enterococci

Pseudomonas aeruginosa

COLOR ATLAS

Fungal Stains

Daniel Caplivski, MD
Edward J. Bottone, PhD

FUNGAL STAINS

Actinomyces (lung biopsy)

Candida albicans (blood)

Alternaria (skin biopsy)

Candida albicans with
pseudohyphae (blood)

Aspergillus (lung biopsy)

Candida as fungal ball (lung biopsy)

Candida (liver biopsy)

Fusarium (skin biopsy)

Cryptococcus (lung biopsy)

Histoplasma capsulatum (lung biopsy)

Cunninghamella (lung biopsy)

Malasezzia (blood)

Mucormycosis (bone marrow)

Pneumocystis (lung biopsy)

Nocardia (lung biopsy)

Rhizomucor (sinus biopsy)

Paracoccidioidomycosis (bone biopsy)

Scedosporium (lung biopsy)

Table 6.11. Endocarditis Prophylaxis for Below-the-Waist (Genitourinary, Gastrointestinal) Procedures Involving an Infected Field*† (cont'd)

Prophylaxis	Reaction to Penicillin	Antibiotic Regimen
IV prophylaxis	None	Ampicillin 2 gm (IV) 30 minutes pre-procedure **plus** Gentamicin 80 mg (IM) or (IV) over 1 hour 60 minutes pre-procedure
	Non-anaphylactoid, anaphylactoid	Vancomycin 1 gm (IV) over 1 hour 60 minutes pre-procedure **plus** Gentamicin 80 mg (IM) or (IV) over 1 hour 60 minutes pre-procedure

* Endocarditis prophylaxis is directed against E. faecalis, the usual SBE pathogen below the waist.
† Seto TB. The case for infectious endocarditis prophylaxis. Arch Intern Med 167:327–330, 2007.
 Harrison JL, Hoen B, Prendergast BD. Antibiotic Prophylaxis for Infective Endocarditis. Lancet 371: 1317–1319, 2008.

TRAVEL PROPHYLAXIS

Travelers may acquire infectious diseases from ingestion of fecally-contaminated water/ food, exchange of infected body secretions, inhalation of aerosolized droplets, direct inoculation via insect bites, or from close contact with infected birds/animals. Recommendations to prevent infection in travelers consist of general travel precautions (Table 6.12), and specific travel prophylaxis regimens (Table 6.13).

Table 6.12. General Infectious Disease Travel Precautions

Exposure	Risk	Precautions
Unsafe water (fecally-contaminated)	Diarrhea/ dysentery, viral hepatitis (HAV)	• Avoid ingestion of unbottled/unpotable water. Be sure bottled water has an unbroken seal and has not been opened/refilled with tap water. • Avoid ice cubes made from water of uncertain of origin/handling, and drinking from unclean glasses. • Drink only pasteurized bottled drinks. Be sure bottles/ cans are opened by you or in your presence. • Avoid drinking unpasteurized/warm milk; beer, wine, and pure alcoholic beverages are safe. • Eat only canned fruit or fresh fruit peeled by you or in your presence with clean utensils. • Avoid eating soft cheeses.

Table 6.12. General Infectious Disease Travel Precautions (cont'd)

Exposure	Risk	Precautions
		• Avoid eating raw tomatoes/uncooked vegetables that may have been exposed to contaminated water. • Avoid using hotel water for tooth brushing/rinsing unless certain of purity. Many hotels use common lines for bath/sink water that is unsuitable for drinking. • Avoid wading/swimming/bathing in lakes or rivers.
Food-borne (fecally-contaminated)	Diarrhea/dysentery	• Eat only seafood/poultry/meats that are freshly cooked and served hot. Avoid eating at roadside stands or small local restaurants with questionable sanitary practices. • "Boil it, peel it, or forget it."
Body fluid secretions	Viral hepatitis (HBV, HCV, etc.), STDs, HIV/other retroviruses	• Do not share utensils/glasses/straws or engage in "risky behaviors" involving body secretion exchange. • Avoid blood transfusion (use blood expanders instead). • Treat dental problems before travel.
Animal bite	Animal bite-associated infections	• Do not pet/play with stray dogs/cats. Rabies and other infections are common in wild (and some urban) animals.
Flying insects	Malaria, arthropod-borne infections	• Avoid flying/biting insects by wearing dark protective clothing (long sleeves/pants) and using insect repellent on clothes/exposed skin, especially during evening hours. • Minimize dawn-to-dusk outdoor exposure. • Use screens/mosquito nets when possible. • Do not use perfume, after shave, or scented deodorants/toiletries that will attract flying insects.

Table 6.13. Travel Prophylaxis Regimens

Exposure	Usual Pathogens	Prophylaxis Regimens	Comments
	E. coli Salmonella Shigella Non-cholera vibrios V. cholerae Aeromonas Plesiomonas Rotavirus Norwalk virus Giardia lamblia Campylobacter	Doxycycline 100 mg (PO) q24h for duration of exposure **or** Any quinolone (PO) for duration of exposure **or** TMP–SMX 1 SS tablet (PO) q24h for duration of exposure	Observe without prophylaxis and treat mild diarrhea symptomatically with loperamide (2 mg). Persons with medical conditions adversely affected by dehydration caused by diarrhea may begin prophylaxis after arrival in country and continue for 1 day after returning home. Should severe diarrhea/dysentery occur, continue/switch to a quinolone, maximize oral hydration, and see a physician if possible. Anti-spasmodics may be used

Table 6.13. Travel Prophylaxis Regimens (cont'd)

Exposure	Usual Pathogens	Prophylaxis Regimens	Comments
Traveler's diarrhea	Yersinia Cryptosporidium Cyclospora Enteroviruses Amebiasis		for symptomatic relief of mild, watery diarrhea but are contraindicated in severe diarrhea/dysentery. Bismuth subsalicylate is less effective than antibiotic prophylaxis. Most cases are due to enterotoxigenic E. coli. TMP–SMX is active against some bacterial pathogens and Cyclospora, but not against E. histolytica or enteroviral pathogens (e.g., Rotavirus, Norwalk agent). Doxycycline is active against most bacterial pathogens and E. histolytica, but misses Campylobacter, Cryptosporidium, Cyclospora, Giardia, and enteroviral pathogens. Rifaxamin only active against E.coli. Antibiotics are inactive against viral/parasitic pathogens causing diarrhea.
Meningococcal meningitis	N. meningitidis	<u>Pre-travel prophylaxis</u> Meningococcal conjugate vaccine 0.5 mL (IM) ≥ 1 month prior to travel to outbreak area <u>Post-exposure prophylaxis</u> See p. 358	Acquired via close face-to-face contact (airborne aerosol/droplet exposure). Vaccine is highly protective against N. meningitidis serotypes A, C, Y, and W-135, but misses B serotype.
Hepatitis A (HAV)	Hepatitis A virus	HAV vaccine 1 mL (IM) prior to travel, then follow with a one-time booster 3, 6 months later	HAV vaccine is better than immune globulin for prophylaxis. Take care to avoid direct/indirect ingestion of fecally contaminated water. HAV vaccine is recommended for travel to all developing countries. Protective antibody titers develop after 2 weeks.
Typhoid fever	S. typhi	ViCPS vaccine 0.5 mL (IM). Booster every 2 yrs for repeat travelers	For the oral vaccine, do not co-administer with antibiotics. Contraindicated in compromised hosts and children < 6 years old.

Table 6.13. Travel Prophylaxis Regimens (cont'd)

Exposure	Usual Pathogens	Prophylaxis Regimens	Comments
		or Oral Ty21a vaccine 1 capsule (PO) q48h × 4 doses. Booster every 5 years for repeat travelers	Take oral capsules with cold water. Degree of protective immunity is limited with vaccine. Some prefer chemoprophylaxis the same as for Traveler's diarrhea (p. 373).
Yellow fever	Yellow fever virus	Yellow fever vaccine 0.5 mL (SC). Booster every 10 years for repeat travelers	Vaccine is often required for travel to or from Tropical South America or Tropical Central Africa. Administer 1 month apart from other live vaccines. Contraindicated in children < 4 months old; caution in children < 1 year old. Reactions may occur in persons with egg allergies. Immunity is probably life long, but a booster every 10 years is needed for vaccination certification by some countries.
Japanese encephalitis (JE)	Japanese encephalitis virus	JE vaccine 1 mL (SC) on days 0, 7, and 14 or 30. Booster schedule not established	Recommended for travelers planning prolonged (> 3 week) visits during the rainy season to rural, endemic areas of Asia (e.g., Eastern Russia, Indian subcontinent, China, Southeast Asia, Thailand, Korea, Laos, Cambodia, Vietnam, Malaysia, Philippines). Administer 3, 2 weeks before exposure. Children < 3 years may be given 0.5 mL (SC) on same schedule as adults.
Rabies	Rabies virus	HDCV, PCEC, or RVA 1 mL (IM) on days 0, 7, and 21 or 28 prior to travel	Avoid contact with wild dogs/ animals during travel. Dose of rabies vaccine for adults and children are the same. A booster dose prior to travel is recommended if antibody levels are measured and are low.

Table 6.13. Travel Prophylaxis Regimens (cont'd)

Exposure	Usual Pathogens	Prophylaxis Regimens	Comments
		or HDCV 0.1 mL (ID) on days 0, 7, and 21 or 28 prior to travel	
Tetanus Diphtheria Pertussis	C. tetani C. diphtheriae B. pertussis	Tdap 0.5 ml (IM)	Tdap preferred to Td since Tdap also boosts pertussis immunity.

Table 6.14. Malaria Prophylaxis

Drug	Area of Exposure	Adult Dose	Comments
Atovaquone/ proguanil (Malarone)	Prophylaxis in all areas	Adult tablets contain 250 mg atovaquone and 100 mg proguanil hydrochloride. 1 adult tablet orally, daily	Begin 1–2 days before travel to malarious areas. Take daily at the same time each day while in the malarious area and for 7 days after leaving such areas. Contraindicated in persons with severe renal impairment (creatinine clearance < 30 mL/min). Atovaquone/ proguanil should be taken with food or a milk drink. Not recommended prophylaxis for pregnant women, and women breastfeeding.
Chloroquine phosphate (Aralen and generic)	Prophylaxis only in areas with chloroquine-sensitive malaria	300 mg base (500 mg salt) orally, once/ week	Begin 1–2 weeks before travel to malarious areas. Take weekly on the same day of the week while in the malarious area and for 4 weeks after leaving such areas.
Doxycycline	Prophylaxis in all areas	100 mg orally, (with food) daily	Begin 1–2 days before travel to malarious areas. Take daily at the same time each day while in the malarious area and for 4 weeks after leaving such areas. Contraindicated in children < 8 years and in pregnancy.

Table 6.14. Malaria Prophylaxis (cont'd)

Drug	Area of Exposure	Adult Dose	Comments
Hydroxy-chloroquine sulfate (Plaquenil)	An alternative to chloroquine for prophylaxis only in areas with chloroquine-sensitive malaria	310 mg base (400 mg salt) orally, once/week	Begin 1–2 weeks before travel to malarious areas. Take weekly on the same day of the week while in the malarious area and for 4 weeks after leaving such areas.
Mefloquine (Larium)	Prophylaxis in areas with mefloquine-sensitive malaria (mefloquine resistance in SE Asia)	228 mg base (250 mg salt) orally, once/week	Begin at least 2 weeks before travel to malarious areas. Take weekly on the same day of the week while in the malarious area and for 4 weeks after leaving such areas. Contraindicated in persons allergic to mefloquine or related compounds (e.g., quinine, quinidine) and in persons with active depression, a recent history of depression, generalized anxiety disorder, psychosis, schizophrenia, other major psychiatric disorders, or seizures. Use with caution in persons with psychiatric disturbances or a previous history of depression. Not recommended for persons with cardiac conduction abnormalities.
Primaquine[†]	Prophylaxis for short-duration travel to areas with principally P. vivax	30 mg base (52.6 mg salt) orally, daily	Begin 1–2 days before travel to malarious areas. Take daily at the same time each day while in the malarious area and for 7 days after leaving such areas. Contraindicated in persons with G6PD deficiency, pregnancy and breast feeding unless the infant being breastfed has a documented normal G6PD level.

Table 6.14. Malaria Prophylaxis (cont'd)

Drug	Area of Exposure	Adult Dose	Comments
Primaquine	Used for presumptive antirelapse therapy (terminal prophylaxis) to decrease the risk for relapses of P. vivax and P. ovale	30 mg base (52.6 mg salt) orally, once/day for 14 days after departure from the malarious area.	Indicated for persons who have had prolonged exposure to P. vivax and P. ovale or both. Contraindicated in persons with G6PD† deficiency. Also contraindicated during pregnancy and lactation unless the infant being breastfed has a documented normal G6PD level.

HDCV = human diploid cell vaccine, PCEC = purified chick embryo cell vaccine, RVA = rabies vaccine absorbed, RIG = rabies immune globulin.
† Glucose-6-phosphate dehydrogenase. Those who take primaquine should have a normal G6PD level before starting the medication.

TETANUS PROPHYLAXIS

Current information suggests that immunity lasts for decades/life-time after tetanus immunization. A tetanus booster should not be routinely given for minor wounds, but is recommended for wounds with high tetanus potential (e.g., massive crush wounds, soil-contaminated wounds, or deep puncture wounds).

Table 6.15. Tetanus Prophylaxis in Routine Wound Management

History of Adsorbed Tetanus Toxoid	Wound Type	Recommendations
Unknown or < 3 doses	Clean, minor wounds	Td‡ or Tdap‡
	Tetanus-prone wounds†	(Td‡ or Tdap‡) plus TIG
≥ 3 doses	Clean, minor wounds	No prophylaxis needed
	Tetanus-prone wounds†	Td‡ if > 10 years since last dose*

DT = diphtheria and tetanus toxoids adsorbed (pediatrics), DTP = diphtheria and tetanus toxoids and pertussis vaccine adsorbed, Td = tetanus and diphtheria toxoids adsorbed (adult), TIG = tetanus immune globulin, Tdap = tetanus and diphtheria toxoids and pertussis vaccine absorbed.
† For example, massive crush wounds; wounds contaminated with dirt, soil, feces, or saliva; deep puncture wounds; or significant burn wounds or frostbite.
‡ For children < 7 years, DTP (DT if pertussis is contraindicated) is preferred to tetanus toxoid alone. For children ≥ 7 years old and adults, Tdap is preferred to Td or tetanus toxoid alone.
* More frequent booster doses are unnecessary and can increase side effects. Protection lasts > 20 yrs
Adapted from: Centers for Disease Control and Prevention. MMWR Rep 40 (RR-10):1–28. 1991.

IMMUNIZATIONS

Immunizations are designed to reduce infections in large populations, and may prevent/ decrease the severity of infection in non-immunized individuals. Compromised hosts with altered immune systems may not develop protective antibody titers to antigenic components of various vaccines. **Immunizations are not fully protective, but are recommended** (depending on the vaccine) for most normal hosts, since some protection is better than none.

Table 6.16. Adult Immunizations

Vaccine	Indications	Dosage	Comments
Bacille Calmette Guérin (BCG)	Possibly beneficial for adults at high-risk of multiple-drug resistant tuberculosis.	Primary: 1 dose (intradermal). Booster not recommended.	Live attenuated vaccine induces a positive PPD which may remain positive for years/life. Contraindicated in immuno-compromised hosts. Injection site infection or disseminated infection are rare.
Hemophilus influenzae (type B)	Consider for patients with splenic dysfunction.	Primary: 0.5 mL dose (IM). Booster not recommended.	Capsular polysaccharide conjugated to diphtheria toxoid. Benefit uncertain. Safety in pregnancy unknown. Mild local reaction in 10%.
Hepatitis A (HAV)	All children beginning age 12 to 23 months and adults at increased risk of HAV.	Primary: 1 mL dose (IM). One-time booster ≥ 6 months later. Booster not routinely recommended.	Inactivated whole virus. Pregnancy risk not fully evaluated. Mild soreness at injection site. Occasional headache/malaise.
Hepatitis B (HBV)	Household/sexual contact with carrier, IV drug use, multiple sex partners (heterosexual), homosexual male activity, blood product recipients, hemodialysis, occupational exposure to blood,	Primary (3 dose series): Recombivax 10 mcg (1 mL) or Engerix-B 20 mcg (1 mL) IM in deltoid at 0, 1, and 6 months. Alternate schedule for Engerix-B: 4 dose series at 0, 1, 2, and 12 months. Booster	Recombinant vaccine comprised of hepatitis B surface antigen. For compromised hosts (including dialysis patients), use specially packaged Recombivax 40-mcg doses (1 mL vial containing 40 mcg/mL). HBsAb titers should be obtained 6 months after 3-dose primary series. Those with non-protective titers (≤ 10 mIU/mL) should receive 1 dose monthly

Table 6.16. Adult Immunizations (cont'd)

Vaccine	Indications	Dosage	Comments
	residents/staff of institutions for developmentally disabled, prison inmates, residence ≥ 6 months in areas of high endemicity, others at high risk.	not routinely recommended.	up to a maximum of 3 doses and retest for HbsAb titers. Pregnancy not a contraindication in high-risk females. Mild local reaction in 10–20%. Occasional fever, headache, fatigue, nausea. Twinrix 1 mL (IM) (combination of Hepatitis A inactivated vaccine and Hepatitis B recombinant vaccine) is available for adults on a 0, 1, and 6-month schedule or 0, 7 days, 21–30 days, and 12 month schedules.
Herpes zoster (VZV)	Adults ≥ 60 years to reduce the frequency of shingles/ prevent post-herpetic neuralgia. Use in those with previous H. zoster is not yet defined. Protection best in 60–69 year group; efficacy decreases with increasing age.	Primary: 0.65 mL (SC). Need for revaccination not yet defined. Vaccine must be stored frozen and used within 30 minutes after thawing.	Duration of protection is at least 4 years. Injection site reactions in 48%. Contraindicated in immunocompromised hosts (with immunosuppressive disorder or receiving immunosuppressive drug) or untreated TB. Not indicated for therapy of H. zoster or post-herpetic neuralgia.
Influenza	All adults.	Annual vaccine. Single 0.5 mL dose (IM) before flu season is optimal, but can be given anytime during flu season. High dose inactivated vaccine indicated for adults ≥ 65 years.	Trivalent inactivated whole and split virus. Contraindications include anaphylaxis to eggs or sensitivity to thimerosal. Mild local reaction in up to 30%. Occasional malaise/myalgia beginning 6–12 hours after vaccination. Neurologic and allergic reactions are rare. For pregnancy, administer in 2nd or 3rd trimester during flu season. A nasally-administered live attenuated influenza vaccine has been approved for healthy individuals aged 5–49 years.

Table 6.16. Adult Immunizations (cont'd)

Vaccine	Indications	Dosage	Comments
Measles	Adults born after 1956 without live-virus immunization or measles diagnosed by a physician or immunologic test. Also indicated for revaccination of persons given killed measles vaccine between 1963–67.	Primary: 0.5 mL dose (SC). A second dose (≥ 1 month later) is recommended for certain adults at increased risk of exposure (e.g., healthcare workers, travelers to developing countries). No routine booster.	Live virus vaccine (usually given in MMR). Contraindicated in compromised hosts, pregnancy, history of anaphylaxis to eggs or neomycin. Ineffective if given 3–11 months after blood products. Side effects include low-grade fever 5–21 days after vaccination (5–15%), transient rash (5%), and local reaction in 4–55% of persons previously immunized with killed vaccine (1963–67).
Meningococcus (invasive disease)	Patients with splenic dysfunction or defects in terminal complement; laboratory workers.	Meningococcal conjugate vaccine 0.5 mL (IM).	Also used in epidemic control of N. meningitides serogroups A, C, Y, and W-135.
Mumps	Non-immune adults.	Primary: 0.5 mL dose (SC). No routine booster.	Live attenuated vaccine (usually given in MMR). Contraindicated in immunocompromised hosts, pregnancy, history of anaphylaxis to eggs or neomycin. Side effects include mild allergic reactions (uncommon), parotitis (rare).
Papilloma (human) Virus (HPV)	Females up to 26 years of age. Contraindicated in pregnancy. Suggested for males up to 26 years of age.	Primary: 0.5 mL (IM). Second dose: 2 months after 1st dose. Third dose: 6 months after 1st dose.	Quadrivalent vaccine used to prevent genital warts (Condyloma accuminata), cervical cancer, AIS, CIN, VIN, VaIN due to HPV types 6, 11, 16, 18. Not indicated for therapy of active genital warts, cervical cancer, CIN, VIN, or VaIN.
Pertussis	Use Tdap instead of Td in booster dose.	A Single Tdap booster dose 0.5 mL (IM). Schedule for subsequent boosters to be determined.	Recommended since adults may get pertussis or transmit it to susceptible infants.

Table 6.16. Adult Immunizations (cont'd)

Vaccine	Indications	Dosage	Comments
Pneumococcus (S. neumoniae)	Immunocompetent hosts ≥ 65 years old, or > 2 years old with diabetes, CSF leaks, or chronic cardiac, pulmonary or liver disease. Also for immunocompromised hosts > 2 years old with functional/anatomic asplenia, leukemia, lymphoma, multiple myeloma, widespread malignancy, chronic renal failure, bone marrow/organ transplant, or on immunosuppressive/ steroid therapy.	Primary: 0.5 mL dose (SC or IM). A one-time booster at 5 years is recommended for immuno compromised hosts > 2 years old and for those who received the vaccine before age 65 for high-risk conditions.	Polyvalent vaccine against 23 strains. Studies are inadequate regarding routine reimmunization. Practitioners should decide their own policy.
Rubella	Non-immune adults, particularly women of childbearing age.	Primary: 0.5 mL dose (SC). No routine booster.	Live virus (RA 27/3 strain) vaccine (usually given in MMR). Contraindicated in immuno-compromised hosts, pregnancy, history of anaphylactic reaction to neomycin. Joint pains and transient arthralgias in up to 40%, beginning 3–25 days after vaccination and lasting 1–11 days; frank arthritis in < 2%.
Tetanus-diphtheria	Adults	Primary: Td two 0.5 mL doses (IM), 1–2 months apart; third dose 6–12 months after second dose. Booster: a single Tdap 0.5 mL (IM) is recommended. Tdap should be substituted for one of the three Td doses.	Adsorbed toxoid vaccine. Contraindicated if hypersensitivity/neurological reaction or severe local reaction to previous doses. Side effects include local reactions, occasional fever, systemic symptoms, Arthus-like reaction in persons with multiple previous boosters, and systemic allergy (rare).

Table 6.16. Adult Immunizations (cont'd)

Vaccine	Indications	Dosage	Comments
Varicella (VZV) chickenpox	Non-immune adolescents and adults, especially healthcare workers and others likely to be exposed.	Primary: Two 0.5 mL doses (SC), 4–8 weeks apart. Vaccine must be stored frozen and used within 30 minutes after thawing and reconstitution. No routine booster.	Live attenuated vaccine. Contraindications include pregnancy, active untreated TB, immunocompromised host, malignancy of bone marrow or lymphatic system, anaphylactic reaction to gelatin/neomycin, or blood product recipient within previous 6 months (may prevent development of protective antibody). Mild febrile illness in 10%. Injection site symptoms in 25–30% (local rash in 3%). Mild diffuse rash in 5%.

REFERENCES AND SUGGESTED READINGS

Andrews WW, Kimberlin DF, Whitley R, Cliver S, Ramsey PS. Valacyclovir therapy to reduce recurrent genital herpes in pregnant women. Am J Obstet Gynecol 194:774–81, 2006.

Antrum RM, Solomkin JS. A review of antibiotic prophylaxis for open fractures. Orthop Rev 16:246–54, 1987.

Batiuk TD, Bodziak KA, Goldman M. Infectious disease prophylaxis in renal transplant patients: a survey of US transplant centers. Clin Transplant 16:1–8, 2002.

Baum SG. Oseltamivir and the influenza alphabet. Clin Infect Dis 43:445–6, 2006.

Bennett JE, Echinocandins for Candidemia in Adults without Neutropenia. New Engl J Med 355:1154–9, 2006.

Bow EJ, Rotstein C, Noskin GA, et al. A Randomized, Open-Label, Multicenter Comparative Study of the Efficacy and Safety of Piperacillin-Tazobactam and Cefepime for the Empirical Treatment of Febrile Neutropenic Episodes in Patients with Hematologic Malignancies. Clin Infect Dis 43:447–59, 2006.

Brantley JS, Hicks L, Sra K, Tyring SK. Valacyclovir for the treatment of genital herpes. Expert Rev Anti-Infect Ther 4:367–76, 2006.

Camann W, Tuomala R. Antibiotic prophylaxis for cesarean delivery: always before skin incision! Int J Obstet Anesth 20:1–2, 2011.

Caple J. Varicella-Zoster Virus vaccine: a review of its use in the prevention of Herpes Zoster in older adults. Drugs of Today 42:249–54, 2006.

Carratala J. Role of antibiotic prophylaxis for the prevention of intravascular catheter-related infection. Clin Microbiol Infect 7 (Suppl 4):83–90, 2001.

Centers for Disease Control and Prevention. Recommended adult immunization schedule—United States, 2012. MMWR, 61(4):1–7, 2012.

Chen LH, Wilson ME, Schlagenhauf P. Prevention of Malaria in Long-term Travelers. JAMA 296:2234–44, 2006.

Chattopadhyay B. Splenectomy pneumococcal vaccination and antibiotic prophylaxis. Br J Hosp Med 41:172–4, 1989.

Colizza S, Rossi S. Antibiotic prophylaxis and treatment of surgical abdominal sepsis. J Chemother 13:193–201, 2001.

Craig AS, Schaffner W. Prevention of hepatitis A with the hepatitis A vaccine. N Engl J Med 350:476–81, 2004.

Cullen M, Steven N, Billingham L, et al. Antibacterial prophylaxis after chemotherapy for solid tumors and lymphomas. N Engl J Med 353:988–98, 2005.

Cunha BA, Gossling HR, Nightingale CH, et al. Penetration of cefazolin and cefradine into bone in patients undergoing total knee arthroplasty. Infection 2: 80–84, 1984.

Cunha BA. Antibiotic tissue penetration. Bulletin of the New York Academy of Medicine 59:443–449, 1983.

Cunha BA, Ristuccia A, Jonas M, et al. Penetration of ceftizoxime and cefazolin into bile and gallbladder wall. Journal of Antimicrobial Chemotherapy 10: 117–120, 1982.

Cunha BA, Pyrtek LJ, Quintiliani R. Prophylactic antibiotics in cholecystectomy. Lancet 1:207–8, 1979.

Cunha BA, Gossling HR, Nightingale C, et al. Penetration characteristics of cefazolin, cephalothin, and cephradine into bone in patients undergoing total hip replacement. Journal of Bone and Surgery 59: 856–859, 1977.

Darouiche RG. Treatment of infections associated with surgical implants. N Engl J Med 350:1422–9, 2004.

De Lall F. Antibiotic prophylaxis in orthopedic prosthetic surgery. J Chemother 13 Spec No 1:48–53, 2001.

De la Camara R. Antifungal prophylaxis in haematology patients. 12:S65–76, 2006.

Diaz-Pedroche C, Lumbreras C, San Juan R, et al. Valganciclovir preemptive therapy for the prevention of cytomegalovirus disease in high-risk seropositive solid-organ transplant recipients. Transplantation 82:30–5, 2006.

Dietrich ES, Bieser U, Frank U, et al. Ceftriaxone versus other cephalosporins for perioperative antibiotic prophylaxis: a meta analysis of 43 randomized controlled trials. Chemotherapy 48:49–56, 2002.

Drew RH, Perfect JR.Use of Polyenes for Prophylaxis for Invasive Fungal Infections. Infections in Medicine 23:S12–24, 2006.

Esposito S. Is single-dose antibiotic prophylaxis sufficient for any surgical procedure? J Chemother 11:556, 2000.

Faix, RG. Immunization during pregnancy. Clin Obstet Gynecol 45:42–58, 2002.

Fennessy BG, O'Sullivan MJ, Fulton GJ, et al. Prospective Study of Use of Perioperative Antimicrobial Therapy in General Surgery. Surgical Infections 7:355–60, 2006.

Fritze D, Englesbe MJ, Campbell DA Jr. Oral antibiotics to prevent surgical site infections following colon surgery. Adv Surg 45:141–153, 2011.

Fry DE. Colon preparation and surgical site infection. Am J Surg 202:225–232, 2011.

Gardner P, Eickhoff T. Immunization in adults in the 1990s. Curr Clin To Infect Dis 15:271–300, 1995.

Gardner P, Peter G. Recommended schedules for routine immunization of children and adults. Infect Dis Clin North Am 15:1–8, 2001.

Gardner P, Schaffner W. Immunization of adults. N Engl J Med 328:1252–8, 1993.

Grabe M. Perioperative antibiotic prophylaxis in urology. Curr Opin Urol 11:81–5, 2001.

Guaschino S, De Santo D, De Seta F. New perspectives in antibiotic prophylaxis for obstetric and gynecological surgery. J Hosp Infect 50 (Suppl A):SS13–6, 2002.

Haines SJ. Antibiotic prophylaxis in neurosurgery. The controlled trials. Neurosurg Clin N Am 3:355–8, 1992.

Hartman BJ. Selective aspects of infective endocarditis: considerations on diagnosis, risk factors, treatment and prophylaxis. Adv Cardiol 39:195–202, 2002.

Hasin T, Davidovitch N, Cohen R, et al. Postexposure Treatment with Doxycycline for the Prevention of Tick-Borne Relapsing Fever. N Engl J Med 355:147–55, 2006.

Hiemenz J, Cagnoni P, et al. Pharmacokinetic and maximum tolerated dose study of micafungin in combination with fluconazole versus fluconazole alone for prophylaxis of fungal infections in adult patients undergoing a bone marrow or peripheral stem cell transplant. Antimicrob Agents Chemother 49:1331–6, 2005.

Higuchi Y, Takesue Y, Yamada Y, et al. A single-dose regimen for antimicrobial prophylaxis to prevent perioperative infection in urological clean and clean-contaminated surgery. J Infect Chemother 17:219–223, 2011.

Hill DR, Ericsson CD, Pearson RD, Keystone JS, et al. The Practice of Travel Medicine: Guidelines by the Infectious Diseases Society of America. Clin Infect Dis 43:1499–539, 2006.

Hornberger H, Robertus K. Cost-Effectiveness of a Vaccine To Prevent Herpes Zoster and Postherpetic Neuralgia in Older Adults. 145:317–25, 2006.

Howdieshell TF, Heffernan D, Dipiro JT. Surgical Infection Society Guidelines for Vaccination after Traumatic Injury. Surgical Infections 7:275–303, 2006.

Jackson LA, Neuzil KM, Yu O et al. Effectiveness of pneumococcal polysaccharide vaccine in older adults. N Engl J Med 348:1747–55, 2003.

Kambaroudis AG, Papadopoulos S, Christodoulidou M, et al. Perioperative use of antibiotics in intra-abdominal surgical infections. Surg Infect (Larchmt) 11:535–544, 2011.

Khoury JA, Storch GA, Bohl DL, et al. Prophylactic verus preemptive oral valganciclovir for the management of cytomegalovirus infection in adult renal transplant recipients. Am J Transplant 6:2134–43, 2006.

Klein A, Miller KB, Sprague K, et al. A randomized, double-blind, placebo controlled trial of valacyclovir prophylaxis to prevent zoster recurrence from months 4 to 24 after BMT. Bone Marrow Transplant, 26:1–6, 2010.

Kotton CN, Kumar D, Caliendo AM, et al. International concensus guidelines on the management cytomegalovirus in solid organ transplanation. Transplantation 89:779–795, 2010

Laftavi MR, Rostami R, Feng L, et al. The role of antibiotic prophylaxis in the new era of immunosuppression. Transplant Proc 43:533–535, 2011.

Lewis RT. Oral versus systemic antibiotic prophylaxis in elective colon surgery: a randomized study and meta-analysis send a message from the 1990s. Can J Surg 45:173–80, 2002.

Musher DM, Rueda-Jaimes AM, Graviss EA, Rodriguez-Barradas MC. Effect of Pneumococcal Vaccination: A Comparison of Vaccination Rates in Patients with Bactermic and Nonbacteremic Pneumococcal Pneumonia. Clin Infect Dis 43:1004–08, 2006.

New York State Department of Health AIDS Institute. HIV Prophylaxis following occupational exposure. October 2012 http://www.hivguidelines.org/clinical-guidelines/post-exposure-prophylaxis/hiv-prophylaxis-following-occupational-exposure/, 2012.

Paul M, Yahav D, Fraser A, et al. Empirical antibiotic monotherapy for febrile neutropenia: systematic review and meta-analysis of randomized controlled trials. J Antimicrob Chemother 57:176–89, 2006.

Pham H, Geraci SA, Burton MJ. Adult immunizations: update on recommendations. Am J Med 124:698–201, 2011.

Phillips P, Chan K, Hogg R, et al. Azithromycin prophylaxis for Mycobacterium avium complex during the era of highly active antiretroviral therapy: evaluation of a provincial program. Clin Infect Dis 34:371–8, 2002.

Pratesi C, Russo D, Dorigo W, et al. Antibiotic prophylaxis in clean surgery: vascular surgery. J Chemother 13 (Spec 1):123–8, 2001.

Rex JH, Sobel JD. Prophylactic antifungal therapy in the intensive care unit. Clin Infect Dis 32:1191–200, 2001.

Rupprecht CE, Gibbons RV. Prophylaxis against rabies. N Engl J Med 351:2626–35, 2004.

Segreti J. Is antibiotic prophylaxis necessary for preventing prosthetic device infection. Infect Dis Clin North Am 13:871–7, 1999.

Seto TB. The case for infectious endocarditis prophylaxis. Arch Intern Med 167:327–330, 2007.

Seymour RA, Whitworth JM. Antibiotic prophylaxis for endocarditis, prosthetic joints, and surgery. Dent Clin North Am 46:635–51, 2002.

Small TN, Cowan MJ. Immunization of hematopoietic stem cell transplant recipients against vaccine-preventable diseases. Expert Rev Clin Immunol 7:193–203, 2011.

Snydman DR. Cytomegalovirus prevention strategies: The case for prophylaxis. Am J Transplant 9:1254, 2009.

Snydman DR. Prevention of cytomegalovirus (CMV) infection and CMV disease in recipients of solid organ transplants: the case for prophylaxis. Clin Infect Dis 40:709–12, 2005.

Sobel JD, Rex JH. Invasive andidiasis: Turning risk into a practical prevention policy? Clin Infect Dis 33:187–190, 2001.

Spira AM. Yellow Fever: An Update on Risks, Presentation, and Prevention. Infections in Medicine 23:385–89, 2006.

Syndman DR. Use of valganciclovir for prevention and treatment of cytomegalovirus disease. Clin Infect Dis, 46:28–29, 2008.

Taub DD, Ershler WB, Janowski M, et al. Immunity from Smallpox Vaccine Persists for Decades: A Longitudinal Study. Am J Med 121:1058–1064, 2008.

Vazquez M, LaRussa PS, Gershon AA, et al. The effectiveness of the varicella vaccine in clinical practice. N Engl J Med 344:955–60, 2001.

Victor JC, Mourfi AS, Sundina TY, et al. Hepatitis A vaccine versus immune globulin for postexposure prophylaxis. N Engl J Med 357:1685–1694, 2007.

Wingard JR. Antifungal chemoprophylaxis after blood and marrow transplantation. Clin Infect Dis 34:1386–90, 2002.

Winston DJ, Busuttil RW. Randomized controlled trial of oral itraconazole solution versus intravenous/oral fluconazole for prevention of fungal infections in liver transplant recipients. Transplantation 74:688–95, 2002.

Wistrom J, Norrby R. Antibiotic prophylaxis of travellers' diarrhoea. Scand J Infect Dis Suppl 70:111–29, 1990.

Zelenitsky SA, Ariano RE, Harding GK, et al. Antibiotic pharmacodynamics in surgical prophylaxis: an association between intraoperative antibiotic concentrations and efficacy. Antimicrob Agents Chemother 46:3026–30, 2002.

GUIDELINES

CDC. Prevention of Perinatal Group B Streptococcal Disease. MMWR, 59:1–31, 2010.

Dykewicz CA. Summary of the guidelines for preventing opportunistic infections among hematopoietic stem cell transplant recipients. Clin Infect Dis 33:139–44, 2001.

Hauser CJ, Adams CA, Eachempati SR. Prophylactic Antibiotic Use in Open Fractures: An Evidence-Based Guideline. Surgical Infections 7:379–405, 2006.

Medical Letter Antimicrobial Prophylaxis for Surgery. Guidelines. Medical Letter 7:47–50, 2009.

TEXTBOOKS

Antibiotic Prophylaxis for Surgical Site Infection Prevention in Adults, 4th ed. Institute for Clinical Systems Improvement, October, 2010.

Brunette GW, Kozarsky PE, Magill AJ, et al. CDC Health Information for International Travel 2010, Mosby Elsevier, 2010.

Brunette GW, Kozarsky P, Magill A. The Yellow Book CDC Health Information for International Travel 2012. Oxford University Press, 2012.

Brusch JL, Endocarditis Essentials. Jones & Bartlett, Sudbury, MA, 2011.

Gorbach SL, Bartlett JG. Blacklow NR Infectious (eds). Diseases, 3rd edition, Lippincott, Williams & Wilkins, Philadelphia, 2004.

Hawker J, Begg N, Blairl, et al. Communicable Disease Control Handbook, 2nd edition, Malden, Massachusetts, Blackwell Publishing, 2005.

Heymann DL. Control of Communicable Disease Manual, 19th edition, American Public Health Association, 2008.

Keystone JS, Kozarski PE, Freedman DO, et al. Travel Medicine. Mosby, Edinburgh, 2004.

Koff R. Hepatitis Essentials. Jones & Bartlett, Sudbury, MA, 2011.

Mandell GL, Bennett JE, Dolin R. Mandell, Douglas, and Bennett's Principles and Practice of Infectious Diseases, 7th edition, Philadelphia, Elsevier, 2010.

Plotkin SA, Orenstein WA Vaccines, 5th edition, Philadelphia, W.B. Saunders, 2004.

Sax PE, Cohen CJ, Kuritzkes DR. HIV Essentials, 5th edition. Jones & Bartlett, Sudbury, MA, 2012.

Yu VL, Merigan Jr, TC, Barriere SL. Antimicrobial Therapy and Vaccines, 2nd edition, Williams & Wilkins, Baltimore, 2005.

Chapter 7

Pediatric Infectious Diseases and Pediatric Drug Summaries

Leonard R. Krilov, MD
George H. McCracken, Jr, MD

This chapter pertains to infectious diseases and antimicrobial agents in the pediatric population. It is organized by clinical syndrome, patient subset, and in some cases, specific organism. Clinical summaries immediately follow each treatment grid. Therapeutic recommendations are based on antimicrobial effectiveness, reliability, cost, safety, and resistance potential. Antimicrobial agents and duration of therapy are listed in the treatment grids; corresponding drug dosages are provided on pages 414–422 and represent the usual dosages for normal renal and hepatic function. Drug dosages in infants/children are generally based on weight, up to adult dosage as maximum. **For any treatment category, i.e., preferred IV therapy, alternate IV therapy, PO therapy recommended drugs are equally effective and not ranked by priority.** Please refer to other pediatric drug references and the manufacturer's package inserts for dosage adjustments, side effects, drug interactions, and other important prescribing information.

"IV-to-PO Switch" in the last column of the shaded title bar in each treatment grid indicates the clinical syndrome can be treated either by IV therapy alone or IV followed by PO therapy, but *not* by PO therapy alone. "PO Therapy or IV-to-PO Switch" indicates the clinical syndrome can be treated by IV therapy alone, PO therapy alone, or IV followed by PO therapy (unless otherwise indicated in the footnotes under each treatment grid). Most patients on IV therapy able to take oral medications should be switched to PO equivalent therapy after clinical improvement.

Empiric Therapy of CNS Infections

Acute Bacterial Meningitis

Subset (age)	Usual Pathogens	Preferred IV Therapy[†]	Alternate IV Therapy[†]
Neonate (0–30 days)	Group B streptococci E. coli Listeria monocytogenes Other gram-negatives (e.g., Citrobacter, Serratia) and gram-positives (e.g., Enterococci)	Ampicillin **plus** cefotaxime*	Ampicillin **plus** gentamicin*
1–3 months	Overlap neonate and > 3 months	Vancomycin **plus either** cefotaxime **or** ceftriaxone*	Ampicillin **plus either** cefotaxime **or** ceftriaxone*
> 3 months	S. pneumoniae N. meningitidis H. influenzae (very rare) Non-typeable H. influenzae (rare)	<u>Before culture results</u>: Vancomycin **plus either** ceftriaxone **or** cefotaxime* <u>After culture results</u> Discontinue vancomycin if penicillin-susceptible S. pneumoniae, N. meningitidis, or H. influenza is isolated	Meropenem* <u>Severe penicillin allergy</u> Vancomycin **plus either** rifampin **or** chloramphenicol*

Acute Bacterial Meningitis (cont'd)

Subset (age)	Usual Pathogens	Preferred IV Therapy[†]	Alternate IV Therapy[†]
CNS shunt infection

(Treat initially for S. epidermidis; if later identified as MSSA, treat accordingly) | S. epidermidis S. aureus (MRSA) | Vancomycin **with or without** rifampin 10 mg/kg (IV or PO) q12h × 7–10 days after shunt removal | Linezolid × 7–10 days after shunt removal

<u>If MSSA isolated</u> Nafcillin **with or without** rifampin 10 mg/kg (PO) q12h × 7–10 days after shunt removal |
| | S. aureus (MSSA) | Nafcillin × 7–10 days after shunt removal | Vancomycin × 7–10 days after shunt removal |
| | Enterobacteriaceae | Cefotaxime **or** ceftriaxone × 7–10 days after shunt removal | Meropenem × 7–10 days after shunt removal |

MRSA/MSSA = methicillin-resistant/sensitive S. aureus. Duration of therapy represents total time IV or IV + PO. Most patients on IV therapy able to take PO meds should be switched to PO therapy after clinical improvement.

† **See pp. 414–422 for drug dosages.**

* Duration of therapy: Group B strep ≥ 14 days (with ventriculitis 4 weeks); E. coli, Citrobacter, Serratia ≥ 21 days; Listeria 10–14 days; Enterococcus ≥ 14 days; S. pneumoniae 10–14 days; H. influenza ≥ 10 days; N. meningitidis 4–7 days.

Acute Bacterial Meningitis (Normal Hosts)

Clinical Presentation: Fever, headache, stiff neck (or bulging anterior fontanelle in infants), irritability, vomiting, lethargy, evolving over hours to 1–2 days. The younger the child, the more nonspecific the presentation (e.g., irritability, lethargy, fever, poor feeding).

Diagnostic Considerations: Diagnosis by CSF chemistries, gram stain, culture. CSF findings are similar to those in adults: pleocytosis (100–5000 WBCs/mm³; predominately PMNs), ↑ protein, ⇉ glucose. Normal CSF values differ by age:

	WBC/mm³ (range); %PMNs	Protein, mg/dL (range)	Glucose, mg/dL (range)
Preterm	9 (0–25); 57% PMNs	115 (65–150)	50 (24–63)
Term newborn	8 (0–22); 61% PMNs	90 (20–170)	52 (34–119)
Child	0 (0–7); 0% PMNs	(5–40)	(40–80)

Modified from *The Harriet Lane Handbook*, 15ᵗʰ edition.

Pitfalls: The younger the child, the more nonspecific the presentation. With prior antibiotic use (e.g., oral therapy for otitis media), partially-treated meningitis is a concern; the addition of bacterial antigen or CIE tests may be of diagnostic value in this setting. Especially in the summer season, rapid viral diagnosis (especially enteroviral PCR) can exclude ABM and prevent unnecessary hospitalization and antibiotic use. HSV PCR can also be helpful in excluding ABM.

Therapeutic Considerations: Meningitic doses of antibiotics are required for the *entire* course of treatment. Repeat lumbar puncture (LP) is indicated at 24–48 hours if not responding clinically or in situations where a resistant organism is a concern (e.g., penicillin-resistant S. pneumonia, or neonate with gram-negative bacillary meningitis). Dexamethasone (0.3 mg/kg IV q12h × 2 days) may reduce neurologic sequelae (e.g., hearing loss) in children ≥ 6 weeks of age when given before/with the first dose of antibiotics.

Prognosis: Varies with causative agent and age at presentation. Overall mortality < 5% in US (higher in developing countries). Morbidity 30–35% with hearing loss the most common neurologic sequella. Incidence of neurologic sequelae: S. pneumoniae > H. influenzae > N. meningitidis. Use of H. influenzae (type B) and pneumococcal conjugate vaccines in routine childhood immunizations has reduced the incidence of meningitis caused by these pathogens, but recent emergence of pneumococcal serotype 19A is responsible for continued cases of meningococcal meningitis. Neonates are at increased risk of mortality and major neurologic sequelae, and there is a significant incidence of brain abscesses in neonates with gram-negative meningitis (especially Citrobacter and Serratia infections).

Acute Bacterial Meningitis (CNS Shunt Infections)
Clinical Presentation: Indolent (lethargy, irritability, vomiting) or acute (high fever, depressed mental status).
Diagnostic Considerations: Diagnosis by CSF gram stain/culture, often obtained by shunt tap.
Pitfalls: Blood cultures are usually negative for shunt pathogens and CSF WBCs may be low.
Therapeutic Considerations: High risk of nafcillin resistance with coagulase-negative staphylococcal infection. The addition of rifampin to vancomycin may improve clearance of bacteria. Removal of prosthetic material is usually necessary to achieve a cure.
Prognosis: Good with removal of prosthetic material.

Encephalitis

Subset	Usual Pathogens	IV Therapy†	IV-to-PO Switch†
Herpes	HSV-1	Acyclovir × 14–21 days	Treat IV only
Arbovirus	WNV, SLE, Powassan encephalitis, EEE, WEE, VEE, JE, CE	No specific therapy	
Mycoplasma	M. pneumoniae	Doxycycline **or** minocycline × 2–4 weeks	Doxycycline **or** minocycline × 2–4 weeks

Encephalitis (cont'd)

Subset	Usual Pathogens	IV Therapy†	IV-to-PO Switch†
Respiratory viruses	Influenza, Enteroviruses, Measles	No specific therapy	

Duration of therapy represents total time IV or IV + PO. Most patients on IV therapy able to take PO meds should be switched to PO therapy after clinical improvement. *WNV = West Nile Virus, SLE = St. Louis encephalitis, EEE = Eastern equine encephalitis, WEE = Western equine encephalitis, VEE = Venezuelan equine encephalitis, JE = Japanese encephalitis, CE = California encephalitis.*
†   **See pp. 414–422 for drug dosages.**

Herpes Encephalitis (HSV-1)
Clinical Presentation: Acute onset of fever and mental status/behavioral changes. High fever with intractable seizures and profoundly depressed sensorium may dominate the clinical picture.
Diagnostic Considerations: Diagnosis by CSF PCR for HSV-1. CSF findings include ↑ RBC/WBC, ↓ glucose, and ↑↑ protein. Classic EEG changes with temporal lobe spikes may be present early. Brain biopsy is rarely, if ever, indicated.
Pitfalls: MRI/CT scan can be normal initially. Delays in diagnosis and therapy adversely affect outcome.
Therapeutic Considerations: HSV is the only treatable viral encephalitis in normal hosts.
Prognosis: Antiviral therapy improves survival, but based on level of consciousness at presentation, mortality is still 10–20%.

Arboviral Encephalitis
Clinical Presentation: Acute onset of fever, headache, altered mental status. Usually seasonal (more common in summer/fall), based on vector/travel history. Can be very severe with high mortality. Symptomatic West Nile encephalitis is rare in children.
Diagnostic Considerations: Serological studies are the primary means of diagnosis. PCR "encephalitis panels" are being developed for clinical use.
Therapeutic Considerations: No specific antiviral therapy. Supportive therapy is crucial.
Pitfalls: Be sure to elicit potential exposures/travel history in children with fever/altered mental status.
Prognosis: Varies with agent. Severe residual deficits and high mortality rates can occur, especially with Eastern Equine encephalitis.

Mycoplasma Encephalitis
Clinical Presentation: Acute onset of fever and mental status changes. Prodromal cough, sore throat, respiratory symptoms may occur.
Diagnostic Considerations: CSF shows mild pleocytosis with a predominance of mononuclear cells, normal or mildly ↓ glucose, and mildly ↑ protein. Mycoplasma IgG/IgM titers are elevated.
Pitfalls: CSF findings can be confused with viral encephalitis.
Therapeutic Considerations: Often self-limited illness even without antibiotic therapy. Doxycycline or minocycline penetrate CNS and can be used in children > 8 years of age. Macrolides may treat pulmonary infection but do not penetrate CNS.
Prognosis: Good. Neurologic sequelae are rare.

Respiratory Virus Encephalitis

Clinical Presentation: Encephalitis may occur during or immediately after an acute respiratory illness. Influenza encephalitis, although rare, may be especially severe with a number of deaths reported every year in previously healthy children and adolescents.

Diagnostic Considerations: Rarely, adenoviruses have been recovered from CSF or brain in cases of encephalitis. Encephalitis has also been described very rarely in association with RSV and parainfluenza infections as well.

Pitfalls: Most cases of encephalitis remain undiagnosed, in part due to failure to consider and test for respiratory viruses.

Therapeutic Considerations: No evidence to date suggests a benefit of anti-influenza therapy in influenza encephalitis.

Prognosis: Generally self-limited with recovery, but death has been reported with influenza encephalitis. Adenovirus encephalitis in immunocompromised hosts may also be severe.

Empiric Therapy of HEENT Infections

Periorbital (Preseptal) Cellulitis/Orbital Cellulitis

Subset	Usual Pathogens	Preferred IV Therapy†	Alternate IV Therapy†	IV-to-PO Switch†
Periorbital cellulitis	S. pneumoniae H. influenzae M. catarrhalis S. aureus	**Combination therapy with** Nafcillin* **plus either** ceftriaxone **or** cefotaxime × 10–14 days	Ampicillin-sulbactam × 10–14 days	Amoxicillin-clavulanate **or** cefuroxime **or** cefpodoxime **or** cefdinir × 10–14 days
Orbital cellulitis	S. pneumoniae H. influenzae M. catarrhalis S. aureus Anaerobes Group A streptococci	**Combination therapy with** Nafcillin **plus** ceftriaxone × 10–14 days	Piperacillin-tazobactam **or** ampicillin-sulbactam **or** ticarcillin-clavulanate × 10–14 days	Amoxicillin-clavulanate **or** cefuroxime **or** cefpodoxime **or** cefdinir × 10–14 days

Duration of therapy represents total time IV or IV + PO. Most patients on IV therapy able to take PO meds should be switched to PO therapy after clinical improvement.

*   Or vancomycin if MRSA likely.

†   See pp. 414–422 for drug dosages.

Clinical Presentation: Periorbital and orbital cellulitis are bacterial infections. Fever, lid swelling, and erythema around the eye often in conjunction with acute sinusitis. In periorbital cellulitis the infection is anterior to the orbital septum. Orbital cellulitis involves the orbit proper, extraocular muscles/nerves, and possibly the orbital nerve. Proptosis and limitation of ocular mobility define orbital cellulitis.

Diagnostic Considerations: CT scan is used to differentiate preseptal from periorbital cellulitis and identify the extent of orbital involvement when present.

Pitfalls: Failure to recognize orbital involvement leading to optic nerve damage or CNS extension/ cavernous sinus thrombosis. CT scan cannot differentiate phlegmon from abscess.

Therapeutic Considerations: Orbital cellulitis is more emergent than periorbital cellulitis and should be treated with IV antibiotics initially. Surgical drainage may be indicated if a well defined abscess is present or in more severe disease.

Prognosis: Good with prompt antimicrobial therapy and ophthalmologic surgery if needed.

Sinusitis

Subset	Usual Pathogens	IV Therapy† (Hospitalized)	PO Therapy or IV-to-PO Switch† (Ambulatory)
Acute	S. pneumoniae H. influenzae M. catarrhalis	Ceftriaxone **or** cefuroxime × 1–2 weeks	Amoxicillin **or** amoxicillin/ clavulanic acid **or** cephalosporin **or** clarithromycin* × 10–14 days **or** azithromycin* × 5 days
Chronic	Same as acute + oral anaerobes	Requires prolonged antimicrobial therapy (2–4 weeks)	

Duration of therapy represents total time IV, PO, or IV + PO. Most patients on IV therapy able to take PO meds should be switched to PO therapy soon after clinical improvement (usually < 72 hrs).
*   Macrolides may be less effective and should be reserved for penicillin- and cephalosporin-allergic patients.
†   **See pp. 414–422 for drug dosages.**

Clinical Presentation: Nasal discharge and cough frequently with headache, facial pain, and low-grade fever lasting > 10–14 days. Can also present acutely with high fever (≥ 104°F) and purulent nasal discharge ± intense headache for ≥ 3 days.

Diagnostic Considerations: Acute sinusitis is a clinical diagnosis. Imaging studies are not routinely indicated. Overlap with acute viral infection and allergic symptoms may make diagnosis difficult.

Pitfalls: Transillumination, sinus tenderness to percussion, and color of nasal mucus are not reliable indicators of sinusitis.

Therapeutic Considerations: Microbiology/antibiotics are similar to acute otitis media, but duration of therapy is 10–14 days. Failure to respond to initial antibiotic therapy suggests a resistant pathogen or an alternative diagnosis. There are insufficient data to support long-course antibiotic treatment. Quinolones not approved for sinusitis.

Prognosis: Good. For frequent recurrences, consider radiologic studies and ENT/allergy consultation.

Otitis Externa

Subset	Usual Pathogens	Topical Therapy
"Swimmer's ear"	Pseudomonas sp. Enterobacteriaceae S. aureus	Polymyxin B plus neomycin **plus** hydrocortisone (eardrops) q6h × 7–10 days **or** Ofloxacin (3% otic solution) q12h × 7–10 days

Clinical Presentation: Ear pain, itching, and sensation of fullness. Pain is exacerbated by tugging on the pinna or tragus of the outer ear. Purulent discharge may be visible in the external ear canal. Fever is generally absent.

Diagnostic Considerations: Otitis externa is a clinical diagnosis. A recent history of swimming or cleaning with cotton swabs is often elicited. Malignant otitis externa, as seen in elderly adults with diabetes mellitus, is extremely rare in children but may be seen in immunocompromised hosts.

Pitfalls: Failure to recognize a ruptured tympanic membrane may lead to a misdiagnosis of otitis externa based on purulence in the canal.

Therapeutic Considerations: Local cleansing (e.g., 2% acetic acid) and topical therapy with corti-cosporin-polymyxin B-neomycin suspension is usually sufficient. Oral antibiotics should be considered for fever/cervical adenitis.

Prognosis: Excellent. Cleansing with 2% acetic acid drops after swimming prevents recurrences.

Acute Otitis Media

Subset	Usual Pathogens	IM Therapy†	PO Therapy†
Initial uncomplicated bacterial infection	S. pneumoniae H. influenzae M. catarrhalis	Ceftriaxone × 1 dose	Amoxicillin × 10 days **or** cefdinir × 10 days** **or** azithromycin (1-, 3-, or 5-day regimen) **or** erythromycin-sulfisoxazole × 10 days** **or** TMP–SMX × 10 days**
Treatment failure or resistant organism*	MRSP Beta-lactamase positive H. influenzae	Ceftriaxone q24h × 3 doses	Amoxicillin/clavulanic acid **or** ES-600†† × 10 days** **or** cephalosporin × 10 days‡*

DRSP = drug-resistant S. pneumoniae. Pediatric doses are provided; acute otitis media is uncommon in adults. For chronic otitis media, prolonged antimicrobial therapy is required.

†   **See pp. 414–422 for drug dosages.**

*   Treatment failure = persistent symptoms and otoscopy abnormalities 48–72 hours after starting initial antimicrobial therapy. For risk factors for DRSP, see Therapeutic Considerations, below. If still fails after recommended therapy, consider clindamycin for resistant S. pneumoniae or tympanocentesis for gram stain and culture.

** In children > 6 years of age with mild-moderate acute otitis media, a 5–7 day course of antimicrobial theory may be adequate.

†† ES-600 = 600 mg amoxicillin/5 mL.

‡   10-day course with either cefuroxime axetil 15 mg/kg (PO) q12h or cefdinir 7 mg/kg (PO) q12h or 14 mg/kg (PO) q24h or cefpodoxime 5 mg/kg (PO) q12h may be used.

Clinical Presentation: Fever, otalgia, hearing loss. Nonspecific presentation is more common in younger children (irritability, fever). Key to diagnosis is examination of the tympanic membrane. Acute otitis media requires evidence of inflammation *and* effusion. Uncommon in adults.

Diagnostic Considerations: Diagnosis is made by finding an opaque, hyperemic, bulging tympanic membrane with loss of landmarks and decreased mobility on pneumatic otoscopy.

Pitfalls: Failure to remove cerumen (inadequate visualization of tympanic membrane) and reliance on history of ear tugging/pain are the main factors associated with overdiagnosis of otitis media. Otitis media with effusion (i.e., tympanic membrane retracted or in normal position with decreased mobility or mobility with negative pressure; fluid present behind the drum but normal in color) usually resolves spontaneously and should not be treated with antibiotics.

Therapeutic Considerations: Risk factors for infection with drug-resistant S. pneumoniae (DRSP) include antibiotic therapy in past 30 days, failure to respond within 48–72 hours of therapy, day care attendance, and antimicrobial prophylaxis. Macrolides and TMP–SMX may predispose to DRSP, and 25% of S. pneumoniae are naturally resistant to macrolides. Quinolones not approved for therapy.

Prognosis: Excellent, but tends to recur. Chronic otitis, cholesteatomas, mastoiditis are rare complications. Tympanostomy tubes/adenoidectomy for frequent recurrences of otitis media are the leading surgical procedures in children.

Mastoiditis

Subset	Usual Pathogens	Preferred IV Therapy†	Alternate IV Therapy†	PO Therapy or IV-to-PO Switch†
Acute	S. pneumoniae S. aureus Group A streptococci H. influenzae	Nafcillin **or** vancomycin (if MRSA suspected) **plus either** ceftriaxone **or** cefotaxime × 10–14 days	Ampicillin-sulbactam × 10–14 days	Amoxicillin-clavulanate **or** cefpodoxime **or** cefdinir × 10–14 days
Chronic	Polymicrobial, including P. aeruginosa, S. aureus, anaerobes, Enterobacteriaceae	Piperacillin **or** ticarcillin × 10–14 days	Meropenem **or** imipenem × 10–14 days	None

Duration of therapy represents total time IV, IV + PO, or PO. Most patients on IV therapy able to take PO meds should be switched to PO therapy after clinical improvement.

† **See pp. 414–422 for drug dosages.**

Clinical Presentation: Fever and otalgia with postauricular swelling/erythema pushing the ear superiorly and laterally. The presentation may be more subtle (e.g., less toxic, less swelling, Bell's palsy alone) in older children partially treated with antibiotics. Concomitant otitis media is rare.

Diagnostic Considerations: Acute mastoiditis is diagnosed clinically, but CT scan is definitive. Tympanocentesis through intact ear drum for aspirate and insertion of tympanostomy tube are helpful for microbiology and drainage, respectively. Chronic mastoiditis is often polymicrobial, including anaerobes and P. aeruginosa. Tuberculosis rarely presents as chronic mastoiditis.

Pitfalls: Do not overlook mastoiditis in older child with unresponsive otitis. Orbital involvement may lead to optic nerve damage or CNS extension/cavernous sinus thrombosis.

Therapeutic Considerations: Treatment is based on microbiology and requires at least 3 weeks of antibiotics.

Prognosis: Good with early treatment.

Pharyngitis

Subset	Usual Pathogens	IV or IM Therapy[†]	PO Therapy or IV-to-PO Switch[†]
Exudative (culture)	Group A streptococci	Benzathine penicillin IM × 1 dose	Penicillin V **or** amoxicillin × 10 days. *Alternate*: azithromycin 12 mg/kg/day × 5 days **or** cephalexin **or** cefadroxil **or** erythromycin **or** clarithromycin **or** clindamycin × 10 days
Asymptomatic carrier	Group A streptococci	No treatment indicated	No treatment indicated
Persistent/recurrent disease	Group A streptococci	Clindamycin	Amoxicillin-clavulanate × 10 days **or combination therapy with either** penicillin V **or** amoxicillin × 10 days plus rifampin added on days 7–10
Exudative, sexually active	N. gonorrhoeae	Ceftriaxone (IM) × 1 dose	Quinolone*
Lemierre's Syndrome (Jugular vein septic thrombophlebitis)[‡]	Fusobacterium necrophorum	Clindamycin (IV) **or** penicillin G (IV) × 4–6 weeks	Clindamycin **or** penicillin VK × 4–6 weeks
Vesicular, ulcerative	Enteroviruses HSV 1 or 2	Primary HSV: Acyclovir × 5–7 days	Primary HSV: Acyclovir **or** valacyclovir × 5–7 days

Duration of therapy represents total time IV, IM, IV + PO, or PO. Most patients on IV therapy able to take PO meds should be switched to PO therapy after clinical improvement.

†   **See pp. 414–422 for drug dosages.**

*   Likely okay in adolescent although licensed only for age > 18 years. See adult section for agents and dosages.

‡   Treat only IV or IV-to-PO switch.

Clinical Presentation: Acute sore throat and fever with tender cervical lymphadenitis. Primary clinical consideration is differentiating Group A streptococci (GAS) from viral/other causes (e.g., adenovirus, enterovirus, respiratory viruses, other strep groups [C, G], Arcanobacterium hemolyticum, M. pneumoniae, C. pneumoniae, EBV). GAS is less likely with concomitant coryza, conjunctivitis, hoarseness, cough, acute stomatitis, discrete oral ulcerations, or diarrhea—children with these manifestations should not be cultured routinely.

Diagnostic Considerations: Laboratory testing for GAS is recommended, since clinical differentiation of viral pharyngitis from GAS is not possible. Rapid tests for GAS antigens are reliable with excellent specificities, but due to variable sensitivities of the assays, a negative rapid test should be confirmed by a throat culture. The accuracy of antigen and culture tests is dependent on obtaining a good throat swab containing pharyngeal/tonsillar secretions.

Pitfalls: Be sure to obtain a good throat swab. Post-treatment testing is generally not recommended unless the patient is at high risk for rheumatic fever (e.g., family history, ongoing outbreak) or is still symptomatic after 10 days of therapy. Asymptomatic GAS carriers do not require antibiotic therapy, but identifying a "true carrier" may be difficult. Eradication of GAS carriage should be considered in the following situations: an outbreak of acute rheumatic fever or post-streptococcal glomerulonephritis; an outbreak of GAS in a closed community; a family history of rheumatic fever; multiple episodes of GAS infection within the family for many weeks despite therapy; family anxiety about the presence of GAS; or tonsillectomy is being considered based on persistent carriage. Eradication is achieved using the same antimicrobial regimen as for "persistent/recurrent disease" (see treatment grid p. 395).

Therapeutic Considerations: Penicillin V (or amoxicillin) is the drug of choice for GAS pharyngitis. Erythromycin is still considered the drug of choice for penicillin-allergic individuals, although macrolide-resistant GAS strains are being reported. First-generation cephalosporins are also useful alternatives. Broader spectrum agents, although likely effective, should not be used routinely. Tetracyclines and sulfonamides do not eradicate GAS pharyngitis. When eradication of carriage is indicated as noted above, clindamycin alone or penicillin plus rifampin may be useful.

Prognosis: Excellent. Rheumatic fever is rare in the US.

Empiric Therapy of Lower Respiratory Tract Infections

Community-Acquired Pneumonia

Subset (age)	Usual Pathogens	IV Therapy[†]	PO Therapy or IV-to-PO Switch[†]
Community-acquired pneumonia *Birth to 20 days*	Group B streptococci, Gram-negative enteric bacteria, CMV	Ampicillin **plus either** gentamicin **or** cefotaxime × 10–21 days	Not applicable

Duration of therapy represents total time IV or IV, PO, or IV + PO. Most patients on IV therapy able to take PO meds should be switched to PO therapy after clinical improvement.

†   **See pp. 414–422 for drug dosages.**

Community-Acquired Pneumonia (cont'd)

Subset (age)	Usual Pathogens	IV Therapy[†]	PO Therapy or IV-to-PO Switch[†]
3 weeks to 3 months	RSV Parainfluenza Human metapneumovirus (hmpv)	None (supportive care)	None
	C. trachomatis S. pneumoniae B. pertussis S. aureus	Cefotaxime **or** ceftriaxone × 10–14 days*. Alternative: ampicillin **or** clindamycin*	<u>Afebrile:</u> Erythromycin × 14 days **or** azithromycin × 5–7 days. <u>Lobar, febrile:</u> Amoxicillin **or** amoxicillin/clavulanic acid **or** cefdinir **or** cefuroxime **or** cefpodoxime × 10–14 days
> 3 months to < 5 years	Viruses (RSV, parainfluenza, influenza, adenovirus, rhinoviruses)	<td colspan="2"><u>RSV:</u> consider ribavirin.[§] For infants at highest risk for severe RSV infection, consider palivizumab 15 mg/kg/month × 1–2 seasons for prevention. <u>Influenza:</u> Oseltamivir (influenza A, B).[¶] Routine immunization for all children > 6 months</td>
	S. pneumoniae H. influenzae M. pneumoniae	Ceftriaxone **or** cefotaxime **or** ertapenem × 10–14 days*	Amoxicillin **or** amoxicillin-clavulanate **or** clarithromycin **or** azithromycin × 10–14 days
5–15 years	M. pneumoniae C. pneumoniae S. pneumoniae	Ceftriaxone **or** cefotaxime **or** ertapenem × 10–14 days*	Erythromycin **or** clarithromycin **or** azithromycin **or** doxycycline (age > 8 years) × 10–14 days
Pertussis	Bordetella spp.[‡] certain Adenoviruses M. pneumoniae C. trachomatis C. pneumoniae	Azithromycin × 5 days **or** erythromycin × 14 days	Erythromycin estolate × 14 days **or** clarithromycin × 7 days **or** azithromycin × 5 days. If macrolide-intolerant: TMP–SMX × 14 days
Tuberculosis	M. tuberculosis	See pp. 400–401	See pp. 400–401

Duration of therapy represents total time IV or IV, PO, or IV + PO. Most patients on IV therapy able to take PO meds should be switched to PO therapy after clinical improvement.

†   **See pp. 414–422 for drug dosages.**

*   If chronic cough of more insidious onset, consider adding IV or PO macrolide (azithromycin, clarithromycin, erythromycin) to cover Pertussis/C. trachomatis (3 weeks–3 months of age), Mycoplasma (3 months–5 years of age), or Mycoplasma/C. pneumoniae (5–15 years of age).

‡   B. pertussis, B. parapertussis, B. bronchiseptica.

§   Use should be limited to the most severely ill with RSV, i.e., transplant patients.

¶   Influenza A strains circulating in 2011–2012 are amantadine resistant.

Community-Acquired Pneumonia

Clinical Presentation: Fever ± dyspnea, cough, tachypnea with infiltrates on chest x-ray.

Diagnostic Considerations: Usual pathogens differ by age. In neonates, pneumonia is typically diffuse and part of early-onset sepsis. In young infants, there is significant overlap between signs and symptoms of bronchiolitis (primarily due to RSVU) and pneumonia. Severe pneumonia is usually due to bacterial infection, although the organism is frequently not isolated (e.g., blood cultures are positive in only 10–20% of children < 2 years of age with bacterial pneumonia). In young infants, Chlamydia trachomatis can be detected by antigen assay or culture of nasopharyngeal (NP) secretions. Mycoplasma pneumonia, diagnosed by cold agglutinins and IgG/IgM serologies, peaks at 5–15 years of age, although cases in children < 5 years have been reported. Respiratory viruses (RSV, influenza, adenoviruses, parainfluenza viruses, hmpv) can also be detected in NP secretions. If child lives in area with high prevalence of tuberculosis, consider tuberculosis in the differential diagnosis of primary pneumonia.

Pitfalls: Reliance on upper airway specimen for gram stain/culture leads to misdiagnosis and mistreatment, as true deep sputum specimen is rarely obtainable in children.

Therapeutic Considerations: Therapy is primarily empiric based on child's age, clinical/epidemiologic features and chest x-ray findings. Mycoplasma requires 2–3 weeks of treatment; C. pneumoniae may require up to 6 weeks of treatment. Routine use of conjugated pneumococcal vaccine (Prevnar) has decreased the incidence of pneumococcal pneumonia.

Prognosis: Varies with pathogen, clinical condition at presentation, and underlying health status. Prognosis is worse in children with chronic lung disease, congenital heart disease, immunodeficiency, neuromuscular disease, hemoglobinopathy.

Lower Respiratory Tract Infections due to Respiratory Viruses

Clinical Presentation: Viruses cause the majority of lower respiratory tract infections (LRTIs) in children. Respiratory syncytial virus (RSV) is the leading cause of LRTI in young infants, manifesting as bronchiolitis/viral pneumonia and causing annual mid-winter epidemics. The risk of secondary bacterial infection (other than possibly otitis media) is very low. Fever is typically low grade and usually improves over 3–5 days, even if hospitalized. Influenza viruses are another major cause of winter epidemic LRTIs in children of all ages. Hospitalization rates in infants under one year of age rival those in the > 65 year old population. Characteristic findings include high fever and diffuse inflammation of the airways. Young infants may have prominent GI symptoms as well. Secondary bacterial infection (otitis media, pneumonia, sepsis) are frequent complications of influenza. Primary influenza pneumonia, encephalopathy, and myocarditis are rare, severe complications. Other respiratory viruses associated with LRTIs in children include parainfluenza type 3 (viral pneumonia), parainfluenza types 1 and 2 (croup), adenoviruses, and the recently identified human metapneumovirus (hmpv). Swine influenza (H_1N_1) in children resembles that in adults with some important differences. In adults and children, leukocytosis rather than leukopenia is the role, otherwise unexplained relative lymphopenia is a cardinal finding in adults but is uncommon in children. In children, lymphocytosis is usual. Atypical lymphocytes are common in children, but are not present in adults with H_1N_1. Thrombocytopenia is common in both children and adults.

Diagnostic Considerations: Viral syndromes are often diagnosed based on clinical assessment alone. For confirmation or in more severe cases, rapid diagnosis by antigen detection (direct fluorescent antibody staining, ELISA, PCR) and/or viral culture are readily available.

Pitfalls: Routine use of corticosteroids or bronchodilators in RSV bronchiolitis are not supported by clinical evidence. Overuse of the diagnosis of "flu" (e.g., stomach flu, summer flu) has led to diluted appreciation for true influenza and its severity. Influenza vaccine has been traditionally underutilized in children. As in adults, a negative rapid influenza diagnostic test does not rule out influenza.

Therapeutic Considerations: For most viral LRTIs treatment is primarily supportive (e.g., adequate hydration, fever control, supplemental oxygen for severe illness). Ribavirin is approved for RSV infection but is very rarely used due to uncertain clinical benefit, high cost, and cumbersome method of administration (prolonged aerosol). For infants at greatest risk of severe RSV disease (e.g., premature infants, infants with underlying chronic lung disease or congenital heart disease), monthly prophylaxis with palivizumab (Synagis) 15 mg/kg/month (IM) decreases RSV hospitalization rates. Per American Academy of Pediatrics guidelines, palivizumab is indicated for infants with chronic lung disease or congenital heart disease who are ≤ 24 months of age at start of RSV season. For premature infants, palivizumab is considered based on a combination of gestational age (GA) and chronological age (CA): GA ≤ 28 weeks plus CA ≤ 12 months; GA 29–32 weeks plus CA ≤ 6 months; GA 33–35 weeks plus CA ≤ 3 months plus sibling < 5 years old or in day care. For the latter group a maximum of 3 doses stopping at > 90 days of age is recommended; for other groups of high-risk infants a maximum of 5 doses through the winter season are recommended.

Annual influenza vaccination is indicated for all individuals > 6 months of age. All circulating influenza A strains are resistant to amantadine. The neuraminidase inhibitors oseltamivir and zanamivir have pediatric indications for treatment and prophylaxis of influenza. (Table 7.1)

Table 7.1. Influenza Antiviral Medication Dosing Recommendations

Antiviral		Treatment	Chemoprophylaxis
Oseltamivir*			
Adults		75-mg capsule twice per day × 5 days	75-mg capsule once per day × 10 days
Children (age, 12 months or older), weight:	15 kg or less	60 mg per day divided into 2 doses	30 mg once per day
	15–23 kg	90 mg per day divided into 2 doses	45 mg once per day
	24–40 kg	120 mg per day divided into 2 doses	60 mg once per day
	> 40 kg	150 mg per day divided into 2 doses	75 mg once per day
Zanamivir			
Adults		Two 5-mg inhalations (10 mg total) twice per day	Two 5-mg inhalations (10 mg total) once per day
Children		Two 5-mg inhalations (10 mg total) twice per day (age, 7 years or older)	Two 5-mg inhalations (10 mg total) once per day (age, 5 years or older)

*   CDC recommends oseltamivir 3 mg/kg (PO) q12h × 5 days for severely ill infants < 12 months.

Prognosis: Most children with viral LRTIs do well and recover without sequelae. Infants hospitalized with RSV infection have higher rates of wheezing episodes over the next 10 years. The highest rates of hospitalization from influenza occur in children < 2 years of age and in the elderly.

Pertussis

Clinical Presentation: Upper respiratory tract symptoms (congestion, rhinorrhea) over 1–2 weeks (catarrhal stage) progressing to paroxysms of cough (paroxysmal stage) lasting 2–4 weeks, often with a characteristic inspiratory whoop, followed by a convalescent stage lasting 1–2 weeks during which cough paroxysms decrease in frequency and severity. Fever is low grade or absent. In children < 6 months, whoop is frequently absent and apnea may occur. Duration of classic pertussis is 6–10 weeks. Older children and adults may present with persistent cough (without whoop) lasting 2–6 weeks. Complications include seizures, secondary bacterial pneumonia, encephalopathy, death; risk of complications is greatest in children < 1 year.

Diagnostic Considerations: Diagnosis is usually based on nature of cough and duration of symptoms. Laboratory diagnosis may be difficult. A positive culture for Bordetella pertussis from a nasopharyngeal swab inoculated on fresh selective media is diagnostic, but the organism is difficult to recover after 3–4 weeks of illness. Direct fluorescent antibody (DFA) staining of nasopharyngeal secretions is available, but sensitivities/specificities are variable to poor. PCR of nasal secretions best rapid diagnostic test for pertussis.

Pitfalls: Be sure to consider pertussis in older children and adults with prolonged coughing illness. Family contacts of index case should receive post-exposure antimicrobial prophylaxis. Virtually all children should be vaccinated against pertussis. A single booster dose of acellular pertussis is recommended at 11–12 years of age (additional guidelines for catch-up for older adolescents and adults up to 64 years of age). "Coccining" to protect young infants from pertussis includes immunizing parents/grandparents (> 65 years) and their caretakers against pertussis. Rare contraindications to pertussis vaccination include anaphylaxis to a prior dose or encephalopathy within 7 days of a dose. Relative precautions to further pertussis immunization include: seizure within 3 days of a dose; persistent, severe, inconsolable crying for ≥ 3 hours within 48 hours of a dose; collapse or shock-like state within 48 hours of a dose; or temperature of ≥ 40.5° C without other cause within 48 hours of a dose.

Therapeutic Considerations: Infants < 6 months frequently require hospitalization. By the paroxysmal stage, antibiotics have minimal effect on the course of the illness but are still indicated to decrease transmission. An association has been made between oral erythromycin and infantile hypertrophic pyloric stenosis in infants < 6 weeks of age; consider an alternative macrolide (azithromycin or clarithromycin) in these cases.

Prognosis: Good. Despite the prolonged course, long-term pulmonary sequelae have not been described after pertussis. Children < 1 year are at greatest risk of morbidity and mortality, although mortality rates remain very low.

Tuberculosis

Subset	Pathogen	PO or IM Therapy (see footnote for drug dosages)
Latent infection (positive PPD, clinically well, negative chest x-ray)	M. tuberculosis	INH × 9 months **or** rifampin × 6 months (if INH-resistant)
Pulmonary and extrapulmonary TB (except meningitis)	M. tuberculosis	INH **plus** rifampin **plus** PZA × 2 months followed by INH **plus** rifampin × 4 months[†]

Duration of therapy represents total time IV or IV, PO, or IV + PO. Most patients on IV therapy able to take PO meds should be switched to PO therapy after clinical improvement.

† If drug resistance is a concern, EMB or streptomycin (IM) is added (4-drug regimen in areas where MDR TB is prevalent) to the initial regimen until drug susceptibilities are determined.

Tuberculosis (cont'd)

Subset	Pathogen	PO or IM Therapy (see footnote for drug dosages)
Meningitis	M. tuberculosis	INH **plus** rifampin **plus** PZA **plus either** streptomycin (IM) **or** ethionamide × 2 months, followed by INH **plus** rifampin × 7–10 months (i.e., 9–12 months total therapy)‡
Congenital	M. tuberculosis	INH **plus** rifampin **plus** PZA **plus** streptomycin (IM)

Duration of therapy represents total time IV or IV, PO, or IV + PO. Most patients on IV therapy able to take PO meds should be switched to PO therapy after clinical improvement.

‡ Plus steroids.

TB Drug	Daily dosage (mg/kg)	Twice weekly dosage (mg/kg)
Isoniazid (INH)	10–15	20–30
Rifampin	10–20	10–20
Ethambutol (EMB)	15–25	50
Pyrazinamide (PZA)	20–40	50
Streptomycin	20–40 (IM)	–
Ethionamide	15–20 (in 2–3 divided doses/day)	–

Alternative drugs (capreomycin, ciprofloxacin, levofloxacin, cycloserine, kanamycin, para-aminosalicylic acid) are used less commonly and should be administered in consultation with an expert in the treatment of tuberculosis.

Tuberculosis

Clinical Presentation: Most children diagnosed with tuberculosis have asymptomatic infection detected by tuberculin skin testing. Symptomatic disease typically presents 1–6 months after infection with fever, growth delay, weight loss, night sweats, and cough. Extrapulmonary involvement may present with meningitis, chronic mastoiditis, lymphadenopathy, bone, joint, or skin involvement. Renal tuberculosis and reactivation cavitary disease are rare in children but may be seen in adolescents.

Diagnostic Considerations: A positive tuberculin skin test indicates likely infection with M. tuberculosis. Tuberculin reactivity develops 2–12 weeks after infection. The definition of a positive skin test reaction is based on age, immune status, risk of exposure, and degree of suspicion of tuberculosis disease. Children < 8 years old cannot produce sputum for AFB smear and culture; specimens for analysis can be obtained by collecting 3 consecutive morning gastric aspirates.

Pitfalls: Tuberculosis may be missed if not considering the diagnosis in children at increased epidemiological risk for exposure. Tuberculous meningitis often presents insidiously with nonspecific irritability and lethargy weeks prior to the development of frank neurological defects.

Therapeutic Considerations: Choice of initial therapy depends on stage of disease and likelihood of resistant organisms (based on index case, geographical region of acquisition). For HIV-infected patients, duration of therapy is prolonged to ≥ 12 months. For tuberculosis meningitis and miliary disease, the addition of corticosteroids to anti-TB therapy is beneficial.

Prognosis: Varies with extent of disease, drug resistance and underlying immune status, but is generally good for pulmonary disease in children. Bone infection may result in orthopedic sequelae (e.g., Pott's disease of the spine with vertebral collapse). The prognosis for meningitis is guarded once focal neurological deficits and persistent depression of mental status occur.

Empiric Therapy of Vascular Infections

Central Venous Catheter (CVC) Infections (Broviac, Hickman, Mediport)

Subset	Usual Pathogens	Preferred IV Therapy[†]	Alternate IV Therapy[†]
Empiric; immuno-compromised host	S. epidermidis S. aureus[¶] Enterobacteriaceae Pseudomonas Viridans Streptococci Enterococcus	Meropenem **or** piperacillin/tazobactam **or** cefepime × 7–14 days	Piperacillin/tazobactam **plus** an aminoglycoside × 7–14 days
Isolate-based	S. aureus *MSSA*	Nafcillin **or** oxacillin for ≥ 2 weeks	Cefazolin **or** vancomycin (preferred if severe beta-lactam allergy) for ≥ 2 weeks
	MRSA	Vancomycin **with or without** gentamicin (for potential synergy) for ≥ 2 weeks	Linezolid **or** quinupristindalfopristin for ≥ 2 weeks (addition of rifampin may be of benefit, for MRSA)
	Enterobacteriaceae Pseudomonas	Piperacillin **or** ticarcillin **with or without** an aminoglycoside* for ≥ 2 weeks	Meropenem **or** imipenem **with or without** an aminoglycoside* for ≥ 2 weeks
	ESBL-producing gram-negative bacilli	Meropenem **or** imipenem **with or without** an aminoglycoside* for ≥ 2 weeks	—

Central Venous Catheter Infections (Broviac, Hickman, Mediport) (cont'd)

Subset	Usual Pathogens	Preferred IV Therapy[†]	Alternate IV Therapy[†]
	Candida	Amphotericin B × 2–6 weeks[‡]	Fluconazole **or** caspofungin **or** liposomal amphotericin B (if renal dysfunction) × 2–6 weeks[‡]

MSSA/MRSA = methicillin-sensitive/resistant S. aureus. Duration of therapy represents total time IV.

[†] **See pp. 414–422 for drug dosages.**
[*] Gentamicin, tobramycin, or amikacin.
[‡] Based on promptness of line removal, clearance of blood cultures, evidence of metastatic foci.
[¶] If severely ill or suspicion of MRSA based on local epidemiology, include vancomycin in initial regimen pending culture results.

Clinical Presentation: Fever ± site tenderness, erythema.

Diagnostic considerations: Quantitative blood cultures from the peripheral blood/vascular catheter are best used to make the diagnosis. However in clinical practice these are not often obtained, and the diagnosis is based on culture results in conjunction with one or more of the following features: local phlebitis or inflammation at the catheter insertion site; embolic disease distal to the catheter; sepsis refractory to appropriate therapy; resolution of fever after device removal; or clustered infections caused by infusion-associated organisms.

Pitfalls: It may be difficult to differentiate infection from contamination in blood cultures, especially with coagulase-negative staphylococci. Multiple positive cultures with the same organism and/or clinical features noted above suggest infection, not colonization. Semiquantitative culture of the catheter tip yielding ≥ 15 colonies may be useful in confirming the diagnosis but requires removal of the device.

Therapeutic Considerations: Indications for catheter removal include septic shock, tunnel infection, failure to respond to treatment within 48–72 hours, or infection with Candida, atypical mycobacteria, or possibly S. aureus. Otherwise attempt to retain the catheter while treating with antibiotics. Localized exit site infections (erythema, induration, tenderness, purulence) within 2 cm of the exit site should be treated topically (e.g., Neosporin, Bacitracin, Bactroban) in conjunction with systemic therapy.

Prognosis: Major complications (septic emboli, endocarditis, vasculitis) are rare with aggressive therapy. Recrudescent infection can occur after therapy/apparent clearance and can often be successfully treated with additional courses of antibiotics; persistence ultimately requires line removal.

Empiric Therapy of Gastrointestinal Infections

Acute Diarrheal Syndromes (Gastroenteritis)

Subset	Usual Pathogens	Preferred Therapy[†]	Alternate Therapy[†]
Community-acquired	Viruses (Rotavirus, Norwalk agent, enteric adenovirus, enteroviruses)	No specific therapy indicated	No specific therapy indicated

Acute Diarrheal Syndromes (Gastroenteritis) (cont'd)

Subset	Usual Pathogens	Preferred Therapy†	Alternate Therapy†
	Salmonella non-typhi	Ceftriaxone (IV) **or** cefotaxime (IV) × 10–14 days*	TMP–SMX (IV or PO) **or** amoxicillin (PO) **or** cefixime (PO) × 10–14 days
	Shigella	Ceftriaxone (IV) **or** azithromycin (PO) × 5 days	TMP–SMX (PO) **or** cefixime (PO) **or** ampicillin (PO) × 5 days
	Campylobacter	Erythromycin (PO) × 7 days **or** azithromycin (PO) × 5 days	Doxycycline (PO) (> 8 year old) × 7 days
	Yersinia enterocolitica	TMP–SMX (PO) × 5–7 days	Cefotaxime (IV) **or** tetracycline (PO) **or** doxycycline (PO) × 5–7 days
Traveler's diarrhea	E. coli	TMP–SMX (PO) × 3 days	Azithromycin (PO) × 3 days
Typhoid (Enteric) fever	Salmonella typhi	Ceftriaxone (IV) **or** cefotaxime (IV) × 10–14 days	TMP–SMX (IV or PO) **or** amoxicillin (PO) **or** cefixime (PO) × 10–14 days
Antibiotic-associated colitis	Clostridium difficile	Metronidazole (PO) × 7–10 days **or** nitazoxanide (PO) × 3 days	Vancomycin (PO) × 7–10 days
Chronic watery diarrhea	Giardia lamblia‡	Metronidazole (PO) × 5–7 days **or** nitazoxanide (PO) × 3 days	Tinidazole (PO) × 1 dose **or** furazolidone (PO) × 7–10 days **or** albendazole × 5–7 days
	Cryptosporidia‡	Nitazoxanide (PO) × 3 days	Human immunoglobulin (PO) **or** bovine colostrum (PO) for immunocompromised hosts
Acute dysentery	E. histolytica	Metronidazole (PO) × 10 days **followed by either** iodoquinol (PO) × 20 days **or** paromomycin (PO) × 7 days	Tinidazole (PO) × 3–5 days **followed by either** iodoquinol (PO) × 20 days **or** paromomycin (PO) × 7 days

Acute Diarrheal Syndromes (Gastroenteritis) (cont'd)

Subset	Usual Pathogens	Preferred Therapy†	Alternate Therapy†
	Shigella**	Ceftriaxone (IV) **or** azithromycin (PO) × 5 days	TMP–SMX (PO) **or** cefixime (PO) **or** ampicillin (PO) × 5 days

†   **See pp. 414–422 for drug dosages.**

*   Therapy only indicated in child < 3 to 6 months of age, immunocompromised host, or toxic appearing child.

**   Mild cases acquire no antibiotic therapy. However, antibiotic therapy shortens durations of symptoms and by decreasing the duration of diarrhea limits potential syneral.

‡   May also present as acute watery diarrhea.

Acute Gastroenteritis (Community-Acquired)

Clinical Presentation: Typically presents with the acute onset of diarrhea with fever. This is not an indication for antibiotic therapy unless illness is severe (≥ 6 unformed stools/day, fever ≥ 102° F, bloody stools). Travel history regarding risk for potential E. coli and parasitic exposures is important.

Diagnostic Considerations: In the absence of blood in the stools viruses are the most common cause of acute community-acquired gastroenteritis. Rotaviruses are the most common cause of acute gastroenteritis in 4–24 month old children. Enteric adenoviruses, Norwalk-like virus, enteroviruses and astroviruses are common causes of gastroenteritis in older children. Commercially available antigen tests using ELISA or latex agglutination techniques are readily available to detect rotavirus. Testing for the other viral agents may not be as readily available. Inflammatory changes (presence of white blood cells and/or blood) in the stool are more consistent with bacterial infection. When requesting stool cultures, it may be necessary to order special conditions/media for the detection of yersinia or E. coli O157.

Pitfalls: Antimotility drugs may worsen the course of illness in children with colitis. Empiric therapy with antibiotics may prolong the carriage of Salmonella or increase the risk for developing hemolytic uremic syndrome (HUS) with E. coli O157 infection. The benefit of antibiotics in treating diarrhea caused by yersinia is also unproven. Thus, antibiotic therapy is not routinely indicated prior to culture results in most instances of diarrheal disease, especially as most such infections are self-limited.

Therapeutic Considerations: As above, pending cultures in the absence of severe symptoms or dysentery antibiotics may not be indicated. Overall, the fluoroquinolones have the most complete spectrum for pathogens causing bacterial diarrhea but are not presently approved for use in children < 18 years of age.

Prognosis: Good. Up to 5–10% of children with E. coli O157 are at risk for hemolytic-uremic syndrome.

Giardiasis (Giardia lamblia)

Clinical Presentation: Giardia lamblia is the most common parasite causing diarrheal illness in children. Giardiasis may present as acute watery diarrhea with abdominal pain and bloating or as a chronic, intermittent illness with foul smelling stools, abdominal distension, and anorexia.

Diagnostic Considerations: Trophozoites or cysts of Giardia lamblia can be identified in direct examination of infected stools with 75%–95% sensitivity on a single specimen. Testing 3 or more stools further increases sensitivity of detection. If giardiasis is suspected with negative stool tests, examination of duodenal contents (Entero- or string test) may be helpful.

Pitfalls: Asymptomatic infection is commonly seen in children in day care; therefore, indications to treat must take into account stool testing results *and* clinical findings.

Therapeutic Considerations: Treatment failures occur commonly, and retreatment with the same initial drug is recommended. Furazolidone is the only pediatric liquid available for treating giardiasis < 3 years of age.

Prognosis: Good.

Cryptosporidiosis

Clinical Presentation: Usually presents as fever, vomiting, and non-bloody, watery diarrhea. Infection may also be asymptomatic. More severe and chronic infection is seen in immunocompromised patients (e.g., HIV infection). Cryptosporidia parasite is resistant to chlorine and maybe transmitted in swimming pools. Transmission can also occur from livestock, and a major outbreak through contamination of a public water supply has been reported.

Diagnostic Considerations: Cryptosporidium cysts are detected by microscopic examination of Kinyoun-stained stool specimens using a sucrose floatation method or formalin-ethyl acetate method to concentrate oocysts. This test is not part of routine stool ova and parasite examination and must be specifically requested. Shedding is intermittent; therefore, 3 stool samples should be submitted for optimal detection.

Pitfalls: The oocysts of cryptosporidium are small and may be missed by an inexperienced examiner. A commercially available ELISA test is available but may have false-positive and false-negative results.

Therapeutic Considerations: Treatment failures are frequent. In immunocompromised hosts oral human immune globulin and bovine colostrum are beneficial. Improvement in CD_4 counts with antiretroviral therapy in HIV-infected patients shortens the clinical illness.

Prognosis: Good. Recovery may take months.

Amebiasis (Entamoeba histolytica)

Clinical Presentation: E. histolytica can lead to a spectrum of clinical illnesses from asymptomatic infection to acute dysentery to fulminant colitis. Disseminated disease, primarily manifest as hepatic abscesses, can also occur. E. histolytica is most prevalent in developing countries and is transmitted by the fecal-oral route.

Diagnostic Considerations: Trophozoites or cysts of E. histolytica can be identified in stool specimens. In more severe disease (amebic colitis, hepatic abscesses), serum antibodies can be detected.

Pitfalls: Treatment with steroids or antimotility drugs can worsen symptoms and should not be used.

Therapeutic Considerations: Treatment is two-staged to eliminate tissue-invading trophozoites and organisms in the intestinal lumen. Surgical drainage of large hepatic abscesses may be beneficial.

Prognosis: Good.

Clostridirim difficile Colitis

Clinical Presentation: Classically occurs in a child receiving antibiotic therapy and presents as diarrhea, cramping, bloody/mucousy stools, abdominal tenderness, fever, and toxicity. It may also present weeks after a course of antibiotics.

Diagnostic Considerations: C. difficile toxin can be detected with commercially available immunoassays. Endoscopic finding of pseudomembranous colitis is the definitive method of diagnosis although rarely indicated.

Pitfalls: C. difficile may be normal flora in infants < 1 year of age and probably does not cause illness in this age group. The finding of C. difficile toxin in an infant should not be equated with cause and additional evaluations should be perused. Antimotility drugs may worsen symptoms and should be avoided.

Therapeutic Considerations: Cessation of antibiotics is recommended if possible in the presence of significant C. difficile colitis. Patients with severe symptoms or persistent diarrhea × 2–3 days after discontinuing antibiotics should then be treated with oral metronidazole or oral vancomycin. Up to ~25% relapse after a single course; re-treatment using the same initial antibiotic is recommended. For persistent infection alternate therapies such as nitazoxanide, rifaximin, tinidazole, oral immune globulin therapy, toxin binders or repopulating intestinal flora may be considered.

Prognosis: Good.

Empiric Therapy of Bone and Joint Infections

Septic Arthritis

Subset	Usual Pathogens	Preferred IV Therapy[†*]	Alternate IV Therapy[†*]	IV-to-PO Switch[†]
Newborns (≤ 3 months)	S. aureus[‡] Group B streptococci Enterobacteriaceae N. gonorrhea	**Combination therapy with** nafcillin **or** vancomycin **plus either** ceftriaxone **or** cefotaxime*	**Combination therapy with** vancomycin **or** clindamycin **plus either** ceftriaxone **or** cefotaxime **or** gentamicin **or** tobramycin*	Not applicable
Child (> 3 months to 14 years)	S. aureus[‡] Group A streptococci S. pneumoniae Gram-negative bacilli N. meningitidis (H. influenza type b in prevaccine era) Kingella	**Combination therapy with** nafcillin **or** vancomycin **plus either** ceftriaxone **or** cefotaxime*	**Combination therapy with** vancomycin **or** clindamycin **plus either** ceftriaxone **or** cefotaxime*	Dicloxacillin **or** cephalexin **or** clindamycin (PO) after 1 week of IV therapy*

†   **See pp. 414–422 for drug dosages.**

*   Total duration of therapy for non-gonococcal septic arthritis ≥ 3 weeks based on clinical response.

‡   If CA-MRSA is suspected based on clinical presentation/local epidemiology, consider empiric coverage for CA-MRSA with clindamycin, TMP–SMX, doxycycline, or vancomycin pending culture results.

Septic Arthritis (cont'd)

Subset	Usual Pathogens	Preferred IV Therapy†*	Alternate IV Therapy†*	IV-to-PO Switch†
Adolescents (sexually active)	As above plus N. gonorrhoeae (typically 2 or 3 joints involved)	**Combination therapy with** nafcillin **or** vancomycin **plus either** ceftriaxone **or** cefotaxime*	If GC isolated and penicillin allergy: Ciprofloxacin **or** ofloxacin **or** spectinomycin	GC arthritis with prompt response to IV therapy may switch to ciprofloxacin **or** ofloxacin **or** cefixime to complete 7 days of total therapy

Duration of therapy represents total time IV or IV + PO. Most patients on IV therapy able to take PO meds should be switched to PO therapy after clinical improvement. Taper to individual drug therapy once organism isolated and sensitivities are available.

† **See pp. 414–422 for drug dosages**.
* Total duration of therapy for non-gonococcal septic arthritis ≥ 3 weeks based on clinical response.
‡ If CA-MRSA is suspected based on clinical presentation/local epidemiology, consider empiric coverage for CA-MRSA with clindamycin, TMP–SMX, doxycycline, or vancomycin pending culture results.

Clinical Presentation: Varies with age of the child. Presentation is often nonspecific in infants (i.e., fever, poor feeding, tachycardia). Physical exam findings can be subtle: asymmetrical tissue folds, unilateral swelling of an extremity, subtle changes in limb/joint position. In older children, signs and symptoms are more localized to the involved joint. Commonly affected joints: hips, elbows, knees.

Diagnostic Considerations: Joint aspiration (large-bore needle) shows 50,000–250,000 WBCs/mm³ with a marked predominance of PMNs. Gram stain/culture of joint fluid confirm the diagnosis. Toxic synovitis, Lyme arthritis, rheumatoid arthritis, traumatic arthritis, and sympathetic effusion from adjacent osteomyelitis can mimic septic arthritis on presentation, but joint fluid has fewer WBCs and cultures are negative. Multiple joint involvement is more typical of rheumatic/Lyme disease. In young infants, persistence of the nutrient artery can lead to osteomyelitis and septic arthritis.

Pitfalls: Septic arthritis of the hip is an emergency concomitant condition requiring prompt joint aspiration and irrigation to minimize the risk of femoral head necrosis, which may occur within 24 hours. Toxic synovitis of the hip, which is treated with anti-inflammatory agents and observation, typically causes less fever, pain, and leukocytosis than septic arthritis; however, at times the two can not be differentiated and aspiration of the joint is indicated. In sexually active adolescents, consider N. gonorrhea and culture aspirate.

Therapeutic Considerations: IV therapy is recommended for at least 3–4 weeks, followed by oral therapy for a total antibiotic course of 4–6 weeks based on clinical response and laboratory parameters (WBC, ESR, CRP). Intra-articular therapy is not helpful. Empiric coverage is broader than for osteomyelitis in children.

Prognosis: Good with prompt joint aspiration and at least 3 weeks of antibiotics.

Acute Osteomyelitis, Osteochondritis, Diskitis

Subset	Usual Pathogens	Preferred IV Therapy†	Alternate IV Therapy†	IV-to-PO Switch or PO Therapy†
Acute osteomyelitis Newborn (0–3 months)	S. aureus§ Gram-negative bacilli Group B streptococci	**Combination therapy with nafcillin or oxacillin plus either** cefotaxime **or** ceftriaxone × 4–6 weeks	Vancomycin **plus either** cefotaxime or ceftriaxone × 4–6 weeks	Not applicable
> 3 months*	S. aureus§ Group A streptococci Gram-negative bacteria (rare) Salmonella (sickle cell disease)	Nafcillin **or** oxacillin **or** cefazolin × 4–6 weeks	Clindamycin **or** ampicillin-sulbactam **or** vancomycin × 4–6 weeks	Cephalexin **or** clindamycin **or** cefadroxil × 4–6 weeks
Osteochondritis	P. aeruginosa S. aureus§	Ticarcillin-clavulanate × 7–10 days after surgery **or** combination therapy with nafcillin plus ceftazidime × 7–10 days after surgery	Piperacillin **or** ciprofloxacin × 7–10 days after surgery	Ciprofloxacin** × 7–10 days after surgery
Diskitis	S. aureus, K. kingae Enterobacteriaceae S. pneumoniae S. epidermidis	PO Therapy: Cephalexin **or** cefadroxil **or** clindamycin × 3–4 weeks or ESR returns to normal††		

Duration of therapy represents total time IV, PO, or IV + PO. Most patients on IV therapy able to take PO meds should be switched to PO therapy soon after clinical improvement.

† **See pp. 414–422 for drug dosages.**
** Not approved for children but might consider in adolescent.
* Treat only IV or IV-to-PO switch.
†† Add gram-negative coverage only if culture proven.
§ If CA-MRSA is suspected based on clinical presentation/local epidemiology, consider empiric coverage for CA-MRSA with clindamycin, TMP–SMX, doxycycline, or vancomycin pending culture results.

Acute Osteomyelitis

Clinical Presentation: Acute onset of fever and pain/decreased movement around the infected area. Can be difficult to localize, especially in younger children. Occurs primarily via hematogenous spread (vs. direct inoculation) to metaphysis of long bones.

Diagnostic Considerations: Acute phase reactants are elevated (ESR, CRP, WBC). X-rays may not reveal osteolytic lesions for > 7 days, but soft tissue swelling and periosteal reaction may be seen as early as 3 days. Bone scan/MRI reveal changes in the first 24 hours, but bone scans are insensitive in neonates. Blood cultures may be positive, especially in younger children. Definitive diagnosis by bone aspirate for gram stain and culture, but empiric therapy is often initiated based on clinical history and the presence of an acute lytic lesion on MRI, bone scan, or x-ray.

Pitfalls: Bony changes on x-ray may not be present initially. It may be difficult to differentiate cellulitis from osteomyelitis, even on bone scan.

Therapeutic Considerations: Initiate empiric therapy by IV route. Treatment is required ≥ 4 weeks, but children with compliant families can complete therapy with high-dose oral antibiotics. With adequate treatment, CPR and ESR normalize over 2 weeks and 4 weeks, respectively.

Prognosis: Good with 4–6 weeks of total therapy. Long-term growth of affected bone may be impaired.

Osteochondritis of the Foot ("Puncture Wound Osteomyelitis")

Clinical Presentation: Tenderness, erythema, and swelling several days to weeks after a nail puncture wound through a sneaker/tennis shoe (Pseudomonas found in foam layer between sole and lining of shoe). Fever and other systemic complaints are rare. Develops in 1–2% of puncture wounds of foot.

Diagnostic Considerations: P. aeruginosa is the primary pathogen, although infection with S. aureus is also a concern.

Pitfalls: Antibiotics surgical of necrotic cartilage.

Therapeutic Considerations: With prompt debridement, 7–10 days of antibiotic therapy is usually sufficient.

Prognosis: Good with debridement and antibiotics.

Diskitis

Clinical Presentation: Typically involves the lumbar region and occurs in children < 6 years old. Presents with gradual onset (over weeks) of irritability and refusal to walk. Fever is low-grade or absent. Older children may be able to localize pain to back, hip, or abdomen. Pain is exacerbated by motion of the spine and can be localized by percussion of the vertebral bodies.

Diagnostic Considerations: ESR is elevated, but WBC count is normal. X-rays are usually normal initially, but later reveal disk space narrowing and sclerosis of the vertebrae. Increased disk space uptake can be seen on bone scan. MRI is very sensitive for assessing disk space involvement.

Therapeutic Considerations: Diskitis is probably a low-grade bacterial infection, but the role of antibiotic therapy is unclear. Bed rest and anti-inflammatory medications are the mainstays of treatment. Immobilization may be required for severe cases. Oral antibiotics are given for 3–4 weeks or until the ESR returns to normal.

Pitfalls: Difficult to isolate an organism, even with needle aspiration of disk space. S. aureus is the most common pathogen, but diskitis can also be caused by coagulase-negative staphylococcus, K. kingae, coliforms, S. pneumoniae.

Prognosis: Fusion of involved vertebrae may occur as the infection resolves. Otherwise, outcome is generally good.

Empiric Therapy of Skin and Soft Tissue Infections

Skin and Soft Tissue Infections

Subset	Usual Pathogens	Preferred IV Therapy[†]	Alternate IV Therapy[†]	PO Therapy or IV-to-PO Switch[†]
Cellulitis, impetigo	S. aureus Group A streptococci	Cefazolin **or** nafcillin **or** oxacillin × 7–10 days	Clindamycin[‡] × 7–10 days	Cephalexin **or** cefadroxil **or** dicloxacillin **or** clindamycin **or** amoxicillin/clavulanate **or** erythromycin **or** azithromycin × 7–10 days
Severe pyodermas abscesses	CA-MRSA	Vancomycin **plus** Clindamycin × 7–14 days	Vancomycin or linezolid × 7–14 days	TMP–SMX **or** doxycycline × 7–14 days**
Animal bite wounds (dog/cat)	Group A streptococci P. multocida Capnocytophaga S. aureus	Ampicillin-sulbactam × 7–10 days	Piperacillin **or** ticarcillin × 7–10 days Penicillin allergy: Clindamycin **plus** TMP–SMX × 7–10 days (dog bites); doxycycline **or** cefuroxime × 7–10 days (cat bites)	Amoxicillin-clavulanate **or** doxycycline × 7–10 days
Human bite wounds	Oral anaerobes E. corrodens Group A streptococci S. aureus	Ampicillin-sulbactam × 5–7 days	Piperacillin **or** ticarcillin × 5–7 days Penicillin allergic patient: Clindamycin **plus** TMP–SMX × 5–7 days	Amoxicillin-clavulanate **or** doxycycline × 5–7 days
Cat scratch disease (CSD)*	Bartonella henselae	Gentamicin × 10–14 days	—	Azithromycin × 5 days **or** TMP–SMX **or** ciprofloxacin **or** rifampin × 10–14 days

† **See pp. 414–422 for drug dosages.**
** In children > 8 years of age.
* No well-controlled trials of antibiotic treatment for CSD to demonstrate benefit.
‡ Preferred therapy for patients in geographic regions with a high prevalence of MRSA or for those with penicillin/cephalosporin allergy.

Skin and Soft Tissue Infections (cont'd)

Subset	Pathogens	IV Therapy†	PO Therapy or IV-to-PO Switch†
Chicken pox *Immuno-compromised host*	VZV	Acyclovir × 7–10 days	Acyclovir **or** valacyclovir × 7–10 days
Immuno-competent host	VZV	Acyclovir × 5 days	Acyclovir **or** valacyclovir × 5 days
H. zoster (Shingles)	VZV	Same as for chicken pox	Acyclovir **or** valacyclovir × 10 days (for individuals ≥ 12 years of age)

Duration of therapy represents total time IV, PO, or IV + PO. Most patients on IV therapy able to take PO meds should be switched to PO therapy soon after clinical improvement.
† **See pp. 414–422 for drug dosages.**

Cellulitis
Clinical Presentation: Erythema, warmth, and tenderness of skin. Impetigo is characterized by a vesiculopapular rash with honey-colored discharge.
Diagnostic Considerations: Primarily a clinical diagnosis. Group A streptococci and Staphylococcus are primary pathogens in healthy children. Wound culture of discharge or leading edge of lesion and gram stain may be helpful.
Pitfalls: Differential diagnosis of cellulitis may include hypersensitivity to insect bites. Herpetic whitlow (HSV) may be mistaken for a bacterial skin or paronychial infection.
Therapeutic Considerations: First generation cephalosporin or semi-synthetic penicillin with anti-staphylococcal activity (i.e., dicloxacillin, nafcillin, oxacillin) are drugs of choice. Increasing incidence of community-acquired MRSA may affect treatment decisions.
Prognosis: Excellent. Impetigo may only require topical treatment/(mupirocin).

Bite Wounds
Clinical Presentation: 80% of animal bite wounds in children are from dogs, and 15%–50% of dog bites become infected. More than 50% of cat bites become infected, and due to their long teeth, there is an increased risk of inoculation into bone/joints with development of osteomyelitis/septic arthritis. Human bite wounds are most prone to infection, and 75%–90% of all human bites become infected.
Diagnostic Considerations: Clinical diagnosis. Culture of wound exudate may yield organism.
Pitfalls: Failure to assess depth of infection, especially with cat bites, may result in late identification of bone/joint infection. Macrolides are ineffective against P. multocida.
Therapeutic Considerations: It is important to cover oral anaerobes, S. aureus, and Group A streptococci in human bite wounds. P. multocida is an important pathogen in cat and dog bite wounds. Facial/hand lesions require plastic surgery. Recurrent debridement may be necessary, especially with human bite wound infections of hand. Assess tetanus immunization status for all bite wounds

(p. 377). For human bites consider the risk of HIV and hepatitis B. For dog bites consider the risk of rabies. Antimicrobial therapy initiated within 8 hours of a bite wound and administered for 2–3 days may decrease the rate of infection.

Prognosis: Good with early debridement and antibiotics.

Cat Scratch Disease (CSD)

Clinical Presentation: Classic presentation is a papular lesion at site of cat scratch with lymphadenitis in the draining region (axillary, epitrochlear, inguinal, cervical most commonly). Frequently associated with fever/malaise 1–2 weeks after scratch. Infection can present with conjunctivitis and ipsilateral preauricular lymph node (Parinaud oculoglandular syndrome). Unusual presentations in normal hosts include encephalitis, hepatitis, microabscesses in liver/spleen, fever of unknown origin, osteolytic lesions.

Diagnostic Considerations: Most often secondary to kitten scratch with Bartonella henselae. Diagnosed using specific serology for antibodies to B. henselae. CSD antigen skin test from pus obtained from aspirated CSD lymph nodes is unlicenced and should not be used.

Pitfalls: Failure to obtain history of kitten exposure. Surgical excision of lymph node is generally not necessary.

Therapeutic Considerations: Most lesions are self-limited and resolve over 2–4 months. There are no well-controlled studies, but antibiotic therapy may be helpful in severe cases with hepatosplenomegaly. Doxycycline, erythromycin, or azithromycin are helpful in immunocompromised hosts.

Prognosis: Very good with spontaneous resolution over 2–4 months.

Chicken Pox/Shingles (VZV)

Clinical Presentation: Primary illness is chicken pox, a generalized pruritic, vesicular rash with fever that erupts in crops of lesions over 3–5 days followed by crusting and recovery. Complications include bacterial superinfection of skin lesions, sepsis, cerebellar ataxia, thrombocytopenia, hepatitis, pneumonia and encephalitis. The disease tends to be more severe in adolescents and adults, particularly if immunocompromised. Primary infection early in pregnancy can rarely result in varicella embryopathy with imb atrophy and CNS malformations in the neonate. Reactivation disease (shingles) may occur in children and in normal hosts and remains localized to a single dermatome. Post-herpetic neuralgia occurs less often in children than adults. Reactivation disease in immunocompromised hosts can spread and re-disseminate.

Diagnostic Considerations: The characteristic eruption of chicken pox occurs in waves—multiple stages appear at the same time, from new papules and vesicles to more advanced larger and crusted lesions—and is unique to varicella. Direct fluorescent antibody staining of a scraped lesion can confirm the diagnosis.

Pitfalls: Initially lesions may be primarily papular, and if the diagnosis is not considered, exposure of others can occur.

Therapeutic Considerations: Antiviral therapy with acyclovir, if started within 24 hours of rash, should be considered for children > 12 years of age, those on steroid or salicylate therapy, and those with underlying chronic pulmonary, skin, or immunosuppressive states. Oral administration is acceptable, although IV therapy may be preferred for immunocompromised hosts at risk of disseminated disease. More severe varicella has been observed in individuals acquiring the infection from a household contact, presumable due to a higher innocuous with closer contact; household contacts may be considered for acyclovir therapy at onset of rash in child. Additionally, individuals ≥ 13 years may develop more extensive varicella than younger children. Immunocompromised children or pregnant women without a history of varicella or immunization may benefit from prophylaxis with varicella zoster immune globulin (VZIG) within 96 hours of varicella exposure. Newborns whose mothers develop chicken pox within 5 days before or 48 hours after delivery and exposed premature infants are also candidates for VZIG. A like-attenuated varicella vaccine has been licensed since 1995 for use in individuals ≥ 12 months of age who have not had chicken pox. A two-dose vaccine schedule is recommended for children ≥ 12 months of age.

Prognosis: Overall prognosis is good with complete recovery and minimal risk of scarring unless immunosuppressed host with disseminated disease. Although rare, Group A streptococcal toxic shock syndrome (manifest as cellulitis or in conjunction with necrotizing fasciitis complicating varicella skin lesions) and Group A streptococcal septicemia, which can occur in the absence of apparent secondarily infected skin lesions, may be fatal complications of varicella in normal children.

Common Pediatric Antimicrobial Drugs

Drug	Dosage in Neonates	Dosage in Infants/Children*
Acyclovir	20 mg/kg (IV) q8h × 14–21 days. Dosing interval may need to be increased for infants < 34 weeks post-maturational age (GA + CA) or if significant renal impairment or liver failure Chronic suppression: 75 mg/kg (PO) q12h	<u>HSV encephalitis</u>: 10 mg/kg (IV) q8h × 12–21 days <u>Primary HSV infection</u>: 10–20 mg/kg (PO) q6h × 5–10 days **or** 5 mg/kg/dose (IV) q8h × 5 days <u>Varicella in immunocompromised hosts</u>: 10 mg/kg (IV) q8h × 7–10 days <u>Varicella in immunocompetent hosts</u>: 20 mg/kg (PO) q6h × 5 days (maximum 800 mg/dose)
Albendazole	Not applicable	400 mg (PO) q24h
Amikacin**	*During first week of life* dosing is based on gestational age (administer IV dose over 30 min) • ≤ 27 weeks (or asphyxia, PDA, or indomethacin): 18 mg/kg (IV) q48h • 28–30 weeks: 18 mg/kg (IV) q36h • 31–33 weeks: 16 mg/kg (IV) q36h • ≥ 34 weeks: 15 mg/kg (IV) q24h	5–7.5 mg/kg (IV or IM) q8h

Drug	Dosage in Neonates			Dosage in Infants/Children*
	After first week of life: Initial dose of 15 mg/kg, then draw serum concentrations 30 min after end of infusion (peak) and 12–24 hours later (trough) to determine dosing interval. Aim for peak of 20–30 mcg/mL and trough of 2–5 mcg/mL			
Amoxicillin	Not indicated			22.5–45 mg/kg (PO) q12h
Amoxicillin-clavulanate	Not indicated			22.5–45 mg/kg (of amoxicillin component) (PO) q12h
Amphotericin B (conventional)	0.5–1 mg/kg (IV over 2–6 hours) q24-48h (Some authorities recommend an initial test dose of 0.1–0.5 mg/kg IV over 2–6 hours)			
Ampicillin	25–50 mg/kg/dose (IV or IM). Severe Group B streptococcal sepsis: 100 mg/kg/dose. Dosing interval is based on gestational age (GA) and chronological age (CA):			25–50 mg/kg (IV or IM) q6h
	GA + CA (weeks)	**CA (days)**	**Interval (hours)**	
	≤ 29	0–28 > 28	12 8	
	30–36	0–14 > 14	12 8	
	≥ 37	0–7 > 7	12 8	
Ampicillin-sulbactam	Not indicated			25–50 mg/kg (of ampicillin component) (IV) q6h
Azithromycin	Not indicated			Otitis media/sinusitis: 30 mg/kg (PO) × 1 dose **or** 10 mg/kg (PO) q24h × 3 days **or** 10 mg/kg (PO) on day 1 followed by 5 mg/kg (PO) q24h on days 2–5 Pharyngitis/tonsillitis: 12 mg/kg (PO) q24h × 5 days

* Dosages are generally based on weight (mg/kg), up to adult dose as maximum.

** Drug can be given IM but absorption may be variable.

Drug	Dosage in Neonates	Dosage in Infants/Children*
		Community-acquired pneumonia (not indicated for moderate or severe disease): 10 mg/kg (PO) × 5 days **or** 10 mg/kg (IV or PO) on day 1 followed by 5 mg/kg (IV or PO) q24h on days 2–5 Skin/soft tissue infections (including Cat Scratch Disease): 10 mg/kg (PO) on day 1 followed by 5 mg/kg (PO) q24h on days 2–5
Aztreonam	30 mg/kg (IV or IM). See *ampicillin* for dosing interval (p. 415)	30 mg/kg (IV or IM) q6-8h
Caspofungin	70 mg/m2 loading dose, then 50 mg/m2 (IV) q24h	70 mg/m2 loading dose, then 50 mg/m2 (IV) q24h
Cefadroxil	Not indicated	15 mg/kg (PO) q12h
Cefazolin	25 mg/kg (IV or IM). See *ampicillin* for dosing interval (p. 415)	25–100 mg/kg/day (IV or IM) divided q8h
Cefdinir	Not indicated	7 mg/kg (PO) q12h or 14 mg/kg (PO) q24h
Cefepime	50 mg/kg (IV) q8-12h	33.3–50 mg/kg (IV or IM) q8h
Cefotaxime	50 mg/kg (IV or IM). (25 mg/kg/dose is adequate for gonococcal infection). See *ampicillin* for dosing interval (p. 415)	25–50 mg/kg (IV or IM) q6–8h
Cefotetan	Not indicated	20–40 mg/kg (IV or IM) q12h
Cefoxitin	25–33 mg/kg/dose (IV or IM). See *ampicillin* for dosing interval (p. 415)	80–160 mg/kg/day (IV or IM) divided q4–8h
Cefpodoxime	Not indicated	5 mg/kg (PO) q12h
Cefprozil	Not indicated	15 mg/kg (PO) q12h
Ceftazidime	30 mg/kg/dose (IV or IM). See *ampicillin* for dosing interval (p. 415)	25–50 mg/kg (IV or IM) q8h
Ceftibuten	Not indicated	9 mg/kg (PO) q24h
Ceftizoxime	Not indicated	50 mg/kg (IV or IM) q6–8h

* Dosages are generally based on weight (mg/kg), up to adult dose as maximum.

Drug	Dosage in Neonates	Dosage in Infants/Children*
Ceftriaxone‡	<u>Sepsis and disseminated gonococcal infection:</u> 50 mg/kg (IV or IM) q24h <u>Meningitis:</u> 100 mg/kg loading dose followed by 80 mg/kg (IV or IM) q24h <u>Uncomplicated gonococcal ophthalmia:</u> 50 mg/kg (maximum 125 mg) as a single dose (IV or IM)	50 mg/kg (IV or IM) q24h. <u>Meningitis:</u> 50 mg/kg (IV or IM) q12h or 100 mg/kg (IV or IM) q24h <u>Acute otitis media:</u> 50 mg/kg (IM) × 1 dose (or 3 doses IM q24h in high-risk patients)
Cefuroxime	Not indicated	10–15 mg/kg (PO) q12h 25–50 mg/kg (IV or IM) q8h
Cephalexin	Not indicated	6.25–25 mg/kg (PO) q6h
Cephalothin	Not indicated	25 mg/kg (IV or IM) q4-6h
Clarithromycin	Not indicated	7.5 mg/kg (PO) q12h
Clindamycin	5.0–7.5 mg (IV or PO). Dosing interval is based on gestational age (GA) and chronological age (CA)	5–10 mg/kg (IV or IM) q6-8h or 10–30 mg/kg/day (PO) divided q6-8h

	GA + CA (weeks)	CA (days)	Interval (hours)	
	< 29	0–28	12	
		> 28	8	
	30–36	0–14	12	
		> 14	8	
	37–44	0–7	8	
		> 7	6	

Drug	Dosage in Neonates	Dosage in Infants/Children*
Dicloxacillin	Not indicated	3.125–25 mg/kg (PO) q6h
Doxycycline	Contraindicated	> 45 kg: 100 mg (PO) q12h ≤ 45 kg: 1.1–2.5 mg/kg (PO) q12h Use only in children > 8 years (unless RMSF) 1–2 mg/kg (IV) q12–24h

*   Dosages are generally based on weight (mg/kg), up to adult dose as maximum.

‡   Do not use in presence of hyperbilirubinemia.

Drug	Dosage in Neonates	Dosage in Infants/Children*
Erythromycin	<u>Chlamydia pneumonitis/conjunctivitis or pertussis:</u> 12.5 mg/kg (PO) q6h (E. estolate preferred) <u>Other infections:</u> E. estolate 10 mg/kg (PO) q8h **or** E. ethylsuccinate 10 mg/kg (PO) q6h <u>Severe infections and PO not possible:</u> 5–10 mg/kg (IV over ≥ 60 min) q6h	10–12.5 mg/kg (PO) q6–8h 5–12.5 mg/kg (IV) q6h
Ertapenem	Not indicated	15 mg/kg (IV) q12h (not to exceed 1 gm/day)
Ethambutol	See p. 401	See p. 401
Ethionamide	See p. 401	See p. 401
Fluconazole	<u>Systemic infection or meningitis:</u> 12 mg/kg (IV over 30 min or PO) × 1 dose, then 6 mg/kg/dose (IV or PO) with dosing interval based on gestational age (GA) and chronological age (CA) (below) <u>Prophylaxis</u> (e.g., extremely low birth weight infants in NICU with high rates of fungal disease): 3 mg/kg/dose (IV or PO) according to dosing interval grid (below) <u>Thrush:</u> 6 mg/kg (PO) × 1 dose, then 3 mg/kg (PO) q24h	10 mg/kg (IV or PO) loading dose followed by 3–6 mg/kg (IV or PO) q24h

GA + CA (weeks)	CA (days)	Interval (weeks)
≤ 29	0–14 > 14	72 48
30–36	0–14 > 14	48 24
37–44	0–7 > 7	48 24

* Dosages are generally based on weight (mg/kg), up to adult dose as maximum.

Drug	Dosage in Neonates	Dosage in Infants/Children*
Gentamicin**	*During first week of life* dosing is based on gestational age (administer IV dose over 30 min): • ≤ 29 weeks (or asphyxia, PDA, or indomethacin): 5 mg/kg (IV) q48h • 30–33 weeks: 4.5 mg/kg (IV) q48h • 34–37 weeks: 4 mg/kg (IV) q36h • ≥ 38 weeks: 4 mg/kg (IV) q24h *After first week of life:* Initial dose of 4 mg/kg, then draw serum concentrations 30 min after end of infusion (peak) and 12–24 hours later (trough) to determine dosing interval. Aim for peak of 5–12 mcg/mL and trough of 0.5–1 mcg/mL	2–2.5 mg/kg (IV or IM) q8h
Imipenem	20–25 mg/kg (IV) q12h	15–25 mg/kg (IV or IM) q6h
Iodoquinol	10–13.3 mg/kg (PO) q8h	10–13.3 mg/kg (PO) q8h
Isoniazid	See p. 401	See p. 401
Linezolid	10 mg/kg (IV) q12h	10 mg/kg (IV) q8h
Liposomal/lipid complex Amphotericin preparations	1–5 mg/kg (IV over 2 hours) q24h	3–6 mg/kg (IV) q24h
Meropenem	20 mg/kg (IV) q12h	10 mg/kg (IV) q8h (skin); 20 mg/kg (IV) q8h (intraabdominal); 40 mg/kg (IV) q8h (meningitis)
Methenamine mandelate	Not indicated	15–25 mg (PO) q6–8h
Metronidazole	15 mg/kg (IV or PO) × 1 dose, then 7.5 mg/kg/dose (IV or PO) with dosing interval based on gestational age (GA) and chronological age (CA):	5–12.5 mg/kg (PO) q8h 15 mg/kg (IV) × 1 dose followed by 7.5 mg/kg (IV) q6h

* Dosages are generally based on weight (mg/kg), up to adult dose as maximum.
** Drug can be given IM but absorption may be variable.

Drug	Dosage in Neonates			Dosage in Infants/Children*
	GA + CA (weeks)	CA (days)	Interval (hours)	
	≤ 29	0–28	24	
		> 28	48	
	30–36	0–14	24	
		> 14	12	
	37–44	0–7	24	
		> 7	12	
Micafungin	Not applicable			4–12 mg/kg (IV) q24 (higher dose for patients < 8 year of age
Mupirocin	Not indicated			Nasal cream: ½ of single use tube into nostril q12h × 5 days; Cream: apply q8h × 5–190 days
Nafcillin	25–50 mg/kg/dose (IV). See *ampicillin* for dosing interval (p. 415)			12.5–50 mg/kg (IV or IM) q6h
Nitazoxanide	Not applicable			Children 1–3 years old: 100 mg (PO) q12h; children 4–11 years old: 200 mg (PO) q12h
Nitrofurantoin	Not indicated			UTI: 1.25–1.75 mg/kg (PO) q6h UTI prophylaxis: 1–2 mg/kg (PO) q24h
Nystatin	Oral: 1 mL (preterm) to 2 mL (term) of 100,000 U/mL suspension applied with swab to each side of mouth q6h until 3 days after resolution of lesions Topical: Apply ointment or cream to affected area q6h until 3 days after resolution of lesions.			Suspension: 4–6 mL swish and swallow 4×/day Troche: 1–2 troches 4–5×/ day
Oxacillin	25–50 mg/kg/dose (IV). See *ampicillin* for dosing interval (p. 415)			25–50 mg/kg (IV or IM) q6h
Paromomycin	Not applicable			10 mg/kg (PO) q8h
Penicillin G	25,000–50,000 IU/kg/dose (IV). See *ampicillin* for dosing interval (p. 415) Meningitis: 75,000–100,000 IU/kg			12,500–75,000 U/kg (IV or IM) q4–6h

*　Dosages are generally based on weight (mg/kg), up to adult dose as maximum.

Drug	Dosage in Neonates	Dosage in Infants/Children*
	(IV) in meningitis (IV).† Q8–12h based on GA + CA, See *ampicillin* for dosing interval (p. 415). Crystalline penicillin G: IM: procaine penicillin G q24 hours. Congenital syphilis: Aqueous penicillin G 50,000 IU/kg (slow IV push) q12h × 7 days, then q8h to complete 10–14 days **or** procaine penicillin G 50,000 IU/kg (IM) q24h × 10–14 days	
Penicillin V	Not indicated	25–50 mg/kg (PO) q6-8h
Piperacillin	50–100 mg/kg/dose (IV or IM). See *ampicillin* for dosing interval (p. 415)	25–75 mg/kg (IV or IM) q6h; may increase to q4h in severe infection, especially with pseudomonas
Piperacillin-tazobactam	Not indicated	100–300 mg/kg/day (IV) (of piperacillin component) divided q6-8h
Pyrazinamide	See p. 401	See p. 401
Quinupristin-dalfopristin	7.5 mg/kg (IV) q12h	7.5 mg/kg (IV) q12h
Rifampin	10–20 mg/kg (PO) q24h **or** 5–10 mg/kg (IV) q24h	20 mg/kg (PO) q24h **or** 10 mg/kg (PO) q12h 10–20 mg/kg/day (IV) divided q12–24h
Streptomycin	See p. 401	See p. 401
Sulfisoxazole	Contraindicated	30–35 mg/kg (PO) q6h Otitis media prophylaxis: 37.5 mg/kg (PO) q12h
Tetracycline	Contraindicated	5–12.5 mg/kg (PO) q6h. Use only in children > 8 years
Ticarcillin	75–100 mg/kg/dose (IV). See *ampicillin* for dosing interval (p. 415)	25–75 mg/kg (IV or IM) q6h
Ticarcillin-clavulanate	75–100 mg/kg/dose (of ticarcillin component) (IV). See *ampicillin* for dosing interval (p. 415)	25–75 mg/kg (of ticarcillin component) (IV or IM) q6h
Tinidazole	Not applicable	50–60 mg/kg (PO) q24h
Tobramycin	Same as gentamicin (p. 419)	2–2.5 mg/kg (IV or IM) q8h

*   Dosages are generally based on weight (mg/kg), up to adult dose as maximum.

Drug	Dosage in Neonates	Dosage in Infants/Children*
Trimethoprim-sulfameth-oxazole (TMP–SMX)	Contraindicated	<u>UTI</u>: 4–5 mg/kg (of trimethoprim component) (PO) q12h <u>Pneumocystis carinii pneumonia (PCP)</u> 5 mg/kg (PO) q6h (typically after initial IV therapy) <u>UTI prophylaxis</u>: 2–4 mg/kg (PO) q24h *IV dosing* <u>PCP or severe infection</u>: 5 mg/kg (of trimethoprim component) (IV) q6h <u>Minor infections</u>: 4–6 mg/kg (of trimethoprim component) (IV) q12h
Vancomycin	<u>Bacteremia</u>: 10 mg/kg/dose (IV) <u>Meningitis</u>: 15 mg/kg/dose (IV). Administer IV dose over 60 min. Dosing interval is based on gestational age (GA) and chronological age (CA):	10–15 mg/kg (IV) q6h

GA + CA (weeks)	CA (days)	Interval (weeks)
≤ 29	0–14	18
	> 14	12
30–36	0–14	12
	> 14	8
37–44	0–7	12
	> 7	8

Drug	Dosage in Neonates	Dosage in Infants/Children*
Voriconazole	Not applicable	7 mg/kg (IV) q12h 8 mg/kg (PO) q12h × 1 day, then 7 mg/kg (PO) q12h

* Dosages are generally based on weight (mg/kg), up to adult dose as maximum.

REFERENCES AND SUGGESTED READINGS

Betts R, Glasmacher A, Maertens J, et al. Efficacy of caspofungin against invasive Candida or invasive Aspergillus infections in neutropenic patients. Cancer 106:466–73, 2006.

Bisno AL, Kaplan EL. Strep throat over and over: How frequent? How real? Mayo Clin Proc 81:1153–4, 2006.

CDC. Outbreak of Swine-Origin Influenza A (H₁N₁) Virus Infection—Mexico, March–April 2009, MMWR Dispatch 58:April 30, 2009.

CDC. Use of rapid influenza diagnostic tests for patients with influenza-like illness during the novel H₁N₁ influenza virus (Swine Flu) outbreak. Swine Influenza Bulletin June 12, 2009.

Cheng VCC, Lau Y-K, Lee K-I, et al. Fatal co-infection with swine origin influenza virus A/H₁N₁ and community-acquired methicillin resistant Staphylococcus aureus. J Infection (Epub ahead of print): 1–5, 2009.

Committee of Infectious Disease. Prevention of varicella: Recommendations for use of varicella vaccine in children, including a recommendation for a routine 2-dose varicella immunization schedule. Pediatrics 120:221–231, 2007.

Dominguez-Cherit G, Lapinsky SE, Macias AE, et al. Critically I11 Patients with 2009 Influenza A (H₁N₁) in Mexico. JAMA 302:1872–1879, 2009.

Ellis JM, Kuti JL, Nicolau DP. Pharmacodynamic evaluation of meropenem and cefotaxime for pediatric meningitis: a report from the OPTAMA program. Pediatr Drugs 8:131–8, 2006.

Fox JW, Marcon MJ, Bonsu BK. Diagnosis of streptococcal pharyngitis by detection of Streptococcus pyogenes in posterior pharyngeal vs oral cavity specimens. Journal of Clin Microbiology 44:2593–94, 2006.

Groll AH, Attarbasehi A, Schuster FR, et al. Treatment with caspofungin in immunocompromised paediatric patients: a multicentre survey. A Antimicrob Chemother 57:527–35, 2006.

Hidron AI, Low CE, Honig EG, et al. Emergence of community-acquired methicillin-resistant Staphylococcus aureus strain USA300 as a cause of necrotizing community-onset pneumonia. Lancet Infect Dis 9:384–392, 2009.

Kaplan SL, Afghani B, Lopez P, et al. Linezolid for the treatment of methicillin-resistant Staphylococcus aureus infections in children. Pediatric Infect Disease 22:S178–185, 2003.

Lehtinen P, Jartti T, Virkki R, et al. Bacterial coinfections in children with viral wheezing. Eur J Clin Microbiol Infect Dis 25:463–9, 2006.

Lorente L, Lorenzo L, Martin MM, Jimenez A, Mora ML. Meropenem by continuous versus intermittent infusion in ventilator-associated pneumonia due to gram-negative bacilli. Ann Pharmacother 40:219–23, 2006.

Louie JK, Acosta M, Winter K, et al. Factors Associated with death or hospitalization due to pandemic 2009 influenza (H₁N₁) infection in California. JAMA 302: 1896–1902, 2009.

Mathys J, DeMeyere M. Acute pharyngitis: no reliability of rapid streptococcal tests and clinical findings. Arch Intern Med 166:2285–86, 2006.

Saiman L, Goldfarb J, Kaplan SL, et al. Safety and tolerability of linezolid in children. Pediatric Infect Disease 22:S193–200, 2003.

GUIDELINES

Bradley J, Byington C, Shah S, et al. The management of community-acquired pneumonia in infants and children older than 3 months of age: clinical practice guidelines by the Pediatric Infectious Diseases Society and the Infectious Diseases Society of America. Clinical Infectious Diseases. 53:617–630, 2011.

CDC Prevention and Control of Influenza with Vaccines. Recommendations of the Advisory Committee on Immunization. Practices (ACIP); MMWR 60:1128–1132, 2011.

CDC Antiviral Agents for Treatment and Chemoprophylaxis of Influenza, MMWR 60:1–24, 2011.

CDC Prevention of perinatal group B streptococcal disease. Revised guidelines from CDC, 2010. MMWR 59:1–32, 2010.

CDC Hospitalized patients with novel influenza A (H₁N₁) infection–California, MMWR 2009. 58:536–541, 2009.

CDC Intensive-care patients with severe novel influenza (H₁N₁) virus infection–Michigan, MMWR 2009. 58:749–752, 2009.

CDC Recommended childhood and adolescent immunization schedule-United States, 2007. MMWR 55: Q1–Q4, January 5, 2007.

Committee of infectious Disease. Prevention of varicella: Recommendations for use of varicella vaccine in children, including a recommendation for a routine 2-dose varicella immunization schedule. Pediatrics 120:221–231, 2007.

Solomkin JS, Mazuski JE, Bradley JS, et al. Diagnosis and management of complicated intra-abdominal infection in adults and children: Guidelines by the Surgical Infection Society and the Infectious Diseases Society of America. Clin Infect Dis 50:133–164, 2010.

TEXTBOOKS

Bradley JS, Nelson JD, Kimberlin DW, et al. (eds). 2012–2013 Nelson's Pediatric Antimicrobial Therapy, 19th Edition, American Academy of Pediatrics, Elk Grove Village, IL, 2012.

Feigin RD, Cherry JD, Demmler GJ, Kaplan SL (eds). Textbook of Pediatric Infectious Diseases. 6th Edition, Philadelphia, Saunders, 2009.

Long SS, Pickering LK, Prober CG (eds). Principles and Practice of Pediatric Infectious Diseases, 4th Edition, Saunders, Philadelphia, 2012.

Pickering LK (ed). Red Book: 2012 Report of the Committee on Infectious Diseases, 29th Edition, American Academy of Pediatrics, Elk Grove Village, IL, 2012.

Remington JS, Klein JO (eds) Infectious Diseases of the Fetus and Newborn 6th Edition, WB Saunders Co., Philadelphia, PA, 2006.

Shah S. Pediatric Infectious Disease Practice. New York: McGraw-Hill, 2009.

Steele RW. Clinical Handbook of Pediatric Infectious Disease 3rd Edition, Informa Healthcare, New York, 2007.

Chapter 8

CHEST X-RAY ATLAS

Burke A. Cunha, MD
Douglas S. Katz, MD
Robert Moore, MD
Daniel S. Siegal, MD

This atlas has been developed to assist in the management of patients who present with respiratory symptoms and chest x-ray abnormalities. Eight common chest x-ray patterns are provided. Common infections and noninfectious etiologies are followed by usual clinical features, which can be used to identify the disorder and help guide empiric/specific therapy.

UNILATERAL FOCAL SEGMENTAL/LOBAR INFILTRATE WITHOUT EFFUSION

Infectious Causes

Causes	Features (may have some, none, or all)			
	History	**Physical**	**Laboratory**	**Chest X-Ray**
S. pneumoniae	Elderly, smokers, COPD, ↓ humoral immunity (multiple myeloma, SLE, CLL, hyposplenism).	Fever, chills, no relative bradycardia. Chest signs related to extent of consolidation.	↑ WBC, ↓ platelets (overwhelming infection/hyposplenism), normal LFTs. Sputum with abundant PMNs and gram-positive diplococci. Blood cultures usually positive.	Consolidation usually limited to one lobe (RLL most common) ± air bronchogram. Pleural effusion very uncommon. Empyema not uncommon. No cavitation.
H. influenzae	Recent contact with H. influenzae URI.	Fever, chills.	↑ WBC. Sputum/pleural effusion with gram-negative pleomorphic bacilli. Blood cultures often positive.	Usually RLL with small/moderate effusion. No empyema. No cavitation.

Infectious Causes (cont'd)

	Features (may have some, none, or all)			
Causes	History	Physical	Laboratory	Chest X-Ray
M. catarrhalis	Chronic/heavy smoker, COPD.	Nonspecific.	Sputum with gram-negative/variable diplococci. Blood cultures negative.	Usually lower lobe ± consolidation. No pleural effusion or cavitation.
K. pneumoniae	Nosocomial pneumonia or history of alcoholism in patient with community-acquired pneumonia.	Fever, chills, signs of alcoholic cirrhosis, signs of consolidation over involved lobe.	↑ WBC, ↓ platelets, ↑ SGOT/SGPT (2° to alcoholism). "Red currant jelly" sputum with PMNs and plump gram-negative encapsulated bacilli.	"Bulging fissure" sign secondary to expanded lobar volume. Empyema rather than pleural effusion. Cavitation in 5–7 days (thick walled).
Legionella	Recent contact with Legionella containing water. Usually elderly. May have watery diarrhea, abdominal pain, mental confusion.	Fever/chills, relative bradycardia. Hepatic/splenic enlargement goes against the diagnosis. ↓ breath sounds if consolidation or pleural effusion.	↑ WBC, ↑ SGOT/SGPT, ↓ PO$_4^-$, ↓ Na$^+$, ↑ CPK, ↑ ESR, ↑ CRP, ↑ ferritin levels, microscopic hematuria, L. pneumophila antigenuria (serotypes 01–06 only) may not be positive early. Mucoid/purulent sputum with few PMNs. Sputum culture for Legionella or sputum DFA (before therapy) is diagnostic. ↑ Legionella titer ≥ 1:256 or ≥ 4-fold rise between acute and convalescent titers.	Rapidly progressive asymmetrical infiltrates clue to Legionella. Consolidation and pleural effusion not uncommon. Cavitation rare.

Infectious Causes (cont'd)

	Features (may have some, none, or all)			
Causes	History	Physical	Laboratory	Chest X-Ray
Psittacosis	Recent bird contact with psittacine birds. Severe headache.	Fever/chills, ± relative bradycardia, Horder's spots on face, epistaxis, ± splenomegaly. Signs of consolidation common.	↑/normal WBC, ↑ LFTs. Sputum with few PMNs. ↑ C. psittaci titers.	Dense infiltrate. Consolidation common. Pleural effusion/cavitation rare.
Q fever	Recent contact with sheep or parturient cats.	Fever/chills, ± relative bradycardia, splenomegaly, ± hepatomegaly.	↑/normal WBC, ↑ LFTs. Sputum with no bacteria/few PMNs (caution–biohazard). Acute Q fever with ↑ in phase II ELISA antigens.	Dense consolidation. Cavitation/pleural effusion rare.

Noninfectious Causes

	Features (may have some, none, or all)			
Causes	History	Physical	Laboratory	Chest X-Ray
Atelectasis	Ineffectual moist recurrent cough characteristic of post-operative atelectasis.	Fevers ≤ 102°F. If large, signs of volume loss (↓ respiratory excursion, ↑ diaphragm, mediastinum shift toward affected side). If small, ↓ breath sounds over affected segment/lobe.	↑ WBC (left shift), normal platelets. Other lab results related to underlying cause of atelectasis.	Segmental infiltrate. RUL/RML atelectasis obscures right heart border. In LUL atelectasis, may be triangular infiltrate extending to upper anterior mediastinum mimicking malignancy. LLL atelectasis causes ↑ density of heart shadow. No cavitation or pleural effusion.

Noninfectious Causes (cont'd)

	Features (may have some, none, or all)			
Causes	History	Physical	Laboratory	Chest X-Ray
Pulmonary embolus/ infarct	Acute onset dyspnea/ pleuritic chest pain. History of lower extremity trauma, stasis or hypercoagulable disorder.	↑ pulse/ respiratory rate.	↑ fibrin split products and D-dimers ± ↑ total bilirubin. Bloody pleural effusion. ECG with RV strain/P-pulmonale (large embolus). Positive V/Q scan and CT pulmonary angiogram.	Normal or show non-specific pleural-based infiltrates resembling atelectasis. Focal segmental/lobar hyperlucency (Westermark's sign) in some. "Hampton's hump" with infarct. Resolving infarcts ↓ in size but maintain shape/density ("melting ice cube").
Lymphoma	Fever, ↓ appetite with weight loss, night sweats, fatigue.	Adenopathy ± splenomegaly.	Normal WBC, ↑ basophils, ↑ eosinophilia, ↓ lymphocytes, ↑ platelets, ↑ ESR, ↑ alkaline phosphatase, ↑$\propto_{1,2}$ globulins on SPEP.	Unilateral or asymmetrical bilateral hilar adenopathy. Lung infiltrate may appear contiguous with hilar adenopathy. No clear channel between mediastinum and hilar nodes. Small pleural effusions rare.
Alveolar cell carcinoma	Fever, ↑ appetite with weight loss, night sweats.	± dullness over lobe with large lower lobe lesions.	Positive cytology by BAL/lung biopsy.	Well/ill-defined circumscribed peripheral infiltrates ± air bronchograms. May be multifocal/ multilobar. Hilar adenopathy present. Stranding to the hilum ("pleural tail" sign). ± pleural effusion if lower lobe infiltrate. No cavitation.

Noninfectious Causes (cont'd)

| Causes | Features (may have some, none, or all) | | | |
	History	Physical	Laboratory	Chest X-Ray
Aspiration pneumonia	Swallowing disorder 2° to CNS/GI disorder; impaired consciousness; recent aspiration 2° to dental, upper GI, or pulmonary procedure.	Unremarkable.	↑ WBC, ↑ ESR.	Infiltrate usually involves superior segments of lower lobes (or posterior segments of upper lobes if aspiration occurred supine). Focal infiltrate initially, which may be followed in 7 days by cavitation/lung abscess.

UNILATERAL FOCAL SEGMENTAL/LOBAR INFILTRATE WITH EFFUSION

Infectious Causes

	Features (may have some, none, or all)			
Causes	History	Physical	Laboratory	Chest X-Ray
Klebsiella pneumoniae	Nosocomial pneumonia or history of alcoholism in patient with community-acquired pneumonia.	Fever, chills, signs of alcoholic cirrhosis, signs of consolidation over involved lobe.	↑ WBC, ↓ platelets, SGOT/SGPT (2° to alcoholism). "Red currant jelly" sputum with PMNs and plump gram-negative encapsulated bacilli.	"Bulging fissure" sign secondary to expanded lobar volume. Empyema rather than pleural effusion. Usually cavitation in 5–7 days (thick walled).
H. influenzae	Recent contact with H. influenzae URI.	Fever, chills.	↑ WBC. Sputum/ pleural effusion with gram-negative pleomorphic bacilli. Blood cultures often positive.	Usually RLL with small/moderate effusion. No empyema. No cavitation.

Infectious Causes (cont'd)

Causes	Features (may have some, none, or all)			
	History	Physical	Laboratory	Chest X-Ray
TB (primary)	Recent TB contact.	Unilateral lower lobe dullness related to size of pleural effusion.	PPD (−)/anergic. Exudative pleural effusion (pleural fluid with ↑ lymphocytes, ↑ glucose, ± RBCs).	Lower lobe infiltrate with small/moderate pleural effusion. No cavitation or apical infiltrates. Hilar adenopathy asymmetrical when present.
Coccidio-mycosis (chronic)	Previous exposure in endemic coccidiomycosis areas. Asymptomatic.	± E. nodosum.	Normal WBC, no eosinophilia in chronic phase. Complement fixation IgG titer ≥ 1:32 indicates active disease.	Thick/thin-walled cavities < 3 cm ± calcifications. Air fluid level rare unless secondarily infected. Cavities usually in anterior segments of upper lobes (vs. posterior segments with TB). No surrounding tissue reaction. Pleural effusion common.
Tularemia	History of recent deer fly, rabbit, or tick exposure. Tularemia pneumonia may complicate any of the clinical presentations of tularemia.	Fever, chills, no relative bradycardia. Chest findings related to extent of infiltrate/ consolidation and pleural effusion.	Normal/↑ WBC, normal LFTs. Sputum/pleural effusion with gram-negative coccobacilli (caution–biohazard). Bloody pleural effusion. Tularemia serology with ↑ microagglutination titer ≥ 1:160 acutely and ≥ 4-fold rise between acute and convalescent titers.	Pleural effusion ± hilar adenopathy.

Infectious Causes (cont'd)

	Features (may have some, none, or all)			
Causes	History	Physical	Laboratory	Chest X-Ray
Adenovirus	Recent URI.	Fever, chills, myalgias. Sore throat and conjunctivitis not always present with adenoviral pneumonia. Chest exam ± signs of consolidation.	↑ adenoviral titers and positive adenoviral cultures of respiratory secretions. Respiratory viral FA panel + for adenovirus.	Ill-defined infiltrate(s) without cavitation ± pleural effusion.
Legionella	Recent contact with Legionella containing water. Usually elderly. May have watery diarrhea, abdominal pain, mental confusion.	Fever/chills, relative bradycardia. Hepatic/splenic enlargement goes against the diagnosis. ↓ breath sounds if consolidation or pleural effusion.	↑ WBC, ↑ SGOT/SGPT, ↓ $PO_4^=$, ↓ Na^+, ↑ CPK, ↑ ESR, ↑ CRP, ↑ ferritin levels, microscopic hematuria, L. pneumophila antigenuria (serotypes 01–06 only) may not be positive early. Mucoid/purulent sputum with few PMNs. Sputum culture for Legionella or sputum DFA (before therapy) is diagnostic. ↑ Legionella titer ≥ 1:256 or ≥ 4-fold rise between acute/convalescent titers.	Rapidly progressive asymmetrical infiltrates clue to Legionella. Consolidation and pleural effusion not uncommon. Cavitation rare.
Group A streptococci	Recent exposure or recent blunt chest trauma ± chest pain.	Fever/chills. Physical signs related to size of pleural effusion.	↑ WBC. Pleural fluid is serosanguineous. Sputum/pleural fluid with gram-positive cocci in pairs/chains. Positive pleural fluid/blood cultures.	Unilateral infiltrate may be obscured by large pleural effusion. No empyema. No cavitation.

Infectious Causes (cont'd)

	Features (may have some, none, or all)			
Causes	History	Physical	Laboratory	Chest X-Ray
Rhodococcus equi	Insidious onset of fever, dyspnea, chest pain, ± hemoptysis. Immuno-suppressed patients with ↓ cell-mediated immunity or exposure to cattle, horses, pigs.	Unremarkable.	Normal/↑ WBC. Sputum/pleural fluid with gram-positive pleomorphic weakly acid-fast bacilli. Sputum, pleural fluid, blood cultures positive for R. equi.	Segmental infiltrate with upper lobe predominance ± cavitation. Air-fluid levels and pleural effusion common.

Noninfectious Causes

	Features (may have some, none, or all)			
Causes	History	Physical	Laboratory	Chest X-Ray
Pulmonary embolus/ infarct	Acute onset dyspnea/ pleuritic chest pain. History of lower extremity trauma, stasis or hypercoagulable disorder.	↑ pulse/ respiratory rate.	↑ fibrin split products and D-dimers ± ↑ total bilirubin. Bloody pleural effusion. ECG with RV strain/P-pulmonale (large embolus). Positive V/Q scan and CT pulmonary angiogram.	Normal or show non-specific pleural-based infiltrates resembling atelectasis. Focal segmental/ lobar hyperlucency (Westermark's sign) in some. "Hampton's hump" with infarct. Resolving infarcts ↓ in size but maintain shape/density ("melting ice cube").

Noninfectious Causes (cont'd)

Causes	Features (may have some, none, or all)			
	History	Physical	Laboratory	Chest X-Ray
Lymphoma	Fever, ↓ appetite with weight loss, night sweats, fatigue.	Adenopathy ± splenomegaly.	Normal WBC, ↑ basophils, ↑ eosinophilia, ↓ lymphocytes, ↑ platelets, ↑ ESR, ↑ alkaline phosphatase, ↑$\propto_{1,2}$ globulins on SPEP.	Unilateral or asymmetrical bilateral hilar adenopathy. Lung infiltrate may appear contiguous with hilar adenopathy. No clear channel between mediastinum and hilar nodes. Small pleural effusions rare.
Alveolar cell carcinoma	Fever, ↑ appetite with weight loss, night sweats.	± dullness over lobe with large lower lobe lesions.	Positive cytology by BAL/lung biopsy.	Well/ill-defined circumscribed peripheral infiltrates ± air bronchograms. May be multifocal/ multilobar. Hilar adenopathy present. Stranding to the hilum ("pleural tail" sign). ± pleural effusion if lower lobe infiltrate. No cavitation.
Radiation pneumonitis	History of mantle radiation for lymphoma, lung cancer, or breast cancer.	Nonspecific.	Nonspecific.	Symmetrical infiltrates in the distribution of radiation therapy after 1 month. Infiltrates have "straight edges"± air bronchograms. Fibrosis common over radiation field after 9–12 months. Usually no pleural effusions (small, if present).

UNILATERAL ILL-DEFINED INFILTRATES WITHOUT EFFUSION

Infectious Causes

| Causes | Features (may have some, none, or all) | | | |
	History	Physical	Laboratory	Chest X-Ray
Mycoplasma pneumoniae	Prolonged dry/ nonproductive cough. No laryngitis. Mild sore throat/ear. Watery diarrhea.	Usually fevers ≤102°F without relative bradycardia. Myalgias, bullous myringitis or otitis, non-exudative pharyngitis, E. multiforme. Chest exam with rales and no signs of consolidation or effusion.	Normal/↑ WBC; normal platelets, LFTs, $PO_4^=$, CPK. ↑ cold agglutinins (early). ↑ IgM (not IgG) Mycoplasma pneumoniae titers. Respiratory secretions culture positive for Mycoplasma pneumoniae.	Ill-defined usually lower lobe indistinct infiltrates. No consolidation or air bronchograms. Small/ no pleural effusion.

Infectious Causes (cont'd)

| Causes | Features (may have some, none, or all) | | | |
	History	Physical	Laboratory	Chest X-Ray
Chlamydophilia (Chlamydia) pneumoniae	Prolonged "mycoplasma-like" illness with laryngitis.	Low-grade fevers, myalgias, non-exudate pharyngitis, laryngitis. No relative bradycardia, ear findings, or rash. Chest exam without signs of consolidation or pleural effusion.	↑ WBC, normal platelets, normal LFTs. No cold agglutinins. ↑ IgM (not IgG) C. pneumoniae titers. Respiratory secretions culture positive for C. pneumoniae.	Ill-defined, usually lower lobe indistinct infiltrate(s). May be "funnel shaped." No consolidation, cavitation, or pleural effusion.
Adenovirus	Recent URI.	Fever, chills, myalgias. Sore throat and conjunctivitis not always present with adenoviral pneumonia. Chest exam ± signs of consolidation.	↑ adenoviral titers and positive adenoviral cultures of respiratory secretions. Respiratory viral FA panel + for adenovirus.	Ill-defined infiltrate(s) without cavitation ± pleural effusion.
Legionella	Recent contact with Legionella containing water. Usually elderly. May have watery diarrhea, abdominal pain, mental confusion.	Fever/chills, relative bradycardia. Hepatic/splenic enlargement goes against the diagnosis. ↓ breath sounds if consolidation or pleural effusion.	↑ WBC, ↑ SGOT/SGPT, ↓ PO_4^-, ↓ Na^+, ↑ CPK, ↑ ESR, ↑ CRP, ↑ ferritin levels, microscopic hematuria, L. pneumophila antigenuria (serotypes 01–06 only) may not be positive early. Mucoid/purulent sputum with few PMNs. Sputum culture for Legionella or sputum DFA (before therapy) is diagnostic. ↑ Legionella titer ≥ 1:256 or ≥ 4-fold rise between acute/convalescent titers.	Rapidly progressive asymmetrical infiltrates clue to Legionella. Consolidation and pleural effusion not uncommon. Cavitation rare.

Infectious Causes (cont'd)

	Features (may have some, none, or all)			
Causes	History	Physical	Laboratory	Chest X-Ray
Psittacosis	Recent bird contact with psittacine birds. Severe headache.	Fever/chills, ± relative bradycardia, ± Horder's spots on face, epistaxis, ± splenomegaly. Signs of consolidation common.	↑/normal WBC, ↑ LFTs. Sputum with few PMNs. ↑ C. psittaci titers.	Dense infiltrate. Consolidation common. Pleural effusion/ cavitation rare.
Q fever	Recent contact with sheep or parturient cats.	Fever/chills, ± relative bradycardia, splenomegaly, ± hepatomegaly.	↑/normal WBC, ↑ LFTs. Sputum with no bacteria/few PMNs (caution–biohazard). Acute Q fever with ↑ in phase II ELISA antigens.	Dense consolidation. Cavitation/ pleural effusion rare.
Nocardia	Fevers, night sweats, fatigue, ↓ cell-mediated immunity (e.g., HIV, organ transplants, PAP, immunosup-pressive therapy).	Unremarkable.	Normal/↑ WBC, ↑ ESR. Sputum with gram-positive AFB.	Dense large infiltrates. May cavitate and mimic TB, lymphoma, or squamous cell carcinoma. No calcification ± pleural effusion.

Infectious Causes (cont'd)

| | Features (may have some, none, or all) | | | |
Causes	History	Physical	Laboratory	Chest X-Ray
Actinomycosis	Recent dental work.	± chest wall sinus tracts.	Normal/↑ WBC, ↑ ESR. Sputum with gram-positive filamentous anaerobic bacilli.	Dense infiltrates extending to chest wall. No hilar adenopathy. Cavitation rare. ± pleural effusion rare.
Cryptococcus neoformans	Exposure to air conditioner or pigeons.	Unremarkable.	Normal WBC. Cryptococcal serology with ↑ C. neoformans antigen levels.	Dense lower nodular mass lesions. No calcification or cavitation. ± pleural effusion.
Aspiration pneumonia	Swallowing disorder 2° to CNS/GI disorder; impaired consciousness; recent aspiration 2° to dental, upper GI, or pulmonary procedure.	Unremarkable.	↑ WBC, ↑ ESR.	Infiltrate usually involves superior segments of lower lobes (or posterior segments of upper lobes if aspiration occurred supine). Focal infiltrate initially, which may be followed in 7 days by cavitation/lung abscess.

Noninfectious Causes

	Features (may have some, none, or all)			
Causes	**History**	**Physical**	**Laboratory**	**Chest X-Ray**
Bronchogenic carcinoma	Fever, ↓ appetite with weight loss, cough ± hemoptysis. Cough with copious clear/mucoid sputum in large cell anaplastic carcinoma. Increased risk in smokers, aluminum/uranium miners, cavitary lung disease (adeno-carcinoma), previous radiation therapy from lymphoma/breast cancer.	Paraneoplastic syndromes especially with small (oat) cell/squamous cell carcinoma ± hypertrophic pulmonary osteoarthro-pathy.	Normal/↑ WBC, ↑ platelets, ↑ ESR, findings related to underlying malignancy, ± clubbing.	Small/squamous cell carcinomas present as central lesions/hilar masses. Adenocarcinoma/large cell anaplastic carcinomas are usually peripheral initially. "Tumor tendrils" extending into surrounding lung tissue is characteristic. No calcifications (may be present on chest CT). Cavitation with squamous cell carcinoma. ± pleural effusions.
Lymphangitic metastases	History of breast, thyroid, pancreas, cervical, prostate, or lung carcinoma.	Findings related to underlying malignancy.	Normal/↑ WBC, ↑ ESR.	Interstitial indistinct pulmonary infiltrates (may be reticulonodular) with lower lobe predominance Usually unilateral but may be bilateral. No consolidation or cavitation ± pleural effusions.
Lung contusion	Recent closed chest trauma, chest pain.	Chest wall contusion over infiltrate.	↑ WBC (left shift).	Patchy ill-defined infiltrate(s) ± rib fractures/pneumothorax in area of infiltrate. Infiltrate clears within 1 week.

Noninfectious Causes (cont'd)

	Features (may have some, none, or all)			
Causes	History	Physical	Laboratory	Chest X-Ray
Congestive heart failure	Coronary heart disease, valvular heart disease, cardiomyopathy.	No/low-grade fevers ↑ pulse and respiratory rate, positive jugular venous distension and hepatojugular reflex, cardio-megaly, S_3, ascites, hepatomegaly, pedal edema.	↑ WBC (left shift), normal platelets, mildly ↑ SGOT/SGPT.	Cardiomegaly, pleural effusion (R > [R + L] > L). Kerley B lines with vascular redistribution to upper lobes. Typically bilateral rather than unilateral.
Alveolar cell carcinoma	Fever, ↑ appetite with weight loss, night sweats.	± dullness over lobe with large lower lobe lesions.	Positive cytology by BAL/lung biopsy.	Well/ill-defined circumscribed peripheral infiltrates ± air bronchograms. May be multifocal/multilobar. Hilar adenopathy present. Stranding to the hilum ("pleural tail" sign). ± pleural effusion if lower lobe infiltrate. No cavitation.
Lymphoma	Fever, ↓ appetite with weight loss, night sweats, fatigue.	Adenopathy ± splenomegaly.	Normal WBC, ↑ basophils, ↑ eosinophilia, ↓ lymphocytes, ↑ platelets, ↑ ESR, ↑ alkaline phosphatase, ↑$\propto_{1,2}$ globulins on SPEP.	Unilateral or asymmetrical bilateral hilar adenopathy. Lung infiltrate may appear contiguous with hilar adenopathy. No clear channel between media-stinum and hilar nodes. Small pleural effusions rare.

Noninfectious Causes (cont'd)

Causes	Features (may have some, none, or all)			
	History	Physical	Laboratory	Chest X-Ray
Pulmonary hemorrhage	History of closed chest trauma or hemorrhagic disorder.	↑ WBC (left shift), ↑ pulse rate, respiratory rate. Signs of closed chest trauma.	Anemia plus findings secondary to underlying hemorrhagic disorder.	Localized or diffuse fluffy alveolar infiltrate(s). No cavitation, consolidation, or effusion.
Systemic lupus erythematosus (SLE)	Fatigue, chest pain. History of SLE.	Fever/ myalgias, alopecia, malar rash, "cytoid bodies" in retina, painless oral ulcers, synovitis, splenomegaly, generalized adenopathy, Raynaud's phenomenon.	↑ ANA, ↑ DS-DNA, ↓ C_3, polyclonal gammopathy on SPEP, ↑ ferritin. Pleural fluids with ↑ ANA, ↓ C_3.	Migratory ill-defined non-segmental infiltrates ± small pleural effusions. No consolidation or cavitation.
Aspiration pneumonia	Swallowing disorder 2° to CNS/GI disorder; impaired consciousness; recent aspiration 2° to dental, upper GI, or pulmonary procedure.	Unremarkable.	↑ WBC, ↑ ESR.	Infiltrate usually involves superior segments of lower lobes (or posterior segments of upper lobes if aspiration occurred supine). Focal infiltrate initially, which may be followed in 7 days by cavitation/lung abscess.

UNILATERAL ILL-DEFINED INFILTRATES WITH EFFUSION

Infectious Causes

	Features (may have some, none, or all)			
Causes	History	Physical	Laboratory	Chest X-Ray
TB (primary)	Recent TB contact.	Unilateral lower lobe dullness related to size of pleural effusion.	PPD anergic. Exudative pleural effusion (pleural fluid with ↑ lymphocytes, ↑ glucose, ± RBCs).	Lower lobe infiltrate with small/moderate pleural effusion. No cavitation or apical infiltrates. Hilar adenopathy asymmetrical when present.
Nocardia	Fevers, night sweats, fatigue, ↓ cell-mediated immunity (e.g., HIV, organ transplant, PAP, immuno-suppressive therapy).	Unremarkable.	Normal/↑ WBC, ↑ ESR. Sputum with gram-positive AFB.	Dense large infiltrates. May cavitate and mimic TB, lymphoma, or squamous cell carcinoma. No calcification ± pleural effusion.

Infectious Causes (cont'd)

Causes	Features (may have some, none, or all)			
	History	Physical	Laboratory	Chest X-Ray
Legionella	Recent contact with Legionella containing water. Usually elderly. May have watery diarrhea, abdominal pain, mental confusion.	Fever/chills, relative bradycardia. Hepatic/splenic enlargement goes against the diagnosis. ↓ breath sounds if consolidation or pleural effusion.	↑ WBC, ↑ SGOT/SGPT, ↓ PO_4^-, ↓ Na^+, ↑ CPK, ↑ ESR, ↑ CRP, ↑ ferritin levels, microscopic hematuria, L. pneumophila antigenuria (serotypes 01–06 only) may not be positive early. Mucoid/purulent sputum with few PMNs. Sputum culture for Legionella or sputum DFA (before therapy) is diagnostic. ↑ Legionella titer ≥ 1:256 or ≥ 4-fold rise between acute/convalescent titers.	Rapidly progressive asymmetrical infiltrates clue to Legionella. Consolidation and pleural effusion not uncommon. Cavitation rare.

Noninfectious Causes

Causes	Features (may have some, none, or all)			
	History	Physical	Laboratory	Chest X-Ray
Lymphangitic metastases	History of breast, thyroid, pancreas, cervical, prostate, or lung carcinoma.	Findings related to underlying malignancy.	Normal/ ↑ WBC, ↑ ESR.	Interstitial indistinct pulmonary infiltrates (may be reticulonodular) with lower lobe predominance Usually unilateral but may be bilateral. No consolidation or cavitation ± pleural effusions.

Noninfectious Causes (cont'd)

	Features (may have some, none, or all)			
Causes	History	Physical	Laboratory	Chest X-Ray
Pulmonary embolus/ infarct	Acute onset dyspnea/ pleuritic chest pain. History of lower extremity trauma, stasis or hypercoagulable disorder.	↑ pulse/ respiratory rate.	↑ fibrin split products and D-dimers ± ↑ total bilirubin. Bloody pleural effusion. ECG with RV strain/ P-pulmonale (large embolus). Positive V/Q scan and CT pulmonary angiogram.	Normal or show non-specific pleural-based infiltrates resembling atelectasis. Focal segmental/lobar hyperlucency (Westermark's sign) in some. "Hampton's hump" with infarct. Resolving infarcts ↓ in size but maintain shape/density ("melting ice cube").
Lymphoma	Fever, ↓ appetite with weight loss, night sweats, fatigue.	Adenopathy ± splenomegaly.	Normal WBC, ↑ basophils, ↑ eosinophilia, ↓ lymphocytes, ↑ platelets, ↑ ESR, ↑ alkaline phosphatase, ↑∝$_{1,2}$ globulins on SPEP.	Unilateral or asymmetrical bilateral hilar adenopathy. Lung infiltrate may appear contiguous with hilar adenopathy. No clear channel between mediastinum and hilar nodes. Small pleural effusions rare.

Noninfectious Causes (cont'd)

	Features (may have some, none, or all)			
Causes	**History**	**Physical**	**Laboratory**	**Chest X-Ray**
Bronchogenic carcinoma	Fever, ↓ appetite with weight loss, cough ± hemoptysis. Cough with copious clear/ mucoid sputum in large cell anaplastic carcinoma. Increased risk in smokers, aluminum/ uranium miners, cavitary lung disease (adeno- carcinoma), previous radiation therapy from lymphoma/ breast cancer.	Paraneoplastic syndromes especially with small (oat) cell/ squamous cell carcinoma ± hypertrophic pulmonary osteoarthropathy.	Normal/↑ WBC, ↑ platelets, ↑ ESR, findings related to underlying malignancy, ± clubbing.	Small/squamous cell carcinomas present as central lesions/ hilar masses. Adenocarcinoma/ large cell anaplastic carcinomas are usually peripheral initially. "Tumor tendrils" extending into surrounding lung tissue is characteristic. No calcifications (may be present on chest CT). Cavitation with squamous cell carcinoma. ± pleural effusions.
Alveolar cell carcinoma	Fever, ↑ appetite with weight loss, night sweats.	± dullness over lobe with large lower lobe lesions.	Positive cytology by BAL/lung biopsy.	Well/ill-defined circumscribed peripheral infiltrates ± air bronchograms. May be multifocal/ multilobar. Hilar adenopathy present. Stranding to the hilum ("pleural tail" sign). ± pleural effusion if lower lobe infiltrate. No cavitation.

Noninfectious Causes (cont'd)

	Features (may have some, none, or all)			
Causes	History	Physical	Laboratory	Chest X-Ray
Metastatic carcinoma	History of breast, thyroid, renal cell, colon, pancreatic cancer or osteogenic sarcoma.	Findings related to underlying malignancy and, when present, to bone, hepatic, CNS metastases.	Secondary to effects of primary neoplasm, metastases, paraneoplastic syndrome.	Nodular lesions that vary in size. Metastatic lesions are usually well circumscribed with lower lobe predominance. Usually no bronchial obstruction (obstruction suggests colon, renal, or melanoma metastases). Usually no cavitation (except for squamous cell metastases). Calcification usually suggests osteosarcoma (rarely adenocarcinoma). Pleural effusion rare (except for breast cancer).

BILATERAL INFILTRATES WITHOUT EFFUSION

Infectious Causes

| | Features (may have some, none, or all) | | | |
Causes	History	Physical	Laboratory	Chest X-Ray
Influenza (human, avian, swine)	Acute onset of fever, myalgias, headache, fatigue, sore throat, rhinorrhea, dry cough, ± pleuritic chest pain.	↑ respiratory rate, cyanosis in severe cases.	↓ WBC, ↓ platelets, few/no atypical lymphocytes, ↑ A-a gradient. Influenza in respiratory secretions by culture/viral FA panel.	Early normal/ near normal appearance. (< 48 hours) Later (> 48 hours) diffuse patchy bilateral interstitial infiltrates. No focal/segmental infiltrates unless secondary bacterial pneumonia present. ± small pleural effusions.

Infectious Causes (cont'd)

Causes	Features (may have some, none, or all)			
	History	**Physical**	**Laboratory**	**Chest X-Ray**
SARS	Acute onset of fever, myalgia, dry cough ± diarrhea.	↑ respiratory rate, cyanosis in severe cases.	N/↓ WBC, N/↓ platelets, ↓ pO_2, ↑ A-a gradient.	Culture of SARS – CoV from respiratory secretions.
HSV-1	Fever. Often presents in normal hosts as "failure to wean" from ventilator.	Unremarkable.	↑ WBC, ↓ pO_2, ↑ A-a gradient. HSV-1 in respiratory secretions by culture/viral FA panel. Cytology + for cytopathic effects (CPE) of HSV.	Minimal bilateral diffuse infiltrates without cavitation or effusion.
RSV	Recent URI contact, dry cough, wheezing.	Mild lower respiratory tract infection in normal host. Moderate/severe pneumonia in organ transplants.	Normal WBC; ↓ pO_2/↑ A-a gradient in severe RSV. RSV in respiratory secretions by culture/viral FA panel.	Near normal chest x-ray or bilateral symmetrical patchy infiltrates. Consolidation uncommon. No cavitation or effusion.
VZV	VZV pneumonia occurs 2–3 days after rash. ↑ risk with pregnancy, smoking.	Healing vesicles, dry cough. Mild pneumonia in normal hosts. Moderate/severe pneumonia in organ transplants.	↑ WBC, ↑ platelets, ↑ basophils; ↓ pO_2/↑ A-a gradient in severe chickenpox pneumonia. ↑ VZV titers.	Minimal diffuse fluffy interstitial infiltrates. Diffuse small calcifications may develop years later. No calcification of hilar nodes (in contrast to TB/histoplasmosis).

Infectious Causes (cont'd)

Causes	\multicolumn{4}{c}{Features (may have some, none, or all)}			
	History	Physical	Laboratory	Chest X-Ray
CMV	↓ cell-mediated immunity (HIV, organ transplants, immunosuppressive therapy). Increasing dyspnea over 1 week.	Fever ≤ 102°F.	↓ pO$_2$, ↑ A-a gradient, ↑ LDH (PCP). PCP cysts or CMV "Cowdry Owl eye" inclusion bodies in respiratory secretions or transbronchial/ open lung biopsy.	Most HIV patients with PCP also have underlying CMV. Organ transplants with CMV usually do not have underlying PCP.
P (carinii) jiroveci (PCP)	↓ cell-mediated immunity (e.g., HIV, immuno-suppressive therapy). Increasing dyspnea over 1 week. Chest pain with shortness of breath suggests pneumothorax.	↓ breath sounds bilaterally. Other findings depend on size/location of pneumothorax (if present).	Normal/↑ WBC (left shift), ↑ lymphocytes, ↑ LDH. ↓ pO$_2$, ↓ DL$_{CO}$, ↑ A-a gradient. PCP cysts in sputum/ respiratory secretions.	Bilateral perihilar symmetrical patchy infiltrates ± pneumothorax. No calcification, cavitation, or pleural effusion.
TB (reactivation)	Fevers, night sweats, normal appetite with weight loss, cough ± hemoptysis.	± bilateral apical dullness.	Normal WBC, ↑ platelets, ↑ ESR (≤ 70 mm/h). Positive PPD. AFB in sputum smear/ culture.	Slowly progressive bilateral infiltrates. No pleural effusion. Usually in apical segment of lower lobes or apical/ posterior segments of upper lobes. Calcifications common.

Infectious Causes (cont'd)

Causes	Features (may have some, none, or all)			
	History	Physical	Laboratory	Chest X-Ray
Legionella	Recent contact with Legionella containing water. Usually elderly. May have watery diarrhea, abdominal pain, mental confusion.	Fever/chills, relative bradycardia. Hepatic/splenic enlargement goes against the diagnosis. ↓ breath sounds if consolidation or pleural effusion.	↑ WBC, ↑ SGOT/SGPT, ↑ pO$_4$", ↓ Na$^+$, ↑ CPK, ↑ ESR, ↑ CRP, ↑ ferritin levels, microscopic hematuria, L. pneumophila antigenuria (serotypes 01–06 only) may not be positive early. Mucoid/purulent sputum with few PMNs. Sputum culture for Legionella or sputum DFA (before therapy) is diagnostic. ↑ Legionella titer ≥ 1:256 or ≥ 4-fold rise between acute/convalescent titers.	Rapidly progressive asymmetrical infiltrates clue to Legionella. Consolidation and pleural effusion not uncommon. Cavitation rare.
Psittacosis	Recent bird contact with psittacine birds. Severe headache.	Fever/chills, ± relative bradycardia, ± Horder's spots on face, epistaxis, ± splenomegaly. Signs of consolidation common.	↑/normal WBC, ↑ LFTs. Sputum with few PMNs. Positive C. psittaci serology.	Dense infiltrate. Consolidation common. Pleural effusion/cavitation rare.

Infectious Causes (cont'd)

	Features (may have some, none, or all)			
Causes	History	Physical	Laboratory	Chest X-Ray
Q fever	Recent contact with sheep or parturient cats.	Fever/chills, ± relative bradycardia, splenomegaly, ± hepatomegaly.	↑/normal WBC, ↑ LFTs. Sputum with no bacteria/few PMNs (caution– biohazard). Acute Q fever with ↑ in phase II ELISA antigens.	Dense consolidation. Cavitation/pleural effusion rare.
Nosocomial pneumonia (hematogenous)	Fever/pulmonary symptoms ≥ 7 days in hospital. Increased risk with antecedent heart failure in previous 1–2 weeks.	Bilateral rales ± purulent respiratory secretions (tracheobronchitis).	↑ WBC (left shift). Blood cultures positive for pulmonary pathogens. Respiratory secretions with WBCs ± cultures positive for P. aeruginosa, Acinetobacter, Enterobacter, Klebsiella, or Serratia (represents colonization, *not* lower respiratory tract/lung pathogens). Definitive diagnosis by lung biopsy/ culture.	Bilateral symmetrical diffuse infiltrates. May be focal/ segmental in aspiration nosocomial pneumonia. ↑ lung volumes (vs. ARDS). Klebsiella cavitation in 3–5 days; P. aeruginosa cavitation in 72 hours. No pleural effusion.

Noninfectious Causes

	Features (may have some, none, or all)			
Causes	History	Physical	Laboratory	Chest X-Ray
Adult respiratory distress syndrome (ARDS)	Intubated on ventilator, multi-organ system failure.	± rales.	↑ WBC (left shift), normal ESR, ↓ pO$_2$, ↓ D$_L$CO, ↑ A-a gradient.	Bilateral fluffy infiltrates appearing ≥ 12 hours after profound hypoxemia. No cardiomegaly or pleural effusion. Reduced lung volumes (vs. nosocomial pneumonia or CHF). Bilateral consolidation ≥ 48 hours after appearance of infiltrates.
Goodpasture's Syndrome	Often preceded by a URI. Most common in 20–30 year old adults. Fever, weight loss, fatigue, cough, hemoptysis, hematuria.	Findings secondary to iron deficiency anemia.	↑ WBC, anemia, ↑ creatinine, urine with RBCs/RBC casts. Positive pANCA. Linear IgG pattern on alveolar/ glomerular basement membrane.	Bilateral fine reticulonodular infiltrates predominantly in lower lobes. No cavitation.
Wegener's granulomatosis	Most common in middle-aged adults. Cough, fever, fatigue.	Findings of chronic sinusitis, bloody nasal discharge.	↑ WBC, anemia, ↑ platelets, ↑ ESR, ↑ RF, negative ANA, proteinuria, hematuria. Positive cANCA.	Bilateral asymmetrical nodular infiltrates of varying size with irregular margins. Cavitation common. Inner lining of cavities irregular. Air-fluid levels rare. ± pleural effusions. No calcifications.
Pulmonary hemorrhage	History of closed chest trauma or hemorrhagic disorder.	↑ WBC (left shift), ↑ pulse rate, ↑ respiratory rate. Signs of closed chest trauma.	Anemia plus findings secondary to underlying hemorrhagic disorder.	Localized or diffuse fluffy alveolar infiltrates. No cavitation, consolidation, or effusion.

Noninfectious Causes (cont'd)

| Causes | Features (may have some, none, or all) | | | |
	History	Physical	Laboratory	Chest X-Ray
Chronic renal failure	Chronic renal failure on dialysis.	Findings related to uremia.	Normal/↑ WBC (left shift) plus findings related to renal failure.	Bilateral symmetrical fluffy perihilar infiltrates (butterfly pattern) ± pleural effusions. No cardiomegaly (unlike CHF), but large pericardial effusion can mimic cardiomegaly.
Lung contusion	Recent closed chest trauma, chest pain.	Chest wall contusion over infiltrate.	↑ WBC (left shift).	Patchy ill-defined infiltrate(s) ± rib fractures/pneumothorax in area of infiltrate. Infiltrate clears within 1 week.
Fat emboli	1–2 days post-long bone fracture/trauma.	↑ respiratory rate.	Urinalysis with "Maltese crosses."	Bilateral predominantly peripheral lower lobe infiltrates. Usually clears within 1 week.
Loeffler's Syndrome	Drug or parasitic exposure.	Unremarkable.	Normal WBC, ↑ eosinophilia, ↑ ESR.	Characteristic "reversed bat-wing" pattern (i.e., peripheral infiltrates). Upper lobe predominance.
Sarcoidosis (Stage III)	Dyspena, fatigue, nasal stuffiness.	Waxy/ yellowish papules on face/ upper trunk. Funduscopic exam with "candle wax drippings."	↑ ESR, normal LFTs, ↑ creatinine (if renal involvement), ↑ ACE levels, hypercalciuria, hypercalcemia, polyclonal gammopathy on SPEP. Anergic.	Bilateral nodular infiltrates of variable size without hilar adenopathy. Cavitation/ pleural effusion rare.

Noninfectious Causes (cont'd)

	Features (may have some, none, or all)			
Causes	History	Physical	Laboratory	Chest X-Ray
Alveolar cell carcinoma	Fever, ↑ appetite with weight loss, night sweats.	± dullness over lobe with large lower lobe lesions.	Positive cytology by BAL/lung biopsy.	Well/ill-defined circumscribed peripheral infiltrates ± air bronchograms. May be multifocal/multilobar. Hilar adenopathy present. Stranding to the hilum ("pleural tail" sign). ± pleural effusion if lower lobe infiltrate. No cavitation.
Metastatic carcinoma	History of breast, thyroid, renal cell, colon, pancreatic cancer or osteogenic sarcoma.	Findings related to underlying malignancy and, when present, to bone, hepatic, CNS metastases.	Secondary to effects of primary neoplasm, metastases, paraneoplastic syndrome.	Nodular lesions that vary in size. Metastatic lesions are usually well circumscribed with lower lobe predominance. Usually no bronchial obstruction (obstruction suggests colon, renal, or melanoma metastases). Usually no cavitation (except for squamous cell metastases). Calcification usually suggests osteosarcoma (rarely adenocarcinoma). Pleural effusion rare (except for breast cancer).
Lymphoma	Fever, ↓ appetite with weight loss, night sweats, fatigue.	Adenopathy ± splenomegaly.	Normal WBC, ↑ basophils, ↑ eosinophilia, ↓ lymphocytes, ↑ platelets, ↑ ESR, ↑ alkaline phosphatase, ↑ $\propto_{1, 2}$ globulins on SPEP.	Unilateral or asymmetrical bilateral hilar adenopathy. Lung infiltrate may appear contiguous with hilar adenopathy. No clear channel between mediastinum and hilar nodes. Small pleural effusions rare.

Noninfectious Causes (cont'd)

Causes	Features (may have some, none, or all)			
	History	Physical	Laboratory	Chest X-Ray
Leukostasis (AML)	Untreated acute myelogenous leukemia (AML).	Fever, sternal tenderness, petechiae, ecchymosis.	↑ WBC (≥ 100 K/mm³) with blasts in peripheral smear/bone marrow, ↓ platelets.	Diffuse symmetrical fluffy infiltrates without pleural effusion.
Drug-induced	Exposure to chemo-therapeutic agents (e.g., BCNU, busulfan, methotrexate, cyclophospham-ide, bleomycin) or other drugs (e.g., nitro-furantoin, sulfasalazine, amiodarone, opiates, cocaine).	Unremarkable.	Normal WBC ± ↑ eosinophilia, normal/↑ ESR/LFTs. Eosinophils in pleural effusion.	Bilateral coarse symmetrical patchy infiltrates/fibrosis ± pleural effusions. Hilar adenopathy only with drug-induced pseudolymphoma (secondary to dilantin). No cavitation.
Idiopathic pulmonary hemosiderosis (IPH)	Hemoptysis ± cough.	Findings of iron deficiency anemia.	Iron deficiency anemia. Hemosiderin in alveolar macrophages and urine.	Diffuse, bilateral ill-defined opacities or multiple "stellate" shaped infiltrates that clear between attacks. Recent hemorrhage may be superimposed on a fine reticular pattern that occurs after repeated bleeds.

Noninfectious Causes (cont'd)

| Causes | Features (may have some, none, or all) | | | |
	History	Physical	Laboratory	Chest X-Ray
Bronchiolitis obliterans with organizing pneumonia (BOOP)	Fever, dyspnea, cough.	Unremarkable.	↑ WBC (left shift), ↑ LDH, ↓ pO$_2$, ↑ A-a gradient.	Classically bilateral patchy peripheral infiltrates. Often lower lobe predominance. No cavitation or pleural effusion.
Pulmonary alveolar proteinosis (PAP)	Asymptomatic if not infected with Nocardia.	Unremarkable.	Normal/↑ WBC, ↑ LDH.	Bilateral granular or peripheral infiltrates in butterfly pattern. No hilar adenopathy, cardiomegaly, or pleural effusion.

BILATERAL INFILTRATES
WITH EFFUSION

Infectious Causes

	Features (may have some, none, or all)			
Causes	**History**	**Physical**	**Laboratory**	**Chest X-Ray**
Legionella	Recent contact with Legionella containing water. Usually elderly. May have watery diarrhea, abdominal pain, mental confusion.	Fever/chills, relative bradycardia. Hepatic/splenic enlargement goes against the diagnosis. ↓ breath sounds if consolidation or pleural effusion.	↑ WBC, ↑ SGOT/SGPT, ↑ PO₄⁻, ↓ Na⁺, ↑ CPK, ↑ ESR, ↑ CRP, ↑ ferritin levels, microscopic hematuria, L. pneumophila antigenuria (serotypes 01–06 only) may not be positive early. Mucoid/purulent sputum with few PMNs. Sputum culture for Legionella or sputum DFA (before therapy) is diagnostic. ↑ Legionella titer ≥ 1:256 or ≥ 4-fold rise between acute/convalescent titers.	Rapidly progressive asymmetrical infiltrates clue to Legionella. Consolidation and pleural effusion not uncommon. Cavitation rare.

Infectious Causes (cont'd)

	Features (may have some, none, or all)			
Causes	History	Physical	Laboratory	Chest X-Ray
Hantavirus (HPS)	Subacute onset, shortness of breath, substernal chest discomfort. Interim improvement followed by rapid deterioration.	↑ respiratory rate, cyanosis in severe cases.	↓ WBC, ↓ platelets ↓ pO_2, ↑ A-a gradient. ↑ hantavirus titers.	Large pleural effusions.
Measles	Recent airborne exposure.	Measles rash, Koplik's spots.	Normal/↑ WBC (left shift), normal/↓ platelets, ↑ LFTs, ↑ CPK, normal/↓ pO_2. If ↓ pO_2, then ↑ A-a gradient. ↑ IgM measles titer. Warthin-Finkeldey cells in respiratory secretions.	Bilateral diffuse fine reticulonodular infiltrates ± hilar adenopathy. Lower lobe predominance. Consolidation/ pleural effusion uncommon. No cavitation. Focal infiltrate indicates superimposed bacterial pneumonia.
Strongyl-oides	Strongyloides exposure. 1/3 asymptomatic; 2/3 with fever, dyspnea, cough. Hyperinfection syndrome with abdominal pain, diarrhea ± GI bleed.	With hyperinfection syndrome, fever, ↓ BP, abdominal tenderness ± rebound, ± meningitis.	↑ WBC (left shift), ↑ eosinophilia, ± anemia. Blood/CSF cultures positive for enteric gram-negative bacilli. Rhabditiform larvae in sputum/stool.	Diffuse hilar patchy infiltrates without consolidation or cavitation. Eosinophilic pleural effusion common.

Noninfectious Causes

Causes	Features (may have some, none, or all)			
	History	Physical	Laboratory	Chest X-Ray
Congestive heart failure	Coronary heart disease, valvular heart disease, cardiomyopathy.	No/low grade fevers, ↑ pulse/respiratory rate, positive jugular venous distension and hepatojugular reflex, cardiomegaly, S₃, ascites, hepatomegaly, pedal edema.	↑ WBC (left shift), normal platelets, mildly ↑ SGOT/SGPT.	Cardiomegaly, pleural effusion (R > [R + L] > L). Kerley B lines with vascular redistribution to upper lobes. Typically bilateral rather than unilateral.
Chronic renal failure	Chronic renal failure on dialysis.	Findings related to uremia.	Normal/↑ WBC (left shift) plus findings related to renal failure.	Bilateral symmetrical fluffy perihilar infiltrates (butterfly pattern) ± pleural effusions. No cardiomegaly (unlike CHF), but large pericardial effusion can mimic cardiomegaly.
SLE	Fatigue, chest pain. History of SLE.	Fever/myalgias, alopecia, malar rash, "cytoid bodies" in retina, painless oral ulcers, synovitis, splenomegaly, generalized adenopathy, Raynaud's phenomenon.	↑ ANA, ↑ DS-DNA, ↓ C₃, polyclonal gammopathy on SPEP, ↑ ferritin. Pleural fluids with ↑ ANA, ↓ C₃.	Migratory ill-defined non-segmental infiltrates. No signs of consolidation or cavitation. ± small pleural effusions.

Noninfectious Causes (cont'd)

	Features (may have some, none, or all)			
Causes	History	Physical	Laboratory	Chest X-Ray
Goodpasture's Syndrome	Often preceded by a URI. Most common in 20–30 year old adults. Fever, weight loss, fatigue, cough, hemoptysis, hematuria.	Findings secondary to iron deficiency anemia.	↑ WBC, anemia, ↑ creatinine, urine with RBCs/RBC casts. Positive pANCA. Linear IgG pattern on alveolar/ glomerular basement membrane.	Bilateral fine reticulonodular infiltrates predominantly in lower lobes. No cavitation.
Wegener's granulomatosis	Most common in middle-aged adults. Cough, fever, fatigue.	Findings of chronic sinusitis, bloody nasal discharge.	↑ WBC, anemia, ↑ platelets, ↑ ESR, ↑ RF, negative ANA, proteinuria, hematuria. Positive cANCA.	Bilateral asymmetrical nodular infiltrates of varying size with irregular margins. Cavitation common. Inner lining of cavities irregular. Air-fluid levels rare. ± pleural effusions. No calcifications.
Sarcoidosis (Stage III)	Dyspnea, fatigue, nasal stuffiness.	Waxy/ yellowish papules on face/ upper trunk. Funduscopic exam with "candle wax drippings."	↑ ESR, normal LFTs, ↑ creatinine (if renal involvement), ↑ ACE levels, hypercalciuria, hypercalcemia, polyclonal gammopathy on SPEP. Anergic.	Bilateral nodular infiltrates of variable size without hilar adenopathy. Cavitation/pleural effusion rare.

Noninfectious Causes (cont'd)

	Features (may have some, none, or all)			
Causes	History	Physical	Laboratory	Chest X-Ray
Lymphoma	Fever, ↓ appetite with weight loss, night sweats, fatigue.	Adenopathy ± splenomegaly.	Normal WBC, ↑ basophils, ↑ eosinophilia, ↓ lymphocytes, ↑ platelets, ↑ ESR, ↑ alkaline phosphatase, ↑∝$_{1,2}$ globulins on SPEP.	Unilateral or asymmetrical bilateral hilar adenopathy. Lung infiltrate may appear contiguous with hilar adenopathy. No clear channel between mediastinum and hilar nodes. Small pleural effusions rare.
Lymphangitic metastases	History of breast, thyroid, pancreas, cervical, prostate, or lung carcinoma.	Findings related to underlying malignancy.	Normal/ ↑ WBC, ↑ ESR.	Interstitial indistinct pulmonary infiltrates (may be reticulonodular) with lower lobe predominance Usually unilateral but may be bilateral. No consolidation or cavitation ± pleural effusions.
Drug-induced	Exposure to chemotherapeutic agents (e.g., BCNU, busulfan, methotrexate, cyclophosphamide, bleomycin) or other drugs (e.g., nitrofurantoin, sulfasalazine, amiodarone, opiates, cocaine).	Unremarkable.	Normal WBC ± ↑ eosinophilia, normal/↑ ESR/ LFTs. Eosinophils in pleural effusion.	Bilateral coarse symmetrical patchy infiltrates/ fibrosis ± pleural effusions. Hilar adenopathy only with drug-induced pseudolymphoma (secondary to dilantin). No cavitation.

CAVITARY INFILTRATES
(THICK-WALLED)

Infectious Causes Based on Speed of Cavitation

Speed of Cavitation	Causes
Very rapid cavitation (3 days)	S. aureus, P. aeruginosa
Rapid cavitation (5–7 days)	K. pneumoniae
Slow cavitation (> 7 days)	Pyogenic lung abscess, septic pulmonary emboli
Chronic cavitation	TB (reactivation), histoplasmosis (reactivation), sporotrichosis, melioidosis, nocardia, actinomycosis, Rhodococcus equi, amebic abscess, alveolar echinococcosis (hydatid cysts)

Infectious Causes

| Causes | Features (may have some, none, or all) | | | |
	History	Physical	Laboratory	Chest X-Ray
S. aureus	Fever, cough, dyspnea. Recent/ concurrent influenza pneumonia.	↓ breath sounds ± cyanosis.	↑ WBC (left shift), ↓ pO$_2$, ↑ A-a gradient. Sputum positive for S. aureus. ↑ IgM influenza titers.	Multiple thick-walled cavitary lesions super-imposed on normal looking lung fields or early minimal infiltrates of influenza.
P. aeruginosa	Nosocomial pneumonia usually on ventilator. Nearly always rapidly fatal.	Unremarkable.	↑ WBC (left shift). Respiratory secretions culture ± for P. aeruginosa. Blood cultures positive for P. aeruginosa (hematogenous nosocomial pneumonia).	Bilateral diffuse infiltrates with rapid cavitation (≤ 72 hours).
Klebsiella pneumoniae	Nosocomial pneumonia or history of alcoholism in patient with community-acquired pneumonia.	Fever, chills, signs of alcoholic cirrhosis, signs of consolidation over involved lobe.	↑ WBC, ↓ platelets, ↑ SGOT/SGPT (2° to alcoholism). "Red currant jelly" sputum with PMNs and plump gram-negative encapsulated bacilli.	"Bulging fissure" sign secondary to expanded lobar volume. Empyema rather than pleural effusion. Usually cavitation in 5–7 days (thick walled).
Pyogenic lung abscess	Recent aspiration. Fevers, chills, weight loss. Swallowing disorder secondary to CNS/GI disorder.	Foul (putrid lung abscess) breath.	↑ WBC, ↑ ESR. Sputum with normal oropharyngeal anaerobic flora in putrid lung abscess.	Thick-walled cavity in portion of lung dependent during aspiration (usually basilar segment of lower lobes if aspiration occurred supine). Cavitation occurs > 7 days.

Infectious Causes (cont'd)

Causes	Features (may have some, none, or all)			
	History	Physical	Laboratory	Chest X-Ray
Septic pulmonary emboli	Usually IV drug abuser with fever/ chills. Tricuspid regurgitation murmur or recent OB/GYN surgical procedure.	Fever > 102°F. Tricuspid valve regurgitant murmur with cannon A waves in neck.	Blood cultures positive for acute bacterial endocarditis pathogens.	Multiple peripheral nodules of varying size. Lower lobe predominance. Cavitation > 7 days characteristic of septic pulmonary emboli.
TB (reactivation)	Fevers, night sweats, normal appetite with weight loss, cough ± hemoptysis.	± bilateral apical dullness.	Normal WBC, ↑ platelets, ↑ ESR (≤ 70 mm/h). Positive PPD. AFB in sputum smear/ culture.	Slowly progressive bilateral infiltrates. No pleural effusion. Usually in apical segment of lower lobes or apical/ posterior segments of upper lobes. Calcifications common.
Histoplas-mosis (reactivation)	Fever, night sweats, cough, weight loss, histoplasmosis exposure (river valleys of Central/ Eastern United States).	± E. nodosum; otherwise unremarkable.	Normal WBC, normal/ ↑ eosinophilia, anemia, ↑ platelets, PPD negative. Immunodiffusion test with positive H precipitin band (diagnostic of active/chronic histoplasmosis).	Unilateral/ bilateral multiple patchy infiltrates with upper lobe predilection. Bilateral hilar adenopathy uncommon. Calcifications common. No pleural effusion. Chest x-ray resembles reactivation TB.

Infectious Causes (cont'd)

	Features (may have some, none, or all)			
Causes	**History**	**Physical**	**Laboratory**	**Chest X-Ray**
Sporotrichosis	Fever, cough, weight loss. ± hemoptysis. Antecedent lympho-cutaneous or skeletal sporotrichosis, rare.	Only if secondary to residual of lympho-cutaneous sporotrichosis, ± E. nodosum.	Normal WBC. No eosinophilia.	Unilateral > bilateral upper lobe nodular densities. Thick or thin-walled cavities. No hilar adenopathy. No pleural effusion.
Melioidosis	Past travel to Asia (usually > 10 years). Fever, cough, hemoptysis. ↑ risk of reactivation/ dissemination with DM, alcoholics, renal failure, leukemias/ lymphomas, steroids, immuno-suppressives. May occur in normal hosts.	Unremarkable.	↑ WBC (left shift), anemia, ↑ ESR, PPD negative. GNBs with bipolar "safety pin" staining in sputum. Sputum/ blood cultures positive for B. (Pseudomonas) pseudomallei.	Resembles reactivation TB, but infiltrates nodular/ diffuse (septicemic) or cavitary (chronic) predominantly in middle/lower lung fields. ± air fluid level. No pleural effusion.
Nocardia	Fevers, night sweats, fatigue, ↓ cell-mediated immunity (e.g., HIV, organ transplants, PAP, immuno-suppressive therapy).	Unremarkable.	Normal/↑ WBC, ↑ ESR. Sputum with gram-positive AFB.	Dense large infiltrates. May cavitate and mimic TB, lymphoma, or squamous cell carcinoma. No calcification ± pleural effusion.
Actinomycosis	Recent dental work.	± chest wall sinus tracts.	Normal/↑ WBC, ↑ ESR. Sputum with Gram-positive filamentous anaerobic bacilli.	Dense infiltrates extending to chest wall. No hilar adenopathy. Cavitation ± pleural effusion rare.

Infectious Causes (cont'd)

	Features (may have some, none, or all)			
Causes	History	Physical	Laboratory	Chest X-Ray
Rhodococcus equi	Insidious onset of fever, dyspnea, chest pain, ± hemoptysis. Immuno-suppressed patients with ↓ cell-mediated immunity or exposure to cattle, horses, pigs.	Unremarkable.	Normal/↑ WBC. Sputum/pleural fluid with gram-positive pleomorphic weakly acid-fast bacilli. Sputum, pleural fluid, blood cultures positive for R. equi.	Segmental infiltrate with upper lobe predominance ± cavitation. Air-fluid levels and pleural effusion common.
Amebic cysts	Hepatic amebic abscess. Remote history of usually mild amebic dysentery.	± hepato-megaly.	Normal WBC and ESR. ↑ E. histolytica HI titers.	Well-circumscribed cavitary lesions adjacent to right diaphragm. ± calcifications. Sympathetic pleural effusion above hepatic amebic abscess.
Alveolar echinoco-ccosis (hydatid cysts)	Symptoms related to cyst size/location: 1/3 asymptomatic; 2/3 with fever, malaise, chest pain ± hemoptysis. RUQ abdominal pain may occur.	Hepatomegaly common.	Normal/↑ WBC, no eosinophilia, ↑ alkaline phosphate/SGPT with hepatic cysts. Abdominal ultrasound/CT with calcified hepatic irregularly shaped cysts ("Swiss cheese" calcification characteristic). ↑ E. multilocularis IHA titers.	RLL usual location (hepatic cysts penetrate diaphragm into RLL). Nodules are 70% solitary, 30% multiple. Pleural effusion rare. Endocyst membrane on surface of cyst fluid ("water lilly" sign) is characteristic.

Noninfectious Causes

| Causes | Features (may have some, none, or all) | | | |
	History	Physical	Laboratory	Chest X-Ray
Wegener's granulomatosis	Most common in middle-aged adults. Cough, fever, fatigue.	Findings of chronic sinusitis, bloody nasal discharge.	↑ WBC, anemia, ↑ platelets, ↑ ESR, ↑ RF, negative ANA, proteinuria, hematuria. Positive cANCA.	Bilateral asymmetrical nodular infiltrates of varying size with irregular margins. Cavitation common. Inner lining of cavities irregular. Air-fluid levels rare. ± pleural effusions. No calcifications.
Squamous cell carcinoma	Long-term smoking history.	Clubbing, hypertrophic pulmonary osteoarthropathy ± findings 2° to superior vena caval syndrome and CNS/bone metastases.	↑ Ca^{++} (without bone metastases).	Unilateral perihilar mass lesion. Cavitation common. No pleural effusion.
Lymphoma	Fever, ↓ appetite with weight loss, night sweats, fatigue.	Adenopathy ± splenomegaly.	Normal WBC, ↑ basophils, ↑ eosinophilia, ↓ lymphocytes, ↑ platelets, ↑ ESR ↑ alkaline phosphatase, ↑∝$_{1, 2}$ globulins on SPEP.	Unilateral or asymmetrical bilateral hilar adenopathy. Lung infiltrate may appear contiguous with hilar adenopathy. No clear channel between mediastinum and hilar nodes. Small pleural effusions rare.

Noninfectious Causes (cont'd)

	Features (may have some, none, or all)			
Causes	History	Physical	Laboratory	Chest X-Ray
Metastatic carcinoma	History of breast, thyroid, renal cell, colon, pancreatic cancer or osteogenic sarcoma.	Findings related to underlying malignancy and, when present, to bone, hepatic, CNS metastases.	Secondary to effects of primary neoplasm, metastases, paraneoplastic syndrome.	Nodular lesions that vary in size. Metastatic lesions are usually well-circumscribed with lower lobe predominance. Usually no bronchial obstruction (obstruction suggests colon, renal, or melanoma metastases). Usually no cavitation (except for squamous cell metastases). Calcification usually suggests osteosarcoma (rarely adenocarcinoma). Pleural effusion rare (except for breast cancer).
Rheumatoid nodules	Usually in severe rheumatoid arthritis (RA); ± history of silicosis.	Findings secondary to RA. Rheumatoid nodules on exterior surfaces of arms.	Normal WBC, ↑ ESR, ↑ ANA, ↑ RF (high titer). Pleural fluid with ↓ glucose.	Lung nodules are round and well-circumscribed, predominantly in lower lobes and typically superimposed on interstitial lung disease ("rheumatoid lung"). Cavitation is common. ± pulmonary fibrosis, pleural effusion. Silicosis + RA nodules = Caplan's syndrome.

CAVITARY INFILTRATES
(THIN-WALLED)

Infectious Causes

	Features (may have some, none, or all)			
Causes	History	Physical	Laboratory	Chest X-Ray
Atypical TB	Often occurs in setting of previous lung disease.	Unremarkable.	Normal WBC, ↑ ESR. Weakly positive PPD. Positive sputum AFB/culture.	Multiple cavitary lesions ± calcifications usually involving both lungs. Resembles reactivation TB except that cavities are thin-walled. No pleural effusion.
Coccidiomycosis (reactivation)	Previous exposure in endemic coccidiomycosis areas (e.g., Southwest USA). Asymptomatic.	± E. nodosum.	Normal WBC. Eosinophilia acutely but not in chronic phase, and eosinophils in pleural fluid. CF IgG titer ≥ 1:32 indicates active disease.	Thick/thin walled cavities (< 3 cm) usually in anterior segments of lower lobes ± calcifications/bilateral hilar adenopathy. Air-fluid levels rare unless secondarily infected. Pleural effusion rare.

Infectious Causes (cont'd)

Causes	Features (may have some, none, or all)			
	History	Physical	Laboratory	Chest X-Ray
Paragonimiasis	Ingestion of fresh-water crabs/crayfish. Acute symptoms (< 6 months): fevers, abdominal pain, diarrhea followed by episodes of pleuritic chest pain. Chronic symptoms (> 6 months): fevers, night sweats, cough ± hemoptysis. Asymptomatic in some.	Wheezing, ± urticaria (acutely).	↑ WBC, eosinophilia. Eosinophils in pleural fluid. Sputum with Charot-Leyden crystals. Sputum/feces with operculated P. Westermani eggs.	Cavitary patchy or well-defined infiltrates predominantly in mid-lung fields. Hydropneumothorax common. Calcifications and pleural effusion common.
Sporotrichosis	Fever, cough, weight loss. ± hemoptysis. Antecedent lymphocutaneous or skeletal sporotrichosis, rare.	Only if secondary to residual of lympho-cutaneous sporotrichosis, ± E. nodosum.	Normal WBC. No eosinophilia.	Unilateral > bilateral upper lobe nodular densities. Thick or thin-walled cavities. No hilar adenopathy. No pleural effusion.
Pneumatoceles	Common in S. aureus pneumonia in children. Fever, cough, dyspnea. ± antecedent influenza.	Unremarkable unless pneumatocele ruptures, then signs of pneumothorax.	↑ WBC (left shift), ↓ pO_2 (secondary to influenza).	Multiple thin-walled cavities in areas of S. aureus pneumonia. Common in children; rare in adults.

Noninfectious Causes

	Features (may have some, none, or all)			
Causes	History	Physical	Laboratory	Chest X-Ray
Emphysema (blebs/cyst)	Long history of smoking. Rupture of apical bleb common in males > 30 years. Pneumonia rare in severe emphysema (vs. chronic bronchitis) but may occur early in unaffected areas of lung.	Asthenic "pink puffers." Barrel chest. Diaphragmatic excursions < 2 cm.	Normal WBC, ↓ pO_2.	↓ lung markings ("vanishing lung") ± blebs. Hyperlucent lungs with upper lobe predominance. Flattened diaphragms, vertically elongated cardiac silhouette, ↑ retrocardiac and retrosternal airspaces. No infiltrates or pleural effusions. (In upper lobe emphysema, no vascular redistribution to upper lobes with CHF).
Bronchogenic cyst	Congenital anomaly. Usually asymptomatic. Cough if symptomatic.	Unremarkable unless secondarily infected, then signs 2° to mediastinal abscess.	Normal WBC/ESR.	Circumscribed cystic lesion originates in lung but appears high in mediastinum. If filled with fluid, appears as solitary tumor. If near the trachea, may rupture into bronchus/trachea and cyst may contain air. If communicates openly with bronchus, appears as thin-walled cavitary nodule. If infected, presents as mediastinal abscess.
Cystic bronchiectasis	Recurrent pulmonary infections with purulent sputum ± hemoptysis.	Unremarkable unless dextrocardia with sinusitis (Kartagener's syndrome).	↑ WBC, normal ESR.	Bilateral large cystic lucencies at lung bases. Upper lobes relatively spared (unless secondary chronic aspiration). Thickened bronchial markings at bases. Bronchiectasis of cystic fibrosis predominantly involves upper lobes.

Noninfectious Causes (cont'd)

Causes	Features (may have some, none, or all)			
	History	Physical	Laboratory	Chest X-Ray
Sequestered lung	Usually asymptomatic. Productive cough ± hemoptysis if communicates with bronchus or if infected.	Unremarkable.	Normal WBC, ↑ ESR.	Solid nodule unless communicates with bronchus, then thin-walled cavity ± air fluid levels. Usually posterior based segment of lower lobes (LLL > RLL). If > 3 cm, presents as mass lesion.
Histiocytosis X (eosinophilic granuloma, Langerhan's cell histiocytosis)	Patients usually 20–40 years. Usually asymptomatic. Fever, cough, dyspnea in some. Diabetes insipidus rare.	Hepato-splenomegaly, skin lesions, hemoptysis (rare).	Normal WBC, eosinophilia.	Pneumothorax superimposed on diffuse pulmonary fibrosis. Cystic bone lesions. Usually mid/upper lung fields with nodules/ thin-walled cysts or infiltrates. No hilar adenopathy or pleural effusion.

REFERENCES AND SUGGESTED READINGS

Burgener FA, Kormano M. Differential Diagnosis in Conventional Radiology, 2nd ed. Stuttgart, Georg Thieme Verlag, 1991.

Chapman S, Nakielny R. Aids to Radiological Differential Diagnosis, 2nd ed. London, Bailliere Tindall, 1990.

Conn RB, Borer WZ, Snyder JW. Current Diagnosis 9. Philadelphia, W. B. Saunders Company, 1997.

Crapo JD, Glassroth J, Karlinsky JB, King TE. Baum's Textbook of Pulmonary Diseases, 7th ed. Philadelphia, Lippincott Williams & Wilkins, 2004.

Cunha BA. Pneumonia Essentials, 3rd ed. Jones & Bartlett, Sudbury MA, 2010.

Eisenberg RL. Clinical Imaging. An Atlas of Differential Diagnosis, 2nd ed. Gaithersburg, Aspen Publishers, Inc., 1992.

Gorbach SL, Bartlett JG, Blacklow NR. Infectious Diseases, 3rd ed. Philadelphia, Lippincott Williams & Wilkins, 2004.

Karetzky M, Cunha BA, Brandstetter RD. The Pneumonias. New York, Springer-Verlag, 1993.

Kasper L, Braunwald E, Fauci AS, Hauser SL, Longo DL, Jameson JL. Harrison's Principles of Internal Medicine, 17th ed. New York, The McGraw Hill Companies, 2008.

Levison ME. The Pneumonias: Clinical Approaches to Infectious Diseases of the Lower Respiratory Tract. Boston, John Wright, PSG Inc., 1984.

Lillington GA, Jamplis RW. A Diagnostic Approach to Chest Diseases, 2nd ed. Baltimore, The Williams & Wilkins Company, 1977.

Mandell GL, Bennet JE, Dolin R. Mandell, Douglas, and Bennett's Principles and Practice of Infectious Diseases, 7th ed., Elsevier, 2010.

Murray JF, Nadel JA. Textbook of Respiratory Medicine, 3rd ed. Philadelphia, W.B. Saunders Company, 2000.

Raoof S, Feigin D, Sung A, et al. Interpretation of Plain Chest Roentgenogram. Chest 141:545–558, 2012.

Teplick JE, Haskin ME. Roentgenologic Diagnosis, 3rd ed. Philadelphia, W. B. Saunders Company, 1976.

Wright FW. Radiology of the Chest and Related Conditions. London, Taylor & Francis, 2002.

Chapter 9

Infectious Disease Differential Diagnosis

Cheston B. Cunha, MD

Infectious diseases often present with important findings on physical diagnosis and laboratory evaluation. In this chapter, findings of key infectious diseases and noninfectious diseases likely to be considered in the differential diagnosis are presented. Tropical infections are also included since this book is also for international use.

Table 9.1. Fever Curves

Finding	Causes
Morning (am) temperature spikes	<u>Infectious</u>: TB, typhoid fever, Whipple's disease <u>Noninfectious</u>: PAN
Relative tachycardia	<u>Infectious</u>: gas gangrene, myocarditis (Coxsackie, RMSF, typhus, diptheria, trichinosis, VLM, influenza) <u>Noninfectious</u>: Hyperthyroidism, hypoxia, cardiac arrhythmias, anxiety, pulmonary emboli
Relative bradycardia	<u>Infectious</u>: typhoid fever, typhus, leptospirosis, Legionnaire's disease, Q fever, psittacosis, RMSF, babesiosis, ehrlichiosis, yellow fever, dengue fever, arboviral hemorrhagic fevers <u>Noninfectious</u>: drug fever, CNS lesions, β-blockers, verapamil, diltiazem, lymphoma, factitious fever
Single fever spikes	<u>Infectious</u>: Transient bacteremia <u>Noninfectious</u>: Blood/blood product transfusions
Double quotidian fevers	<u>Infectious</u>: kala-azar, right sided GC ABE, miliary TB, mixed malarial infections <u>Noninfectious</u>: adult Still's disease, antipyretics
Camelback fever pattern	<u>Infectious</u>: Colorado tick fever, dengue fever, leptospirosis, brucellosis, LCM, yellow fever, poliomyelitis, smallpox, rat-bite fever (Spirillum minus), chikungunya fever, rift valley fever, african hemorrhagic fevers (Marburg, Ebola, Lassa, etc), echovirus (echo 9) <u>Noninfectious</u>: antipyretics

Table 9.2. General Appearance Abnormalities

Finding	Causes
Hypotension/shock	<u>Infectious</u>: anthrax, plague, typhus, **GI sources**: colon (perforation, colitis, abscess); **GU sources**: cystitis (only in SLE, DM, alcoholism, multiple myeloma, Vibrio vulnificus, CLL, steroids); obstruction: relative (BPH), unilateral (partial), or bilateral/ureteral (partial/total); kidney (acute pyelonephritis, renal abscess, perinephric abscess, renal calculi); prostate (acute prostatitis, prostatic abscess). **Other sources**: CVC infection, TSS (S. aureus, group A streptococci, C. sordellii), dengue fever, SARS, HPS, influenza (human, avian, swine), CAP with decreased/absent splenic function, or severe cardiopulmonary disease, influenza/ILI with CA-MRSA (PVL+)
	<u>Noninfectious</u>: myocardial infarction, pulmonary embolism, acute pancreatitis, relative adrenal insufficiency, GI bleed, overzealous diuresis, inadequate volume replacement or hypotonic fluid replacement, aortic dissection, abdominal aneurysm rupture, rectus sheath hematoma
Soft tissue crepitance	<u>Infectious</u>: mixed aerobic/anaerobic infection*
	<u>Noninfectious</u>: subcutaneous emphysema, recent surgery in area of crepitance
Bullae	<u>Infectious</u>: gas gangrene (hemorrhagic), S. aureus > group A streptococci, V. vulnificus (hemorrhagic), necrotizing fasciitis, bullous impetigo
	<u>Noninfectious</u>: pemphigus, pemphigoid, dermatitis herpetiformis, TEN, porphyria, contact dermatitis, E. multiforme, DM, barbiturates
Generalized edema/nephrotic syndrome	<u>Infectious</u>: malaria (P. malariae), trichinosis, VZV, yellow fever, influenza A, HBV, HIV, EBV, CMV, 2° syphilis, leprosy
	<u>Noninfectious</u>: drugs, lymphomas, thiamine deficiency (wet beri-beri), kwashiorkor, post-streptococcal glomerulonephritis, DM, PAN, Henoch-Schönlein purpura, SLE, constrictive pericarditis, tricuspid regurgitation, IVC obstruction, myxedema, sickle cell disease, amyloidosis, α-1 antitrypsin deficiency, nail-patella syndrome, Wegener's granulomatosis, sarcoidosis, renal vein thrombosis
Erythroderma	<u>Infectious</u>: human T-cell leukemia virus 1 (HTLV-1), TSS, scarlet fever, dengue fever
	<u>Noninfectious</u>: psoriasis, lymphoma, atopic dermatitis, contact dermatitis, exfoliative dermatitis, drugs, ichthyosis, erythroleukemia, pityriasis, dermatomyositis, Kawasaki's disease
Hyperpigmentation	<u>Infectious</u>: kala-azar, Whipple's disease, histoplasmosis
	<u>Noninfectious</u>: hemochromatosis, PBC, Addison's disease, drugs – brown (bleomycin), blue/gray (busulfan, fluorouracil, chlorpromazine), purple/gray (amiodarone), blue/gray (minocycline)

* Versus gas gangrene (minimal/no gas on muscle auscultation).

Table 9.2. General Appearance Abnormalities (cont'd)

Finding	Causes
Jaundice	<u>Infectious</u>: yellow fever, EBV, leptospirosis, ascariasis (in bile/pancreatic duct), viral hemorrhagic fevers, viral hepatitis
	<u>Noninfectious</u>: hepatobiliary malignancy, benign biliary obstruction, PBC, cirrhosis, hemolytic anemias, alcoholic hepatitis, drugs, Gilbert's syndrome, pancreatic carcinoma
Vitiligo	<u>Infectious</u>: leprosy, yaws, pinta, HIV
	<u>Noninfectious</u>: DM, hyperthyroidism, hypothyroidism, Hashimoto's thyroiditis
Lizard/elephant skin	<u>Infectious</u>: onchocerciasis
	<u>Noninfectious</u>: ichthyosis
Urticaria	<u>Infectious</u>: strongyloides, dracunculiasis, HBV, F. hepatica, schistosomal dermatitis
	<u>Noninfectious</u>: insect bites/stings, drugs, malignancies, cholinergic urticaria, serum sickness, urticarial vasculitis, cryoglobulinemia, systemic mastocytosis
Rash (only below waist)	<u>Infectious</u>: Parvovirus B19 (stocking/glove)
	<u>Noninfectious</u>: Henoch-Schönlein purpura (HSP)

Table 9.3. Head Abnormalities

Finding	Causes
Prematurely gray hair	<u>Infectious</u>: HIV
	<u>Noninfectious</u>: smoking, pernicious anemia
Temporal muscle wasting	<u>Infectious</u>: HIV
	<u>Noninfectious</u>: myotonic dystrophy
Facial swelling (edema)	<u>Infectious</u>: arboviral hemorrhagic fevers, trichinosis, leprosy, EEE, onchocerciasis
	<u>Noninfectious</u>: angioneurotic edema, nephrotic syndrome, acute glomerulonephritis, leukemic infiltrates, amyloidosis
Severe seborrheic dermatitis	<u>Infectious</u>: HIV
	<u>Noninfectious</u>: CGD
Facial red spots	<u>Infectious</u>: psittacosis (Horder's spots)
	<u>Noninfectious</u>: Campbell de Morgan spots

Table 9.3. Head Abnormalities (cont'd)

Finding	Causes
Localized alopecia	<u>Infectious</u>: leprosy, Tinea capitis, smallpox, blastomycosis, VZV, TB (cutaneous)
	<u>Noninfectious</u>: SLE, DM, scleroderma, common variable immune deficiency (CVID)
Generalized alopecia	<u>Infectious</u>: post-malaria, post-typhoid fever, post-kala-azar, post-yellow fever, 2° syphilis, HIV
	<u>Noninfectious</u>: nutritional deficiencies, drugs, hyperthyroidism
Total/partial eyebrow loss	<u>Infectious</u>: leprosy, syphilis
	<u>Noninfectious</u>: iatrogenic, hereditary, hypothyroidism, hypopituitarism
Long eyelashes	<u>Infectious</u>: kala-azar, trypanosomiasis
	<u>Noninfectious</u>: hereditary, drugs, HIV drugs
Lacrimal gland enlargement *unilateral*	<u>Infectious</u>: Chagas' disease
	<u>Noninfectious</u>: malignancies
bilateral	<u>Infectious</u>: TB
	<u>Noninfectious</u>: Sjogren's syndrome, RA, SLE, sarcoidosis
Facial erythema	<u>Infectious</u>: facial cellulitis, erysipelas, TB (lupus vulgaris), arboviral hemorrhagic fevers
	<u>Noninfectious</u>: dermatomyositis, drugs, rosacea, carcinoid syndrome, SLE
Parotid enlargement	<u>Infectious</u>: mumps, Chagas' disease, rat bite fever (Streptobacillus moniliformis), meliodosis
	<u>Noninfectious</u>: Sjogren's syndrome, sarcoidosis, cirrhosis
Scalp nodules	<u>Infectious</u>: myiasis, onchocerciasis
	<u>Noninfectious</u>: bony exostoses, malignancies, benign cysts, pyogenic granuloma, Kimura's disease

Table 9.4. Eye Abnormalities

Finding	Causes
Bilateral upper lid edema	<u>Infectious</u>: EBV (Hoagland's sign)
	<u>Noninfectious</u>: bilateral eye irritation
Bilateral lid edema	<u>Infectious</u>: trichinosis, meningococcemia, adenovirus
	<u>Noninfectious</u>: Wegener's granulomatosis

Table 9.4. Eye Abnormalities (cont'd)

Finding	Causes
Heliotrope eyelid discoloration	<u>Infectious</u>: cholera (early), influenza A (severe)
	<u>Noninfectious</u>: dermatomyositis
Periorbital edema *unilateral*	<u>Infectious</u>: Chagas' disease, loiasis, gnathostomiasis, sparganosis
	<u>Noninfectious</u>: insect bites, unilateral eye irritation
bilateral	<u>Infectious</u>: RMSF, trichinosis, tularemia, dengue fever
	<u>Noninfectious</u>: allergies, Insect bites, dermatomyositis
Argyll-Robertson pupils	<u>Infectious</u>: syphilis
	<u>Noninfectious</u>: sarcoidosis
Iritis	<u>Infectious</u>: onchocerciasis, 2° syphilis, relapsing fever, leprosy
	<u>Noninfectious</u>: SLE, dermatomyositis, Behçet's syndrome, Reiter's syndrome, RA
Conjunctivitis *unilateral*	<u>Infectious</u>: TB, HSV, tularemia, adult inclusion conjunctivitis, Chagas' disease, LGV, CSD, loiasis, ocular myiasis, diphtheria, adenovirus (types 8, 19)
	<u>Noninfectious</u>: SLE, eye irritation
bilateral	<u>Infectious</u>: TSS, measles, rubella, meningococcemia, gonorrhea, adenovirus (type 3), plague, RMSF, sparganosis, LGV, listeria, relapsing fever, pertussis, influenza, microsporidia, HHV-6, arboviral hemorrhagic fevers, dengue hemorrhagic fever
	<u>Noninfectious</u>: Kawasaki's disease, Reiter's syndrome, Steven-Johnson syndrome, adult Still's disease, eye irritation
Hemorrhagic conjunctivitis *unilateral*	<u>Infectious</u>: adenovirus (type 8, 19)
	<u>Noninfectious</u>: trauma
bilateral	<u>Infectious</u>: trichinosis, pertussis, leptospirosis, Coxsackie A (type 24), adenovirus (type 11), enterovirus (type 70), arboviral hemorrhagic fevers
	<u>Noninfectious</u>: trauma
Subconjunctival hemorrhage	<u>Infectious</u>: SBE, trichinosis, meningococcemia, pertussis, leptospirosis, RMSF
	<u>Noninfectious</u>: severe anemia, Kawasaki's disease
Conjunctival suffusion	<u>Infectious</u>: RMSF, leptospirosis, relapsing fever, ehrlichiosis, HPS, influenza (human, avian), arboviral hemorrhagic fevers, St.LE
	<u>Noninfectious</u>: bilateral eye irritation

Table 9.4. Eye Abnormalities (cont'd)

Finding	Causes
Episcleritis	<u>Infectious</u>: TB, leprosy, 2° syphilis, Lyme disease
	<u>Noninfectious</u>: sarcoidosis, RA, adult Still's disease, SLE, PAN, TA, RE
Scleral nodules	<u>Infectious</u>: loiasis, sparganosis, leprosy, tularemia, TB
	<u>Noninfectious</u>: RA, vitamin A deficiency (Bitot's spots), sarcoidosis
Dry eyes	<u>Infectious</u>: measles
	<u>Noninfectious</u>: vitamin A deficiency, SLE, Sjogren's syndrome, RA, sarcoidosis
Watery eyes	<u>Infectious</u>: bacterial conjunctivitis, adenovirus
	<u>Noninfectious</u>: PAN, allergenic conjunctivitis
Uveitis	<u>Infectious</u>: TB, histoplasmosis, leprosy, syphilis, malaria, HSV, VZV, EBV, TSS, typhus, LGV, CMV, African trypanosomiasis, brucellosis, leptospirosis, RMSF, CSD
	<u>Noninfectious</u>: adult Still's disease, SLE, PAN, sarcoidosis, Behçet's syndrome, Reiter's syndrome, RA, relapsing polychondritis, ankylosing spondylitis, Kawasaki's disease, Wegener's granulomatosis
Corneal haziness	<u>Infectious</u>: adenovirus, leprosy, trachoma, onchocerciasis
	<u>Noninfectious</u>: vitamin A deficiency, cataracts
Keratitis	<u>Infectious</u>: HSV, congenital syphilis, acanthamoeba, TB, toxoplasmosis, histoplasmosis, CMV, trachoma, microsporidia, nocardia, leprosy, onchocerciasis, meliodosis
	<u>Noninfectious</u>: Behçet's syndrome, Reiter's syndrome, Steven-Johnson syndrome, vitamin A deficiency
Corneal ulcers	<u>Infectious</u>: HSV, listeria, acanthamoeba, tularemia, shigella, RMSF
	<u>Noninfectious</u>: trauma, Wegener's granulomatosis
Endophthalmitis	<u>Infectious</u>: TB, candida, aspergillus, toxocara, serratia, S. pneumoniae
	<u>Noninfectious</u>: retinoblastoma
Chorioretinitis	<u>Infectious</u>: toxoplasmosis, CMV, onchocerciasis, congenital syphilis, histoplasmosis, TB, WNE, coccidiomycosis, leptospirosis
	<u>Noninfectious</u>: sarcoidosis, SLE, PAN
Cytoid bodies (cotton wool spots)	<u>Infectious</u>: CSD, HIV, CMV, SBE
	<u>Noninfectious</u>: SLE, adult Still's disease, PAN, atrial myxoma, Wegener's granulomatosis, TA

Table 9.4. Eye Abnormalities (cont'd)

Finding	Causes
Roth spots	<u>Infectious</u>: SBE, psittacosis, RMSF, malaria
	<u>Noninfectious</u>: PAN, SLE, DM, severe anemia, leukemia, cholesterol emboli syndrome, atrial myxoma, TA, Takayasu's arteritis
Periphlebitis (candle wax drippings)	<u>Infectious</u>: CMV, leptospirosis (Weil's syndrome)
	<u>Noninfectious</u>: sarcoidosis

Table 9.5. Ear Abnormalities

Finding	Causes
Acute deafness	<u>Infectious</u>: ABM, mumps (aseptic meningitis), RMSF, typhus, brucellosis, Lassa fever
	<u>Noninfectious</u>: sound/barotrauma
External ear lesions	<u>Infectious</u>: cutaneous leishmaniasis (Chiclero ulcer), leprosy, Kaposi's sarcoma
	<u>Noninfectious</u>: relapsing polychondritis, eczema, carcinoma, contact dermatitis, sarcoidosis, SLE, gout (tophi), keloids, actinic keratosis

Table 9.6. Nasal Abnormalities

Finding	Causes
Purple nose tip	<u>Infectious</u>: Kaposi's sarcoma, TB (Bazin's erythema induratum)
	<u>Noninfectious</u>: vasculitis, lymphoma, drugs, sarcoidosis
Nose tip gangrene	<u>Infectious</u>: Staphylococcus aureus ABE (emboli)
	<u>Noninfectious</u>: SLE, vasculitis
Epistaxis	<u>Infectious</u>: psittacosis, typhoid fever, nasal diphtheria, Colorado tick fever, TBRF, influenza, dengue hemorrhagic fever, arboviral hemorrhagic fevers, acute renal failure, leprosy, leptospirosis, VZV, TB, rhinosporidium, mucocutaneous leishmaniasis
	<u>Noninfectious</u>: Local trauma, sinus malignancies, von Willebrand's disease, polycythemia vera, Waldenstrom's macroglobulinemia, relapsing polychondritis
Nasal septal perforation	<u>Infectious</u>: leprosy, 2° syphilis, mucocutaneous leishmaniasis, blastomycosis, pinta, yaws
	<u>Noninfectious</u>: cocaine, lethal midline granuloma, Wegener's granulomatosis, miasis

Table 9.7. Mouth Abnormalities

Finding	Causes
Trismus	<u>Infectious</u>: tetanus
	<u>Noninfectious</u>: temporomandibular joint dislocation/arthritis, trigeminal neuralgia
Herpes labialis	<u>Infectious</u>: HSV, pneumococcal pneumonia, meningococcal meningitis, malaria
	<u>Noninfectious</u>: contact dermatitis (may mimic H. labialis)
Angular chelitis	<u>Infectious</u>: 2° syphilis, HIV
	<u>Noninfectious</u>: riboflavin deficiency, trauma, contact dermatitis, anemia
Gingivitis	<u>Infectious</u>: trench mouth
	<u>Noninfectious</u>: Wegener's granulomatosis
Tongue tenderness	<u>Infectious</u>: relapsing fever
	<u>Noninfectious</u>: vitamin deficiencies, pernicious anemia
Tongue ulcers	<u>Infectious</u>: histoplasmosis, HSV, syphilis
	<u>Noninfectious</u>: aphthous ulcers, chemotherapy, radiation therapy
Leukoplakia	<u>Infectious</u>: HIV (hairy), syphilis
	<u>Noninfectious</u>: lichen planus
Oral ulcers *solitary*	<u>Infectious</u>: syphilis, CMV, histoplasmosis, TB, Leishmania braziliensis
	<u>Noninfectious</u>: squamous cell carcinoma, Behçet's syndrome, Wegener's granulomatosis
multiple	<u>Infectious</u>: HSV, HFM disease, herpangina, brucellosis, Lassa fever, African tick bite fever
	<u>Noninfectious</u>: SLE, celiac disease, aphthous ulcers, squamous cell carcinoma, Behçet's syndrome, FAPA syndrome, hyper IgE (Job's) syndrome E. multiforme, RE, cyclic neutropenia, Sweet's syndrome
Frenal ulcer	<u>Infectious</u>: pertussis
	<u>Noninfectious</u>: trauma
Palatal petechiae	<u>Infectious</u>: Group A streptococci, EBV, CMV, HSV, VZV, toxoplasmosis, rubella, HIV, tularemia
	<u>Noninfectious</u>: thrombocytopenia (2° to any cause), platelet dysfunction disorders, DIC, Ehlers-Danlos syndrome, Marfan's syndrome

Table 9.7. Mouth Abnormalities (cont'd)

Finding	Causes
Palatal perforation	<u>Infectious</u>: congenital syphilis, myiasis
	<u>Noninfectious</u>: Post-surgical, midline granuloma, cocaine
Palatal vesicles	<u>Infectious</u>: ***Anterior:*** HSV, VZV, hand-foot-mouth disease (Coxsackie A). ***Posterior:*** herpangina (Coxsackie A)
	<u>Noninfectious</u>: bullous pemphigus, Steven-Johnson syndrome (drug-induced)
Uvular edema	<u>Infectious</u>: Group A streptococci
	<u>Noninfectious</u>: Franklin's disease, drugs, angioneurotic edema
Crimson crescents	<u>Infectious</u>: chronic fatigue syndrome (CFS), HIV
	<u>Noninfectious</u>: None
Tonsillar membranes	<u>Infectious</u>: diphtheria, Arcanobacterium hemolyticum
	<u>Noninfectious</u>: None
Tonsillar ulcers	<u>Infectious</u>: tularemia (oropharyngeal), 1° syphilis, Vincent's angina, TB
	<u>Noninfectious</u>: carcinoma, T-cell lymphoma, AML
Hoarseness	<u>Infectious</u>: laryngeal TB, C. pneumoniae, respiratory viruses, pertussis
	<u>Noninfectious</u>: recurrent laryngeal nerve paralysis, laryngeal cancer

Table 9.8. Neck Abnormalities*

Finding	Causes
Enlarged greater auricular nerve	<u>Infectious</u>: leprosy
	<u>Noninfectious</u>: none
Bull neck	<u>Infectious</u>: diphtheria, mumps, Ludwig's angina, pertussis, group A streptococcal suppurative lymphangitis
	<u>Noninfectious</u>: angioneurotic edema, subcutaneous emphysema
Jugular vein tenderness	<u>Infectious</u>: suppurative jugular thrombophlebitis (Lemierre's syndrome)
	<u>Noninfectious</u>: thrombophlebitis
Neck sinus tract	<u>Infectious</u>: actinomycosis, TB, atypical TB
	<u>Noninfectious</u>: branchial cleft cyst, CGD
Superior vena cava syndrome	<u>Infectious</u>: actinomycosis
	<u>Noninfectious</u>: lymphoma, squamous cell carcinoma

*   See Table 9.13 for cervical adenopathy (p. 488).

Table 9.9. Chest Abnormalities

Finding	Causes
Shoulder tenderness	<u>Infectious</u>: subdiaphragmatic abscess, septic arthritis (shoulder)
	<u>Noninfectious</u>: squamous cell carcinoma (Pancoast's tumor), bursitis
Sternal tenderness	<u>Infectious</u>: sternal osteomyelitis (post-open heart surgery)
	<u>Noninfectious</u>: metastatic carcinoma, pre-leukemia, acute leukemia, myeloproliferative disorder, trauma
Costochondral tenderness	<u>Infectious</u>: costochondritis (Coxsackie B)
	<u>Noninfectious</u>: trauma, plasmacytoma
Trapezius tenderness	<u>Infectious</u>: subdiaphragmatic abscess
	<u>Noninfectious</u>: fibromyalgia
Chest wall sinuses	<u>Infectious</u>: TB, actinomycosis, blastomycosis, abscess, M. fortuitum-chelonei (post-breast implant surgery), sternal osteomyelitis (post-sternotomy)
	<u>Noninfectious</u>: bronchogenic carcinoma
Spontaneous pneumothorax	<u>Infectious</u>: TB, PCP, Legionnaire's disease, lung abscess, pertussis
	<u>Noninfectious</u>: histiocytosis X (eosinophilic granuloma, Langerhan's cell histiocytosis), osteogenic sarcoma, emphysema, ARDS
Diffuse wheezing	<u>Infectious</u>: RSV, influenza, HMPV, HBOV, C. pneumoniae, M. pneumoniae, acute shistosomiasis (S. mansoni > S. haematobium)
	<u>Noninfectious</u>: pulmonary emboli, LVF, asthma, Churg-Strauss granulomatosis, carcinoid syndrome, asthmatic bronchitis, angioedema
Chest dullness *consolidation*	<u>Infectious</u>: bacterial pneumonia, psittacosis, nocardia, Q fever
	<u>Noninfectious</u>: large cell carcinoma
pleural effusion	<u>Infectious</u>: group A streptococci, tularemia, H. influenzae, 1° TB
	<u>Noninfectious</u>: Meig's syndrome, pancreatitis, CHF, malignancies, pulmonary embolism

Table 9.10. Back Abnormalities

Finding	Causes
Spinal tenderness	<u>Infectious</u>: vertebral osteomyelitis, typhoid fever, TB, brucellosis, SBE
	<u>Noninfectious</u>: malignancies, multiple myeloma
D'espine's sign	<u>Infectious</u>: bilateral pneumonia (consolidation), TB
	<u>Noninfectious</u>: sarcoidosis, large cell carcinoma, lymphoma
Unilateral CVA tenderness	<u>Infectious</u>: pyelonephritis, renal/perinephric abscess
	<u>Noninfectious</u>: trauma

Table 9.11. Heart Abnormalities

Finding	Causes
Tachycardia	<u>Infectious</u>: myocarditis (Coxsackie, RMSF, typhus, diphtheria, trichinosis, Toxocara canis/cati (VLM), influenza, dengue), gas gangrene
	<u>Noninfectious</u>: hypovolemia, hypoxia, anxiety, hyperthyroidism, MI, pulmonary embolism, CHF, Kawasaki's disease, substance withdrawal, myocarditis (idiopathic giant cell)
Heart block *Acute*	<u>Infectious</u>: Lyme disease, ABE with paravalvular/septal abscess, diptheria, myocarditis (Coxsackie, influenza, RMSF)
	<u>Noninfectious</u>: acute (inferior) MI, drugs, myocarditis (idiopathic giant cell)
Chronic	<u>Infectious</u>: Chagas' disease
	<u>Noninfectious</u>: AV nodal ablation, sarcoidosis, Lev's/Lenegre's disease
Pericardial effusion	<u>Infectious</u>: viral pericarditis, TB pericarditis, dengue
	<u>Noninfectious</u>: SLE, uremia, malignancy
Heart murmur	<u>Infectious</u>: SBE, 3° syphilis
	<u>Noninfectious</u>: valvular heart disease, severe anemia, Takayasu's arteritis, SLE (Libman-Sacks), endomyocardial fibroelastosis, atrial myxoma, marantic endocarditis

Table 9.12. Abdominal Abnormalities

Finding	Causes
Abdominal wall tenderness	<u>Infectious</u>: leptospirosis, abdominal wall cellulitis/abscess, trichinosis
	<u>Noninfectious</u>: trauma, rectus sheath hematoma
Abdominal wall sinus tract	<u>Infectious</u>: TB, abscess, ameboma, actinomycosis
	<u>Noninfectious</u>: carcinomas
Rose spots	<u>Infectious</u>: typhoid fever, shigella, trichinosis, rat bite fever, brucellosis, leptospirosis
	<u>Noninfectious</u>: Campbell de Morgan spots
Abdominal tenderness (2° to pancreatitis)	<u>Infectious</u>: Coxsackie virus, echovirus, mumps, ascariasis, EBV, CMV, HBV, HSV, VZV, HIV
	<u>Noninfectious</u>: EtOH, cholelithiasis (+ common pancreatitis duct), tauma, post-ERCP, hyperlipidemia (types I, IV, V), hypertriglyceridemia, TPN, hypercalcemia, SLE, PAN, posterior penetrating duodenal ulcer, drugs (steroids, azathioprine, diuretics, furosemide, thiazides, L-asparaginase, valproic acid, pentamidine)

Table 9.12. Abdominal Abnormalities (cont'd)

Finding	Causes
Right upper quadrant tenderness	<u>Infectious</u>: cholangitis, cholecystitis, pylephlebitis, splenic flexure diverticulitis, emphysematous cholecystitis (Clostridia sp.), hepatic abscess (amebic, echinococcal, bacterial), right lower lobe CAP, brucellosis, leptospirosis, typhoid fever, viral hepatitis, dengue, malaria <u>Noninfectious</u>: burns, post-partum, ptosed right kidney, acute pancreatitis, Kawasaki's disease, cholesterol emboli syndrome, acalculous cholecystitis PAN, SLE, total parenteral nutrition, ceftriaxone (pseudocholelithiasis)
Right upper quadrant tympany	<u>Infectious</u>: peritonitis (2° to organ perforation) <u>Noninfectious</u>: post-abdominal surgery
Right upper quadrant mass	<u>Infectious</u>: bacterial abscess, echinococcal cysts, amebic abscess <u>Noninfectious</u>: ptosed right kidney, Reidel's lobe, hepatoma, malignancies, distended gallbladder (Couvoisier's sign)
Right lower quadrant tenderness	<u>Infectious</u>: shigella, typhoid fever, typhoidal EBV, typhoidal tularemia, parvovirus B19, TB, ameboma, typhlitis, actinomycetoma, pseudoappendicitis (scarlet fever), Legionnaires' disease, yersinia, campylobacter, measles (pre-eruptive), RMSF, PID, syphilis (luetic crisis), brucellosis <u>Noninfectious</u>: appendicitis, RE, ectopic pregnancy, diverticulitis, hyper IgE (Job's) syndrome, DM crisis, porphyria, pancreatitis, SLE
Left upper abdominal quadrant tenderness (splenic tenderness)	<u>Infectious</u>: SBE, brucellosis, typhoid fever, malaria, splenic abscess, EBV, CMV, HHV-6 <u>Noninfectious</u>: splenic infarct
Abdominal wall nodules	<u>Infectious</u>: leprosy <u>Noninfectious</u>: lipomas, panniculitis, metastatic disease, sarcoidosis
Periubilical purpura (thumbprint sign)	<u>Infectious</u>: strongyloides (hyperinfection syndrome) <u>Noninfectious</u>: retroperitoneal hemorrhage (Cullen's sign)

Table 9.12. Abdominal Abnormalities (cont'd)

Finding	Causes
Hepatomegaly	<u>Infectious</u>: viral hepatitis, bacterial liver abscess, amebic abscess, ehrlichiosis, babesiosis, brucellosis, leptospirosis (Weil's syndrome), arboviral hemorrhagic fevers, typhus, typhoid fever, malaria, Q fever, EBV, CMV, HIV
	<u>Noninfectious</u>: alcoholic cirrhosis, cholangiocarcinoma, carcinoma of pancreas, constrictive pericarditis, pericholangitis, veno-occlusive disease, autoimmune hepatitis, α-1antitrypsin deficiency, cystic fibrosis, fatty liver, hemangiomas, jejunoileal bypass, Reye's syndrome, multiple myeloma, hepatocellular carcinoma, metastatic carcinoma*, parenteral hyperalimentation (TPN)
Splenomegaly	<u>Infectious</u>: ***Mildly enlarged spleen:*** malaria, dengue fever, kala-azar, dengue, SBE, ehrlichiosis, babesiosis, typhoid fever, typhus, leptospirosis (Weil's syndrome), viral hepatitis, EBV, CMV, ARS, relapsing fever, syphilis, toxoplasmosis, psittacosis, brucellosis, Q fever, CSD, schistosomiasis, RE, trypanosomiasis, histoplasmosis, TB, splenic abscess, HIV, hydatid cysts, colorado tick fever; ***Moderately enlarged spleen:*** malaria, kala-azar; ***Massively enlarged spleen:*** malaria, kala-azar
	<u>Noninfectious</u>: ***Mildly enlarged spleen:*** SLE, sarcoidosis, Felty's syndrome, hemochromatosis, Wilson's disease, Budd-Chiari syndrome, megaloblastic anemia, iron deficiency anemia, systemic mastocytosis, angioblastic lymphadenopathy, splenic cysts, splenic trauma/hemorrhage, histiocytosis X (Langerhan's eosinophilic granuloma), hyperthyroidism, serum sickness, amyloidosis, berylliosis, Kawasaki's disease ***Moderately enlarged spleen:*** portal hypertension, hemolytic anemias, myeloproliferative disorders, CLL, Gaucher's disease, Niemann-Pick disease; ***Massively enlarged spleen:*** CML, hairy cell leukemia, lymphoma, myelofibrosis
Hepatosple-nomegaly	<u>Infectious</u>: malaria, typhoid fever, toxocara (visceral larval migrans), psittacosis, brucellosis, trypanosomiasis, kala-azar, 2° syphilis, EBV, CMV, acute HIV, schistosomiasis, toxoplasmosis, relapsing fever, RMSF, typhus, CSD, histoplasmosis, TB, dengue, babesiosis, ehrlichiosis, Q fever
	<u>Noninfectious</u>: hypernephroma, CGD, sarcoidosis
Ascites	<u>Infectious</u>: TB peritonitis, shistosomiasis, filariasis, spontaneous bacterial peritonitis, dengue, Whipple's disease
	<u>Noninfectious</u>: malignancies, Budd-Chiari syndrome, tricuspid regurgitation, constrictive pericarditis, inferior vena cava syndrome, FMF, Henoch-Schönlein purpura, SLE, portal hypertension, pancreatic/bile ascites, CHF, Meig's syndrome

* Usually from lung, colon, pancreas, kidney, breast, stomach, or esophagus.

Table 9.13. Lymph Node Abnormalities

Finding	Causes
Preauricular adenopathy	<u>Infectious</u>: ipsilateral conjunctivitis, tularemia, anterior scalp infections, rat bite fever (Spirillum minus)
	<u>Noninfectious</u>: lymphoma
Occipital adenopathy	<u>Infectious</u>: posterior scalp infections, CSD, rubella
	<u>Noninfectious</u>: lymphoma
Anterior cervical adenopathy	<u>Infectious</u>: group A streptococcal pharyngitis, viral pharyngitis, mouth/dental infections, TB (scrofula), HHV-6, toxoplasmosis, CSD, brucellosis
	<u>Noninfectious</u>: head/neck cancer, Kawasaki's disease, lymphoma, SLE, Kikuchi's disease, Rosai-Dorfman disease
Posterior cervical adenopathy *unilateral*	<u>Infectious</u>: toxoplasmosis, African trypanosomiasis (Winterbottom's sign)
	<u>Noninfectious</u>: posterior scalp infection, Kawasaki's disease, lymphoma, Kikuchi's disease, Rosai-Dorfman disease
bilateral	<u>Infectious</u>: EBV, HHV-6, CMV, Chagas' disease
	<u>Noninfectious</u>: lymphoma, Kawasaki's disease, Rosai-Dorfman disease, sarcoidos
Supraclavicular adenopathy	<u>Infectious</u>: TB, CSD
	<u>Noninfectious</u>: intra-abdominal malignancy (Virchow's sign), Kikuchi's disease
Infraclavicular adenopathy	<u>Infectious</u>: african trypanosomiasis, CSD
	<u>Noninfectious</u>: lymphoma
Epitrochlear adenopathy	<u>Infectious</u>: 2° syphilis, CSD, brucellosis
	<u>Noninfectious</u>: sarcoidosis, IVDA
Axillary adenopathy	<u>Infectious</u>: CFS (usually left), CSD, B. malayi, rat bite fever (Spirillum minus), brucellosis
	<u>Noninfectious</u>: lymphoma, CLL, sarcoidosis
Ulcer-node syndromes	<u>Infectious</u>: **Ulcer > node:** anthrax, rickettsial fevers (except RMSF), sporotrichosis, cutaneous leishmaniasis (new world). **Node = ulcer:** 1° syphilis, chancroid, tularemia (ulceroglandular), rat bite fever (Spirillum minus). **Node > ulcer:** syphilis, LGV, chancroid, HSV-2
	<u>Noninfectious</u>: lymphoma
Periumbilical nodule	<u>Infectious</u>: intra-abdominal infection
	<u>Noninfectious</u>: malignancy (Sister Joseph's sign)

Table 9.13. Lymph Node Abnormalities (cont'd)

Finding	Causes
Inguinal adenopathy *unilateral*	<u>Infectious</u>: lower extremity infections, bubonic plague, rat bite fever (Spirillum minus), filariasis, leprosy, tularemia, CSD
	<u>Noninfectious</u>: intra-abdominal malignancy, bilateral lower extremity infection, IVDA
bilateral	<u>Infectious</u>: any infection causing generalized adenopathy, B. malayi, HSV-2, syphilis, LGV
	<u>Noninfectious</u>: any disorder causing generalized adenopathy
Generalized lymphadenopathy	<u>Infectious</u>: TB, EBV, HHV-6, CMV, rubella, measles, toxoplasmosis, CSD, LGV, brucellosis, group A streptococci, 2° syphilis, HIV, kala-azar (African), trypanosomiasis, arboviral hemorrhagic fevers, Whipple's disease
	<u>Noninfectious</u>: SLE, RA, adult Still's disease, pseudolymphoma (Dilantin), Kikuchi's disease, Gaucher's disease, sarcoidosis, serum sickness, hyperthyroidism, ALL, CLL, Kimura's disease

Table 9.14. Genitourinary Abnormalities

Finding	Causes
Epididymoorchitis	<u>Infectious</u>: mumps, TB, blastomycosis, melioidosis, brucellosis, leptospirosis, EBV, W. bancrofti, Coxsackie B, S. hematobium, LCM, GC, C. trachomatis (young adults), P. aeruginosa (elderly adults), Colorado tick fever, rat bite fever (Spirillum minus), relapsing fever
	<u>Noninfectious</u>: lymphoma, SLE, PAN, sarcoidosis, FMF, trauma, torsion, malignancy
Scrotal enlargement	<u>Infectious</u>: mumps, W. bancrofti (not B. malayi), Fournier's gangrene
	<u>Noninfectious</u>: hydrocele, testicular torsion
Groin mass	<u>Infectious</u>: onchocerciasis (hanging groins), TB, W. bancrofti, shistosomiasis
	<u>Noninfectious</u>: lymphoma
Perirectal fistula	<u>Infectious</u>: peri-rectal abscess, actinomycosis, LGV
	<u>Noninfectious</u>: RE, malignancies
Perirectal ulcer	<u>Infectious</u>: HSV, amebiasis cutis, 1° syphilis
	<u>Noninfectious</u>: malignancy
Prostate enlargement/ tenderness	<u>Infectious</u>: prostatitis, prostatic abscess*
	<u>Noninfectious</u>: BPH

* Acute: aerobic GNB, VSE/VRE, Ureoplasma urealyticum, C. trachomatis, B. fragilis (post-transrectal biopsy). Chronic: TB, histoplasmosis, blastomycosis, aspergillus, candida, cryptococcus, meliodosis.

Table 9.15. Extremity Abnormalities

Finding	Causes
Digital gangrene	<u>Infectious</u>: SBE, S. aureus bacteremia/ABE (emboli), meningococcemia, RMSF, typhus
	<u>Noninfectious</u>: SLE, vasculitis, peripheral vascular disease
Splinter hemorrhages	<u>Infectious</u>: SBE, ABE, trichinosis
	<u>Noninfectious</u>: trauma, atrial myxoma, acute leukemia, RA, scurvy, mitral stenosis, severe anemia
Clubbing	<u>Infectious</u>: SBE, lung abscess, TB
	<u>Noninfectious</u>: ulcerative colitis (UC), Crohn's disease (RE), cirrhosis, cyanoic congenital heart disease, bronchogenic carcinoma, PBC, celiac disease, hyperthyroidism, hyperparathyroidism, bronchiectasis, hereditary
Dactylitis	<u>Infectious</u>: kala-azar, 2° syphilis, TB
	<u>Noninfectious</u>: sarcoidosis, sickle cell disease, gout, psoriatic arthritis
Tender fingertips	<u>Infectious</u>: SBE, typhoid fever
	<u>Noninfectious</u>: SLE, vasculitis, radial artery occlusion
Lymphangitis	<u>Infectious</u>: group A streptococci, B. malayi, onchocerciasis, melioidosis
	<u>Noninfectious</u>: IVDA
Nodular lymphangitis	<u>Infectious</u>: sporotrichosis, atypical TB, Erysipelothrix rhusiopathiae, kala-azar, coccidiomycosis, histoplasmosis, blastomycosis, nocardia, Pseudoallescheria boydii, cryptococcus, anthrax, group A streptococci, tularemia
	<u>Noninfectious</u>: ganglion cyst (wrist/hand only)
Painless purple palm/sole lesions	<u>Infectious</u>: ABE (Janeway lesions)
	<u>Noninfectious</u>: trauma
Carpal tunnel syndrome	<u>Infectious</u>: TB, leprosy
	<u>Noninfectious</u>: cirrhosis, RA, scleroderma, SLE, DM, hypothyroidism, sarcoidosis, multiple myeloma, amyloidosis
Verrucous hand/arm lesions	<u>Infectious</u>: TB, leprosy, syphilis, sporotrichosis, kala-azar, bartonellosis (verruga peruana)
	<u>Noninfectious</u>: squamous cell carcinoma, sarcoidosis
Edema of the dorsum of hand/foot	<u>Infectious</u>: RMSF, TSS, loiasis, dengue fever
	<u>Noninfectious</u>: trauma, PMR, Kawasaki's disease

Table 9.15. Extremity Abnormalities (cont'd)

Finding	Causes
Wrist swelling	<u>Infectious</u>: loiasis, septic arthritis, parvovirus B$_{19}$, rubella <u>Noninfectious</u>: RA
Arthritis (septic/reactive)	<u>Infectious</u>: septic arthritis, rat bite fever (Streptobacillus moniliformis), Lyme disease, LGV, brucellosis, GC, parvovirus B19, shigella, yersinia, salmonella, campylobacter, Clostridium difficle, mumps, rubella, chikungunya fever, dengue fever, HIV, HBV, Whipple's disease <u>Noninfectious</u>: FMF, RA, pseudogout, SLE, hyper IgD syndrome, lymphoma, Reiter's syndrome, post-streptococcal RF, Poncet's disease, JRA
Papular axillary lesions	<u>Infectious</u>: hydraadenitis suppurativa, 2° syphilis, yaws, blastomycosis <u>Noninfectious</u>: chronic contact dermatitis, acanthosis nigricans, Fox-Fordyce disease, seborrheic dermatitis
Tenosynovitis	<u>Infectious</u>: GC (acute), TB (chronic) <u>Noninfectious</u>: rheumatic diseases
Thigh tenderness (bilateral, anterior)	<u>Infectious</u>: bacteremia (Louria's sign), leptospirosis, ehrlichiosis, endocarditis, parvovirus B$_{19}$ <u>Noninfectious</u>: myositis, vasculitis, sickle cell crisis
Calf tenderness	<u>Infectious</u>: RMSF <u>Noninfectious</u>: myositis
Tender muscles	<u>Infectious</u>: trichinosis <u>Noninfectious</u>: myositis
Thrombophlebitis	<u>Infectious</u>: psittacosis, campylobacter <u>Noninfectious</u>: Behçet's disease, malignancy
Verrucous foot/leg lesions	<u>Infectious</u>: TB, cutaneous leishmaniasis, paracoccidomycosis, sporotrichosis, leprosy, 2° syphilis, mycetoma <u>Noninfectious</u>: lichen planus, squamous cell carcinoma
Foot/leg ulcers	<u>Infectious</u>: M. ulcerans (Buruli ulcer may be anywhere), yaws, cutaneous diphtheria, cutaneous leishmaniasis, TB, rat bite fever (Spirillum minus) <u>Noninfectious</u>: sickle cell (medial malleolar ulcers), DM (only sole of foot/between toes), peripheral vascular disease
Leg edema *unilateral*	<u>Infectious</u>: onchocerciasis, B. malayi (below knee) <u>Noninfectious</u>: malignancy, Milroy's disease

Table 9.15. Extremity Abnormalities (cont'd)

Finding	Causes
bilateral	<u>Infectious</u>: elephantiasis (chronic recurrent erysipelas), Chagas' disease
	<u>Noninfectious</u>: lymphatic obstruction (2° to abdominal/pelvic malignancy), congenital yellow nail syndrome
Nodular arm/leg lesions	<u>Infectious</u>: TB (Bazin's erythema induratum), filariasis, sporotrichosis, cutaneos leishmaniasis, atypical TB, leprosy, HIV
	<u>Noninfectious</u>: erythema nodosum, PAN, thrombophlebitis, panniculitis, nodular vasculitis, Wegener's granulomatosis, Sweet's syndrome, myiasis
Palpable purpura	<u>Infectious</u>: meningococcemia, RMSF
	<u>Noninfectious</u>: vasculitis, cryoglobulinemia, Gardner-Diamond syndrome, Sweet's syndrome
Eschar	<u>Infectious</u>: ecthyma gangrenosum, typhus, rickettsial spotted fevers (except RMSF, rickettsial pox), anthrax, cutaneous diphtheria, African tick bite fever (multiple eschars)
	<u>Noninfectious</u>: burns, drugs, recluse spider bite
Scleroderma (wood hard skin lesions)	<u>Infectious</u>: actinomycosis
	<u>Noninfectious</u>: malignancies, DM
Hyperpigmented shins	<u>Infectious</u>: onchocerciasis
	<u>Noninfectious</u>: DM (dermopathy)
Cutaneous cold abscesses	<u>Infectious</u>: TB, atypical TB
	<u>Noninfectious</u>: hyper IgE (Job's) syndrome, CGD
Purple nodules	<u>Infectious</u>: disseminated cryptococcus, aspergillus, candida, trypanosomiasis, Kaposi's sarcoma, HIV
	<u>Noninfectious</u>: leukemia, lymphoma, melanoma
Painful leg nodules	<u>Infectious</u>: Kaposi's sarcoma
	<u>Noninfectious</u>: erythema nodosum, superficial thrombophlebitis, PAN, panniculitis, osteogenic sarcoma
Migratory rashes	<u>Infectious</u>: hookworms, dracunculiasis, loiasis, gnathostomiasis, strongyloidiasis, sparganosis
	<u>Noninfectious</u>: myiasis
Rash of palms/soles	<u>Infectious</u>: syphilis, RMSF, EBV, scarlet fever, echo 9, smallpox, monkeypox, chickenpox, rat bite fever (Streptobacillus moniliformis), HFM, orf
	<u>Noninfectious</u>: drug rashes

Table 9.15. Extremity Abnormalities (cont'd)

Finding	Causes
Rash (purpuric) of hands/feet	<u>Infectious</u>: parvovirus B19, VZV, EBV, CMV, HHV-6, HHV-7, HBV, Coxsackie, rubella <u>Noninfectious</u>: trauma
Erythema nodosum	<u>Infectious</u>: TB, group A streptococci, EBV, LGV, psittacosis, coccidiomycosis, blastomycosis, histoplasmosis, CSD, yersinia, campylobacter <u>Noninfectious</u>: UC, RE, drugs, sarcoidosis, lymphoma, SLE
Erythema multiforme	<u>Infectious</u>: HSV, M. pneumoniae, Coxsackie B <u>Noninfectious</u>: drugs
Plantar hyperkeratoses	<u>Infectious</u>: 3° syphilis, yaws, pinta, HIV, tungiasis <u>Noninfectious</u>: Reiter's syndrome, arsenic
Desquamation of hands/feet	<u>Infectious</u>: erysipelas, scarlet fever, TSS, severe infections, yaws, leptospirosis, influenza, measles, arboviral hemorrhagic fevers, chickungunya fever <u>Noninfectious</u>: Kawasaki's disease, post-edematous states, radiation therapy, vitamin A excess, pellagra, drugs

Table 9.16. Neurological Abnormalities

Finding	Causes
Mental confusion/ encephalopathy (acute)	<u>Infectious</u>: legionnaire's disease, HSV, HHV-6, RMSF, listeria, mycoplasma meningoencephalitis, amebic meningitis, trichinosis, brain abscess, anthrax, brucellosis, SBE, ABE, HIV, viral encephalitis, CSD, Whipple's disease, Q fever, Colorado tick fever, chikungunya fever, meliodosis <u>Noninfectious</u>: Wernicke's encephalopathy, toxic/metabolic disorders, Behçet's syndrome, SLE, alcoholism, drugs, CHF, chronic renal failure, hepatic encephalopathy, brain tumor, CNS metastases, meningeal carcinomatosis, celiac disease
Nuchal rigidity	<u>Infectious</u>: meningitis (bacterial, fungal, TB, viral) <u>Noninfectious</u>: meningismus, cervical arthritis
General muscle rigidity	<u>Infectious</u>: trichinosis, tetanus, rabies, viral encephalitis, brucellosis <u>Noninfectious</u>: malignancies, malignant neuroleptic syndrome, strychnine poisoning, Parkinson's disease
Transient deafness	<u>Infectious</u>: RMSF, mediterranean spotted fever, murine typhus, S. pneumoniae meningitis, H. influenzae meningitis, mumps, measles, VZV (Ramsey-Hunt Syndrome), EEE, congenital syphilis, brucellosis, Lassa fever <u>Noninfectious</u>: trauma, Susac's syndrome

Table 9.16. Neurological Abnormalities (cont'd)

Finding	Causes
Cranial nerve (CN) abnormalities *unilateral*	Infectious: 6th CN palsy (TB meningitis, N. meningitidis), 7th CN palsy (see Bell's palsy), TBRF, 8th CN palsy (N. meningitidis)
	Noninfectious: 7th CN palsy (neurosarcoidosis, meningeal carcinomatosis), 2nd, 6th CN palsy (Wegener's granulomatosis)
bilateral	Infectious: 6th CN palsy (TB)
	Noninfectious: meningeal carcinomatosis
Optic nerve atrophy	Infectious: 3° syphilis, TB, toxoplasmosis, mumps, measles, rubella
	Noninfectious: sickle cell disease, severe anemia, polycythemia vera, drugs, sarcoidosis, TA, Behçet's syndrome, SLE, PAN, MS, glaucoma
Bell's Palsy	Infectious: Lyme disease, HSV-1, VZV (Ramsay-Hunt syndrome), HIV, St.LE, CSD, mumps, EBV infectious mononucleosis, Mycoplasma pneumoniae, syphilis, otitis media, bacterial meningitis, leprosy
	Noninfectious: sarcoidosis, multiple sclerosis, Guillain-Barre syndrome, B-cell lymphoma, Wegener's granulamatosis, pontine lesions (infarct, tumors, demyelinative lesions), tumor compressing the facial nerve, sphenoid ridge mengiomas, acoustic neuromas, neurofibromatosis (type 2), fibrous dysplasia, osteopetrosis, Paget's disease, scleroderma, Melkersson-Rosenthal syndrome, trauma, drugs (vincristine, HBV vaccination), idiopathic
Anisocoria	Infectious: TB, 3° syphilis, VZV, meningitis, encephalitis, botulism, diphtheria
	Noninfectious: DM, toxins, cavernous sinus thrombosis, glaucoma, brain tumor, intracranial aneurysm
Papilledema	Infectious: meningitis (bacterial, fungal, TB, viral, etc.)
	Noninfectious: pseudotumor cerebri, hypercarbia, brain tumor, DM, subarachnoid bleed, SLE, drugs, central retinal artery occlusion, cavernous sinus thrombosis, hypertensive encephalopathy
Mononeuritis multiplex	Infectious: leprosy, Lyme disease, HIV
	Noninfectious: DM, amyloidosis, sarcoidosis, lymphomatoid granulomatosis, vasculitis
Transverse myelitis	Infectious: HIV, HTLV-1, EBV, CMV, VZV, HSV, polio, rabies, TB, EV 71, epidural abscess, typhus, brucellosis, shistosomiasis, Lyme disease, syphilis, toxoplasmosis
	Noninfectious: MS, malignancies, vaccines, SLE, sarcoidosis
Guillain-Barré syndrome	Infectious: influenza, Campylobacter jejuni, CMV, EBV, VZV, M. pneumoniae, EV 71, brucellosis
	Noninfectious: influenza vaccine
Flaccid paralysis (acute)	Infectious: polio, WNE, CMV, VZV, rabies, botulism, JE, EV 71, Powassan encephalitis (PE), chikungunya fever, brucellosis
	Noninfectious: CVA, tick bite paralysis, hypocalcemic periodic paralysis

Table 9.16. Neurological Abnormalities (cont'd)

Finding	Causes
Hemiplegia/ hemiparesis	<u>Infectious</u>: SBE, subdural empyema, brain abscess, JE, brucellosis, post-VZV
	<u>Noninfectious</u>: TIA, CVA, malignancies, CNS vasculitis, migraine, GCA/TA, SLE, birth control pills, neurosarcoidosis

Table 9.17. WBC Abnormalities

Finding	Causes
Leukocytosis	<u>Infectious</u>: most acute infections
	<u>Noninfectious</u>: most acute noninfectious disease disorders, any major stress, steroids, drug fever, daptomycin
Leukopenia	<u>Infectious</u>: miliary TB, typhoid fever, malaria, tularemia, brucellosis, kala-azar, psittacosis, viral hepatitis, EBV, CMV, HHV-6, VZV, influenza, Colorado tick fever, histoplasmosis, relapsing fever, WNE, VEE, ehrlichiosis
	<u>Noninfectious</u>: drugs, pre/acute leukemias, Felty's syndrome, Gaucher's disease, splenomegaly, pernicious anemia, SLE, cyclic neutropenia, severe combined immunodeficiency disease (SCID), Chediak-Higashi syndrome, sarcoidosis
Relative lymphocytosis	<u>Infectious</u>: Whipple's disease, acute infection (convalescence), TB, brucellosis, pertussis, tularemia, 2° syphilis, histoplasmosis, EBV, CMV, HHV-6, mumps, viral hepatitis, rubella, VZV, kala-azar, toxoplasmosis, RMSF, chickungunya fever, typhoid fever (non-S. typhi > S. typhi)
	<u>Noninfectious</u>: ALL, CLL, lymphomas, carcinomas, multiple myeloma, RA, Hashimoto's thyroiditis, myxedema, adrenal insufficiency, thyrotoxicosis, vasculitis, Dilantin (DPH), p-aminosalicylic acid (PAS), serum sickness
Relative lymphopenia	<u>Infectious</u>: CMV, HHV-6, HHV-8, HIV, miliary TB, Legionella, typhoid fever (S. typhi > non-S. typhi), Q fever, brucellosis, SARS, malaria, babesiosis, influenza (human, avian, swine), RMSF, histoplasmosis, dengue fever, chickungunya fever, ehrlichiosis, parvovirus B19, HPS, WNE, viral hepatitis (early), Whipple's disease
	<u>Noninfectious</u>: cytoxic drugs, steroids, sarcoidosis, SLE, lymphoma, RA, radiation, Wiskott-Aldrich syndrome, severe combine immunodeficiency disease (SCID), common variable immune deficiency (CVID), Di George's syndrome, Nezelof's syndrome, intestinal lymphangiectasia, ataxia-telangiectasia, constrictive pericarditis, tricuspid regurgitation, Kawasaki's disease, idiopathic CD$_4$ cytopenia, acute/chronic renal failure, hemodialysis, myasthenia gravis, celiac disease, alcoholic cirrhosis, coronary bypass, Wegener's granulomatosis, CHF, acute pancreatitis, carcinomas (terminal)

Table 9.17. WBC Abnormalities (cont'd)

Finding	Causes
Monocytosis	<u>Infectious</u>: TB, SBE, RMSF, diphtheria, histoplasmosis, brucellosis, pertussis, kala-azar, 2° syphilis, malaria, typhoid fever, babesiosis, EBV, CMV, recovery from chronic infection
	<u>Noninfectious</u>: sarcoidosis, myeloproliferative disorders, lymphomas, Gaucher's disease, RE, UC, celiac disease, RA, SLE, PAN, TA, post-splenectomy
Atypical lymphocytes†	<u>Infectious</u>: EBV*, CMV*, HHV-6, viral hepatitis, mumps, measles, rubella, VZV, toxoplasmosis, brucellosis, HSV, arboviral hemorrhagic fevers, malaria, dengue, babesiosis, ehrlichiosis
	<u>Noninfectious</u>: drug fever
Immunoblasts	<u>Infectious</u>: HPS
	<u>Noninfectious</u>: lymphomas
Eosinophilia	<u>Infectious</u>: trichinosis, echinococcosis, fascioliasis, paragonimiasis, taenia, Strongyloides stercoralis, hookworm, filariasis, schistosomiasis, Toxocara canis/cati (VLM), histoplasmosis, coccidioidomycosis, filariasis ascariasis, gnathostomiasis, angiostrongyliasis, cysticercosis, Isospora belli, scarlet fever
	<u>Noninfectious</u>: dermatitis herpetiformis, pemphigus vulgaris, eczema, psoriasis, atopic dermatitis, mycosis fungoides, myeloproliferative disorders, polycythemia vera, CML, eosinophilic leukemia, eosinophilic gastritis, acute leukemias, sickle cell anemia, lymphomas, malignancies, Churg-Strauss granulomatosis, urticaria, hyper IgE syndrome (Job's syndrome), Sweet's syndrome, asthma, bronchopulmonary aspergillosis (BPA), angioneurotic edema, serum sickness, eosinophilia-myalgia syndrome, drug fever, dermatomyositis, PAN, allergic vasculitis, Loffler's syndrome, pulmonary infiltrates eosinophilia (PIE) syndrome, Loffler's endocarditis, Addison's disease, sarcoidosis, Wegener's granulomatosis, Goodpasture's syndrome, UC, RE, peritoneal dialysis, radiation, Wiskott-Aldrich syndrome, IgA deficiency, hay fever/allergic rhinitis, allergic vasculitis
Basophilia	<u>Infectious</u>: smallpox, chickenpox (VZV)
	<u>Noninfectious</u>: pre-leukemias, acute leukemias, lymphomas, myeloproliferative disorders, post-splenectomy
WBC inclusions	<u>Infectious</u>: ehrlichiosis (morula: HGA > HME)
	<u>Noninfectious</u>: staining artifacts

*   May have > 20% atypical lymphocytes.
†   Not seen with malignancies. Abnormal lymphocytes (morphologically monotonous) seen with leukemias.

Table 9.18. RBC Abnormalities

Finding	Causes
Schistocytes (microangiopathic hemolytic anemia)	Infectious: meningococcemia (DIC)
	Noninfectious: DIC (due to any cause), TTP, hemolytic uremic syndrome (HUS), "Waring Blender" syndrome (prosthetic valve), malignant hypertension
Spherocytes	Infectious: gas gangrene
	Noninfectious: autoimmune hemolytic anemias, hereditary spherocytosis, severe transfusion reactions, severe burns, cirrhosis
Target cells	Infectious: none
	Noninfectious: post-splenectomy, iron deficiency anemia, cirrhosis, hemoglobulin S or C, thalassemia
RBC inclusions	Infectious: malaria, babesiosis
	Noninfectious: Cabot's rings (severe hemolytic anemia, pernicious anemia), Heinz bodies (GGPD deficiency, drug induced, hereditary anemias), Pappenheimer bodies (thalassemia, sideroblastic anemias, lead poisoning), artifacts
Howell-Jolly bodies[†]	Infectious: fulimant pneumococcal sepsis
	Noninfectious: asplenia/hyposplenism*, congenital asplenia, splenectomy, splenic infarcts, splenic neoplasms, megaloblastic anemias, thalassemia, steroids
Erythrophago-cytosis	Infectious: HIV, HSV, EBV, CMV, adenovirus, parvovirus B19, malaria, babesiosis, toxoplasmosis, kala-azar, histoplasmosis, cryptococcosis, disseminated candidiasis, typhoid fever, syphilis, listeria, SBE, Q fever, leprosy, TB, brucellosis
	Noninfectious: histiocytosis X (eosinophilic granuloma, Langerhans cell histiocytosis), myeloproliferative disorders, SLE, sarcoidosis, RA, lymphomas, acute leukemias, multiple myeloma, Chediak-Higashi syndrome, Dilantin (DPH), familial hemophagocytic histiocytosis
Anemia (acute)	Infectious: Oroya fever, gas gangrene, malaria, babesiosis, CMV
	Noninfectious: ITP, "Waring blender" syndrome (prosthetic heart valve), hemorrhagic/necrotic pancreatitis, drug induced

* Chronic alcoholism, amyloidosis, chronic active hepatitis, IgA deficiency, intestinal lymphangectasia, myeloproliferative disorders, Waldenstrom's macroglobulinemia, NHL, celiac disease, RA, UC, thyroiditis, systemic mastocytosis, sickle cell disease, Fanconi's syndrome, Sezary's syndrome.

† Also "pitted/pocked" RBCs.

Table 9.19. Platelet Abnormalities

Finding	Causes
Thrombocytopenia	<u>Infectious</u>: acute/severe bacterial infections, measles, rubella, dengue, arboviral, hemorrhagic fevers, EBV, CMV, VZV, mumps, influenza (human, avian, swine), typhus, RMSF, WNE, ehrlichiosis, diphtheria, malaria, babesiosis, trypanosomiasis, TSS, histoplasmosis, kala-azar, HIV, miliary TB, relapsing fever, HPS, brucellosis
	<u>Noninfectious</u>: drugs, DIC, fat emboli syndrome, TTP, ITP, hemolytic uremic syndrome, pre/acute/leukemias, lymphomas, carcinomas, myeloproliferative disorders, multiple myeloma, Gaucher's disease, cirrhosis, hemodialysis
Thrombocytosis	<u>Infectious</u>: TB, chronic infections (e.g., osteomyelitis, abscess), SBE, Q fever, M. pneumoniae
	<u>Noninfectious</u>: Malignancies, myeloproliferative disorders, post-splenectomy, lymphomas, Wegener's granulomatosis, vasculitis, TA, PAN, Kawasaki's disease, fosfomycin, miconazole, ceftriaxone, oral cephalosporins, carbapenems, β-lactam/β-lactamase inhibitor combinations, iron therapy

Table 9.20. Pancytopenia

Finding	Causes
Pancytopenia	<u>Infectious</u>: miliary TB, brucellosis, histoplasmosis, ehrlichiosis, parvovirus B19, HBV, CMV, HIV
	<u>Noninfectious</u>: myeloproliferative disorders, drugs, malignancies, Chediak-Higashi syndrome, megaloblastic anemias, Gaucher's disease, hypersplenism, sarcoidosis, SLE, paroxysmal nocturnal hemoglobinuria (PNH), myelophistic anemias, leukemias, lymphoma

Table 9.21. Serum Test Abnormalities

Finding	Causes
Erythrocyte Sedimentation Rate (ESR) *highly elevated (≥100 mm/hr)*	<u>Infectious</u>: SBE, osteomyelitis, abscess, CAP (Leginnaire's disease, Q fever, S. pneumoniae), non-pulmonary TB
	<u>Noninfectious</u>: malignancies, rheumatic disorders, vasculitis, drug fever, PMR/GCA, uremia/chronic renal failure, cirrhosis, Kawasaki's disease, Sweet's syndrome, pulmonary emboli/infarction
subnormal (~0 mm/hr)	<u>Infectious</u>: trichinosis, CFS, ehrlichiosis
	<u>Noninfectious</u>: severe anemia, cachexia, massive hepatic necrosis, DIC, polycythemia vera, hypofibrinogenemia
SPEP (polyclonal gammopathy)	<u>Infectious</u>: HIV, malaria, kala-azar, LGV, rat bite fever, Toxocara canis/cati (VLM), Q fever (chronic)
	<u>Noninfectious</u>: SLE, PAN, cirrhosis, CAH, sarcoidosis, atrial myxoma, Takayasu's arteritis, Rosai-Dorfman disease

Table 9.21. Serum Test Abnormalities (cont'd)

Finding	Causes
SPEP (monoclonal gammopathy)	<u>Infectious</u>: CMV, kala-azar, typhoid fever
	<u>Noninfectious</u>: multiple myeloma, Waldenström's macroglobulinemia, MGUS
Elevated ferritin levels† *acute*	<u>Infectious</u>: legionnaires' disease, WNE, EBV, CMV, MSSA/MRSA ABE, malaria, dengue, DHF, arboviral hemorrhagic fevers, ehlichiosis (HGA)
	<u>Noninfectious</u>: Kawasaki's disease, Rosai-Dorfman disease, hemophagocytic syndrome
chronic	<u>Infectious</u>: HIV, TB, filariasis
	<u>Noninfectious</u>: Malignancies (preleukemias, lymphomas, multiple myeloma, hepatomas, liver/CNS metastases), myeloproliferative disorders, RA, adult Sill's disease, SLE, TA, Kawasaki's disease, chronic renal failure, hemodialysis, liver transplants, hemochromatosis, cirrhosis, α-1 antitrypsin deficiency, CAH, chronic HCV, cholestatic jaundice, sickle cell anemia, multiple blood transfusions, anemia of chronic disease
Elevated cold agglutinins	<u>Infectious</u>: Mycoplasma pneumoniae, EBV, CMV, mumps, measles, malaria, Coxsackie, Q fever, HIV, HCV, influenza, adenovirus, trypanosomiasis
	<u>Noninfectious</u>: lymphomas, CLL, CML, multiple myeloma, Waldenstrom's macroglubulinemia, cold agglutinin disease, paroxysmal nocturnal hemoglobinuria (PNH), SLE, sinus histiocytosis
Monospot (false +)	<u>Infectious</u>: CMV, HSV, HHV-6, malaria, babesiosis, toxoplasmosis, brucellosis, Mediterranean spotted fever (MSF), rubella, mumps, viral hepatitis, Lyme disease, HIV
	<u>Noninfectious</u>: SLE, sarcoidosis, AML, drugs, idiopathic
↑ Lactate dehydrogenase (LDH)	<u>Infectious</u>: malaria, babesiosis, ehrlichiosis, viridans streptococcal SBE, PCP, disseminated histoplasmosis, disseminated TB/MAI, disseminated toxoplasmosis, HPS, oroya fever, gas gangrene, viral myocarditis, rubella, measles, viral hepatitis, CAP/NP, dengue, dengue hemorrhagic fever, arboviral hemorrhagic fevers, trichinosis, SARS, adenovirus, CMV, amebic liver abscess, influenza (human, avian, swine)
	<u>Noninfectious</u>: hemolyzed blood, hemolytic anemia, malignancies, pernicious anemia, megaloblastic anemia, pulmonary emboli, acute MI, renal infarction, muscle injury, liver injury, DIC, SLE pneumonitis, adult Still's disease, "Waring blender" syndrome (prosthetic heart valve), hemorrhagic/necrotic pancreatitis
↑ Procalcitonin levels (PCT)	<u>Infectious</u>: bacterial pneumonias (CAP, NHAP, NP), bacteremias (gram − > gram +), TB, ABM, fungal pneumonias, viral hepatitis, toxoplasmosis, osteomyelitis, SBE*, malaria (P. falciparum)
	<u>Noninfectious</u>: renal insufficiency, alcoholic hepatitis, lung cancer (small cell), thyroid cancer, surgery, trauma, burns, cardiogenic shock, Goodpasture's syndrome shock, GVHD, peritoneal dialysis (PD), hypotension hemorrhagic/ necrotic pancreatitis, normal variant (elderly) BMT, febrile neutropenia, drug fever, immunosuppression/steroids, OKT$_3$ therapy

* Viridans streptococci.

† Not an acute phase reactant when highly/persistently ↑ > 2× normal.

Table 9.22. Liver Test Abnormalities

Finding	Causes
↑ Alkaline phosphatase (AP) *mildly elevated*	<u>Infectious</u>: legionnaires' disease, viral hepatitis, liver abscess, EBV, CMV, Q fever, syphilis (2° or tertiary), TSS, hepatic candidiasis, clonorchiasis, ehrlichiosis, diphtheria, malaria, trypanosomiasis, histoplasmosis, HIV, miliary TB, relapsing fever, HPS
	<u>Noninfectious</u>: drugs, DIC, fat emboli syndrome, TTP, ITP, hemolytic uremic syndrome, pre/acute/leukemias, lymphomas, carcinomas, myeloproliferative disorders, multiple myeloma, Gaucher's disease, cirrhosis, post-hepatic obstruction, alcoholic hepatitis, pregnancy, bone growth (children), osteomalacia, rickets, hyperthyroidism, UC, drug fever, hepatoma, liver metastases, lymphoma, normal variant (elderly)
moderately/highly elevated	<u>Infectious</u>: liver abscess
	<u>Noninfectious</u>: PBC, post-hepatic obstruction, post-necrotic cirrhosis, Paget's disease, osteogenic sarcoma, hepatoma, bone fractures
↑ Serum transaminases (SGOT/SGPT) *mildly elevated*	<u>Infectious</u>: legionella disease, psittacosis, Q fever, relapsing fever, brucellosis, TSS, RMSF, ehrlichiosis, liver abscess, syphilis (2° or tertiary), shigellosis, clonorchiasis, EBV, CMV, HSV-1, VZV (disseminated), HHV-6, anicteric viral hepatitis, gonococcemia, malaria, gram-negative bacteremia, adenovirus, dengue
	<u>Noninfectious</u>: drug fever, cirrhosis, CHF, infarction (myocardial, cerebral, pulmonary), pancreatitis, intrahepatic cholestasis, sickle cell disease, amyloidosis, delirium tremens, intravascular hemolysis, UC, eosinophilia-myalgia syndrome, Kawasaki's disease
highly elevated	<u>Infectious</u>: viral hepatitis, HSV hepatitis, yellow fever, arboviral hemorrhagic fevers, rhabdomyolysis (see p. 503)
	<u>Noninfectious</u>: shock liver, rhabdomyolysis (SGOT > SGPT), exercise, drugs (statins INH, RIF)
↑ Total bilirubin	<u>Infectious</u>: legionnaires' disease, gonococcemia, liver abscess, viral hepatitis, EBV, CMV, pneumococcal bacteremia, malaria
	<u>Noninfectious</u>: hemolysis, Gilbert's syndrome, cirrhosis, alcoholic hepatitis, carcinoma (pancreatic, biliary), choledocholithiasis, amyloidosis, sickle cell disease, Rotor's syndrome, α-1 antitrypsin deficiency, hepatic vein thrombosis, autoimmune (lupoid) hepatitis, hemachromatosis
↑ GGT (GGTP)	<u>Infectious</u>: acute viral hepatitis, EBV
	<u>Noninfectious</u>: alcoholism, cirrhosis, alcoholic hepatitis, PBC, fatty liver, CAH, hepatoma, liver metastases, pancreatitis (acute), myocardial infarction (acute), breast cancer, lung cancer, prostate cancer, melanoma, hypernephroma, obstructive jaundice, cholestasis, CAH

Table 9.23. Rheumatic Test Abnormalities

Finding	Causes
↑ Rheumatoid factors (RF)	Infectious: SBE, TB, syphilis, kala-azar, EBV, typhoid fever Noninfectious: cirrhosis, CAH, ITP, sarcoidosis, silicosis, asbestosis, RA, asthma, scleroderma, Behçet's disease, cryoglobulinemia, MCTD, SLE. Sjögren's, dermatomyositis, PBC, malignancy, normal variant (elderly)
↑ Anti-nuclear antibody titers (ANA)	Infectious: HIV, EBV, CMV, TB, SBE, leprosy, kala-azar, malaria Noninfectious: SLE, scleroderma, MCTD, CREST syndrome, RA, autoimmune (lupoid) hepatitis, CAH, dermatomyositis, autoimmune thyroiditis, ITP, PBC, multiple sclerosis, sarcoidosis, myasthenia gravis, ESRD on HD, normal variant (elderly)
↑ Double stranded DNA (DS-DNA)	Infectious: CMV, EBV Noninfectious: SLE, RA, CAH, PBC
↑ Angiotensin-converting enzyme levels (ACE)	Infectious: TB, leprosy, coccidiomycosis, viral hepatitis Noninfectious: sarcoidosis, allergic alveolitis, hyperparathyroidism, PBC, Gaucher's disease, DM, ESRD, hyperthyroidism, amyloidosis, multiple myeloma, lymphoma, cirrhosis, psoriasis, silicosis, asbestosis, berylliosis
↑ c-ANCA	Infectious: viridans streptococcal SBE, S. bovis SBE, chromomycosis, invasive aspergillosis, invasive amebiasis, Legionnaires' disease, leptospirosis, HIV Noninfectious: crescentic GMN, microscopic polyangitis (MPA), Sweet's syndrome, PAN, UC, RE, SLE, Churg-Strauss granulomatosis, Wegener's granulomatosis, HSP, TA, Kawasaki's disease, sarcoidosis
↑ Anti-smooth muscle antibodies (ASM)	Infectious: Q fever, HCV (chronic), EBV, typhoid fever Noninfectious: autoimmune (lupoid) hepatitis, Wilson's disease, PBC, normal variant (elderly)

Table 9.24. Urinary Abnormalities

Finding	Causes
Pyuria*§	Infectious: TB, leptospirosis, brucellosis, TSS, diphtheria, candida, GC, trichomonas, cystitis, pyelonephritis, prostatitis, acute urethral syndrome, partially treated UTI, medullary abscess, chlamydia/mycoplasma NGU, balanitis, acute appendicitis, St.LE. Noninfectious: interstitial nephritis, urethral irritation/inflammation, strenuous exercise, SLE, calculi, bladder tumors, chronic interstitial cystitis, RE, diverticulitis, Kawasaki's disease, sarcoidosis

* Gross pus suggests ruptured renal abscess.
§ WBC casts suggest SLE, nephritis, or acute pyelonephritis.

Table 9.24. Urinary Abnormalities (cont'd)

Finding	Causes
Hematuria *gross*	<u>Infectious</u>: ABE (renal septic emboli), malaria (P. falciparum), yellow fever, adenoviral cystitis (type 11), BKV (transplants)
	<u>Noninfectious</u>: renal malignancy, bladder malignancy, BPH, papillary necrosis, trauma
microscopic	<u>Infectious</u>: SBE, renal TB, schistosomiasis (S. hematobium), S. saprophyticus, HPS, legionnaire's disease, Q fever, BKV (transplants), EBV
	<u>Noninfectious</u>: trauma, prostatitis, malignancy, malignant hypertension, PAN, rug reactions, calculi, urethral stricture, renal vein thrombosis, hydronephrosis, polycystic kidney disease, malakoplakia, strenuous exercise, renal infarction, sarcoidosis
Proteinuria	<u>Infectious</u>: TB, HBV, syphilis, malaria (black water fever), brucellosis, SBE, chronic pyelonephritis, leprosy, shistosomiasis, any acute infection
	<u>Noninfectious</u>: strenuous exercise, post-streptococcal GMN, malignant hypertension, ATN, amyloidosis, sickle cell disease, polycystic kidneys, scleroderma, sarcoidosis, PAN, Wegener's granulomatosis, Goodpasture's syndrome, multiple myeloma, lymphomas, renal neoplasm, renal trauma
Urinary pH *alkaline*	<u>Infectious</u>: Corynebacterium urealyticum, klebsiella (rare), proteus, providencia, S. saprophyticus, Ureaplasma urealyticum
	<u>Noninfectious</u>: systemic alkalosis, postprandial "alkaline tide," alkalinization therapy, old urine, vegetarian diet
acidic	<u>Infectious</u>: TB
	<u>Noninfectious</u>: acidification therapy, systemic acidosis, ketosis
↓ Specific gravity (1.023 – 1.030)	<u>Infectious</u>: pyelonephritis[†]
	<u>Noninfectious</u>: diabetes insipidus, tubo-interstitial renal diseases, sickle cell disease
Nitrite positive	<u>Infectious</u>: most uropathogens**
	<u>Noninfectious</u>: none
Leukocyte esterase[†‡]	<u>Infectious</u>: acute cystitis, acute pyelonephritis
	<u>Noninfectious</u>: inflammation anywhere in the upper/lower GU tract

†   Cystitis is associated with a normal specific gravity. The transient decrease in specific gravity of pyelonephritis corrects to normal following effective treatment.
**   Negative urinary nitrite occurs with group B streptococci, group D enterococci, (VSE/VRE) S. saprophyticus, S. aureus, Acinetobacter sp., Gardnerella sp., Corynebacterium urealyticum, Burkholderia sp., Pseudomonas sp., Candida sp.
‡   ≥ 5 WBCs = positive.

Table 9.24. Urinary Abnormalities (cont'd)

Finding	Causes
Eosinophiluria‡	<u>Infectious</u>: Shistosoma hematobium
	<u>Noninfectious</u>: cholesterol emboli syndrome, HSP, drug induced interstital nephritis, renal allograft rejection
Myoglobinuria (2° to rhabdomyolysis)	<u>Infectious</u>: legionnaires' disease, gas gangrene, leptospirosis, Vibrio vulnificus, listeria, S. aureus, group A streptococci, group B streptococci, S. pneumoniae, tularemia, typhoid fever, echovirus, Coxsackie, influenza, adenovirus, EBV, CMV, HSV, VZV, HIV
	<u>Noninfectious</u>: crush injury, excessive exercise, MI, seizures, malignant hyperthermia, dermatomyositis, burns, polymyositis, SLE, diabetic ketoacidosis, McArdle's syndrome, drugs (statins alcohol, cocaine, PCP, neuroleptics, amphetamines, ethylene glycol)
Chyluria	<u>Infectious</u>: W. bancrofti
	<u>Noninfectious</u>: abdominal or chest lymphatic obstruction

‡   ≥ 5 WBCs=positive.

Table 9.25. Pleural Fluid Abnormalities

Pleural Fluid	Causes
Bloody*	<u>Infectious</u>: tularemia, anthrax
	<u>Noninfectious</u>: mesothelioma, pulmonary infarct, carcinoma (pulmonary/metastatic), lymphoma, trauma
Yellow/whitish	<u>Infectious</u>: empyema, hydatid cyst
	<u>Noninfectious</u>: chylous effusion
Brownish	<u>Infectious</u>: empyema, amebic cyst
	<u>Noninfectious</u>: parapneumonic effusion
Yellow-green	<u>Infectious</u>: None
	<u>Noninfectious</u>: rheumatoid lung
pH < 7.2	<u>Infectious</u>: empyema, TB
	<u>Noninfectious</u>: bronchogenic carcinoma (rarely), rheumatoid lung, SLE

*   TB effusions are not grossly bloody, but often contain RBCs.

Table 9.25. Pleural Fluid Abnormalities (cont'd)

Pleural Fluid	Causes
↓ Glucose	<u>Infectious</u>: TB, bacterial, cryptococcosis, coccidiomycosis, mycoplasma, empyema
	<u>Noninfectious</u>: carcinoma, rheumatoid lung, lymphoma, esophageal rupture, parapneumonic effusion
↑ Protein	<u>Infectious</u>: TB
	<u>Noninfectious</u>: carcinoma, lymphoma, rheumatoid lung
↑ Amylase	<u>Infectious</u>: None
	<u>Noninfectious</u>: pancreatitis/pseudocyst, adenocarcinoma, esophageal rupture
Extracellular debris	<u>Infectious</u>: abscesses, anaerobic empyema
	<u>Noninfectious</u>: rheumatoid lung
PMNs	<u>Infectious</u>: bacteria, cryptococcosis, coccidiomycosis, empyema, TB (early)
	<u>Noninfectious</u>: pancreatitis, subdiaphragmatic abscess (sympathetic effusion), CHF, idiopathic
Lymphocytes	<u>Infectious</u>: TB
	<u>Noninfectious</u>: carcinoma, lymphoma, rheumatoid lung, SLE

Pleural Effusion Profiles in Various Diseases

Pleural Fluid	Infectious		Noninfectious		Rheumatoid Effusion	SLE
	TB	Empyema	Malignancy	Mesothelioma		
WBCs (per mm³)	< 5000; lymphocyte predominance	> 10,000; PMN predominance	< 10,000; lymphocyte predominance	↑ PMNs/ lymphocytes	> 10,000; lymphocyte predominance	> 10,000; lymphocyte predominance
Eosinophils	−	−	+	±	−	−
RBCs (per mm³)	< 10,000	−	> 100,000	−	−	−
pH	< 7.2	< 7.2	> 7.2	> 7.2	< 7.2	< 7.2
Glucose	↓↓	Normal/↓	↓	Normal/↓	↓↓↓	Normal

+ present; − absent; ± present or absent; ↑ increased; ↓ decreased.

Table 9.25. Pleural Fluid Abnormalities (cont'd)

Pleural Fluid	Infectious		Noninfectious		Rheumatoid Effusion	SLE
	TB	Empyema	Malignancy	Mesothelioma		
Rheumatoid factor (RF)	↑	–	↑	–	↑	±
Other	< 1% meso-thelial cells; pleural biopsy/culture + for AFB	Purulent; foul odor (2° to anaerobic organisms)	↑ LDH_4/LDH_5; ↓ α-2 globulins; ↑ amylase; cytology + for malignant cells	Very viscous	Turbid greenish yellow; ↓ C_3; ↑↑ protein; epithelioid cells; degen-erated PMNs/amorphous cellular debris	↑ pleural fluid ANA is diagnostic; ↓ pleural fluid C_3

+ present; – absent; ± present or absent; ↑ increased; ↓ decreased.

Table 9.26. CSF Abnormalities

Finding	Causes
RBCs in CSF	<u>Infectious</u>: listeria, leptospirosis[†], TB, amebic meningoencephalitis, HSV, anthrax meningitis <u>Noninfectious</u>: traumatic tap, CNS bleed/tumor
Purulent CSF with negative gram Stain	<u>Infectious</u>: Neisseria meningitidis, Streptococcus pneumoniae <u>Noninfectious</u>: none
CSF with negative gram stain and predominantly PMNs/decreased glucose	<u>Infectious</u>: PTBM, listeria, HSV, TB (early), parameningeal infection, emboli secondary to SBE, amebic meningoencephalitis, CNS syphilis (early) <u>Noninfectious</u>: sarcoidosis, posterior-fossa syndrome/intracranial hemorrhage
CSF with negative gram stain and predominantly *lymphocytes/ normal glucose*	<u>Infectious</u>: PTBM, viral meningitis, Lyme disease, HIV, leptospirosis[†], RMSF, parameningeal infection, TB, fungi, parasitic meningitis <u>Noninfectious</u>: sarcoidosis, meningeal carcinomatosis

† The only disorder with the CSF bilirubin > serum bilirubin.

Table 9.25. CSF Abnormalities (cont'd)

Finding	Causes
lymphocytes/ decreased glucose	<u>Infectious</u>: PTBM, CNS TB, CNS fungi, LCM, mumps, enteroviral meningitis, listeria, leptospirosis†, syphilis
	<u>Noninfectious</u>: neurosarcoidosis, meningeal carcinomatosis
↑ CSF lactic acid levels	<u>Infectious</u>: **< 4 nm/L**, Not acute bacterial meningitis (ABM); **< 4–6 nm/L**, TB, HSV, partially treated bacterial meningitis (PTBM), parameningeal infections; **> 6 nm/L**, acute bacterial meningitis (ABM), cerebral malaria (severe)
	<u>Noninfectious</u>: **< 6 nm/L**, neurosarcoidosis, CNS SLE, cerebral anoxia, hepatic encephalopathy; meningeal carcinomatosis; CNS lymphomas, RBCs
Highly ↑ CSF Protein	<u>Infectious</u>: brain abscess, CNS TB (with subarachnoid block), viral meningitis, viral encephalitis
	<u>Noninfectious</u>: brain tumor, MS, demyelinating CNS diseases
↑ CSF adenosine deaminase (ADA) levels	<u>Infectious</u>: CNS TB, listeria, ABM, neurobrucellosis
	<u>Noninfectious</u>: SAH, CNS malignancy
CSF plasma cells	<u>Infectious</u>: CNS TB, WNE, VZV, HIV, neuroborreliosis, neurosyphilis
	<u>Noninfectious</u>: CNS lymphoma, MS, CNS myeloma, ADEM
CSF eosinophils	<u>Infectious</u>: coccidioidomycosis, neurocysticercosis, gnathostomiasis, angiostrongyliasis, baylisascariasis, shistosomiasis, paragonamiasis, Toxocariasis canis/cati (VLM)
	<u>Noninfectious</u>: CNS lymphomas, CNS leukemias, V-A/VP shunts, myelography (contrast material), CNS vasculitis, drugs (NSAIDs, TMP–SMX), intrathecal drugs

† Leptospirosis is the only disorder with the CSF bilirubin > serum bilirubin.

Chapter 10

Antibiotic Pearls & Pitfalls

Burke A. Cunha, MD

PENICILLIN

- *Penicillin is expensive* because it is made by a single manufacturer.
- There are very few uses for parenteral penicillin therapy today.
- PRSP has been associated with TMP–SMX and macrolides, *not penicillin*.

AMPICILLIN

- Unless treating serious systemic infections due to E. faecalis (VSE), *avoid using ampicillin. Ampicillin use results in increased E. coli resistance.*
- Remember ampicillin is the preferred drug to treat serious systemic infections caused by VSE but is *ineffective against nearly all E. faecium (VRE).*
- Because susceptibility is in part "concentration dependent," *do not assume that susceptibilities of ampicillin or amoxicillin are the same.* On a same-dose basis, amoxicillin achieves twice the concentrations of ampicillin in body fluids (e.g., middle ear fluid, sinus fluid, bronchial fluid, urine).
- Remember that *unlike ampicillin, amoxicillin is infrequently associated with oral thrush or irritative diarrhea.*
- *Amoxicillin 1 gm (PO) q8h* can be used in ampicillin IV-to-PO switch programs since this dose *provides levels comparable to parenteral (IM) ampicillin.*

AMOXICILLIN/CLAVULANIC ACID

- Clavulanic acid is a beta-lactamase inhibitor which, when added to amoxicillin, restores its activity against beta-lactamase—producing strains of H. influenzae.
- The *newer preparations of amoxicillin/clavulanic acid result in less gastrointestinal symptoms and diarrhea* compared to older preparations with more clavulanate.
- *Ineffective against PRSP due to alterations in PBPs which are not β-lactamase mediated.*

ORAL ANTI-STAPHYLOCOCCAL PENICILLINS

* *Do not rely on oral anti-staphylococcal penicillins* such as dicloxacillin for methicillin-sensitive S. aureus (MSSA) infections since they *are erratically/poorly absorbed and not consistently effective.* When treating MSSA infections orally, a first generation cephalosporin (e.g., cephalexin) is preferable.
* *Dicloxacillin is poorly tolerated due to its metallic taste and belching.*

ORAL ANTI-PSEUDOMONAL PENICILLINS

* *Avoid using indanyl carbenicillin for P. aeruginosa UTI's due to the rapid development of resistance with P. aeruginosa.* Use other oral anti-P. aeruginosa agents for P. aeruginosa lower UTI's, e.g., doxycycline, levofloxacin, or fosfomycin.

PARENTERAL FIRST-GENERATION CEPHALOSPORINS

* *Cefazolin has limited activity against H. influenzae.*
* Cefazolin remains *preferred therapy for skin infections due to group A streptococci or MSSA.*
* For treatment of biliary tract infections, cefazolin is active against E. coli and Klebsiella pneumoniae but is *not active against E. faecalis* (VSE).
* *Cefazolin remains useful prophylaxis for cardiothoracic procedures in hospitals with low prevalence of MRSA.*

ORAL FIRST-GENERATION CEPHALOSPORINS

* *Cephalexin suboptimal for respiratory tract infections* i.e., H. influenzae a likely pathogen (otitis media, sinusitis, AECB, community-acquired pneumonia) *since 1st GCs have limited H. influenzae activity.*
* For IV-to-PO switch programs and *cephalexin 1gm (PO) q6h approximates the serum concentrations of parenteral (IM) cefazolin.*
* Oral 3rd GCs do not have the same degree of anti-S. aureus MSSA activity as cephalexin.

PARENTERAL SECOND-GENERATION CEPHALOSPORINS

- Cefoxitin and cefotetan are useful for intra-abdominal infections.
- *Cefuroxime* offers no advantage for bacterial URIs over doxycycline, respiratory quinolones, or 3rd GCs and *does not prevent CNS "seeding" by S. pneumoniae or H. influenzae bacteremia secondary to CAP.*

ORAL SECOND-GENERATION CEPHALOSPORINS

- *Oral second generation cephalosporins* include cefaclor, cefprozil, and cefuroxime are *used primarily to treat URIs.*
- *Cefaclor has limited ability to penetrate into respiratory secretions* limiting its efficacy in URIs.
- Among the oral second generation cephalosporins, *cefprozil has the greatest degree of penetration into respiratory secretions.*

PARENTERAL THIRD-GENERATION CEPHALOSPORINS

- *Except for cefoperazone, 1st, 2nd, 3rd generation cephalosporins have no anti-E. faecalis (VSE) activity.*
- *Except for ceftriaxone,* third generation cephalosporins predispose to C. difficile diarrhea. *Ceftriaxone is associated with non-C. difficile diarrhea* related to changes in colonic flora.
- Be aware that *ceftriaxone is associated with pseudo-biliary lithiasis.* Patients developing right upper quadrant pain on ceftriaxone should be suspected as having drug-induced pseudo/actual cholelithiasis.
- *For CNS infections give third generation cephalosporins in "meningeal doses."*
- *The only third-generation cephalosporin associated with resistance is ceftazidime e.g., P. aeruginosa.*
- *Ceftazidime predisposes to MDR P. aeruginosa, and increases MRSA prevalence.*
- *Ceftazidime associated with ESBL K. pneumoniae, E. coli, or Enterobacter agglomerans.*
- *Ceftazidime little anti-MSSA activity.*
- 3rd GCs *without anti-B. fragilis activity are ceftazidime and ceftriaxone.*
- 3rd GCs *without significant anti-P. aeruginosa activity are cefotaxime, ceftizoxime, and ceftriaxone.*

ORAL THIRD-GENERATION CEPHALOSPORINS

- Oral third generation cephalosporins, i.e., cefdinir, cefditoren, cefixime, cefpodoxime and ceftibuten are often used for their aerobic anti-GNB activity.
- Oral 3rd GCs do not have the same degree of activity against aerobic GNBs as their parenteral counterparts.
- *Oral third generation cephalosporins have less anti-MSSA activity than their parenteral counterparts. The only 3rd GC with good anti-MSSA activity is cefpodoxime.*

PARENTERAL FOURTH-GENERATION CEPHALOSPORIN

- Cefipime (4th GC) is *an anti-Pseudomonal cephalosporin that is often active against* ceftazidime resistant P. aeruginosa strains.

PARENTERAL ANTI-MRSA CEPHALOSPORIN (ABSSSI ONLY)

- Ceftaroline fosamil is the *only cephalosporin active in vivo against both MSSA and MRSA.*

MONOBACTAMS

- *Aztreonam has no gram-positive activity.*
- Although structurally similar to the beta-lactams, *aztreonam is safe in penicillin-allergic patients.*

CARBAPENEMS

- *Avoid imipenem in patients with seizures/CNS disorders* since imipenem may cause seizures. Also, *renal insufficiency increases imipenem's seizure potential.*
- *All carbapenems have anti-pseudomonal activity except for ertapenem.*
- *Ertapenem has no anti-enterococcal activity*, important in biliary/UTIs.
- Avoid IV bolus injections/rapid infusions of doripenem, ertapenem or imipenem. *Only meropenem may be administered as an IV bolus*, important in septic shock.
- *Imipenem susceptibility breakpoints may overestimate imipenem's activity against Acinetobacter baumanni.*

BETA-LACTAMASE INHIBITOR COMBINATIONS

- All beta-lactamase inhibitor combinations are active against Bacteroides fragilis.
- *Piperacillin/tazobactam and sulbactam/ampicillin have the highest degree of anti-E. faecalis (VSE) activity among these antibiotics.*
- *Some strains of MDR Acinetobacter baumannii are susceptible only to sulbactam/ ampicillin.*
- *Preferred for animal or human bites* in penicillin-tolerant patients.
- *Tazobactam does not enhance the anti-pseudomonal activity of piperacillin.*
- *Beta-lactamase inhibitors are not effective against PRSP strains* (resistance mediated by alterations in PBPs, not beta-lactamases).

TETRACYCLINES

- There is virtually no clinical use for conventional tetracycline. *Doxycycline and minocycline, compared to tetracycline have a high degree of activity against key pathogens, e.g., S. pneumoniae, MSSA/MRSA, improved pharmacokinetics, and a "low resistance pontential."*
- *While MRSA may be susceptible to doxycycline in vitro, in vivo it frequently fails or the clinical response is delayed/incomplete. Clinically, minocycline IV/PO for treatment of MSSA/MRSA infections is more effective than doxycycline.*
- *Doxycycline has good CSF preparation and is often used for oral therapy of neuroborreliosis. Minocycline has even better CSF penetration and may be preferable to doxycycline for neuroborreliosis.*
- *At urinary concentrations, doxycycline is effective against P. aeruginosa CAB/lower UTIs, i.e., high urine levels > 300 mcg/ml. However, in vitro testing will report P. aeruginosa resistant to doxycycline.*
- For nearly all non-viral zoonotic infections, *doxycycline is effective except for babesiosis. Although streptomycin/gentamicin preferred for tularemia, doxycycline is also effective.*
- *Oral minocycline is useful to treat serious systemic infections due to MSSA/MRSA i.e., ABE, osteomyelitis, meningitis, etc.*
- *Minocycline is the most cost effective oral anti-MRSA antibiotic.*

CHLORAMPHENICOL

- Chloramphenicol is *one of few drugs that can be given orally to treat acute bacterial meningitis* due to susceptible organisms.
- *Chloramphenicol is the only antibiotic that when given orally results in higher serum concentrations than when given at the same dose intravenously.*
- *Avoid chloramphenicol for the treatment of hepatobiliary infections and UTIs since chloramphenicol is excreted into the bile as an inactivate metabolite, and urinary levels are low.*
- Remember, *aplastic anemia is a rare idiosyncratic side effect associated with oral/topical therapy but not IV therapy.*
- Chloramphenicol-induced aplastic anemia is an idiosyncratic reaction and *serial CBCs are unhelpful in predicting/avoiding aplastic anemia.*
- Serial *CBCs may be obtained to monitor dose-related side effects (anemia)* not idiosyncratic side effects (aplastic anemia).
- *Prolonged chloramphenicol therapy may cause sequential, dose-related suppression of bone marrow elements. Suppressed blood elements return in reverse sequence when chloramphenicol is discontinued.*
- *Chloramphenicol dose-related bone marrow suppression/toxicity is reversible and is not a harbinger of aplastic anemia.*
- *Vacuolization on bone marrow biopsy* specimens in patients receiving chloramphenicol *is a manifestation of chloramphenicol effect, not aplastic anemia.*
- *Chloramphenicol is effective for E. faecium (VRE) systemic infections.*
- Avoid chloramphenicol in neonates (Gray Baby Syndrome) due to immature hepatic enzymes unable to metabolize chloramphenicol.

CLINDAMYCIN

- *Clindamycin misses approximately 15% of coagulase-negative S. epidermidis (CoNS),* the most common pathogen in foreign body/implant-related infections.
- *Clindamycin is one of the few antibiotics able to penetrate/dissolve staphylococcal biofilms.* Clindamycin may be useful adjunctively in treating foreign body associated infections when the prosthetic device cannot be removed.

- The *incidence of C. difficile diarrhea is greater with PO > IV clindamycin.*
- Clindamycin is active against most gram-positive cocci but not group D enterococci.
- Unless resistant, *clindamycin is effective against CA-MRSA but not HA-MRSA/ CO-MRSA* (see Chapter 1, Table 1.11).
- With CA-MRSA, *inducible clindamycin resistance (MLS(B)) should be suspected if erythromycin is resistant and clindamycin is susceptible.* The "D test" will confirm clindamycin resistance.

AMINOGLYCOSIDES

- Among aminoglycosides, *gentamicin has the most anti-gram-positive coccal activity*.
- *Amikacin has the highest degree of P. aeruginosa activity.*
- Gentamicin and tobramycin have 6 loci that may be inactivated by acetylating, acetylating and phosphorylating enzymes. Amikacin has only 1 locus that may be attacked by these enzymes, making P. aeruginosa resistance less likely.
- *Avoid aminoglycoside monotherapy in the treatment of nosocomial pneumonia since aminoglycoside activity is diminished in the presence of tissue hypoxia, WBC debris and local acidosis, which are prominent in nosocomial pneumonia.*
- *Avoid administering aminoglycosides via nebulizer since aerosolized aminoglycosides may predispose to resistance.*
- *Avoid administering aminoglycosides in split-daily doses.* A single daily dose is optimal since aminoglycosides obey "concentration-dependent" killing kinetics.
- When aminoglycosides are given to *patients with renal insufficiency, begin with the usual initial dose, then decrease the maintenance dose in proportion to the degree of renal dysfunction* based on the creatinine clearance.
- *If aminoglycosides are being used for synergy, use half the therapeutic dose (synergy dose).*
- *Aminoglycosides given on a once-daily basis optimize aminoglycoside antibacterial killing while minimizing nephrotoxic potential and eliminate the need for aminoglycoside levels.*
- *Aminoglycoside ototoxicity may occur with extremely high/prolonged peak levels.* Episodic elevated peak levels are not associated with ototoxicity.
- When aminoglycosides are given on a once-daily basis, renal tubular cells have sufficient time between dosing intervals to decrease intracellular levels and thus avoid nephrotoxicity.

- *Do not assess aminoglycoside nephrotoxicity based on the serum creatinine.* Aminoglycoside nephrotoxicity is best *assessed by indicators of renal tubular damage such as urinary renal cast counts.*

- *Limiting aminoglycoside therapy to 2 weeks with split-daily dosing minimizes the risk for aminoglycoside nephrotoxicity.*

- *Aminoglycosides are suboptimal for P. aeruginosa.* Other antibiotics (e.g., meropenem, doripenem, cefepime) are preferred.

- *Aminoglycosides appear to be active against streptococci by in-vitro* susceptibility testing, but *aminoglycosides have no inherent activity against streptococci,* i.e., groups A, B, C, G, D.

- Aminoglycosides (e.g., gentamicin) are *only active against group D enterococci (E. faecalis, VSE) when combined with penicillin or vancomycin.*

- *Avoid, if possible, using aminoglycosides for peritoneal lavage* since the peritoneum provides a very large cross-sectional area for drug absorption, *increasing the risk for neuromuscular blockade/respiratory arrest.*

- For *CNS infections, aminoglycosides must be administered intrathecally* (I.T.) since they do not cross the blood brain barrier in sufficient concentrations to be therapeutic.

TMP–SMX

- Remember, *TMP–SMX has the same spectrum as ceftriaxone* (i.e., no P. aeruginosa coverage).

- *Avoid using TMP–SMX to treat serious systemic K. pneumoniae infections.* K. pneumoniae isolates that are sensitive to TMP–SMX *in-vitro* are often ineffective *in-vivo.*

- *In patients with hypersensitivity reactions to TMP–SMX, it is always the sulfa component, not the TMP component, which is responsible.* If continued treatment is desired with TMP–SMX, therapy may be completed with the TMP component alone.

- *Although TMP–SMX is inactive against most streptococci, it is an excellent antibiotic against MSSA.*

- *TMP–SMX is active against CA-MRSA but only variably active against HA-MRSA and CO-MRSA* (see Chapter 1, Table 1.11).

- For the *treatment of hydradenitis suppurativa due to MSSA, TMP–SMX is preferred* antibiotic because of its ability to penetrate deep into infected sebaceous glands.

- For aerobic GNB bacteremias (other than P. aeruginosa), use TMP–SMX 10 mg/kg/day (IV/PO) given in 4 equally divided doses q6h.
- *For CNS penetration and the treatment of unusual organisms (e.g., PCP), use TMP–SMX at dose of 20 mg/kg/day (IV/PO) given in 4 equally divided doses q6h.*
- *Avoid TMP–SMX in the treatment of respiratory tract infections since it is associated with PSRP/MDRSP.*

QUINOLONES

- *Levofloxacin at a dose of 750 mg IV/PO is preferred to ciprofloxacin for treatment of serious systemic P. aeruginosa infections.*
- *With the exception of ciprofloxacin quinolones do not lower the seizure threshold/cause seizures.*
- *Avelox is the only quinolone with a hepatobiliary mode of excretion; dose does not need to be modified and renal insufficiency but concentrations in the urine for lower UTIs may be suboptimal.*
- *For meningococcal prophylaxis, quinolones are equally effective* (quinolones penetrate well into respiratory secretions/have a high degree of anti-meningococcal activity).
- The "*respiratory quinolones*", e.g., moxifloxacin, levofloxacin have a high degree of bioavailability which makes them *ideal to treat systemic infections PO or as part of IV to PO switch therapy*. Respiratory quinolones have anti-TB activity (an option in treating MDR TB).
- *Ciprofloxacin has less activity against S. pneumoniae and S. aureus than moxifloxacin or levofloxacin.*
- Quinolones have some degree of anti-E. faecalis (VSE) but have no E. faecium (VRE) activity. *Among the quinolones, moxifloxacin has the highest degree of anti-VSE activity.*

NITROFURANTOIN

- *Nitrofurantoin is an ideal oral agent to treat cystitis.* (CrCl > 60 ml/min).
- *If the CrCL < 30 ml/min, nitrofurantoin should not be used to treat lower UTIs/CAB.*
- If treatment of CAB is desired, i.e., in some compromised hosts, e.g., diabetics, SLE, myeloma, CLL, steroids, neutropenia, *nitrofurantoin is an ideal oral agent and is active against the usual CAB pathogens, i.e., coliforms and group D enterococci (VSE/VRE).*
- Nitrofurantoin is active *against all aerobic GNB uropathogens except P. aeruginosa, Serratia marcesens, and Proteus sp.*

VANCOMYCIN

- If vancomycin is combined with a nephrotoxic drug and nephrotoxicity occurs, it *should be ascribed to the nephrotoxic drug* and not vancomycin.

- Vancomycin is a *"concentration-dependent"* drug (with MSSA/MRSA with MICs > 1 mcg/ml), but a *"time dependent"* drug (with MSSA/MRSA MICs < 1 mcg/ml).

- Since vancomycin obeys *"concentration-dependent"* killing kinetics for relatively resistant MSSA/MRSA and is not nephrotoxic, 30 mg/kg/day may be used for serious systemic infections.

- *No need for vancomycin levels for usual vancomycin dosing.* However, vancomycin levels may be useful in patients with unusually high volume of distribution (V_d) (e.g., edema/ascites, trauma, burns).

- Vancomycin "tolerance" is *common among staphylococci and enterococci.*

- Vancomycin is *bacteriostatic* against E. faecalis (VSE).

- Avoid vancomycin for empiric coverage of CVC infections. *Treat potential CVC infection with catheter removal*, not antibiotics.

- Vancomycin therapy *may select out heteroresistant S. aureus* (hVISA) due to *cell wall thickening* ("permeability-mediated" resistance).

- In CAP with PRSP bacteremia, *avoid vancomycin for CNS coverage since CSF penetration is inadequate in the absence of meningeal inflammation.*

- Because of its large molecular size, *vancomycin does not penetrate well into most tissues* (synovial fluid, bone, etc).

- *Vancomycin IV predisposes to VRE*, but PO vancomycin does *not*.

LINEZOLID

- Linezolid is highly active against the major gram-positive pathogens, including MSSA, MRSA, VSE, and VRE.

- Linezolid is *equally efficacious when administered PO or IV*.

- Unlike vancomycin, *linezolid does not increase E. faecium* (VRE) prevalence.

- Because linezolid is eliminated by hepatic mechanisms, no dosing adjustment is necessary in renal insufficiency.

- Linezolid is *one of the few PO antibiotics that can be used to treat CNS infections*.

- Linezolid is *more cost effective than IV vancomycin* when the total cost of IV vancomycin administration is calculated (cost of the PICC line + cost of the surgical procedure for PICC line insertion + cost of CXR to verify PICC line position + cost associated with home IV therapy + monitoring cost of vancomycin, e.g., serial creatinines + physician cost for PICC line removal + costs related to the diagnosis/consequence of vancomycin side effects).

QUINUPRISTIN/DALFOPRISTIN

- Quinupristin/dalfopristin is active against E. faecium (VRE) but *not E. faecalis (VSE)*.
- Quinupristin/dalfopristin is highly effective against MSSA and MRSA and is a *therapeutic alternative if other antibiotics fail/cannot be used to treat MSSA/MRSA* infections.

DAPTOMYCIN

- Daptomycin is more *active against MSSA/MRSA than Group D enterococci* (VSE/VRE). *If daptomycin is used to treat VSE/VRE, a higher dose may be required.*
- Daptomycin is *inactivated by calcium in alveolar surfactant fluid* and should *not* be used for pneumonias.
- Following vancomycin therapeutic failures with MSSA/MRSA bacteremias/ABE, *daptomycin resistance may occur during therapy*.
- *An initial dose of gentamicin may increase intracellular entry/effectiveness of daptomycin* when treating MSSA/MRSA infections.

TIGECYCLINE

- Tigecycline may be given safely to patients with penicillin or sulfa drug allergy but *avoid in patients with tetracycline allergy*.
- Tigecycline (hepatobiliary elimination) does *not need to be adjusted in renal insufficiency*.
- Tigecycline *is not* a substrate or inhibitor of the cytochrome P450 system and is particularly useful in patients on multiple cardiac or HIV drugs.
- Tigecycline is highly active against *MDR K. pneumoniae* and may be the *only antibiotic effective against such strains*.
- Tigecycline is one of only two antibiotics effective against the nearly pan-resistant strains of NDM-1.

MACROLIDES

- *Macrolides have been largely responsible for PRSP and MDRSP.* Use instead doxycycline or a "respiratory quinolone."
- IV erythromycin lactobionate is the macrolide *most* likely to be associated with QTc prolongation. Macrolides with lower serum levels (e.g., azithromycin) are not associated with QTc prolongation.
- Macrolides may cause an "irritative" diarrhea but *not* C. difficile diarrhea.
- Erythromycin estolate may cause cholestatic jaundice in adults but not in children.
- Due to widespread group A streptococci and MSSA resistance to macrolides, *avoid* macrolides for the treatment of skin/soft tissue infections.

METRONIDAZOLE

- Metronidazole (IV) is *preferred therapy* for C. difficile *colitis*.
- Metronidazole (PO) *frequently fails and is inferior to PO vancomycin* for C. difficile *diarrhea*.
- A underecognized/untoward effect of metronidazole (PO) use for C. difficile *diarrhea* is *increased VRE* prevalence.
- Metronidazole has a long serum half life ($t_{1/2}$) of approximately 7 hr which permits *once daily dosing*, i.e., 1 g (IV) q24h. Except for C. difficile *colitis*, there is little rationale for dosing metronidazole 500 mg (IV) on a q6 or q8h basis.
- Metronidazole is *one of the few hepatically eliminated antibiotics that requires a dosing adjustment in severe renal in sufficiency* (CrCl < 10 ml/min.).
- For cIAIs *don't combine metronidazole and moxifloxacin* (no rationale for double B. fragilis coverage).

TELAVANCIN

- *Lipoglycopeptide with long $t_{1/2}$ (8 hrs) with normal renal function which permits once daily (q24h) dosing.*
- Telavancin is not removed by HD (protein binding = 90%), but *like some other antibiotics, may have decreased efficacy with CrCl < 50 ml/min.*

- *Useful for cSSSIs due to MSSA, MRSA, VSE (not VRE), groups A, B streptococci and S. anginosus group.*
- *Falsely elevated INR, PT, PTT may occur with telavancin.*
- *Infuse telavancin 10 mg/kg (IV) slowly over 1 hour*. Steady-state concentrations are achieved by the 3rd dose.

FOSFOMYCIN

- Fosfomycin is highly active against *most* MDR GNS uropathogens and may be used *orally* to treat lower UTIs/CAB due to susceptible organisms.
- *Fosfomycin is one of the few oral antibiotics effective against most MDR GNB uropathogens. Misses some strains of MDR Enterobacter sp., Klebsiella pneumoniae, and P. aeruginosa.*
- *Longer fosfomycin treatment courses may be needed to eradicate some MDR GNB uropathogens.*
- *Achieves very high urinary concentrations (> 2000 mcg/ml) which minimizes the potential for GNB resistance.*
- *Synergistic with quinolones against GNBs/MDROs.*

POLYMYXIN B/COLISTIN

- The increased prevalence of resistant aerobic GNBs has resulted in increased use of colisitin for MDR *P. aeruginosa*, MDR *E. coli*, MDR *Enterobacter sp.*, MDR *Acinetobacter baumanii*, MDR *Klebsiella pneumoniae*.
- *Polymyxin B and colistin have same spectrum of activity, but differ in activity, e.g., polymyxin B has greater activity against P. aeruginosa than colistin.*
- Polymyxin B and colistin are active against most aerobic GNBs but no activity *against Proteus, Providencia, Morganella, Serratia, or B. cepacia.*
- *Gram + organisms and Gram – cocci are naturally resistant to polymyxin B and colistin.*
- *Colistin is one of the very few antibiotics effective against the nearly pan-resistant strains of NDM-1.*
- *Colistin is one of the very few antibiotics for GNBs that may be given at each HD (q48h)*. HD dose: 2 mg/kg (IV) q48h (no post-HD dose needed).

Chapter 11

Antimicrobial Drug Summaries

**Burke A. Cunha, MD, Damary C. Torres, PharmD,
Jean E. Hage, MD, David W. Kubiak, PharmD,
Nardeen Mickail, MD, Arthur Gran, MD,
Sigridh Muñoz-Gomez, MD, Cheston B. Cunha, MD,
John H. Rex, MD, Mark H. Kaplan, MD**

This section contains prescribing information pertinent to the clinical use of antimicrobial agents in adults, as compiled from a variety of sources. *Antimicrobial agents for pediatric infectious diseases are described in Chapter 7*. The information provided is not exhaustive, and the reader is referred to other drug information references and the manufacturer's product literature for further information. Clinical use of the information provided and any consequences that may arise from its use are the responsibilities of the prescribing physician. The authors, editors, and publisher do not warrant or guarantee the information contained in this section, and do not assume and expressly disclaim any liability for errors or omissions or any consequences that may occur from such. **The use of any drug should be preceded by careful review of the package insert, which provides indications and dosing approved by the U.S. Food and Drug Administration. This information can be obtained on the website provided at the end of the reference list for each drug summary.**

Drugs are listed alphabetically by generic name; trade names follow in parentheses. To search by trade name, consult the index. Each drug summary contains the following information:

Usual dose. Represents the usual dose to treat most susceptible infections in adult patients with normal hepatic and renal function. Dosing for special situations is listed under the comments section; additional information can be found in Chapters 2, 4, 5 and the manufacturer's product literature. Loading doses for doxycycline, fluconazole, itraconazole, voriconazole, caspofungin, and other antimicrobials are described in either the usual dose or comments section. **Meningeal doses of antimicrobials used for CNS infection are described at the end of the comments section.**

Peak serum levels. Refers to the peak serum concentrations (mcg/ml) after the usual dose is administered. Peak serum level is useful in calculating the "kill ratios," the ratio of peak serum level to minimum inhibitory concentration (MIC) of the organism. **The higher the "kill ratio," the more effective the "dose dependent" antimicrobial is likely to be against a particular organism.**

Bioavailability. Refers to the percentage of the dose reaching the systemic circulation from the site of administration (PO or IM). **For PO antibiotics, bioavailability refers to the percentage of dose**

adsorbed from the GI tract. For IV antibiotics, "not applicable" appears next to bioavailability, since the entire dose reaches the systemic circulation. Antibiotics with high bioavailability (> 90%) are ideal for IV to PO switch therapy.

Excreted unchanged. Refers to the percentage of drug excreted unchanged, and **provides an indirect measure of drug concentration in the urine/feces. Antibiotics excreted unchanged in the urine in low concentration are unlikely to be useful for urinary tract infections.**

Serum half-life (normal/ESRD). The serum half-life ($t_{1/2}$) is the time (in hours) in which serum concentration falls by 50%. **Serum half-life is useful in determining dosing interval**. If the half-life of drugs eliminated by the kidneys is prolonged in end-stage renal disease (ESRD), then the total daily dose is reduced in proportion to the degree of renal dysfunction. If the half-life in ESRD is similar to the normal half-life, then the total daily dose does not change.

Plasma protein binding. Expressed as the **percentage of drug reversibly bound to serum albumin. It is the unbound (free) portion of a drug that equilibrates with tissues and imparts antimicrobial activity. Plasma protein binding is not typically a factor in antimicrobial effectiveness unless binding exceeds 95%.** Decreases in serum albumin (nephrotic syndrome, liver disease) or competition for protein binding from other drugs or endogenously produced substances (uremia, hyperbilirubinemia) will increase the percentage of free drug available for antimicrobial activity, and may require a decrease in dosage. Increases in serum binding proteins (trauma, surgery, critical illness) will decrease the percentage of free drug available for antimicrobial activity, and may require an increase in dosage.

Volume of distribution (V_d). Represents the apparent volume into which the drug is distributed, and is calculated as the amount of drug in the body divided by the serum concentration (in liters/kilogram). V_d is related to total body water distribution (V_d H_2O = 0.7 L/kg). Hydrophilic (water soluble) drugs are restricted to extracellular fluid and have a $V_d \leq 0.7$ L/kg. In contrast, **hydrophobic (highly lipid soluble) drugs penetrate most fluids/tissues of the body and have a large V_d.** Drugs that are concentrated in certain tissues (e.g., liver) can have a V_d greatly exceeding total body water. V_d is affected by organ profusion, membrane diffusion/permeability, lipid solubility, protein binding, and state of equilibrium between body compartments. **For hydrophilic drugs, increases in V_d may occur with burns, heart failure, dialysis, sepsis, cirrhosis, or mechanical ventilation**; decreases in V_d may occur with trauma, hemorrhage, pancreatitis (early), or GI fluid losses. Increases in V_d may require an increase in total daily drug dose for antimicrobial effectiveness; decreases in V_d may require a decrease in drug dose. **In addition to drug distribution, V_d reflects binding avidity to cholesterol membranes and concentration within organ tissues (e.g., liver).**

Mode of elimination. Refers to the primary route of inactivation/excretion of the antibiotic, which **impacts dosing adjustments in renal/hepatic failure.**

Dosage adjustments. Each grid provides dosing adjustments based on renal and hepatic function. **In renal insufficiency** (*for **renally eliminated antibiotics***), **the initial dose is the same as with normal renal function**; but the **maintenance dose is decreased ~ ↓ CrCl** (see antibiotic drug summaries for specific dosing recommendations). **Antimicrobial dosing for hemodialysis (HD)/ peritoneal dialysis (PD) patients (between HD/PD) is the same as a CrCl < 10 mL/min. Some antimicrobial agents require a supplemental dose immediately after hemodialysis (post–HD)/ peritoneal dialysis (post–PD).** Following the post–HD or post–PD supplemental dose, antimicrobial dosing should resume as for a CrCl < 10 mL/min. "No change" indicates no change from the usual dose. "Avoid" indicates the drug should be avoided in the setting described. "None" indicates no supplemental dose is required. "No information" indicates there are insufficient data from which to make a dosing recommendation. **Dosing recommendations are based on pharmacokinetic data, published studies, and experience.** CVVH dosing recommendations represent general guidelines, since antibiotic removal is dependent on area/type of filter, ultrafiltration rates, and sieving coefficients; replacement dosing should be individualized and guided by serum levels, if possible. **Creatinine clearance (CrCl) is used to gauge the degree of renal insufficiency, and can be estimated by the following calculation: CrCl (mL/min) = [(140 − age) × weight (kg)] / [72 × serum creatinine (mg/dL)]. The calculated value is multiplied by 0.85 for females**. It is important to recognize that due to age-dependent decline in renal function, elderly patients with "normal" serum creatinines may have low CrCls requiring dosage adjustments. (For example, a 70-year-old, 50-kg female with a serum creatinine of 1.2 mg/dL has an estimated CrCl of 34 mL/min.)

Slow extended daily dialysis (SLEDD) is now being used in some critical care patients. It is less likely to remove molecules > 1000 Daltons as compared to CVVH. Assuming a dialysate flow rate of 100 mL/min and a blood flow rate of 200 mL/min clearances during dialysis are about 82-98 mL/min using a Fresenius AV600 polysulfone hemodialyzer. However increasing the flow rate to 300 mL/min increases the clearance during dialysis to 170 mL/min. Therefore, doses during SLEDD may be the same as for normal renal function. **Clearances for SLEDD are comparable to CVVH except over a shorter period, so when no information is available, dosage adjustments can be made as for CVVH.** If needed, post-SLEDD doses should be given depending on the antibiotic.

"Antiretroviral Dosage Adjustment" grids indicate recommended dosage adjustments when protease inhibitors (PIs) and non-nucleoside reverse transcriptase inhibitor (NNRTIs) are combined or used in conjunction with rifampin or rifabutin.

Drug interactions. Refers to common/important drug-drug interactions, compiled from various sources. If a specific drug interaction is well-documented (e.g., antibiotic × with lovastatin), than other drugs from the same drug class (e.g., atorvastatin) may also be listed, based on theoretical considerations. Drug interactions may occur as a consequence of altered absorption (e.g., metal ion chelation of tetracycline), altered distribution (e.g., sulfonamide displacement of barbiturates from serum albumin), altered excretion (e.g., probenecid competition with penicillin for active transport in the kidney), altered metabolism (e.g., rifampin–induced hepatic P-450 metabolism of theophylline/ warfarin; chloramphenicol inhibition of phenytoin metabolism).

Adverse side effects. Common/important side effects are indicated.

Allergic potential. Described as low or high. **Refers to the likelihood of a hypersensitivity reaction** to a particular antimicrobial.

Safety in pregnancy. Designated by the U.S. Food and Drug Administration's (USFDA) use-in-**pregnancy letter code** (Table 11.3).

Comments. Includes other useful information for each antimicrobial agent.

Cerebrospinal fluid penetration. Expressed as a **percentage relative to serum concentration**. If an antimicrobial is used for CNS infections, the meningeal dose is indicated directly above CSF penetration. No meningeal dose is given if CSF penetration is inadequate for treatment of meningitis due to susceptible organisms.

Biliary tract penetration. Expressed as a percentage relative to peak serum concentrations. Percentages > 100% reflect concentrations within the biliary system. This information is useful for estimating biliary tract concentrations.

Table 11.1 Selected Substrates, Inhibitors, and Inducers of Cytochrome P450 Isoenzymes

	Substrates	Inhibitors	Inducers
CYP1A2	Theophylline	Erythromycin	None
CYP2C9	Phenytoin, warfarin	Erythromycin, INH, metronidazole, amiodarone	TMX-SMX, RIF, phenobarbital, carbamazepine
CYP3A4	Cyclosporine, tacrolimus, simvastatin, diltiazem	Erythromycin, amiodarone	None
OATI	Oseltamivir, cidofovir	Probenecid	None
PGP	Quinolones, itraconazole, digoxin	Cyclosporine, tacrolimus	RIF

OAT-1 = organic anion transporter-1; TMP–SMX = trimethoprim sulfamethoxazole; RIF = rifampin; INH = isoniazid.

Table 11.2 Antibiotics and Cytochrome P450 Isoenzymes

Antibiotics that are not involved in CYP450 system	Antibiotics that are involved in CYP450 system either as inducer or inhibitor
Tigecycline, daptomycin, clindamycin, linezolid, vancomycin, minocycline, cephalosporins, carbapenems, nitrofurantoin, colistin, penicillins, oxacillin, aztreonam, moxifloxacin, aminoglycosides	Nafcillin, quinupristin/dalfopristin, macrolides, telithromycin, fluoroquinolones (except moxifloxacin), all azoles, rifampin, INH, TMP–SMX, tetracycline, doxycycline, metronidazole, chloramphenicol

Table 11.3 USFDA Use-in-Pregnancy Letter Code

Category	Interpretation
A	**Controlled studies show no risk.** Adequate, well-controlled studies in pregnant women have not shown a risk to the fetus in any trimester of pregnancy.
B	**No evidence of risk in humans.** Adequate, well-controlled studies in pregnant women have not shown increased risk of fetal abnormalities despite adverse findings in animals, or, in the absence of adequate human studies, animal studies show no fetal risk. The chance of fetal harm is remote, but remains a possibility.
C	**Risk cannot be ruled out.** Adequate, well-controlled human studies are lacking, and animal studies have shown a risk to the fetus or are lacking. There is a chance of fetal harm if the drug is administered during pregnancy, but potential benefit from use of the drug may outweigh potential risk.
D	**Positive evidence of risk.** Studies in humans or investigational or post-marketing data have demonstrated fetal risk. Nevertheless, potential benefit from use of the drug may outweigh potential risk. For example, the drug may be acceptable if needed in a life-threatening situation or serious disease for which safer drugs cannot be used or are ineffective.

Table 11.3 USFDA Use-in-Pregnancy Letter Code

Category	Interpretation
X	**Contraindicated in pregnancy.** Studies in animals or humans or investigational or post-marketing reports have demonstrated positive evidence of fetal abnormalities or risk which clearly outweigh any possible benefit to the patient.

Lipid-Associated Formulations of Amphotericin B. There are 3 licensed lipid-associated formulations of amphotericin B (LFAB) (Table 11.4). Although closely related in some ways, these formulations have distinct properties and must be understood separately. The principal advantage of the LFAB over amphotericin B deoxycholate (AMBD) is greater safety. In general, the rates of both acute infection-related toxicities (fever, chills, etc.) and chronic therapy-associated toxicities (principally nephrotoxicity) are reduced with LFAB. However, the LFAB can produce all of the toxicities of AMBD (and in selected patients, LFAB have been more toxic than AMBD). Overall, (L-Amb) (AmBisome) and ABLC (Abelcet) appear to be safer than ABCD (Amphotec, Amphocil). Whichever formulation is selected for therapy, it is important to specify its name carefully when prescribing. The phrase "lipid amphotericin B" should be avoided due to its imprecision. Patients who are tolerating one formulation may develop all the standard infusion-related toxicities if switched inadvertently to a new formulation. In general (and in contrast to the usual preference for generic names), use of trade names is the clearest way to specify the choice of drug in this category. In this handbook, the phrase "lipid-associated formulation of amphotericin B" suggests use of any of the 3 formulations. The issues surrounding the selection of an LFAB for an individual patient are summarized in Table 11.4 (see comments).

Table 11.4 Lipid-Associated Formulations of Amphotericin B

Generic name (abbreviation)	Trade names	Licensed (IV) dosages in the United States	Comments
Amphotericin B lipid complex (ABLC)	Abelcet	5 mg/kg/d	Reliable choice; long history of use.
Liposomal amphotericin B (L-Amb)	AmBisome	3 mg/kg/d (empiric therapy) 3–5 mg/kg/d (systemic fungal infections) 6 mg/kg/d (cryptococcal meningitis in HIV patients)	Reliable choice; best studied (L-Amb); well-supported dosing recommendations by indication; probably the least nephrotoxic; good data to support increasing the dose safely.
Amphotericin B colloidal dispersion, amphotericin B cholesteryl sulfate complex (ABCD)	Amphotec, Amphocil	3–4 mg/kg/d	Infusion-related toxicities have limited its use.

Abacavir (Ziagen) ABC

Drug Class: Antiretroviral NRTI (nucleoside reverse transcriptase inhibitor).

Usual Dose: 300 mg (PO) q12h.

Pharmacokinetic Parameters:

Peak serum level: 3 mcg/mL
Bioavailability: 83%
Excreted unchanged (urine): 1.2%
Serum half-life (normal/ESRD): 1.5/8 hrs
Plasma protein binding: 50%
Volume of distribution (V_d): 0.86 L/kg

Primary Mode of Elimination: Hepatic

Dosage Adjustments*

CrCl < 10 mL/min	No change
Post–HD dose	None
Post–PD dose	None
CVVH/CVVHD/ CVVHDF dose	No change
Mild hepatic insufficiency	200 mg (PO) q12h
Moderate—severe hepatic insufficiency	Avoid

Drug Interactions: Methadone (↑ methadone clearance with abacavir 600 mg bid); ethanol (↑ abacavir serum levels/half-life and may ↑ toxicity).

Adverse Effects: *Abacavir may cause severe hypersensitivity reactions which may be fatal (see comments); usually during the first 4–6 weeks of therapy;* Patients who carry the HLA-B*5701 allele are at high risk for experiencing a hypersensitivity reaction to abacavir. Discontinue abacavir as soon as a hypersensitivity reaction is suspected. Regardless of HLA-B*5701 status, permanently discontinue abacavir if hypersensitivity cannot be ruled out, even when other diagnoses are possible. Following a hypersensitivity reaction to abacavir, never restart abacavir or any other abacavir-containing product. Report cases of hypersensitivity syndrome to Abacavir Hypersensitivity Registry at 1-800-270-0425. Drug fever/rash, abdominal pain/diarrhea, nausea, vomiting, anorexia, bad dreams/sleep disorders, weakness, headache, ↑ SGOT/ SGPT, hyperglycemia, hypertriglyceridemia, lactic acidosis with hepatic steatosis (rare, but potentially life-threatening toxicity with use of NRTI's).

Allergic Potential: High (~5%)

Safety in Pregnancy: C

Comments: Discontinue abacavir and *do not restart in patients with signs/symptoms of hypersensitivity reaction*, which may include fever, rash, fatigue, nausea, vomiting, diarrhea, abdominal pain, anorexia, respiratory symptoms. Ethanol increases abacavir levels by 41%. When combined with didanosine rapid emergence of cross resistance via mutations to K65R, L74V, Y11F, and M184V occurs leading to failure of drug efficacy. Use with caution in patients with serious risk of coronary disease.

Cerebrospinal Fluid Penetration: 27–33%

REFERENCES:

Bedimo RJ, Westfall AO, Drechsler H, et al. Abacavir use and risk of acute myocardial infarction and cerebrovascular events in the highly active antiretroviral therapy era. Clin Infect Dis 53:83–94, 2011.

Carr A, Workman C, Smith DE, et al. Abacavir substitution for nucleoside analogs in patients with HIV lipoatrophy. A randomized trial. JAMA 288:207–15, 2002.

"Usual dose" assumes normal renal/hepatic function. * For renal insufficiency, give usual dose × 1 followed by maintenance dose per CrCl. For dialysis patients, dose the same as for CrCl < 10 mL/min and give supplemental (post-HD/PD dose) immediately after dialysis. CrCl = creatinine clearance; CVVH = continuous veno-venous hemofiltration; HD/PD = hemodialysis/peritoneal dialysis.

Katalama C, Clotet B, Plettenberg A, et al. The role of abacavir (AVC, 1592) in antiretroviral therapy-experiences patients: results from randomized, double-blind, trial. CNA3002 European Study Team. AIDS 14:781–9, 2000.

Keating MR. Antiviral agents. Mayo Clin Proc 67:160–78, 1992.

Nishijima T, Tsukada K, Teruya K, et al. Efficacy and safety of once-daily ritonavir-based antiretroviral therapy in low-body weight treatment-naïve patients with HIV infections. AIDS 13;26:649–51, 2012.

Panel on Antiretroviral Guidelines for Adults and Adolescents. Department of Health and Human Services. Guidelines for the use of antiretroviral agents in HIV-infected adults and adolescents. http://aidsinfo.nih.gov/ConsentFiles/AdultandAdolescentGL.pdf, 2012.

Sax PE, Tierney C, Collier AC, et al. Abacavir/lamivudine versus tenofovir DF/emtricitabine as part of combination regimens for initial treatment of HIV: final results. J Infect Dis 204:1191–201, 2011.

Staszewski S, Keiser P, Mantaner J, et al. Abacavir-lamivudine-zidovudine vs. indinavir-lamivudine-zidovudine in antiretroviral-naive HIV-infected adults: a randomized equivalence trial. JAMA 285:1155–63, 2001.

Thompson MA, Aberg JA, Cahn P, et al. Antiretroviral treatment of adult HIV infection: 2012 recommendations of the International Antiviral society — USA panel. JAMA 308:387–402, 2012.

Website: www.TreatHIV.com

Abacavir + Lamivudine (Epzicom) ABC/3TC

Drug Class: Antiretroviral NRTI combination.
Usual Dose: Epzicom tablet = abacavir 600 mg + lamivudine 300 mg. Usual dose: 1 tablet q24h.
Pharmacokinetic Parameters:
Peak serum level: 4.06/2.04 mcg/L
Bioavailability: 86/86%
Excreted unchanged (urine): 1.2/71%
Serum half-life (normal/ESRD): (1.5/8)/(5-7/20) hrs
Plasma protein binding: 50/36%
Volume of distribution (V_d): 0.86/1.3 L/kg
Primary Mode of Elimination: Hepatic/Renal
Dosage Adjustments*

CrCl < 50 mL/min	Avoid
Post–HD dose	Avoid
Post–PD dose	Avoid
CVVH/CVVHD/CVVHDF dose	Avoid
Mild hepatic insufficiency	Contraindicated
Moderate–severe hepatic insufficiency	Contraindicated

Drug Interactions: Methadone (↑ methadone clearance with abacavir 600 mg bid); ethanol (↑ abacavir serum levels/half-life; may ↑ toxicity); didanosine, zalcitabine (↑ risk of pancreatitis); TMP–SMX (↑ lamivudine levels); zidovudine (↑ zidovudine levels).

Adverse Effects: Abacavir may cause severe hypersensitivity reactions that may be fatal (see comments), usually during the first 4–6 weeks of therapy; Patients who carry the HLA-B*5701 allele are at high risk for experiencing a hypersensitivity reaction to abacavir. Discontinue Abacavir as soon as a hypersensitivity reaction is suspected. Regardless of HLA-B*5701 status, permanently discontinue Abacavir if hypersensitivity cannot be ruled out, even when other diagnoses are possible. Following a hypersensitivity reaction to abacavir, NEVER restart Abacavir or any other abacavir-containing product. Drug fever, rash, abdominal pain, diarrhea, nausea, vomiting, anorexia, anemia, leukopenia, photophobia, depression, insomnia, weakness, headache, cough, nasal complaints, dizziness,

---

"Usual dose" assumes normal renal/hepatic function. * For renal insufficiency, give usual dose × 1 followed by maintenance dose per CrCl. For dialysis patients, dose the same as for CrCl < 10 mL/min and give supplemental (post-HD/PD dose) immediately after dialysis. CrCl = creatinine clearance; CVVH = continuous veno-venous hemofiltration; HD/PD = hemodialysis/peritoneal dialysis.

peripheral neuropathy, myalgias, ↑ AST/
ALT, hyperglycemia, hypertriglyceridemia,
pancreatitis, lactic acidosis with hepatic
steatosis (rare, but potentially life-
threatening toxicity with the NRTI's). Immune
reconstitution syndrome and redistribution/
accumulation of body fat have been reported
in patients treated with combination
antiretroviral therapy.
Allergic Potential: High (~5%)/Low
Safety in Pregnancy: C
Comments: In patients with signs/symptoms of
hypersensitivity reactions discontinue and do not
restart, which may include fever, rash, fatigue,
nausea, vomiting, diarrhea, abdominal pain,
anorexia, respiratory symptoms. **Potential cross
resistance with didanosine.** When combined
with didanosine rapid emergence of cross
resistance via mutations to K65R, L74V,
Y115F, and M184V occurs leading to failure
of drug efficacy. Severe acute exacerbations
of hepatitis B have been reported in patients
who are co-infected with hepatitis B virus (HBV)
and HIV and have discontinued epivir.
Hepatic function should be monitored closely for at least
several months in patients who discontinue
epivir.
Cerebrospinal Fluid Penetration: 27–33/15%

REFERENCES:
Panel on Antiretroviral Guidelines for Adults and
  Adolescents. Department of Health and Human
  Services. Guidelines for the use of antiretroviral
  agents in HIV-infected adults and adolescents.
  http://aidsinfo.nih.gov/ConsentFiles/
  AdultandAdolescentGL.pdf, 2012.
Thompson MA, Aberg JA, Cahn P, et al. Antiretroviral
  treatment of adult HIV infection: 2012 recommen-
  dations of the International Antiviral society — USA
  panel. JAMA 308:387–402, 2012.
Website: www.epzicom.com

Abacavir + Lamivudine + Zidovudine (Trizivir) ABC/3TC/ZDV

Drug Class: Antiretroviral NRTI combination.
Usual Dose: Trizivir tablet = abacavir 300 mg +
lamivudine 150 mg + zidovudine 300 mg. Usual
dose = 1 tablet (PO) q12h.
Pharmacokinetic Parameters:
Peak serum level: 3/1.5/1.2 mcg/mL
Bioavailability: 86/86/64%
Excreted unchanged (urine): 1.2/90/16%
*Serum half-life (normal/ESRD): [1.5/6/1.1] /
8/20/2.2] hrs*
Plasma protein binding: 50/36/20%
Volume of distribution (V_d): 0.86/1.3/1.6 L/kg
Primary Mode of Elimination: Hepatic/renal
Dosage Adjustments*

CrCl < 50 mL/min	Avoid
Post–HD or Post–PD	Avoid
CVVH/CVVHD/ CVVHDF dose	Avoid
Moderate–severe hepatic insufficiency	Avoid

Drug Interactions: Amprenavir, atovaquone
(↑ zidovudine levels); clarithromycin
(↓ zidovudine levels); cidofovir (↑ zidovudine
levels, flu-like symptoms); doxorubicin
(neutropenia); stavudine (antagonistic to
zidovudine; avoid combination); TMP–SMX
(↑ lamivudine and zidovudine levels); zalcitabine
(↓ lamivudine levels). May exacerbate
neutropenia in combination with gangciclovir.
Adverse Effects: *Abacavir may cause severe/
fatal rash/hypersensitivity reaction;* Patients
who carry the HLA-B*5701 allere are at high

"Usual dose" assumes normal renal/hepatic function. * For renal insufficiency, give usual dose × 1 followed by
maintenance dose per CrCl. For dialysis patients, dose the same as for CrCl < 10 mL/min and give supplemental
(post-HD/PD dose) immediately after dialysis. CrCl = creatinine clearance; CVVH = continuous veno-venous
hemofiltration; HD/PD = hemodialysis/peritoneal dialysis.

risk for experiencing a hypersensitivity reaction to abacavir. Discontinue abacavir as soon as a hypersensitivity reaction is suspected. Regardless of HLA-B*5701 status, permanently discontinue abacavir if hypersensitivity cannot be ruled out, even when other diagnoses are possible. Following a hypersensitivity reaction to abacavir, never restart abacavir or any other abacavir-containing product. Most common (> 5%): nausea, vomiting, diarrhea, anorexia, insomnia, fever/chills, headache, malaise/fatigue. Others (less common): peripheral neuropathy, myopathy, steatosis, pancreatitis. Lab abnormalities: anemia, leukopenia, mild hyperglycemia, ↑ LFTs, ↑ CPK, ↑ aldolase, hypertriglyceridemia. Immune reconstitution syndrome and redistribution/accumulation of body fat have been reported in patients treated with combination antiretroviral therapy.

Allergic Potential: High (~5%)
Safety in Pregnancy: C
Comments: Avoid in patients with CrCl < 50 mL/min. HBV hepatitis may relapse if lamivudine is discontinued.

REFERENCES:

McDowell JA, Lou Y, Symonds WS, et al. Multiple-dose pharmacokinetics and pharmacodynamics of abacavir alone and in combination with zidovudine in human immunodeficiency virus-infected adults. Antimicrob Agents Chemother 44:2061–7, 2000.

Panel on Antiretroviral Guidelines for Adults and Adolescents. Department of Health and Human Services. Guidelines for the use of antiretroviral agents in HIV-infected adults and adolescents. http://aidsinfo.nih.gov/ConsentFiles/AdultandAdolescentGL.pdf, 2012.

Thompson MA, Aberg JA, Cahn P, et al. Antiretroviral treatment of adult HIV infection: 2012 recommendations of the International Antiviral society — USA panel. JAMA 308:387–402, 2012.

Website: www.TreatHIV.com

Acyclovir (Zovirax)

Drug Class: Antiviral (see comments).
Usual Dose:
HSV-1/2: Herpes labialis: 400 mg (PO) 5x/day × 5 days. Genital herpes: *Initial therapy.* 200 mg (PO) 5x/day × 10 days. *Recurrent/intermittent therapy* (< 6 episodes/year): 200 mg (PO) 5x/day × 5 days. *Chronic suppressive therapy* (> 6 episodes/year): 400 mg (PO) q12h × 1 year. Mucosal/genital herpes: 5 mg/kg (IV) q8h × 7 days or 400 mg (PO) 5x/day × 7 days. Nosocomial pneumonia 5 mg/kg (IV) q8h × 10 days or 400 mg (PO) 5x/day × 7 days. Meningitis/encephalitis: 10 mg/kg (IV) q8h × 10 days or 800 mg (PO) 5x/day × 10 days.
VZV: Chickenpox: 10 mg/kg (IV) q8h × 5 days or 800 mg (PO) q6h × 5 days. VZV pneumonia: 5–10 mg/kg (IV) q8h × 10 days (normal hosts) 10 mg/kg (IV) q8h × 10 days (compromised hosts). Herpes zoster (shingles): *Dermatomal/Disseminated:* 10 mg/kg (IV) q8h × 7–10 days or 800 mg (PO) 5x/day × 7–10 days. VZV meningitis/encephalitis: 10 mg/kg (IV) q8h × 10 days or 800 mg (PO) 5x/day × 10 days.

Pharmacokinetic Parameters:
Peak serum level: 7.7 mcg/mL
Bioavailability: 30%
Excreted unchanged (urine): 70%
Serum half-life (normal/ESRD): 3/5 hrs
Plasma protein binding: 30%
Volume of distribution (V_d): 0.7 L/kg
Primary Mode of Elimination: Renal
Dosage Adjustments* for HSV/VZV

CrCl 10–25 mL/min	No change/ 800 mg (IV/PO) q8h
CrCl < 10 mL/min	400 mg (IV/PO) q12h/ 800 mg (IV/PO) q12h

"Usual dose" assumes normal renal/hepatic function. * For renal insufficiency, give usual dose × 1 followed by maintenance dose per CrCl. For dialysis patients, dose the same as for CrCl < 10 mL/min and give supplemental (post-HD/PD dose) immediately after dialysis. CrCl = creatinine clearance; CVVH = continuous veno-venous hemofiltration; HD/PD = hemodialysis/peritoneal dialysis.

Post–HD dose	None
Post–PD dose	None
CVVH/CVVHD/ CVVHDF dose	5 mg/kg(IV) q24h/ 10 mg/kg(IV) q24h 400 mg (PO) q8h/ 800 mg (PO) q8h
Moderate—severe hepatic insufficiency	No change

Drug Interactions: Cimetidine, probenecid, theophylline (↑ acyclovir levels); nephrotoxic drugs (↑ nephrotoxicity); zidovudine (lethargy); theophylline (↑ levels).

Adverse Effects: Seizures/tremors (dose related), encephalopathy, crystalluria, ATN. HUS (only with HIV) Base dose on ideal body weight in the elderly to minimize adverse effects.

Allergic Potential: Low

Safety in Pregnancy: B

Comments: Na^+ content = 4 mEq/g. CSF levels may be increased with probenecid.

Highly active against HSV and VZV. Some activity against CMV. No activity against EBV, RSV or adenoviruses.

Meningeal dose = HSV or VZV encephalitis dose.

Cerebrospinal Fluid Penetration: 20%

REFERENCES:

Gupta R, Wald A, Krantz E, et al. Valacyclovir and acyclovir for suppression of shedding of herpes simplex virus in the genital tract. J Infect Dis 190:1374–81, 2004.

Henao-Martinez AF, Weinberg A, Waldman WJ, et al. Successful treatment of acyclovir-resistant herpes simplex virus type 2 proctitis with leflunomide in an HIV-infected man. J Clin Virol 54:276–278, 2012.

Keating MR. Antiviral Agents. Mayo Clin Proc 67:160–78, 1992.

Mugwanya K, Baeten JM, Mugo NR, et al. High-dose valacyclovir HSV-2 suppression results in greater reduction in plasma HIV-1 levels compared with standard dose acyclovir among HIV-1/HSV-2 coinfected persons: a randomized, crossover trial. J Infect Dis 204:1912–1017, 2011.

Owens RC, Ambrose PG. Acyclovir. Antibiotics for Clinicians 1:85–93, 1997.

Vanpouille C, Lisco A, Introini A, et al. Exploiting the anti-HIV-1 activity of acyclovir: suppression of primary and drug-resistant HIV isolates and potentiation of the activity by ribavirin. Antimicrob Agents Chemother 56:2604–2611, 2012.

Vanpouille C, Lisco A, Margolis L. Acyclovir: a new use for an old drug. Curr Opin Infect Dis 22:583–587, 2009.

Whitley RJ, Gnann JW Jr. Acyclovir: a decade later. N Engl J Med 327:782–3, 1992.

Website: www.pdr.net

Adefovir dipivoxil (Hepsera)

Drug Class: Antihepatitis B drug.

Usual Dose: 10 mg (PO) q24h.

Pharmacokinetic Parameters:

Peak serum level: 18 ng/mL

Bioavailability: 59%

Excreted unchanged (urine): 45%

Serum half-life (normal/ESRD): 7.5/9 hrs

Plasma protein binding: 4%

Volume of distribution (V_d): 0.4 L/kg

Primary Mode of Elimination: Renal

Dosage Adjustments*

CrCl ≥ 50 mL/min	10 mg (PO) q24h
CrCl 20–50 mL/min	10 mg (PO) q48h
CrCl 10–20 mL/min	10 mg (PO) q72h
Hemodialysis	10 mg (PO) q7days
Post–HD or PD dose	10 mg (PO)

"Usual dose" assumes normal renal/hepatic function. * For renal insufficiency, give usual dose × 1 followed by maintenance dose per CrCl. For dialysis patients, dose the same as for CrCl < 10 mL/min and give supplemental (post-HD/PD dose) immediately after dialysis. CrCl = creatinine clearance; CVVH = continuous veno-venous hemofiltration; HD/PD = hemodialysis/peritoneal dialysis.

| CVVH/CVVHD/ CVVHDF dose | 10 mg (PO) q72h |
| Moderate—severe hepatic insufficiency | No change |

Drug Interactions: No significant interaction with lamivudine, TMP–SMX, acetaminophen, ibuprofen.

Adverse Effects: Asthenia, headache, abdominal pain, nausea, flatulence, diarrhea, dyspepsia.

Allergic Potential: Low

Safety in Pregnancy: C

Comments: May be taken with or without food. Does not inhibit CP450 isoenzymes. Do not discontinue abruptly to avoid exacerbation of HBV hepatitis.

Cerebrospinal Fluid Penetration: No data

REFERENCES:

Buti M, Esteban R. Adefovir dipivoxil. Drugs of Today 39:127–35, 2003.

Cundy KC, Burditch-Crovo P, Walker RE, et al. Clinical pharmacokinetics of adefovir in human HIV-1 infected patients. Antimicrob Agents Chemother 35:2401–2405, 1995.

Lu H, Geng DY, Shen F, et al. Optimization of adefovir dipivoxil therapy in chronic hepatitis B according to baseline predictors and on-treatment HBV DNA: a 5-Year prospective study. Virol J 8:444, 2011.

Segovia MC, Chacra W, Gordon SC. Adefovir dipivoxil in chronic hepatitis B: history and current uses. Expert Opin Pharmacother 13:245–254, 2012.

Sheng YJ, Liu JY, Tong SW, et al. Lamivudine plus adefovir combination therapy versus entecavir monotherapy for lamivudine-resistant chronic hepatitis B: a systematic review and meta-analysis. Virol J 8:393, 2011.

Yang HJ, Lee JH, Kim YJ, et al. Antiviral efficacy of combination therapy with entecavir and adefovir for entecavir/lamivudine-resistant hepatitis B virus with or without adefovir resistance. J Med Virol 84:424–430, 2012.

Website: www.hepsera.com

Amantadine (Symmetrel)

Drug Class: Antiviral (influenza A).

Usual Dose: 200 mg (PO) q24h.

Pharmacokinetic Parameters:

Peak serum level: 0.5 mcg/mL

Bioavailability: 90%

Excreted unchanged (urine): 90%

Serum half-life (normal/ESRD): 16/192 hrs

Plasma protein binding: 67%

Volume of distribution (V_d): 6.6 L/kg

Primary Mode of Elimination: Renal

Dosage Adjustments*

CrCl > 30 mL/min	100 mg (PO) q24h
CrCl 15–30 mL/min	100 mg (PO) q48h
CrCl < 15 mL/min	200 mg (PO) q week
Post–HD	None
Post–PD	None
CVVH/CVVHD/ CVVHDF dose	100 mg (PO) q48h
Moderate—severe hepatic insufficiency	No change

Drug Interactions: Alcohol (↑ CNS effects); benztropine, trihexyphenidyl (↑ interacting drug effect: dry mouth, ataxia); CNS stimulants (additive stimulation); digoxin (↑ digoxin levels); trimethoprim (↑ amantadine and trimethoprim levels); scopolamine (↑ scopolamine effect: blurred vision, slurred speech, toxic psychosis).

Adverse Effects: Confusion/delusions, insomnia, dysarthria, ataxia, anticholinergic effects (blurry vision, dry mouth, orthostatic hypotension, urinary retention, constipation), livedo reticularis, may ↑ QT_c interval.

Allergic Potential: Low

Safety in Pregnancy: C

"Usual dose" assumes normal renal/hepatic function. * For renal insufficiency, give usual dose × 1 followed by maintenance dose per CrCl. For dialysis patients, dose the same as for CrCl < 10 mL/min and give supplemental (post-HD/PD dose) immediately after dialysis. CrCl = creatinine clearance; CVVH = continuous veno-venous hemofiltration; HD/PD = hemodialysis/peritoneal dialysis.

Comments: May precipitate heart failure. Avoid co-administration with anticholinergics, MAO inhibitors, or antihistamines. Resistant to amantadine, widespread may improve peripheral airway function/oxygenation in ventilated patients with severe influenza (human, avian, swine). *Highly active against influenza A. No activity against other viruses.*

Cerebrospinal Fluid Penetration:
Non-inflamed meninges = 15%
Inflamed meninges = 20%

REFERENCES:
Cunha BA, Amantadine may be lifesaving in severe influenza A. Clin Infect Dis 43:1372–3, 2006.
Gubareva LV, Kaiser L, Hayden FG. Influenza virus neuraminidase inhibitors. Lancet 355:827–5, 2000.
Jackson RJ, Cooper KL, Tappenden P, et al. Oseltamivir, zanamivir and amantadine in the prevention of influenza: A systematic review. J Infect 62:14–25, 2011.
Kawai N, Ikematsu H, Iwaki N, et al. Factors influencing the effectiveness of oseltamivir and amantadine for the treatment of influenza: A multicenter study from Japan of the 2002–2003 influenza season. Clin Infect Dis 40:1309–16, 2005.
Keyers LA, Karl M, Nafziger AN, et al. Comparison of central nervous system adverse effects of amantadine and rimantadine used as sequential prophylaxis of influenza A in elderly nursing home patients. Arch Intern Med 160:1485–8, 2000.
Website: www.pdr.net

Amikacin (Amikin)

Drug Class: Aminoglycoside.
Usual Dose: 1 gm or 15 mg/kg (IV) q24h (preferred to q12h dosing).
Spectrum: (see *Susceptibility Profiles* pp. 198–202).
Resistance Potential: Low
Pharmacokinetic Parameters:
Peak serum level 65–75 mcg/mL (q24h dosing): 20–30 mcg/mL (q12h dosing)

Bioavailability: Not applicable
Excreted unchanged (urine): 95%
Serum half-life (normal/ESRD): 2/50 hrs
Plasma protein binding: < 5%
Volume of distribution (V_d): 0.25 L/kg
Primary Mode of Elimination: Renal
Dosage Adjustments*

CrCl 50–80 mL/min	500 mg (IV) q24h or 7.5 mg/kg (IV) q24h
CrCl 10–50 mL/min	500 mg (IV) q48h or 7.5 mg/kg (IV) q48h
CrCl < 10 mL/min	250 mg (IV) q48h or 3.75 mg/kg (IV) q48h
Post–HD dose	500 mg (IV) or 7.5 mg/kg (IV)
Post–HFHD dose	500 mg (IV) or 7.5 mg/kg (IV)
Post–PD dose	250 mg (IV) or 3.75 mg/kg (IV)
CVVH/CVVHD/ CVVHDF dose	500 mg (IV) q48h or 7.5 mg/kg (IV)
Moderate—severe hepatic insufficiency	No change

Drug Interactions: Amphotericin B, cephalothin, cyclosporine, enflurane, methoxyflurane, NSAIDs, polymyxin B, radiographic contrast, vancomycin (↑ nephrotoxicity); cis-platinum (↑ nephrotoxicity, ↑ ototoxicity); loop diuretics (↑ ototoxicity); neuromuscular blocking agents (↑ apnea, prolonged paralysis); non-polarizing muscle relaxants (↑ apnea).

Adverse Effects: Neuromuscular blockade with rapid infusion/absorption. Nephrotoxicity only with prolonged/extremely high serum trough levels; may cause reversible non–oliguric renal failure (ATN). Ototoxicity associated

---

"Usual dose" assumes normal renal/hepatic function. * For renal insufficiency, give usual dose × 1 followed by maintenance dose per CrCl. For dialysis patients, dose the same as for CrCl < 10 mL/min and give supplemental (post-HD/PD dose) immediately after dialysis. CrCl = creatinine clearance; CVVH = continuous veno-venous hemofiltration; HD/PD = hemodialysis/peritoneal dialysis.

with prolonged/extremely high peak serum levels (usually irreversible): Cochlear toxicity (1/3 of ototoxicity) manifests as decreased high frequency hearing, but deafness is unusual. Vestibular toxicity (2/3 of ototoxicity) develops before ototoxicity (typically manifests as tinnitus).

Allergic Potential: Low
Safety in Pregnancy: D
Comments: Synergy dose: 500 mg (IV) q24h or 7.5 mg/kg (IV) q24h. **Single daily dosing virtually eliminates nephrotoxic/ ototoxic potential.** Incompatible with solutions containing β-lactams, erythromycin, chloramphenicol, furosemide, sodium bicarbonate. IV infusion should be given slowly over 30 minutes. May be given IM. Intraperitoneal infusion ↑ risk of neuromuscular blockade. Avoid intratracheal/ aerosolized intrapulmonary instillation, which may predispose to antibiotic resistance. V_d increases with edema/ascites, trauma, burns, cystic fibrosis; may require ↑ dose. V_d decreases with dehydration, obesity; may require ↓ dose. **Renal cast counts are the best indicator of aminoglycoside nephrotoxicity, not serum creatinine.** Dialysis removes ~ 50% of amikacin from serum. **CAPD dose:** 10–20 mg/L in dialysate (IP) with each exchange.

Therapeutic Serum Concentrations (for therapeutic efficacy, *not toxicity*): Peak (q24h/q12h dosing): 65–75/20–30 mcg/mL Trough (q24h/q12h dosing): 0/4–8 mcg/mL
Intrathecal (IT) dose: 10–40 mg (IT) q24h.
Cerebrospinal Fluid Penetration:
Non-Inflamed meninges = 15%
Inflamed meninges = 20%
Bile Penetration: 30%

REFERENCES:
Cunha BA. Aminoglycosides: Current role in antimicrobial therapy. Pharmacotherapy 8:334–50, 1988.
Cunha BA. New uses for older antibiotics: nitrofurantoin, amikacin, colistin, polymyxin B, doxycycline, and minocycline revisited. Med Clin North Am 90:1089–107, 2006.
Cunha BA. Pseudomonas aeruginosa: Resistance and therapy. Semin Respir Infect 17:231–9, 2002.
Edson RS, Terrel CL. The Aminoglycosides. Mayo Clin Proc 74:519–28, 1999.
Fulnecky E, Wright D, Scheld WM, et al. Amikacin and colistin for treatment of Acinetobacter baumanni meningitis. Journal of Infection 51;e249–e251, 2005.
Layeux B, Taccone FS, Fagnoul D, et al. Amikacin monotherapy for sepsis caused by panresistant Pseudomonas aeruginosa. Antimicrob Agents Chemother 54:4939–4941, 2010.
Le J, McKee B, Srisupha-Olarn W, Burgess Ds. In vitro activity of carbapenems alone and in combination with amikacin against KPC-producing Klebsiella pneumoniae. J Clin Med Res 3:106–110, 2011.
Pankuch GA, Seifert H, Appelbaum PC. Activity of doripenem with and without levofloxacin, amikacin, and colistin against Pseudomonas aeruginosa and Acinetobacter baumannii. Diagn Microbiol Infect Dis 67:191–197, 2010.
Taccone FS, de Backer D, Laterre PF, et al. Pharmacokinetics of a loading dose of amikacin in septic patients undergoing continuous renal replacement therapy. Int J Antimicrob Agents 37:531–535, 2011.
Taccone FS. Optimizing amikacin regimens in septic patients. Int J Antimicrob Agents. 39:264–264, 2012.

Amoxicillin (Amoxil, A-cillin, Polymox, Trimox, Wymox)

Drug Class: Aminopenicillin.
Usual Dose: 1 gm (PO) q8h.
Spectrum: (see *Susceptibility Profiles* pp. 186–190).

"Usual dose" assumes normal renal/hepatic function. * For renal insufficiency, give usual dose × 1 followed by maintenance dose per CrCl. For dialysis patients, dose the same as for CrCl < 10 mL/min and give supplemental (post-HD/PD dose) immediately after dialysis. CrCl = creatinine clearance; CVVH = continuous veno-venous hemofiltration; HD/PD = hemodialysis/peritoneal dialysis.

Resistance Potential: Low

Pharmacokinetic Parameters:

Peak serum level: 14 mcg/mL

Bioavailability: 90%

Excreted unchanged (urine): 60%

Serum half-life (normal/ESRD): 1.3/16 hrs

Plasma protein binding: 20%

Volume of distribution (V_d): 0.26 L/kg

Primary Mode of Elimination: Renal

Dosage Adjustments*

CrCl 50–80 mL/min	500 mg (PO) q8h
CrCl 10–50 mL/min	500 mg (PO) q12h
CrCl < 10 mL/min	500 mg (PO) q24h
Post–HD or post–PD	500 mg
CVVH/CVVHD/CVVHDF dose	500 mg (PO) q24h
Moderate—severe hepatic insufficiency	No change

Drug Interactions: Allopurinol (↑ risk of rash).

Adverse Effects: Drug fever/rash, ↑ SGOT/SGPT.

Allergic Potential: High

Safety in Pregnancy: B

Comments: ↑ risk of rash with EBV infectious mononucleosis. No irritative diarrhea with 1 gm (PO) q8h dose due to nearly complete proximal GI absorption. Na^+ content = 2.7 mEq/g.

Cerebrospinal Fluid Penetration:

Non-inflamed/Inflamed meninges = 1%/8%

Bile Penetration: 3000%

(also see ***Antibiotic Pearls & Pitfalls*** p. 508).

REFERENCES:

Addo-Yobo E, Chisaka N, Hassan M, et al. Oral amoxicillin versus injectable penicillin for severe pneumonia in children age 3 to 59 months: a randomized multicentre equivalency study. Lancet 364:1141–48, 2004.

Camacho MT, Casal J, AGuilar L, et al. Very high resistance to amoxicillin in Streptococcus pneumoniae: an epidemiological fact or a technical issue? Journal of Chemotherapy 18:303–06, 2006.

Cunha BA. Oral antibiotic therapy of serious systemic infections. Med Clin N Am 90:1197–1222, 2006.

Cunha BA. The aminopenicillins. Urology 40:186–190, 1992.

Curtin-Wirt C, Casey JR, Murray PC, et al. Efficacy of penicillin vs. amoxicillin in children with group A beta hemolytic streptococcal tonsillopharyngitis. Clin Pediatr 42:219–24, 2003.

Dhaon NA. Amoxicillin tablets for oral suspension in the treatment of acute otitis media: a new formulation with improved convenience. Adv Ther 21:87–95, 2004.

File Jr. TM, Clinical implications and treatment of multiresistant Streptococcus pneumoniae pneumonia. Clin Microbiol Infect 12:31–41, 2006.

Garbutt JM, Banister C, Spitznagel E, et al. Amoxicillin for acute rhinosinusitis: a randomized controlled trail. JAMA 15:685–92, 2012.

Moreillon P, Wilson WR, Leclercq R, et al. Single-dose oral amoxicillin or linezolid for prophylaxis of experimental endocarditis due to vancomycin-susceptible and vancomycin-resistant Enterococcus faecalis. Antimicrob Agents Chemother 51:1661–1665, 2007.

Piglansky L, Leibovitz E, Raiz S, et al. Bacteriologic and clinical efficacy of high dose amoxicillin for therapy of acute otitis media in children. Pediatr Infect Dis J 22:405–13, 2003.

Ready D, Lancaster H, Qureshi F, et al. Effect of amoxicillin use on oral microbiota in young children. Antimicrob Agents Chemother 48:2883–7, 2004.

Website: www.pdr.net

Amoxicillin/Clavulanic Acid (Augmentin)

Drug Class: Aminopenicillin/β-lactamase inhibitor.

Usual Dose: 500/125 mg (PO) q8h or 875/125 mg (PO) q12h for severe infections or respiratory tract infections.

"Usual dose" assumes normal renal/hepatic function. * For renal insufficiency, give usual dose × 1 followed by maintenance dose per CrCl. For dialysis patients, dose the same as for CrCl < 10 mL/min and give supplemental (post-HD/PD dose) immediately after dialysis. CrCl = creatinine clearance; CVVH = continuous veno-venous hemofiltration; HD/PD = hemodialysis/peritoneal dialysis.

Spectrum: (see *Susceptibility Profiles* pp. 186–190).

Resistance Potential: Low

Pharmacokinetic Parameters:

Peak serum level: 10.0/2.2 mcg/mL
Bioavailability: 90/60%
Excreted unchanged (urine): 80/40%
Serum half-life (normal/ESRD): [1.3/16]/[½] hrs
Plasma protein binding: 18/25%
Volume of distribution (V_d): 0.26/0.3 L/kg

Primary Mode of Elimination: Renal

Dosage Adjustments* (based on 500 mg q8h)

CrCl 10–50 mL/min	500/125 mg (PO) q12h
CrCl < 10 mL/min	250/125 mg (PO) q24h
Post–HD dose	250/125 mg (PO)
Post–PD dose	250/125 mg (PO)
CVVH/CVVHD/CVVHDF dose	500/125 mg (PO) q24h
Moderate—severe hepatic insufficiency	No change

Drug Interactions: Allopurinol (↑ risk of rash).

Adverse Effects: Drug fever/rash, diarrhea, ↑ SGOT/SGPT. Rash potential same as ampicillin.

Resistance Potential: Low

Allergic Potential: High

Safety in Pregnancy: B

Comments: ↑ risk of rash with EBV infectious mononucleosis. **875/125 mg formulation should not be used in patients with CrCl < 30 mL/min.**

Cerebrospinal Fluid Penetration:

Non-Inflamed meninges = 1%

Inflamed meninges = 1%

Bile Penetration: 3000%

(also see *Antibiotic Pearls & Pitfalls* p. 508).

REFERENCES:

Cunha BA. Amoxicillin/clavulanic acid in respiratory infections: microbiologic and pharmacokinetic considerations. Clinical Therapeutics 14:418–25, 1992.

Donowitz GR, Mandell GL. Beta-lactam antibiotics. N Engl J Med 318:419–26 and 318:490–500, 1993.

Fernandez-Sabe N, Carratala J, Dorca J, et al. Efficacy and safety of sequential amoxicillin-clavulanate in the treatment of anaerobic lung infections. Eur J Clin Microbiol Infect Dis 22:185–7, 2003.

File TM Jr, Lode H, Kurz H, et al. Double-blind, randomized study of the efficacy and safety of oral pharmacokinetically enhanced amoxicillin-clavulanic (2,000/125 milligrams) versus those of amoxicillin-clavulanic (875/125 milligrams), both given twice daily for 7 days, in treatment of bacterial community-acquired pneumonia adults. Antimicrob Agents Chemother 48:3323–31, 2004.

Malingoni MA, Song J, Herrington J, et al. Randomized controlled trial of moxifloxacin compared with piperacillin-tazobactam and amoxicillin-clavulanate for the treatment of complicated intra-abdominal infections. Ann Surg 244:204–11, 2006.

Scaglione F, Caronzolo D, Pintucci JP, et al. Measurement of cefaclor and amoxicillin-clavulanic acid levels in middle-ear fluid in patients with acute otitis media. Antimicrob Agents Chemother 47:2987–9, 2003.

Vons C, Barry C, Maitre S, et al. Amoxicillin plus clavulanic acid versus appendicectomy for treatment of acute uncomplicated appendicitis: an open-label, non-inferiority, randomized controlled trial. Lancet 377:1573–1579, 2011.

Wright AJ, Wilkowske CJ. The penicillins. Mayo Clin Proc 66:1047–63, 1991.

Website: www.augmentin.com

Amoxicillin/Clavulanic Acid ES-600 (Augmentin ES-600)

Drug Class: Aminopenicillin/β-lactamase inhibitor.

Usual Dose: 90 mg/kg/day oral suspension in 2 divided doses (see comments).

Spectrum: (see *Susceptibility Profiles* pp. 186–190).

"Usual dose" assumes normal renal/hepatic function. * For renal insufficiency, give usual dose × 1 followed by maintenance dose per CrCl. For dialysis patients, dose the same as for CrCl < 10 mL/min and give supplemental (post-HD/PD dose) immediately after dialysis. CrCl = creatinine clearance; CVVH = continuous veno-venous hemofiltration; HD/PD = hemodialysis/peritoneal dialysis.

Resistance Potential: Low
Pharmacokinetic Parameters:
Peak serum level: 15.7/1.7 mcg/mL
Bioavailability: 90/60%
Excreted unchanged (urine): 70/40%
*Serum half-life (normal/ESRD): [1.4/16]/
[1.1/2] hrs*
Plasma protein binding: 18%/25%
Volume of distribution (V_d): 0.26/0.3 L/kg
Primary Mode of Elimination: Renal
Dosage Adjustments*

CrCl < 30 mL/min	Avoid
Moderate—severe hepatic insufficiency	Use with caution

Drug Interactions: Allopurinol (↑ risk of rash).
Adverse Effects: Drug fever/rash, diarrhea,
↑ SGOT/SGPT. Rash potential same as ampicillin.
Allergic Potential: High
Safety in Pregnancy: B
Comments: 5 mL contains 600 mg amoxicillin and
42.9 mg clavulanatic acid. Take at start of meal
to minimize GI upset. **Do not substitute 400 mg
or 200 mg/5 mL formulation for ES-600.** Not
for children < 3 months or > 40 kg. Contains
phenylalanine.
Volume of ES-600 to provide 90 mg/kg/day:

Weight	Volume (q12h)	Weight	Volume (q12h)
8 kg	3.0 mL	24 kg	9.0 mL
12 kg	4.5 mL	28 kg	10.5 mL
16 kg	6.0 mL	32 kg	12.0 mL
20 kg	7.5 mL	36 kg	13.5 mL

Cerebrospinal Fluid Penetration:
Non-Inflamed meninges = 1%
Inflamed meninges = 1%

Bile Penetration: 3000%
(also see *Antibiotic Pearls & Pitfalls*
p. 508).

REFERENCES:
Chung KP, Huang YT, Lee LN, et al. Alarmingly
decreasing rates of amoxicillin-clavulanate
susceptibility among clinical isolates of Haemophilus
influenzae from 2001 to 2009 in a medical center in
Taiwan. J Infect 62:185–187, 2011.
Easton J, Noble S, Perry CM. Amoxicillin/clavulanic acid:
a review of its use in the management of paediatric
patients with acute otitis media. Drugs 63:311–40,
2003.
Ghaffar F, Muniz LS, Katz K, et al. Effects of large
dosages of amoxicillin/clavulanate or azithromycin
on nasopharyngeal carriage of Streptococcus
pneumoniae, Haemophilus influenzae,
nonpneumococcal alpha-hemolytic streptococci, and
Staphylococcus aureus in children with acute otitis
media. Clin Infect Dis 34:1301–9, 2002.
Website: www.augmentin.com

Amoxicillin/Clavulanic Acid XR (Augmentin XR)

Drug Class: Aminopenicillin/β-lactamase
inhibitor.
Usual Dose: 2000/125 mg (2 tablets) (PO)
q12h (see comments).
Spectrum: (see *Susceptibility Profiles*
pp. 186–190).
Resistance Potential: Low
Pharmacokinetic Parameters:
Peak serum level: 17/2 mcg/mL
Bioavailability: 90/60%
Excreted unchanged (urine): 70/40%
Serum half-life (normal/ESRD): [1.3/16]/[½] hrs
Plasma protein binding: 18/25%
Volume of distribution (V_d): 0.26/0.3 L/kg
Primary Mode of Elimination: Renal

"Usual dose" assumes normal renal/hepatic function. * For renal insufficiency, give usual dose × 1 followed by maintenance dose per CrCl. For dialysis patients, dose the same as for CrCl < 10 mL/min and give supplemental (post-HD/PD dose) immediately after dialysis. CrCl = creatinine clearance; CVVH = continuous veno-venous hemofiltration; HD/PD = hemodialysis/peritoneal dialysis.

Dosage Adjustments*

CrCl > 30 mL/min	No change
CrCl < 30 mL/min	Avoid
Post–HD/PD dose	Avoid
CVVH/CVVHD/ CVVHDF dose	Avoid
Moderate–severe hepatic insufficiency	Use with caution

Drug Interactions: Allopurinol (↑ risk of rash);
may ↓ effectiveness of oral contraceptives.
Adverse Effects: Drug fever, rash, diarrhea,
↑ SGOT/SGPT, nausea, abdominal pain.
Allergic Potential: High
Safety in Pregnancy: B
Comments: Amoxicillin/clavulanic acid XR
is a time-released formulation. Do not crush
tablets. XR formulation contains a different
ratio of amoxicillin/clavulanic acid so other
formulations cannot be interchanged. 2 tablets
(1000/62.5 mg per tablet) 2000/125 mg per
dose. **2 gm amoxicillin effective against
most strains of PRSP**. Take with food (not
high fat meal) to increase absorption.
Cerebrospinal Fluid Penetration:
Non-Inflamed meninges = 1%
Inflamed meninges = 1%
Bile Penetration: 3000%
(also see **Antibiotic Pearls & Pitfalls**
p. 508).

REFERENCES:

Augmentin XR. Med Lett Drugs Ther. 45:5–6, 2003.

Benninger MS. Amoxicillin/clavulanate potassium
extended release tablets: a new antimicrobial
for the treatment of acute bacterial sinusitis and
community-acquired pneumonia. Expert Opin
Pharmacother. 4:1839–46, 2003.

File Jr TM, Jacobs M, Poole M, et al. Outcome of treatment
of respiratory tract infections due to Streptococcus
pneumoniae, including drug-resistant strains, with
pharmacokinetically enhanced amoxicillin/clavulatate.
International J Antimicrobial Agents 20:235–247, 2002.

Kaye C, Allen A, Perry S, et al. The clinical
pharmacokinetics of a new pharmacokinetically
enhanced formulation of amoxicillin/clavulatate. Clin
Therapeutics 23:578–584, 2001.

Website: www.augmentin.com

Amphotericin B (Fungizone)

Drug Class: Antifungal.
Usual Dose: 0.5–0.8 mg/kg (IV) q24h.
Pharmacokinetic Parameters:
Peak serum level: 1–2 mcg/mL
Bioavailability: Not applicable
Excreted unchanged (urine): 5%
Serum half-life (normal/ESRD): 15/48 days
Plasma protein binding: 90%
Volume of distribution (V_d): 4 L/kg
Primary Mode of Elimination: Metabolized
Dosage Adjustments*

CrCl 10–50 mL/min	No change
Post–HD or post–PD dose	None
Post–HFHD dose	No change
CVVH/CVVHD/ CVVHDF dose	No change
Moderate–severe hepatic insufficiency	No change

Drug Interactions: Adrenocorticoids
(hypokalemia); aminoglycosides, cyclosporine,
polymyxin B (↑ nephrotoxicity); digoxin (↑ digitalis
toxicity due to hypokalemia); flucytosine
(↑ flucytosine levels if amphotericin B produces
renal dysfunction); neuromuscular blocking agents
(↑ neuromuscular blockade due to hypokalemia).
Adverse Effects: Fevers/chills, flushing
thrombophlebitis, bradycardia, seizures,
hypotension, distal renal tubular acidosis
(↓ K$^+$/↓ Mg^{++}), anemia, pancreatitis. If renal

"Usual dose" assumes normal renal/hepatic function. * For renal insufficiency, give usual dose × 1 followed by
maintenance dose per CrCl. For dialysis patients, dose the same as for CrCl < 10 mL/min and give supplemental
(post-HD/PD dose) immediately after dialysis. CrCl = creatinine clearance; CVVH = continuous veno-venous
hemofiltration; HD/PD = hemodialysis/peritoneal dialysis.

insufficiency is secondary to amphotericin, either ↓ daily dose by 50%, give dose every other day, or switch to an amphotericin lipid formulation.

Allergic Potential: Low

Safety in Pregnancy: B

Comments: Higher doses (1–1.5 mg/kg q24h) may be needed in life-threatening situations but are nephrotoxic and should only be administered under expert supervision. Do not co-administer in same IV with other drugs. Give by slow IV infusion over 2 hours initially. Aggressive hydration (1–2 liters/d) may reduce nephrotoxicity. **Test dose unnecessary.** Amphotericin B with granulocyte colony stimulating factor (GCSF) may result in ARDS. Amphotericin B with pentamidine may cause acute tubular necrosis in HIV patients. **Fevers/chills may be reduced by meperidine, aspirin, NSAIDs, hydrocortisone or acetamino-phen, if given 30–60 minutes before infusion. Bladder irrigation dose:** 50 mg/L until cultures are negative.

Highly active against Candida (↓ susceptibility to C. glabrata, C. krusei), Cryptococcus, Histoplasmosis, Blastomycosis, Sporotrichosis, Penicillum marneffei, Paracoccidiomycosis, Coccidiomycosis. Some activity against Fusarium, Naegleria, Leishmania, Malassezia or Mucor. No activity against C. lusitaniae, Pseudoallescheria/Scedosporium or Trichosporon.

Meningeal dose = usual dose plus 0.5 mg 3–5x/week (IT) via Ommaya reservoir.

Cerebrospinal Fluid Penetration: < 10%

REFERENCES:

Arikan S, Lozano-Chiu M, Paetznick V, et al. In vitro synergy of caspofungin and amphotericin B against Aspergillus and Fusarium spp. Antimicrob Agents Chemother 46:245–7, 2002.

Barchiesi F, Maracci M, Baldassarri I, et al. Tolerance to amphotericin B in clinical isolates of Candida tropicalis. Diagn Microbiol Infect Dis 50:179–85, 2004.

Chocarro Martinez A, Gonzalez A, Garcia I. Caspofungin versus amphotericin B for the treatment of candidal esophagtis. Clin Infect Dis 35:107; discussion 107–8, 2002.

Cruz JM, Peacock JE Jr., Loomer L, et al. Rapid intravenous infusion of amphotericin B: A pilot study. Am J Med 93:123–30, 1992.

Deray G. Amphotericin B nephrotoxicity. J Antimicrob Chemother 49 Suppl 1:37–41, 2002.

Ellis D. Amphotericin B: spectrum and resistance. J Antimicrob Chemother 49 Suppl 1:7–10, 2002.

Gallis HA, Drew RH, Pickard WW. Amphotericin B: 30 years of clinical experience. Rev Infect Dis 12:308–29, 1990.

Gubbins PO, Heldenbrand S. Clinically relevant drug interactions of current antifungal agents. Mycoses 53:95–113, 2010.

Lewis, RE, Wiederhold NP, Klepser ME. In vitro pharmacodynamics amphotericin B, itraconazole, and voriconazole against aspergillus, fusarium, and scedosporium spp. Antimicrob Agents and Chemotherapy 49:945–951, 2005.

Lyman CA, Walsh TJ. Systemically administered antifungal agents: A review of their clinical pharmacology and therapeutic applications. Drugs 44:9–35, 1992.

Menzies D, Goel K, Cunha BA. Amphotericin B. Antibiotics for Clinicians 2:73–6, 1998.

Miceli MH, Diaz JA, Lee SA. Emerging opportunistic yeast infections. Lancet Infectious Diseases 11:142–151, 2011.

Moosa MY, Alangaden GJ, Manavathu E. Resistance to amphotericin B does not emerge during treatment for invasive aspergillosis. J Antimicrob Chemother 49:209–13, 2002.

Nivoix Y, Zamfir A, Lutun P, Kara F, et al. Combination of caspofungin and an azole or an amphotericin B formulation in invasive fungal infections. J Infect 52:67–74, 2006.

Pagano L, Valentini CG, Fianchi L, et al. Treatment strategies for invasive aspergillosis in neutropenic patients: voriconazole or liposomal amphotericin-B? J Chemother 23:5–8, 2011.

Pappas PG, Chetchotisakd P, Larsen RA, et al. A phase II randomized trial of amphotericin B alone or combined with fluconazole in the treatment of HIV-associated cryptococcal meningitis. Clin Infect Dis 48:1775–1784, 2009.

Perfect JR. "Amphoterrible": In the era of broad-spectrum azoles and candins. Infections in Medicine. 23:S2, 2006.

Perfect JR, Dismukes WE, Dromer F, et al. Clinical Practice guidelines for the management of cryptococcal disease: 2010 update by the Infectious Disease Society of America. Clin Infect Dis 50:291–322, 2010.

Safdar A, Ma J, Saliba F, et al. Drug-induced nephrotoxicity caused by amphotericin B lipid complex and liposomal amphotericin B: a review and meta-analysis. Medicine (Baltimore) 89:236–244, 2010.

Website: www.pdr.net

Amphotericin B Lipid Complex (Abelcet) ABLC

Drug Class: Antifungal (see p. 525).
Usual Dose: 5 mg/kg (IV) q24h.
Pharmacokinetic Parameters:
Peak serum level: 1.7 mcg/mL
Bioavailability: Not applicable
Excreted unchanged (urine): 5%
Serum half-life (normal/ESRD): 173/173 hrs
Plasma protein binding: 90%
Volume of distribution (V_d): 131 L/kg
Primary Mode of Elimination: Metabolized
Dosage Adjustments*

CrCl < 50 mL/min	No change
Post–HD/PD dose	None
Post–HFHD dose	None
CVVH/CVVHD/CVVHDF dose	No change
Moderate–severe hepatic insufficiency	No change

Drug Interactions: Adrenocorticoids (hypokalemia); aminoglycosides, cyclosporine, polymyxin B (↑ nephrotoxicity); digoxin (↑ digitalis toxicity due to hypokalemia); flucytosine (↑ flucytosine effect); neuromuscular blocking agents (↑ neuromuscular blockade due to hypokalemia).
Adverse Effects: Fevers/chills, flushing thrombophlebitis, bradycardia, seizures, hypotension, distal renal tubular acidosis (↓ K⁺/↓ Mg⁺⁺), anemia. Fewer/less severe side effects and less nephrotoxicity than amphotericin B. Renal toxicity is dose-dependent (use caution).
Allergic Potential: Low
Safety in Pregnancy: B
Comments: See p. 525. Useful in patients unable to tolerate amphotericin B or in patients with amphotericin B nephrotoxicity. Infuse at 2.5 mg/kg/hr.
Highly active against Candida (↓ susceptibility to C. glabrata, C. krusei), Cryptococcus, Histoplasmosis, Blastomycosis, Sporotrichosis, Penicillum marneffei, Paracoccidiomycosis, Coccidiomycosis. Some activity against Fusarium, Naegleria, Leishmania, Malassezia or Mucor. No activity against C. lusitaniae, Pseudoallescheria/Scedosporium or Trichosporon.
Cerebrospinal Fluid Penetration: < 10%

REFERENCES:

Arikan S, Rex JH. Lipid-based antifungal agents: current status. Curr Pharm Des 7:393–415, 2001.

Arnold TM, Dotson E, Sarosi GA, et al. Traditional and emerging antifungal therapies. Proc Am Thorac Soc 7:222–228, 2010.

Dupont B. Overview of the lipid formulations of amphotericin B. J Antimicrob Chemother 49 Suppl 1:31–6, 2002.

Hiemenz JW, Walsh TJ. Lipid formulations of amphotericin B: Recent progress and future directions. Clin Infect Dis 2:133–44, 1996.

"Usual dose" assumes normal renal/hepatic function. * For renal insufficiency, give usual dose × 1 followed by maintenance dose per CrCl. For dialysis patients, dose the same as for CrCl < 10 mL/min and give supplemental (post-HD/PD dose) immediately after dialysis. CrCl = creatinine clearance; CVVH = continuous veno-venous hemofiltration; HD/PD = hemodialysis/peritoneal dialysis.

Miceli MH, Diaz JA, Lee SA. Emerging opportunistic yeast infections. Lancet Infectious Diseases 11:142–151, 2011.

Mondal S, Bhattacharya P, Ali N. Current diagnosis and treatment of visceral leishmaniasis. Expert Rev Anti Infect Ther 8:919–944, 2010.

Website: www.pdr.net

Amphotericin B Liposomal (AmBisome)

Drug Class: Antifungal (see p. 525).
Usual Dose: 3–6 mg/kg (IV) q24h (see comments).
Pharmacokinetic Parameters:
Peak serum level: 17–83 mcg/mL
Bioavailability: Not applicable
Excreted unchanged (urine): 5%
Serum half-life (normal/ESRD): 153 hrs/no data
Plasma protein binding: 90%
Volume of distribution (V_d): 131 L/kg
Primary Mode of Elimination: Metabolized
Dosage Adjustments*

CrCl < 50 mL/min	No change
Post–HD/PD dose	None
Post–HFHD dose	None
CVVH/CVVHD/ CVVHDF dose	No change
Moderate—severe hepatic insufficiency	No change

Drug Interactions: Adrenocorticoids (hypokalemia); aminoglycosides, cyclosporine, polymyxin B (↑ nephrotoxicity); digoxin (↑ digitalis toxicity due to hypokalemia); flucytosine (↑ flucytosine effect); neuromuscular blocking agents (↑ neuromuscular blockade due to hypokalemia).
Adverse Effect: Fevers/chills, flushing, thrombophlebitis, bradycardia, seizures, hypotension, distal renal tubular acidosis (↓ K*/↓ Mg**), anemia.
Allergic Potential: Low
Safety in Pregnancy: B
Comments: See p. 525. Less nephrotoxicity than amphotericin B and other amphotericin lipid preparations. **Empiric therapy of fungemia dose:** 3 mg/kg (IV) q24h can be used. **Suspected/ known Aspergillus dose:** 5 mg/kg (IV) q24h. **Cryptococcal meningitis dose:** 6 mg/kg (IV) q24h. *Highly active against Candida (↓ susceptibility to C. glabrata, C. krusei), Cryptococcus, Histoplasmosis, Blastomycosis, Sporotrichosis, Penicillum marneffei, Paracoccidiomycosis, Coccidiomycosis. Some activity against Fusarium, Naegleria, Leishmania, Malassezia or Mucor. No activity against C. lusitaniae, Pseudoallescheria/Scedosporium or Trichosporon.*
Cerebrospinal Fluid Penetration: < 10%

REFERENCES:

Chopra R. AmBisome in the treatment of fungal infections: the UK experience. J Antimicrob Chemother 49 Suppl 1:43–7, 2002.

Chu P, Sadullah S. The current role of amphotericin B lipid complex in managing systemic fungal infections. Curr Med Res Opin 25:3011–3020, 2009.

Hiemenz JW, Walsh TJ. Lipid formulations of amphotericin B: Recent progress and future directions. Clin Infect Dis 2:133–44, 1996.

Kuse ER, Chetchotisakd P, da Cunha CA, et al. Micafungin versus liposomal amphotericin B for candidaemia and invasive candidosis: a phase III randomised double-blind trial. Lancet 369:1519–1527, 2007.

Lequaglie C. Liposomal amphotericin B (AmBisome): efficacy and safety of low-dose therapy in pulmonary fungal infections. J Antimicrob Chemother 49 Suppl 1:49–50, 2002.

Miceli MH, Diaz JA, Lee SA. Emerging opportunistic yeast infections. Lancet Infectious Diseases 11:142–151, 2011.

"Usual dose" assumes normal renal/hepatic function. * For renal insufficiency, give usual dose × 1 followed by maintenance dose per CrCl. For dialysis patients, dose the same as for CrCl < 10 mL/min and give supplemental (post-HD/PD dose) immediately after dialysis. CrCl = creatinine clearance; CVVH = continuous veno-venous hemofiltration; HD/PD = hemodialysis/peritoneal dialysis.

Safdar A, Ma J, Saliba F, et al. Drug-induced nephrotoxicity caused by amphotericin B lipid complex and liposomal amphotericin B: a review and meta-analysis. Medicine (Baltimore) 89:236–244, 2010.
Website: www.ambisome.com

Amphotericin B Cholesteryl Sulfate Complex (Amphotec), ABCD (amphotericin B colloidal dispersion)

Drug Class: Antifungal (see p. 525).
Usual Dose: 3–4 mg/kg (IV) q24h.
Pharmacokinetic Parameters:
Peak serum level: 2.9 mcg/mL
Bioavailability: Not applicable
Excreted unchanged (urine): 5%
Serum half-life (normal/ESRD): 39/29 hrs
Plasma protein binding: 90%
Volume of distribution (V_d): 4 L/kg
Primary Mode of Elimination: Metabolized
Dosage Adjustments*

CrCl < 50 mL/min	No change
Post–HD/PD dose	None
Post–HFHD dose	None
CVVH/CVVHD/CVVHDF dose	None
Moderate–severe hepatic insufficiency	No change

Drug Interactions: Adrenocorticoids (hypokalemia); aminoglycosides, cyclosporine, polymyxin B (↑ nephrotoxicity); digoxin (↑ digitalis toxicity due to hypokalemia); flucytosine (↑ flucytosine effect); neuromuscular blocking agents (↑ neuromuscular blockade due to hypokalemia).
Adverse Effects: Fevers/chills, flushing, thrombophlebitis, bradycardia, seizures,

hypotension, distal renal tubular acidosis (↓ K+/↓ Mg++), anemia. Fewer/less severe side effects/less nephrotoxicity vs. amphotericin B.
Allergic Potential: Low
Safety in Pregnancy: B
Comments: See p. 525. Reconstitute in sterile water, not dextrose, saline or bacteriostatic water. Do not co-administer with in same IV line with other drugs. Give by slow IV infusion over 2 hours (1 mg/kg/hr). Test dose unnecessary.
Highly active against Candida
(↓ susceptibility to C. glabrata C. krusei),
Cryptococcus, Histoplasmosis, Blastomycosis,
Sporotrichosis, Penicillum marneffei,
Paracoccidiomycosis, Coccidiomycosis.
Some activity against Fusarium, Naegleria,
Leishmania, Malassezia or Mucor.
No activity against C. lusitaniae,
Pseudoallescheria/Scedosporium or
Trichosporon.
Cerebrospinal Fluid Penetration: < 10%

REFERENCES:
De Marie S. Clinical use of liposomal and lipid-complexed amphotericin B. J Antimicrob Chemother 33:907–16, 1994.
Rapp RP, Gubbins PO, Evans ME. Amphotericin B lipid complex. Ann Pharmacother 31:1174–86, 1997.
Safdar A, Ma J, Saliba F, et al. Drug-induced nephrotoxicity caused by amphotericin B lipid complex and liposomal amphotericin B: a review and meta-analysis. Medicine (Baltimore) 89:236–244, 2010.
Website: www.pdr.net

Ampicillin (various)

Drug Class: Aminopenicillin.
Usual Dose: 2 gm (IV) q4h, 500 mg (PO) q6h.
Spectrum: (see *Susceptibility Profiles* pp. 186–190.)
Resistance Potential: High (MSSA, aerobic GNBs)

"Usual dose" assumes normal renal/hepatic function. * For renal insufficiency, give usual dose × 1 followed by maintenance dose per CrCl. For dialysis patients, dose the same as for CrCl < 10 mL/min and give supplemental (post-HD/PD dose) immediately after dialysis. CrCl = creatinine clearance; CVVH = continuous veno-venous hemofiltration; HD/PD = hemodialysis/peritoneal dialysis.

Pharmacokinetic Parameters:
Peak serum level: 48 (IV)/5 (PO) mcg/mL
Bioavailability: 50%
Excreted unchanged (urine): 90%
Serum half-life (normal/ESRD): 0.8/10 hrs
Plasma protein binding: 20%
Volume of distribution (V_d): 0.25 L/kg
Primary Mode of Elimination: Renal
Dosage Adjustments*

CrCl 50–80 mL/min	1 gm (IV) q4h
	500 mg (PO) q6h
CrCl 10–50 mL/min	1 gm (IV) q8h
	250 mg (PO) q8h
CrCl < 10 mL/min	1 gm (IV) q12h
	250 mg (PO) q12h
Post–HD dose	1 gm (IV)
	500 mg (PO)
Post–PD dose	1 gm (IV)
	250 mg (PO)
CVVH/CVVHD/ CVVHDF dose	1 gm (IV) q8h
	250 mg (PO) q12h
Moderate—severe hepatic insufficiency	No change

Drug Interactions: Allopurinol (↑ frequency of rash); warfarin (↑ INR).
Adverse Effects: Drug fever/rash, nausea, GI upset, irritative diarrhea, ↑ SGOT/SGPT, ↑ incidence of rash vs. penicillin (in patients with EBV, HIV, lymphocytic leukemias, or allopurinol), C. difficile diarrhea/colitis.
Allergic Potential: High
Safety in Pregnancy: B
Comments: Incompatible in solutions containing amphotericin B, heparin, corticosteroids, erythromycin, aminoglycosides, or metronidazole.
Na^+ content = 2.9 mEq/g.
Meningeal dose = 2 gm (IV) q4h.

Cerebrospinal Fluid Penetration:
Non-Inflamed meninges = 1%
Inflamed meninges = 10%
Bile Penetration: 3000%
(also see ***Antibiotic Pearls & Pitfalls*** p. 508).

REFERENCES:
Sakoulas G, Bayer AS, Pogliano J, et al. Ampicillin enhances daptomycin- and cationic host defense peptide-mediated killing of ampicillin- and vancomycin-resistant Enterococcus faecium. Antimicrob Agents Chemother. 56:838–844, 2012.
Wright AJ. The penicillins. Mayo Clin Proc 74:290–307, 1999.

Ampicillin/Sulbactam (Unasyn)

Drug Class: Aminopenicillin/β-lactamase inhibitor.
Usual Dose: 1.5–3 gm (IV) q6h (see comments).
Spectrum: (see ***Susceptibility Profiles*** pp. 186–190).
Resistance Potential: Low (pseudoresistance with E. coli/Klebsiella)
Pharmacokinetic Parameters:
Peak serum level: 109-150/48-88 mcg/mL
Bioavailability: Not applicable
Excreted unchanged (urine): 80/80%
Serum half-life (normal/ESRD): [1/9]/[1/9] hrs
Plasma protein binding: 28/38%
Volume of distribution (V_d): 0.25/0.38 L/kg
Primary Mode of Elimination: Renal/hepatic
Dosage Adjustments* (based on 3 gm (IV) q6h)

CrCl 30–80 mL/min	1.5 gm (IV) q6h
CrCl 15–30 mL/min	1.5 gm (IV) q12h
CrCl < 15 mL/min	1.5 gm (IV) q24h
Post–HD dose	1.5 gm (IV)

"Usual dose" assumes normal renal/hepatic function. * For renal insufficiency, give usual dose × 1 followed by maintenance dose per CrCl. For dialysis patients, dose the same as for CrCl < 10 mL/min and give supplemental (post-HD/PD dose) immediately after dialysis. CrCl = creatinine clearance; CVVH = continuous veno-venous hemofiltration; HD/PD = hemodialysis/peritoneal dialysis.

Post–PD dose	None
CVVH/CVVHD/ CVVHDF dose	1.5–3 gm (IV) q12h
Moderate—severe hepatic insufficiency	No change

Drug Interactions: Probenecid (↑ ampicillin/ sulbactam levels); allopurinol (↑ rash).

Adverse Effects: Drug fever/rash, ↑ SGOT/SGPT, hemolytic anemia, C. difficile diarrhea/colitis.

Allergic Potential: High

Safety in Pregnancy: B

Comments: Mild/moderate infection dose: 1.5 gm (IV) q6h.

Meningeal dose: 4.5 gm (IV) q6h (for susceptible strains of MDR Acinetobacter baumanii meningitis).

Na+ content = 4.2 mEq/g.

Cerebrospinal Fluid Penetration: 30%

Bile Penetration: 900%

(also see **Antibiotic Pearls & Pitfalls** p. 508).

REFERENCES:

Itokazu GS, Danziger LH. Ampicillin-sulbactam and ticarcillin-clavulanic acid: A comparison of their in vitro activity and review of their clinical efficacy. Pharmacotherapy 11:382–414, 1991.

Jain R, Danziger LH. Multidrug-resistant Acinetobacter infections: an emerging challenge to clinicians. Ann Pharmacother 38:1449–59, 2004.

Sensakovic JW, Smith LG. Beta-lactamase inhibitor combinations. Med Clin North Am 79:695–704, 1995.

Swenson JM, Killgore GE, Tenover FC. Antimicrobial susceptibility testing of Acinetobacter spp. by NCCLS broth microdilution and disk diffusion methods. J Clin Microbiol 42:5102–8, 2004.

Wood GC, Hanes SD, Croce MA, et al. Comparison of ampicillin-sulbactam and imipenem-cilastatin for the treatment of Acinetobacter ventilator-associated pneumonia. Clin Infect Dis 34:1425–30, 2002.

Wright AJ. The penicillins. Mayo Clin Proc 73:290–307, 1999.

Website: www.pdr.net

Amprenavir (Agenerase) APV

Drug Class: Antiretroviral protease inhibitor.

Usual Adult Dose: 1200 mg (PO) q12h (capsules) or 1400 mg (PO) q12h (solution); age 13–16 years < 50 kg or pediatrics 4–12 years: 20 mg/kg (PO) q12h (capsules) or 1.5 ml/kg (PO) q12h (15 mg/mL solution). Maximum dose 2400 mg/d (capsules), 2800 mg/d (oral solution).

Pharmacokinetic Parameters:

Peak serum level: 7.6 mcg/mL
Bioavailability: No data
Excreted unchanged (urine): 1%
Serum half-life (normal/ESRD): 7-10/7-10 hrs
Plasma protein binding: 90%
Volume of distribution (V_d): 6.1 L/kg

Primary Mode of Elimination: Hepatic

Dosage Adjustments*

CrCl > 10 mL/min	No change
CrCl < 10 mL/min	No change (avoid solution)
Post-HD/PD dose	No change
CVVH/CVVHD/ CVVHDF dose	No change
Moderate hepatic insufficiency	450 mg (PO) q12h (capsules)
Severe hepatic insufficiency	300 mg (PO) q12h (capsules)

Antiretroviral Dosage Adjustments

Delavirdine	Avoid
Didanosine buffered solution	Take amprenavir 1 hour before or after
Efavirenz	No data

"Usual dose" assumes normal renal/hepatic function. * For renal insufficiency, give usual dose × 1 followed by maintenance dose per CrCl. For dialysis patients, dose the same as for CrCl < 10 mL/min and give supplemental (post-HD/PD dose) immediately after dialysis. CrCl = creatinine clearance; CVVH = continuous veno-venous hemofiltration; HD/PD = hemodialysis/peritoneal dialysis.

Indinavir	No data
Lopinavir/ritonavir	May ↓ lopinavir levels
Nelfinavir	No data
Nevirapine	No data
Ritonavir	Limited data for amprenavir 600 mg q12h + ritonavir 100 mg q12h (or amprenavir 1200 mg q24h + ritonavir 200 mg q24h)
Saquinavir	No data
Rifampin	Avoid
Rifabutin	Rifabutin 150 mg q24h or 300 mg 2–3x/week

Drug Interactions: Antiretrovirals, rifabutin, rifampin (see dose adjustment grid, above); bepridil, cisapride, ergotamine, statins, benzodiazepines, St. John's wort, pimozide, sildenafil, methadone (avoid if possible); carbamazepine, phenobarbital, phenytoin (may ↓ amprenavir levels, monitor anticonvulsant levels); H$_2$ blockers, proton pump inhibitors (↓ amprenavir levels).

Adverse Effects: Rash, Stevens-Johnson Syndrome (rare), GI upset, headache, depression, taste perversion, diarrhea, perioral paresthesias, hyperglycemia (including worsening diabetes, new-onset diabetes, DKA), ↑ cholesterol/triglycerides (evaluate risk for coronary disease/pancreatitis), fat redistribution, ↑ SGOT/SGPT, possible increased bleeding in hemophilia.

Allergic Potential: High. Amprenavir is a sulfonamide; use with caution in sulfa allergy

Safety in Pregnancy: C

Comments: Can be taken with or without food, but avoid high fat meals (may ↓ absorption). High vitamin E content. Capsules and solution are not interchangeable on a mg per mg basis. Decrease dosage in moderate or severe liver disease; use with caution. Oral solution contains propylene glycol: avoid in pregnancy, hepatic/renal failure, patients taking disulfiram or metronidazole, or children < 4 years old. Effective antiretroviral therapy consists of three antiretrovirals (same/different classes) GlaxoSmithKline discontinued production and sale of amprenavir in the United States in order to focus on production of the amprenavir prodrug, fosamprenavir. This action was not taken because of concerns about safety or efficacy of amprenavir. Amprenavir may continue to be available in some countries outside the United States.

REFERENCES:

Adkins JC, Faulds D. Amprenavir. Drugs 55:837–42, 1998.

Croteau D, Letendre S, Best BM, et al. Therapeutic amprenavir concentrations in cerebrospinal fluid. Antimicrob Agents Chemother 56:1985–9, 2012.

Kappelhoff BS, Crommentuyn KM, de Maat MM, et al. Practical guidelines to interpret plasma concentrations of antiretroviral drugs. Clin Pharmacokinet 43:845–53, 2004.

Panel on Antiretroviral Guidelines for Adults and Adolescents. Department of Health and Human Services. Guidelines for the use of antiretroviral agents in HIV-infected adults and adolescents.

Thompson MA, Aberg JA, Cahn P, et al. Antiretroviral treatment of adult HIV infection: 2010. recommendations of the international AIDS society – USA panel. JAMA 304:321–333, 2010.

"Usual dose" assumes normal renal/hepatic function. * For renal insufficiency, give usual dose × 1 followed by maintenance dose per CrCl. For dialysis patients, dose the same as for CrCl < 10 mL/min and give supplemental (post-HD/PD dose) immediately after dialysis. CrCl = creatinine clearance; CVVH = continuous veno-venous hemofiltration; HD/PD = hemodialysis/peritoneal dialysis.

Anidulafungin (Eraxis, Ecalta)

Drug Class: Echinocandin antifungal.
Usual Dose: 200 mg (IV) × 1 dose, then 100 mg (IV) q24h.
Pharmacokinetic Parameters:
Peak serum level: 4.2 mg/L (100/50 mg dose)/7.2 mg/L (200/100 mg dose)
Bioavailability: Not applicable
Excreted unchanged (urine): < 1%
Serum half-life (normal/ESRD): 40–50 hours/40–50 hours
Plasma protein binding: 99%
Volume of distribution (V_d): 30–50L
Primary Mode of Elimination: Fecal (30%)
Dosage Adjustments*

CrCl < 50 mL/min	No change
Post–HD dose	None
Post–PD dose	None
CVVH/CVVHD/CVVHDF dose	No change
Moderate—severe hepatic insufficiency	No change

Drug Interactions: No significant interactions.
Adverse Effects: ↑ SGOT/SGPT/GGTP/alkaline phosphatase. Histamine-related reactions (rash, urticaria, pruritus, fever, dyspnea and hypotension) if infusion > 1.1 mg/min.
Allergic Potential: Histamine-related symptoms
Safety in Pregnancy: C
Comments: Not an inducer, inhibitor, or substrate of CYP450 system. Rate of infusion should not exceed 1.1 mg/min. Incompatible with other drugs. Do not infuse with other medications. Use reconstituted vials within 24 hours. Infusion solution should be stored at 25°C/77°F.

Highly active against Candida albicans, non-albicans Candida (↓ susceptibility to C. parasilosis).
Some activity against Aspergillus.
No activity against Cryptococcus, Fusarium, Pseudoallescheria/Scedosporium, Trichosporon, Rhodotorula or Mucor.
Cerebrospinal Fluid Penetration: No data

REFERENCES:

Bennett JE, Echinocandins for candidemia in adults without neutropenia. N Engl J Med 355:1154–9, 2006.

Cohen-Wolkowiez M, Benjamin Jr. DK, Steinbach WJ, Smith PB. Anidulafungin: A new Echinocandin for the Treatment of Fungal Infections. Drugs of Today. 42:533–44, 2006.

de la Torre P, Reboli AC. Anidulafungin: a new echinocandin for candidal infections. Expert Rev Anti Infect Ther 5:45–52, 2007.

Dowell JA, Schranz J, Baruch A, Foster G. Safety and pharmacokinetics of coadministered voriconazole and andigulafungin. J Clin Pharmacol 45:1373–82, 2005.

Dowell JA, Stogniew M, Krause D, et al. Anidulafungin does not require dosage in subjects with varying degrees of hepatic or renal impairment. J Clin Pharmacol 47:461–470, 2007.

Dowell JA, Stogniew M, Krause D, et al. Lack of pharmacokinetic interaction between anidulafungin and tacrolimus. J Clin Pharmacol 47:305–314, 2007.

Garber G, Laverdiere M, Libman M, et al. Anidulafungin versus fluconazole for invasive candidiasis. N Engl J Med 356:2472–2482, 2007.

Kofia G, Ruhnke M. Pharmacology and metabolism of anidulafungin, caspofungin and micafungin in the treatment of invasive candidosis: review of the literature. Eur J Med Res 16:159–166, 2011.

Miceli MH, Diaz JA, Lee SA. Emerging opportunistic yeast infections. Lancet Infectious Diseases 11:142–151, 2011.

Morrison VA. Echinocandin antifungals: review and update. Expert Rev Anti Infect Ther 4:325–42, 2006.

Nir-Paz R, Moses AE. Anidulafungin and fluconazole for candidiasis. N Engl J Med 357:1347–1348, 2007.

"Usual dose" assumes normal renal/hepatic function. * For renal insufficiency, give usual dose × 1 followed by maintenance dose per CrCl. For dialysis patients, dose the same as for CrCl < 10 mL/min and give supplemental (post-HD/PD dose) immediately after dialysis. CrCl = creatinine clearance; CVVH = continuous veno-venous hemofiltration; HD/PD = hemodialysis/peritoneal dialysis.

Paderu P, Garcia-Effron G, Balashov S, et al. Serum differentially alters the antifungal properties of echinocandin drugs. Antimicrob Agents Chemother 51:2253–2256, 2007.

Patel PN, Charneski L. Anidulafungin (Eraxis) for Fungal Infections. Pharmacy and Therapeutics 31:644–53, 2006.

Pfaller MA, Diekema DJ, Boyken L. Effectiveness of anidulafungin in eradicating candida species in invasive candidiasis. Antimicrob Agents Chemother 49:4795–97, 2005.

Raasch RH. Anidulafungin: review of a new echinocandin antifungal agent. Expert Rev Anti Infect Ther 2:499–508, 2004.

Reboli AC, Rotstein C, Pappas PG, et al. Anidulafungin versus fluconazole for invasive candidiasis. N Engl J Med 356:2472–2482, 2007.

Theuretzbacher U. Pharmacokinetics/pharmacodynamics of echinocandins. Eur J Clin Microbiol Infect Dis 23:805–12, 2004.

Turner MS, Drew RH, Perfect JR. Emerging echinocandins for treatment of invasive fungal infections. Expert Opin Emerg Drugs 11:231–50, 2006.

Vazquez JA, Sobel JD. Anidulafungin: a novel echinocandin. Clin Infect Dis 43:215–22, 2006.

Wiederhold NP, Lewis RE. The echinocandin antifungals: an overview of the pharmacology, spectrum and clinical efficacy. Expert Opin Investig Drugs 12:1313–33, 2003.

Wilke M. Treatment and prophylaxis of invasive candidiasis with anidulafungin, caspofungin, and micafungin and its impact on use and costs: review of the literature. Eur J Med Res 16:180–186, 2011.

Website: www.eraxisrx.com

Atazanavir (Reyataz) ATV

Drug Class: Antiretroviral protease inhibitor.
Usual Dose: 300 mg (PO) q24h with ritonavir 100 mg (PO) q24h or 400 mg (PO) q24h with food if unable to tolerate ritonavir.
Treatment Experienced Patients: 300 mg with ritonavir 100 mg once daily with food.

Pharmacokinetic Parameters:
Peak serum level: 3152 ng/mL; with ritonavir: 5233 ng/mL
Bioavailability: No data
Excreted unchanged (urine) (urine/feces): 7%/20%
Serum half-life (normal/ESRD): 6.5 hrs; with ritonavir: 8.6 hrs/no data
Plasma protein binding: 86%
Volume of distribution (V$_d$): No data
Primary Mode of Elimination: Hepatic
Dosage Adjustments*

CrCl < 50 mL/min	No change
Post–HD or PD dose	None
CVVH/CVVHD/CVVHDF dose	No change
Moderate hepatic insufficiency	300 mg (PO) q24h without ritonavir
Severe hepatic insufficiency	Avoid

Antiretroviral Dosage Adjustments

Delavirdine	No data
Didanosine	Give atazanavir 2 hrs before didanosine with food
Efavirenz	Treatment naive: atazanavir 400 mg q24h + ritonavir 100 mg q24h + efavirenz 600 mg q24h Treatment experienced: not recommended
Indinavir	Avoid combination
Nevirapine	No data
Ritonavir	Atazanavir 300 mg/d + ritonavir 100 mg/d as single daily dose with food

----

"Usual dose" assumes normal renal/hepatic function. * For renal insufficiency, give usual dose × 1 followed by maintenance dose per CrCl. For dialysis patients, dose the same as for CrCl < 10 mL/min and give supplemental (post-HD/PD dose) immediately after dialysis. CrCl = creatinine clearance; CVVH = continuous veno-venous hemofiltration; HD/PD = hemodialysis/peritoneal dialysis.

Saquinavir	↑ saquinavir (soft-gel) levels; no information
Rifampin	Avoid
Rifabutin	150 mg q48h or 3x/week

Drug Interactions: Antacids or buffered medications (↓ atazanavir levels; give atazanavir 2 hours before or 1 hour after); H₂-receptor blockers (↓ atazanavir levels). In treatment-naïve patients taking an H₂-receptor antagonist, give either atazanavir 400 mg once daily with food at least 2 hours before and at least 10 hours after the H₂-receptor antagonist, or give atazanavir 300 mg once daily with ritonavir 100 mg once daily with food, without the need for separation from the H₂-receptor antagonist. In treatment-experienced patients, give atazanavir 300 mg once daily with ritonavir 100 mg once daily with food at least 2 hours before and at least 10 hours after the H₂-receptor antagonist); antiarrhythmics (↑ amiodarone, systemic lidocaine, quinidine levels; prolongs PR interval; monitor antiarrhythmic levels); antidepressants (↑ tricyclic antidepressant levels; monitor levels); calcium channel blockers (↑ calcium channel blocker levels; ↑ PR interval; ↓ diltiazem dose by 50%; use with caution; consider ECG monitoring); clarithromycin (↑ clarithromycin and atazanavir levels; consider 50% dose reduction; consider alternate agent for infections not caused by MAI); cyclosporine, sirolimus, tacrolimus (↑ immunosuppressant levels; monitor levels); ethinyl estradiol, norethindrone (↑ oral contraceptive levels; use lowest effective oral contraceptive dose); lovastatin, simvastatin (↑ risk of myopathy, rhabdomyolysis; avoid combination); sildenafil (↑ sildenafil levels; do not give more than

25 mg q48h); tadalafil (max. 10 mg/72 hours); vardenafil (max. 2.5 mg/72 hours); St. John's wort (avoid combination); warfarin (↑ warfarin levels; monitor INR); tenofovir (tenofovir reduces systemic exposure to atazanavir).
Contraindications: atazanavir include cisapride, pimozide, rifampin, irinotecan, midazolam, triazolam, lovastatin, simvastatin, bepridil, some ergot derivatives, indinavir, PPIs, St. John's wort, rifapentine, boceprevir.
Adverse Effects: Abdominal pain, nausea, vomiting, headache, diarrhea, asthenia, anorexia, and dizziness.
Allergic Potential: Low
Safety in Pregnancy: B
Comments: Monitor LFTs in patients with HBV, HCV. Take 400 mg (two 200-mg capsules) once daily with food. Bioavailability is enhanced with food. Monitor LFTs in patients with HBV, HCV. In moderate liver disease reduce dose to 200 mg once daily. It is not recommended in patients with severe liver impairment.

REFERENCES:

Cossarini F, Salpietro S, Galli L, et al. Monotheraphy with atazanavir as a simplification strategy: results from an observational study. J Acquir Immune Defic Syndr 60:101–3, 2012.

Foca E, Ripamonti D, Motta D, et al. Unboosted atazanavir for treatment of HIV infection: rationale and recommendations for use. Drugs 72:1161–73, 2012.

Gandhi M, Ameli N, Bacchetti P, et al. Atazanavir concentration in hair in the strongest predictor of outcomes on antiretroviral therapy. Clin Infect Dis 52:1267–1275, 2011.

Havlir DV, O'Marro SD. Atazanavir: new option for treatment of HIV infection. Clin Infect Dis 38:1599–604, 2004.

Hughes PJ, Cretton-Scott E, Teague A, et al. Protease inhibitors for patients with HIV-1 infection. Pharm Ther 36:332–344, 2011.

Panel on Antiretroviral Guidelines for Adults and Adolescents. Department of Health and Human Services. Guidelines for the use of antiretroviral agents in HIV-infected adults and adolescents. http://aidsinfo.nih.gov/ConsentFiles/AdultandAdolescentGL.pdf, 2012.

Piliero PJ. Atazanavir: a novel HIV-1 protease inhibitor. Expert Opin Investig Drugs 11:1295–301, 2002.

Thompson MA, Aberg JA, Cahn P, et al. Antiretroviral treatment of adult HIV infection: 2012 recommendations of the International Antiviral society — USA panel. JAMA 308:387–402, 2012.

Atovaquone (Mepron)

Drug Class: Antiprotozoal.
Usual Dose: **PCP treatment dose:** 750 mg (PO) q12h with food. **PCP prophylaxis dose:** 1500 mg (PO) q24h with food.
Pharmacokinetic Parameters:
Peak serum level: 12–24 mcg/mL
Bioavailability: 30% (47% with food; food ↑ bioavailability by 2-fold)
Excreted unchanged (feces): 94%
Serum half-life (normal/ESRD): 2.9/2.9 days
Plasma protein binding: 99.9%
Volume of distribution (V$_d$): 0.6 L/kg
Primary Mode of Elimination: Hepatic
Dosage Adjustments*

CrCl < 80 mL/min	No change
Post–HD/PD dose	None
CVVH/CVVHD/CVVHDF dose	No change
Mild-moderate hepatic insufficiency	No change
Severe hepatic insufficiency	No change

Drug Interactions: Rifabutin, rifampin (↓ atovaquone effect); zidovudine (↑ zidovudine

levels). Rifampin decreases atovaquone levels by 50%.
Adverse Effects: Rash, nausea, diarrhea, headache, fever, cough, anemia, leukopenia, ↑ SGOT/SGPT, ↑ amylase.
Allergic Potential: Low
Safety in Pregnancy: C
Comments: **Active against T. gondii, PCP, Plasmodia, and Babesia**. Take with food.
Cerebrospinal Fluid Penetration: < 1%

REFERENCES:

Artymowicz RJ, James VE. Atovaquone: A new anti-pneumocystis agent. Clin Pharmacol 12:563–70, 1993.

Baggish AL, Hill DR. Antiparasitic agent atovaquone. Antimicrob Agents Chemother 46:1163–73, 2002.

Bonoan JT, Johnson DH, Schoch PE, Cunha BA. Life threatening babesiosis treated by exchange transfusion with azithromycin and atovaquone. Heart & Lung 27:42–8, 1998.

Haile LG, Flaherty JF. Atovaquone: a review. Ann Pharmacother 27:1488–94, 1993.

Tommasi C, Bellagamba R, Tempestilli M, et al. Marked increase in etravirine and saquinavir plasma concentrations furring atovaquone/proguanil prophylaxis. Malar J 21:141, 2011.

Wormser GP, Prasad A, Neuhaus E, et al. Emergence of resistance to azithromycin-atovaquone in immunocompromised patients with babesia microti infection. Clin Infect Dis 50:381–386, 2010.

Atovaquone + Proguanil (Malarone)

Drug Class: Antimalarial.
Usual Dose: Malaria prophylaxis: 1 tablet (250 mg/100 mg) (PO) q24h for 2 days before entering endemic area, daily during exposure, and daily × 1 week post-exposure. Malaria

---

treatment: 4 tablets (1000 mg/400 mg) (PO) as single dose × 3 days.

Pharmacokinetic Parameters:
Peak serum level: 38 mcg/mL
Bioavailability: 23/90%
Excreted unchanged (feces): 94/50%
Serum half-life (normal/ESRD):
[60/60]/[21/no data] hrs
Plasma protein binding: 99/75%
Volume of distribution (V_d): 3.5/42 L/kg

Primary Mode of Elimination: Metabolized

Dosage Adjustments*

CrCl > 30 mL/min	No change
CrCl 10–30 mL/min	Avoid (for prophylaxis)
CrCl < 10 mL/min	Avoid (for prophylaxis)
Post–HD/PD dose	Avoid
CVVH/CVVHD/ CVVHDF dose	Avoid
Mild-moderate hepatic insufficiency	No change
Severe hepatic insufficiency	No change

Drug Interactions: Chloroquine (↑ incidence of mouth ulcers); metoclopramide, rifabutin, rifampin, tetracycline (↓ atovaquone + proguanil effect); ritonavir (↑ or ↓ atovaquone + proguanil effect); typhoid vaccine (↓ typhoid vaccine effect).

Adverse Effects: Headache, dizziness, nausea, vomiting, diarrhea, abdominal pain, anorexia, myalgias, fever.

Allergic Potential: Low

Safety in Pregnancy: C

Comments: Malarone tablet = 250 mg atovaquone + 100 mg proguanil. **Effective against chloroquine sensitive/resistant strains of P. falciparum, but not P. ovale, P. vivax, or P. malariae**. Dosage may be decreased in patients with diarrhea. Take with food/milk.

Cerebrospinal Fluid Penetration: < 1%

REFERENCES:

[No authors listed.] Atovaquone/proguanil (Malarone) for malaria. Med Lett Drugs Ther 42:109–11, 2000.

Camus D, Djossou F, Schithuis HJ, et al. Atovaquone-proguanil versus chloroquine-proguanil for malaria prophylaxis in nonimmune pediatric travelers: results of an international, randomized, open-label study. Clin Infect Dis 38:1716–23, 2004.

Looareesuwan S, Chulay JD, Canfield CJ. Malarone (atovaquone and proguanil hydrochloride): a review of its clinical development for treating malaria. Malarone clinical trials study group. Am J Trop Med Hyg 60:533–41, 1999.

Marra F, Salzman JR, Ensom MH. Atovaquone-proguanil for prophylaxis and treatment of malaria. Ann Pharmacother 37:1266–75, 2003.

McKeage K, Scott L. Atovaquone/proguanil: a review of its use for the prophylaxis of Plasmodium falciparum malaria. Drugs 63:597–623, 2003.

Thapar MM, Ashton M, Lindegardh N, et al. Time-dependent pharmacokinetics and drug metabolism of atovaquone plus proguanil (Malarone) when taken as chemoprophylaxis. Eur J Clin Pharmacol 15:19–27, 2002.

Website: www.pdr.net

Azithromycin (Zithromax)

Drug Class: Macrolide (Azolide).

Usual Dose: 500 mg (IV/PO) × 1 dose, then 250 mg (IV/PO) q24h (see comments).

Spectrum: (see *Susceptibility Profiles* pp. 186–190).

Resistance Potential: High (S. pneumoniae, GAS, MSSA)

"Usual dose" assumes normal renal/hepatic function. * For renal insufficiency, give usual dose × 1 followed by maintenance dose per CrCl. For dialysis patients, dose the same as for CrCl < 10 mL/min and give supplemental (post-HD/PD dose) immediately after dialysis. CrCl = creatinine clearance; CVVH = continuous veno-venous hemofiltration; HD/PD = hemodialysis/peritoneal dialysis.

Pharmacokinetic Parameters:
Peak serum level: 1.1 (IV)/0.2 (PO) mcg/mL
Bioavailability: 35%
Excreted unchanged (urine): 6%
Serum half-life (normal/ESRD): 68/68 hrs
Plasma protein binding: 50%
Volume of distribution (V_d): 31 L/kg
Primary Mode of Elimination: Hepatic
Dosage Adjustments*

CrCl 10–50 mL/min	No change
CrCl < 10 mL/min	Use with caution
Post–HD/PD dose	None
CVVH/CVVHD/ CVVHDF dose	No change
Moderate—severe hepatic insufficiency	No change

Drug Interactions: Amiodarone,
carbamazepine, cisapride, clozapine,
corticosteroids, midazolam, triazolam, valproic
acid (not studied/not reported); cyclosporine
(↑ cyclosporine levels with toxicity); digoxin
(↑ digoxin levels); pimozide (may ↑ QT interval,
torsade de pointes).
Adverse Effects: ↑ incidence cardiac/
non-cardiac sudden deaths after 5 days
of therapy. Nausea, GI upset, non-C. difficile
diarrhea. May ↑ QT_c interval.
Allergic Potential: Low
Safety in Pregnancy: B
Comments: Bioavailability is decreased by food.
C. trachomatis urethritis dose: 1 gm (PO) ×
1 dose.
N. gonorrhoea urethritis dose: 2 gm (PO) ×
1 dose.

MAI prophylaxis dose: 1200 mg (PO) weekly.
MAI therapy dose: 600 mg (PO) q24h.

Cerebrospinal Fluid Penetration: < 10%
Bile Penetration: > 3000%

REFERENCES:
Alvarez-Elcoro S, Enzler MJ. The macrolides:
  Erythromycin, clarithromycin and azithromycin. Mayo
  Clin Proc 74:613–34, 1999.
Bergman M, Huikko S, Huovinen P, et al. Macrolide and
  azithromycin use are linked to increased macrolide
  resistance in Streptococcus pneumoniae. Antimicrob
  Agents Chemother 50:3646–3650, 2006.
Centers for Disease Control. Neisseria gonorrhoeae with
  reduced susceptibility to azithromycin. Morb Mortal
  Wkly Rep 60:579–581, 2011.
Chandra R, Liu P, Breen JD, et al. Clinical pharmacokinetics and gastrointestinal tolerability of a novel
  extended-release microsphere formulation of
  azithromycin. Clin Pharmacokinet 46:247–259, 2007.
Cochereau I, Goldschmidt P, Goepogui A, et al. Efficacy
  and safety of short duration azithromycin eye
  drops versus azithromycin single oral dose for the
  treatment of trachoma in children: a randomized,
  controlled, double-masked clinical trial. Br J
  Ophthalmol 91:667–672, 2007.
Cunha BA. Macrolides, doxycycline, and
  fluoroquinolones in the treatment of Legionnaires'
  Disease. Antibiotics for Clinicians 2:117–8, 1998.
Daneman N, McGeer A, Green K, et al. Macrolide
  resistance in bacteremic pneumococcal disease.:
  Implications for patient management. Clin Infect Dis
  43:432–438, 2006.
DuPont HL. Azithromycin for the self-treatment of
  traveler's diarrhea. Clin Infect Dis 44:347–349, 2007.
Fisher AJ. Azithromycin and bronchiolitis obliterans
  syndrome after lung transplantation: is prevention is
  better than cure? Eur Respir J 37:10–12, 2011.
Frenck RW, Mansour A, Nakhla I, et al. Short-course
  azithromycin for the treatment of uncomplicated
  typhoid fever in children and adolescents. Clin Infect
  Dis 38:951–7, 2004.
Geisler WM. Management of uncomplicated Chlamydia
  trachomatis infections in adolescents and adults:
  evidence reviewed for the 2006 Centers for Disease
  Control and Prevention sexually transmitted diseases
  treatment guidelines. Clin Infect Dis 44(S3):S77–S83,
  2007.

"Usual dose" assumes normal renal/hepatic function. * For renal insufficiency, give usual dose × 1 followed by maintenance dose per CrCl. For dialysis patients, dose the same as for CrCl < 10 mL/min and give supplemental (post-HD/PD dose) immediately after dialysis. CrCl = creatinine clearance; CVVH = continuous veno-venous hemofiltration; HD/PD = hemodialysis/peritoneal dialysis.

Griffin AT, Peyrani P, Wiemken T, et al. Macrolides versus quinolones in Legionella pneumonia: results from the Community-Acquired Pneumonia Organization international study. Int J Tuberc Lung Dis 14:495–499, 2010.

Hook EW III, Behets F, Van Damme E, et al. A phase III equivalence trial of azithromycin versus benzathine penicillin for treatment of early syphilis. J Infect Dis 201:1729–1735, 2010.

Jain R, Danzinger LH. The macrolide antibiotics: a pharmacokinetic and pharmacodynamic overview. Curr Pharm Des 10:3045–53, 2004.

Jenkins SG, Farrell DJ. Increase in Pneumococcus Macrolide Resistance, United States. Emerging Infect Dis 15:1260–1264, 2009.

Kim Y-S, Yun H-J, Shim SK, et al. A comparative trial of a single dose of azithromycin versus doxycycline for the treatment of mild scrub typhus. Clin Infect Dis 39:1329–35, 2004.

Magbanua JP, Goh BT, Michel CE, et al. Chlamydia trachomatis variant not detected by plasmid based nucleic acid amplification tests: molecular characterization and failure of single dose azithromycin. Sex Transm Infect 83:339–343, 2007.

Malhotra-Kumar S, Lammens C, Coenen S, et al. Effect of azithromycin and clarithromycin therapy on pharyngeal carriage of macrolide-resistant streptococci in healthy volunteers: a randomized, double-blind, placebo-controlled study. Lancet 369:482–490, 2007.

Mena LA, Mroczkowski TF, Nsuami M, et al. A randomized comparison of azithromycin and doxycycline for the treatment of Mycoplasma genitalium – positive urethritis in men. Clin Infect Dis 48:1649–1654, 2009.

Paradisi F, Corti G. Azithromycin. Antibiotics for Clinicians 3:1–8, 1999.

Phillips P, Chan K, Hogg R, et al. Azithromycin prophylaxis for Mycobacterium avium complex during the era of highly active antiretroviral therapy: evaluation of a provincial program. Clin Infect Dis 34:371–8, 2002.

Pichichero ME, Hoeger WJ, Casey JR. Azithromycin for the treatment of pertussis. Pediatr Infect Dis J 22:847–9, 2003.

Plouffe JF, Breiman RF, Fields BS, et al. Azithromycin in the treatment of Legionella pneumonia in patients requiring hospitalization. Clin Infect Dis 37:1475–80, 2003.

Saiman L, Marshall BC, Mayer-Hamblett N, et al. Azithromycin in patients with cystic fibrosis chronically infected with Pseudomonas aeruginosa: a randomized controlled trial. JAMA. 290:1749–5, 2003.

Savaris RF, Teixeira LM, Torres TG, et al. Comparing ceftriaxone plus azithromycin or doxycycline for pelvis inflammatory disease: a randomized controlled trial Obstet Gynecol 110:53–60, 2007.

Schlossberg D. Azithromycin and clarithromycin. Med Clin N Amer 79:803–816, 1995.

Suzuki S, Yamazaki T, Narita M. Clinical evaluation of macrolide-resistant Mycoplasma pneumoniae. Antimicrobial Agents and Chemotherapy. 50:709–12, 2006.

Swainston Harrison T, Keam SJ. Azithromycin extended release: a review of its use in the treatment of acute bacterial sinusitis and community-acquired pneumonia in the US. Drugs 773–79, 2007.

To KK, Chan KH, Fung YF, et al. Azithromycin treatment failure in macrolide-resistant Mycoplasma pneumoniae pneumonia. Eur Respir J 36:969–971, 2010.

Toltzis P, Dul M, Blumer J. Change in pneumococcal susceptibility to azithromycin during treatment for acute otitis media. Pediatr Infect Dis 26:647–649, 2007.

Topic A, Skerk V, Puntaric A, et al. Azithromycin: 1.0 or 3.0 gram dose in the treatment of patients with asymptomatic urogenital chlamydial infections. Journal of Chemotherapy 18:115–16, 2006.

Videler WJ, Badia L, Harvey RJ. Lack of efficacy of long-term, low-dose azithromycin in chronic rhinosinusitis: a randomized controlled trial. Allergy 66:1457–1468, 2011.

Wilson R, Wells AU. Azithromycin in bronchiectasis: when should it be used? Lancet. 380:627–629, 2012.

Wormser GP, Prasad A, Neuhaus E, et al. Emergence of resistance to azithromycin-atovaquone in immunocompromised patients with Babesia microti infection. Clin Infect Dis 50:381–386, 2010.

Zuckerman JM, Qamar F, Bono BR. Review of macroliders (azithromycin, clarithromycin), ketolids (telithromycin) and glycylcyclines (tigecycline). Med Clin North Am 95:761–791, 2011.

Website: www.zithromax.com

- -

"Usual dose" assumes normal renal/hepatic function. * For renal insufficiency, give usual dose × 1 followed by maintenance dose per CrCl. For dialysis patients, dose the same as for CrCl < 10 mL/min and give supplemental (post-HD/PD dose) immediately after dialysis. CrCl = creatinine clearance; CVVH = continuous veno-venous hemofiltration; HD/PD = hemodialysis/peritoneal dialysis.

Aztreonam (Azactam)

Drug Class: Monobactam.
Usual Dose: 2 gm (IV) q8h (see comments).
Spectrum: (see *Susceptibility Profiles* pp. 198–202).
Resistance Potential: Low
Pharmacokinetic Parameters:
Peak serum level: 204 mcg/mL
Bioavailability: Not applicable
Excreted unchanged (urine): 60–70%
Serum half-life (normal/ESRD): 1.7/7 hrs
Plasma protein binding: 56%
Volume of distribution (V_d): 0.2 L/kg
Primary Mode of Elimination: Renal
Dosage Adjustments* (based on 2 gm IV q8h)

CrCl 10–50 mL/min	1 gm (IV) q8h
CrCl < 10 mL/min	500 mg (IV) q8h
Post–HD dose	500 mg (IV)
Post–PD dose	500 mg (IV)
CVVH/CVVHD/ CVVHDF dose	1–2 gm (IV) q12h
Moderate hepatic insufficiency	No change
Severe hepatic insufficiency	No change

Drug Interactions: None.
Adverse Effects: None.
Allergic Potential: Low
Safety in Pregnancy: B
Comments: Incompatible in solutions containing vancomycin or metronidazole. **No cross allergenicity with penicillins, β-lactams; safe to use in penicillin allergic patients. CAPD dose:** 1 gm (IP), then 250 mg/L of dialysate (IP) with each exchange. Meningeal dose = 2 gm (IV) q6h.
Cerebrospinal Fluid Penetration:

Non-Inflamed meninges = 1%
Inflamed meninges = 40%
Bile Penetration: 300%
(also see *Antibiotic Pearls & Pitfalls* p. 511).

REFERENCES:
Assael BM. Aztreonam inhalation solution for suppressive treatment of chronic Pseudomonas aeruginosa lung infection in cystic fibrosis. Expert Rev Anti Infect Ther 9:967–973, 2011.
Brogden RN, Heal RC. Aztreonam: A review of its antibacterial activity, pharmacokinetic properties, and therapeutic use. Drugs 31:96–130, 1986.
Critchley IA, Sahm DF, Kelly LJ, et al. In vitro synergy studies using aztreonam and fluoroquinolone combinations against six species of Gram-negative bacilli. Chemotherapy 49:44–8, 2003.
Cunha BA. Aztreonam: A review. Urology 41:249–58, 1993.
Cunha BA. Cross allergenicity of penicillin with carbapenems and monobactams. J Crit Illness 13:344, 1998.
Fleming DR, Ziegler C, Baize T, et al. Cefepime versus ticarcillin and clavulanate potassium and aztreonam for febrile neutropenia therapy in high-dose chemotherapy patients. Am J Clin Oncol 26:285–8, 2003.
Gasink LB, Neil OF, Nachamkin I, et al. Risk factors for the impact of infection or colonization with aztreonam-resistant Pseudomonas aeruginosa. Infection Control and Hospital Epidemiology 28:1175–1180, 2007.
Hellinger WC, Brewer NS. Carbapenems and monobactams: Imipenem, meropenem, and aztreonam. Mayo Clin Proc 74:420–34, 1999.
Johnson, Cunha BA. Aztreonam. Med Clin North Am 79:733–43, 1995.
Jordan EF, Nye MB, Luque AE. Successful treatment of Pasteurella multocida meningitis with aztreonam. Scand J Infect Dis 39:72–74, 2007.
Zeitler K, Salvas B, Stevens V, et al. Aztreonam lysine for inhalation: new formulation of an old antibiotic. Am J Health Syst Pharm 69:107–115, 2012.
Website: www.elan.com/Products/

"Usual dose" assumes normal renal/hepatic function. * For renal insufficiency, give usual dose × 1 followed by maintenance dose per CrCl. For dialysis patients, dose the same as for CrCl < 10 mL/min and give supplemental (post-HD/PD dose) immediately after dialysis. CrCl = creatinine clearance; CVVH = continuous veno-venous hemofiltration; HD/PD = hemodialysis/peritoneal dialysis.

Boceprevir (Victrelis)

Drug Class: NS3/4A PI for HCV (genotype 1).
Usual Dose: 800 mg (PO) q7–9h with food
(+ ribavirin and peginterferon alfa).
Pharmacokinetic Parameters:
Peak serum level: 1723 mcg/L
Bioavailability: No data
Excreted unchanged: 3%
Serum half-life (normal/ESRD): 3/3 hrs
Plasma protein binding: 75%
Volume of distribution (V_d): 772 L
Primary Mode of Elimination: hepatic
Dosage Adjustments*

CrCl <10 mL/min	No change
Post–HD dose	None
Post–PD dose	None
CVVH/CVVHD/ CVVHDF dose	No change
Hepatic insufficiency	No change

Drug Interactions: Strong inhibitor of
and metabolized via CYP3A4/5. Digoxin,
trazodone, azole antifungals, colchicines,
dihydropiridine calcium channel blockers,
inhaled corticosteroids, bosentan,
atorvastatin, immunosuppressant
(↑ levels) warfarin and HIV PI (↑/↓ levels)
ethynil estradiol (↓ levels).
Contraindications: Alfuzosin,
**carbamazepine, phenobarbital, phenytoin,
rifampin, ergot derivatives, cisapride,
St. John's Wort, lovastatin, simvastatin,
drosperinone, Revatio or Adcirca,
pimozide, triazolam, inhaled salmeterol,**
Ritonavir boosted atazanavir, lopinavir,
darunavir (↓ trough levels); lopinavir/ritonavir
boosted darunavir (↓ boceprevir levels).

Adverse Effects: Nausea, vomiting,
dysgeusia, dry mouth, diarrhea, fatigue, chills
asthenia, decreased appetite, arthralgia,
dizziness, insomnia, irritability, exertional
dyspnea, alopecia, dry skin, rash, anemia,
neutropenia.
Allergic Potential: Low
Safety in Pregnancy: B for boceprevir, X for
ribavirin, (see ribavirin Drug Summary)
**Comments: Do not use as monotherapy,
only use with ribavirin and peginterferon
alfa.** No data in decompensated cirrhosis,
organ transplant, HIV, HBV coinfection or
children < 18 yo. Counsel patients if missed
dose is less than 2 hours before next dose
is due, skip missed dose. If missed dose is
more than 2 hours from next scheduled
dose, patient should take missed dose and
resume normal dosing schedule. Hormonal
contraceptives may not be reliable during
Incivek and for 2 weeks after discontinuation.
Adjust dose for decrease in hemoglobin,
neutrophils and/or platelets (see ribavirin Drug
Summary).

REFERENCES:
Bacon BR, Gordon SC, Lawitz E, et al. Boceprevir for
previously treated chronic HCV genotype 1 infection.
N Engl J Med 31:1207–1217, 2011.
Charlton M. Boceprevir (Victrelis) for HCV: V is for victory
and very complex. Hepatology 54:1882–1886, 2011.
Foote BS, Spooner LM, Belliveau PP. Boceprevir: a
protease inhibitor for the treatment of chronic
hepatitis C. Ann Pharmacother 45:1085–1093, 2011.
Hsu CS, Kao JH. Boceprevir for chronic HCV genotype 1
infection. N Engl J Med 45:176–177, 2011.
Kwo PY, Zhao R. Boceprevir: a user's guide. Clin Liver
Dis 15:15:537–553, 2011.
Limaye AR, Draganov PC, Cabrera R. Boceprevir for
chronic HCV genotype 1 infection. N Engl J Med 14:
176, 2011.

"Usual dose" assumes normal renal/hepatic function. * For renal insufficiency, give usual dose × 1 followed by
maintenance dose per CrCl. For dialysis patients, dose the same as for CrCl < 10 mL/min and give supplemental
(post-HD/PD dose) immediately after dialysis. CrCl = creatinine clearance; CVVH = continuous veno-venous
hemofiltration; HD/PD = hemodialysis/peritoneal dialysis.

Poordaj F, McCone J Jr, Bacon BR, et al. Boceprevir for Untreated chronic HCV genotype 1 infection. N Engl J Med 31:1195–1206, 2011.

Razonable R. Antiviral Drugs for Viruses Other Than Human Immunodeficiency Virus. Mayo Clinic Proceedings 86:1009–1026, 2011.

Capreomycin (Capastat)

Drug Class: Anti-TB drug.
Usual Dose: 1 gm (IM) q24h.
Pharmacokinetic Parameters:
Peak serum level: 30 mcg/mL
Bioavailability: Not applicable
Excreted unchanged (urine): 50%
Serum half-life (normal/ESRD): 5/30 hrs
Plasma protein binding: No data
Volume of distribution (V_d): 0.4 L/kg
Primary Mode of Elimination: Renal
Dosage Adjustments*

CrCl 50–80 mL/min	500 mg (IM) q24h
CrCl 10–50 mL/min	500 mg (IM) q48h
CrCl < 10 mL/min	500 mg (IM) q72h
Post–HD dose	500 mg (IM)
Post–PD dose	None
CVVH/CVVHD/CVVHDF dose	500 mg (IM) q48h
Moderate hepatic insufficiency	No change
Severe hepatic insufficiency	No change

Drug Interactions: None.
Adverse Effects: Eosinophilia, leukopenia, drug fever/rash, ototoxicity (vestibular), nephrotoxicity (glomerular/tubular).
Allergic Potential: Moderate

Safety in Pregnancy: C
Comments: Pain/phlebitis at IM injection site. Additive toxicity with aminoglycosides/viomycin.
Cerebrospinal Fluid Penetration: < 10%

REFERENCES:
Caminero JA, Sotgiu G, Zumla A, et al. Best drug treatment for multidrug-resistant and extensively drug-resistant tuberculosis. Lancet Infect Dis 10:621–629, 2010.

Davidson PT, Le HQ. Drug treatment of tuberculosis - 1992. Drugs 43:651–73, 1992.

Furin J, Nardell EA. Multidrug-resistant tuberculosis: an update on the best regimens. J Respir Dis 27:172–82, 2006.

Iseman MD. Treatment of multidrug resistant tuberculosis. N Engl J Med 329:784–91, 1993.

Website: www.pdr.net

Caspofungin (Cancidas)

Drug Class: Echinocandin antifungal.
Usual Dose: *Loading Dose* 70 mg (IV) × 1 dose, then *Maintenance Dose:* 50 mg (IV) q24h (see comments).
Pharmacokinetic Parameters:
Peak serum level:
70 mg: 12.1 (single dose)/14.83 mcg/mL (multiple dose)
50 mg: 7.6/8.7 mcg/mL (multiple dose)
Bioavailability: Not applicable
Excreted unchanged (urine): 1.4%
Serum half-life (normal/ESRD): 10/10 hrs
Plasma protein binding: 97%
Volume of distribution (V_d): No data
Primary Mode of Elimination: Hepatic
Dosage Adjustments*

CrCl < 10 mL/min	No change
Post–HD/PD dose	None

"Usual dose" assumes normal renal/hepatic function. * For renal insufficiency, give usual dose × 1 followed by maintenance dose per CrCl. For dialysis patients, dose the same as for CrCl < 10 mL/min and give supplemental (post-HD/PD dose) immediately after dialysis. CrCl = creatinine clearance; CVVH = continuous veno-venous hemofiltration; HD/PD = hemodialysis/peritoneal dialysis.

CVVH/CVVHD/ CVVHDF dose	None
Moderate hepatic insufficiency	35 mg (IV) q24h (maintenance dose after 70 mg (IV) loading dose)
Severe hepatic insufficiency	Use with caution

Drug Interactions: Carbamazepine, rifampin, dexamethasone, efavirenz, nelfinavir, nevirapine, phenytoin (↓ caspofungin levels; ↑ caspofungin maintenance dose to 70 mg/ day); cyclosporine (↑ caspofungin levels, ↑ SGOT/SGPT; co-administration is discouraged unless careful monitoring can be ensured and unless the benefit of caspofungin outweighs the risk of hepatotoxicity); tacrolimus (↓ tacrolimus levels, ↑ SGOT/SGPT).

Adverse Effects: Drug fever/rash.

Allergic Potential: Low

Safety in Pregnancy: C

Comments: Administer by slow IV infusion over 1 hour; do not give IV bolus. Do not mix/co-infuse with glucose solutions.

Highly-resistant organisms dose: 70 mg (IV) q24h. Esophageal candidiasis dose: begin therapy with 50 mg dose.

Highly active against Candida albicans and non-albicans Candida, Hansenula.

Some activity against C. parapsilosis, Aspergillus. No activity against Cryptococcus, Fusarium, Pseudoallescheria/Scedosporium, Rhodotorula, Trichosporon, or Mucor.

Cerebrospinal Fluid Penetration: 20%

REFERENCES:

Arathoon EG, Gotuzzo E, Noriega LM, et al. Randomized, double-blind, multicenter study of caspofungin versus amphotericin B for treatment of oropharyngeal and esophageal candidiasis. Antimicrob Agents Chemother 46:451–7, 2002.

Armstrong-James D, Stebbing J, John L, et al. A trial of caspofungin salvage treatment in PCP pneumonia. Thorax 66:537–538, 2011.

Barchiesi F, Spreghini E, Tomassetti S, et al. Efficacy of caspofungin against invasive Candida or invasive Aspergillus infections in neutropenic patients. Antimicrob Agents Chemother 50:2719–27, 2006.

Bennett JE, Echinocandins for candidemia in adults without neutropenia. N Engl J Med 355:1154–9, 2006.

Betts RF, Nucci M, Talwar D, et al. A multicenter, double-blind trial of a high-dose caspofungin treatment regimen versus a standard caspofungin treatment regimen for adult patients with invasive candidiasis. Clin Infect Dis 48:1676–1684, 2009.

Betts RF, Glasmacher A, Maertens J, et al. Efficacy of caspofungin against invasive Candida or invasive Aspergillus infections in neutropenic patients. Cancer 106:466–73, 2006.

Colombo AL, Ngai AL, Bourque M, et al. Caspfungin use in patients with invasive candidiasis caused by common non-albicans Candida species: review of the caspofungin database. Antimicrob Agents Chemother 54:1864–1871, 2010.

Deresinski SC, Stevens DA. Caspofungin. Clin Infect Dis 36:1445–57, 2003.

Falagas ME, Ntziora F, Betsi GI, et al. Caspofungin for the treatment of fungal infections: a systematic review of randomized controlled trials. Int J Animicrob Agents 29:136–143, 2007.

Glasmacher A, Cornely OA, Orlopp K, et al. Caspofungin treatment in severely ill, immunocompromised patients: a case-documentation study of 118 patients. J Antimicrob Chemother 57:127–34, 2006.

Hiemenz JW, Raad II, Maertens JA, et al. Efficacy of caspofungin as salvage therapy for invasive aspergillosis compared to standard therapy in a historical cohort. Eur J Clin Microbiol Infect Dis 29:1387–1394, 2010.

Hope WW, Shoham S, Walsh TJ. The pharmacology and clinical use of caspofungin. Expert Opin Drug Metab Toxicol 3:263–274, 2007.

Keating G, Figgitt D. Caspofungin: a review of its use in esophageal candidiasis, invasive candidiasis and invasive aspergillosis. Drugs 63:2235–63, 2003.

- -

"Usual dose" assumes normal renal/hepatic function. * For renal insufficiency, give usual dose × 1 followed by maintenance dose per CrCl. For dialysis patients, dose the same as for CrCl < 10 mL/min and give supplemental (post-HD/PD dose) immediately after dialysis. CrCl = creatinine clearance; CVVH = continuous veno-venous hemofiltration; HD/PD = hemodialysis/peritoneal dialysis.

Kofia G, Ruhnke M. Pharmacology and metabolism of anidulafungin, caspofungin, and micafungin in the treatment of invasive candidosis: review of the literature. Eur J Med Res 16:159–166, 2011.

Lomaestro BM. Caspofungin. Hospital Formulary 36:527–36, 2001.

Lortholary O, Desnos-Ollivier M, Sitbon K, et al. Recent exposure to caspofungin or fluconazole influences the epidemiology of candidemia: a prospective multicenter study involving 2,441 patients. Antimicrob Agents Chemother 55:532–538, 2011.

Maertens J, Raad I, Petrikkos G, et al. Efficacy and safety of caspofungin for treatment of invasive aspergillosis in patients refractory to or intolerant of conventional antifungal therapy. Clin Infect Dis 39:1563–71, 2004.

Mattiuzzi GN, Alvarado G, Giles FJ, et al. Open-label, randomized comparison of itraconazole versus caspofungin for prophylaxis in patients with hematologic malignancies. Antimicrob Agents Chemother 50:143–7, 2006.

Miceli MH, Diaz JA, Lee SA. Emerging opportunistic yeast infections. Lancet Infectious Diseases 11:142–151, 2011.

Mora-Duarte J, Betts R, Rotstein C, et al. Comparison of caspofungin and amphotericin B for invasive candidiasis. N Engl J Med 347:2020–9, 2002.

Morrison VA. Echinocandin antifungals: review and update. Expert Rev Anti Infect Ther 4:325–42, 2006.

Nevado J, De Alarcon A, Hernandez A. Caspofungin: a new therapeutic option for fungal endocarditis. Clin Microbiol Infect 11:248, 2005.

Nguyen TH, Hoppe-Tichy T, Geiss HK, et al. Factors influencing caspofungin plasma concentrations in patients of a surgical intensive care unit. J Antimicrob Chemother 60:100–106, 2007.

Nivoix Y, Zamfir A, Lutun P, Kara F, et al. Combination of caspofungin and an azole or an amphotericin B formulation in invasive fungal infections. J Infect 52:67–74, 2006.

Pappas PG, Rotstein CM, Betts RF, et al. Micafungin versus caspofungin for treatment of candidemia and other forms of invasive candidiasis. Clin Infect Dis 45:883–893, 2007.

Pfaller MA, Messer SA, Boyken L, et al. Caspofungin activity against clinical isolates of fluconazole-resistant Candida. J Clin Microbiol 41:5729–31, 2003.

Sobel JD, Bradshaw SK, Lipka CJ, et al. Caspofungin in the treatment of symptomatic candiduria. Clin Infect Dis 44:e46–e49, 2007.

Steinmann J, Buer J, Rath PM. Caspofungin: cross-reactivity in the Aspergillus antigen assay. J Clin Microbiol 48:2313, 2010.

Walsh TJ, Teppler H, Donowitz GR, et al. Caspofungin versus liposomal amphotericin B for empirical antifungal therapy in patients with persistent fever and neutropenia. N Engl J Med 351:1391–402, 2004.

Wiederhold NP, Najvar LK, Bocanegra RA, et al. Caspofungin dose escalation for invasive candidiasis due to resistant Candida albicans. Antimicrob Agents Chemother 55:3254–3260, 2011.

Wilke M. Treatment and prophylaxis of invasive candidiasis with anidulafungin, caspofungin, and micafungin and its impact on use and costs: review of the literature. Eur J Med Res 16:180–186, 2011.

Winkler M, Pratschke J, Schulz U, et al. Caspofungin for post solid organ transplant invasive fungal disease: results of a retrospective observational study. Transpl Infect Dis 12:230–237, 2010.

Website: www.cancidas.com

Cefaclor (Ceclor)

Drug Class: 2nd generation oral cephalosporin.
Usual Dose: 500 mg (PO) q8h.
Spectrum: (see *Susceptibility Profiles* pp. 191–197).
Resistance Potential: Low
Pharmacokinetic Parameters:
Peak serum level: 13 mcg/mL
Bioavailability: 80%
Excreted unchanged (urine): 60–85%
Serum half-life (normal/ESRD): 0.8/3 hrs

"Usual dose" assumes normal renal/hepatic function. * For renal insufficiency, give usual dose × 1 followed by maintenance dose per CrCl. For dialysis patients, dose the same as for CrCl < 10 mL/min and give supplemental (post-HD/PD dose) immediately after dialysis. CrCl = creatinine clearance; CVVH = continuous veno-venous hemofiltration; HD/PD = hemodialysis/peritoneal dialysis.

Plasma protein binding: 25%
Volume of distribution (V_d): 0.30 L/kg

Primary Mode of Elimination: Renal
Dosage Adjustments*

CrCl < 10 mL/min	250 mg (PO) q8h
Post–HD dose	250 mg (PO)
Post–PD dose	None
CVVH/CVVHD/CVVHDF dose	No change
Moderate–severe hepatic insufficiency	No change

Drug Interactions: None.
Adverse Effects: Drug fever/rash, C. difficile diarrhea/colitis.
Allergic Potential: High
Safety in Pregnancy: B
Comments: Limited penetration into respiratory secretions. **Ceclor CD 500 mg (PO) q12h is equivalent to cefaclor 250 mg (PO) q8h, not cefaclor 500 mg (PO) q8h. Ceclor CD 500 mg (PO) q12h is equivalent to 250 mg (PO) q8h of cefaclor.**
Cerebrospinal Fluid Penetration: < 10%
Bile Penetration: 60%
(also see **Antibiotic Pearls & Pitfalls** p. 510).

REFERENCES:

Cazzola M, Di Perna F, Boveri B. Interrelationship between the pharmacokinetics and pharmacodynamics of cefaclor advanced formulation in patients with acute exacerbation of chronic bronchitis. J Chemother 12:216–22, 2000.

Mazzei T, Novelli A, Esposito S, et al. New insight into the clinical pharmacokinetics of cefaclor: Tissue penetration. J Chemother 12:53–62, 2000.

Meyers BR. Cefaclor revisited. Clin Ther 22:154–66, 2000.

Website: www.pdr.net

Cefadroxil (Duricef, Ultracef)

Drug Class: 1st generation oral cephalosporin.
Usual Dose: 1000 mg (PO) q12h.
Spectrum: (see **Susceptibility Profiles** pp. 191–197).
Resistance Potential: Low
Pharmacokinetic Parameters:
Peak serum level: 16 mcg/mL
Bioavailability: 99%
Excreted unchanged (urine): 85%
Serum half-life (normal/ESRD): 0.5/22 hrs
Plasma protein binding: 20%
Volume of distribution (V_d): 0.31 L/kg
Primary Mode of Elimination: Renal
Dosage Adjustments*

CrCl 10–25 mL/min	500 mg (PO) q24h
CrCl < 10 mL/min	500 mg (PO) q36h
Post–HD dose	500 mg (PO)
Post–PD dose	250 mg (PO)
CVVH/CVVHD/CVVHDF dose	500 mg (PO) q24h
Moderate hepatic insufficiency	No change
Severe hepatic insufficiency	No change

Drug Interactions: None.
Adverse Effects: Drug fever/rash, C. difficile diarrhea/colitis.
Allergic Potential: High
Safety in Pregnancy: B
Comments: Penetrates oral/respiratory secretions well.
Cerebrospinal Fluid Penetration: < 10%
Bile Penetration: 20%
(also see **Antibiotic Pearls & Pitfalls** p. 509).

"Usual dose" assumes normal renal/hepatic function. * For renal insufficiency, give usual dose × 1 followed by maintenance dose per CrCl. For dialysis patients, dose the same as for CrCl < 10 mL/min and give supplemental (post-HD/PD dose) immediately after dialysis. CrCl = creatinine clearance; CVVH = continuous veno-venous hemofiltration; HD/PD = hemodialysis/peritoneal dialysis.

REFERENCES:

Bucko AD, Hunt BJ, Kidd SL, et al. Randomized, double-blind, multicenter comparison of oral cefditoren 200 or 400 mg BID with either cefuroxime 250 mg BID or cefadroxil 500 mg BID for the treatment of uncomplicated skin and skin-structure infections. Clin Ther 24:1134–47, 2002.

Cunha BA. Antibiotics selection for the treatment of sinusitis, otitis media, and pharyngitis. Infect Dis Pract 7:S324–S326, 1998.

Gustaferro CA, Steckelberg JM. Cephalosporins: Antimicrobic agents and related compounds. Mayo Clin Proc 66:1064–73, 1991.

Website: www.pdr.net

Cefamandole (Mandol)

Drug Class: 2nd generation cephalosporin.
Usual Dose: 2 gm (IV) q6h.
Resistance Potential: High (H. influenzae, Enterobacter sp.)
Pharmacokinetic Parameters:
Peak serum level: 240 mcg/mL
Bioavailability: Not applicable
Excreted unchanged (urine): 85%
Serum half-life (normal/ESRD): 1/11 hrs
Plasma protein binding: 76%
Volume of distribution (V_d): 0.29 L/kg
Primary Mode of Elimination: Renal
Dosage Adjustments*

CrCl 50–80 mL/min	1 gm (IV) q6h
CrCl 10–50 mL/min	1 gm (IV) q6h
CrCl < 10 mL/min	1 gm (IV) q12h
Post–HD dose	1 gm (IV)
Post–PD dose	1 gm (IV)
CVVH/CVVHD/CVVHDF dose	1 gm (IV) q6h
Moderate—severe hepatic insufficiency	No change

Drug Interactions: Alcohol (disulfiram-like reaction); antiplatelet agents, heparin, thrombolytics, warfarin (↑ risk of bleeding).
Adverse Effects: Drug fever/rash, ↑ INR.
Allergic Potential: High
Safety in Pregnancy: B
Comments: Incompatible in solutions with Mg++ or Ca++. **Contains MTT side chain, but no increase in clinical bleeding.**
Cerebrospinal Fluid Penetration: < 10%
Bile Penetration: 300%
(also see ***Antibiotic Pearls & Pitfalls*** p. 510).

REFERENCES:

Cunha BA, Klimek JJ, Qunitiliani R. Cefamandole nafate in respiratory and urinary tract infections. Curr Ther Res 25:584–9, 1971.

Gentry LO, Zeluff BJ, Cooley DA. Antibiotic prophylaxis in open-heart surgery: A comparison of cefamandole, cefuroxime, and cefazolin. Ann Thorac Surg 46:167–71, 1988.

Cefazolin (Ancef, Kefzol)

Drug Class: 1st generation cephalosporin.
Usual Dose: 1 gm (IV) q8h.
Spectrum: (see ***Susceptibility Profiles*** pp. 191–197).
Resistance Potential: Low
Pharmacokinetic Parameters:
Peak serum level: 185 mcg/mL
Bioavailability: Not applicable
Excreted unchanged (urine): 96%
Serum half-life (normal/ESRD): 1.8/40 hrs
Plasma protein binding: 85%
Volume of distribution (V_d): 0.2 L/kg
Primary Mode of Elimination: Renal
Dosage Adjustments*

CrCl 35–55 mL/min	1 gm (IV) q12h
CrCl 10–35 mL/min	500 mg (IV) q12h

"Usual dose" assumes normal renal/hepatic function. * For renal insufficiency, give usual dose × 1 followed by maintenance dose per CrCl. For dialysis patients, dose the same as for CrCl < 10 mL/min and give supplemental (post-HD/PD dose) immediately after dialysis. CrCl = creatinine clearance; CVVH = continuous veno-venous hemofiltration; HD/PD = hemodialysis/peritoneal dialysis.

CrCl < 10 mL/min	500 mg (IV) q24h
Post–HD dose	1 gm (IV)
Post–HFHD dose	2 gm (IV)
Post–PD dose	500 mg (IV)
CVVH/CVVHD/ CVVHDF dose	500 mg (IV) q12h
HD q 48–72h dose	2 gm (IV) q HD*
Moderate–severe hepatic insufficiency	No change

*Give at end of HD.

Drug Interactions: None.
Adverse Effects: Drug fever/rash, AIHA.
Allergic Potential: High
Safety in Pregnancy: B
Comments: Incompatible in solutions containing erythromycin, aminoglycosides, cimetidine, theophylline.
Cerebrospinal Fluid Penetration: < 10%
Bile Penetrations: 300%
(also see **Antibiotic Pearls & Pitfalls** p. 509).

REFERENCES:
Adembri C, Ristori R, Chelazzi C, et al. Cefazolin bolus and continuous administration for elective cardiac surgery: improved pharmacokinetic and pharmacodynamic parameters. J Thorac Cardiovasc Surg 140:471–475, 2010.
Cunha BA, Hamid N, Kessler H, Parchuri S. Daptomycin cure after cefazolin treatment failure of Methicillin-sensitive Staphylococcus aureus (MSSA) tricuspid valve acute bacterial endocarditis from a peripherally inserted central catheter (PICC) line. Heart & Lung. 34:442–7, 2005.
Cunha BA, Gossling HR, Pasternak HS, et al. Penetration of cephalosporins into bone. Infection 12:80–4, 1984.
Gentry LO, Zeluff BJ, Cooley DA. Antibiotic prophylaxis in open-heart surgery: A comparison of cefamandole, cefuroxime, and cefazolin. Ann Thorac Surg 46:167–71, 1988.

Kelkar PS, Li JTC. Cephalosporin allergy. N Engl J Med 345:804–809, 2001.
Marshall WF, Blair JE. The cephalosporins. Mayo Clin Proc 74:187–95, 1999.
Nightingale CH, Klimek JJ, Quintiliani R. Effect of protein binding on the penetration of nonmetabolized cephalosporins into atrial appendage and pericardial fluids in open-heart surgical patients. Antimicrob Agents Chemother 17:595–8, 1980.
Quintiliani R, Nightingale CH. Cefazolin. Ann Intern Med 89:650–6, 1978.
Turnidge JD. Cefazolin and Enterobacteriaceae: rationale for revised susceptibility testing breakpoints. Clin Infect Dis 52:917–924, 2011.

Cefdinir (Omnicef)

Drug Class: 3rd generation oral cephalosporin.
Usual Dose: 600 mg (PO) q24h.
Spectrum: (see **Susceptibility Profiles** pp. 191–197).
Resistance Potential: Low
Pharmacokinetic Parameters:
Peak serum level: 2.9 mcg/mL
Bioavailability: 16% (tab) / 25%(suspension)
Excreted unchanged (urine): 11–18%
Serum half-life (normal/ESRD): 1.7/3 hrs
Plasma protein binding: 70%
Volume of distribution (V_d): 0.35 L/kg
Primary Mode of Elimination: Renal
Dosage Adjustments*

CrCl < 30 mL/min	300 mg (PO) q24h
Post–HD dose	300 mg (PO)
Post–PD dose	None
CVVH/CVVHD/ CVVHDF dose	300 mg (PO) q24h
Moderate–severe hepatic insufficiency	No change

"Usual dose" assumes normal renal/hepatic function. * For renal insufficiency, give usual dose × 1 followed by maintenance dose per CrCl. For dialysis patients, dose the same as for CrCl < 10 mL/min and give supplemental (post-HD/PD dose) immediately after dialysis. CrCl = creatinine clearance; CVVH = continuous veno-venous hemofiltration; HD/PD = hemodialysis/peritoneal dialysis.

Drug Interactions: Probenecid (↑ cefdinir levels).
Adverse Effects: Drug fever/rash, C. difficile diarrhea/colitis.
Allergic Potential: High
Safety in Pregnancy: B
Comments: Good activity against bacterial respiratory pathogens. Available as capsules or suspension. **CAP dose:** 300 mg (PO) q12h; **Other respiratory infections dose:** 600 mg (PO) q24h.
Cerebrospinal Fluid Penetration: < 10% (also see *Antibiotic Pearls & Pitfalls* p. 511).

REFERENCES:

Cefdinir: A new oral cephalosporin. Med Lett Drugs Therap 40:85–7, 1998.

Fogarty CM, Bettis RB, Griffin TJ, et al. Comparison of a 5 day regimen of cefdinir with a 10 day regimen of cefprozil for treatment of acute exacerbations of chronic bronchitis. J Antimicrob Chemother 45:851–8, 2000.

Guay DR. Cefdinir: an advanced-generation, broad-spectrum oral cephalosporin. Clin Ther 24:473–89, 2002.

Hedrick JA. Community-acquired upper respiratory tract infections and the role of third-generation oral cephalosporins. Expert Rev Anti Infect Ther 8:15–21, 2010.

Perry CM, Scott LJ. Cefdinir: a review of its use in the management of mild-to-moderate bacterial infections. Drugs 64:1433–64, 2004.

Website: www.omnicef.com

Cefditoren (Spectracef)

Drug Class: 3rd generation oral cephalosporin.
Usual Dose: 400 mg (PO) q12h.
Spectrum: (see *Susceptibility Profiles* pp. 191–197).
Resistance Potential: Low
Pharmacokinetic Parameters:
Peak serum level: 1.8 mcg/mL

Bioavailability: 16%
Excreted unchanged (urine): 20%
Serum half-life (normal/ESRD): 1.5/5 hrs
Plasma protein binding: 88%
Volume of distribution (V_d): 0.13 L/kg
Primary Mode of Elimination: Renal
Dosage Adjustments*

CrCl 50–80 mL/min	No change
CrCl 30–50 mL/min	200 mg (PO) q12h
CrCl < 30 mL/min	200 mg (PO) q24h
Post–HD dose	200 mg (PO)
Post–PD dose	None
CVVH/CVVHD/ CVVHDF dose	200 mg (PO) q24h
Moderate–severe hepatic insufficiency	No change

Drug Interactions: H₂ receptor antagonists, Al⁺⁺, Mg⁺⁺) antacids (↓ absorption of cefditoren); Probenecid (↓ elimination of cefditoren).
Adverse Effects: Drug fever/rash, C. difficile diarrhea/colitis.
Allergic Potential: Low
Safety in Pregnancy: B
Comments: Serum concentrations increased ~ 50% if taken without food. ↑ elimination of carnitine; do not use in carnitine deficiency or hereditary carnitine metabolism disorder. **Contains Na+ caseinate; avoid in patients with casein hypersensitivity.**
Cerebrospinal Fluid Penetration: < 1%
Bile Penetration: 200%
(also see *Antibiotic Pearls & Pitfalls* p. 511).

REFERENCES:

Alvarez-Sala JL, Kardos P, et al. Martinez-Beltran et al. Clinical and bacteriological efficacy in treatment of acute exacerbations of chronic bronchitis with

---

"Usual dose" assumes normal renal/hepatic function. * For renal insufficiency, give usual dose × 1 followed by maintenance dose per CrCl. For dialysis patients, dose the same as for CrCl < 10 mL/min and give supplemental (post-HD/PD dose) immediately after dialysis. CrCl = creatinine clearance; CVVH = continuous veno-venous hemofiltration; HD/PD = hemodialysis/peritoneal dialysis.

cefditoren-pivoxil versus cefuroxime-axetil. Antimicrob Agents and Chemother 50:1762–67, 2006.

Balbisi EA. Cefditoren, a new aminothiazolyl cephalosporin. Pharmacotherapy 22:1278–93, 2002.

Chow J, Russel M, Bolk S. et al. Efficacy of cefditoren pivoxil vs. amoxicillin-clavulanic in acute maxillary sinusitis. Presented at the 40th Interscience Conference on Antimicrobial Agents and Chemotherapy; Abstract 835, Toronto, ON 2000.

Clark CL, Nagai K, Dewasse BE, et al. Activity of cefditoren against respiratory pathogens. J Antimicrob Chemother 50:33–41, 2002.

Darkes MJ, Plosker GL. Cefditoren pivoxil. Drugs 62:319–36, 2002.

Guay DR. Review of cefditoren, an advanced-generation, broad-spectrum oral cephalosporin. Clin Ther 23:1924–37, 2002.

Tempera G, Furneri PM, Carlone NA, et al. Antibiotic susceptibility of respiratory pathogens recently isolated in Italy: focus on cefditoren. J Chemother 22:153–159, 2010.

Wellington K, Curran MP. Cefditoren pivoxil: a review of its use in the treatment of bacterial infections. Drugs 64:2597–618, 2004.

Website: www.pdr.net

Cefepime (Maxipime)

Drug Class: 4th generation cephalosporin.
Usual Dose: 2 gm (IV) q12h (see comments).
Spectrum: (see *Susceptibility Profiles* pp. 191–197).
Resistance Potential: Low
Pharmacokinetic Parameters:
Peak serum level: 163 mcg/mL
Bioavailability: Not applicable
Excreted unchanged (urine): 80%
Serum half-life (normal/ESRD): 2.2/18 hrs
Plasma protein binding: 20%
Volume of distribution (V_d): 0.29 L/kg
Primary Mode of Elimination: Renal
Dosage Adjustments*

CrCl 30–60 mL/min	2 gm (IV) q12h
CrCl 10–30 mL/min	2 gm (IV) q24h
CrCl < 10 mL/min	1 gm (IV) q24h
Post–HD dose	2 gm (IV)
Post–HFHD dose	2 gm (IV)
Post–PD dose	1 gm (IV)
CAPD	2 gm (IV) q48h
CVVH/CVVHD/ CVVHDF dose	1 gm (IV) q12h
HD q 48–72h dose	2 gm (IV) q HD*
Moderate–severe hepatic insufficiency	No change

*Give at end of HD.
Drug Interactions: None.
Adverse Effects: Drug fever/rash, C. difficile diarrhea/colitis.
Allergic Potential: Moderate
Safety in Pregnancy: B
Comments: For proven serious systemic P. aeruginosa infections, febrile neutropenia, or cystic fibrosis, use 2 gm (IV) q8h. For aerobic GNB bacteremias use 2 gm (IV) q12h. Meningeal dose = 2 gm (IV) q8h.
Cerebrospinal Fluid Penetration:
Non-Inflamed meninges = 1%
Inflamed meninges = 15%
Bile Penetration: 10%
(also see *Antibiotic Pearls & Pitfalls* p. 511).

REFERENCES:
Akhabue E, Synnestvedt M, Weiner MG, et al. Cefepime-resistant Pseudomonas aeruginosa. Emerg Infect Dis 17:1037–1043, 2011.

Ambrose PF, Owens RC Jr, Garvey MJ, et al. Pharmacodynamic considerations in the treatment of moderate to severe pseudomonal infections with cefepime. J Antimicrob Chemother 49:445–53, 2002.

Al-Hassan MN, Eckel-Passow JE, Baddour LM. Cefepime effectiveness in Gram-negative bloodstream infections. J Antimicrob Chemother 66:1156–1160, 2011.

Badaro R, Molinar F, Seas c, et al. A multicenter comparative study of cefepime versus broad-spectrum antibacterial therapy in moderate and severe bacterial infections. Braz J Infect Dis 6: 206–18, 2002.

Bazan JA, Martin SI, Kaye KM. Newer beta-lactam antibiotics: doripenem, ceftobiprole, ceftaroline fosamil, and cefepime. Med Clin North Am 95:743–760, 2011.

Boselli E, Breilh D, Duflo F, et al. Steady-state plasma and intrapulmonary concentrations of cefepime administered in continuous infusion in critically ill patients with severe nosocomial pneumonia. Crit Care Med 31:2102–6, 2003.

Bow EJ, Rotstein C, Noskin GA, et al. A Randomized, open-label, multicenter comparative study of the efficacy and safety of piperacillin-tazobactam and cefepime for the empirical treatment of febrile neutropenic episodes in patients with hematologic malignancies. Clin Infect Dis 43:447–59, 2006.

Chapman TM, Perry CM. Cefepime: a review of its use in the management of hospitalized patients with pneumonia. Am J Respir Med 2:75–107, 2003.

Cheatham SC, Shea KM, Healy DP, et al. Steady-state pharmacokinetics and pharmacodynamics of cefepime administered by prolonged infusion in hospitalized patients. Int J Antimicrob Agents 37:46–50, 2011.

Cornely OA, Bethe U, Seifert H, et al. A randomized monocentric trial in febrile neutropenic patients: ceftriaxone and gentamicin vs cefepime and gentamicin. Ann Hematol 81:37–43, 2002.

Cunha BA. Pseudomonas aeruginosa: Resistance and therapy. Semin Respir Infect 17:231–9, 2002.

Cunha BA, Gill MV. Cefepime. Med Clin North Am 79:721–32, 1995.

Durand-Maugard C, Lemaire-Hurtel A, Gras-Champel V, et al. Blood and CSF monitoring of cefepime-induced neurotoxicity: nine case reports. J Antimicrob Chemother 1093:1297–1298, 2012.

Gangireddy VG, Mitchell LC, Coleman T. Cefepime neurotoxicity despite renal adjusted dosing. Scand J Infect Dis 43:827–829, 2011.

Grover SS, Sharma M, Chattopadhya D, Kapoor H, et al. Phenotypic and genotypic detection of ESBL mediated cephalosporin resistance in Klebsiella pneumoniae: Emergence of high resistance against cefepime, the fourth generation. Journal of Infection 53:279–88, 2006.

Lee SY, Kuti JL, Nicolau DP. Cefepime pharmacodynamics in patients with extended spectrum beta-lactamase (ESBL) and non-ESBL infections. J Infect 54:463–468, 2007.

Montalar J, Segura A, Bosch C, et al. Cefepime monotherapy as an empirical initial treatment of patients with febrile neutropenia. Med Oncol 19:161–6, 2002.

Moreno E, Davila I, Laffond E, et al. Selective immediate hypersensitivity to cefepime. J Investig Allergol Clin Immunol 17:52–54, 2007.

Perez KK, Hughes DW, Maxwell PR, et al. Cefepime for Gram-negative bacteremia in long-term hemodialysis: a single-center experience. Am J Kidney Dis 59:740–742, 2012.

Spriet I, Meersseman W, De Troy E, et al. Meropenem–valproic acid interaction in patients with cefepime-associated status epilepticus. Am J Health Syst Pharm 64:54–58, 2007.

Tam VH, McKinnon PS, Akins RL, et al. Pharmacodynamics of cefepime in patients with gram-negative infections. J Antimicrob Chemother 50:425–8, 2002.

Tam VH, McKinnon PS, Akins RL, et al. Pharmacokinetics and pharmacodynamics of cefepime in patients with various degrees of renal function. Antimicrob Agents Chemother 47:1853–61, 2003.

Yahave D, Paul M, Fraser A, et al. Efficacy and safety of cefepime: a systematic review and meta-analysis. Lancet Infect Dis 7:338–348, 2007.

Wilson FP, Bachhuber MA, Caroff D, et al. Low cefepime concentrations during high blood and dialysate flow continuous venovenous hemodialysis. Antimicrob Agents Chemother 56:2178–2180, 2012.

Website: www.elan.com/Products/

"Usual dose" assumes normal renal/hepatic function. * For renal insufficiency, give usual dose × 1 followed by maintenance dose per CrCl. For dialysis patients, dose the same as for CrCl < 10 mL/min and give supplemental (post-HD/PD dose) immediately after dialysis. CrCl = creatinine clearance; CVVH = continuous veno-venous hemofiltration; HD/PD = hemodialysis/peritoneal dialysis.

Cefixime (Suprax)

Drug Class: 3rd generation oral cephalosporin.
Usual Dose: 400 mg (PO) q12h.
Spectrum: (see *Susceptibility Profiles* pp. 191–197).
Resistance Potential: Low
Pharmacokinetic Parameters:
Peak serum level: 3.7 mcg/mL
Bioavailability: 50%
Excreted unchanged (urine): 50%
Serum half-life (normal/ESRD): 3.1/11 hrs
Plasma protein binding: 65%
Volume of distribution (V_d): 0.1 L/kg
Primary Mode of Elimination: Renal
Dosage Adjustments*

CrCl 20–50 mL/min	400 mg (PO) q24h
CrCl < 20 mL/min	200 mg (PO) q24h
Post–HD dose	400 mg (PO)
Post–PD dose	200 mg (PO)
CVVH/CVVHD/ CVVHDF dose	200 mg (PO) q12h
Moderate hepatic insufficiency	No change
Severe hepatic insufficiency	No change

Drug Interactions: Carbamazepine (↑ carbamazepine levels).
Adverse Effects: Drug fever/rash, C. difficile diarrhea/colitis.
Allergic Potential: High
Safety in Pregnancy: B

Comments: **PRNG dose:** 400 mg (PO) × 1 dose. Also useful for quinolone-resistant GC.
Little/no activity against S. aureus (MSSA).
Cerebrospinal Fluid Penetration: < 10%
Bile Penetration: 800%
(also see *Antibiotic Pearls & Pitfalls* p. 511).

REFERENCES:

Chisholm SA, Mouton JW, Lewis DA, et al. Cephalosporin MIC creep among gonococci: time for a pharmacodynamic rethink? J Antimicrob Chemother 65:2141–2148, 2010.

Quintiliani R. Cefixime in the treatment of patients with lower respiratory tract infections: results of US clinical trials. Clinical Therapeutics 18:373–90, 1996.

Update to CDC's Sexually Transmitted Diseases Treatment Guidelines, 2006: fluoroquinolones no longer recommended for treatment of gonococcal infections. MMWR 56:332–336, 2007.

Website: www.pdr.net

Cefoperazone (Cefobid)

Drug Class: 3rd generation cephalosporin.
Usual Dose: 2 gm (IV) q12h.
Spectrum: (see *Susceptibility Profiles* pp. 191–197).
Resistance Potential: Low
Pharmacokinetic Parameters:
Peak serum level: 240 mcg/mL
Bioavailability: Not applicable
Excreted unchanged (urine): 20%
Serum half-life (normal/ESRD): 2.4/2.4 hrs
Plasma protein binding: 90%
Volume of distribution (V_d): 0.17 L/kg

"Usual dose" assumes normal renal/hepatic function. * For renal insufficiency, give usual dose × 1 followed by maintenance dose per CrCl. For dialysis patients, dose the same as for CrCl < 10 mL/min and give supplemental (post-HD/PD dose) immediately after dialysis. CrCl = creatinine clearance; CVVH = continuous veno-venous hemofiltration; HD/PD = hemodialysis/peritoneal dialysis.

Primary Mode of Elimination: Hepatic
Dosage Adjustments*

CrCl < 10 mL/min	No change
Post–HD dose	None
Post–PD dose	None
CVVH/CVVHD/CVVHDF dose	No change
Moderate hepatic insufficiency	No change
Severe hepatic insufficiency	1 gm (IV) q12h

Drug Interactions: Alcohol (disulfiram-like reaction); antiplatelet agents, heparin, thrombolytics, warfarin (↑ risk of bleeding).
Adverse Effects: Drug fever/rash. ↑ **INR due to MTT side chain, but no increase in clinical bleeding. Prophylactic vitamin K unnecessary.**
Allergic Potential: Low
Safety in Pregnancy: B
Comments: **One of the few antibiotics to penetrate into an obstructed biliary tract.** May be administered IM. **Concentration dependent serum half life.**
Meningeal dose = 2 gm (IV) q8h.
Cerebrospinal Fluid Penetration:
Non-Inflamed meninges = 1%
Inflamed meninges = 10%
Bile Penetration: 1200% (also see **Antibiotic Pearls & Pitfalls** p. 510).

REFERENCES:

Cunha BA. 3rd generation cephalosporins: A review. Clin Ther 14:616–52, 1992.

Klein NC, Cunha BA. Third-generation cephalosporins. Med Clin North Am 79:705–19, 1995.

Marshall WF, Blair JE. The cephalosporins. Mayo Clin Proc 74:187–95, 1999.

Oie S, Uematsu T, Sawa A, et al. In vitro effects of combinations of antipseudomonal agents against seven strains of multidrug-resistant Pseudomonas aeruginosa. J Antimicrob Chemother 52:911–4, 2004.

Website: www.pdr.net

Cefotaxime (Claforan)

Drug Class: 3rd generation cephalosporin.
Usual Dose: 2 gm (IV) q6h.
Spectrum: (see **Susceptibility Profiles** pp. 191–197).
Resistance Potential: Low
Pharmacokinetic Parameters:
Peak serum level: 214 mcg/mL
Bioavailability: Not applicable
Excreted unchanged (urine): 20–36%; 15–25% excreted as active metabolite
Serum half-life (normal/ESRD): 1/15 hrs
Plasma protein binding: 37%
Volume of distribution (V_d): 0.25 L/kg
Primary Mode of Elimination: Renal
Dosage Adjustments*

CrCl 10–50 mL/min	1 gm (IV) q12h
CrCl < 10 mL/min	1 gm (IV) q24h
Post–HD dose	1 gm (IV)
Post–PD dose	1 gm (IV)
CVVH/CVVHD/CVVHDF dose	2 gm (IV) q12h
Moderate hepatic insufficiency	No change
Severe hepatic insufficiency	No change

"Usual dose" assumes normal renal/hepatic function. * For renal insufficiency, give usual dose × 1 followed by maintenance dose per CrCl. For dialysis patients, dose the same as for CrCl < 10 mL/min and give supplemental (post-HD/PD dose) immediately after dialysis. CrCl = creatinine clearance; CVVH = continuous veno-venous hemofiltration; HD/PD = hemodialysis/peritoneal dialysis.

Drug Interactions: None.
Adverse Effects: Drug fever/rash, C. difficile diarrhea/colitis.
Allergic Potential: Moderate
Safety in Pregnancy: B
Comments: Incompatible in solutions containing sodium bicarbonate, metronidazole, or aminoglycosides. **Desacetyl metabolite** ($t_{1/2}$ = 1.5 hrs) **synergistic with cefotaxime against S. aureus/B. fragilis.**
Meningeal dose = 3 gm (IV) q6h.
Cerebrospinal Fluid Penetration:
Non-Inflamed meninges = 1%
Inflamed meninges = 10%
Bile Penetration: 75%
(also see *Antibiotic Pearls & Pitfalls* p. 510).

REFERENCES:
Brogden RN, Spencer CM. Cefotaxime: A reappraisal of its antibacterial activity and pharmacokinetic properties and a review of its therapeutic efficacy when administered twice daily for the treatment of mild to moderate infections. Drugs 53:483–510, 1987.
File Jr. TM, Clinical implications and treatment of multiresistant Streptococcus pneumoniae pneumonia. Clin Microbiol Infect 12:31–41, 2006.
Klein NC, Cunha BA. Third-generation cephalosporins. Med Clin North Am 79:705–19, 1995.
Marshall WF, Blair JE. The cephalosporins. Mayo Clin Proc 74:187–95, 1999.
Patel KB, Nicolau DP, Nightingale CH, et al. Comparative serum bactericidal activities of ceftizoxime and cefotaxime against intermediately penicillin-resistant Streptococcus pneumoniae. Antimicrob Agents Chemother 40:2805–8, 1996.
Website: www.pdr.net

Cefotetan (Cefotan)

Drug Class: 2nd generation cephalosporin (Cephamycin).
Usual Dose: 2 gm (IV) q12h.

Spectrum: (see *Susceptibility Profiles* pp. 191–197).
Resistance Potential: Low
Pharmacokinetic Parameters:
Peak serum level: 237 mcg/mL
Bioavailability: Not applicable
Excreted unchanged (urine): 50–80%
Serum half-life (normal/ESRD): 4/10 hrs
Plasma protein binding: 88%
Volume of distribution (V_d): 0.17 L/kg
Primary Mode of Elimination: Renal
Dosage Adjustments*

CrCl 30–80 mL/min	2 gm (IV) q12h
CrCl 10–30 mL/min	2 gm (IV) q24h
CrCl < 10 mL/min	2 gm (IV) q48h
Post–HD dose	1 gm (IV)
Post–PD dose	1 gm (IV)
CVVH/CVVHD/CVVHDF dose	750 mg (IV) q12h
Moderate—severe hepatic insufficiency	No change

Drug Interactions: Alcohol (disulfiram-like reaction); antiplatelet agents, heparin, thrombolytics, warfarin (↑ risk of bleeding).
Adverse Effects: Drug fever/rash, hemolytic anemia, C. difficile diarrhea/colitis. ↑ **INR due to MTT side chain, but no increase in clinical bleeding.**
Allergic Potential: Low
Safety in Pregnancy: B
Comments: Less effective than cefoxitin against B. fragilis D.O.T strains.
Cerebrospinal Fluid Penetration: < 10%
Bile Penetration: 20% (also see *Antibiotic Pearls & Pitfalls* p. 510).

"Usual dose" assumes normal renal/hepatic function. * For renal insufficiency, give usual dose × 1 followed by maintenance dose per CrCl. For dialysis patients, dose the same as for CrCl < 10 mL/min and give supplemental (post-HD/PD dose) immediately after dialysis. CrCl = creatinine clearance; CVVH = continuous veno-venous hemofiltration; HD/PD = hemodialysis/peritoneal dialysis.

REFERENCES:
Moes GS, MacPherson BR. Cefotetan-induced
  hemolytic anemia: A case report and a review of
  the literature. Arch Pathol Lab Med 124:1344–6,
  2000.
Ray EK, Warkentin TE, O'Hoski PL. Delayed onset of
  life-threatening immune hemolysis after perioperative
  antimicrobial prophylaxis with cefotetan. Can J Surg
  43:461–2, 2000.
Stroncek D, Procter JL, Johnson J. Drug-induced
  hemolysis: cefotetan-dependent hemolytic
  anemia mimicking an acute intravascular immune
  transfusion reaction. Am J Hematol 64:67–70,
  2000.
Website: www.pdr.net

Cefoxitin (Mefoxin)

Drug Class: 2nd generation cephalosporin
(Cephamycin).
Usual Dose: 2 gm (IV) q6h.
Spectrum: (see *Susceptibility Profiles*
pp. 191–197).
Resistance Potential: Low
Pharmacokinetic Parameters:
Peak serum level: 221 mcg/mL
Bioavailability: Not applicable
Excreted unchanged (urine): 85%
Serum half-life (normal/ESRD): 1/21 hrs
Plasma protein binding: 75%
Volume of distribution (V_d): 0.12 L/kg
Primary Mode of Elimination: Renal
Dosage Adjustments*

CrCl 30–50 mL/min	2 gm (IV) q12h
CrCl 10–30 mL/min	1 gm (IV) q12h
CrCl < 10 mL/min	1 gm (IV) q24h
Post–HD dose	2 gm (IV)

Post–PD dose	1 gm (IV)
CVVH/CVVHD/ CVVHDF dose	2 gm (IV) q12h
Moderate hepatic insufficiency	No change
Severe hepatic insufficiency	No change

Drug Interactions: None.
Adverse Effects: Drug fever/rash, C. difficile
diarrhea/colitis.
Allergic Potential: Low
Safety in Pregnancy: B
Comments: Effective against B. fragilis,
including D.O.T. strains (B. distasonis, B. ovatus,
B. thetaiotaomicron).
Cerebrospinal Fluid Penetration: < 10%
Bile Penetration: 250%
(also see *Antibiotic Pearls & Pitfalls* p. 510).

REFERENCES:
da Costa Darini AL, Palazzo IC. Cefoxitin does not
  include production of penicillin binding protein 2a in
  methicillin-susceptible Staphylococcus aureus strains.
  J Clin Microbiol 42:4412, 2004.
Donowitz GR, Mandell GL. Beta-lactam antibiotics.
  N Engl J Med 318:419–26 and 318:490–500, 1993.
Hansen EA, Cunha BA. Cefoxitin. Antibiotics for
  Clinicians 5:33–41, 2001.
Marshall WF Blair JE. The cephalosporins. Mayo Clin
  Proc 74:187–95, 1999.
Website: www.pdr.net

Cefpodoxime (Vantin)

Drug Class: 3rd generation oral cephalosporin.
Usual Dose: 200 mg (PO) q12h (see comments).
Spectrum: (see *Susceptibility Profiles*
pp. 191–197).

"Usual dose" assumes normal renal/hepatic function. * For renal insufficiency, give usual dose × 1 followed by
maintenance dose per CrCl. For dialysis patients, dose the same as for CrCl < 10 mL/min and give supplemental
(post-HD/PD dose) immediately after dialysis. CrCl = creatinine clearance; CVVH = continuous veno-venous
hemofiltration; HD/PD = hemodialysis/peritoneal dialysis.

Resistance Potential: Low
Pharmacokinetic Parameters:
Peak serum level: 2.3 mcg/mL
Bioavailability: 50%
Excreted unchanged (urine): 30%
Serum half-life (normal/ESRD): 2.3/9.8 hrs
Plasma protein binding: 21–33%
Volume of distribution (V_d): 0.9 L/kg
Primary Mode of Elimination: Renal
Dosage Adjustments*

CrCl 30–80 mL/min	No change
CrCl < 30 mL/min	200 mg (PO) q24h
Post–HD dose	200 mg (PO)
Post–PD dose	200 mg (PO)
CVVH/CVVHD/ CVVHDF dose	200 mg (PO) q12h
Moderate hepatic insufficiency	No change
Severe hepatic insufficiency	No change

Drug Interactions: None.
Adverse Effects: Drug fever/rash, C. difficile diarrhea/colitis pulmonary infiltrates with eosinophilia, ↑ SGOT/SGPT.
Allergic Potential: High
Safety in Pregnancy: B
Comments: Only oral 3rd generation cephalosporin active against S. aureus (MSSA).
PPNG dose: 400 mg (PO) × 1 dose.
cSSSI dose: 400 mg (PO) q12h.
Cerebrospinal Fluid Penetration: < 10%
Bile Penetration: 100%
(also see **Antibiotic Pearls & Pitfalls** p. 511).

REFERENCES:
Adam D, Bergogne-Berezin E, Jones RN. Symposium on cefpodoxime proxetil: A new third generation oral cephalosporin. Drugs 42:1–66, 1991.
Cohen R. Clinical efficacy of cefpodoxime in respiratory tract infection. J Antimicrob Chemother 50(Suppl):23–7, 2002.
Liu P, Muller M, Grant M, et al. Interstitial tissue concentrations of cefpodoxime. J Antimicrob Chemother 50(Suppl):19–22, 2002.
Schatz BS, Karavokiros KT, Taeubel MA, et al. Comparison of cefprozil, cefpodoxime proxetil, loracarbef, cefixime, and ceftibuten. Ann Pharmacother 30:258–68, 1996.
Website: www.pdr.net

Cefprozil (Cefzil)

Drug Class: 2nd generation oral cephalosporin.
Usual Dose: 500 mg (PO) q12h.
Spectrum: (see **Susceptibility Profiles** pp. 191–197).
Resistance Potential: Low
Pharmacokinetic Parameters:
Peak serum level: 10 mcg/mL
Bioavailability: 95%
Excreted unchanged (urine): 60%
Serum half-life (normal/ESRD): 1.3/5.9 hrs
Plasma protein binding: 36%
Volume of distribution (V_d): 0.23 L/kg
Primary Mode of Elimination: Renal
Dosage Adjustments*

CrCl < 30 mL/min	250 mg (PO) q12h
Post–HD dose	500 mg (PO)
Post–PD dose	250 mg (PO)
CVVH/CVVHD/ CVVHDF dose	500 mg (PO) q24h

"Usual dose" assumes normal renal/hepatic function. * For renal insufficiency, give usual dose × 1 followed by maintenance dose per CrCl. For dialysis patients, dose the same as for CrCl < 10 mL/min and give supplemental (post-HD/PD dose) immediately after dialysis. CrCl = creatinine clearance; CVVH = continuous veno-venous hemofiltration; HD/PD = hemodialysis/peritoneal dialysis.

Moderate hepatic insufficiency	No change
Severe hepatic insufficiency	No change

Drug Interactions: None.
Adverse Effects: Drug fever/rash, C. difficile diarrhea/colitis.
Allergic Potential: Low
Safety in Pregnancy: B
Comments: Penetrates oral/respiratory secretions well. No resistance.
Cerebrospinal Fluid Penetration: < 10% (also see **Antibiotic Pearls & Pitfalls** p. 510).

REFERENCES:

Cunha BA. New antibiotics for the treatment of acute exacerbations of chronic bronchitis. Adv Ther 13:313–23, 1996.

Gainer RB 2nd. Cefprozil: A new cephalosporin; its use in various clinical trials. South Med J 88:338–46, 1995.

Marshall WF Blair JE. The cephalosporins. Mayo Clin Proc 74:187–95, 1999.

Schatz BS, Karavokiros KT, Taeubel MA, et al. Comparison of cefprozil, cefpodoxime, proxetil, loracarbef, cefixime, and ceftibuten. Ann Pharmacother 30:258–68, 1996.

Website: www.pdr.net

Ceftaroline fosamil (Teflaro)

Drug class: Anti-MRSA cephalosporin*.
Usual dose: 600 mg (IV) q12h.
Spectrum: (see **Susceptibility Profiles** pp. 191–197).
Resistance Potential: Low
Pharmacokinetic Parameters:

Peak serum level: 19 mcg/mL
Bioavailability: not applicable
Excreted unchanged: 64%
Serum half-life (normal/ESRD): 2.7 hours / 6.16 hours
Plasma protein binding: 20%
Volume of distribution (V_d): 20.3 L/kg
Primary Mode of Elimination: Renal
Dosage of Ceftaroline fosamil in Patients with Renal Impairment

CrCl[a] > 50	No change
CrCl > 30 to ≤ 50	400 mg (IV) (over 1 hour) q12h
CrCl ≥ 15 to ≤ 30	300 mg (IV) (over 1 hour) q12h
End-stage renal disease, including hemodialysis[b]	200 mg (IV) (over 1 hour) q12h[c]

[a]Creatinine clearance (CrCl) estimated using the Cockcroft-Gault formula.
[b]End-stage renal disease is defined as CrCl < 15 mL/min.
[c]Ceftaroline fosamil is hemodialyzable and ceftaroline fosamil should be administered after hemodialysis on hemodialysis days.

Drug Interactions: No significant interactions.
Warnings & Precautions: hypersensitivity (including anaphylaxis), C. difficile associated diarrhea, direct Coombs test.
Serious Adverse Events: respiratory and infection system organ classes.
Adverse Reactions: diarrhea, nausea, rash, constipation, vomiting, increased transanimases, hypokalemia, phlebitis.
Safety in Pregnancy: B

---

* Ceftaroline fosamil is approved for MRSA in ABSSSI and has not been evaluated in clinical trials for any other MRSA infections.Ceftaroline fosamil is also approved for ABSSSI caused by methicillin-susceptible S. aureus, S. pyogenes, S. agalactiae, E. coli, K. pneumoniae and K. oxytoca and CAP caused by S. pneumoniae, S. aureus (methicillin-susceptible isolates only), H. influenzae, K. pneumoniae, K. oxytoca and E. coli. "Usual dose" assumes normal renal/hepatic function.

Comments: The only cephalosporin effective against MRSA *in vivo*. Not an inducer, inhibitor or substrate of CYP450 system. Infuse over 1 hour.

References:

Biek D, Critchley IA, Riccobene TA, et al. Ceftaroline fosamil: a novel broad-spectrum cephalosporin with expanded anti-Gram-positive activity. J Antimicrob Chemother 65:9–16, 2010.

Casapao AM, Steed ME, Levine DP, et al. Ceftaroline fosamil for community-acquired bacterial pneumonia and acute bacterial skin and skin structure infection. Expert Opin Pharmacother 13:1177–1186, 2012.

Corey GR, Wilcox M, Talbot GH, et al. Integrated analysis of CANVAS 1 and 2: phase 3, multicenter, randomized, double-blind studies to evaluate the safety and efficacy of ceftaroline versus vancomycin plus aztreonam in complicated skin and skin-structure infection. Clin Infect Dis 51:641–650; 2010.

File TM Jr, Low DE, Edckburg PB, et al. Efficacy and safety of ceftaroline fosamil versus ceftriaxone in patients with community-acquired pneumonia. Clin Infect Dis 51:1395–1405, 2011.

Ho TT, Cadena J, Childs LM, et al. Methicillin-resistant Staphylococcus aureus bacteremia and endocarditis treated with ceftaroline salvage therapy. J Antimicrob Chemother 67:1267–1270, 2012.

Kaushik D, Rathi S, Jain A. Ceftaroline: a comprehensive update. Int J Antimicrob Agents 37:389–395, 2011.

Laudano JB, Ceftaroline fosamil: a new broad-spectrum cephalosporin. J Antimicrob Chemother 66:11–18, 2011.

Lim L, Sutton E, Brown J. Ceftaroline: A new broad-spectrum cephalosporin. Am J Health Syst Pharm 15:491–4198, 2011.

Mendes RE, Tsakris A, Sader HS, et al. Characterization of methicillin-resistant Staphylococcus aureus displaying increased MICs of ceftaroline. J Antimicrob Chemother 67:1231–1234, 2012.

Nannini Ec, Stryjewskin ME, Corey GR. Ceftaroline for complicated skin and skin-structure infections. Expert Opin Pharmacother 11:1197–1206, 2010.

Panagiotidis G, Backstrom T, Asker-Hagelberg C, et al. Effect of ceftaroline on normal human intestinal microflora. Antimicrob Agents Chemother 54:1811–1814, 2010.

Poon H, Chang MH, Fung HB. Ceftaroline fosamil: a cephalosporin with activity against methicillin-resistant Staphylococcus aureus. Clin Ther 34:743–765, 2012.

Saravolatz LD, Pawlak J, Johnson L. In vitro activity of ceftaroline against community-associated methicillin-resistant, vancomycin-intermediate, vancomycin-resistant, and daptomycin-nonsusceptible Staphylococcus aureus isolates. Antimicrob. Agents Chemother 54:3027–3030, 2010.

Saravolatz LD, Stein GE, Johnson LB. Ceftaroline: A novel cephalosporin with activity against methicillin-resistant Staphylococcus aureus. Clin Infect Dis 52:1156–1163, 2011.

Watkins RR. Successful treatment of osetomyelitis from methicillin-resistant Staphylococcus aureus with ceftaroline. Infectious Disease in Clinical Practice 21:1;48–49, 2013.

Zainah H, Vazquez JA. Use of ceftaroline in complicated methicillin-resistant Staphylococcus aureus bacteremia. Infectious Disease in Clinical Practice 21:1;58–60, 2013.

Zhanel GG, Sniezek G, Schweizer F, et al. Ceftaroline: a novel broad-spectrum cephalosporin with activity against methicillin-resistant Staphylococcus aureus. Drugs 69:809–831, 2009.

Ceftazidime (Fortaz, Tazicef, Tazidime)

Drug Class: 3rd generation cephalosporin.
Usual Dose: 2 gm (IV) q8h (see comments).
Spectrum: (see *Susceptibility Profiles* pp. 191–197).
Resistance Potential: High (P. aeruginosa, Klebsiella pneumoniae; ↑ prevalence of MRSA)
Pharmacokinetic Parameters:
Peak serum level: 170 mcg/mL
Bioavailability: Not applicable
Excreted unchanged (urine): 80–90%
Serum half-life (normal/ESRD): 1.9/21 hrs
Plasma protein binding: 10%
Volume of distribution (V_d): 0.36 L/kg
Primary Mode of Elimination: Renal
Dosage Adjustments*

CrCl 30–80 mL/min	2 gm (IV) q12h
CrCl 10–30 mL/min	2 gm (IV) q24h
CrCl < 10 mL/min	1 gm (IV) q48h
Post–HD dose	1 gm (IV)
Post–PD dose	500 mg (IV)
CVVH/CVVHD/ CVVHDF dose	2 gm (IV) q12h
HD q48–72h dose	2 gm (IV) q HD*
Moderate hepatic insufficiency	No change
Severe hepatic insufficiency	No change

*Give at end of HD.
Drug Interactions: None.
Adverse Effects: Phlebitis, Drug fever/rash, C. difficile diarrhea/colitis.
Allergic Potential: High
Safety in Pregnancy: B
Comments: Incompatible in solutions containing vancomycin or aminoglycosides. *Use increases MRSA prevalence and P. aeruginosa resistance. Potent inducer of Klebsiella/Enterobacter/E. coli ESBLs.*
CAPD dose: 125 mg/L of dialysate (I.P.) with each exchange.
Meningeal dose = 2 gm (IV) q8h.
Cerebrospinal Fluid Penetration:
Non-Inflamed meninges = 1%
Inflamed meninges = 20%
Bile Penetration: 50%
(also see *Antibiotic Pearls & Pitfalls* p. 510).

REFERENCES:
Briscoe-Dwyer L. Ceftazidime. Antibiotics for Clinicians 1:41–8, 1997.
Fortaleza CM, Freire MP, de Carvalho Ramos M. Risk factors for recovery of imipenem- or ceftazidime-resistant Pseudomonas aeruginosa among patients admitted to a teaching hospital in Brazil. Infection Control and Hosp Epidemiol 27:901–06, 2006.
Klein NC, Cunha BA. Third-generation cephalosporins. Med Clin North Am 79:705–19, 1995.
Lu Q, Yang J, Liu Z, et al. Nebulized ceftazidime and amikacin in ventilator-associated pneumonia caused by Pseudomonas aeruginosa. Am J Respir Crit Care Med. 184:106–115, 2011.
Nicolau DP, Nightingale CH, Banevicius MA, et al. Serum bactericidal activity of ceftazidime: Continuous infusion versus intermittent injections. Antimicrob Agents Chemother 40:61–4, 1996.
Owens JC, Jr, Ambrose PG, Quintiliani R. Ceftazidime to cefepime formulary switch: Pharmacodynamic rationale. Conn Med 61:225–7, 1997.
Rains CP, Bryson HM, Peters DH. Ceftazidime: An update of its antibacterial activity, pharmacokinetic properties, and therapeutic efficacy. Drugs 49:577–617, 1995.
Website: www.pdr.net

Ceftibuten (Cedax)

Drug Class: 3rd generation oral cephalosporin.
Usual Dose: 400 mg (PO) q24h.
Spectrum: (see *Susceptibility Profiles* pp. 191–197).
Resistance Potential: Low
Pharmacokinetic Parameters:
Peak serum level: 18 mcg/mL
Bioavailability: 80%
Excreted unchanged: 56% (urine); 39% (fecal)
Serum half-life (normal/ESRD): 2.4/22 hrs
Plasma protein binding: 65%
Volume of distribution (V_d): 0.2 L/kg
Primary Mode of Elimination: Renal
Dosage Adjustments*

| CrCl 30–50 mL/min | 200 mg (PO) q24h |
| CrCl < 30 mL/min | 100 mg (PO) q24h |

"Usual dose" assumes normal renal/hepatic function. * For renal insufficiency, give usual dose × 1 followed by maintenance dose per CrCl. For dialysis patients, dose the same as for CrCl < 10 mL/min and give supplemental (post-HD/PD dose) immediately after dialysis. CrCl = creatinine clearance; CVVH = continuous veno-venous hemofiltration; HD/PD = hemodialysis/peritoneal dialysis.

Post–HD dose	400 mg (PO)
Post–PD dose	200 mg (PO)
CVVH/CVVHD/ CVVHDF dose	200 mg (PO) q24h
Moderate hepatic insufficiency	No change
Severe hepatic insufficiency	No change

Drug Interactions: None.
Adverse Effects: Drug fever/rash.
Allergic Potential: High
Safety in Pregnancy: B
Comments: Little/no activity against
S. aureus/S. pneumoniae.
Cerebrospinal Fluid Penetration: < 10%
(also see *Antibiotic Pearls & Pitfalls* p. 511).

REFERENCES:
Andrews JW, Wise R, Baldwin DR, et al. Concentrations of ceftibuten in plasma and the respiratory tract following a single 400 mg oral dose. Int J Antimicrob Agents 5:141–144, 1995.
Guay DR. Ceftibuten: A new expanded-spectrum oral cephalosporin. Ann Pharmacother 31:1022–33, 1997.
Owens RC Jr, Nightingale CH, Nicolau DP. Ceftibuten: An overview. Pharmacother 17:707–20, 1997.
Wiseman LR, Balfour JA. Ceftibuten: A review of its antibacterial activity, pharmacokinetic properties and clinical efficacy. Drugs 47:784–808, 1994.
Website: www.pdr.net

Ceftizoxime (Cefizox)

Drug Class: 3rd generation cephalosporin.
Usual Dose: 2 gm (IV) q8h (see comments).
Spectrum: (see *Susceptibility Profiles* pp. 191–197).
Resistance Potential: Low
Pharmacokinetic Parameters:
Peak serum level: 132 mcg/mL

Bioavailability: Not applicable
Excreted unchanged (urine): 90%
Serum half-life (normal/ESRD): 1.7/35 hrs
Plasma protein binding: 30%
Volume of distribution (V_d): 0.32 L/kg
Primary Mode of Elimination: Renal
Dosage Adjustments*

CrCl 50–80 mL/min	1 gm (IV) q8h
CrCl 10–50 mL/min	1 gm (IV) q12h
CrCl < 10 mL/min	1 gm (IV) q24h
Post–HD dose	1 gm (IV)
Post–PD dose	1 gm (IV)
CVVH/CVVHD/ CVVHDF dose	1 gm (IV) q12h
Moderate hepatic insufficiency	No change
Severe hepatic insufficiency	No change

Drug Interactions: None.
Adverse Effects: Drug fever/rash, C. difficile diarrhea/colitis.
Allergic Potential: High
Safety in Pregnancy: B
Comments: PRNG dose: 500 mg (IM) ×
1 dose.
Meningeal dose = 3 gm (IV) q6h.
Cerebrospinal Fluid Penetration:
Non-Inflamed meninges = 1%
Inflamed meninges = 10%
Bile Penetration: 50%
(also see *Antibiotic Pearls & Pitfalls* p. 510).

REFERENCES:
Klein NC, Cunha BA. Third-generation cephalosporins. Med Clin North Am 79:705–19, 1995.

"Usual dose" assumes normal renal/hepatic function. * For renal insufficiency, give usual dose × 1 followed by maintenance dose per CrCl. For dialysis patients, dose the same as for CrCl < 10 mL/min and give supplemental (post-HD/PD dose) immediately after dialysis. CrCl = creatinine clearance; CVVH = continuous veno-venous hemofiltration; HD/PD = hemodialysis/peritoneal dialysis.

Donowitz GR, Mandell GL. Beta-lactam antibiotics. N Engl J Med 318:419–26 and 318:490–500, 1993.

Marshall WF, Blair JE. The cephalosporins. Mayo Clin Proc 74:187–95, 1999.

Website: www.pdr.net

Ceftriaxone (Rocephin)

Drug Class: 3rd generation cephalosporin.
Usual Dose: 1–2 gm (IV) q24h (see comments).
Spectrum: (see *Susceptibility Profiles* pp. 191–197).
Resistance Potential: Low
Pharmacokinetic Parameters:
Peak serum level: 151–257 mcg/mL
Bioavailability: Not applicable
Excreted unchanged (urine/feces): 33–67%
Serum half-life (normal/ESRD): 8/16 hrs
Plasma protein binding: 90%
Volume of distribution (V_d): 0.08–0.3 L/kg
Primary Mode of Elimination: Renal/hepatic
Dosage Adjustments*

CrCl < 10 mL/min	No change
Post–HD dose	None
Post–HFHD dose	None
Post–PD dose	None
CVVH/CVVHD/CVVHDF dose	No change
Moderate hepatic insufficiency	No change
Severe hepatic insufficiency	No change (max dose: 2 gm/d)

Drug Interactions: May cause intravascular precipitation when co-administered with calcium-containing solutions/products.

Adverse Effects: Drug fever/rash, non-C. difficile diarrhea, pseudobiliary lithiasis, hemolytic anemia, may interfere with platelet aggregation, thrombocytosis.
Allergic Potential: High
Safety in Pregnancy: B. **Avoid near term in 3rd trimester** (↑ incidence of kernicterus in newborns)
Cerebrospinal Fluid Penetration:
Non-Inflamed meninges = 1%
Inflamed meninges = 10%
Bile Penetration: 500%
(also see *Antibiotic Pearls & Pitfalls* p. 510).

REFERENCES:

Araz N, Okan V, Demirci M, et al. Pseudolithiasis due to ceftriaxone treatment for meningitis in children: report of 8 cases. Tohoku J Exp Med 211:285–290, 2007.

Borg R, Dotevall L, Hagberg L, et al. Intravenous ceftriaxone compared with oral doxycycline for the treatment of Lyme neuroborreliosis. Scand J Infect Dis 37:449–454, 2005.

Cunha BA, Klein NC. The selection and use of cephalosporins: A review. Adv Ther 12:83–101, 1995.

Dietrich ES, Bieser U, Frank U, et al. Ceftriaxone versus other cephalosporins for perioperative antibiotic prophylaxis: a meta analysis of 43 randomized controlled trials. Chemotherapy 48:49–56, 2002.

Faella F, Pagliano P, Fusco U, Attanasio V, Conte M. Combined treatment with ceftriaxone and linezolid of pneumococcal meningitis: a case series including penicillin-resistant strains. Clin Micrbiol Infect 12:391–4, 2006.

Feurle GE, Junga NS, Marth T. Efficacy of ceftriaxone or meropenem as initial therapies in Whipple's disease. Gastroenterology 138:478–486, 2010.

File TM Jr. Clinical implications and treatment of multiresistant Streptococcus pneumoniae pneumonia. Clin Microbiol Infect 12:31–41, 2006.

File TM Jr, Low DE, Edckburg PB, et al. Efficacy and safety of ceftaroline fosamil versus ceftriaxone in patients with community-acquired pneumonia. Clin Infect Dis 51:1395–1405, 2011.

"Usual dose" assumes normal renal/hepatic function. * For renal insufficiency, give usual dose × 1 followed by maintenance dose per CrCl. For dialysis patients, dose the same as for CrCl < 10 mL/min and give supplemental (post-HD/PD dose) immediately after dialysis. CrCl = creatinine clearance; CVVH = continuous veno-venous hemofiltration; HD/PD = hemodialysis/peritoneal dialysis.

Freeman CD, Nightingale CH, Nicolau DP, et al. Serum bactericidal activity of ceftriaxone plus metronidazole against common intra-abdominal pathogens. Am J Hosp Pharm 51:1782–7, 1994.

Grassi C. Ceftriaxone. Antibiotics for Clinicians 2:49–57, 1998.

Klein NC, Cunha BA. Third generation cephalosporins. Med Clin North Am 79:705–19, 1995.

Lamb HM, Ormrod D, Scott LJ, et al. Ceftriaxone: an update of its use in the management of community-acquired and nosocomial infections. Drugs 62:1041–89, 2002.

Marshall WF, Blair JE. The cephalosporins. Mayo Clin Proc 74:187–95, 1999.

Pichichero ME. Use of selected cephalosporins in penicillin-allergic patients: a paradigm shift. Diagn Microbiol Infect Dis 57:13S–18S, 2007.

Roberts JA, Boots R, Rickard CM, et al. Is continuous infusion ceftriaxone better than once-a-day dosing in intensive care? A randomized controlled pilot study. J Antimicrob Chemother 59:285–291, 2007.

Savaris RF, Teixeira LM, Torres TG, et al. Comparing ceftriaxone plus azithromycin or doxycycline for pelvic inflammatory disease: a randomized controlled trial. Obstet Gynecol 110:53–60, 2007.

Shelburne SA 3rd, Greenburg SB, Aslam S, et al. Successful ceftriaxone therapy of endocarditis due to penicillin non-susceptible viridans streptococci. J Infect 54:e108–e110, 2007.

Woodfield JC, Van Rij AM, Pettigrew RA, et al. A comparison of the prophylactic efficacy of ceftriaxone and cefotaxime in abdominal surgery. Am J Surg 185:45–9, 2003.

Website: www.rocheusa.com/products/rocephin

Spectrum: (see *Susceptibility Profiles* **pp. 191–197**).
Resistance Potential: Low
Pharmacokinetic Parameters:
Peak serum level: 100 (IV)/7 (PO) mcg/mL
Bioavailability: 52%
Excreted unchanged (urine): 89%
Serum half-life (normal/ESRD): 1.2/17 hrs
Plasma protein binding: 50%
Volume of distribution (V_d): 0.15 L/kg
Primary Mode of Elimination: Renal
Dosage Adjustments*

CrCl 20 –80 mL/min	No change
CrCl 10–20 mL/min	750 mg (IV) q12h 500 mg (PO) q12h
CrCl < 10 mL/min	750 mg (IV) q24h 250 mg (PO) q24h
Post–HD dose	750 mg (IV) 250 mg (PO)
Post–PD dose	750 mg (IV) 250 mg (PO)
CVVH/CVVHD/ CVVHDF dose	1 gm (IV) q12h 500 mg (PO) q12h
Moderate hepatic insufficiency	No change
Severe hepatic insufficiency	No change

Cefuroxime (Kefurox, Zinacef, Ceftin)

Drug Class: 2nd generation IV/oral cephalosporin.
Usual Dose: 1.5 gm (IV) q8h; 500 mg (PO) q12h (see comments).

Drug Interactions: None.
Adverse Effects: Drug fever/rash, C. difficile diarrhea/colitis.
Allergic Potential: High
Safety in Pregnancy: B
Comments: Oral preparation penetrates oral/respiratory secretions well. **PPNG dose:** 1 gm

---

"Usual dose" assumes normal renal/hepatic function. * For renal insufficiency, give usual dose × 1 followed by maintenance dose per CrCl. For dialysis patients, dose the same as for CrCl < 10 mL/min and give supplemental (post-HD/PD dose) immediately after dialysis. CrCl = creatinine clearance; CVVH = continuous veno-venous hemofiltration; HD/PD = hemodialysis/peritoneal dialysis.

(IM) × 1 dose. **Ineffective for H. influenzae meningitis prophylaxis or therapy.**
Cerebrospinal Fluid Penetration: < 10% (also see **Antibiotic Pearls & Pitfalls** p. 510).

REFERENCES:

Alvarez-Sala JL, Kardos P, Martinez-Beltran, et al. Clinical and bacteriological efficacy in treatment of acute exacerbations of chronic bronchitis with cefditoren-pivoxil versus cefuroxime-axetil. Antimicrob Agents and Chemother 50:1762–67, 2006.

Bucko AD, Hunt BJ, Kidd SL, et al. Randomized, double-blind, multicenter comparison of oral cefditoren 200 or 400 mg BID with either cefuroxime 250 mg BID or cefadroxil 500 mg BID for the treatment of uncomplicated skin and skin-structure infections. Clin Ther 24:1134–47, 2002.

Gentry LO, Zeluff BJ, Cooley DA. Antibiotic prophylaxis in open-heart surgery: A comparison of cefamandole, cefuroxime, and cefazolin. Ann Thorac Surg 46:167–71, 1988.

Marshall WF, Blair JE. The cephalosporins. Mayo Clin Proc 74:187–95, 1999.

Perry Cm, Brogden RN. Cefuroxime axetil. A review of its antibacterial activity, pharmacokinetic properties, and therapeutic efficacy. Drugs 52:125–58, 1996.

Website: www.pdr.net

Cephalexin (Keflex)

Drug Class: 1st generation oral cephalosporin.
Usual Dose: 500 mg (PO) q6h.
Spectrum: (see **Susceptibility Profiles** pp. 191–197).
Resistance Potential: Low
Pharmacokinetic Parameters:
Peak serum level: 18 mcg/mL
Bioavailability: 99%
Excreted unchanged (urine): > 90%
Serum half-life (normal/ESRD): 0.7/16 hrs
Plasma protein binding: 10%
Volume of distribution (V_d): 0.35 L/kg

Primary Mode of Elimination: Renal
Dosage Adjustments*

CrCl 10–50 mL/min	500 mg (PO) q12h
CrCl < 10 mL/min	500 mg (PO) q24h
Post–HD dose	500 mg (PO)
Post–PD dose	250 mg (PO)
CVVH/CVVHD/ CVVHDF dose	250 mg (PO) q8h
Moderate hepatic insufficiency	No change
Severe hepatic insufficiency	No change

Drug Interactions: None.
Adverse Effects: Drug fever/rash, C. difficile diarrhea/colitis.
Allergic Potential: High
Safety in Pregnancy: B
Comments: Highly active against S. aureus (MSSA) and Group A streptococci. **Limited activity against H. influenzae.**
Cerebrospinal Fluid Penetration: < 10%
Bile Penetration: 200%
(also see **Antibiotic Pearls & Pitfalls** p. 509).

REFERENCES:

Chow M, Quintiliani R, Cunha BA, et al. Pharmacokinetics of high dose oral cephalosporins. J Pharmacol 19:185–194, 1979.

Cunha BA. Cephalexin remains preferred oral antibiotic therapy for uncomplicated cellulitis. Am J Med 121:e11–15, 2008.

Cunha BA. Oral antibiotic therapy of serious systemic infections. Med Clin N Am 90:1197–1222, 2006.

Marshall WF Blair JE. The cephalosporins. Mayo Clin Proc 74:187–95, 1999.

Smith GH. Oral cephalosporins in perspective. DICP 24:45–51, 1990.

Website: www.pdr.net

"Usual dose" assumes normal renal/hepatic function. * For renal insufficiency, give usual dose × 1 followed by maintenance dose per CrCl. For dialysis patients, dose the same as for CrCl < 10 mL/min and give supplemental (post-HD/PD dose) immediately after dialysis. CrCl = creatinine clearance; CVVH = continuous veno-venous hemofiltration; HD/PD = hemodialysis/peritoneal dialysis.

Chloramphenicol (Chloromycetin)

Drug Class: No specific class.
Usual Dose: 500 mg (IV/PO) q6h.
Spectrum: (see *Susceptibility Profiles* pp. 186–190).
Resistance Potential: Low
Pharmacokinetic Parameters:
Peak serum level: 9 mcg/mL
Bioavailability: 90%
Excreted unchanged (urine): 10%
Serum half-life (normal/ESRD): 2.5/3 hrs
Plasma protein binding: 50%
Volume of distribution (V_d): 1 L/kg
Primary Mode of Elimination: Hepatic
Dosage Adjustments*

CrCl < 50 mL/min	No change
Post–HD dose	500 mg (IV/PO)
Post–PD dose	None
CVVH/CVVHD/ CVVHDF dose	No change
Moderate–severe hepatic insufficiency	No change

Drug Interactions: Barbiturates (↑ barbiturate effect, ↓ chloramphenicol effect); cyclophosphamide (↑ cyclophosphamide toxicity); cyanocobalamin, iron (↓ response to interacting drug); warfarin (↑ INR); phenytoin (↑ phenytoin toxicity); rifabutin, rifampin (↓ chloramphenicol levels); sulfonylureas (↑ sulfonylurea effect, hypoglycemia).
Adverse Effects:
Dose–related bone marrow suppression
Reversible. Bone marrow aspirate shows vacuolated WBCs ("chloramphenicol effect," not toxicity). Does not precede aplastic anemia

Idiosyncratic bone marrow toxicity
Irreversible aplastic anemia. May occur after only one dose; monitoring with serial CBCs is useless. Very rare. Usually associated with IM, intraocular, or oral administration. Rarely, if ever, with IV chloramphenicol.
Allergic Potential: Low
Safety in Pregnancy: A
Comments: Incompatible in solutions containing diphenylhydantoin, methylprednisone, aminophylline, ampicillin, gentamicin, erythromycin, vancomycin. **Dose-related marrow suppression is common, and reversible.** Hepatic toxicity related to prolonged/high doses (> 4 gm/d). **Oral administration results in higher serum levels than IV administration.** Do not administer IM. Chloramphenicol is inactivated in bile. **Urinary concentrations are therapeutically ineffective.**
Meningeal dose = usual dose.
Cerebrospinal Fluid Penetration:
Non-Inflamed meninges = 90%
Inflamed meninges = 90%
Bile Penetration: 0%
(also see *Antibiotic Pearls & Pitfalls* p. 513).

REFERENCES:
Ariyal A, Basnyat B, Koirala S, et al. Gatifloxacin versus chloramphenicol for uncomplicated enteric fever: an open-label, randomized, controlled trial. Lancet Infect Dis 11:445–454, 2011.
Cunha BA. New uses of older antibiotics. Postgrad Med 100:68–88, 1997.
Cunha BA. Oral antibiotic therapy of serious systemic infections. Med Clin N Am 90:1197–1222, 2006.
Feder HM Jr, Osier C, Maderazo EG. Chloramphenicol: A review of its use in clinical practice. Rev Infect Dis 3:479–91, 1981.

"Usual dose" assumes normal renal/hepatic function. * For renal insufficiency, give usual dose × 1 followed by maintenance dose per CrCl. For dialysis patients, dose the same as for CrCl < 10 mL/min and give supplemental (post-HD/PD dose) immediately after dialysis. CrCl = creatinine clearance; CVVH = continuous veno-venous hemofiltration; HD/PD = hemodialysis/peritoneal dialysis.

Kasten MJ. Clindamycin, metronidazole, and
  chloramphenicol. Mayo Clin Proc 74:825–33, 1999.
Safdar A, Bryan CS, Stinson S, et al. Prosthetic valve
  endocarditis due to vancomycin-resistant Enterococcus
  faecium: treatment with chloramphenicol plus
  minocycline. Clin Infect Dis 34:61–3, 2002.
Smilack JD, Wilson WE, Cocerill FR 3rd. Tetracycline,
  chloramphenicol, erythromycin, clindamycin, and
  metronidazole. Mayo Clin Proc 66:1270–80, 1991.
Wareham DW, Wilson P. Chloramphenicol in the 21st
  century. Hosp Med 63:157–61, 2002.
Website: www.pdr.net

Cidofovir (Vistide)

Drug class: Antiviral (see comments).
Usual dose: 5 mg/kg (IV) weekly for 2 weeks,
then 5 mg/kg every 2 weeks (for CMV retinitis
in HIV patients, patients must have all of the
following: SrCr < 1.5 mg/dL, CrCl > 55 mL/min,
urine protein < 100 mg/dL).
Pharmacokinetic Parameters:
Peak serum level: 19.6 mcg/mL
Bioavailability: not applicable
Excreted unchanged: 1%
Serum half-life (normal/ESRD): 2.2 h/no data
Plasma protein binding: 6%
Volume of distribution (V_d): 0.54 l/kg
Primary Mode of Elimination: Renal
Dosage Adjustments*

Cr increase of 0.3–0.4 mg/dL above baseline	3 mg/kg (IV) (see usual dose for duration)
Cr increase of ≥ 0.5 mg/dL or + 3 proteinuria	Discontinue cidofovir
Moderate—severe hepatic insufficiency	No change

Drug Interactions: Amphotericin B,
aminoglycosides, foscarnet, pentamidine,
tenofovir, zidovudine (↑ nephrotoxicity).
Adverse Effects: Nephrotoxicity; neutropenia;
nausea, vomiting associated with probenecid,
take with food; metabolic acidosis; decreased
intraocular pressure; anterior uveitis and iritis.
Contraindications: if CrCl < 55 ml/min.
Allergic Potential: Low for cidofovir, high for
probenecid.
Safety in Pregnancy: C
Comments: All patients should receive
probenecid (2 g (PO) 3 hours before infusion
start, then 1 g at 2 and again at 8 hours after
completion of cidofovir infusion, take with
food to minimize nausea and vomiting) and
hydration with at least 1 L of normal saline
with each dose of cidofovir; infuse over 1 hour;
monitor neutrophils, growth factor support
may be needed; contraindicated in severe
hypersensitivity to probenecid or other sulfa
drugs; direct ocular injection is contraindicated;
effective contraception required for male and
female patients. ***Highly active against CMV
and HSV. Some activity against BK virus, JC
virus, VZV, and adenoviruses. No activity
against HHV-6, EBV, RSV, or influenza
viruses.***
Cerebrospinal Fluid Penetration: < 1%

REFERENCES:
Ganguly N, Clough LA, Dubois LK, et al. Low-dose
  cidofovir in the treatment of symptomatic BK
  virus infection in patients undergoing allogenic
  hematopoietic stem cell transplantation: a
  retrospective analysis of an algorithmic approach.
  Transpl Infect Dis 12:406–411, 2010.
Hua DK, Howard K, Craig JC, et al. Cost-effectiveness
  of cidofovir treatment of polyomavirus nephropathy
  in kidney transplant recipients. Transplantation
  27:188–94, 2012.

"Usual dose" assumes normal renal/hepatic function. * For renal insufficiency, give usual dose × 1 followed by
maintenance dose per CrCl. For dialysis patients, dose the same as for CrCl < 10 mL/min and give supplemental
(post-HD/PD dose) immediately after dialysis. CrCl = creatinine clearance; CVVH = continuous veno-venous
hemofiltration; HD/PD = hemodialysis/peritoneal dialysis.

Lurrain NS, Chou S. Antiviral drug resistance of human cytomegalovirus, Clin Microbiol Rev 23:689–712, 2010.

Pallet N, Burgard M, Quamouss O, et al. Cidofovir may be deleterious in BK virus-associated nephropathy. Transplantation 89:1542–1544, 2010.

Ciprofloxacin (Cipro)

Drug Class: Fluoroquinolone.
Usual Dose: 400 mg (IV) q12h; 500–750 mg (PO) q12h (see comments).
Spectrum: (see *Susceptibility Profiles* pp. 198–202).
Resistance Potential: High (S. pneumoniae, E. coli, P. aeruginosa; ↑ prevalence of MRSA)
Pharmacokinetic Parameters:
Peak serum level: 4.6 (IV)/2.9 (PO) mcg/mL
Bioavailability: 70%
Excreted unchanged (urine): 70%
Serum half-life (normal/ESRD): 4/8 hrs
Plasma protein binding: 20–40%
Volume of distribution (V_d): 2.5 L/kg
Primary Mode of Elimination: Renal
Dosage Adjustments*

CrCl 30–50 mL/min	400 mg (IV) q12h 500 mg (PO) q12h
CrCl < 30 mL/min	400 mg (IV) q24h 500 mg (PO) q24h
Post–HD dose	200–400 mg (IV) 250–500 mg (PO)
Post–PD dose	200–400 mg (IV) 250–500 mg (PO)
CVVH/CVVHD/ CVVHDF dose	400 mg (IV) q12h 250 mg (PO) q12h
Moderate hepatic insufficiency	No change
Severe hepatic insufficiency	No change

Drug Interactions: Al++, Ca++, Fe++, Mg++, Zn++ antacids, citrate/citric acid, dairy products (↓ absorption of ciprofloxacin only if taken together); caffeine, cyclosporine, theophylline (↑ interacting drug levels); cimetidine (↑ ciprofloxacin levels); foscarnet (↑ risk of seizures); oral hypoglycemics (slight ↑ or ↓ in blood glucose); NSAIDs (may ↑ risk of seizures/ CNS stimulation); phenytoin (↑ or ↓ phenytoin levels); probenecid (↑ ciprofloxacin levels); warfarin (↑ INR).
Adverse Effects: Drug fever/rash, C. difficile diarrhea/colitis, headache, dizziness, insomnia, malaise, seizures. FQ use has an increased risk of tendinitis/tendon rupture. Risk is highest in the elderly, those on steroids, and those with heart, lung or renal transplants. May ↑ QT$_c$. Vitamins C and E (↓ ciprofloxacin levels).
Allergic Potential: Low
Safety in Pregnancy: C
Comments: Enteral feeding decreases ciprofloxacin absorption ≥ 30%. Use with caution in patients with severe renal insufficiency or seizure disorder. Administer 2 hours before or after H$_2$ antagonists, omeprazole, sucralfate, calcium, iron, zinc, multivitamins, or aluminum/ magnesium containing medications. Administer ciprofloxacin (IV) as an intravenous infusion over 1 hour. **Nosocomial pneumonia dose:** 400 mg (IV) q8h.
↑ incidence of C. difficile diarrhea/colitis with PPIs (for patients on PPIs during FQ therapy, D/C PPIs or switch to H$_2$ blocker for duration of FQ therapy).
Cerebrospinal Fluid Penetration:
Non-Inflamed meninges = 10%
Inflamed meninges = 26%
Bile Penetration: 3000%
(also see *Antibiotic Pearls & Pitfalls* p. 516).

"Usual dose" assumes normal renal/hepatic function. * For renal insufficiency, give usual dose × 1 followed by maintenance dose per CrCl. For dialysis patients, dose the same as for CrCl < 10 mL/min and give supplemental (post-HD/PD dose) immediately after dialysis. CrCl = creatinine clearance; CVVH = continuous veno-venous hemofiltration; HD/PD = hemodialysis/peritoneal dialysis.

REFERENCES:

Davis R, Markham A, Balfour JA. Ciprofloxacin: An updated review of its pharmacology, therapeutic efficacy, and tolerability. Drugs 51:1019–74, 1996.

Didier JP, Villet R, Huggler E, et al. Impact of ciprofloxacin exposure on Staphylococcus aureus genomic alterations linked with emergence of rifampin resistance. Antimicrob Agents Chemother 55:1946–1952, 2011.

Fantin B, Duval X, Massias L, et al. Ciprofloxacin dosage and emergence of resistance in human commensal bacteria. Journal of Infect Dis 200: 390–398, 2009.

Howell MD, Novack V, Grgurich P, et aJ. Iatrogenic gastric acid suppression and the risk of nosocomial Clostridium difficile infection. Arch Intern Med 170:784–790, 2010.

Lewis GJ, Fang Z, Gooch M, et al. Decreased resistance of Pseudomonas aeruginosa with restriction of ciprofloxacin in a large teaching hospitals intensive care and intermediate care units. Infect Control Hosp Epidemiol 33:368–73, 2012.

Linsky A, Gupta K, LawlerEV, et al. Proton pump inhibitors and risk for recurrent Clostridium difficile infection. Arch Intern Med 170:772–778, 2010.

Masadeh MM, Mhaidat NM, Alzoubi KH, et al. Ciprofloxacin-induced antibacterial activity is reversed by vitamin E and vitamin C. Curr Microbiol 64:457–62, 2012.

Miliani K, L'Heriteau, F, Lacave L, et al. Imipenem and ciprofloxacin consumption as factors associated with high incidence rates of resistance Pseudomonas aeruginosa in hospitals in northern France. J Hosp Infect 77:343–347, 2011.

Sanders CC. Ciprofloxacin: In vitro activity, mechanism of action, resistance. Rev Infect Dis 10:516–27, 1998.

Sandberg T, Skoog G, Hermansson AB, et al. Ciprofloxacin for 7 days versus 14 days in women with acute pyelonephritis: a randomized, open-label and double-blind, placebo-controlled, non-inferiority trail. Lancet 4:484–90, 2012.

Website: www.cipro.com

Ciprofloxacin Extended-Release (Cipro XR)

Drug Class: Fluoroquinolone.

Usual Dose: 500 mg or 1000 mg (PO) q24h (see comments).

Spectrum: (see *Susceptibility Profiles* pp. 198–202).

Resistance Potential: High (S. pneumoniae, E. coli, P. aeruginosa; ↑ prevalence of MRSA)

Pharmacokinetic Parameters (500/1000 mg):

Peak serum level: 1.59/3.11 mcg/mL

Bioavailability: 70%

Excreted unchanged (urine): 50–70%; 22% excreted as active metabolite

Serum half-life: 6.6/6.3 hrs

Plasma protein binding: 20–40%

Volume of distribution (V_d): 2.5 L/kg

Primary Mode of Elimination: Renal

Dosage Adjustments*

CrCl < 30 mL/min	No change for 500 mg dose; reduce 1000 mg dose to 500 mg (PO) q24h
Post–HD/PD dose	500 mg (PO)
CVVH/CVVHD/ CVVHDF dose	same as for CrCl < 30 mL/min
Moderate–severe hepatic insufficiency	No change

Drug Interactions: Al⁺⁺, Ca⁺⁺, Fe⁺⁺, Mg⁺⁺, Zn⁺⁺ antacids, citrate/citric acid, dairy products, didanosine (↓ absorption of ciprofloxacin only if taken together); caffeine,

---

"Usual dose" assumes normal renal/hepatic function. * For renal insufficiency, give usual dose × 1 followed by maintenance dose per CrCl. For dialysis patients, dose the same as for CrCl < 10 mL/min and give supplemental (post-HD/PD dose) immediately after dialysis. CrCl = creatinine clearance; CVVH = continuous veno-venous hemofiltration; HD/PD = hemodialysis/peritoneal dialysis.

cyclosporine, theophylline (↑ interacting drug levels); cimetidine (↑ ciprofloxacin levels); foscarnet (↑ risk of seizures); insulin, oral hypoglycemics (slight ↑ or ↓ in blood glucose); NSAIDs (may ↑ risk of seizures/ CNS stimulation); phenytoin (↑ or ↓ phenytoin levels); probenecid (↑ ciprofloxacin levels); warfarin (↑ INR).

Adverse Effects: Drug fever/rash, C. difficile diarrhea/colitis, seizures. FQ use has an increased risk of tendinitis/tendon rupture. Risk in highest in the elderly, those on steroids, and those with heart, lung or renal transplants.

Allergic Potential: Low

Safety in Pregnancy: C

Comments: Uncomplicated UTI (acute cystitis) dose: 500 mg (PO) q24h; **complicated UTI/acute uncomplicated pyelonephritis dose:** 1000 mg (PO) q24h. May be administered with or without food. Administer at least 2 hours before or 6 hours after H$_2$ antagonists, omeprazole, sucralfate, calcium, iron, zinc, multivitamins, or aluminum/ magnesium containing medications.

↑ incidence of C. difficile diarrhea/colitis with PPIs (for patients on PPIs during FQ therapy, D/C PPIs or switch to H$_2$ blocker for duration of FQ therapy).

Cerebrospinal Fluid Penetration:

Non-Inflamed meninges = 10%

Inflamed meninges = 26%

Bile Penetration: 3000%

(also see *Antibiotic Pearls & Pitfalls* p. 516).

REFERENCES:

Davis R, Markham A, Balfour JA. Ciprofloxacin: An updated review of its pharmacology, therapeutic efficacy, and tolerability. Drugs 51:1019–74, 1996.

Website: www.ciproxr.com

Clarithromycin (Biaxin)

Drug Class: Macrolide.

Usual Dose: 500 mg (PO) q12h.

Spectrum: (see *Susceptibility Profiles* pp. 186–190).

Resistance Potential: High (S. pneumoniae, GAS, MSSA)

Pharmacokinetic Parameters:

Peak serum level: 1–4 mcg/mL

Bioavailability: 50%

Excreted unchanged (urine): 20%

Serum half-life (normal/ESRD): 3–7/4 hrs

Plasma protein binding: 70%

Volume of distribution (V$_d$): 3 L/kg

Primary Mode of Elimination: Hepatic

Dosage Adjustments*

CrCl < 30 mL/min	250 mg (PO) q12h
Post–HD dose	500 mg (PO)
Post–PD dose	None
CVVH/CVVHD/ CVVHDF dose	No change
Moderate–severe hepatic insufficiency	No change

Drug Interactions: Amiodarone, procainamide, sotalol, astemizole, terfenadine, cisapride, pimozide (may ↑ QT interval, torsade de pointes); carbamazepine (↑ carbamazepine levels, nystagmus, nausea, vomiting, diarrhea); cimetidine, digoxin, ergot alkaloids, midazolam, triazolam, phenytoin, ritonavir, tacrolimus, valproic acid (↑ interacting drug levels); clozapine, corticosteroids (not studied); cyclosporine (↑ cyclosporine levels with toxicity); efavirenz (↓ clarithromycin levels); rifabutin, rifampin (↓ clarithromycin levels, ↑ interacting drug levels); statins (↑ risk of rhabdomyolysis);

"Usual dose" assumes normal renal/hepatic function. * For renal insufficiency, give usual dose × 1 followed by maintenance dose per CrCl. For dialysis patients, dose the same as for CrCl < 10 mL/min and give supplemental (post-HD/PD dose) immediately after dialysis. CrCl = creatinine clearance; CVVH = continuous veno-venous hemofiltration; HD/PD = hemodialysis/peritoneal dialysis.

theophylline (↑ theophylline levels, nausea, vomiting, seizures, apnea); warfarin (↑ INR); zidovudine (↓ zidovudine levels).

Adverse Effects: Nausea, vomiting, GI upset, **Non-C. difficile diarrhea,** abdominal pain. May ↑ QT_c; avoid with other medications that prolong the QT_c interval and in patients with cardiac arrhythmias/heart block.

Allergic Potential: Low

Safety in Pregnancy: C

Comments: Peculiar "aluminum sand" taste sensation on swallowing.

Cerebrospinal Fluid Penetration: < 10%

Bile Penetration: 7000%

(also see **Antibiotic Pearls & Pitfalls** p. 519).

REFERENCES:

Alcaide F, Calatayud L, Santin M, et al. Comparative in vitro activities of linezolid, telithromycin, clarithromycin, levofloxacin, moxifloxacin and four conventional antimycobacterial drugs against mycobacterium kansasii. Antimicrob Agents Chemother 48:4562–5, 2004.

Alvarez-Elcoro S, Enzler MJ. The macrolides: Erythromycin, clarithromycin and azithromycin. Mayo Clin Proc 4:613–34, 1999.

Benson CA, Williams PL, Cohn DL, and the ACTG 196/CPCRA 009 Study Team. Clarithromycin or rifabutin alone or in combination for primary prophylaxis of Mycobacterium avium complex disease in patients with AIDS: A randomized, double-blinded, placebo-controlled trial. J Infect Dis 181:1289–97, 2000.

Berg HF, Tjhie JH, Scheffer GJ, et al. Emergence and persistence of macrolide resistance in oropharyngeal flora and elimination of nasal carriage of Staphylococcus aureus after therapy with slow-release clarithromycin: a randomized, double-blind, placebo-controlled study. Antimicrob Agents Chemother 48:4138–8, 2004.

Bergman M, Huikko S, Huovinen P, et al. Macrolide and azithromycin use are linked to increased macrolide resistance in Streptococcus pneumoniae. Antimicrob Agents Chemother 50:3646–3650, 2006.

Daneman N, McGeer A, Green K, et al. Macrolide resistance in bacteremic pneumococcal disease.: Implications for patient management. Clin Infect Dis 43:432–438, 2006.

Dean NC, Sperry P, Wikler M, et al. Comparing clarithromycin in pneumonia symptom resolution and process of care. Antimicrob Agents Chemother 50:1164–69, 2006.

Jain R, Danzinger LH. The macrolide antibiotics: a pharmacokinetic and pharmacodynamic overview. Curr Pharm Des 10:3045–53, 2004.

Jenkins SG, Farrell DJ. Increase in pneumococcus macrolide resistance, United States. Emerging Infect Dis 15:1260–1264, 2009.

Kafetzis DA, Chantzi F, Tigaani G, et al. Safety and tolerability of clarithromycin administered to children at higher-than-recommended doses. Eur J Clin Microbiol Infect Dis 26:99–103, 2007.

Kraft M, Cassell AGH, Jpak J, et al. Mycoplasma pneumoniae and Chlamydia pneumoniae in asthma: effect of clarithromycin. Chest 121:1782–8, 2002.

Malfertheiner P, Bazzoli F, Delchier JC, et al. Helicobacter pylori eradication with a capsule containing bismuth subcitrate potassium, metronidazole, and tetracycline given with omeprazole versus clarithromycin-based triple therapy: a randomized open-label, non-inferiority, phase 3 trial. Lancet 33:905–913, 2011.

McConnell SA, Amsden GW. Review and comparison of advanced-generation macrolides clarithromycin and dirithromycin. Pharmacotherapy 19:404–15, 1999.

Ozsoylar G, Sayin A, Bolay H. Clarithromycin monotherapy-induced delirium. J Antimicrob Chemother 59:331, 2007.

Periti P, Mazzei T. Clarithromycin: Pharmacokinetic and pharmacodynamic interrelationships and dosage regimen. J Chemother 11:11–27, 1999.

Portier H, Filipecki J, Weber P, et al Five day clarithromycin modified release versus 10 day penicillin V for group A streptococcal pharyngitis: a multi-centre, open-label, randomized study. J Antimicrob Chemother 49:337–44, 2002.

Rodvold KA. Clinical pharmacokinetics of clarithromycin. Clin Pharmacokinet 37:385–98, 1999.

Schlossberg D. Azithromycin and clarithromycin. Med Clin North Am 79:803–16, 1995.

"Usual dose" assumes normal renal/hepatic function. * For renal insufficiency, give usual dose × 1 followed by maintenance dose per CrCl. For dialysis patients, dose the same as for CrCl < 10 mL/min and give supplemental (post-HD/PD dose) immediately after dialysis. CrCl = creatinine clearance; CVVH = continuous veno-venous hemofiltration; HD/PD = hemodialysis/peritoneal dialysis.

Stein GE, Schooley S. Serum bactericidal activity of extended-release clarithromycin against macrolide-resistant strains of Streptococcus pneumoniae. Pharmacotherapy 22:593–6, 2002.

Svensson M, Strom M, Nelsson M et al. Pharmacodynamic effects of nitroimidazoles alone and in combination with clarithromycin on Helicobacter pylori. Antimicrob Agents Chemother 46:2244–8, 2002.

Tartaglione TA. Therapeutic options for the management and prevention of Mycobacterium avium complex infection in patients with acquired immunodeficiency syndrome. Pharmacotherapy 16:171–82, 1996.

Website: www.biaxin.com

Clarithromycin XL (Biaxin XL)

Drug Class: Macrolide.
Usual Dose: 1 gm (PO) q24h.
Spectrum: (see *Susceptibility Profiles* pp. 186–190).
Resistance Potential: High (S. pneumoniae, GAS, MSSA)
Pharmacokinetic Parameters:
Peak serum level: 3 mcg/mL
Bioavailability: 50%
Excreted unchanged (urine): 20%; 10–15% excreted as active metabolite
Serum half-life (normal/ESRD): 4/4 hrs
Plasma protein binding: 70%
Volume of distribution (V_d): 3 L/kg
Primary Mode of Elimination: Hepatic
Dosage Adjustments*

CrCl < 30 mL/min	500 mg (PO) q24h
Post–HD dose	None
Post–PD dose	None
CVVH/CVVHD/ CVVHDF dose	No change

Moderate hepatic insufficiency	No change
Severe hepatic insufficiency	No change

Drug Interactions: Amiodarone, procainamide, sotalol, astemizole, terfenadine, cisapride, pimozide (may ↑ QT interval, torsade de pointes); carbamazepine (↑ carbamazepine levels, nystagmus, nausea, vomiting, diarrhea); cimetidine, digoxin, ergot alkaloids, midazolam, triazolam, phenytoin, ritonavir, tacrolimus, valproic acid (↑ interacting drug levels); clozapine, corticosteroids (not studied); cyclosporine (↑ cyclosporine levels with toxicity); efavirenz (↓ clarithromycin levels); rifabutin, rifampin (↓ clarithromycin levels, ↑ interacting drug levels); statins (↑ risk of rhabdomyolysis); theophylline (↑ theophylline levels, nausea, vomiting, seizures, apnea); warfarin (↑ INR); zidovudine (↓ zidovudine levels).
Adverse Effects: Nausea, vomiting **Non-C. difficile diarrhea.** May ↑ QT$_c$; avoid with other medications that prolong the QT$_c$ interval and in patients with cardiac arrhythmias/heart block.
Allergic Potential: Low
Safety in Pregnancy: C
Comments: Two 500 mg tablets of XL preparation permits once daily dosing and decreases GI intolerance.
Cerebrospinal Fluid Penetration: < 10%
Bile Penetration: 7000%
(also see *Antibiotic Pearls & Pitfalls* p. 519).

REFERENCES:

Adler JL, Jannetti W, Schneider D, et al. Phase III, randomized, double-blind study of clarithromycin extended-release and immediate-release formulations in the treatment of patients with acute exacerbation of chronic bronchitis. Clin Ther 22:1410–20, 2000.

"Usual dose" assumes normal renal/hepatic function. * For renal insufficiency, give usual dose × 1 followed by maintenance dose per CrCl. For dialysis patients, dose the same as for CrCl < 10 mL/min and give supplemental (post-HD/PD dose) immediately after dialysis. CrCl = creatinine clearance; CVVH = continuous veno-venous hemofiltration; HD/PD = hemodialysis/peritoneal dialysis.

Anzueto A, Fisher CL Jr, Busman T. Comparison of the efficacy of extended-release clarithromycin tablets and amoxicillin/clavulanate tablets in the treatment of acute exacerbation of chronic bronchitis. Clin Ther 23:72–86, 2000.

Bergman M, Huikko S, Huovinen P, et al. Macrolide and azithromycin use are linked to increased macrolide resistance in Streptococcus pneumoniae. Antimicrob Agents Chemother 50:3646–3650, 2006.

Daneman N, McGeer A, Green K, et al. Macrolide resistance in bacteremic pneumococcal disease.: Implications for patient management. Clin Infect Dis 43:432–438, 2006.

Gotfried HM. Clarithromycin (Biaxin) extended-release tablet: a therapeutic review. Expert Rev Anti Infect Ther 1:9–20, 2004.

Jenkins SG, Farrell DJ. Increase in pneumococcus macrolide resistance, United States. Emerging Infect Dis 15:1260–1264, 2009.

Laine L, Estrada R, Trujillo M, et al. Once-daily therapy for H. pylori infection: Randomized comparison of four regimens. Am J Gastroenterol 94:962–6, 1999.

Mandell LA, Wunderink RG, Anzuetto A, et al. Infectious Diseases Society of America/American Thoracic Society consensus guidelines on the management of community-acquired pneumonia in adults. Clin Infect Dis 44:S27–72, 2007.

Nalepa P, Dobryniewska M, Busman T, et al. Short-course therapy of acute bacterial exacerbation of chronic bronchitis: a double-blind, randomized, multicenter comparison of extended-release versus immediate-release clarithromycin. Curr Med Res Opin 19:411–20, 2003.

Website: biaxinxl.com

Clindamycin (Cleocin)

Drug Class: Lincosamide.
Usual Dose: 600 mg (IV) q8h; 150–300 mg (PO) q6h.
Spectrum: (see *Susceptibility Profiles* pp. 186–190).
Resistance Potential: Low
Pharmacokinetic Parameters:
Peak serum level: 2.5–10 mcg/mL

Bioavailability: 90%
Excreted unchanged (urine): 10%; 3.6% excreted as active metabolite
Serum half-life (normal/ESRD): 2.4/4 hrs
Plasma protein binding: 90%
Volume of distribution (V_d): 1 L/kg
Primary Mode of Elimination: Hepatic
Dosage Adjustments*

CrCl < 10 mL/min	No change
Post–HD/PD dose	None
CVVH/CVVHD/CVVHDF dose	No change
Moderate—severe hepatic insufficiency	No change

Drug Interactions: Muscle relaxants, neuromuscular blockers (↑ apnea, respiratory paralysis); kaolin (↓ clindamycin absorption); theophylline (↑ theophylline levels, seizures).
Adverse Effects: C. difficile diarrhea/colitis, neuromuscular blockade.
Allergic Potential: Low
Safety in Pregnancy: B
Comments: *Anti-spasmodics contraindicated in C. difficile diarrhea.* C. difficile diarrhea more common with PO vs. IV clindamycin. *Clindamycin misses some Peptostreptococci, Fusobacteria, non-perfringens Clostridia, and Prevotella.*
Cerebrospinal Fluid Penetration: < 10%
Bile Penetration: 300%
(also see *Antibiotic Pearls & Pitfalls* p. 513).

REFERENCES:
Back EE, O'Grady EJ, Back JD. High rates of perinatal group B Streptococcus clindamycin and erythromycin resistance in an upstate New York Hospital. Antimicrob Agents Chemother 56:739–742, 2012.

"Usual dose" assumes normal renal/hepatic function. * For renal insufficiency, give usual dose × 1 followed by maintenance dose per CrCl. For dialysis patients, dose the same as for CrCl < 10 mL/min and give supplemental (post-HD/PD dose) immediately after dialysis. CrCl = creatinine clearance; CVVH = continuous veno-venous hemofiltration; HD/PD = hemodialysis/peritoneal dialysis.

Coyle EA, Cha R, Rybak MJ. Influences of linezolid, penicillin, and clindamycin, alone and in combination, on streptococcal pyrogenic exotoxin a release. Antimicrob Agents Chemother 47:1752–5, 2003.

Cunha BA. Oral Antibiotic Therapy of Serious Systemic Infections. Med Clin N Am 90:1197–1222, 2006.

Czekaj J, Dinh A, Moldovan A, et al. Efficacy of a combined oral clindamycin-rifampicin regimen for therapy of staphylococcal osteoarticular infections. Scand J Infect Dis 43:962–967, 2011.

Falagas ME, Gorbach SL. Clindamycin and metronidazole. Med Clin North Am 79:845–67, 1995.

Kasten MJ. Clindamycin, metronidazole, and chloramphenicol. Mayo Clin Proc 74:825–33, 1999.

Klepser ME, Nicolau DP, Quintiliani R, et al. Bactericidal activity of low-dose clindamycin administered at 8- and 12-hour intervals against Streptococcus pneumoniae and Bacteroides fragilis. Antimicrob Agents Chemother 41:630–5, 1997.

Lell B, Dremsner PG. Clindamycin as an antimalarial drug: review of clinical trials. Antimicrob Agents Chemother 46:2315–20, 2002.

Levin TP, Suh B, Axelrod P, et al. Potential clindamycin resistance in clindamycin-susceptible, erythromycin-resistant staphylococcus aureus: Report of a clinical failure. Antimicrob Agents Chemother 49:1222–24, 2005.

Patel M, Waites KB, Moser SA, et al. Prevalence of inducible clindamycin resistance among community- and hospital-associated Staphylococcus aureus isolates. Journal of Clinical Microbiology 44:2481–84, 2006.

Website: www.pdr.net

Colistin/Polymyxin E
Colistin methanesulfonate
(Coly-Mycin M)

Drug Class: Cell membrane altering antibiotic.
Usual Dose: 1.7 mg/kg (IV) q8h.
Spectrum: (see *Susceptibility Profiles* pp. 198–202).
Resistance Potential: Low
Pharmacokinetic Parameters:
Peak serum level: 5 mcg/mL

Bioavailability: Not applicable
Excreted unchanged (urine): 90%
Serum half-life (normal/ESRD): 3.5/48–72 hrs
Plasma protein binding: < 10%
Volume of distribution (V_d): 0.09 L/kg
Primary Mode of Elimination: Renal
Dosage Adjustments*

CrCl 40–60 mL/min	2.5 mg/kg (IV) q12h
CrCl 10–40 mL/min	2.5 mg/kg (IV) q24h
CrCl < 10 mL/min	1.5 mg/kg (IV) q36h
Post–HD dose	None
Post–PD dose	None
CVVH/CVVHD/CVVHDF dose	2.5 mg/kg (IV) q48h
Mild hepatic insufficiency	No change
Moderate—severe hepatic insufficience	No change

Drug Interactions: Neuromuscular blocking agents (↑ neuromuscular blockade); nephrotoxic drugs (↑ nephrotoxic potential).
Adverse Effects: Dose dependent/reversible nephrotoxic potential (acute tubular necrosis). Paresthesias, vertigo, dizziness, slurred speech, blurry vision, respiratory arrest.
Allergic Potential: Low
Safety in Pregnancy: C
Comments: 1 mg = 12,500 U. Colistin (Polymyxin E) has **less nephrotoxic potential than previously thought. Useful for MDR P. aeruginosa and Acinetobacter species.** For P. aeruginosa or Acinetobacter meningitis *also give amikacin 10–40 mg (IT) q24h or colistin 10 mg (IT) q24h.* **Intrathecal colistin dose:** 10 mg (IT) Q24h. **Nebulizer dose:** 80 mg in saline q8h; for recurrent infection use 160 mg q8h (freshly prepare solution and use within 24 hours). If possible, avoid aerosolized colistin,

---

"Usual dose" assumes normal renal/hepatic function. * For renal insufficiency, give usual dose × 1 followed by maintenance dose per CrCl. For dialysis patients, dose the same as for CrCl < 10 mL/min and give supplemental (post-HD/PD dose) immediately after dialysis. CrCl = creatinine clearance; CVVH = continuous veno-venous hemofiltration; HD/PD = hemodialysis/peritoneal dialysis.

which may result in pulmonary/systemic toxicity due to the polymyxin E1 metabolite. **Continuous infusion dose:** give ½ of daily dose (IV) over 5–10 min, then give remaining ½ dose (in D5W or NS) 1 hour after initial dose over next 24 hours. **Cerebrospinal Fluid Penetration:** < 25% (also see *Antibiotic Pearls & Pitfalls* p. 520).

REFERENCES:

Berlana D, Llop JM, Fort E, et al. Use of colistin in the treatment of multidrug resistant gram-negative infections. Am J Health Syst Pharm 62:39–47, 2005.

Cai Y, Chai D, Wang R, et al. Colistin resistance of Acinetoacter baumannii: clinical reports, mechanisms and antimicrobial strategies. J Antimicrob Chemother 67:1607–15, 2012.

Cascio A, Conti A, Sinardi L, et al. Post-neurosurgical multidrug-resistant Acinetobacter baumannii meningitis successfully treated with intrathecal colistin. A new case and a systematic review of the literature. Int J Infect Dis 14:e572–9,2010.

Cheng CY, Sheng WH, Wang JT, et al. Safety and efficacy of intravenous colistin (colistin methanesulphonate) for severe multidrug-resistant Gram-negative bacterial infections. Int J Antimicrob Agents 35:297–300, 2010.

Couet W, Gregoire N, Marchan S, et al. Colistin pharma-cokinetics: the fog is lifting. Clin Microbiol Infect 18: 30–39, 2012.

Cunha BA. New uses for older antibiotics: nitrofurantoin, amikacin, colistin, polymyxin B, doxycycline, and minocycline revisited. Med Clin North Am 90:1089–1107, 2006.

Daikos GL, Skiada A, Pavleas J, et al. Serum bactericidal activity of three different dosing regimens of colistin with implications for optimum clinical use. J Chemother 22:175–178, 2010.

Deryke CA, Crawford AJ, Uddin N, et al. Colistin dosing and nephrotoxicity in a large community teaching hospital. Antimicrob Agents Chemother 54:4503–4505, 2010.

Durakovic N, Radojcic V, Boban A, et al. Efficacy and safety of colistin in the treatment of infections caused by multidrug-resistance Pseudomonas aeruginosa in patients with hematologic malignancy: a match pair analysis. Intern Med 50:1009–1013, 2011.

Falagas ME, Rafailidis PL. Colistin in ventilator-associated pneumonia. Clin Infect Dis 54:681–3, 2012.

Falagas ME, Rafailidis PI, Kasiakou SK, et al. Effectiveness and nephrotoxicity of colistin monotherapy vs colistin-meropenem combination therapy for multidrug-resistant Gram-negative bacterial infections. Clin Micrbiol Infect 12:1227–30, 2006.

Falagas ME, Rafailidis PI. Nephrotoxicity of colistin: new insight into an old antibiotic. Clin Infect Dis 48:1729–1731, 2009.

Falagas ME, Rafailidis PI, Ioannidou E, et al. Colistin therapy for microbiologically documented multi drug-resistant Gram-negative bacterial infections: a retrospective cohort study of 258 patients. Int J Antimicrob Agents 35:194–199, 2010.

Hachem RY, Chemaly RF, Ahmar CA, et al. Colistin is effective in treatment of infections caused by multidrug-resistant Pseudomonas aeruginosa in cancer patients. Antimicrob Agents Chemother 51:1905–1911, 2007.

Hartzell JD, Neff R, Ake J, et al. Nephrotoxicity associated with intravenous colistin (colistimethate sodium) treatment at a tertiary care medical center. Clin Infect Dis 48:1724–1728, 2009.

Horton J, Pankey GA. Polymyxin B, colistin, and sodium colistimethate. Med Clin North Am 66:135–42, 1982.

Humphries RM, Kelesidis T, Dien Bard J, et al. Successful treatment of pan-resistant Klebsiella pneumoniae pneumonia and bacteraemia with a combination of high-dose tigecycline and colistin. J Med Microbiol 59:1383–1386, 2010.

Imberti R. Intravenous colistimethate administration and colistin lung tissue concentrations. Intensive Care Med 36:1795, 2010.

Kempf M, Djouhri-Bouktab L, Brunel JM, et al. Synergistic activity of sulbactam combined with colistin against colistin-resistant Acinetobacter baumannii. Int J Antimicrob Agents 39:180–1, 2012.

Koch-Weser G, Sidel VW, Federman EB, et al. Adverse effects of sodium colistimethate. Ann Intern Med 72:857–68, 1970.

Kofteridis DP, Alexopoulou C, Valachis A, et al. Aerosolized plus intravenous colistin versus intravenous colistin alone for the treatment of ventilator-associated pneumonia: a matched case-control study. Clin Infect Dis 51: 1238–1244, 2010.

"Usual dose" assumes normal renal/hepatic function. * For renal insufficiency, give usual dose × 1 followed by maintenance dose per CrCl. For dialysis patients, dose the same as for CrCl < 10 mL/min and give supplemental (post-HD/PD dose) immediately after dialysis. CrCl = creatinine clearance; CVVH = continuous veno-venous hemofiltration; HD/PD = hemodialysis/peritoneal dialysis.

Kwa AL, Falagas ME, Michalopoulos A, et al. Benefits of aerosolized colistin for ventilator-associated pneumonia: absence of proof versus proof of absence? Clin Infect Dis 52:1278–1279, 2011.

Levin AS, Baron AA, Penco J, et al. Intravenous colistin as therapy for nosocomial infections caused by multidrug resistant Pseudomonas aeruginosa and Acinetobacter baumannii. Clin Infect Dis 28: 1008–11, 1999.

Liang W, Liu XR, Huang, J, et al. Activities of colistin- and minocycline-based combinations against extensive drug resistant Acinetobacter baumannii isolates from intensive care unit patients. BMC Infect Dis 11:109, 2011.

Linden PK, Kusne S, Coley K, et al. Use of parenteral colistin for the treatment of serious infection due to antimicrobial-resistant Pseudomonas aeruginosa. Clin Infect Dis 37:154–60, 2003.

Marchand S, Frat JP, Petitpas F, et al. Removal of colistin during intermittent haemodialysis in two critically ill patients. J Antimicrob Chemother 65:1836–1837, 2010.

Markantonis SL, Markou N, Fousteri M, et al. Penetration of colistin into cerebrospinal fluid. Antimicrob Agents Chemother 53:4907–4910, 2009.

Oliveira MS, Prado GV, Costa SF, et al. Polymyxin B and colistimethate are comparable as to efficacy and renal toxicity. Diagn Microbiol Infect Dis 65:431–434, 2009.

Ozbek B, OtUk G. In vitro activities of tigecycline alone and in combination with colistin su fate or sulbactam against carbapenem-susceptible and -resistant Acinetobacter baumannii strains isolated from Intensive Care Units. Int J Antimicrob Agents 36:191–192, 2010.

Paul M, Bishara J, Levcovich A, et al. Effectiveness and safety of colistin: prospective comparative cohort study. J Antimicrob Chemother 65:1019–1027, 2010.

Papagelopoulos PJ, Mavrogenis AF, Giannitsioti E, et al. Management of a multidrug-resistant Pseudomonas aeruginosa infected knee arthroplasty using colistin. A care report and review of the literature. J Arthroplasty 22:457–463, 2007.

Plachouras D, Giamerllos-Bourboulis EJ, Kentepozidis N, et al. In vitro postantibiotic effect of colistin on multidrug-resistant Acinetobacter baumannii. Diagn Microbiol Infect Dis 57:419–422, 2007.

Rattanaumpawan P, Ungprasert P, Thamlikitkul V. Risk factors for colistin-associated nephrotoxicity. J Infect 62:187–190, 2011.

Reed MD, Stern RC, O'Riordan MA, et al. The pharmacokinetics of colistin in patients with cystic fibrosis. J Clin Pharmacol 41:645–54, 2001.

Rynn C, Wooton M, Bowker KE, et al. In vitro assessment of colistin's antipseudomonal antimicrobial interactions with other antibiotics. Clin Microbiol Infect 5:32–6, 1999.

Santamaría C, Mykietiuk A, Temporiti E, et al. Nephrotoxicity associated with the use of intravenous colistin. Scand J Infect Dis 41:767–769, 2009.

Stein A, Raoult D. Colistin: an antimicrobial for the 21st century? Clin Infect Dis 35:901–2, 2002.

Tan TY, Ng SY. Comparison of Etest, Viteck and agar dilution for susceptibility testing of colistin. Clin Microbiol Infect 13:541–544, 2007.

Tarchini G. Nephrotoxicity associated with intravenous colistin. Clin Infect Dis 49:1773, 2009.

Van Leeuwen DH. A closer look at aerosolized colistin. Clin Infect Dis 52:1472–1473, 2011.

Wahby K, Chopra T, Chandrasekar P. Intravenous and Inhalational colistin-induced respiratory failure. Clin Infect Dis 50:e38–40, 2010.

Yahav D, Farbman L, Leibovici L, et al. Colistin: New lessons on an old antibiotic. Clin Microbiol Infect 18:18–29, 2012.

Cycloserine (Seromycin)

Drug Class: Anti-TB drug.
Usual Dose: 250 mg (PO) q12h.
Pharmacokinetic Parameters:
Peak serum level: 20 mcg/mL
Bioavailability: 90%
Excreted unchanged (urine): 65%

Serum half-life (normal/ESRD): 10–25 hrs/no data
Plasma protein binding: No data
Volume of distribution (V_d): 0.2 L/kg
Primary Mode of Elimination: Renal
Dosage Adjustments*

CrCl 10–50 mL/min	250 mg (PO) q12–24h
CrCl < 10 mL/min	250 mg (PO) q24h
Post–HD dose	None
Post–PD dose	250 mg (PO)
CVVH/CVVHD/CVVHDF dose	No change
Moderate—severe hepatic insufficiency	No change

Drug Interactions: Alcohol (seizures); ethambutol, ethionamide (drowsiness, dizziness); phenytoin (↑ phenytoin levels).
Adverse Effects: Peripheral neuropathy, seizures (dose related), psychosis/delirium.
Allergic Potential: Low
Safety in Pregnancy: C
Comments: Avoid in patients with seizures. Ethambutol, ethionamide, or ethanol may increase CNS toxicity.
Meningeal dose = usual dose.
Cerebrospinal Fluid Penetration:
Non-Inflamed meninges = 90%
Inflamed meninges = 90%

REFERENCES:

[No authors listed.] Drugs for tuberculosis. Med Lett Drugs Ther 35:99–101, 1993.

Davidson PT, Le HQ. Drug treatment of tuberculosis 1992. Drugs 43:651–73, 1992.

Furin J, Nardell EA. Multidrug-resistant tuberculosis: An update on the best regimens. J Respir Dis 27:172–82, 2006.

Iseman MD. Treatment of multidrug resistant tuberculosis. N Engl J Med 329:784–91, 1993.

Dapsone

Drug Class: Antiparasitic, anti-leprosy, anti-PCP drug.
Usual Dose: 100 mg (PO) q24h (see comments).
Pharmacokinetic Parameters:
Peak serum level: 1.8 mcg/mL
Bioavailability: 85%
Excreted unchanged (urine): 10%
Serum half-life (normal/ESRD): 25/30 hrs
Plasma protein binding: 80%
Volume of distribution (V_d): 1.2 L/kg
Primary Mode of Elimination: Hepatic/renal
Dosage Adjustments*

CrCl < 10 mL/min	No change
Post–HD dose	None
Post–PD dose	None
CVVH/CVVHD/CVVHDF dose	No change
Moderate hepatic insufficiency	No change
Severe hepatic insufficiency	No data

Drug Interactions: Didanosine (↓ dapsone absorption); oral contraceptives (↓ oral contraceptive effect); pyrimethamine, zidovudine (↑ bone marrow suppression); rifabutin, rifampin (↓ dapsone levels); trimethoprim (↑ dapsone and trimethoprim levels, methemoglobinemia).
Adverse Effects: Drug fever/rash, nausea, vomiting, hemolytic anemia in G6PD deficiency, methemoglobinemia.
Allergic Potential: High
Safety in Pregnancy: C
Comments: **Useful in sulfa (SMX) allergic patients.** Avoid, if possible, in G6PD deficiency or hemoglobin M deficiency.

"Usual dose" assumes normal renal/hepatic function. * For renal insufficiency, give usual dose × 1 followed by maintenance dose per CrCl. For dialysis patients, dose the same as for CrCl < 10 mL/min and give supplemental (post-HD/PD dose) immediately after dialysis. CrCl = creatinine clearance; CVVH = continuous veno-venous hemofiltration; HD/PD = hemodialysis/peritoneal dialysis.

PCP prophylaxis dose: 100 mg (PO) q24h.
PCP therapy dose: 100 mg (PO) q24h.
Cerebrospinal Fluid Penetration: < 50%

REFERENCES:

East J, Blanton LS. Symptomatic hyperbilirubinemia secondary to dapsone-induced hemolysis and atazanavir therapy. Antimicrob Chemother 67:465–8, 2012.

El-Sadr WM, Murphy RI, Yurik TM, et al. Atovaquone compared with dapsone to the prevention of Pneumocystis carinii in patients with HIV infection who cannot tolerate trimethoprim, sulfonamides, or both. N Engl J Med 339:1889–95, 1998.

Medina I, Mills J, Leoung G, et al. Oral therapy for Pneumocystis carinii pneumonia in the acquired immunodeficiency syndrome. A controlled trial of trimethoprim-sulfamethoxazole versus trimethoprim-dapsone. N Engl J Med 323:776–82, 1990.

Podzamczer D, Salazar A, Jiminez J, et al. Intermittent trimethoprim-sulfamethoxazole compared with dapsone-pyrimethamine for the simultaneous primary prophylaxis of Pneumocystis pneumonia and toxoplasmosis in patients infected with HIV. Ann Intern Med 122:755–61, 1995.

Website: www.pdr.net

Daptomycin (Cubicin)

Drug Class: Lipopeptide.
Usual Dose: Complicated skin/skin structure infections: 4 mg/kg (IV) q24h. Bacteremia, endocarditis: 6 mg/kg (IV) q24h. Bacteremia, endocarditis unresponsive to 6 mg/kg (IV) q24h × 3 days: 12 mg/kg (IV) q24h.
Spectrum: (see *Susceptibility Profiles* pp. 198–202).
Resistance Potential: Low
Pharmacokinetic Parameters:
Peak serum level:
4 mg/kg = 58 mcg/mL; 6 mg/kg = 99 mcg/mL.

Bioavailability: Not applicable
Excreted unchanged (urine): 80%
Serum half-life (normal/ESRD): 8.1/29.8 hrs
Plasma protein binding: 92%
Volume of distribution (V$_d$): 0.096 L/kg
Primary Mode of Elimination: Renal
Dosage Adjustments*

CrCl > 30 mL/min	No change
CrCl < 30 mL/min	4 mg/kg (IV) q48h or 6 mg/kg (IV) q48h or 12 mg/kg (IV) q48h
Post–HD dose	None
Post–PD dose	None
CVVH/CVVHD/ CVVHDF dose	8 mg/kg (IV) q48h
HD q 48–72h dose	10 mg/kg (IV) q HD*
Moderate—severe hepatic insufficiency	No change

*Give at end of HD.
Drug Interactions: Warfarin/statin (no significant interaction in small number of volunteers; consider temporary suspension of statins during daptomycin use).
Adverse Effects: Constipation, nausea, headache. Rarely, ↑ CPK; in clinical trials, same or less (0.2%) than comparators; monitor for muscle pain/weakness and CPK weekly. Eosinophilic pneumonia (rare and reversible when drug discontinued). False-positive ↑ INR.
Allergic Potential: No data
Safety in Pregnancy: B
Comments: Concentration-dependent killing may be enhanced with an initial dose of gentamicin. Antecedent vancomycin (↑ cell wall thickness of staphylococci) predisposes to daptomycin resistance (penetration mediated resistance). ↑ daptomycin MICs with strains of

---

"Usual dose" assumes normal renal/hepatic function. * For renal insufficiency, give usual dose × 1 followed by maintenance dose per CrCl. For dialysis patients, dose the same as for CrCl < 10 mL/min and give supplemental (post-HD/PD dose) immediately after dialysis. CrCl = creatinine clearance; CVVH = continuous veno-venous hemofiltration; HD/PD = hemodialysis/peritoneal dialysis.

S. aureus may be ↓ by adding a β–lactam (to ↑ cell wall permeability) for staphylococci add nafcillin to daptomycin; for enterococci add ampicillin to daptomycin. **High-dose daptomycin 12 mg/kg (IV) q24h has been used for MSSA/MRSA bacteremias/ABE unresponsive to other an-tistaphylococcal drugs without toxicity.** Post-antibiotic effect (PAE) up to 6 hours. For rapid effect or need to limit infusion volume, daptomycin *may be given IV push over 5 minutes* (500 mg dose given in 10 mL; 1 g dose given in 20 mL). Cannot be given IM.

Cerebrospinal Fluid Penetration: ~ 5% (also see *Antibiotic Pearls & Pitfalls* p. 518).

REFERENCES:

Alder JD. Daptomycin: a new drug class for the treatment of gram-positive infections. Drugs Today 41:81–90, 2005.

Bassetti M, Nicco E, Ginocchio F, et al. High-dose daptomycin in documented Staphylococcus aureus infections. Int J Antimicrob Agents 36:459–461, 2010.

Bhavnani SM, Prakhya A, Hammel JP, et al. Cost-Effectiveness of daptomycin versus vancomycin and gentamicin for patients with methicillin-resistant Staphylococcus aureus bacteremia and/or endocarditis. Clin Infect Dis 49:691–698, 2009.

Benevuto M, Benziger DP, Yankelev S, Vigliani G. Pharmacokinetics and tolerability of daptomycin at doses up to 12 milligrams per kilogram of body weight once daily in healthy volunteers. Antimicrobial Agents and Chemotherapy 50: 3245–49, 2006.

Burkhardt O, Kielstein JT. A simplified three-times weekly daptomycin dosing regimen for chronic hemodialysis patients. Expert Rev Anti Infect Ther 8:11–14, 2010.

Cai T, Mazzoli S, Malossino G, et al. A potential role for daptomycin in enterococcal infections: what is evidence? J Antimicrob Chemother 66:1195–1196, 2011.

Cantón R, Ruiz-Garbajosa P, Chaves RL, Johnson AP. A potential role for daptomycin in enterococcal infections: what is the evidence? J Antimicrob Chemother 65:1126–1136, 2010.

Cervera C, Casteneda X, Pericas JM, et al. Clinical utility of daptomycin in infective endocarditis caused by Gram-positive cocci. Int J Antimicrob Agents 38:365–370, 2011.

Chaftari AM, Hachem R, Mulanovich V, et al. Efficacy and safety of daptomycin in the treatment of Gram-positive catheter-related bloodstream infections in cancer patients. Int J Antimicrob Agents 36:182–186, 2010.

Crompton JA, North DS, McConnell SA, et al. Safety and efficacy of daptomycin in the treatment of osteomyelitis: results from the CORE Registry. J Chemother 21:414–420; 2009.

Crompton JA, North DS, Yoon M, et al. Outcomes with daptomycin in the treatment of Staphylococcus aureus infections with a range of vancomycin MICs. J Antimicrob Chemother 65:1784–1791, 2010.

Cunha BA, Mickail N, Eisenstein L. E. faecalis vancomycin sensitive enterococci (VSE) Bacteremia unresponsive to vancomycin successfully treated with high dose daptomycin. Heart & Lung 36: 456–461, 2007.

Cunha BA, Eisenstein LE, Hamid NS. Pacemaker-induced Staphylococcus aureus mitral valve acute bacterial endocarditis complicated by persistent bacteremia from a coronary stent: Cure with prolonged/high-dose daptomycin without toxicity. Heart & Lung 35:207–11, 2006.

Cunha BA. Persistent S. aureus bacteremia: clinical pathway for diagnosis and treatment. Antibiotics for Clinicians 10:S39–46, 2006b.

Cunha BA. Staphylococcal aureus acute bacterial endocarditis (abe): clinical pathway for diagnosis and treatment. Antibiotics for Clinicians 10:S29–33, 2006a.

Cunha BA, Hamid N, Kessler H, Parchuri S. Daptomycin cure after cefazolin treatment failure of methicillin-sensitive Staphylococcus aureus (MSSA) tricuspid valve acute bacterial endocarditis from a peripherally inserted central catheter (PICC) line. Heart & Lung 34:442–7, 2005.

"Usual dose" assumes normal renal/hepatic function. * For renal insufficiency, give usual dose × 1 followed by maintenance dose per CrCl. For dialysis patients, dose the same as for CrCl < 10 mL/min and give supplemental (post-HD/PD dose) immediately after dialysis. CrCl = creatinine clearance; CVVH = continuous veno-venous hemofiltration; HD/PD = hemodialysis/peritoneal dialysis.

De Rosa FG, Mollaretti O, Cometto C, et al. Early experience with high-dosage daptomycin for prosthetic infections. Clin Infect Dis 49:1772–1773, 2009.

Dhand A, Bayer AS, Pogliano J, et al. Use of antistaphylococcal beta-lactams to increase daptomycin activity in eradicating persistent bacteremia due to methicillin-resistant Staphylococcus aureus: role of enhanced daptomycin binding. Clin Infec Dis 53:158–163, 2011.

Doan TL, DePetrillo J, Singer C. Daptomycin-induced eosinophilia without pulmonary involvement. Am J Health Syst Pharm 67:2107–2109, 2010.

Dretler R, Branch T. MRSA knee infection treated successfully with daptomycin after two failed prolonged high-dose courses of vancomycin. Infect Dis Clin Pract 13:327–329, 2005.

Falagas ME, Giannopoulou KP, Ntziora F, et al. Daptomycin for endocarditis and/or bacteremia: a systematic review of the experimental and clinical evidence. J Antimicrob Chemother 60:7–19, 2007.

Figueroa DA, Mangini E, Amodio-Groton M, et al. Safety of high-dose intravenous daptomycin treatment: three-year cumulative experience in a clinical program. Clin Infect Dis 15;49:177–80, 2009.

Gallagher JC, Perez ME, Marino EA, et al. Daptomycin therapy for vancomycin-resistant enterococcal bacteremia: a retrospective case series of 30 patients. Pharmacotherapy 29:792–799, 2009.

Hair PI, Keam SJ. Daptomycin: a review of its use in the management of complicated skin and soft-tissue infections and Staphylococcus aureus bacteremia. Drugs 67:1483–1512, 2007.

Hayes D Jr, Anstead MI, Kuhn RJ. Eosinophilic pneumonia induced by daptomycin. J Infect 54:e211–e213, 2007.

Kanafani ZA, Boucher H, Fowler V, et al. Daptomycin compared to standard therapy for the treatment of native valve endocarditis. Enferm Infecc Microbiol Clin 28:498–503, 2010.

King EA, McCoy D, Desai S, et al. Vancomycin-resistant enterococcal bacteraemia and daptomycin: J Antimicrob Chemother 66:2112–2118, 2011.

Kosmidis C, Levine DP. Daptomycin: pharmacology and clinical use. Expert Opin Pharmacother 11:615–625, 2010.

Kullar R, Davis SL, Levine DP, et al. High-dose daptomycin for treatment of complicated gram-positive infections: a large, multicenter, retrospective study. Pharmacotherapy 31:527–536, 2011.

Lichterfeld M, Ferraro MJ, Davis BT. High-dose daptomycin for the treatment of endocarditis caused by Staphylococcus aureus with intermediate susceptibility to glycopeptides. Int J Antimicrob Agents 35:96, 2010.

Miller BA, Gray A, Leblanc TW, et al. Acute eosinophilic pneumonia secondary to daptomycin: a report of three cases. Clin Infect Dis 50:e63–68, 2010.

Mohan S, McDermott BP, Cunha BA. Methicillin-resistant Staphylococcus aureus (MRSA) prosthetic valve endocarditis (PVE) with paravalvular abscess treated with daptomycin. Heart & Lung 34:69–71, 2005.

Nguyen MH, Eels SJ, Tan J, et al. Pharmacokinetics of daptomycin during cardiopulmonary bypass surgery: A prospective, open-label investigation. Antimicrob Agents Chemother 55:2499–2505, 2011.

Patel JB, Jevitt LA, Hageman J, et al. An association between reduced susceptibility to daptomycin and reduced susceptibility to vancomycin in Staphylococcus aureus. Clin Infect Dis 42:1652–3, 2006.

Patel N, Cardone K, Grabe DW, et al. Use of pharmacokinetic and pharmacodynamic principles to determine optimal administration of daptomycin in patients receiving standardized thrice-weekly hemodialysis. Antimicrob Agents Chemother 55:1677–1683, 2011.

Ritchie ND. Lovering AM, Seaton RA. Daptomycin in synovial fluid during treatment of methicillin-resistant Staphylococcus aureus septic arthritis. J Antimicrob Chemother 65:1314–1315, 2010.

Schutt AC, Bohm NM. Multidrug-resistant Enterococcus faecium endocarditis treated with combination tigecycline and high-dose daptomycin. Ann Pharmacother 43:2108–2112, 2009.

Stewart PS, Davison WM, Steenbergen JN. Daptomycin rapidly penetrates a Staphylococcus epidermidis biofilm. Antimicrob Agents Chemother 53:3505–3507, 2009.

Tascini C, Congiorni G, Cori A, et al. Cardiovascular implantable electronic device endocarditis treated with daptomycin with or without transvenous removal. Heart & Lung 41:24–30, 2012.

"Usual dose" assumes normal renal/hepatic function. * For renal insufficiency, give usual dose × 1 followed by maintenance dose per CrCl. For dialysis patients, dose the same as for CrCl < 10 mL/min and give supplemental (post-HD/PD dose) immediately after dialysis. CrCl = creatinine clearance; CVVH = continuous veno-venous hemofiltration; HD/PD = hemodialysis/peritoneal dialysis.

Traunmüller F, Schintler MV, Metzler J, et al. Soft tissue and bone penetration abilities of daptomycin in diabetic patients with bacterial foot infections. J Antimicrob Chemother 65:1252–1257, 2010.

Van Hai SJ, Paterson DL, Gosbell IB. Emergence of daptomycin resistance following vancomycin-unresponsive Spaphylococcus aureus bacteraenia in daptomycin- native patient—a review of the literature. Eur J Clin Microbol Infec Dis 30:603–610, 2011.

Vilay AM, Grio M, Depestel DD, et al. Daptomycin pharmacokinetics in critically ill patients receiving continuous venovenous hemodialysis. Crit Care Med 39:19–25, 2011.

Wu G, Abraham T, Rapp J, et al. Daptomycin: evaluation of a high-dose treatment strategy. Int J Antimicrob Agents 38:192–196, 2011.

Website: www.cubist.com

Darunavir (Prezista) DRV

Drug Class: Antiretroviral protease inhibitor.
Usual Dose: Treatment naive / treatment experienced with no darunavir resistance-associated substitutions: 800 mg (PO) q24h with ritonavir 100 mg (PO) q24h. Treatment experienced / genotyping not available: 600 mg (PO) q12h with ritonavir 100 mg (PO) q12h.

Pharmacokinetic Parameters:
Peak serum level: 3578 ng/mL
Bioavailability: 37% (alone) 82% (with ritonavir)
Excreted unchanged: 41.2% (feces), 7.7% (urine)
Serum half-life (normal/ESRD): 15/15 hrs
Plasma protein binding: 95%
Volume of distribution (V_d): not studied
Primary Mode of Elimination: Fecal/renal
Dosage Adjustments*

| CrCl 10–50 mL/min | No change |
| CrCl < 10 mL/min | No data |

Post–HD dose	No change
Post–PD dose	No change
CVVH/CVVHD/CVVHDF dose	No change
Mild–moderate hepatic insufficiency	No change
Severe hepatic insufficiency	Use with caution

Antiretroviral Dosage Adjustments

Efavirenz	No data
Nevirapine	No change
Didanosine	1 hour before or 1 hour after darunavir
Tenofovir	No change
Fosamprenavir	No change
Indinavir	No data
Lopinavir/ritonavir	Avoid
Saquinavir	Avoid
Rifabutin	150 mg (PO) qod

Drug Interactions: Indinavir, ketaconazole, nevirapine, tenofovir (↑ darunavir levels); lopinavir/ritonavir, saquinavir, efavirenz (↓ darunavir levels); concomitant administration of darunavir/ritonavir with agents highly-dependent on CYP3A for clearance, astemizole, cisapride, dihydroergotamine, ergonovine, ergotamine, methylergonovine, midazolam, pimozide, terfenadine, midazolam, triazolam (may ↓ darunavir levels and ↓ effectiveness); sildenafil, vardenafil, tadalafil (↑ PDE-5 inhibitors; sildenafil do not exceed 25 mg in 48 hrs, vardenafil do not exceed

2.5 mg in 72 hrs, or tadalafil do not exceed 10 mg in 72 hrs); clarithromycin (↑ QT_c).

Adverse Effects: Rash, diarrhea, nausea, headache, nasopharyngitis drug induced hepatitis. Use with caution in patients with preexisting liver disease. New-onset or exacerbations of pre-exisiting diabetes mellitus and hyperglycemia, and increased bleeding in hemophiliacs (class effect). Immune reconstitution syndrome.

Contraindicated: lovastatin, simvastatin, atorvastatin (> 20 mg/day), rifapentine, boceprevir, telaprevir.

Allergic Potential: High (see comments)

Safety in Pregnancy: C

Comments: Always take with food (increases AUC, Cmax by approximately 30%). Must be given with ritonavir to boost bioavailability. Darunavir contains a sulfonamide moiety (as do fosamprenavir and tipranavir); use with caution in patients with sulfonamide allergies. astemizole, terfenadine, ergot derivatives dihydroergotamine, ergonovine, ergotamine, methylergonovine, cisapride, pimozide, midazolam, triazolam, are contraindicated with darunavir. Phenobarbital, phenytoin, carbamazepine, or products containing St. John's wort, rifampin. Lovostatin and simavastatin may be taken with caution.

Cerebrospinal Fluid Penetration: No data

REFERENCES:

De Meyer S, Azijn H, Surleraux D, et al. TMC114, a novel human immunodeficiency virus type 1 protease inhibitor active against protease inhibitor-resistant viruses, including a broad range of clinical isolates. Antimicrob Agents Chemother 49:2314–2321, 2005.

Dominique L. N. G, Surleraux T, Abdellah Tahri T, et al. Discovery and selection of TMC114, a next generation HIV-I protease inhibitor. J Med Chem 48:1813–1822, 2005.

Okoli C, Siccardi M, Thomas-William S, et al. Once Daily maraviroc 300 mg or 150 mg in combination with ritonavir-boosted darunavir 800/100 mg. J Antimicrob Chemother 67: 671–4, 2012.

Panel on Antiretroviral Guidelines for Adults and Adolescents. Department of Health and Human Services. Guidelines for the use of antiretroviral agents in HIV-infected adults and adolescents. http://aidsinfo.nih.gov/ConsentFiles/AdultandAdolescentGL.pdf, 2012.

Patterson K, Jennings S, Falcon R, et al. Darunavir, ritonavir, etravirine pharmacokinetics in the cervicovaginal fluid and blood plasma of HIV-infected women. Antimicrob Agents Chemother 55:1120–2, 2011.

Sorbera LA, Castaner J, Bayes M. Darunavir: Anti-HIV agent HIV protease inhibitor. Drugs of the Future 30:441–449, 2005.

Thompson MA, Aberg JA, Cahn P, et al. Antiretroviral treatment of adult HIV infection: 2012 recommendations of the International Antiviral Society — USA panel. JAMA 308:387–402, 2012.

Delavirdine (Rescriptor) DLV

Drug Class: Antiretroviral NNRTI (non-nucleoside reverse transcriptase inhibitor).

Usual Dose: 400 mg (PO) q8h.

Pharmacokinetic Parameters:

Peak serum level: 35 mcg/mL

Bioavailability: 85%

Excreted unchanged (urine): 5%

Serum half-life (normal/ESRD): 5.8 hrs/no data

Plasma protein binding: 98%

Volume of distribution (V_d): 0.5 L/kg

Primary Mode of Elimination: Hepatic

Dosage Adjustments*

CrCl 50–80 mL/min	No change
CrCl 10–50 mL/min	No change
CrCl < 10 mL/min	No change

"Usual dose" assumes normal renal/hepatic function. * For renal insufficiency, give usual dose × 1 followed by maintenance dose per CrCl. For dialysis patients, dose the same as for CrCl < 10 mL/min and give supplemental (post-HD/PD dose) immediately after dialysis. CrCl = creatinine clearance; CVVH = continuous veno-venous hemofiltration; HD/PD = hemodialysis/peritoneal dialysis.

Post–HD dose	None
Post–PD dose	None
CVVH/CVVHD/CVVHDF dose	No change
Moderate hepatic insufficiency	Use with caution
Severe hepatic insufficiency	Use with caution

Antiretroviral Dosage Adjustments

Amprenavir	Increased agenerase levels
Efavirenz	No data
Indinavir	Indinavir 600 mg q8h
Lopinavir/ritonavir	No data
Nelfinavir	No information (monitor for neutropenia)
Nevirapine	No data
Ritonavir	Delavirdine: no change; ritonavir: No data
Saquinavir soft-gel	Saquinavir soft-gel 800 mg q8h (monitor transaminases)
Rifampin, rifabutin	Avoid
Statins	Avoid

Drug Interactions: With antiretrovirals adjust according to table above. Avoid in combination with rifabutin rifampin. Contraindicated with astemizole, terrenadine, Dihydroergotamine, ergonovine, ergotamine, methylergonovine, Cisapride, Pimozide, Alprazolam, midazolam, triazolam. Phenytoin may decrease delaviridine levels. Clarithromycin, dapsone nefedipine, warfarin cause increase in interacting drug levels. Sildenaril (do not exceed 25 mg in 48 hrs), tadalafil (max 10mg/72 hrs); vardenafil (max 2.5 mg/72hrs). St. John's wort substantially reduces delaviridine levels.

Adverse Effects: Drug fever/rash, Stevens–Johnson Syndrome (rare), headache, nausea/vomiting, diarrhea, ↑ SGOT/SGPT. May cause immune reconstitution syndrome.

Allergic Potential: High

Safety in Pregnancy: C

Comments: May be taken with or without food, but food decreases absorption by 20%. May disperse four 100-mg tablets in > 3 oz. water to produce slurry; 200-mg tablets should be taken as intact tablets and not used to make an oral solution. Separate dosing with ddI or antacids by 1 hour.

Cerebrospinal Fluid Penetration: 0.4%

REFERENCES:

Been-Tiktak AM, Boucher CA, Brun-Vezinet F, et al. Efficacy and safety of combination therapy with delavirdine and zidovudine: A European/Australian phase II trial. Intern J Antimicrob Agents 11:13–21, 1999.

Conway B. Initial therapy with protease inhibitor-sparing regimens: Evaluation of nevirapine and delavirdine. Clin Infect Dis 2:130–4, 2000.

Demeter LM, Shafer RW, Meehan PM, et al. Delavirdine susceptibilities and associated reverse transcriptase mutations in human immunodeficiency virus type 1 isolates from patients in a phase I/II trial of delavirdine monotherapy (ACTG260). Antimicrob Agents Chemother 44:794–7, 2000.

Justesen US, Klitgaard NA, Brosen K, et al. Dose-dependent pharmacokinetics of delavirdine in combination with amprenavir in healthy volunteers. J Antimicrob Chemother 54:206–10, 2004.

Thompson MA, Aberg JA, Cahn P, et al. Antiretroviral treatment of adult HIV infection: 2010 recommendations of the international AIDS society – USA panel. JAMA 304:321–333, 2010.

Website: rescriptor.com

"Usual dose" assumes normal renal/hepatic function. * For renal insufficiency, give usual dose × 1 followed by maintenance dose per CrCl. For dialysis patients, dose the same as for CrCl < 10 mL/min and give supplemental (post-HD/PD dose) immediately after dialysis. CrCl = creatinine clearance; CVVH = continuous veno-venous hemofiltration; HD/PD = hemodialysis/peritoneal dialysis.

Didanosine EC (Videx) ddI

Drug Class: Antiretroviral NRTI (nucleoside reverse transcriptase inhibitor).

Usual Dose: 400 mg (PO) q24h for > 60 kg; 250 (PO) q24h for < 60 kg.

Pharmacokinetic Parameters:
Peak serum level: 29 mcg/mL
Bioavailability: 42%
Excreted unchanged (urine): 60%
Serum half-life (normal/ESRD): 1.6/4.1 hrs
Plasma protein binding: ≤ 5%
Volume of distribution (V_d): 1.1 L/kg

Primary Mode of Elimination: Renal

Dosage Adjustments*

CrCl 10–59 mL/min	125 mg (PO) q24h
CrCl < 10 mL/min	125 mg (PO) q24h: > 60 kg Avoid: < 60 kg
Post–HD dose	None
Post–PD dose	None
CVVH/CVVHD/ CVVHDF dose	150 mg (PO) q24h [100 mg (PO) q24h]
Moderate hepatic insufficiency	No change
Severe hepatic insufficiency	No change

Drug Interactions: Alcohol, lamivudine, pentamidine and valproic acid increase the risk of pancreatitis. Patients on tenofovir should have didanosine dose reduced to 250 mg/24 hrs. Concomitant use with tenofovir increases risk of virologic failure. The appropriate dose of didanosine when taken with tenofovir has not been determined in patients with creatinine clearance of ≤ 60 ml/min.

Peripheral neuropathy is enhanced by stavudine, INH, metronidazole, ntirofuantoin, vincristine and zalcitabine. Dapsone levels are dramatically reduced by powder form especially and increase risk of PCP. Decreases levels of cipro floxacin delavirdine, indinavir. Methadone will decrease didanosine levels. Coadministration of didanosine with ribavirin is not recommended.

Adverse Effects: Fatal and non-fatal pancreatitis have occured during therapy with didanosine used alone or in combination regimens. Tenofovir can increase this risk as well. Lactic acidosis and severe hepatomegaly with steatosis can also occur especially in pregnant women. Combination with stavuidine potentiates this risk and should be avoided especially in pregnancy and in patients with concomitant HCV/HBV. Other effects include diarrhea, peripheral neuropathy, rash and abdominal pain, anemia, leukopenia, alopecia. Depigmentation and optic neuritis have occured. Patients with underlying liver disease are at increased risk of hepatic toxicity.

Allergic Potential: Low

Safety in Pregnancy: B
Avoid in pregnancy as it may cause fatal pancreatitis

Comments: Available as buffered powder for oral solution and enteric-coated extended-release capsules (Videx EC 400 mg PO q24h). Take 30 minutes before or 2 hours after meal (food decreases serum concentrations by 49%). Avoid in patients with alcoholic cirrhosis/history of pancreatitis. Use with caution in combination with tenofovir, which can potentiate risk of pancreatitis and require a significant dose reduction of ddI. Avoid use with ribavirin.

Cerebrospinal Fluid Penetration: 20%

"Usual dose" assumes normal renal/hepatic function. * For renal insufficiency, give usual dose × 1 followed by maintenance dose per CrCl. For dialysis patients, dose the same as for CrCl < 10 mL/min and give supplemental (post-HD/PD dose) immediately after dialysis. CrCl = creatinine clearance; CVVH = continuous veno-venous hemofiltration; HD/PD = hemodialysis/peritoneal dialysis.

REFERENCES:

Barreiro P, Corbaton A, Nunez M, et al. Tolerance of didanosine as enteric-coated capsules versus buffered tablets. AIDS Patient Care STDS 18:329–31, 2004.

Negredo E, Molto J, Munoz-Moreno JA, et al. Safety and efficacy of once-daily didanosine, tenofovir and nevirapine as a simplification antiretroviral approach. Antivir Ther 9:335–42, 2004.

Panel on Antiretroviral Guidelines for Adults and Adolescents. Department of Health and Human Services. Guidelines for the use of antiretroviral agents in HIV-infected adults and adolescents. http://aidsinfo.nih.gov/ConsentFiles/AdultandAdolescentGL.pdf, 2012.

Perry CM, Balfour JA. Didanosine: An update on its antiviral activity, pharmacokinetic properties, and therapeutic efficacy in the management of HIV disease. Drugs 52:928–62, 1996.

Rathbun RC, Martin ES 3rd. Didanosine therapy in patients intolerant of or failing zidovudine therapy. Ann Pharmacother 26:1347–51, 1992.

Thompson MA, Aberg JA, Cahn P, et al. Antiretroviral treatment of adult HIV infection: 2012 recommendations of the International Antiviral society — USA panel. JAMA 308:387–402, 2012.

Website: www.pdr.net

Doripenem (Doribax)

Drug Class: Carbapenem.
Usual Dose: 1 gm (IV) q8h.
Spectrum: (see *Susceptibility Profiles* pp. 198–202).
Resistance potential: Low
Pharmacokinetic Parameters:
Peak serum level: 23 mcg/mL
Bioavailability: Not applicable
Excreted unchanged (urine): 40%
Serum half-life (normal/ESRD): 1/6.20hrs
Plasma protein binding: 8.1%
Volume of distribution (V_d): 16.8 L/kg
Primary Mode of Elimination: Renal

Dosage Adjustments*

CrCl 30–50 mL/min	1 gm (IV) q12h
CrCl 10–30 mL/min	500 mg (IV) q12h
CrCl < 10 mL/min	500 mg (IV) q24h
Post–HD dose	250 mg (IV)
Post–HFHD dose	500 mg (IV)
Post–PD dose	500 mg (IV)
CVVH/CVVHD/ CVVHDF dose	500 mg (IV) q12h
Moderate hepatic insufficiency	No change
Severe hepatic insufficiency	No change

Drug Interactions: Valproic acid (↓ valproic acid levels).
Adverse Effects: Headache, nausea, diarrhea, rash, phlebitis, pneumonitis if administered by inhalation (do *not* give by inhalation).
Allergic Potential: Anaphylaxis (rare)
Safety in Pregnancy: B
Comments: cSSSIs, cIAIs, or UTIs dose: 500 mg (IV) q8h. Infuse over 1 hour. *MDR P. aeruginosa, MDR Acinetobacter baumannii/ nosocomial pneumonia dose:* 1 gm (IV) q8h. **For NP/VAP, infuse IV over 4 hours. Unlike meropenem, doripenem should most be used for meningitis.**
Cerebrospinal Fluid Penetration: < 1%
Bile Penetration: 117%
(also see *Antibiotic Pearls & Pitfalls* p. 511).

REFERENCES:

Anderson DL. Doripenem. Drugs for Today 42:399–404, 2006.

"Usual dose" assumes normal renal/hepatic function. * For renal insufficiency, give usual dose × 1 followed by maintenance dose per CrCl. For dialysis patients, dose the same as for CrCl < 10 mL/min and give supplemental (post-HD/PD dose) immediately after dialysis. CrCl = creatinine clearance; CVVH = continuous veno-venous hemofiltration; HD/PD = hemodialysis/peritoneal dialysis.

Betriu C, Gómez M, López-Fabal F, et al. Activity of doripenem against extended-spectrum beta-lactamase-producing Enterobacteriaceae and Pseudomonas aeruginosa isolates. Eur J Clin Microbiol Infect Dis 29:1179–1181, 2010.

Castanheira M, RN Jones, DM Livermore. Antimicrobial activities of doripenem and other carbapenems against Pseudomonas aeruginosa, other nonfermentative bacilli, and Aeromonas spp. Diagn. Microbiol Infect Dis 63:426–433, 2012.

Cirillo I, Vaccaro N, Balis D, et al. Influence of continuous venovenous hemofiltration and continuous venovenous hemodiafiltration on the disposition or doripenem. Antimicrob Agents Chemother 55:1187–1193, 2011.

Hellwig TR, Onisk ML, Chapman BA. Potential interaction between valproic acid and doripenem. Curr Drug Saf 6:54–58, 2011.

Lister PD. Carbapenems in the USA: focus on doripenem. Expert Rev Anti Infect Ther 5:793–809, 2007.

Pankuch GA, Seifert H, Appelbaum PC. Activity of doripenem with and without levofloxacin, amikacin, and colistin against Pseudomonas aeruginosa and Acinetobacter baumannii. Diagn Microbiol Infect Dis 67:191–197, 2010.

Paterson DL, DePestel DD. Doripenem. Clin Infect Dis 49:291–298, 2009.

Toya T, Nannya Y, Narukawa K, et al. A comparative analysis of meropenem and doripenem in febrile patients with hematologic malignancies: a single-center retrospective study. Jpn J Infect Dis 65:228–32, 2012.

Doxycycline (Vibramycin, Vibra-tabs)

Drug Class: 2nd generation IV/PO tetracycline.
Usual Dose: 100 mg (IV/PO) q12h or 200 mg (IV/PO) q24h (PI dose). For *serious systemic infections,* begin with a **Loading Regimen:** 200 mg (IV/PO) q12h × 3 days **(PK dose),** then continue at same dose (for acute/serious infections) or decrease to 100 mg (IV/PO) q12h (for subacute/chronic infections) to complete therapy.

Spectrum: (see *Susceptibility Profiles* pp. 186–190).
Resistance Potential: Low
Pharmacokinetic Parameters:
Peak serum level: 100/200 mg = 4/8 mcg/mL
Bioavailability: 93%
Excreted unchanged (urine): 40%
Serum half-life (normal/ESRD): 18–22/18–22 hrs
Plasma protein binding: 93%
Volume of distribution (V_d): 0.75 L/kg
Primary Mode of Elimination: Hepatic
Dosage Adjustments*

CrCl < 10 mL/min	No change
Post–HD or PD dose	None
CVVH/CVVHD/CVVHDF dose	No change
Moderate—severe hepatic insufficiency	No change

Drug Interactions: Antacids, Al^{++}, Ca^{++}, Fe^{++}, Mg^{++}, Zn^{++}, multivitamins, sucralfate (↓ doxycycline absorption); barbiturates, carbamazepine, phenytoin (↓ doxycycline half-life); bicarbonate (↓ doxycycline absorption, ↑ doxycycline clearance); warfarin (↑ INR).
Adverse Effects: Nausea if not taken with food. Phlebitis if given IV in inadequate volume. Avoid in pregnancy and children < 8 years. Photosensitivity rare.
Allergic Potential: Low
Safety in Pregnancy: D
Comments: May be protective against C. difficle. Absorption minimally effected by iron, bismuth, milk, or antacids containing Ca^{++}, Mg^{++}, or Al^{++}. Serum half-life increases with multiple doses. **For MSSA, CA/HA–MRSA. Use minocycline instead of doxycycline.** Meningeal dose = 200 mg (IV/PO) q12h.

PI = package insert
PK = pharmacokinetic dose

Cerebrospinal Fluid Penetration:
Non-Inflamed meninges = 25%
Inflamed meninges = 25%
Bile Penetration: 3000%
(also see ***Antibiotic Pearls & Pitfalls*** p. 512).

REFERENCES:

Berman B, Perez OA, Zell D. Update on rosacea and anti-inflammatory-dose doxycycline. Drugs Today 43:27–34, 2007.

Bernadino ALF, Kaushal D, Philipp MT. The antibiotics doxycycline and minocycline inhibit the inflammatory responses to the lyme disease spirochete Borrelia burgdorferi. Journal of Infectious Diseases 199:1379–1388, 2009.

Borg R, Dotevall L, Hagberg L, et al. Intravenous ceftriaxone compared with oral doxycycline for the treatment of Lyme neuroborreliosis. Scand J Infect Dis 37:449–454, 2005.

Cunha BA. Doxycycline re-revisited. Arch Intern Med 159:1006–7, 1999.

Cunha BA. Doxycycline. Antibiotics for Clinicians 3:21–33, 1999.

Cunha BA, Domenico PD, Cunha CB. Pharmacodynamics of doxycycline. Clin Micro Infect Dis 6:270–3, 2000.

Cunha BA. Doxycycline for community-acquired pneumonia. Clin Infect Dis 37:870, 2003.

Cunha BA. New uses for older antibiotics: nitrofurantoin, amikacin, colistin, polymyxin B, doxycycline, and minocycline revisited. Med Clin North Am 90:1089–107, 2006.

Cunha BA. Oral antibiotic therapy of serious systemic infections. Med Clin N Am 90:1197–1222, 2006.

Cunha BA. Doxycycline for nursing home acquired pneumonia (NHAP). Scandinavian Journal of Infectious Disease 41:77–78, 2009.

Cunha BA, Minocycline versus doxycycline for methicillin-resistant Staphylococcus aureus (MRSA): in vitro susceptibility versus in vivo effectiveness. Int J Antimicrob Agents 35:517–8, 2012.

Cunha BA. Oral doxycycline for non-systemic urinary tract infections (UTIs) due to P. aeruginosa and other Gram negative uropathogens. Eur J Clin Microbiol Infect Dis 31:2865–8, 2012.

Del Rosso JQ, Webster GF, Jackson M, et al. Two randomized phase III clinical trials evaluating anti-inflammatory dose doxycycline (40-mg doxycycline, USP capsules) administered once daily for treatment of rosacea. J Am Acad Dermatol 56:791–802, 2007.

Doernberg SB, Winston LG, Deck LH, et al. Does Doxycycline protect against development of clostridium difficile infection? Clin Infect Dis 55:615–20, 2012.

Haggerty CL, Ness RB. Newest approaches to treatment of pelvic inflammatory disease: a review of recent randomized clinical trials. Clin Infect Dis 44:953–960, 2007.

Hasin T, Davidovitch N, Cohen R, et al. Postexposure treatment with doxycycline for the prevention of tick-borne relapsing fever. N Engl J Med 355:147–55, 2006.

Johnson JR. Doxycycline for treatment of community-acquired pneumonia. Clin Infect Dis 35:632, 2002.

Jones RN, Sader HS, Fritsche TR. Doxycycline use for community-acquired pneumonia: contemporary in vitro spectrum of activity against Streptococcus pneumoniae. Diagn Microbiol Infect Dis 49:147–9, 2004.

Karkkonen K, Stiernstedt SH, Karisson M. Follow-up of patients treated with oral doxycycline for Lyme neuroborreliosis. Scand J Infect Dis 33:259–262, 2001.

Mouratidis PX, Colston KW, Dalgleish AG. Doxycycline induces caspase-dependent apoptosis in human pancreatic cancer cells. Int J Cancer 120:743–752, 2007.

Naini AE, Harandi AA, Morghtaderi J, et al. Doxycycline: a pilot study to reduce diabetic proteinuria. Am J Nephrol 27:269–273, 2007.

Preshaw PM, Grainger P, Bradshaw MH, et al. Subantimicrobial dose doxycycline in the treatment of recurrent oral aphthous ulceration: a pilot study. J Oral Pathol Med 36:235–240, 2007.

Psomas KC, Brun M, Causse A, et al. Efficacy of a ceftriaxone and doxycycline in the treatment of early syphilis. Magn Reson Imaging 30:271–82, 2012.

Ranjbar M, Keramat F, Mamani M, et al. Comparison between doxycycline-rifampin-amikacin and doxycycline-rifampin regimens in the treatment of brucellosis. Int J Infect Dis 11:152–156, 2007.

Raoult D. Doxycycline for Mansonella perstans Infection. N Engl J Med 362:272–273, 2010.

PI = package insert
PK = pharmacokinetic dose

Roushan MRH, Mohraz M, Hajiahmadi M, et al. Efficacy of gentamycin plus doxycycline versus streptomycin plus doxycycline in the treatment of brucellosis in humans. Clin Infect Dis 42:1075–80, 2006.

Schwartz BS, Graber CJ, Diep BA, et al. Doxycycline, not minocycline, induces its own resistance in multidrug-resistant community-associated methicillin-resistant Staphylococcus aureus clone USA300. Clin Infect Dis 48:1483–1484, 2009.

Shea KW, Ueno Y, Abumustafa F, Cunha BA. Doxycycline activity against Streptococcus pneumoniae. Chest 107:1775–6, 1995.

Shkap R, Amir J, et al. Absence of tooth staining with doxycycline treatment in young children. Clin Pediatr 46:121–126, 2007.

Tan KR, Magill AJ, Parise ME, et al. Doxcycycline for malaria chemoprophylaxis and treatment: report from the CDC expert meeting on malaria chemoprophylaxis. Am J Trop Med Hyg 84:517–531, 2011.

Teh B, Grayson ML, Johnson PD, et al. Doxycycline vs. macrolides in combination therapy for treatment of community-acquired pneumonia. Clin Microbiol Infect 18:71–3, 2012.

Turner JD, Mand S, Debrah AY, et al. A randomized, double-blind clinical trial of a 3-week course of doxycycline plus albendazole and ivermectin for the treatment of Wuchereria bancrofti infection. Clin Infect Dis 42:1081–9, 2006.

Volovitz B, Shkap R, Amir J, et al. Absence of tooth staining with doxycycline treatment in young children. Clin Pediatr 46:121–126, 2007.

Efavirenz (Sustiva) EFV

Drug Class: Antiretroviral NNRTI (non-nucleoside reverse transcriptase inhibitor).
Usual Dose: 600 mg (PO) q24h.
Pharmacokinetic Parameters:
Peak serum level: 12.9 mcg/mL
Bioavailability: Increased with food
Excreted unchanged (urine): 14–34%
Serum half-life (normal/ESRD): 40–55 hrs/no data
Plasma protein binding: 99%
Volume of distribution (V_d): No data

Primary Mode of Elimination: Hepatic
Dosage Adjustments*

CrCl < 60 mL/min	No change
Post–HD or PD dose	None
CVVH/CVVHD/CVVHDF dose	No change
Moderate—severe hepatic insufficiency	No change

Antiretroviral Dosage Adjustments

Delavirdine	No data
Indinavir	Indinavir 1000 mg q8h
Lopinavir/ritonavir (l/r)	Consider l/r 533/133 mg q12h in PI-experienced patients
Nelfinavir	No change
Nevirapine	No data
Ritonavir	Ritonavir 600 mg q12h (500 mg q12h for intolerance)
Saquinavir	Avoid use as sole PI
Rifampin	No change
Rifabutin	Rifabutin 450–600 mg q24h or 600 mg 2–3x/week if not on protease inhibitor
Telaprevir increase teleprevie 1125 mg q7–9h	
Voriconazole: give efavirenz 300 mg q24h, voriconazole 400 mg q12h	

"Usual dose" assumes normal renal/hepatic function. * For renal insufficiency, give usual dose × 1 followed by maintenance dose per CrCl. For dialysis patients, dose the same as for CrCl < 10 mL/min and give supplemental (post-HD/PD dose) immediately after dialysis. CrCl = creatinine clearance; CVVH = continuous veno-venous hemofiltration; HD/PD = hemodialysis/peritoneal dialysis.

Drug Interactions: Antiretrovirals, rifabutin, rifampin (see dose adjustment grid, above); astemizole, terfenadine, cisapride, ergotamine, midazolam, carbamazepine, phenobarbital, phenytoin (monitor anticonvulsant levels; use with caution); verapamil, diltiazem (↓ calcium channel blocker levels) caspofungin, itraconazole, posaconazole (↓ anti fungal levels); methadone, clarithromycin (↓ interacting drug levels; titrate methadone dose to effect; consider using azithromycin instead of clarithromycin).
Contraindications: Triazolam, rifapentine, boceprevir.
Adverse Effects: Drug fever/rash, CNS symptoms (nightmares, dizziness, neuropsychiatric symptoms, difficulty concentrating, somnolence), ↑ SGOT/SGPT, E. multiforme/Stevens-Johnson Syndrome (rare), false positive cannabinoid test.
Allergic Potential: High
Safety in Pregnancy: D
Comments: Rash/CNS symptoms usually resolve spontaneously over 2–4 weeks. Take at bedtime. Avoid taking after high fat meals (levels ↑ 50%). 600-mg dose available as single tablet.
Cerebrospinal Fluid Penetration: 1%

REFERENCES:

Haas DW, Fessel WJ, Delapenha RA, et al. Therapy with efavirenz plus indinavir in patients with extensive prior nucleoside reverse-transcriptase inhibitor experience: A randomized, double-blind, placebo-controlled trial. J Infect Dis 183:392–400, 2001.

la Porte CJ, de Graaff-Teulen MJ, Colbers EP, et al. Effect of efavirenz treatment on the pharmacokinetics of nelfinavir boosted by ritonavir in healthy volunteers. Br J Clin Pharmacol 58:632–40, 2004.

Marzolini C, Telenti A, Decosterd LA, et al. Efavirenz plasma levels can predict treatment failure and central nervous system side effects in HIV-1-infected patients. AIDS 15:71–5, 2001.

McComsey GA, Kitch D, Sax PE, et al. Peripheral and central fat changes in subjects randomized to abacavir-lamivudine or tenofovir-emtricitabine with atazanavir-ritonavir or efavirenz: ACTG Study A5224s. Clin Infect Dis 53:185–96, 2011.

Panel on Antiretroviral Guidelines for Adults and Adolescents. Department of Health and Human Services. Guidelines for the use of antiretroviral agents in HIV-infected adults and adolescents. http://aidsinfo.nih.gov/ConsentFiles/AdultandAdolescentGL.pdf, 2012.

Thompson MA, Aberg JA, Cahn P, et al. Antiretroviral treatment of adult HIV infection: 2012 recommendations of the International Antiviral Society — USA panel. JAMA 308:387–402, 2012.

Young J, Schafer J, Fux CA, et al. Renal function in patients with HIV starting therapy with tenofovir and either efavirenz, lopinavir or atazanavir. AIDS 26:567–75, 2012.

Website: www.sustiva.com

Efavirenz + Emtricitabine + Tenofovir disoproxil fumarate (Atripla) EFV/FTC/TDF

Drug Class: Antiretroviral agent.
Usual Dose: 1 tablet (efavirenz 600 mg/emtricitabine 200 mg/tenofovir 300 mg) (PO) q24h on an empty stomach.
Pharmacokinetic Parameters:
Peak serum level: 4.0/1.8 mcg/mL/296 ng/mL
Bioavailability: NR/93%/25%
Excreted unchanged: < 1% unchanged and 14–30% as metabolites/86%/32%
Serum half-life (normal/ESRD): (40–55 hrs/~10 hrs on hemodialysis)/(10 hrs/extended)/(17 hrs/ no data)
Plasma protein binding: 99/< 4/< 0.7%
Volume of distribution (V_d): NR/NR/1.2 L/kg
Primary Mode of Elimination: Hepatic/renal/renal

"Usual dose" assumes normal renal/hepatic function. * For renal insufficiency, give usual dose × 1 followed by maintenance dose per CrCl. For dialysis patients, dose = same as for CrCl < 10 mL/min and give supplemental (post-HD/PD dose) immediately after dialysis. CrCl = creatinine clearance; CVVH = continuous veno-venous hemofiltration; HD/PD = hemodialysis/peritoneal dialysis.

Dosage Adjustments*

CrCl 50–80 mL/min	No change
CrCl 10–50 mL/min	Avoid
CrCl < 10 mL/min	Avoid
Post–HD dose	Avoid
Post–PD dose	Avoid
CVVH/CVVHD/CVVHDF dose	Avoid
Mild hepatic insufficiency	No data
Moderate–severe hepatic insufficiency	No data

Antiretroviral Dosage Adjustments

Fosamprenavir/ritonavir	An additional 100 mg/day (300 mg total) of ritonavir is recommended when ATRIPLA is administered with fosamprenavir/ritonavir q24h. No change in ritonavir dose when ATRIPLA is administered with fosamprenavir/ritonavir q12h
Atazanavir	Atazanavir 300 mg q24h Ritonavir 100 mg q12h
Indinavir	Indinavir 1000 mg q8h
Lopinavir/ritonavir	Increase lopinavir/ritonavir to 600/150 mg (3 tablets) q12h
Ritonavir	No data
Saquinavir	Avoid
Didanosine	Avoid

Rifabutin	Rifabutin 450–600 mg q24h or 600 mg 2–3x/week if not on protease inhibitor
Rifampin	No data

Drug Interactions: Antiretrovirals, rifabutin (see dose adjustment grid above); astemizole, cisapride, ergotamine, methylergonovine, midazolam, triazolam, St John's Wort (↓ efavirenz levels), voriconazole (↓ voriconazole levels; avoid); caspofungin (↓ caspofungin levels); carbamazepine, phenytoin, phenobarbital (monitor anticonvulsant levels; use with caution; potential for ↓ efavirenz levels); statins (may ↓ statin levels); methadone, (↓ methadone levels); clarithromycin (may ↓ clarithromycin effectiveness, consider using azithromycin). Should not be administered concurrently with astemizole, cisapride, midazolam, triazolam, or ergot derivatives. Significantly reduces voriconazole drug levels.

Adverse Effects: Dizziness, insomnia, impaired concentration, somnolence, abnormal dreaming, euphoria, confusion, agitation, amnesia, hallucinations, stupor, abnormal thinking, and depersonalization. Psychiatric symptoms of depression suicidal ideation, nonfatal suicide attempts, aggressive behavior, paranoid reactions, and manic reactions. Mild to moderate skin rash, Steven's Johnson syndrome. Pancreatitis can occur. Increase in lipids and cholesterol. Immune reconstitution Syndrome and redistribution/accumulation of body fat have been reported in patients treated with combination antiretroviral therapy.

Allergic Potential: High

Safety in Pregnancy: D

Comments: Rash/CNS effects usually resolve in a few weeks. Take at bedtime on empty

---

"Usual dose" assumes normal renal/hepatic function. * For renal insufficiency, give usual dose × 1 followed by maintenance dose per CrCl. For dialysis patients, dose the same as for CrCl < 10 mL/min and give supplemental (post-HD/PD dose) immediately after dialysis. CrCl = creatinine clearance; CVVH = continuous veno-venous hemofiltration; HD/PD = hemodialysis/peritoneal dialysis.

stomach. High fat meals can ↑ efavirenz by 50%. Use with caution in patients with history of seizures (↑ risk of convulsions). May cause false positive tests for cannabanoids.

Cerebrospinal Fluid Penetration: 1%

REFERENCES:

Cooper DA, Heera J, Goodrich J, et al. Maraviroc versus efavirenz, both in combination with zidovudine-lamivudine, for the treatment of antiretroviral-naïve subjects with CCR5-tropic HIV-1 infection. J Infect Dis 201:803–813, 2010.

Gallant JE, DeJesus E, Arribas JR, et al: Tenofovir DF, emtricitabine, and efavirenz vs. zidovudine, lamivudine, and efavirenz for HIV. N Engl J Med 354:251–260, 2006.

Panel on Antiretroviral Guidelines for Adults and Adolescents. Department of Health and Human Services. Guidelines for the use of antiretroviral agents in HIV-infected adults and adolescents. http://aidsinfo.nih.gov/ConsentFiles/AdultandAdolescentGL.pdf, 2012.

Thompson MA, Aberg JA, Cahn P, et al. Antiretroviral treatment of adult HIV infection: 2012 recommendations of the International Antiviral Society — USA panel. JAMA 308:387–402, 2012.

Website: www.atripla.com

Elvitegravir + Cobicistat + Emtricitabine + Tenofovir disoproxil fumarate (Stribild) EVS/COBI/FTC/TDF

Drug class Antiretroviral agent: Integrase strand transfer inhibitor (elvitagravir 150 mg), pharmacokinetic enhancer (cobicistat 150 mg), and 2 nucleos(t)ide analog HIV-1 reverse transcriptase inhibitors (emtricitabine 200 mg and tenofovir disoproxil fumarate 300 mg)

Usual dose: 1 tablet once daily with food

Pharmacokinetic Parameters:

Peak serum level: 1.7/1.1/1.9/0.45 mcg/mL
Bioavailability: Increased with food

Excreted unchanged: minimal for elvitegravir and cobicistat, ~ 100% for emtricitabine and tenofovir disoproxil fumarate
Serum half-life (normal/ESRD): 9/3/12/11 (not recommended in renal failure)
Plasma protein binding: 98/98/4/0.7%
Volume of distribution (V_d): No data

Primary Mode of Elimination: Hepatic (elvitegravir and cobicistat); Renal (emtricitabine and tenofovir disoproxil fumarate)

Dosage Adjustments*

CrCl < 50 mL/min	Avoid
Post-HD dose	Avoid
Post-PD dose	Avoid
CVVH dose	Avoid
Severe hepatic insufficiency	Avoid

Drug Interactions: Inhibitor of CYP3A, CYP2D6 and CYP2C9; and p-glycoprotein; metabolized by CYP3A and CYP2D6; antacids (may ↓ elvitegravir absorption)

Contraindications: nephrotoxic drugs

Adverse Effects: nausea, diarrhea, new onset/worsening of renal failure, decreased bone mineral density redistribution/accumulation of body fat, immune reconstitution syndrome, lactic acidosis and hepatomegaly

Allergic Potential: not available

Safety in Pregnancy: B

Comments: not approved for HIV patients co-infected with HBV

References:

DeJesus E, Rockstroh JK, Henry K, et al. Co-formulated elvitegravir, cobicistat, emtricitabine, and tenofovir disoproxil fumarate versus ritonavirboosted atazanavir plus co-formulated emtricitabine and tenofovir disoproxil fumarate for initial treatment of HIV-1 infection: a randomised, double-blind, phase 3, non-inferiority trial. Lancet 379:2429–38, 2012.

"Usual dose" assumes normal renal/hepatic function. * For renal insufficiency, give usual dose × 1 followed by maintenance dose per CrCl. For dialysis patients, dose the same as for CrCl < 10 mL/min and give supplemental (post-HD/PD) dose immediately after dialysis. CrCl = creatinine clearance; CVVH = continuous veno-venous hemofiltration; HD/PD = hemodialysis/peritoneal dialysis.

Desimmie BA, Schrijvers R, Debyser Z. Elvitegravir: a once daily alternative to raltegravir. Lancet Infect Dis 12:3–5, 2012.

Olin JL, Spooner LM, Klibanov OM. Elvitegravir/ Cobicistat/Emtricitabine/Tenofovir Disoproxil Fumarate Single Tablet for HIV-1 Infection Treatment. Ann Pharmacotherapy 46: epub November 7, 2012.

Sax PE, DeJesus E, Mills A, et al. Co-formulated elvitegravir, cobicistat, emtricitabine, and tenofovir versus co-formulated efavirenz, emtricitabine, and tenofovir for initial treatment of HIV-1 infection: a randomised, double-blind, phase 3 trial, analysis of results after 48 weeks. Lancet 379:2439–48, 2012.

Website: www.pdr.net

Emtricitabine (Emtriva) FTC

Drug Class: Antiretroviral NRTI (nucleoside reverse transcriptase inhibitor).

Usual Dose: 200 mg (PO) q24h.

Pharmacokinetic Parameters:

Peak serum level: 1.8 mcg/mL

Bioavailability: 93%

Excreted unchanged (urine): 86%

Serum half-life (normal/ESRD): 10 hrs/ extended

Plasma protein binding: 4%

Primary Mode of Elimination: Renal

Dosage Adjustments*

CrCl ≥ 50 mL/min	200 mg (PO) q24h
CrCl 30–49 mL/min	200 mg (PO) q48h
CrCl 15–29 mL/min	200 mg (PO) q72h
CrCl < 15 mL/min	200 mg (PO) q96h
Post–HD dose	200 mg (PO)
Post–PD dose	200 mg (PO)

| CVVH/CVVHD/ CVVHDF dose | 200 mg (PO) q72h |
| Moderate—severe hepatic insufficiency | No change |

Drug Interactions: No significant interactions with indinavir, stavudine, zidovudine, famciclovir, tenofovir.

Adverse Effects: Lactic acidosis hepatomegaly with steatosis, post-treatment exacerbation of hepatitis B. Headache, diarrhea, nausea and rash as well as abdominal pain, fatigue, dizziness abnormal dreams. Rare cases of skin hyperpigmentation on palms and soles. Immune reconstitution syndrome may occur.

Allergic Potential: Low

Safety in Pregnancy: B

Comments: May be taken with or without food. Does not inhibit CYP450 enzymes. Mean intracellular half-live of 39 hours. Potential cross-resistance to lamivudine and zalcitabine. Low affinity for DNA polymerase-gamma. Should not be coadministered with drugs containing lamivudine.

Cerebrospinal Fluid Penetration: No data

REFERENCES:

Dando TM, Wagstaff AJ. Emtricitabine/tenofovir disoproxil fumarate. Drugs 64:2075–82, 2004.

Gallant JE, DeJesus D, Arribas JR, et al. Tenofovir DF, emtricitabine, and efavirenz vs. zidovudine, lamivudine, and efavirenz for HIV. N Engl J Med 354:251–60, 2006.

Lim SG, Ng TN, Kung N, et al. A double-blind placebo-controlled study of emtricitabine in chronic hepatitis B. Arch Intern Med 166:49–56, 2006.

Panel on Antiretroviral Guidelines for Adults and Adolescents. Department of Health and Human Services. Guidelines for the use of antiretroviral agents in HIV-infected adults and adolescents. http://aidsinfo.nih.gov/ConsentFiles/AdultandAdolescentGL.pdf, 2012.

"Usual dose" assumes normal renal/hepatic function. * For renal insufficiency, give usual dose × 1 followed by maintenance dose per CrCl. For dialysis patients, dose the same as for CrCl < 10 mL/min and give supplemental (post-HD/PD dose) immediately after dialysis. CrCl = creatinine clearance; CVVH = continuous veno-venous hemofiltration; HD/PD = hemodialysis/peritoneal dialysis.

Saag MS. Emtricitabine, a new antiretroviral agent with activity against HIV and hepatitis B virus. Clin Infect Dis 42:128–31, 2006.

Sax PE, Tierney C, Collier AC, et al. Abacavir/lamivudine versus tenofovir DF/emtricitabine as part of combination regimens for initial treatment of HIV: final results. J Infect Dis 204:1191–201, 2011.

Thompson MA, Aberg JA, Cahn P, et al. Antiretroviral treatment of adult HIV infection: 2012 recommendations of the International Antiviral Society — USA panel. JAMA 308:387–402, 2012.

Website: www.emtriva.com

Emtricitabine + Tenofovir disoproxil fumarate (Truvada) FTC/TDF

Drug Class: Antiretroviral NRTI (nucleoside reverse transcriptase inhibitor) + nucleotide analogue.

Usual Dose: One tablet (PO) q24h (each tablet contains 200 mg of emtricitabine + 300 mg of tenofovir).

Pharmacokinetic Parameters:
Peak serum level: 1.8/0.3 mcg/L
Bioavailability: 93%/27% if fasting (39% with high fat meal)
Excreted unchanged (urine): 86/32%
Serum half-life (normal/ESRD): (10 hrs/ extended)/(17 hrs/no data)
Plasma protein binding: 4/0.7–7.2%
Volume of distribution (V_d): no data/1.3 L/kg

Primary Mode of Elimination: Renal/Renal
Dosage Adjustments*

CrCl ≥ 50 mL/min	No change
CrCl 30–49 mL/min	One capsule (PO) q48h
CrCl 15–29 mL/min	Avoid
CrCl < 15 mL/min	Avoid
Post–HD dose	Avoid

Post–PD dose	Avoid
CVVH/CVVHD/ CVVHDF dose	Avoid
Moderate—severe hepatic insufficiency	No change

Drug Interactions: No significant interactions with indinavir, stavudine, zidovudine, famciclovir, lamivudine, lopinavir/ritonavir, efavirenz, methadone, oral contraceptives. Tenofovir ↑ didanosine levels which may result in severe pancreatitis. Tenofovir reduces systemic exposure to atazanavir; whenever the two are co-administered, the recommended dose of atazanavir is 300 mg once daily with ritonavir 100 mg once daily. Atazanavir may increase tenofovir levels. Avoid coadministration with didanosine.

Adverse Effects: Headache, diarrhea, nausea, vomiting, GI upset, rash, lactic acidosis with hepatic steatosis (rare but potentially life-threatening with NRTI's). Decreases bone mineral density. May result in flare of hepatitis after stopping medication in patients with chronic hepatitis B infection. Cases of osteomalacia and renal tubular acidosis have occurred. Renal dysfunction is more common in diabetic patients. Immune reconstitution syndrome and redistribution/accumulation of body fat have been reported in patients treated with combination antiretroviral therapy.

Allergic Potential: Low

Safety in Pregnancy: B

Comments: May be taken with or without food. Does not inhibit CYP450 enzymes. Mean intracellular half-life with emtricitabine is 39 hours. Potential cross-resistance to lamivudine, zalcitabine, abacavir, didanosine. Low affinity for DNA polymerase-gamma.

Cerebrospinal Fluid Penetration: No data

"Usual dose" assumes normal renal/hepatic function. * For renal insufficiency, give usual dose × 1 followed by maintenance dose per CrCl. For dialysis patients, dose the same as for CrCl < 10 mL/min and give supplemental (post-HD/PD dose) immediately after dialysis. CrCl = creatinine clearance; CVVH = continuous veno-venous hemofiltration; HD/PD = hemodialysis/peritoneal dialysis.

REFERENCES:

Dando TM, Wagstaff AJ. Emtricitabine/tenofovir disoproxil fumarate. Drugs 64:2075–82, 2004.

Panel on Antiretroviral Guidelines for Adults and Adolescents. Department of Health and Human Services. Guidelines for the use of antiretroviral agents in HIV-infected adults and adolescents. http://aidsinfo.nih.gov/ConsentFiles/AdultandAdolescentGL.pdf, 2012.

Thompson MA, Aberg JA, Cahn P, et al. Antiretroviral treatment of adult HIV infection: 2012 recommendations of the International Antiviral Society — USA panel. JAMA 308:387–402, 2012.

Website: www.truvada.com

Emtricitabine/Rilpivirine/Tenofovir (Complera) FTC/RPV/TDF

Drug Class: 2 NRTI/1 NNRTI.
Usual Dose: 1 tablet (PO) q24h (contains 200 mg emtricitabine, 25 mg rilpivirine, 300 mg tenofovir).
Pharmacokinetic Parameters:
Peak serum level: 1.8/1/0.3 mcg/L
Bioavailability: 93/No data/25%
Excreted unchanged: 86/1/75%
Serum half-life (normal): 10/50/17 hrs
Plasma protein binding: unknown/99/1%
Volume of distribution (V_d): no data/no data/no data
Primary Mode of Elimination: Renal/hepatic/renal
Dosage Adjustments*

CrCl < 50 mL/min	Avoid
Post-HD dose	Avoid
Post-PD dose	Avoid
CVVH/CVVHD/CVVHDF dose	Avoid

Mild—moderate hepatic insufficiency	No change
Severe hepatic insufficiency	No data

Drug Interactions: Do not administer with other NNRTIs. Antacid and H2 blockers should be separated. Any drug that induces or inhibits CYP3A has the potential to increase or decrease rilpivirine levels and should only be used if benefit outweighs risk, clarithromycin (↓ clarithromycin levels).
Contraindications: carbamazepine, oxycarbazepine, phenobarbital, phenytoin, rifabutin, rifampin, rifapentine, proton pump inhibitors, dexamethasone (except single dose), **St. John's Wort.**
Adverse Effects: Nausea, diarrhea, fatigue, headache, dizziness, depression, insomnia, abnormal dreams, rash, **lactic acidosis/severe hepatomegaly with steatosis and post-treatment acute exacerbation of hepatitis B**, immune reconstitution syndrome, fat redistribution syndrome.
Allergic Potential: Low
Safety in Pregnancy: B
Comments: Monitor BMD in patients at risk for pathological fractures. *Not approved for patients con-infected with HBV and HIV.*
Cerebrospinal Fluid Penetration: No data

REFERENCES:

Molina JM, Cahn P, Ginsztejn B, et al. Rilipivirine versus efavirenz with tenofovir and emtricitabine in treatment-naïve adults infected with HIV-1 (ECHO): a phase 3 randomised double-blind active-controlled trial. Lancet Inf Dis 378:238–246, 2011.

Panel on Antiretroviral Guidelines for Adults and Adolescents. Department of Health and Human Services. Guidelines for the use of antiretroviral agents in HIV-infected adults and adolescents. http://aidsinfo.nih.gov/ConsentFiles/AdultandAdolescentGL.pdf, 2012.

"Usual dose" assumes normal renal/hepatic function. * For renal insufficiency, give usual dose × 1 followed by maintenance dose per CrCl. For dialysis patients, dose the same as for CrCl < 10 mL/min and give supplemental (post-HD/PD dose) immediately after dialysis. CrCl = creatinine clearance; CVVH = continuous veno-venous hemofiltration; HD/PD = hemodialysis/peritoneal dialysis.

Thompson MA, Aberg JA, Cahn P, et al. Antiretroviral treatment of adult HIV infection: 2012 recommendations of the International Antiviral Society — USA panel. JAMA 308:387–402, 2012.

Enfuvirtide (Fuzeon) ENF, T20

Drug Class: Antiretroviral fusion inhibitor.
Usual Dose: 90 mg (SC) q12h.
Pharmacokinetic Parameters:
Peak serum level: 4.9 mcg/mL
Bioavailability: 84.3%
Serum half-life (normal/ESRD): 3.8 hrs/no data
Plasma protein binding: 92%
Volume of distribution (V_d): 5.5 L
Primary Mode of Elimination: Metabolized
Dosage Adjustments*

CrCl > 35 mL/min	No change
CrCl < 35 mL/min	No change
Post–HD dose	No change
Post–PD dose	No change
CVVH/CVVHD/ CVVHDF dose	No change
Moderate—severe hepatic insufficiency	No change

Drug Interactions: No clinically significant interactions with other antiretrovirals. Does not inhibit CYP450 enzymes.
Adverse Effects: Local injection site reactions are common. Diarrhea, nausea, fatigue may occur. Laboratory abnormalities include mild/transient eosinophilia. Pneumonia may occur, but cause is unclear and may not be due to drug therapy. Pancreatitis, myalgia, conjunctivitis (rare).
Allergic Potential: Hypersensitivity reactions may occur, including fever, chills, hypotension,

rash, ↑ serum transaminases. Do not rechallenge following a hypersensitivity reaction
Safety in Pregnancy: B
Comments: Enfuvirtide interferes with entry of HIV-1 into cells by blocking fusion of HIV-1 and CD_4 cellular membranes by binding to HR1 in the gp41 subunit of the HIV-1 envelope glycoprotein. Additive/synergistic with NRTI's, NNRTI's, and PI's, and no cross resistance to other antiretrovirals in cell culture. Reconstitute in 1.1 mL of sterile water. SC injection should be given into upper arm, anterior thigh, or abdomen. Rotate injection sites; do not inject into moles, scars, bruises. After reconstitution, use immediately or refrigerate and use within 24 hours (no preservatives added).

REFERENCES:
Coleman CI, Musial, BL, Ross, J. Enfuvirtide: the first fusion inhibitor for the treatment of patients with HIV-1 infection. Formulary 38:204–222, 2003.
Kilby JM, Lalezari JP, Eron JJ, et al. The safety, plasma pharmacokinetics, and antiviral activity of subcutaneous enfuvirtide (T-20), a peptide inhibitor of gp41-mediated virus fusion, in HIV-infected adults. AIDS Res Hum Retroviruses 18:685–93, 2002.
Lalezari JP, Henry K, O'Hearn M, et al. TORO 1 Study Group. Enfuvirtide, an HIV-1 fusion inhibitor, for drug-resistant HIV infection in North and South America. N Engl J Med 348:2175–85, 2003.
Leen C, Wat C, Nieforth K. Pharmacokinetics of enfuvirtide in a patient with impaired renal function. Clin Infect Dis 4:339–55, 2004.
Panel on Antiretroviral Guidelines for Adults and Adolescents. Department of Health and Human Services. Guidelines for the use of antiretroviral agents in HIV-infected adults and adolescents. http://aidsinfo.nih.gov/ConsentFiles/AdultandAdolescentGL.pdf, 2012.

"Usual dose" assumes normal renal/hepatic function. * For renal insufficiency, give usual dose × 1 followed by maintenance dose per CrCl. For dialysis patients, dose the same as for CrCl < 10 mL/min and give supplemental (post-HD/PD dose) immediately after dialysis. CrCl = creatinine clearance; CVVH = continuous veno-venous hemofiltration; HD/PD = hemodialysis/peritoneal dialysis.

Thompson MA, Aberg JA, Cahn P, et al. Antiretroviral treatment of adult HIV infection: 2012 recommendations of the International Antiviral society — USA panel. JAMA 308:387–402, 2012.
Website: www.fuzeon.com

Entecavir (Baraclude)

Drug Class: Antiviral (nucleoside analogue).
Usual Dose: 0.5 mg (PO) q24h; 1 mg (PO) q24h for lamivudine-refractory patients or with decompensated liver disease.
Pharmacokinetic Parameters:
Peak serum level: 4.2 ng/mL (for 0.5 mg dose)
Bioavailability: Similar for tablet and oral solution
Excreted unchanged (urine): 62–73%
Serum half-life (normal/ESRD): 128–139 hrs
Plasma protein binding: No information
Volume of distribution (V_d): No information
Primary Mode of Elimination: Renal
Dosage Adjustments* (based on 0.5 mg dose)

CrCl > 50 mL/min	No change
CrCl 30–50 mL/min	0.25 mg (PO) q24h
CrCl 10–30 mL/min	0.15 mg (PO) q24h
CrCl < 10 mL/min	0.05 mg (PO) q24h
Post-HD	0.05 mg (PO or 0.5 mg (PO) q week)
Post–PD	0.05 mg (PO)
Moderate–severe hepatic insufficiency	No change

Drug Interactions: Cyclosporin, tacrolimus (may ↑ entecavir levels).
Adverse Effects: Fatigue, headache, upper respiratory tract infection, upper abdominal pain, ↑ ALT, cough, nausea.

Allergic Potential: No information
Safety in Pregnancy: C
Comments: Used to treat chronic hepatitis B infection. Effective in lamivudine-resistant patients. Administer on an empty stomach. Available as tablets and oral solution.

REFERENCES:
Honkoop P, De Man RA. Entecavir: a potent new antiviral drug for hepatitis B. Expert Opin Investig Drugs 12:683–8, 2003.
Keating GM. Entecavir: a review of its use in the treatment of chronic hepatitis B in patients with decompensated liver disease. Drugs 24:2511–29, 2011.
Marzella N. Entecavir (Baraclude) for the treatment of chronic hepatitis B virus (HBV) infection. Pharmacy & Therapeutics 31:313–20, 2006.
[No authors listed]. Entecavir: A new nucleoside analogue for the treatment of chronic Hepatitis B. Drugs for Today 43:201–220, 2007.
Petersen J, Ratziu, Buti M, et al. Entecavir plus tenofovir combination as recur therapy in pre-treated chronic hepatitis B patients: an international multicenter cohort study. J Hepatol 56:520–6, 2012.
Pol S, Lampertico, P. First-line treatment of chronic hepatitis B with entecavir or tenofovir in 'real-life' setting; from clinical trials to clinical practice. J viral Hepat 19:377–86, 2012.
Rivkin A. A review of entecavir in the treatment of chronic hepatitis B infection. Curr Med Res Opin 21:1845–56, 2005.
Scotto G, D'Addiego G, Giammario A, et al. Tenofovir plus entecavir as rescue therapy for multidrug-resistant chronic hepatitis B. Liver Int 32:171–2, 2012.
Sherman M, Yurdaydin C, et al. Entecavir therapy for lamivudine-refractory chronic hepatitis B: improved virologic, biochemical, and serology outcomes through 96 weeks. Hepatology 48:99–108, 2008.
Tsai Mc, Lee CM, Chiu KW, et al. A comparison of telbivudine and entecavir for chronic hepatitis B in real-world clinical practice. J Antimicrob Chemother 67:696–9, 2012.

"Usual dose" assumes normal renal/hepatic function. * For renal insufficiency, give usual dose × 1 followed by maintenance dose per CrCl. For dialysis patients, dose the same as for CrCl < 10 mL/min and give supplemental (post-HD/PD dose) immediately after dialysis. CrCl = creatinine clearance; CVVH = continuous veno-venous hemofiltration; HD/PD = hemodialysis/peritoneal dialysis.

Yang HJ, Lee JH, Kim YJ, et al. Antiviral efficacy of combination therapy with entecavir and adefovir for entecavir/lamivudine-resistant hepatitis B virus with or without adefovir resistance. J Med Virol 84:424–430, 2012.
Website: www.baraclude.com

Ertapenem (Invanz)

Drug Class: Carbapenem.
Usual Dose: 1 gm (IV/IM) q24h.
Spectrum: (see *Susceptibility Profiles* pp. 198–202).
Resistance Potential: Low
Pharmacokinetic Parameters:
Peak serum level: 150 mcg/mL
Bioavailability: 90% (IM)
Excreted unchanged (urine): 40%; 40% excreted as active metabolite
Serum half-life (normal/ESRD): 4/14 hrs
Plasma protein binding: 95%
Volume of distribution (V_d): 0.12 L/kg
Primary Mode of Elimination: Renal
Dosage Adjustments*

CrCl 30–80 mL/min	No change
CrCl < 30 mL/min	500 mg (IV) q24h
Post–HD dose	If dosed < 6 h prior to HD, give 150 mg (IV)
Post–PD dose	No information
CVVH/CVVHD/ CVVHDF dose	500 mg (IV) q24h
Moderate – Severe hepatic insufficiency	No change

* If dosed > 6 h prior to HD, no Post–HD needed.

Drug Interactions: Not a substrate/inhibitor of cytochrome P-450 enzymes; probenecid (↓ clearance of ertapenem). Valproic acid (↓ seizure threshold).
Adverse Effects: Mild headache, infrequent nausea or diarrhea. No seizures. Probenecid (↓ clearance of ertapenem).
Allergic Potential: Low
Safety in Pregnancy: B
Comments: Concentration-dependent protein binding. Compared to imipenem or meropenem, **ertapenem has little activity against VSE, Acinetobacter or P. aeruginosa.** For deep muscle (IM) injection, mix 1 gm with 3.2 mL of 1% lidocaine. **Probably safe to use in penicillin allergic patients.**
Cerebrospinal Fluid Penetration: 5–20%
Bile Penetration: 10%
(also see *Antibiotic Pearls & Pitfalls* p. 511).

REFERENCES:
Beovic B, Kreft S, Seme K, et al. Does ertapenem alter the susceptibility of Pseudomonas aeruginosa to carbapenems? J Chemother 23:216–220, 2011.
Boselli E, Breilh D, Djabarouti S, et al. Diffusion of ertapenem into bone and synovial tissues. J Antimicrob Chemother 60:893–896, 2007.
Cardone KE, Grabe DW, Kulawy RW, Et al. Ertapenem pharmacokinetics and pharmacodynamics during continuous ambulatory peritoneal dialysis. Antimicrob Agents Chemother 56:725–30, 2012.
Collins VL, Marchaim D, Pogue JM, et al. Efficacy of ertapenem for treatment of bloodstream infections caused by extended-spectrum-B-lactamase-producing Enterobacteriaceae. Antimicrob Agents Chemother 56:2173–7, 2012.
Congeni BL. Ertapenem. Expert Opin Pharmacother 11:669–672, 2010.
Cunha BA, Lenopoli S, Hage JE. Klebsiella pneumoniae septic wrist arthritis successfully treated with ertapenem and levofloxacin. J Chemother 23:376–7, 2011.

"Usual dose" assumes normal renal/hepatic function. * For renal insufficiency, give usual dose × 1 followed by maintenance dose per CrCl. For dialysis patients, dose the same as for CrCl < 10 mL/min and give supplemental (post-HD/PD dose) immediately after dialysis. CrCl = creatinine clearance; CVVH = continuous veno-venous hemofiltration; HD/PD = hemodialysis/peritoneal dialysis.

Curran M, Simpson D, Perry C. Ertapenem: a review of its use in the management of bacterial infections. Drugs 63:1855–78, 2003.

Fong JJ, Rose L, Radigan EA. Clinical outcomes with ertapenem as a first-line treatment option of infections caused by extended-spectrum b-lactamase producing gram-negative infections. Ann Pharmacother 46:347–52, 2012.

Graham DR, Lucasti C, Malafaia O, et al. Ertapenem once daily versus piperacillin-tazobactam 4 times per day for treatment of complicated skin and skin-structure infections in adults: results of a prospective, randomized, double-blind multicenter study. Clin Infect Dis 34:1460–8, 2002.

Hyle EP, Ferraro MJ, Silver M, et al. Ertapenem-resistant enterobacteriaceae: risk factors for acquisition and outcomes. Infect Control Hosp Epidemiol 31:1242–1249, 2010.

Itani KMF, Wilson SE, Awad SS, et al. Ertapenem versus cefotetan prophylaxis in elective colorectal surgery. N Engl J Med 355:2640–51, 2006.

Liao FF, Huang YB, Chen CY. Decrease in serum valproic acid levels during treatment with ertapenem. Am J Health Syst Pharm 67:1260–1264, 2010.

Lipsky BA, Armstrong DG, Citron DM, et al. Ertapenem versus piperacillin/tazobactam for diabetic foot infections (SIDESTEP): prospective, randomized, controlled, double-blinded, multicentre trial. Lancet 366:1695–703, 2005.

Livermore DM, Sefton AM, Scott GM. Properties and potential of ertapenem. J Antimicrob Chemother 52:331–44, 2003.

Mody RM, Erwin DP, Summers AM, et al. Ertapenem susceptibility of extended spectrum beta-lactamase-producing organisms. Ann Clin Microbiol Antimicrob 6:6, 2007.

Murcia JM, González-Comeche J, Marín A, et al. Clinical response to ertapenem in severe community-acquired pneumonia: a retrospective series in an elderly population. Clin Microbiol Infect 15:1046–1050, 2009.

Namias N, Solomkin JS, Jensen EH, et al. Randomized, multicenter, double-blind study of efficacy, safety, and tolerability of intravenous ertapenem versus piperacillin/tazobactam in treatment of complicated intra-abdominal infections in hospitalized adults. Surg Infect 8:15–28, 2007.

Orsi GB, Garcia-Fernandezx A, Giordano V, et al. Risk factors and clinical significance of ertapenem-resistant Klebsiella pneumoniae in hospitalized patients. J Hosp Infect 78:54–58, 2011.

Teppler H, Gesser RM, Friedland Ir, et al. Safety and tolerability of ertapenem. J Antimicrob Chemother 53:75–81, 2004.

Tice AD, Turpin RS, Hoey CT, et al. Comparative costs of ertapenem and piperacillin-tazobactam in the treatment of diabetic foot infections. Am J Health Syst Pharm 64:1080–1086, 2007.

Virdier MC, Seguin P, Le Touvet B, et al. Ertapenem in plasma and peritoneal fluid from patients with severe intra-abdominal infections. J Antimicrob Chemother 66:1934–1936, 2011.

Yakovlev SV, Stratchounskin LS, Woods GL, et al. Ertapenem versus cefepime for initial empirical treatment of pneumonia acquired in skilled-care facilities or in hospitals outside the intensive care unit. Eur J Clin Micro Inf Dis 25:633–641, 2006.

Website: www.invanz.com

Erythromycin lactobionate, base (various)

Drug Class: Macrolide.

Usual Dose: 1 gm (IV) q6h; 500 mg (PO) q6h (Take without food).

Spectrum: (see *Susceptibility Profiles* pp. 186–190).

Resistance Potential: High (S. pneumoniae, GAS, MSSA)

Pharmacokinetic Parameters:

Peak serum level: 12 (IV);1.2 (PO) mcg/mL

Bioavailability: 50%

Excreted unchanged (urine): 5%; 5% exerted as active metabolite

Serum half-life (normal/ESRD): 1.4/5.4 hrs

Plasma protein binding: 80%

Volume of distribution (V_d): 0.5 L/kg

"Usual dose" assumes normal renal/hepatic function. * For renal insufficiency, give usual dose × 1 followed by maintenance dose per CrCl. For dialysis patients, dose the same as for CrCl < 10 mL/min and give supplemental (post-HD/PD dose) immediately after dialysis. CrCl = creatinine clearance; CVVH = continuous veno-venous hemofiltration; HD/PD = hemodialysis/peritoneal dialysis.

Primary Mode of Elimination: Hepatic

Dosage Adjustments*

CrCl < 10 mL/min	No change
Post–HD/PD dose	None
CVVH/CVVHD/ CVVHDF dose	No change
Moderate—severe hepatic insufficiency	No change

Drug Interactions: Amiodarone, procainamide, sotalol, astemizole, terfenadine, cisapride, pimozide (↑ QTc); carbamazepine (↑ carbamazepine levels), nystagmus, nausea, vomiting, diarrhea; avoid combination); cimetidine, digoxin, ergot alkaloids, felodipine, midazolam, triazolam, phenytoin, ritonavir, tacrolimus, valproic acid (↑ interacting drug levels); clozapine (↑ clozapine levels; CNS toxicity); corticosteroids (↑ corticosteroid effect); cyclosporine (↑ cyclosporine levels with toxicity); efavirenz (↓ erythromycin levels); rifabutin, rifampin (↓ erythromycin levels, ↑ interacting drug levels); statins (↑ risk of rhabdomyolysis); theophylline (↑ theophylline levels, nausea, vomiting, seizures, apnea); warfarin (↑ INR); zidovudine (↓ zidovudine levels).

Adverse Effects: Nausea, vomiting, GI upset, irritative diarrhea, abdominal pain, phlebitis. May ↑ QTc; avoid with other medications that prolong the QTc interval and in patients with cardiac arrhythmias/heart block.

Allergic Potential: Low

Safety in Pregnancy: B

Comments: Do not mix erythromycin with B/C vitamins, glucose solutions, cephalothin, tetracycline, chloramphenicol, heparin, or warfarin. Increases GI motility and QTc interval.

Limited anti-Legionella activity.

S. pneumoniae resistance prevalent.

Cerebrospinal Fluid Penetration: < 10% (also see **Antibiotic Pearls & Pitfalls** p. 519).

REFERENCES:

Alvarez-Elcoro S, Enzler MJ. The macrolides: Erythromycin, clarithromycin and azithromycin. Mayo Clin Proc 74:613–34, 1999.

Amsden GW. Erythromycin, clarithromycin, and azithromycin: Are the differences real? Clinical Therapeutics 18:572, 1996.

Bergman M, Huikko S, Huovinen P, et al. Macrolide and azithromycin use are linked to increased macrolide resistance in Streptococcus pneumoniae. Antimicrob Agents Chemother 50:3646–3650, 2006.

Cunha BA. The virtues of doxycycline and the evils of erythromycin. Adv Ther 14:172–80, 1997.

Daneman N, McGeer A, Green K, et al. Macrolide resistance in bacteremic pneumococcal disease.: Implications for patient management. Clin Infect Dis 43:432–438, 2006.

Gagliotti C, Nobilio L, Milandri M, et al. Macrolide Prescriptions and Erythromycin Resistance or Streptococcus pyogenes. Clin Infect Dis 42:1153–6, 2006.

Jain R, Danzinger LH. The macrolide antibiotics: a pharmacokinetic and pharmacodynamic overview. Curr Pharm Des 10:3045–53, 2004.

Jenkins SG, Farrell DJ. Increase in pneumococcus macrolide resistance, United States. Emerging Infect Dis 15:1260–1264, 2009.

Mandell LA, Wunderink RG, Anzuetto A, et al. Infectious Diseases Society of America/American Thoracic Society consensus guidelines on the management of community-acquired pneumonia in adults. Clin Infect Dis 44:S27–72, 2007.

Smilack JD, Wilson WE, Cocerill FR 3rd. Tetracycline, chloramphenicol, erythromycin, clindamycin, and metronidazole. Mayo Clin Proc 66:1270–80, 1991.

Suzuki S, Yamazaki T, Narita M. Clinical evaluation of macrolide-resistant Mycoplasma pneumoniae. Antimicrobial Agents and Chemotherapy 50:709–12, 2006.

Website: www.pdr.net

"Usual dose" assumes normal renal/hepatic function. * For renal insufficiency, give usual dose × 1 followed by maintenance dose per CrCl. For dialysis patients, dose the same as for CrCl < 10 mL/min and give supplemental (post-HD/PD dose) immediately after dialysis. CrCl = creatinine clearance; CVVH = continuous veno-venous hemofiltration; HD/PD = hemodialysis/peritoneal dialysis.

Ethambutol (Myambutol) EMB

Drug Class: Anti-TB drug.
Usual Dose: 15 mg/kg (PO) q24h (see comments).
Pharmacokinetic Parameters:
Peak serum level: 2–5 mcg/mL
Bioavailability: 80%
Excreted unchanged (urine): 50%
Serum half-life (normal/ESRD): 4/10 hrs
Plasma protein binding: 20%
Volume of distribution (V_d): 2 L/kg
Primary Mode of Elimination: Renal/hepatic
Dosage Adjustments*

CrCl < 30 mL/min	15 mg/kg (PO) 3×/week
CrCl 15–30 mL/min	15 mg/kg (PO) q36h
Post-HD/PD dose	None
CVVH/CVVHD/CVVHDF dose	15 mg/kg (PO) q36h
Moderate—severe hepatic insufficiency	No change

Drug Interactions: Aluminum salts, didanosine buffer (↓ ethambutol and interacting drug absorption).
Adverse Effects: Drug fever/rash, ↓ visual acuity, central scotomata, color blindness (red-green), metallic taste, mental confusion, peripheral neuropathy, ↑ uric acid.
Allergic Potential: Low
Safety in Pregnancy: C
Comments: Optic neuritis may occur with high doses (≥ 15 mg/kg/day). **TB D.O.T. dose:** 4 gm (PO) 2 ×/week or 3 gm (PO) 3 ×/week. **MAI dose:** 15 mg/kg (PO) q24h (with azithromycin 500 mg [PO] q24h).

Meningeal dose = 25 mg/kg (PO) q24h.
Cerebrospinal Fluid Penetration:
Non-Inflamed meninges = 1%
Inflamed meninges = 40%

REFERENCES:
Chaisson RE, Keiser P, Pierce M, et al. Clarithromycin and ethambutol with or without clofazimine for the treatment of bacteremic Mycobacterium avium complex disease in patients with HIV infection. AIDS 11:311–317, 1997.
Davidson PT, Le HQ. Drug treatment of tuberculosis 1992. Drugs 43:651–73, 1992.
[No authors listed]. Drugs for tuberculosis. Med Lett Drugs Ther 35:99–101, 1993.
McIllerson H, Wash P, Burger A, et al. Determinants of rifampin, isoniazid, pyrazinamide and ethambutol pharmacokinetics in a cohort of tuberculosis patients. Antimicrob Agents Chemother 50:1170–77, 2006.
Perlman DC, Segal Y, Rosenkranz S, et al. The clinical pharmacokinetics of rifampin and ethambutol in HIV-infected persons with tuberculosis. Clinical Infectious Disease 41:1638–47, 2005.
Schlossberg D. Treatment of multi-drug resistant tuberculosis. Antibiotics for Clinicians 9:317–21, 2005.
Van Scoy RE, Wilkowske CJ. Antituberculous agents. Mayo Clin Proc 67:179–87, 1992.

Ethionamide (Trecator)

Drug Class: Anti-TB drug.
Usual Dose: 500 mg (PO) q12h.
Pharmacokinetic Parameters:
Peak serum level: 5 mcg/mL
Bioavailability: 99%
Excreted unchanged (urine): 1%
Serum half-life (normal/ESRD): 2/9 hrs
Plasma protein binding: 30%
Volume of distribution (V_d): No data
Primary Mode of Elimination: Renal/hepatic

"Usual dose" assumes normal renal/hepatic function. * For renal insufficiency, give usual dose × 1 followed by maintenance dose per CrCl. For dialysis patients, dose the same as for CrCl < 10 mL/min and give supplemental (post-HD/PD dose) immediately after dialysis. CrCl = creatinine clearance; CVVH = continuous veno-venous hemofiltration; HD/PD = hemodialysis/peritoneal dialysis.

Dosage Adjustments*

CrCl < 40 mL/min	No change
Post-HD/PD dose	No information
CVVH/CVVHD/CVVHDF dose	No information
Moderate hepatic insufficiency	No change
Severe hepatic insufficiency	500 mg (PO) q24h

Drug Interactions: Cycloserine (↑ neurologic toxicity); ethambutol (↑ GI distress, neuritis, hepatotoxicity); INH (peripheral neuritis, hepatotoxicity); pyrazinamide, rifampin (hepatotoxicity).

Adverse Effects: ↑ SGOT/SGPT, headache, nausea/vomiting, abdominal pain, tremor, olfactory abnormalities, alopecia, gynecomastia, hypoglycemia, impotence, neurotoxicity (central/peripheral neuropathy).

Allergic Potential: Low

Safety in Pregnancy: C

Comments: Additive toxicity with thiacetazone.

Meningeal dose = usual dose.

Cerebrospinal Fluid Penetration: 100%

REFERENCES:

Davidson PT, Le HQ. Drug treatment of tuberculosis 1992. Drugs 43:651–73, 1992.

[No authors listed.] Drugs for tuberculosis. Med Lett Drugs Ther 35:99–101, 1993.

Furin J, Nardell EA. Multidrug-resistant tuberculosis: An update on the best regimens. J Respir Dis 27:172–82, 2006.

Iseman MD. Treatment of multidrug resistant tuberculosis. N Engl J Med 329:784–91, 1993.

Schlossberg D. Treatment of multi-drug resistant tuberculosis. Antibiotics for Clinicians 9:317–321, 2005.

Etravirine (Intelence) ETR

Drug Class: NNRTI.

Usual Dose: 200 mg (PO) q12h (take with meals).

Pharmacokinetic Parameters:

Peak serum level: 2.97 mcg/mL
Bioavailability: no data
Excreted unchanged: 0%
Serum half-life (normal/ESRD): 41/41 hrs
Plasma protein binding: 99%
Volume of distribution (V_d): No data

Primary Mode of Elimination: Hepatic

Dosage Adjustments*

CrCl < 30 mL/min	No change
Post-HD dose	None
Post-PD dose	None
CVVH/CVVHD/CVVHDF dose	No change
Moderate hepatic insufficiency	No change
Severe hepatic insufficiency	use with caution

Drug Interactions: Do not administer with drugs that are inducers, inhibitors or substrates of CYP 3A4, 2C9 and/or 2C19 (tipranavir/ritonavir, atazanavir/ritonavir, protease inhibitors without ritonavir and/or NNRTIs), clarithromycin (↓ clarithromycin levels), statins (↓ statin levels), atovaquone/proguanil (↓ atovaquone/proguanil levels).

Contraindications: carbamazepine, phenytoin, phenobarbital, St. John's wort, rifapentine, atazanavir, efavirenz, fosamprenavir, nevirapine, rilpivirine, tipranavir.

Adverse Effects: Rash, peripheral neuropathy, immune reconstitution syndrome, fat redistribution.

Allergic Potential: Low

"Usual dose" assumes normal renal/hepatic function. * For renal insufficiency, give usual dose × 1 followed by maintenance dose per CrCl. For dialysis patients, dose the same as for CrCl < 10 mL/min and give supplemental (post-HD/PD dose) immediately after dialysis. CrCl = creatinine clearance; CVVH = continuous veno-venous hemofiltration; HD/PD = hemodialysis/peritoneal dialysis.

Safety in Pregnancy: B
Comments: Severe, life-threatening and fatal skin reactions (Steven-Johnson Syndrome, toxic epidermal necrolysis, hypersensitivity reaction and erythema multiforme). Doesn't ↓ methadone levels. If etravirine given with ritonavir–boosted protease inhibitor, rifabutin is contraindicated. Otherwise rifabutin can be given at 300 mg q24h.

REFERENCES:
Panel on Antiretroviral Guidelines for Adults and Adolescents. Department of Health and Human Services. Guidelines for the use of antiretroviral agents in HIV-infected adults and adolescents. http://aidsinfo.nih.gov/ConsentFiles/AdultandAdolescentGL.pdf, 2012.
Patterson K, Jennings S, Falcon R, et al. Darunavir, ritonavir, etravirine pharmacokinetics in the cervicovaginal fluid and blood plasma of HIV-infected women. Antimicrob Agents Chemother 55:1120–2, 2011.
Thompson MA, Aberg JA, Cahn P, et al. Antiretroviral treatment of adult HIV infection: 2012 recommendations of the International Antiviral Society — USA panel. JAMA 308:387–402, 2012.

Famciclovir (Famvir)

Drug Class: Antiviral (see comments).
Usual Dose:
HSV-1/2: Herpes labialis: 500 mg (PO) q12h × 7 days. Genital herpes: Initial therapy: 1 g (PO) q12h × 1 day. Recurrent/intermittent therapy (< 6 episodes/year): normal host: 125 mg (PO) q12h × 5 days; HIV-positive: 500 mg (PO) q12h × 7 days. Chronic suppressive therapy (> 6 episodes/year): 250 mg (PO) q12h × 1 year.
Meningitis/encephalitis: 500 mg (PO) q8h × 10 days.

VZV: Chickenpox: 500 mg (PO) q8h × 5 days. Herpes zoster (shingles) (dermatomal/disseminated): 500 mg (PO) q8h × 7–10 days.
VZV Pneumonia: 500 mg (PO) q8h ×7–10 days.
Pharmacokinetic Parameters:
Peak serum level: 3.3 mcg/mL
Bioavailability: 77%
Excreted unchanged (urine): 60%
Serum half-life (normal/ESRD): 2.5/13 hrs
Plasma protein binding: 20%
Volume of distribution (V_d): 1.1 L/kg
Primary Mode of Elimination: Renal
Dosage Adjustments for HSV/VZV* (based on 250 mg [PO] q8h/500 mg [PO] q8h)

CrCl 40–60 mL/min	No change/500 mg (PO) q12h
CrCl 20–40 mL/min	125 mg (PO) q24h/ 500 mg (PO) q24h
CrCl < 20 mL/min	125 mg (PO) q24h/ 250 mg (PO) q24h
Post–HD dose	125 mg (PO)/ 250 mg (PO)
Post–PD dose	None
CVVH/CVVHD/ CVVHDF dose	125 mg (PO) q24h/ 500 mg (PO) q24h
Moderate hepatic insufficiency	No change
Severe hepatic insufficiency	Use with caution

Drug Interactions: Digoxin (↑ digoxin levels).
Adverse Effects: Headache, seizures/tremors (dose related), nausea, diarrhea.
Allergic Potential: Low
Safety in Pregnancy: B

"Usual dose" assumes normal renal/hepatic function. * For renal insufficiency, give usual dose × 1 followed by maintenance dose per CrCl. For dialysis patients, dose the same as for CrCl < 10 mL/min and give supplemental (post-HD/PD dose) immediately after dialysis. CrCl = creatinine clearance; CVVH = continuous veno-venous hemofiltration; HD/PD = hemodialysis/peritoneal dialysis.

Comments: 99% converted to penciclovir in liver/GI tract. *Highly active against HSV, VZV, and HHV-6. Some activity against CMV. No activity against EBV, RSV or adenoviruses.*
Meningeal dose = VZV dose.
Cerebrospinal Fluid Penetration: 50%

REFERENCES:
Luber AD, Flaherty JF Jr. Famciclovir for treatment of herpesvirus infections. Ann Pharmacother 30:978–85, 1996.
Website: www.famvir.com

Fluconazole (Diflucan)

Drug Class: Antifungal.
Usual Dose: *Loading Dose (LD) = twice the maintenance dose × 1 dose* followed by the *Maintenance Dose (MD)*.
Candidemia:
    LD = 800 mg (IV/PO) × 1 then
    MD = 400 mg (IV/PO) q24h
Mucocutaneous Candidiasis:
    LD = 400 mg (IV/PO) × 1 then
    MD = 200 mg (IV/PO) q24h
Candida esophagitis:
    LD = 200 mg (IV/PO) × 1 then
    MD = 100 mg (IV/PO) q24h
Candiduria:
    LD = 200 mg (IV/PO) × 1 then
    MD = 100 mg (IV/PO) q24h
Pharmacokinetic Parameters:
Peak serum level: 6.7 mcg/mL
Bioavailability: 90%
Excreted unchanged (urine): 80%; 11% excreted as active metabolite
Serum half-life (normal/ESRD): 27/100 hrs
Plasma protein binding: 12%
Volume of distribution (V_d): 0.7 L/kg
Primary Mode of Elimination: Renal

Dosage Adjustments*

CrCl < 50 mL/min	100 mg (IV/PO) q24h
Post–HD dose	200 mg (IV/PO)
Post–PD dose	200 mg (IV/PO)
CVVH/CVVHD/ CVVHDF dose	200–400 mg (IV/PO) q24h
Moderate hepatic insufficiency	No change
Severe hepatic insufficiency	No change

Drug Interactions: Astemizole, cisapride, terfenadine, amiodarone (may ↑ QT interval, torsades de pointes); cyclosporine, oral hypoglycemics, tacrolimus, theophylline, zidovudine (↑ interacting drug levels with possible toxicity); hydrochlorothiazide (↑ fluconazole levels); phenytoin, rifabutin, rifampin (↓ fluconazole levels, ↑ interacting drug levels); warfarin (↑ INR).
Adverse Effects: Not hepatotoxic. Hypokalemia.
Allergic Potential: Low
Safety in Pregnancy: C
Comments: Not effective against most non-albicans Candida. *Highly active against C. albicans, C. tropicalis, C. parasilosis, and C. lusitaniae. Moderately active against Cryptococcus, Histoplasmosis, Blastomycosis, Sporotrichosis, Penicillum marneffei, Paracoccidiomycosis and Coccidiomycosis. Some (dose dependent) activity against C. glabrata. No activity against C. krusei, C. guilliermondii, C. rugosa, Mucor, Fusarium, Pseudoallescheria/Scedosporium, Trichosporon, Malassezia, Hansenula, Geotrichum, Rhodotorula or Aspergillus.*
Meningeal dose = 400 mg (IV/PO) q24h.

"Usual dose" assumes normal renal/hepatic function. * For renal insufficiency, give usual dose × 1 followed by maintenance dose per CrCl. For dialysis patients, dose the same as for CrCl < 10 mL/min and give supplemental (post-HD/PD dose) immediately after dialysis. CrCl = creatinine clearance; CVVH = continuous veno-venous hemofiltration; HD/PD = hemodialysis/peritoneal dialysis.

Cerebrospinal Fluid Penetration:
Non-Inflamed meninges = 50–90%
Inflamed meninges = 50–90%

REFERENCES:

Cha R, Sobel JD. Fluconazole for the treatment of candidiasis: 15 years experience. Expert Rev Anti Infect Ther 2:357–66, 2004.

Clancy CJ, Yu VL, Morris AJ, et al. Fluconazole MIC and fluconazole dose/MIC ratio correlate with therapeutic response among patients with candidemia. Antimicrobial Agents and Chemotherapy 49:3171–3177, 2005.

Hamza OJM, Matee MIN, Bruggemann RJM, et al. Single-dose fluconazole versus standard 2-week therapy for oropharyngeal candidiasis in HIV-infected patients: a randomized, double-blind, double-dummy trial. Clin Infect Dis 47:1270–1276, 2008.

Goa KL, Barradell LB. Fluconazole: An update of its pharmacodynamics and pharmacokinetic properties and therapeutic use in major superficial and systemic mycoses in immunocompromised patients. Drugs 50:658–90, 1995.

Kowalsky SF, Dixon DM. Fluconazole: A new antifungal agent. Clin Pharmacol 10:179–94, 1991.

Miceli MH, Diaz JA, Lee SA. Emerging opportunistic yeast infections. Lancet Infectious Diseases 11: 142–151, 2011.

Nussbaum JC, Jackson A, Namarika D, et al. Combination flucytosine and high-dose fluconazole compared with fluconazole monotherapy for the treatment of Cryptococcal meningitis: a randomized trial in Malawi. Clin Infect Dis 50:338–344, 2010.

Pappas PG, Chetchotisakd P, Larsen RA, et al. A phase II randomized trial of amphotericin B alone or combined with fluconazole in the treatment of HIV-associated cryptococcal meningitis. Clin Infect Dis 48:1775–1784, 2009.

Perfect JR, Dismukes WE, Dromer F, et al. Clinical practice guidelines for the management of cryptococcal disease: 2010 update by the Infectious Disease Society of America. Clin Infect Dis 50:291–322, 2010.

Rex JH, Pappas PG, Karchmer AW, et al. National Institute of Allergy and Infectious Diseases Mycoses Study Group. A randomized and blinded multicenter trial of high-dose fluconazole plus placebo versus fluconazole plus amphotericin B as therapy for candidemia and its consequences in nonneutropenic subjects. Clin Infect Dis 36:1221–8, 2003.

Sabatelli F. Patel R, Mann PA, et al. In vitro activities of posaconazole, fluconazole, itraconazole, voriconazole, and amphotericin B against a large collection of clinically important molds and yeasts. Antimicrob Agents Chemother 50:2009–15, 2006.

Smego RA jr, Ahmad H. The role of fluconazole in the treatment of Candida endocarditis: a meta-analysis. Medicine 90:237–249, 2011.

Sousa AQ, Frutuoo MS, Moraes EA, et al. High-dose oral fluconazole therapy effective for cutaneous leishmaniasis due to Leishmania (Vianna) braziliensis. Clin Infect Dis 53:693–695, 2011.

Terrell CL. Antifungal agents: Part II. The azoles. Mayo Clin Proc 74:78–100, 1999.

Zhai B, Zhou H, Yang L, et al. Polymyxin B, in combination with fluconazole, exerts a potent fungicidal effect. J Antimicrob Chemother 65:931–938, 2010.

Website: www.diflucan.com

Flucytosine (Ancobon) 5-FC

Drug Class: Antifungal.
Usual Dose: 25 mg/kg (PO) q6h.
Pharmacokinetic Parameters:
Peak serum level: 3.5 mcg/ml
Bioavailability: 80%
Excreted unchanged (urine): 90%
Serum half-life (normal/ESRD): 4/85 hrs
Plasma protein binding: 4%
Volume of distribution (V_d): 0.6 L/kg
Primary Mode of Elimination: Renal
Dosage Adjustments*

CrCl 20–40 mL/min	37.5 mg/kg (PO) q12h
CrCl 10–20 mL/min	37.5 mg/kg (PO) q18h

"Usual dose" assumes normal renal/hepatic function. * For renal insufficiency, give usual dose × 1 followed by maintenance dose per CrCl. For dialysis patients, dose the same as for CrCl < 10 mL/min and give supplemental (post-HD/PD dose) immediately after dialysis. CrCl = creatinine clearance; CVVH = continuous veno-venous hemofiltration; HD/PD = hemodialysis/peritoneal dialysis.

CrCl < 10 mL/min	37.5 mg/kg (PO) q24h
Post–HD dose	37.5 mg/kg (PO)
Post–PD dose	1 gm (PO)
CVVH/CVVHD/ CVVHDF dose	37.5 mg/kg (PO) q18h
Moderate—severe insufficiency	No change

Drug Interactions: Cytarabine (↓ flucytosine effect); zidovudine (neutropenia).
Adverse Effects: Leukopenia, anemia, thrombocytopenia, nausea, vomiting, abdominal pain, ↑ SGOT/SGPT, drug fever/ rashes.
Allergic Potential: High
Safety in Pregnancy: C
Comments: Always use in combination with amphotericin B for cryptococcal meningitis.
Highly active against Cryptococcus neoformans. Some activity against C. albicans. No activity against other yeasts/fungi.
Meningeal dose = usual dose.
Cerebrospinal Fluid Penetration:
Non-Inflamed meninges = 100%
Inflamed meninges = 100%

REFERENCES:
Lyman CA, Walsh TJ. Systemically administered antifungal agents. A review of their clinical pharmacology and therapeutic applications: Part I. Amphotericin B preparations and flucytosine. Mayo Clin Proc 73:1205–25, 1998.
Mosquera J, Shartt A, Moore CB, et al. In vitro interaction of terbinafine with itraconazole, fluconazole, amphotericin B and 5-flucytosine against Aspergillus spp. J Antimicrob Chemother 50:189–94, 2002.
Nussbaum JC, Jackson A, Namarika D, et al. Combination Flucytosine and High-Dose Fluconazole Compared with Fluconazole Monotherapy for the Treatment of Cryptococcal Meningitis: A Randomized Trial in Malawi. Clin Infect Dis 50:338–344, 2010.
Pfaller MA, Messer SA, Boyken L, et al. In vitro activities of 5-fluorocytosine against 8,803 clinical isolates of Candida spp.: Global assessment of primary resistance using National Committee for Clinical Laboratory Standards susceptibility testing methods. Antimicrob Agents Chemother 46:3518–3521, 2002.
Perfect JR, Dismukes WE, Dromer F, et al. Clinical practice guidelines for the management of cryptococcal disease: 2010 update by the Infectious Disease Society of America. Clin Infect Dis 50:291–322, 2010.
Te Dorsthorst DT, Verweij PE, Meletidis J, et al. In vitro interaction of flucytosine combined with amphotericin B or fluconazole against thirty-five yeast isolates determined by both the fractional inhibitory concentration index and the response surface approach. Antimicrob Agents Chemother 46:2982–9, 2002.
Wintermeyer SM, Mahata MC. Stability of flucytosine in an extemporaneously compounded oral liquid. Am J Health Syst Pharm 53:407–9, 1996.
Website: www.pdr.net

Fosamprenavir (Lexiva) FPV

Drug Class: Antiretroviral protease inhibitor.
Usual Dose: 1400 mg (PO) q24h plus ritonavir 200 mg (PO) q24h or 700 mg (PO) q12h plus ritonavir 100 mg (PO) q12h. For PI-experienced patients: 700 mg (PO) q12h plus ritonavir 100 mg (PO) q12h.
Pharmacokinetic Parameters:
Peak serum level: 4.8 mcg/mL
Bioavailability: No data
Excreted unchanged (urine) (urine): 1%
Serum half-life (normal/ESRD): 7 hrs/no data

Plasma protein binding: 90%
Volume of distribution (V_d): 6.1 L/kg
Primary Mode of Elimination: Hepatic
Dosage Adjustments*

CrCl 50–80 mL/min	No change
CrCl 10–50 mL/min	No change
CrCl < 10 mL/min	No change
Post-HD or PD dose	No change
CVVH/CVVHD/ CVVHDF dose	No change
Mild-moderate hepatic insufficiency (Child-Pugh score 5–8)	700 mg (PO) q12h without ritonavir; 450 mg (PO) q12h with ritonavir
Severe hepatic insufficiency (Child-Pugh score 9–12)	350 mg (PO) q12h without ritonavir; 300 mg (PO) q12h with ritonavir

Antiretroviral Dosage Adjustments

Didanosine	Administer didanosine 1 hour apart
Delavirdine	Avoid
Efavirenz	Fosamprenavir 700 mg q12h + ritonavir 100 mg q12h + efavirenz; fosamprenavir 1400 mg q24h + ritonavir 200 mg q24h + efavirenz; no data for fosamprenavir 1400 mg q12h + efavirenz
Indinavir	No data
Lopinavir/ ritonavir	Avoid
Nelfinavir	No information
Nevirapine	Avoid
Saquinavir	No information
Rifampin	Avoid
Rifabutin	Reduce usual rifabutin dose by 50% (or 75% if given with fosamprenavir plus ritonavir; max. 150 mg q48h)

Drug Interactions: Antiretrovirals (see dose adjustment grid, above). Contraindicated with: ergot derivatives, cisapride, midazolam, triazolam, pimozide, (flecainide and propafenone if administered with ritonavir). Dose reduction (of other drug): atorvastatin, rifabutin, sildenafil, vardenafil, ketoconazole, itraconazole. colchicine (↑ colchicine levels) Concentration monitoring (of other drug): amiodarone, systemic lidocaine, quinidine, warfarin (INR), tricyclic antidepressants, cyclosporin, tacrolimus, sirolimus. H₂ blockers and proton pump inhibitors interfere with absorption. Sildenafil (do not give > 25 mg/48 hrs); tadalafil (max. 10 mg/72 hrs); vardenafil (max. 2.5 mg/72 hrs). Clarithromycin (↑ QTc). May increase methadone effect/decrease methadone dose.
Contraindications: Rifapentine, telaprevir, do not coadminister with: rifampin, lovastatin, simvastatin, St. John's wort, delavirdine.
Adverse Effects: Rash, Stevens-Johnson Syndrome (rare), GI upset, headache, depression, diarrhea, hyperglycemia (including worsening diabetes, new-onset diabetes, DKA), ↑ cholesterol/triglycerides (evaluate risk for coronary disease/pancreatitis), fat redistribution, ↑ SGOT/SGPT, possible increased bleeding in hemophilia. Immune reconstitution syndrome.
Allergic Potential: High. Fosamprenavir is a sulfonamide; use with caution in patients with sulfonamide allergies
Safety in Pregnancy: C

"Usual dose" assumes normal renal/hepatic function. * For renal insufficiency, give usual dose × 1 followed by maintenance dose per CrCl. For dialysis patients, dose the same as for CrCl < 10 mL/min and give supplemental (post-HD/PD dose) immediately after dialysis. CrCl = creatinine clearance; CVVH = continuous veno-venous hemofiltration; HD/PD = hemodialysis/peritoneal dialysis.

Comments: Usually given in conjunction with ritonavir. May be taken with or without food. Fosamprenavir is a prodrug that is rapidly hydrolyzed to amprenavir by gut epithelium during absorption. Amprenavir inhibits CYP3A4. Fosamprenavir contains a sulfonamide moiety (as do darunavir and tipranavir). Fosamprenavir without ritonavir is no longer recommended in treatment naive patients due to increased development to resistance as well as cross-resistance to darunavir.

REFERENCES:

Blick G, Greiger-Zanlungo P, Gret S, et al. Long-term efficacy and safety of once- daily fosamprenavir 1400 mg boosted by ritonavir 100 mg: the BOLD100 study. Int J STD AIDS 23:18–22, 2012

Hughes PJ, Cretton-Scott E, Teague A, et al. Protease inhibitors for patients with HIV-1 infection. Pharm Ther 36:332–344, 2011.

Panel on Antiretroviral Guidelines for Adults and Adolescents. Department of Health and Human Services. Guidelines for the use of antiretroviral agents in HIV-infected adults and adolescents. http://aidsinfo.nih.gov/ConsentFiles/AdultandAdolescentGL.pdf, 2012.

Thompson MA, Aberg JA, Cahn P, et al. Antiretroviral treatment of adult HIV infection: 2012 recommendations of the International Antiviral Society — USA panel. JAMA 308:387–402, 2012.

Website: www.TreatHIV.com

Foscarnet (Foscavir)

Drug Class: Antiviral (see comments).
Usual Dose: <u>HSV:</u> 40 mg/kg (IV) q12h × 2–3 weeks; <u>CMV:</u> *Induction Dose:* 90 mg/kg (IV) q12h × 2 weeks, then *Maintenance Dose:* 90–120 mg/kg (IV) q24h until cured. *Relapse/reinduction dose:* 120 mg/kg (IV) q24h × 2 weeks.
Pharmacokinetic Parameters:
Peak serum level: 150 mcg/ml
Bioavailability: Not applicable

Excreted unchanged (urine): 85%
Serum half-life (normal/ESRD): 2–4/25 hrs
Plasma protein binding: 17%
Volume of distribution (V_d): 0.5 L/kg
Primary Mode of Elimination: Renal /hepatic
Dosage Adjustments*

Induction	
CrCl 50–80 mL/min	40–50 mg/kg (IV) q8h
CrCl 20–50 mL/min	20–30 mg/kg (IV) q8h
CrCl < 20 mL/min	Avoid
Maintenance	
CrCl 50–80 mL/min	60–70 mg/kg (IV) q24h
CrCl 20–50 mL/min	65–80 mg/kg (IV) q48h
CrCl < 20 mL/min	Avoid
Post–HD dose	60 mg/kg (IV)
Post–HF HD dose	60 mg/kg (IV)
Post–PD dose	None
CVVH/CVVHD/CVVHDF dose	Induction: 20–30 mg/kg (IV) q8h; maintenance: 65–80 mg/kg (IV) q48h
Mod. hepatic insufficiency	No change
Severe hepatic insufficiency	No change

Infusion pump must be used. Adequate hydration is recommended to prevent renal toxicity
† Higher doses may be considered for early reinduction due to progression of CMV retinitis, and for patients showing excellent tolerance.

Drug Interactions: Ciprofloxacin (↑ risk of seizures); amphotericin B, aminoglycosides,

---

"Usual dose" assumes normal renal/hepatic function. * For renal insufficiency, give usual dose × 1 followed by maintenance dose per CrCl. For dialysis patients, dose the same as for CrCl < 10 mL/min and give supplemental (post-HD/PD dose) immediately after dialysis. CrCl = creatinine clearance; CVVH = continuous veno-venous hemofiltration; HD/PD = hemodialysis/peritoneal dialysis.

cis-platinum, cyclosporine, ritonavir, saquinavir (↑ nephrotoxicity); pentamidine IV (severe hypocalcemia reported; do not combine); zidovudine (↑ incidence/severity of anemia).

Adverse Effects: Major side effects include nephrotoxicity and tetany (from ↓ Ca++). Others include anemia, nausea, vomiting, GI upset, headache, seizures, peripheral neuropathy, hallucinations, tremors, nephrogenic DI, ↓ Ca++, ↓ Mg++, ↓ PO$_4$=, oral/genital ulcers.

Allergic Potential: Low

Safety in Pregnancy: C

Comments: Renal failure prevented/minimized by adequate hydration. Dilute with 150 cc normal saline per 1 gm foscarnet. Do not mix with other types of solutions. Administer by IV slow infusion ≤ 1 mg/kg/min using an infusion pump. **Highly active against CMV and HHV-6. Some activity against EBV, HSV and VZV. No activity against RSV or adenoviruses.**

Meningeal dose = usual dose.

Cerebrospinal Fluid Penetration:
Non-Inflamed meninges = 90%
Inflamed meninges = 100%

REFERENCES:

Mattes FM, Hainsworth EG, Geretti AM, et al. A randomized, controlled trial comparing ganciclovir plus foscarnet (each at half dose) preemptive therapy of cytomegalovirus infection in transplant recipients. J Infect Dis 189:1355–61, 2004.

Website: www.pdr.net

Fosfomycin (Monurol)

Drug Class: Urinary antiseptic.

Usual Dose: 3 gm (PO) q24h.

Spectrum: (see *Susceptibility Profiles* pp. 198–202).

Resistance Potential: Low

Pharmacokinetic Parameters:
Peak serum level: 26 mcg/ml
Bioavailability: 37%
Excreted unchanged (urine): 60%; 40% excreted as active metabolite
Serum half-life (normal/ESRD): 5.7/50 hrs
Plasma protein binding: 3%
Volume of distribution (V$_d$): 2 L/kg

Primary Mode of Elimination: Renal

Dosage Adjustments*

CrCl 10–50 mL/min	No change
CrCl < 10 mL/min	Use with caution
Post–HD dose	3 gm (PO)
Post–PD dose	1 gm (PO)
CVVH/CVVHD/CVVHDF dose	No change
Moderate—severe hepatic insufficiency	No change

Drug Interactions: Antacids, metoclopramide (↓ fosfomycin effect).

Adverse Effects: Nausea, vomiting, diarrhea, GI upset, ↑ SGOT/SGPT, thrombocytosis.

Allergic Potential: Low

Safety in Pregnancy: B

Comments: Take without food. **Useful for cystitis/CAB,** not pyelonephritis/urosepsis. Treat cystitis as single dose in females. **Only oral antibiotic active against MDR P. aeruginosa, MDR Klebsiella pneumoniae, and MDR Acinetobacter baumanii in urine** (*cystitis/CAB*). Treatment of MDR GNB cystitis/CAB (change Foley *before* beginning therapy). (also see *Antibiotic Pearls & Pitfalls* p. 520).

"Usual dose" assumes normal renal/hepatic function. * For renal insufficiency, give usual dose × 1 followed by maintenance dose per CrCl. For dialysis patients, dose the same as for CrCl < 10 mL/min and give supplemental (post-HD/PD dose) immediately after dialysis. CrCl = creatinine clearance; CVVH = continuous veno-venous hemofiltration; HD/PD = hemodialysis/peritoneal dialysis.

REFERENCES:

Auer S, Wojna A, Hell M. Oral treatment options for ambulatory patients with urinary tract infections caused by extended-spectrum-beta-lactamase-producing Escherichia coli. Antimicrob Agents Chemother 54:4006–4008, 2010.

Dinh A, Salomon J, Bru JP, et al. fosfomycin: efficacy against infections caused by multidrug-resistant bacteria. Scand J infect Dis 44:182–9, 2012.

Estebanez A, Pascual R, Gil V, et al. Fosfomycin in a single dose versus a 7-day course of amoxicillin-clavulanate for the treatment of asymptomatic bacteriuria during pregnancy. Eur J Clin Microbiol Infect Dis 28:1457–1464, 2009.

Falafas ME, Kastoris AC, Kapaskelis AM, et al. Fosfomycin for the treatment of multidrug-resistant, including extended-spectrum β-lactamase producing, Enterobacteriaceae infections: a systematic review. Lancet Infect Dis 10:43–50, 2010.

Karageorgopoulos DE, Wang R, Yu XH, et al. Fosfomycin evaluation of the published evidence on the emergence of antimicrobial resistance in Gram-negative pathogens. J Antimicrob Chemother 67:225–68, 2012.

Liu HY, Lin HC, Lin YC, et al. Antimicrobial susceptibilities of urinary extended-spectrum beta-lactamase-producing Escherichia coli and Klebsiella pneumoniae to fosfomycin and nitrofurantoin in a teaching hospital in Taiwan. J Microbiol Immunol Infect 44:364–368, 2011.

Livermore Dm, Warner M, Mushtaq S, et al. What remains against carbapenem-resistant Enterbacteriaceae? Evaluation of chloramphenicol, ciprofloxacin, colistin, fosfomycin, minocycline, nitrofurantoin, temocillin and tigecycline. In J Antimicrob Agents 37:415–419, 2011.

Website: www.pdr.net

Ganciclovir (Cytovene)

Drug Class: Antiviral (see comments), nucleoside inhibitor/analogue.
Usual Dose: *Induction Dose:* 5 mg/kg (IV) q12h × 2 weeks; *Maintenance Dose:* 5 mg/kg (IV) q24h or 1 gm (PO) q8h.

Pharmacokinetic Parameters:
Peak serum level: 8.3 (IV)/1.2 (PO) mcg/ml
Bioavailability: 5%
Excreted unchanged (urine): 90%
Serum half-life (normal/ESRD): 3.6/28 hrs
Plasma protein binding: 1%
Volume of distribution (V_d): 0.74 L/kg
Primary Mode of Elimination: Renal
Dosage Adjustments*

CrCl 50–70 mL/min	2.5 mg/kg (IV) q12h (induction); 2.5 mg/kg (IV) q24h (maintenance); 500 mg (PO) q8h
CrCl 25–50 mL/min	2.5 mg/kg (IV) q24h (induction); 1.25 mg/kg (IV) q24h (maintenance); 500 mg (PO) q12h
CrCl 10–25 mL/min	1.25 mg/kg (IV) q24h (induction); 0.625 mg/kg (IV) q24h (maintenance); 500 mg (PO) q24h
CrCl < 10 mL/min	1.25 mg/kg (IV) 3x/week (induction); 0.625 mg/kg (IV) 3x/week (maintenance); 500 mg (PO) 3x/week
Post–HD dose	1.25 mg/kg (IV) (induction); 0.625 mg/kg (IV) (maintenance); 500 mg (PO)
Post–PD dose	Same dose as Post–HD
CVVH/CVVHD/CVVHDF dose	Same dose as CrCl 50–70 mL/min

"Usual dose" assumes normal renal/hepatic function. * For renal insufficiency, give usual dose × 1 followed by maintenance dose per CrCl. For dialysis patients, dose the same as for CrCl < 10 mL/min and give supplemental (post-HD/PD dose) immediately after dialysis. CrCl = creatinine clearance; CVVH = continuous veno-venous hemofiltration; HD/PD = hemodialysis/peritoneal dialysis.

Moderate hepatic insufficiency	No change
Severe hepatic insufficiency	No change

Drug Interactions: Cytotoxic drugs (may produce additive toxicity: stomatitis, bone marrow depression, alopecia); imipenem (↑ risk of seizures); probenecid (↑ ganciclovir levels); zidovudine (↓ ganciclovir levels, ↑ zidovudine levels, possible neutropenia); didanosine (↑ didanosine levels); cyclosporine, amphotericin, (↑ nephrotoxicity); mycophenolate mofetil (↑ mycophenolate mofetil and ganciclovir levels in renal insufficiency); tenofovir (↑ tenofovir, ganciclovir levels).

Adverse Effects: Headaches, hallucinations, seizures/tremor (dose related), drug fever/rash, diarrhea, nausea/vomiting, GI upset, leukopenia, thrombocytopenia, anemia, retinal detachment. Ventricular arrhythmias (VT/torsades de pointes).

Allergic Potential: High

Safety in Pregnancy: C

Comments: *Induction* dose usually given IV. *Maintenance* dose may be given IV or PO. For PO therapy use valganciclovir (not PO ganciclovir). Reduce dose with neutropenia/thrombocytopenia. Bioavailability increased with food: 5% fasting; 6–9% with food; 28–31% with fatty food. ***Highly active against CMV, HHV-6, and HSV. Some activity against VZV, EBV, and adenoviruses. No activity against RSV.*** Meningeal dose = usual dose.

Cerebrospinal Fluid Penetration: 70%

REFERENCES:

Jacobsen T, Sipointis N. Drug interactions and toxicities associated with the antiviral management of cytomegalovirus infection. Am J Health Syst Pharm 67:1417–1425, 2010.

Matthews T, Boehme R. Antiviral activity and mechanism of action of ganciclovir. Rev Infect Dis 10:490–4, 1988.

Singh N. Preemptive therapy for cytomegalovirus with oral ganciclovir after liver transplantation. Transplantation 73:1977–78, 2002.

Tayebi-Khosroshahi H, Makhdami N, Heris HK, et al. Universal prophylaxis with ganciclovir preparation is not necessary in all kidney allograft recipients. Transplant Proc 43:547–50, 2011.

Tokimasa S, Hara J, Osugi Y, et al. Ganciclovir is effective for prophylaxis and treatment of human herpesvirus-6 in allogeneic stem cell transplantation. Bone Marrow Transplant 29:595–8, 2002.

Website: www.rocheusa.com/Products/

Gentamicin (Garamycin)

Drug Class: Aminoglycoside.

Usual Dose: 240 mg or 5 mg/kg (IV) q24h (preferred over q8h dosing) (see comments).

Spectrum: (see *Susceptibility Profiles* pp. 198–202).

Resistance Potential: High (P. aeruginosa, aerobic GNBs)

Pharmacokinetic Parameters:
Peak serum levels: 4–8 mcg/ml (q8h dosing);
* 16–24 mcg/ml (q24h dosing)*
Bioavailability: Not applicable
Excreted unchanged (urine): 95%
Serum half-life (normal/ESRD): 2.5/48 hrs
Plasma protein binding: < 5%
Volume of distribution (V_d): 0.3 L/kg

Primary Mode of Elimination: Renal

Dosage Adjustments*

CrCl 50–80 mL/min	120 mg (IV) q24h or 2.5 mg/kg (IV) q24h
CrCl 10–50 mL/min	120 mg (IV) q48h or 2.5 mg/kg (IV) q48h

"Usual dose" assumes normal renal/hepatic function. * For renal insufficiency, give usual dose × 1 followed by maintenance dose per CrCl. For dialysis patients, dose the same as for CrCl < 10 mL/min and give supplemental (post-HD/PD dose) immediately after dialysis. CrCl = creatinine clearance; CVVH = continuous veno-venous hemofiltration; HD/PD = hemodialysis/peritoneal dialysis.

CrCl < 10 mL/min	80 mg (IV) q48h or 1.25 mg/kg (IV) q48h
Post–HD dose	80 mg (IV) or 1 mg/kg (IV)
Post–PD dose	40 mg (IV) or 0.5 mg/kg (IV)
Post–HFHD dose	120 mg (IV) or 2.5 mg/kg
Post-dose	120 mg (IV) or 2.5 mg/kg (IV)
CVVH/CVVHD/CVVHDF dose	120 mg (IV) q48h or 2.5 mg/kg (IV)
Moderate hepatic insufficiency	No change
Severe hepatic insufficiency	No change

Drug Interactions: Amphotericin B, cephalothin, cyclosporine, enflurane, methoxyflurane, NSAIDs, polymyxin B, radiographic contrast, vancomycin (↑ nephrotoxicity); cis-platinum (↑ nephrotoxicity, ↑ ototoxicity); loop diuretics (↑ ototoxicity); neuromuscular blocking agents, magnesium sulfate (↑ apnea, prolonged paralysis); non-polarizing muscle relaxants (↑ apnea).

Adverse Effects: Neuromuscular blockade with rapid infusion/absorption. Nephrotoxicity only with prolonged/extremely high serum trough levels; may cause reversible non-oliguric renal failure (ATN). Ototoxicity associated with prolonged/extremely high peak serum levels (usually irreversible): Cochlear toxicity (1/3 of ototoxicity) manifests as decreased high frequency hearing, but deafness is unusual. Vestibular toxicity (2/3 of ototoxicity) develops before ototoxicity, and typically manifests as tinnitus.

Safety in Pregnancy: D

Comments: Synergy dose: 2.5 mg/kg (IV) q24h or 120 mg (IV) q24h. **Single daily dosing virtually eliminates nephrotoxic/ototoxic potential.** Incompatible with solutions containing β-lactams, erythromycin, chloramphenicol, furosemide, sodium bicarbonate. IV infusion should be given slowly over 1 hour. **May be given IM. Avoid intraperitoneal infusion due to risk of neuromuscular blockade.** Avoid intratracheal/aerosolized intrapulmonary instillation, which predisposes to antibiotic resistance. V_d increases with edema/ascites, trauma, burns, cystic fibrosis; may require ↑ dose. V_d decreases with dehydration, obesity; may require ↓ dose. **Renal cast counts are the best indicator of aminoglycoside nephrotoxicity, not serum creatinine.** Dialysis removes ~ 1/3 of gentamicin from serum. **CAPD dose:** 2–4 mg/L dialysate (IP) with each exchange.

Therapeutic Serum Concentrations (for therapeutic efficacy, *not toxicity*):
Peak (q24h/q8h dosing) = 16–24/8–10 mcg/ml
Trough (q24h/q8h dosing) = 0/1–2 mcg/ml
Intrathecal (IT) dose: 5 mg (IT) q24h.
Cerebrospinal Fluid Penetration:
Non-Inflamed meninges = 0%
Inflamed meninges = 20%
Bile Penetration: 30%
(also see ***Antibiotic Pearls & Pitfalls*** p. 514).

REFERENCES:
Bhavnani SM, Prakhya A, Hammel JP, et al. Cost-Effectiveness of daptomycin versus vancomycin and gentamicin for patients with methicillin-resistant Staphylococcus aureus bacteremia and/or endocarditis. Clin Infect Dis 49:691–698, 2009.

Bruss JB. Lack of evidence associating nephrotoxicity with low-dose gentamicin for Staphylococcus aureus bacteremia and endocarditis. Clin Infect Dis 49:806, 2009.

"Usual dose" assumes normal renal/hepatic function. * For renal insufficiency, give usual dose × 1 followed by maintenance dose per CrCl. For dialysis patients, dose the same as for CrCl < 10 mL/min and give supplemental (post-HD/PD dose) immediately after dialysis. CrCl = creatinine clearance; CVVH = continuous veno-venous hemofiltration; HD/PD = hemodialysis/peritoneal dialysis.

Cosgrove SE, Vigliani GA, Campion M, et al. Initial low-dose gentamicin for Staphylococcus aureus bacteremia and endocarditis is nephrotoxic. Clin Infect Dis 48:713–721, 2009.

Cunha BA. Aminoglycosides: Current role in antimicrobial therapy. Pharmacotherapy 8:334–50, 1988.

Edson RS, Terrell CL. The aminoglycosides. Mayo Clin Proc 74:519–28, 1999.

Freeman CD, Nicolau DP, Belliveau PP, et al. Once-daily dosing of aminoglycosides: Review and recommendations for clinical practice. J Antimicrob Chemother 39:677–86, 1997.

Hassoun A, Spera R, Dunkel J. Tularemia and once-daily gentamicin. Antimicrob Agents Chemother 50:824, 2006.

Krol V, Cunha BA, Schoch PE, Klein NC. Appropriateness of empiric gentamicin and vancomycin therapy for bacteremias in chronic dialysis outpatient units in the era of antibiotic resistance. J Chemother 18:490–3, 2006.

Roushan MRH, Mohraz M, Hajiahmadi M, et al. Efficacy of gentamicin plus doxycycline versus streptomycin plus doxycycline in the treatment of brucellosis in humans. Clin Infect Dis 42:1075–1080, 2006.

Snydman, DR, McDermott LA, Jacobus NV. Evaluation of in vitro interaction of daptomycin with gentamicin or beta-lactam antibiotics against Staphylococcus aureus and Enterococci by FIC index and timed-kill curves. J Chemother 17:614–21, 2005.

Griseofulvin (Fulvicin, Grifulvin, Ultra, Gris-PEG, Grisactin)

Drug Class: Antifungal.
Usual Dose: 500 mg-1 gm (PO) q24h (microsize); 330–375 mg (PO) q24h (ultramicrosize).
Pharmacokinetic Parameters:
Peak serum level: 1–2 mcg/mL
Bioavailability: 50%
Excreted unchanged (urine): 1%
Serum half-life (normal/ESRD): 9/22 hrs
Plasma protein binding: 84%
Volume of distribution (V_d): No data
Primary Mode of Elimination: Hepatic
Dosage Adjustments*

CrCl < 10 mL/min	No change
Post–HD or PD dose	None
CVVH/CVVHD/ CVVHDF dose	No change
Moderate hepatic insufficiency	No change
Severe hepatic insufficiency	Use with caution

Drug Interactions: Alcohol (↑ griseofulvin toxicity); barbiturates (↓ griseofulvin levels); oral contraceptives, warfarin (↓ interacting drug levels).
Adverse Effects: Photosensitivity reactions, rash, headache, nausea, vomiting, diarrhea, angular stomatitis, glossitis, leukopenia.
Allergic Potential: Moderate
Safety in Pregnancy: C
Comments: May exacerbate SLE/acute intermittent porphyria. Take microsize griseofulvin with fatty meal to ↑ absorption to ~ 70%. Ultramicrosize griseofulvin is absorbed 1.5 times better than microsize griseofulvin.

REFERENCES:
Trepanier EF, Amsden GW. Current issues in onychomycosis. Ann Pharmacotherapy 32:204–14, 1998.
Website: www.pdr.net

"Usual dose" assumes normal renal/hepatic function. * For renal insufficiency, give usual dose × 1 followed by maintenance dose per CrCl. For dialysis patients, dose the same as for CrCl < 10 mL/min and give supplemental (post-HD/PD dose) immediately after dialysis. CrCl = creatinine clearance; CVVH = continuous veno-venous hemofiltration; HD/PD = hemodialysis/peritoneal dialysis.

Imipenem/Cilastatin (Primaxin)

Drug Class: Carbapenem.
Usual Dose: 1 gm (IV) q6h (see comments).
Spectrum: (see *Susceptibility Profiles* pp. 198–202).
Resistance Potential: High (P. aeruginosa, ↑ prevalence of MRSA)

Pharmacokinetic Parameters:
Peak serum level: 42–116 mcg/ml
Bioavailability: Not applicable
Excreted unchanged (urine): 70%
Serum half-life (normal/ESRD): 1/4 hrs
Plasma protein binding: 20% / 40% (cilastatin)
Volume of distribution (V_d): 0.2 L/kg
Primary Mode of Elimination: Renal
Dosage Adjustments*

CrCl 40–70 mL/min	500 mg (IV) q6h
CrCl 20–40 mL/min	250 mg (IV) q8h
CrCl < 20 mL/min[†]	250 mg (IV) q12h
Post–HD dose	250 mg (IV)
Post–PD dose	250 mg (IV)
CVVH/CVVHD/CVVHDF dose	500 mg (IV) q8h
Moderate hepatic insufficiency	No change
Severe hepatic insufficiency	No change

† Avoid if CrCl ≤ 5 mL/min unless dialysis is instituted within 48 hours.

Drug Interactions: Cyclosporine (↑ cyclosporine levels); ganciclovir (↑ risk of seizures); probenecid (↑ imipenem levels); valproic acid (↓ seizure threshold).
Adverse Effects: Seizures, phlebitis.
Allergic Potential: Low
Safety in Pregnancy: C
Comments: Imipenem:cilastatin (1:1). Infuse 1 gm (IV) over 40–60 minutes. Imipenem is renally metabolized by dehydropeptidase I; cilastatin is an inhibitor of this enzyme, effectively preventing the metabolism of imipenem. Imipenem/cilastatin can be given IM (IM absorption: imipenem 75%; cilastatin 100%). *Fully susceptible organisms dose: 500 mg (IV) q6h; Less susceptible organisms (e.g., P. aeruginosa) dose:* 1 gm (IV) q6-8h. Incompatible in solutions containing vancomycin or metronidazole. *Seizures more likely in renal insufficiency/high doses (> 2 gm/d)*. Inhibits endotoxin release from gram-negative bacilli. **Very low incidence of cross reactions with β-lactams.**
Cerebrospinal Fluid Penetration:
Non-Inflamed meninges = 10%
Inflamed meninges = 15%
Bile Penetration: 1%
(also see *Antibiotic Pearls & Pitfalls* p. 511).

REFERENCES:
Balfour JA, Bryson HM, Brogden RN. Imipenem/cilastatin: An update of its antibacterial activity, pharmacokinetics, and therapeutic efficacy in the treatment of serious infections. Drugs 51:99–136, 1996.
Barza M. Imipenem: First of a new class of beta-lactam antibiotics. Ann Intern Med 103:552–60, 1985.
Fish DN, Teitelbaum, I, Abraham E. Pharmacokinetics and pharmacodynamics of imipenem during continuous renal replacement therapy in critically ill patients. Antimicrobial Agents and Chemotherapy 49:2421–2428, 2005.

"Usual dose" assumes normal renal/hepatic function. * For renal insufficiency, give usual dose × 1 followed by maintenance dose per CrCl. For dialysis patients, dose the same as for CrCl < 10 mL/min and give supplemental (post-HD/PD dose) immediately after dialysis. CrCl = creatinine clearance; CVVH = continuous veno-venous hemofiltration; HD/PD = hemodialysis/peritoneal dialysis.

Garbino J, Villiger P, Caviezel A, et al. A randomized prospective study of cefepime plus metronidazole with imipenem-cilastatin in the treatment of intra-abdominal infections. Infection 35:161–166, 2007.

Helinger WC, Brewer NS. Carbapenems and monobactams: Imipenem, meropenem, and aztreonam. Mayo Clin Proc 74:420–34, 1999.

Lamoth F, Erard V, Asner S, et al. High imipenem blood concentrations associated with toxic encephalopathy in a patient with mild renal dysfunction. Int J Antimicrob Agents 34:386–388, 2009.

Lautenbach E, Weiner MG, Nachamkin I, et al. Imipenem resistance among Pseudomonas aeruginosa Isolates: risk factors for infection and impact of resistance on clinical and economic outcomes. Infection Control and Hosp Epidemiol 27:893–900, 2006.

Maravi-Poma E, Gener J, Alvarez-Lerma F, et al. Spanish group for the study of septic complications in severe acute pancreatitis. Early antibiotic treatment (prophylaxis) of septic complications in severe acute necrotizing pancreatitis: a prospective, randomized, multicenter study comparing two regimens with imipenem-cilastatin. Intensive Care Med 29:1974–80, 2003.

Miliani K, L'Heriteau F, Lacave L, et al. Imipenem and ciprofloxacin consumption as factors associated with high incidence rates of resistance Pseudomonas aeruginosa in hospitals in northern France. J Hosp Infect 77:343–347, 2011.

Saltoglu N, Dalkiran A, Tetiker T, et al. Piperacillin/tazobactam versus imipenem/cilastatin for severe diabetic foot infections: a prospective, randomized clinical trial in a university hospital. Clin Microbiol Infect 16:1252–1257, 2010.

Website: www.pdr.net

Indinavir (Crixivan) IDV

Drug Class: Antiretroviral protease inhibitor.
Usual Dose: 800 mg (PO) q8h or 800 mg (PO) q12h with ritonavir 100–200 mg (PO) q12h.

Pharmacokinetic Parameters:
Peak serum level: 252 mcg/mL
Bioavailability: 65% (77% with food)
Excreted unchanged (urine): < 20%
Serum half-life (normal/ESRD): 2 hrs/no data
Plasma protein binding: 60 %
Volume of distribution (V_d): No data
Primary Mode of Elimination: Hepatic
Dosage Adjustments*

CrCl < 10 mL/min	No change
Post–HD dose	None
Post–PD dose	None
CVVH/CVVHD/CVVHDF dose	No change
Moderate hepatic insufficiency	600 mg (PO) q8h
Severe hepatic insufficiency	400 mg (PO) q8h

Antiretroviral Dosage Adjustments

Atazanavir	Avoid
Didanosine	Administer didanosine 1 hour apart
Delavirdine	Indinavir 600 mg q8h
Efavirenz	Indinavir 1000 mg q8h
Lopinavir/ritonavir	Indinavir 600 mg q12h
Nelfinavir	Limited data for indinavir 1200 mg q12h + nelfinavir 1250 mg q12h
Nevirapine	Indinavir 1000 mg q8h
Ritonavir	Indinavir 800 mg q12h + ritonavir 100–200 mg q12h
Saquinavir	No information

"Usual dose" assumes normal renal/hepatic function. * For renal insufficiency, give usual dose × 1 followed by maintenance dose per CrCl. For dialysis patients, dose the same as for CrCl < 10 mL/min and give supplemental (post-HD/PD dose) immediately after dialysis. CrCl = creatinine clearance; CVVH = continuous veno-venous hemofiltration; HD/PD = hemodialysis/peritoneal dialysis.

| Rifampin | Avoid combination |
| Rifabutin | Indinavir 1000 mg q8h; rifabutin 150 mg q24h or 300 mg 2–3x/week |

Drug Interactions: Antiretrovirals, rifabutin, rifampin (see dose adjustment grid, above); astemizole, terfenadine, benzodiazepines, cisapride, ergot alkaloids, statins, calcium channel blockers (↑ calcium channel blocker levels); carbamazepine, phenobarbital, phenytoin (↓ indinavir levels, ↑ anticonvulsant levels; monitor); tenofovir (↓ indinavir levels, ↑ tenofovir levels); clarithromycin, erythromycin, telithromycin (↑ indinavir and macrolide levels); didanosine (administer indinavir on empty stomach 1 hour apart); ethinyl estradiol, norethindrone (↑ interacting drug levels; no dosage adjustment); grapefruit juice (↓ indinavir levels); itraconazole, ketoconazole (↑ indinavir levels); sildenafil (↑ or ↓ sildenafil levels; do not exceed 25 mg in 48 hrs), tadalafil (max. 10 mg/72 hrs), vardenafil (max 2.5 mg/72 hrs); theophylline (↓ theophylline levels); fluticasone nasal spray (avoid concomitant use).

Contraindications: rifapentine, St. John's wort
Adverse Effects: Nephrolithiasis, nausea, vomiting, diarrhea, anemia, leukopenia, headache, insomnia, hyperglycemia (including worsening diabetes, new-onset diabetes, DKA), ↑ SGOT/SGPT, ↑ indirect bilirubin (2° to drug-induced Gilbert's syndrome; inconsequential), fat redistribution, lipid abnormalities (evaluate risk of coronary disease/pancreatitis), abdominal pain, night sweats, possible ↑ bleeding in hemophilia, dry skin, chelitis, paronychiae.
Allergic Potential: Low
Safety in Pregnancy: C

Comments: Renal stone formation may be prevented/minimized by adequate hydration (1–3 liters water daily); ↑ risk of nephrolithiasis with alcohol. Take 1 hour before or 2 hours after meals (may take with skim milk or low fat meal). Separate dosing with ddI by 1 hour.
Cerebrospinal Fluid Penetration: 16%

REFERENCES:
Antinori A, Giancola MI, Griserri S, et al. Factors influencing virological response to antiretroviral drugs in cerebrospinal fluid of advanced HIV-1-infected patients. AIDS 16:1867–76, 2002.

Deeks SG, Smith M, Holodniy M, et al. HIV-1 protease inhibitors: A review for clinicians. JAMA 277:145–53, 1997.

DiCenzo R, Forrest A, Fischl MA, et al. Pharmacokinetics of indinavir and nelfinavir in treatment-naive, human immunodeficiency virus-infected subjects. Antimicrob Agents Chemother 48:918–23, 2004.

Hughes PJ, Cretton-Scott E, Teague A, et al. Protease inhibitors for patients with HIV-1 infection. Pharm Ther 36:332–344, 2011.

Justesen US, Andersen AB, Klitgaard NA, et al. Pharmacokinetic interaction between rifampin and the combination of indinavir and low-dose ritonavir in HIV-infected patients. Clin Infect Dis 38:426–9, 2004.

McDonald CK, Kuritzkes DR. Human immunodeficiency virus type 1 protease inhibitors. Arch Intern Med 157:951–9, 1997.

Panel on Antiretroviral Guidelines for Adults and Adolescents. Department of Health and Human Services. Guidelines for the use of antiretroviral agents in HIV-infected adults and adolescents. http://aidsinfo.nih.gov/ConsentFiles/AdultandAdolescentGL.pdf, 2012.

Thompson MA, Aberg JA, Cahn P, et al. Antiretroviral treatment of adult HIV infection: 2012 recommendations of the International Antiviral Society — USA panel. JAMA 308:387–402, 2012.

Website: www.crixivan.com

"Usual dose" assumes normal renal/hepatic function. * For renal insufficiency, give usual dose × 1 followed by maintenance dose per CrCl. For dialysis patients, dose the same as for CrCl < 10 mL/min and give supplemental (post-HD/PD dose) immediately after dialysis. CrCl = creatinine clearance; CVVH = continuous veno-venous hemofiltration; HD/PD = hemodialysis/peritoneal dialysis.

Isoniazid (INH)

Drug Class: Anti–TB drug.
Usual Dose: 300 mg (PO) q24h or 5 mg/kg (see comments).
Pharmacokinetic Parameters:
Peak serum level: 7 mcg/ml
Bioavailability: 90%
Excreted unchanged (urine): 50–70%
Serum half-life (normal/ESRD): 1/1 hr
Plasma protein binding: 15%
Volume of distribution (V_d): 0.75 L/kg
Primary Mode of Elimination: Hepatic
Dosage Adjustments*

CrCl < 10 mL/min	No change
Post–HD dose	300 mg
Post–PD dose	300 mg
CVVH/CVVHD/CVVHDF dose	None
Moderate hepatic insufficiency	No change
Severe hepatic insufficiency	Use with caution

Drug Interactions: Alcohol, rifampin (↑ risk of ↑ SGOT/SGPT); alfentanil (↑ duration of alfentanil effect); aluminum salts (↓ isoniazid absorption); carbamazepine, phenytoin (↑ interacting drug levels); itraconazole (↓ itraconazole levels); warfarin (↑ INR).
Adverse Effects: ↑ SGOT/SGPT, drug fever/rash, age-dependent hepatotoxicity (after age 60), drug-induced ANA/SLE, hemolytic anemia, neuropsychiatric changes in the elderly. Transient/reversible ↑ SGOT/SGPT frequently occur early

(< 3 weeks) after INH use. If ↑ SGOT/SGPT, monitor levels twice weekly until levels peak, then monitor levels weekly until levels return to within normal range. D/C INH if ↑ SGOT/SGPT ≥ 10 × upper limit of normal. Fulminant hepatic failure (rare).
Allergic Potential: Low
Safety in Pregnancy: C
Comments: Administer with 50 mg of pyridoxine daily to prevent peripheral neuropathy. Increased blood pressure/rash with tyramine–containing products, e.g., cheese/wine. ↑ hepatotoxicity in slow acetylators.
Slow acetylator dose: 150 mg (PO) q24h.
TB D.O.T. dose: 15 mg/kg or 900 mg (PO) 3x/week.
Meningeal dose = usual dose.
Cerebrospinal Fluid Penetration:
Non-Inflamed meninges = 90%
Inflamed meninges = 90%

REFERENCES:
CDC. Severe Isoniazid-associated liver injuries among persons being treated for latent tuberculosis infection. MMWR 59:224–229, 2010.
Colebunders R, Apers L, Shamputa IC. Treatment of multidrug-resistant tuberculosis. Lancet 10:1240, 2004.
Ena J, Valls V. Short-course therapy with rifampin plus isoniazid, compared with standard therapy with isoniazid, for latent tuberculosis infection: A meta-analysis. Clin Infect Dis 40:670–6, 2005.
McIllerson H, Wash P, Burger A, et al. Determinants of rifampin, isoniazid, pyrazinamide and ethambutol pharmacokinetics in a cohort of tuberculosis patients. Antimicrob Agents Chemother 50:1170–77, 2006.
Schaller A, Sun Z, Yang Y, et al. Salicylate reduces susceptibility of Mycobacterium tuberculosis to multiple antituberculosis drugs. Antimicrob Agents Chemother 46:2533–9, 2002.
Schlossberg D. An approach to drug-induced liver injury during tuberculosis therapy. Infect Dis Clin Pract 18:107–108, 2010.

"Usual dose" assumes normal renal/hepatic function. * For renal insufficiency, give usual dose × 1 followed by maintenance dose per CrCl. For dialysis patients, dose the same as for CrCl < 10 mL/min and give supplemental (post-HD/PD dose) immediately after dialysis. CrCl = creatinine clearance; CVVH = continuous veno-venous hemofiltration; HD/PD = hemodialysis/peritoneal dialysis.

Schlossberg D. Treatment of multi-drug resistant tuberculosis. Antibiotics for Clinicians 9:317–321, 2005.

Van Scoy RE, Wilkowske CJ. Antituberculous agents. Mayo Clin Proc 67:179–87, 1992.

Itraconazole (Sporanox)

Drug Class: Antifungal.

Usual Dose: 200 mg (PO, capsules or solution, solution produces better absorption) q12h or q24h **(take *without* food)** depending on disease; due to enhanced drug delivery, IV therapy begins with 200 mg IV q12h × 2 days (4 doses) and then continues with only 200 mg (IV) q24h; PO follow-up to IV therapy for serious infection is at 200 mg PO q12h. Each IV dose should be infused over 1 hour (see comments).

Pharmacokinetic Parameters:

Peak serum level: 2.8 mcg/ml

Bioavailability: 55% (capsules)/90% (solution- **take without food***)*

Excreted unchanged (urine): 1%

Serum half-life (normal/ESRD): 21–64/35 hrs

Plasma protein binding: 99.8%

Volume of distribution (V_d): 10 L/kg

Primary Mode of Elimination: Hepatic; metabolized predominantly by the cytochrome P450 3A4 isoenzyme system (CYP3A4)

Dosage Adjustments*

CrCl > 30 mL/min	No change
CrCl < 30 mL/min	No change for (PO); avoid (IV) due to ↑ cyclodextrin
Post–HD dose	100 mg (IV/PO)
Post–PD dose	None
CVVH/CVVHD/ CVVHDF dose	No change

Moderate hepatic insufficiency	No change†
Severe hepatic insufficiency	Use with caution

† ↑ $t_{1/2}$ of itraconazole in patients with hepatic insufficiency should be considered when given with medications metabolized by P450 isoenzymes. Also see Adverse Effects for information regarding patients who develop liver dysfunction.

Drug Interactions: *Itraconazole may ↑ plasma levels of:* alfentanil, buspirone, busulfan, carbamazepine, cisapride, cyclosporine, digoxin, dihydropyridines, docetaxel, dofetilide, methylprednisolone, oral hypoglycemics (↑ risk of hypoglycemia), pimozide, quinidine, rifabutin, saquinavir, sirolimus, tacrolimus, trimetrexate, verapamil, vinca alkaloids, warfarin; alprazolam, diazepam, midazolam, triazolam (↑ sedative/hypnotic effects); atorvastatin, lovastatin, simvastatin (↑ risk of rhabdomyolysis); indinavir, ritonavir, saquinavir; coadministration of oral midazolam, triazolam, lovastatin, or simvastatin with itraconazole is contraindicated; coadministration of cisapride, pimozide, quinidine, amiodarone, or dofetilide with itraconazole is contraindicated due to the risk of ↑ QT_c/life-threatening ventricular arrhythmias. *Decreased itraconazole levels may occur with:* antacids, carbamazepine, H_2-receptor antagonists, isoniazid, nevirapine, phenobarbital, phenytoin, proton pump inhibitors, rifabutin, rifampin; coadministration of rifampin with itraconazole is not recommended. *Increased itraconazole levels may occur with:* clarithromycin, erythromycin, indinavir, ritonavir.

Adverse Effects: ≥ 2%: nausea, diarrhea, vomiting, headache, abdominal pain, bilirubinemia, rash, ↑ SGPT/SGOT, hypokalemia,

---

"Usual dose" assumes normal renal/hepatic function. * For renal insufficiency, give usual dose × 1 followed by maintenance dose per CrCl. For dialysis patients, dose the same as for CrCl < 10 mL/min and give supplemental (post-HD/PD dose) immediately after dialysis. CrCl = creatinine clearance; CVVH = continuous veno-venous hemofiltration; HD/PD = hemodialysis/peritoneal dialysis.

↑ serum creatinine. Rarely, itraconazole has been associated with serious hepatotoxicity (liver failure/death). If liver disease develops, discontinue treatment, perform liver function testing, and reevaluate risk/benefit of further treatment. Use itraconazole with caution in patients with ↑ liver enzymes, active liver disease, or previous drug-induced hepatotoxicity. Life-threatening ventricular arrhythmias/sudden death have occurred in patients using cisapride, pimozide, or quinidine concomitantly with itraconazole; coadministration of these drugs with itraconazole is contraindicated. Use itraconazole with caution in patients with ventricular dysfunction. IV itraconazole may cause transient, asymptomatic ↓ in ejection fraction for ≤ 12 hours. If CHF develops, consider discontinuation of itraconazole.

Allergic Potential: Low

Safety in Pregnancy: C

Comments: *Oral itraconazole:* Requires gastric acidity for absorption. When antacids are required, administer ≥ 1 hour before or 2 hours after itraconazole capsules. Oral solution is better absorbed without food; capsules are better absorbed with food. Capsule bioavailability is food dependent: 40% fasting/90% post-prandial. For oral therapy, bioavailability of 10 ml of solution without food = 100 mg capsule with food. Administer with a cola beverage in patients with achlorhydria or taking H₂-receptor antagonists/other gastric acid suppressors. While oral solution and capsules can be interchanged for treatment of systemic disease if adequate blood levels are achieved, oral solution produces more reliable blood levels and is definitely preferred for oral/esophageal candidiasis where the local effect of the solution on the infection seem helpful.

IV itraconazole: Hydroxypropyl-β-cyclodextrin stabilizer in IV formulation accumulates in renal failure. IV itraconazole should not be used in patients with CrCl < 30 mL/min; if possible, use the oral preparation. Infuse 60 ml of dilute solution (3.33 mg/ml = 200 mg itraconazole, pH ~ 4.8) IV over 60 minutes, using infusion set provided. After administration, flush the infusion set with 15–20 ml of normal saline injection. The compatibility of IV itraconazole with flush solutions other than normal saline is unknown. *Highly active against C. albicans, non-albicans Candida, Cryptococcus, Histoplasmosis, Blastomycosis, Paracoccidiomycosis, Sporotrichosis. Active against dermatophytes. No activity against Pseudoallescheria/Scedosporium, Fusaria or Mucor.*

Cerebrospinal Fluid Penetration: < 10%

Bile Penetration: 3–18%

REFERENCES:

Boogaerts M, Winston DJ, Bow EJ, et al. Intravenous and oral itraconazole versus intravenous amphotericin B deoxycholate as empirical antifungal therapy for persistent fever in neutropenic patients with cancer who are receiving broad-spectrum antibacterial therapy. A randomized controlled trial. Ann Intern Med 135:412–22, 2001.

Bruggemann RJM, Alffenaar JWC, Blijlevens NMA, et al. Clinical relevance of the pharmoacokinetic interactions of azole antifungal drugs with coadministered agents. Clin Infect Dis 48:1441–1458, 2009.

Calvopina M, Guevara AG, Armijos RX, et al. Itraconazole in the treatment of New World mucocutaneous leishmaniasis. Int J Dermatol 43:659–63, 2004.

Caputo R. Itraconazole (Sporanox) in superficial and systemic fungal infections. Expert Rev Anti Infect Ther 1:531–42, 2004.

Conte JE Jr, Golden JA, Kipps J, et al. Intrapulmonary pharmacokinetics and pharmacodynamics of itraconazole and 14-hydroxyitraconazol steady state. Antimicrob Agents Chemother 48:3823–7, 2004.

"Usual dose" assumes normal renal/hepatic function. * For renal insufficiency, give usual dose × 1 followed by maintenance dose per CrCl. For dialysis patients, dose the same as for CrCl < 10 mL/min and give supplemental (post-HD/PD dose) immediately after dialysis. CrCl = creatinine clearance; CVVH = continuous veno-venous hemofiltration; HD/PD = hemodialysis/peritoneal dialysis.

Dominguez-Gil Hurle A, Sanchez Navarro A, Garcia Sanchez MJ. Therapeutic drug monitoring of itraconazole and the relevance of pharmacokinetic interactions. Clin Microbiol and Infection 12:S97–106, 2006.

Glasmacher A, Prentice A. Current experience with itraconazole in neutropenic patients: a concise overview of pharmacological properties in use in prophylactic and empirical antifungal therapy. Clin Microbiol and Infection 12:S84–90, 2006.

Go J, Cunha BA. Itraconazole. Antibiotics for Clinicians 3:61–70, 1999.

Horousseau JL, Dekker AW, et al. Itraconazole oral solution for primary prophylaxis of fungal infections in patients with hematological malignancy and profound neutropenia: a randomized, double-blind, double-placebo, multicenter trial comparing itraconazole and amphotericin B. Antimicrob Agents Chemother 44:1887–93, 2000.

Marks DI, Pagliuca A, Kibbler CC, et al. Voriconazole versus itraconazole for antifungal prophylaxis following allogeneic haematopoietic stem cell transplantation. Br J Haematol 155:318–327, 2011.

Mattiuzzi GN, Alvarado G, Giles FJ, et al. Open-label, randomized comparison of itraconazole versus caspofungin for prophylaxis in patients with hematologic malignancies. Antimicrob Agents Chemother 50:143–7, 2006.

Phillips EJ. Itraconazole was as effective as amphotericin B for fever and neutropenia in cancer and led to fewer adverse events. ACP J Club 136:58, 2002.

Rubin MA, Carroll KC, Cahill BC. Caspofungin in combination with itraconazole for the treatment of invasive aspergillosis in humans. Clin Infect Dis 34:1160–1, 2002.

Sabatelli F. Patel R, Mann PA, et al. In vitro activities of posaconazole, fluconazole, itraconazole, voriconazole, and amphotericin B against a large collection of clinically important molds and yeasts. Antimicrob Agents Chemother 50:2009–15, 2006.

Terrell CL. Antifungal agents Part II. The azoles. Mayo Clin Proc 74:78–100, 1999.

Urunsak M, Ilkit M, Evruke C, et al. Clinical and mycological efficacy of single-day oral treatment with itraconazole (400 mg) in acute vulvovaginal candidosis. Mycoses 47:422–7, 2004.

Winston DJ. Itraconazole vs. fluconazole for antifungal prophylaxis in allogeneic stem-cell transplant patients 12:S91–96, 2006.

Winston DJ, Busuttil RW. Randomized controlled trial of oral itraconazole solution versus intravenous/oral fluconazole for prevention of fungal infections in liver transplant recipients. Transplantation 74:688–95, 2002.

Website: www.pdr.net

Ketoconazole (Nizoral)

Drug Class: Antifungal.
Usual Dose: 200 mg (PO) q24h.
Pharmacokinetic Parameters:
Peak serum level: 3.5 mcg/ml
Bioavailability: 82%
Excreted unchanged (urine): 2–4%
Serum half-life (normal/ESRD): 6/20 hrs
Plasma protein binding: 99%
Volume of distribution (V_d): 2 L/kg
Primary Mode of Elimination: Hepatic
Dosage Adjustments*

CrCl < 40 mL/min	No change
Post–HD dose	None
Post–PD dose	None
CVVH/CVVHD/CVVHDF dose	No change
Moderate hepatic insufficiency	Use with caution
Severe hepatic insufficiency	Avoid

Drug Interactions: Astemizole, cisapride, terfenadine, amiodarone (may ↑ QT interval, torsades de pointes); carbamazepine, INH

"Usual dose" assumes normal renal/hepatic function. * For renal insufficiency, give usual dose × 1 followed by maintenance dose per CrCl. For dialysis patients, dose the same as for CrCl < 10 mL/min and give supplemental (post-HD/PD dose) immediately after dialysis. CrCl = creatinine clearance; CVVH = continuous veno-venous hemofiltration; HD/PD = hemodialysis/peritoneal dialysis.

(↓ ketoconazole levels); cimetidine, famotidine, nizatidine, ranitidine, omeprazole, INH (↓ ketoconazole absorption); cyclosporine, digoxin, loratadine, tacrolimus (↑ interacting drug levels with possible toxicity); didanosine (↓ ketoconazole levels); midazolam, triazolam (↑ interacting drug levels, ↑ sedative effects); oral hypoglycemics (severe hypoglycemia); phenytoin, rifabutin, rifampin (↓ ketoconazole levels, ↑ interacting drug); statins (↑ statin levels; rhabdomyolysis reported); warfarin (↑ INR).

Adverse Effects: Nausea, vomiting, abdominal pain, pruritus.

Allergic Potential: Low

Safety in Pregnancy: C

Comments: Dose-dependent reduction in gonadal (androgenic) function. Decreased cortisol production with doses ≥ 800 mg/day, but **does not result in adrenal insufficiency**. Give oral doses with citric juices.

Highly active against dermatophytes, Malassezia, Candida albicans. Some activity against Aspergillus, Coccidiomycosis, Paracoccidiomycosis, Histoplasmosis. No activity against Pseudoallescheria/ Scedosporium, Fusaria or Mucor.

Cerebrospinal Fluid Penetration: < 10%

REFERENCES:

Allen LV. Ketoconazole oral suspension. US Pharm 18:98–9, 1993.

Kaur IP, Kakkar S. Topical delivery of antifungal agents. Expert Opin Drug Deliv 7:1303–1327, 2010.

Terrell CL. Antifungal agents: Part II. The azoles. Mayo Clin Proc 74:78–100, 1999.

Zhao Y, Li L, Wang JJ, et al. Cutaneous malasseziasis: four case reports of atypical dermatitis and onychomycosis caused by Malassezia. Int J Dermatol 49:141–145, 2010.

Website: www.pdr.net

Lamivudine (Epivir) 3TC

Drug Class: Antiretroviral NRTI (nucleoside reverse transcriptase inhibitor); antiviral (HBV).

Usual Dose: 150 mg (PO) q12h or 300 mg (PO) q24h (HIV); 100 mg (PO) q24h (HBV).

Pharmacokinetic Parameters:

Peak serum level: 1.5 mcg/mL
Bioavailability: 86%
Excreted unchanged (urine): 71%
Serum half-life (normal/ESRD): 5–7/20 hrs
Plasma protein binding: 36%
Volume of distribution (V_d): 1.3 L/kg

Primary Mode of Elimination: Renal

Dosage Adjustments* (HIV/HBV dose)

CrCl 30–50 mL/min	150 mg (PO) q24h /100 mg (PO), then 50 mg (PO) q24h
CrCl 15–30 mL/min	100 mg (PO) q24h /100 mg (PO), then 25 mg (PO) q24h
CrCl 5–15 mL/min	50 mg (PO) q24h /35 mg (PO), then 15 mg (PO) q24h
CrCl < 5 mL/min	25 mg (PO) q24h /35 mg (PO), then 10 mg (PO) q24h
Post–HD dose	25 mg (PO)/10 mg (PO)
Post–PD dose	None
CVVH/CVVHD/ CVVHDF dose	100 mg (PO) q24h /100 mg (PO), then 25 mg (PO) q24h
Moderate hepatic insufficiency	No change
Severe hepatic insufficiency	Use with caution

"Usual dose" assumes normal renal/hepatic function. * For renal insufficiency, give usual dose × 1 followed by maintenance dose per CrCl. For dialysis patients, dose the same as for CrCl < 10 mL/min and give supplemental (post-HD/PD dose) immediately after dialysis. CrCl = creatinine clearance; CVVH = continuous veno-venous hemofiltration; HD/PD = hemodialysis/peritoneal dialysis.

Drug Interactions: Didanosine, zalcitabine (↑ risk of pancreatitis); TMP–SMX (↑ lamivudine levels); zidovudine + lamivudine not recommended.

Adverse Effects: Lamivudine tablets and oral solution used to treat HIV infection contain a higher dose of lamivudine than Epivir-HBV® tablets and oral solution used to treat chronic hepatitis B. Severe acute exacerbations of hepatitis B have been reported in patients who are co-infected with hepatitis B virus (HBV) and HIV and have discontinued lamivudine. Hepatic function should be monitored closely for at least several months in patients who discontinue lamivudine. Most common include headache, dizziness, malaise, nausea nasal congestion, cough, rash, neuropathy, leucopenia. Pancreatitis and or lactic acidosis with hepatic steatosis (rare but potentially life threatening toxicity with NRTI's). Immune reconstitution syndrome can occur.

Allergic Potential: Low

Safety in Pregnancy: C

Comments: Potential cross resistance with didanosine. Prevents development of AZT resistance and restores AZT susceptibility. May be taken with or without food. Although effective against HBV, lamivudine is no longer a first-line option because of the development of resistance in 70% of treated patients.

Cerebrospinal Fluid Penetration: 15%

REFERENCES:

Diaz-Brito V, Leon A, Knobel H, et al. Post-exposure prophylaxis for HIV-infection: a clinical trail comparing lopinavir/ritonavir versus atazanavir each with zidovudine/lamivudine. Antivir Ther 17:337–46, 2012.

Leung N. Lamivudine for chronic hepatitis B. Expert Rev Anti Infect Ther 2:173–80, 2004.

Liaw YF, Sung JY, Chow WC, et al. Lamivudine for patients with chronic hepatitis B and advanced liver disease. N Engl J Med 351:1521–31, 2004.

Marrone A, Zampino R, D'Onofrio M, et al. Combined interferon plus lamivudine treatment in young patients with dual HBV (HbeAg positive) and HCV chronic infection. J Hepatol 41:1064–5, 2004.

Nishijima T, Tsukada K, Teruya K, et al. Efficacy and safety of once-daily ritonavir-based antiretroviral therapy in low-body weight treatment-naïve patients with HIV infections. AIDS 13;26:649–51 2012.

Panel on Antiretroviral Guidelines for Adults and Adolescents. Department of Health and Human Services. Guidelines for the use of antiretroviral agents in HIV-infected adults and adolescents. http://aidsinfo. nih.gov/ConsentFiles/AdultandAdolescentGL.pdf, 2012.

Perry CM, Faulds D. Lamivudine. A review of its antiviral activity, pharmacokinetic properties and therapeutic efficacy in the management of HIV infection. Drugs 53:657–80, 1997.

Sax PE, Tierney C, Collier AC, et al. Abacavir/lamivudine versus tenofovir DF/emtricitabine as part of combination regimens for initial treatment of HIV: final results. J Infect Dis 204:1191–201, 2011.

Schmilovitz-Weiss H, Ben-Ari Z, Sikuler E, et al. Lamivudine treatment for acute severe hepatitis B: a pilot study. Liver Int 24:547–51, 2004.

Sheng YJ, Liu JY, Tong SW, et al. Lamivudine plus adefovir combination therapy versus entecavir monotherapy for lamivudine-resistant chronic hepatitis B: a systematic review and meta-analysis. Virol J. 8:393, 2011.

Thompson MA, Aberg JA, Cahn P, et al. Antiretroviral treatment of adult HIV infection: 2012 recommendations of the International Antiviral Society — USA panel. JAMA 308:387–402, 2012.

Website: www.TreatHIV.com

Lamivudine + Zidovudine (Combivir) 3TC/ZDV

Drug Class: Antiretroviral NRTI's combination.

Usual Dose: Combivir tablet = 150 mg lamivudine + 300 mg zidovudine. Usual dose = 1 tablet (PO) q12h.

"Usual dose" assumes normal renal/hepatic function. * For renal insufficiency, give usual dose × 1 followed by maintenance dose per CrCl. For dialysis patients, dose the same as for CrCl < 10 mL/min and give supplemental (post-HD/PD dose) immediately after dialysis. CrCl = creatinine clearance; CVVH = continuous veno-venous hemofiltration; HD/PD = hemodialysis/peritoneal dialysis.

Pharmacokinetic Parameters:

Peak serum level: 2.6/1.2 mcg/mL

Bioavailability: 82/60%

Excreted unchanged (urine): 86/64%

Serum half-life (normal/ESRD): [6/1.1]/[20/2.2] hrs

Plasma protein binding: <36/<38%

Volume of distribution (V_d): 1.3/1.6 L/kg

Primary Mode of Elimination: Renal

Dosage Adjustments*

CrCl 50–80 mL/min	No change
CrCl 10–50 mL/min	Avoid
CrCl < 10 mL/min	Avoid
Post–HD dose	Avoid
Post–PD dose	Avoid
CVVH/CVVHD/CVVHDF dose	Avoid
Moderate hepatic insufficiency	Avoid
Severe hepatic insufficiency	Avoid

Drug Interactions: Atovaquone (↑ zidovudine levels); stavudine (antagonist to stavudine; avoid combination); ganciclovir, doxorubicin (neutropenia); tipranavir (↓ zidovudine levels); TMP–SMX (↑ lamivudine and zidovudine levels); vinca alkaloids (neutropenia).

Adverse Effects: Zidovudine, has been associated with hematologic toxicity including neutropenia and severe anemia. Prolonged use of zidovudine has been associated with symptomatic myopathy. Lactic acidosis and severe hepatomegaly with steatosis, including fatal cases. Severe acute exacerbations of hepatitis B have been reported in patients who are co-infected with hepatitis B virus (HBV) and HIV and have discontinued lamivudine. Nausea, vomiting, diarrhea, anorexia, insomnia fever/chills, headache, malaise/fatigue, peripheral neuropathy and pancreatitis. Immune reconstitution syndrome and redistribution/accumulation of body fat have been reported in patients treated with combination antiretroviral therapy.

Allergic Potential: Low

Safety in Pregnancy: C.

Cerebrospinal Fluid Penetration:
Lamivudine = 12%; Zidovudine = 60%

REFERENCES:

[No authors listed.] Drugs for AIDS and associated infections. Med Lett Drug Ther 35:79–86, 1993.

Hirsch MS, D'Aquila RT. Therapy for human immunodeficiency virus infection. N Engl J Med 328:1685–95, 1993.

McLeod GX, Hammer SM. Zidovudine: Five years later. Ann Intern Med 117:487–510, 1992.

Panel on Antiretroviral Guidelines for Adults and Adolescents. Department of Health and Human Services. Guidelines for the use of antiretroviral agents in HIV-infected adults and adolescents. http://aidsinfo.nih.gov/ConsentFiles/AdultandAdolescentGL.pdf, 2012.

Thompson MA, Aberg JA, Cahn P, et al. Antiretroviral treatment of adult HIV infection: 2012 recommendations of the International Antiviral Society — USA panel. JAMA 308:387–402, 2012.

Website: www.TreatHIV.com

Leflunomide (Arava)

Drug Class: CMV, antiviral.

Usual Dose: 100 mg/day (PO) × 3 days, then 20 mg (PO) q24h.

Pharmacokinetic Parameters:

Peak serum level: 8 mcg/mL

Bioavailability: 80%

Excreted unchanged: 0%

Serum half-life (normal/ESRD): 14 days/no data

Plasma protein binding: 99%

Volume of distribution (V_d): 0.13 L/kg

Primary Mode of Elimination: Hepatic/renal

"Usual dose" assumes normal renal/hepatic function. * For renal insufficiency, give usual dose × 1 followed by maintenance dose per CrCl. For dialysis patients, dose the same as for CrCl < 10 mL/min and give supplemental (post-HD/PD dose) immediately after dialysis. CrCl = creatinine clearance; CVVH = continuous veno-venous hemofiltration; HD/PD = hemodialysis/peritoneal dialysis.

Dosage Adjustments*

CrCl 15–30 mL/min	Use with caution
CrCl < 15 mL/min	Use with caution
Post–HD dose	Use with caution
Post–PD dose	Use with caution
CVVH/CVVHD/ CVVHDF dose	Use with caution
Moderate–severe hepatic insufficiency	Avoid if ↑ SGOT/ SGPT > 2 × n or pre-existing liver disease

Drug Interactions: May inhibit CYP 2C9; rifampin (↑ levels of active metabolite, M1); hepatotoxic drugs hepatotoxicity.

Adverse Effects: Headache, nausea, diarrhea, hypertension; ↑ SGOT/SGPT bone marrow suppression, rash, Stevens-Johnson Syndrome, toxic epidermal necrolysis, interstitial lung disease.

Allergic Potential: Low

Safety in Pregnancy: X

Comments: Alternate therapy of CMV infection after 1st line therapies fail; do not use with pre-existing liver disease; metabolized to active metabolite (M1); not recommended in patients with severe, uncontrolled infections, bone marrow dysplasia or severe immunodeficiency, prolonged administration leads to significant accumulation, (drug elimination procedure with cholestyramine described in PI). Screen for TB before starting leflunomide; avoid live vaccinations while on leflunomide; monitor LFT's and CBCs. *Discontinue if ↑ SGOT/SGPT > 3 × n.*

REFERENCES:

Avery RK, et al. Utility of leflunomide in the treatment of complex cytomegalovirus syndromes. Transplantation 90:419–26, 2010.

Chacko B, John GT. Leflunomide for cytomegalovirus: bench to bedside. Transpl Infest Dis 14:111–20, 2012.

Chon WJ, Josephson MA. Leflunomide in renal transplantation. Expert Rev Clin Immunol 7:273–281, 2011.

Henao-Martinez AF, Weinberg A, Waldman WJ, et al. Successful treatment of acyclovir-resistant herpes simplex virus type 2 proctitis with leflunomide in an HIV-infected man. J Clin Virol 54:276–278, 2012.

John GT, et al. Leflunomide therapy for cytomegalovirus disease in renal allograft recipients. Transplantation 77:1460–61, 2004.

Levofloxacin (Levaquin)

Drug Class: Respiratory fluoroquinolone.

Usual Dose: 500–750 mg (IV/PO) q24h (see comments).

Spectrum: (see *Susceptibility Profiles* pp. 198–202).

Resistance Potential: Low

Pharmacokinetic Parameters:

Peak serum level: 5–8 mcg/ml

Bioavailability: 99%

Excreted unchanged (urine): 87%

Serum half-life (normal/ESRD): 7 hrs/40 hrs

Plasma protein binding: 30%

Volume of distribution (V_d): 1.3 L/kg

Primary Mode of Elimination: Renal

Dosage Adjustments* (based on 750 mg/500 mg (IV/PO) q24h)

CrCl > 50 mL/min	No change
CrCl 20–50 mL/min	750 mg (IV/PO) q48h /500 mg (IV/PO), then 250 mg (IV/PO) q24h
CrCl < 20 mL/min	750 mg (IV/PO), then 500 mg (IV/PO) q48h /500 mg (IV/PO), then 250 mg (IV/PO) q48h
HD/CAPD dose	500 mg (IV/PO) q48h
Post–HD dose	mg (IV/PO)

"Usual dose" assumes normal renal/hepatic function. * For renal insufficiency, give usual dose × 1 followed by maintenance dose per CrCl. For dialysis patients, dose the same as for CrCl < 10 mL/min and give supplemental (post-HD/PD dose) immediately after dialysis. CrCl = creatinine clearance; CVVH = continuous veno-venous hemofiltration; HD/PD = hemodialysis/peritoneal dialysis.

Post–HFHD dose	250 mg (IV/PO)
Post–PD dose	250 mg (IV/PO)
CVVH/CVVHD/ CVVHDF dose	500 mg (IV/PO) q48h/250 mg (IV/PO) q24h
HD q 48–72h dose	500 mg (IV/PO) q HD*
Moderate hepatic insufficiency	No change
Severe hepatic insufficiency	No change

*Give at end of HD.

Drug Interactions: Al^{++}, Fe^{++}, Mg^{++}, Zn^{++} antacids (↓ absorption of levofloxacin if taken together); NSAIDs (CNS stimulation); probenecid (↑ levofloxacin levels); warfarin (↑ INR).

Adverse Effects: Does not cause seizures. Headache, insomnia, nausea, constipation, C. difficile diarrhea/colitis. FQ use has an increased risk of tendinitis/tendon rupture. Risk in highest in the elderly, those on steroids, and those with heart, lung, or renal transplants.

Allergic Potential: Low

Safety in Pregnancy: C

Comments: Take 2 hours before or after aluminum/magnesium-containing antacids. Does not increase digoxin concentrations. May ↑ QTc interval, particularly in patients with predisposing conditions or medications e.g., amiodarone.

Acute bacterial sinusitis dose: 750 mg (PO) q24h × 5 days. **CAP dose:** 750 mg (IV/PO) q24h × 5 days. **Nosocomial pneumonia dose:** 750 mg (IV/PO) q24h × 7–14 days. **cSSSI dose:** 750 mg (IV/PO) q24h × 7–14 days. **TB dose** (alternate drug in MDR TB regimen): 500 mg (PO) q24h.

Complicated UTI/acute pylonephritis dose: 750 mg (IV/PO) q24h × 5 days.

↑ incidence of C. difficile diarrhea/colitis with PPIs (for patients on PPIs during FQ therapy, D/C PPIs or switch to H_2 blocker for duration of FQ therapy).

Cerebrospinal Fluid Penetration: 16%

Bile Penetration: 100%

(also see **Antibiotic Pearls & Pitfalls** p. 516).

REFERENCES:

Alvarez-Lerma F, Grau S, Alvarez-Beltran. Levofloxacin in the treatment of ventilator-associated pneumonia. Clin Microbiol Infect 12:81–92, 2006.

Benko R, Matuz M, Doro P, et al. Pharmacokinetics and pharmacodynamics of levofloxacin in critically ill patients with ventilator-associated pneumonia. Int J Antimicrob Agents 30:162–168, 2007.

Bucaneve G, Micozzi A, Menichetti F, et al. Levofloxacin to prevent bacterial infection in patients with cancer and neutropenia. N Engl J Med 353:977–87, 2005.

Cunha BA, Lenopoli S, Hage JE. Klebsiella pneumoniae septic wrist arthritis successfully treated with ertapenem and levofloxacin. J Chemother 23:376–7.

File TM Jr, Milkovich G, Tennenberg AM, et al. Clinical implications of 750 mg, 5-day levofloxacin for the treatment of community-acquired pneumonia. Curr Med Res Opin 20:1473–81, 2004.

Garcia-Vazquez E, Mensa J, Sarasa M, et al. Penetration of levofloxacin into the anterior chamger (aqueous humour) of the human eye after intravenous administration. Eur J Clin Microbiol Infect Dis 26:137–140, 2007.

Glasheen JJ, Prochazka AV. The safety of levofloxacin in patients on warfarin. Am J Med 120:e13, 2007.

Klausner HA, Brown P, Peterson J, et al. Double-blind, randomized comparison of levofloxacin 750 mg once daily for 5 days versus ciprofloxin for 10 days in the treatment of acute pyelonephritis. Curr Med Res Opin 23:2637–2645, 2007.

Kuriyama T, Williams DW, Yanagisawa M, et al. Antimicrobial susceptibility of 800 anaerobic isolates from patients with dentoalveolar infection to 13 oral antibiotics. Oral Microbiol Immunol 22:285–288, 2007.

Lee CK, Boyle MP, Diener-West M, et al. Levofloxacin pharmacokinetics in adult cystic fibrosis. Chest 131:796–802, 2007.

"Usual dose" assumes normal renal/hepatic function. * For renal insufficiency, give usual dose × 1 followed by maintenance dose per CrCl. For dialysis patients, dose the same as for CrCl < 10 mL/min and give supplemental (post-HD/PD dose) immediately after dialysis. CrCl = creatinine clearance; CVVH = continuous veno-venous hemofiltration; HD/PD = hemodialysis/peritoneal dialysis.

Marchetti F, Viale P. Current and future perspectives for levofloxacin in severe Pseudomonas aeruginosa infections. J Chemotherapy 15:315–322, 2003.

Maurin M, Raoult D. Bacteriostatic and bactericidal activity of levofloxacin against Rickettsia rickettsii, Rickettsia conorii, 'Israel spotted fever group rickettsii' and Coxiella burnetii. Journal of Antimicrobial Chemotherapy 39:725–30, 1997.

Nightingale CH, Grant EM, Quintiliani R. Pharmacodynamics and pharmacokinetics of levofloxacin. Chemotherapy 46:6–14, 2000.

Nista EC, Candelli M, Zocco, MA, et al. Levofloxacin-based triple therapy in first-line treatment for Helicobacter pylori eradication. Am J Gastroenterol 101:1985–90, 2006.

Ogrendik M. Levofloxacin treatment in patients with rheumatoid arthritis receiving methotrexate. South Med J 100:135–139, 2007.

Pankey GA, Ashcraft DS. In vitro synergistic/additive activity of levofloxacin with meropenem against Stenotrophomonas maltophilia. Diagn Microbiol Infect Dis 67:297–300, 2010.

Pankuch GA, Seifert H, Appelbaum PC. Activity of doripenem with and without levofloxacin, amikacin, and colistin against Pseudomonas aeruginosa and Acinetobacter baumannii. Diagn Microbiol Infect Dis 67:191–197, 2010.

Pea F, Marioni G, Pavan F, et al. Penetration of levofloxacin into paranasal sinuses mucosa of patients with chronic rhinosinusitis after a single 500 mg oral dose. Pharmacol Res 55:38–41, 2007.

Poole M, Anon J, Paglia M, et al. A trial of high dose, short-course levofloxacin for the treatment of acute bacterial sinusitis. Otolaryngol Head Neck Surg 134:10–17, 2006.

Pugh RJ, Cooke RPD, Dempsey G. Short course antibiotic therapy for Gram-negative hospital-acquired pneumonia in the critically ill. J of Hosp Infect 74:337–343, 2010.

Samonis G, Koutsounaki E, Karageorgopoulos DE, et al. Empirical therapy with ceftazidime combined with levofloxacin or once-daily amikacin for febrile neutropenia in patients with neoplasia: a prospective comparative study. Eur J Clin Microbiol Infect Dis. 31:1389–1398, 2012.

Tsuruoka S, Yokota N, Hayasaka T, et al. Pharmacokinetics of multiple-dose levofloxacin in hemodialysis patients. Am J Kidney Dis 58:498–499, 2011.

Website: www.levaquin.com

Linezolid (Zyvox)

Drug Class: Oxazolidinone.
Usual Dose: 600 mg (IV/PO) q12h.
Spectrum: (see *Susceptibility Profiles* pp. 198–202).
Resistance Potential: Low
Pharmacokinetic Parameters:
Peak serum level: 15–21 mcg/ml
Bioavailability: 100% (IV and PO)
Excreted unchanged (urine): 30%
Serum half-life (normal/ESRD): 6.4/7.1 hrs
Plasma protein binding: 31%
Volume of distribution (V_d): 0.64 L/kg
Primary Mode of Elimination: Hepatic/metabolized
Dosage Adjustments*

CrCl < 10 mL/min	No change
Post–HD dose	600 mg (IV/PO)
Post–PD dose	None
CVVH/CVVHD/CVVHDF dose	No change
Moderate hepatic insufficiency	No change
Severe hepatic insufficiency	Use with caution

Drug Interactions: Pseudoephedrine, tyramine-containing foods (↑ risk of hypertensive crisis); serotonergic agents, e.g., SSRIs, MAOIs, St. John's wort, ritonavir (↑ risk of serotonin

---

"Usual dose": assumes normal renal/hepatic function. * For renal insufficiency, give usual dose × 1 followed by maintenance dose per CrCl. For dialysis patients, dose the same as for CrCl < 10 mL/min and give supplemental (post-HD/PD) dose immediately after dialysis. CrCl = creatinine clearance; CVVH = continuous veno-venous hemofiltration; HD/PD = hemodialysis/peritoneal dialysis.

syndrome). Serotonin syndrome: fever, delerium, hypertension, tremor/clonus, hyperreflexia.

Adverse Effects: Mild, readily reversible thrombocytopenia, anemia, or leukopenia occurs usually after ≥ 2 weeks of therapy. Lactic acidosis (rare), optic/peripheral neuropathy (> 28 days of therapy, rare). If used for > 4 weeks, ↑ risk of myelosuppression or blindness (irreversible) particularly in those with optic nerve disorders or glaucoma. Monitor visual function if symptomatic or therapy ≥ 2 weeks; monitor CBC weekly if therapy > 2 weeks.

Allergic Potential: Low

Safety in Pregnancy: C

Comments: *Ideal for IV-to-PO switch programs*. Unlike vancomycin, *linezolid use does not increase VRE prevalence*. Unlike quinupristin/dalfopristin, linezolid is active against E. faecalis (VSE). **Effective oral therapy for MRSA, MRSE, and E. faecium (VRE) infections.** *Alternate therapy for Nocardia and Listeria infections*.

Meningeal dose = usual dose.

Cerebrospinal Fluid Penetration: 70%

Bile Penetration: 200%

(also see *Antibiotic Pearls & Pitfalls* p. 517).

REFERENCES:

Aeziokoro CO, Cannon JP, Pachucki CT, et al. The effectiveness and safety of oral linezolid for the primary and secondary treatment of osteomyelitis. J Chemother 17:643–50, 2005.

Bassetti M, Vitale F, Melica G, et al. Linezolid in the treatment of gram-positive prosthetic joint infections. J Antimicrob Chemother 55:387–390, 2005.

Cannon JP, Pachucki CT, Aneziokoro CO and Lentino JR. The effectiveness and safety of oral linezolid as primary or secondary treatment of bloodstream infections. Infect Dis Clin Pract14:221–226, 2006.

Carroll W, Choi H, Min S, et al. Rhabdonyolsis in patient treated with linezolid for extensively drug-resistant tuberculosis. Clin Infect Dis 54:1624–7, 2012.

Castro P, Soriano A, Escrich C, Villalba G, et al. Linezolid treatment of ventriculoperitoneal shunt infection without implant removal. Eur J Clin Microbiol Infect Dis 24:603–06, 2005.

Chang KC, Leung CC, Daley CL. Linezolid for multidrug-resistant tuberculosis. Lancet Infect Dis 12:502–3, 2012.

Colli A, Compodonico R, Gherli T. Early switch from vancomycin to oral linezolid for treatment of gram-positive heart valve endocarditis. Ann Thorac Surg 84:87–91, 2007.

Conte JE Jr, Golden JA, Dipps J, et al. Intrapulmonary pharmacokinetics of linezolid. Antimicrob Agents Chemother 46:1475–80, 2000.

Cunha BA. Antimicrobial therapy of multidrug-resistant Streptococcus pneumoniae, vancomycin-resistant enterococci, and methicillin-resistant Staphylococcus aureus. Med Clin N Am 90:1165–82, 2006.

Cunha BA. Oral antibiotic therapy of serious systemic infections. Med Clin N Am 90:1197–1222, 2006.

Estes KS, Derendorf H. Comparison of the pharmacokinetic properties of vancomycin, linezolid, tigecycline, and daptomycin. Eur J. Med Res 15:533–543, 2010.

Falagas ME, Manta KG, Ntziora F, et al. Linezolid for the treatment of patients with endocarditis: a systematic review of published evidence. J Antimicrob Chemother 58:273–280, 2006.

Falagas ME, Siempos II, Vardakas KZ. Linezolid versus glycopeptide or B-lactam for treatment of Gram-positive bacterial infections: meta-analysis of randomized controlled trials. Lancet Infect Dis 8:53–66, 2008.

Hill EE, Herijgers P, Herregods MC, Peetermans WE. Infective endocarditis treated with linezolid: case report and literature review. Eur J Clin Microbiol Infect Dis 25:202–4, 2006.

Hoyo I, Martinez-Pastor J, Garcia-Ramiro S, et al. Decreased serum linezolid concentrations in two patients receiving linezolid and rifampicin due to bone infections. Scand J Infect Dis 44:548–50, 2012.

Joson J, Grover C, Downer C, et al. Successful treatment of methicillin-resistant Staphylococcus aureus mitral valve endocarditis with sequential linezolid and telavancin monotherapy following daptomycin failure. J Antimicrob Chemother 66:2186–2188, 2011.

Johnson JR. Linezolid versus vancomycin for methicillin-resistant Staphylococcus aureus infections. Clin Infect Dis 36:236–7, 2003.

Kaka AS, Rueda AM, Shelburne SA 3rd, Hamill RJ. Bactericidal activity of orally available agents against methicillin-resistant Staphylococcus aureus. J Antimicrob Chemother 58:680–3, 2006.

Kalil AC, Puumala S, Stoner J. Is linezolid superior to vancomycin for complicated skin and soft tissue infections due to methicillin-resistant Staphylococcus aureus? Antimicrob Agents Chemother 50:1910–1911, 2006.

Kruse AJ, Peederman SM, Bet PM, Debets-Oseenkopp YJ. Successful treatment with linezolid of meningitis due to methicillin-resistant Staphylococcus epidermidis refractory to vancomycin treatment. Eur J Clin Microb Infect 215:135–7, 2006.

Kutscha-Lissberg F, Hebler U, Muhr G, et al. Linezolid penetration into bone and joint tissues infected with methicillin-resistant staphylococci. Antimicrob Agents Chemother 47:3964–6, 2003.

Lauridsen TK, Bruun LE, Rasmussen RV, et al. Linezolid as rescue treatment for left-sided infective endocarditis: an observational, retrospective, multicenter study. Eur J Clin Microbiol Infect Dis 31:2567–2574, 2012.

Lawrence KR, Adra M, Gillman PK. Serotonin toxicity associated with the use of linezolid: a review of postmarketing data. Clin Infect Dis 42:1578–83, 2006.

Leonard SN, Szeto YG, Zolotarev M, et al. Comparative in vitro acitivity of telavancin, vancomycin, and linezolid against heterogeneously vancomycin-intermediate Staphycoccus aureus (h VISA). Int J Antimicrob 37:558–561, 2011.

Manfredi R, Sabbatani S, Marinacci G, Salizzoni E, Chiodo F. Listeria monocytogenes meningitis and multiple brain abscesses in an immunocompetent host. favorable response to combination linezolid-meropenem treatment. J Chemother 18:331–33, 2006.

Moreillon P, Wilson WR, Leclercq R, et al. Single-dose oral amoxicillin or linezolid for prophylaxis of experimental endocarditis due to vancomycin-susceptible and vancomycin-resistant Enterococcus faecalis. Antimicrob Agents Chemother 51:1661–1665, 2007.

Moylett EH, Pacheco SE, Brown-Elliott BA, et al. Clinical experience with linezolid for the treatment of nocardia infection. Clin Infect Dis 36:313–8, 2003.

Myrianthefs P, Markantonis SL, Vlachos K, et al. Serum and cerebrospinal fluid concentrations of linezolid in neurosurgical patients. Antimicrob Agents Chemother 50:3971–76, 2006.

Nathani N, Iles P, Elliott TS. Successful treatment of MRSA native valve endocarditis with oral linezolid therapy: a case report. J Infect 51:213–215, 2005.

Nguyen S, Pasquet A, Legout L, et al. Efficacy and tolerance of rifampin-linezolid compared with rifampin-cotrimoxazole combinations in prolonged oral therapy for bone and joint infections. Clin Microbiol Infect Dis 15:1163–1169, 2009.

Park IN, Hong SB, Oh YM, Kim MN, et al. Efficacy and tolerability of daily-half dose linezolid in patients with intractable multidrug-resistant tuberculosis. J Antimicrob Chemther 58:701–4, 2006.

Ravindran V, John J, Kaye GC, et al. Successful use of oral linezolid as a single active agent in endocarditis unresponsive to conventional antibiotic therapy. J Infect 47:164–6, 2003.

Rao N, Ziran BH, Hall RA, et al. Successful treatment of chronic bone and joint infections with oral linezolid. Clin Orthop 427:67–71, 2004.

Schecter GF, Scott C, True L, et al. Linezolid in the treatment of multidrug-resistant tuberculosis. Clin Infect Dis 50:49–55, 2010.

Siegel RE. Linezolid to decrease length of stay in the hospital for patients with methicillin-resistant Staphylococcus aureus infection. Clin Infect Dis 36:124–5, 2003.

Souli M, Pontikis K, Chryssouli Z, et al. Successful treatment of right-sided prosthetic valve endocarditis due to methicillin-resistant teicoplanin-heteroresistant Staphylococcus aureus with linezolid. Eur J Clin Microbiol Infect Dis 24:760–762, 2005.

"Usual dose" assumes normal renal/hepatic function. * For renal insufficiency, give usual dose × 1 followed by maintenance dose per CrCl. For dialysis patients, dose the same as for CrCl < 10 mL/min and give supplemental (post-HD/PD dose) immediately after dialysis. CrCl = creatinine clearance; CVVH = continuous veno-venous hemofiltration; HD/PD = hemodialysis/peritoneal dialysis.

Stein GE, Schooley SL, Havlichek DH, et al. Outpatient intravenous antibiotic therapy compared with oral linezolid in patients with skin and soft tissue infections: a pharmacoeconomic analysis. Infectious Dis in Clin Practice 16:235–240, 2008.

Stevens DL, Herr D, Lampiris H, et al. Linezolid versus vancomycin for the treatment of methicillin-resistant Staphylococcus aureus infections. Clin Infect Dis 34:1481–90, 2002.

Taylor JJ, Wilson JW, Estes LL. Linezolid and serotonergic drug Interactions: a retrospective survey. Clin Infect Dis 43:180–7, 2006.

Valerio M, Pedromingo M, Munoz P, et al. Potential protective role of linezolid against Clostridium difficile infection. Int J Antimicrob Agents 39:414–9, 2012.

Villani P, Pegazzi MB, Marubbi F, et al. Cerebrospinal fluid linezolid concentrations in postneurosurgical central nervous system infections. Antimicrob Agents Chemother 46:936–7, 2002.

Xu HB, Jiang RH, Li L, et al. Linezolid in the treatment of MDR-TB: a retrospective clinical study. Int J Tuberc Lung Dis 16:358–63, 2012.

Website: www.zyvox.com

Lopinavir + Ritonavir (Kaletra) LPV/RTV

Drug Class: Antiretroviral protease inhibitor combination.
Usual Dose: Therapy-naive: 400/100 mg q12h or 800/200 mg q24h (if <3 lopinavir resistance—associated substitutions).
Pharmacokinetic Parameters:
Peak serum level: 9.6/≤ 1 mcg/mL
Bioavailability: No data
Excreted unchanged (urine): 3%
Serum half-life (normal/ESRD): 5–6/5–6 hrs
Plasma protein binding: 99%
Volume of distribution (V_d): No data/ 0.44 L/kg
Primary Mode of Elimination: Hepatic
Dosage Adjustments*

CrCl < 10 mL/min	No change
Post–HD dose	None
Post–PD dose	None
CVVH/CVVHD/CVVHDF dose	No change
Moderate hepatic insufficiency	No change
Severe hepatic insufficiency	Avoid

Antiretroviral Dosage Adjustments

Fosamprenavir	Avoid
Delavirdine	No data
Efavirenz	Consider lopinavir/ ritonavir 500/125 mg q12h
Indinavir	Indinavir 600 mg q12h
Nelfinavir	Same as for efavirenz
Nevirapine	Same as for efavirenz
Rifabutin	Max. dose of rifabutin 150 mg qod or 3 times per week
Saquinavir	Saquinavir 1000 mg q12h

Drug Interactions: Antiretrovirals, rifabutin, (see dose adjustment grid, above); Rifampin may reduce lopinavir levels leading to drug failure and should be avoided. Sidenafil, tadalafil, and virdenafil levels will be greatly increased and their dosage must be decreased. Antiarhythmics such as amiodarone, bepredil, lidocaine and quinidine may increase levels. Once daily dosing not recommended in pregnancy or for patients receiving efavirenz, nevirapine,

"Usual dose" assumes normal renal/hepatic function. * For renal insufficiency, give usual dose × 1 followed by maintenance dose per CrCl. For dialysis patients, dose the same as for CrCl < 10 mL/min and give supplemental (post-HD/PD dose) immediately after dialysis. CrCl = creatinine clearance; CVVH = continuous veno-venous hemofiltration; HD/PD = hemodialysis/peritoneal dialysis.

fosamprenavir, nelfinavir, carbamazepine, phenytoin, or phenobarbital. Tacrolimus, cyclosporine and rapamycin levels can be altered leading to increased toxicity. Methadone levels may be decreased leading to withdrawal reactions. Fluticasone levels may increase leading to Cushing like syndrome, astemizole, terfenadine, benzodiazepines, cisapride, ergotamine, flecainide, pimozide, propafenone, rifampin, statins, tenofovir (↓ lopinavir levels, ↑ tenofovir levels). ↓ effectiveness of oral contraceptives. Insufficient data on other drug interactions listed for ritonavir alone. At end of drug interaction add lopinavir/resolution contains alcohol and can lead to a disulfram reaction when administered with metronidazole clarithromycin (↑ QT$_c$).

Contraindications: St. John's wort, boceprevir, telaprevir, rifapentine.

Adverse Effects: Diarrhea (very common), headache, nausea, vomiting, asthenia, ↑ SGOT/SGPT, hepatotoxicity, abdominal pain, pancreatitis, paresthesias, hyperglycemia (including worsening diabetes, new-onset diabetes, DKA), ↑ cholesterol/triglycerides (evaluate risk for coronary disease, pancreatitis), ↑ CPK, ↑ uric acid, fat redistribution, possible increased bleeding in hemophilia. Oral solution contains 42.4% alcohol. Immune reconstitution syndrome and redistribution/accumulation of body fat have been reported in patients treated with combination antiretroviral therapy.

Allergic Potential: Low

Safety in Pregnancy: C

Comments: Tablet formulation does not require refrigeration and may be taken with or without food. With oral solution, Lopinavir serum concentrations with moderately fatty meals are increased 54%.

REFERENCES:

Decloedt EH, McIlleron H, Smith P, et al. Pharmacokinetics of lopinavir in HIV-infected adults receiving rifampin with adjusted does of lopinavir-ritonavir tablets. Antimicrob Agents Chemother 55:3195–3200, 2011.

Diaz-Brito V, Leon A, Knobel H, et al. Post-exposure prophylaxis for HIV-infection: a clinical trail comparing lopinavir/ritonavir versus atazanavir each with zidovudine/lamivudine. Antivir Ther 17:337–46, 2012.

Panel on Antiretroviral Guidelines for Adults and Adolescents. Department of Health and Human Services. Guidelines for the use of antiretroviral agents in HIV-infected adults and adolescents. http://aidsinfo.nih.gov/ConsentFiles/AdultandAdolescentGL.pdf, 2012.

Thompson MA, Aberg JA, Cahn P, et al. Antiretroviral treatment of adult HIV infection: 2012 recommendations of the International Antiviral Society — USA panel. JAMA 308:387–402, 2012.

Young J, Schafer J, Fux CA, et al. Renal function in patients with HIV starting therapy with tenofovir and either efavirenz, lopinavir or atazanavir. AIDS 26:567–75, 2012

Website: www.kaletra.com

Loracarbef (Lorabid)

Drug Class: 2nd generation oral cephalosporin.

Usual Dose: 400 mg (PO) q12h (see comments).

Spectrum: (see *Susceptibility Profiles* pp. 191–197).

Resistance Potential: Low

Pharmacokinetic Parameters:

Peak serum level: 14 mcg/mL

Bioavailability: 90%

Excreted unchanged (urine): 90%

Serum half-life (normal/ESRD): 1.2/32 hrs

Plasma protein binding: 25%

Volume of distribution (V$_d$): 0.35 L/kg

Primary Mode of Elimination: Renal

"Usual dose" assumes normal renal/hepatic function. * For renal insufficiency, give usual dose × 1 followed by maintenance dose per CrCl. For dialysis patients, dose the same as for CrCl < 10 mL/min and give supplemental (post-HD/PD dose) immediately after dialysis. CrCl = creatinine clearance; CVVH = continuous veno-venous hemofiltration; HD/PD = hemodialysis/peritoneal dialysis.

Dosage Adjustments*

CrCl 10–50 mL/min	200 mg (PO) q24h
CrCl < 10 mL/min	200 mg (PO) q72h
Post–HD dose	400 mg (PO)
Post–PD dose	200 mg (PO)
CVVH/CVVHD/ CVVHDF dose	200 mg (PO) q12h
Moderate hepatic insufficiency	No change
Severe hepatic insufficiency	No change

Drug Interactions: None.
Adverse Effects: Drug fever/rash, C. difficile diarrhea/colitis.
Allergic Potential: Low
Safety in Pregnancy: B
Comments: Take 1 hour before or 2 hours after meals. **CAP dose:** 400 mg (PO) q12h.
Sinusitis/tonsillitis dose: 200 mg (PO) q12h.
Cerebrospinal Fluid Penetration: < 10% (also see *Antibiotic Pearls & Pitfalls* p. 510).

REFERENCES:
Bandak SI, Turnak MR, Allen BS, et al. Assessment of the susceptibility of Streptococcus pneumoniae to cefaclor and loracarbef in 13 cases. J Chemother 12:299–305, 2000.
Gooch WM 3rd, Adelglass J, Kelsey DK, et al. Loracarbef versus clarithromycin in children with acute otitis media with effusion. Clin her 21:711–22, 1999.
Paster RZ, McAdoo MA, Keyserling CH. A comparison of a five-day regimen of cefdinir with a seven-day regimen of loracarbef for the treatment of acute exacerbations of chronic bronchitis. Int J Clin Pract 64:293–9, 2000.
Vogel F, Ochs HR, Wettich K, et al. Effect of step-down therapy of ceftriazone plus loracarbef versus parenteral therapy of ceftriaxone on the intestinal microflora in patients with community-acquired pneumonia. Clin Microbiol Infect 7:376–9, 2001.
Website: www.pdr.net

Maraviroc (Selzentry) MVC

Drug Class: HIV-1 chemokine receptor 5 (CCR5) antagonist.
Usual Dose: 150 mg, 300 mg, or 600 mg (PO) q12h, depending on concomitant medications (see below), in CCR5-tropic HIV-1 isolates. Available in 150 mg and 300 mg tablets.
Pharmacokinetic Parameters:
Peak serum level: 266–618 mcg/mL
Bioavailability: 23–33%
Excreted unchanged: 20% (urine); 76% (feces)
Serum half-life (normal/ESRD): 14–18 hrs/not studied
Plasma protein binding: 76%
Volume of distribution (V_d): 194 L
Primary Mode of Elimination: Fecal/renal
Dosage Adjustments*

CrCl > 30 mL/min with potent CYP3A4 inhibitor	150 mg (PO) q12h
CrCl > 30 mL/min with potent CYP3A4 inducer but no inhibitor	600 mg (PO) q12h
CrCl < 30 mL/min with potent CYP3A4 inducer or inhibitor	Avoid
CrCl < 30 mL/min without potent CYP3A4 inducer or inhibitor	300 mg (PO) q12h

---

"Usual dose" assumes normal renal/hepatic function. * For renal insufficiency, give usual dose × 1 followed by maintenance dose per CrCl. For dialysis patients, dose the same as for CrCl < 10 mL/min and give supplemental (post-HD/PD dose) immediately after dialysis. CrCl = creatinine clearance; CVVH = continuous veno-venous hemofiltration; HD/PD = hemodialysis/peritoneal dialysis.

Post–HD dose	None
Post–PD dose	None
CVVH/CVVHD/CVVHDF dose	No data
Moderate hepatic insufficiency with potent CYP3A4 inhibitor	Use with caution
Severe hepatic insufficiency	Avoid

Antiretroviral Dosage Adjustments

Protease inhibitors (except tipranavir/ritonavir), delavirdine, ketoconazole, itraconazole, clarithromycin, nefazodone, telithromycin	150 mg (PO) q12h
Tipranavir/ritonavir, nevirapine, all NRTIs and enfuvirtide	300 mg (PO) q12h
Efavirenz, rifampin, etravirine, carbamazepine, phenobarbital, phenytoin	600 mg (PO) q12h

Drug Interactions: Maraviroc is a substrate of CYP3A and P-glycoprotein and is likely to be modulated by inhibitors and inducers of these enzymes/transporters.

Adverse Effects: Hepatotoxicity has been reported. A systemic allergic reaction (e.g., pruritic rash, eosinophilia, or elevated IgE) prior to the development of hepatotoxicity may occur. Other Adverse Effects: cough, infection, upper respiratory tract infection, rash, pyrexia, dizziness, abdominal pain, musculoskeletal symptoms (joint/muscle pain). Orthostatic hypotension with severe renal insufficiency.

Allergic Potential: Low

Safety in Pregnancy: B

Comments: Indicated for treatment-experienced adult patients infected with only cellular chemokine receptor (CCR) 5-tropic HIV-1 virus detectable who have evidence of viral replication and HIV-1 strains resistant to multiple antiretroviral agents. Used in combination with other antiretroviral agents. Phenotype test is needed to confirm infection with CCR5-tropic HIV-1 (also known as "R5 virus"). May increase risk of infection (especially HSV) and neoplasms.

Cerebrospinal Fluid Penetration: No data

REFERENCES:

Brown KC, Patterson KB, Malone SA, et al. Single and multiple dose pharmacokinetics of maraviroc in saliva, semen, and rectal tissue of healthy HIV-negative men. J Infect Dis 203:1484–1490, 2011.

Lazzarin A, Than S, Valluri SR, et al. Safety profile of maraviroc in patients coinfected with HIV-1 and hepatitis B or C included in the maraviroc expanded access program. HIV Clin Trials 13:83–9, 2012.

Okoli C, Siccardi M, Thomas-William S, et al. Once Daily maraviroc 300 mg or 150 mg in combination with ritonavir-boosted darunavir 800/100 mg. J Antimicrob Chemother 67: 671–4, 2012.

Panel on Antiretroviral Guidelines for Adults and Adolescents. Department of Health and Human Services. Guidelines for the use of antiretroviral agents in HIV-infected adults and adolescents. http://aidsinfo.nih.gov/ConsentFiles/AdultandAdolescentGL.pdf, 2012.

Parra J, Portilla J, Pulido F, et al. Clinical utility of maraviroc. Clin Drug Investig 31:527–42, 2011.

Thompson MA, Aberg JA, Cahn P, et al. Antiretroviral treatment of adult HIV infection: 2012 recommendations of the International Antiviral Society — USA panel. JAMA 308:387–402, 2012.

Wasmuth JC, Rockstroh Jk, Hardy WD. Drug safety evauation of maraviroc for the treatment of HIV infection. Expert Opin Drug Saf 11: 161–74, 2012.

Website: www.selzentry.com

"Usual dose" assumes normal renal/hepatic function. * For renal insufficiency, give usual dose × 1 followed by maintenance dose per CrCl. For dialysis patients, dose the same as for CrCl < 10 mL/min and give supplemental (post-HD/PD dose) immediately after dialysis. CrCl = creatinine clearance; CVVH = continuous veno-venous hemofiltration; HD/PD = hemodialysis/peritoneal dialysis.

Meropenem (Merrem/Meronem)

Drug Class: Carbapenem.
Usual Dose: 1 gm (IV) q8h (see comments).
Spectrum: (see *Susceptibility Profiles* pp. 198–202).
Resistance Potential: Low
Pharmacokinetic Parameters:
Peak serum level: 49 mcg/ml
Bioavailability: Not applicable
Excreted unchanged (urine): 70%
Serum half-life (normal/ESRD): 1/7 hrs
Plasma protein binding: 2%
Volume of distribution (V_d): 0.35 L/kg
Primary Mode of Elimination: Renal
Dosage Adjustments* (based on 1 gm dose; for 500 mg dosing use half of dose shown in grid)

CrCl 25–50 mL/min	1 gm (IV) q12h
CrCl 10–25 mL/min	500 mg (IV) q12h
CrCl < 10 mL/min	500 mg (IV) q24h
Post–HD dose	500 mg (IV)
Post–HFHD dose	500 mg (IV)
Post–PD dose	500 mg (IV)
CVVH/CVVHD/CVVHDF dose	1 gm (IV) q12h
HD q 48–72h dose	2 gm (IV) q HD*
Moderate hepatic insufficiency	No change
Severe hepatic insufficiency	No change

*Give at end of HD.

Drug Interactions: Probenecid (↑ meropenem half-life by 40%), Valproic acid (↓ seizure threshold).

Adverse Effects: Rarely, mild infusion site inflammation. No seizures. **No cross allergenicity with penicillins/β-lactams; safe to use in patients with a history of penicillin anaphylactic/other allergic reactions.**
Allergic Potential: Low
Safety in Pregnancy: B
Comments: *MDR GNBs, cystic fibrosis/ meningitis dose: 2 gm (IV) q8h;* **uSSSIs or UTIs dose:** 500 mg (IV) q8h. Inhibits endotoxin release from gram-negative bacilli. **Meropenem is the *only carbapenem that may be given by IV bolus injection over 3–5 minutes*.** Na⁺Content = 3.92 mEq/g.
Meningeal dose = 2 gm (IV) q8h.
Cerebrospinal Fluid Penetration:
Non-Inflamed meninges = 10%
Inflamed meninges = 15%
Bile Penetration:
Without obstruction = 75%
With obstruction = 40%
(also see *Antibiotic Pearls & Pitfalls* p. 511).

REFERENCES:
Berman SJ, Fogarty CM, Fabian T, et al. Meropenem monotherapy for the treatment of hospital-acquired pneumonia: results of a multicenter trial. J Chemother 16:362–71, 2004.

Cheng AC, Fisher DA, Anstey NM, et al. Outcomes of patients with melioidosis treated with meropenem. Antimicrob Agents Chemother 48:1763–5, 2004.

Conte JE Jr, Golden JA, Kelley MG, Zurlinden E. Intrapulmonary pharmacokinetics and pharmacodynamics of meropenem. Int J Antimicrob Agents 26:449–56, 2005.

Cunha BA. The safety of meropenem in elderly and renally impaired patients. Intern J Antimicrob Ther 10:109–117, 1998.

Cunha BA. The use of meropenem in critical care. Antibiotics for Clinicians 4:59–66, 2000.

Cunha BA. Pseudomonas aeruginosa: resistance and therapy. Semin Respir Infect 17:231–9, 2002.

"Usual dose" assumes normal renal/hepatic function. * For renal insufficiency, give usual dose × 1 followed by maintenance dose per CrCl. For dialysis patients, dose the same as for CrCl < 10 mL/min and give supplemental (post-HD/PD dose) immediately after dialysis. CrCl = creatinine clearance; CVVH = continuous veno-venous hemofiltration; HD/PD = hemodialysis/peritoneal dialysis.

Cunha BA. Meropenem: Current uses in critical care. Antibiotics for Clinicians 11:433–444, 2007.

Cunha BA. Meropenem: lack of cross reactivity in penicillin allergic patients. Journal of Chemotherapy 20:233–237, 2008.

Doh K, Woo H, Hur J, et al. Population pharmacokinetics of meropenem in burn patients. J Antimicrob Chemother 65:2428–2435, 2010.

Hagihara M, Kuti JL, Nicolau DP. Predicting doripenem susceptibility based on meropenem and imipenem interpretation for Pseudomonas aeruginosa. Diagn Microbiol Infect Dis 72:58–62, 2012.

Kitzes-Cohen R, Farin D, Piva G, et al. Pharmacokinetics and pharmacodynamics of meropenem in critically ill patients. Int J Antimicrob Agents 19:105–10, 2002.

Louie A, Grasso C, Bahniuk N, et al. The combination of meropenem and levofloxacin is synergistic with respect to both Pseudomonas aeruginosa kill rate and resistance suppression. Antimicrob Agents Chemother 54:2646–2654, 2010.

Manfredi R, Sabbatani S, Marinacci G, et al. Listeria monocytogenes meningitis and multiple brain abscesses in an immunocompetent host. Favorable response to combination linezolid-meropenem treatment. Journal of Chemotherapy 18:331–33, 2009.

Mattoes HM, Kuti JL, Drusano GL, et al. Optimizing antimicrobial pharmacodynamics: dosage strategies for meropenem. Clin Ther 26:1187–98, 2004.

Pankey GA, Ashcraft DS. In vitro synergistic/additive activity of levofloxacin with meropenem against Stenotrophomonas maltophilia. Diagn Microbiol Infect Dis 67:297–300, 2010.

Perez-Simon JA, Garcia-Escobar I, Martinez J, et al. Antibiotic prophylaxis with meropenem after allogeneic stem cell transplantation. Bone Marrow Transplant 33:183–7, 2004.

Romano A, Viola M, Gueant-Rodriquez R, et al. Tolerability of meropenem in patients with IgE-mediated hypersensitivity of penicillins. Ann Intern Med 146:266–69, 2007.

Scheetz MH, Bolon MK, Esterly JS, et al. Life-years gained with meropenem over ciprofloxacin in penicillin-allergic patients with gram-negative bacilli sepsis: results of a probabilistic model. Pharmacotherapy 31:469–79, 2011.

Sodhi M, Axtell SS, Callahan J, et al. Is it safe to use carbapenems in patients with a history of allergy to penicillin? J Antimicrob Chemother 54:1155–7, 2004.

Taccone FS, Cotton F, Roisin S, et al. Optimal meropenem concentrations to treat multidrug-resistant Pseudomonas aeruginosa septic shock. Anitimicrob Agents Chemother 56:2129–31, 2012.

Toya T, Nannya Y, Narukawa K, et al. A comparative analysis of meropenem and doripenem in febrile patients with hematologic malignancies: a single-center retrospective study. Jpn J Infect Dis 65:228–32, 2012.

Yamada Y, Ikawa K, Nakamura K, et al. Prostatic penetration of meropenem after intravenous administration in patients undergoing transurethral resection fo the prostate. J Chemother 23:179–180, 2011.

Website: www.MerremIV.com

Methenamine hippurate (Hiprex, Urex) Methenamine mandelate (Mandelamine)

Drug Class: Urinary antiseptic.

Usual Dose: 1 gm (PO) q6h (hippurate); 1 gm (PO) q6h (mandelate).

Spectrum: All gram + and gram − uropathogens.

Resistance Potential: None

Pharmacokinetic Parameters:

Peak serum level: Not applicable

Bioavailability: 90%

Excreted unchanged (urine): 90%

Serum half-life (normal/ESRD): 4 hrs/no data

Plasma protein binding: Not applicable

Volume of distribution (V_d): Not applicable

Primary Mode of Elimination: Renal

Dosage Adjustments*

CrCl 50–80 mL/min	Avoid
CrCl 10–50 mL/min	Avoid
CrCl < 10 mL/min	Avoid

PI = package insert
PK = pharmacokinetic dose

Post–HD dose	Avoid
Post–PD dose	Avoid
CVVH/CVVHD/CVVHDF dose	Avoid
Moderate hepatic insufficiency	No change
Severe hepatic insufficiency	Avoid

Drug Interactions: Acetazolamide, sodium bicarbonate, thiazide diuretics (↓ antibacterial effect if ↑ urinary pH ≥ 5.5).
Adverse Effects: GI upset.
Allergic Potential: Low
Safety in Pregnancy: C
Comments: Take with food to decrease GI upset. Effectiveness depends on maintaining an acid urine (pH ≤ 5.5) with acidifying agents (e.g., ascorbic acid). **Useful only for catheter-associated bacteriuria (CAB)**, not UTIs. **Forms formaldehyde in acid urine; resistance does not develop.**

REFERENCES:
Cunha BA, Comer JB, Pharmacokinetic considerations in the treatment of urinary tract infections. Conn Med 43:347–53, 1979.
Klinge D, Mannisto P, Mantyla R, et al. Pharmacokinetics of methenamine in healthy volunteers. J Antimicrob Chemother 9:209–16, 1982.
Musher DM, Griffith DP. Generation of formaldehyde from methenamine: Effect of pH and concentration, and antibacterial effect. Antimicrob Agents Chemother 6:708–11, 1974.
Musher DM, Griffith DP, Templeton GB, Further observations of the potentiation of the antibacterial effect of methenamine by acetohydroxamic acid. J Infect Dis 133:564–67, 1976.
Schiotz HA, Guttu K, Value of urinary prophylaxis with methenamine in gynecologic surgery. Acta Obstet Gynecol Scand 81:743–6, 2002.

Metronidazole (Flagyl)

Drug Class: Nitroimidazole antiparasitic/antibiotic PK dose
Usual Dose: PI dose: 1 gm (IV) q24h; PK dose: 500 mg (IV/PO) q6–8h (see comments).
Spectrum: (see *Susceptibility Profiles* pp. 186–190).
Resistance Potential: Low (H. pylori, Gardnerella, Prevotella)
Pharmacokinetic Parameters:
Peak serum level: 26 (IV)/12 (PO) mcg/mL
Bioavailability: 100%
Excreted unchanged (urine): 20%
Serum half-life (normal/ESRD): 8/14 hrs
Plasma protein binding: 20%
Volume of distribution (V_d): 0.25–0.85 L/kg
Primary Mode of Elimination: Hepatic
Dosage Adjustments*

CrCl 10–50 mL/min	No change
CrCl < 10 mL/min	500 mg (IV) q24h/250 mg (PO) q12h
Post–HD dose	1 gm (IV) 500 mg (PO)
Post–PD dose	1 gm (IV) 500 mg (PO)
CVVH/CVVHD/CVVHDF dose	No change
Mild-moderate hepatic insufficiency	No change
Severe hepatic insufficiency	500 mg (IV/PO) q24h

Drug Interactions: Alcohol (disulfiram-like reaction); disulfiram (acute toxic psychosis); warfarin (↑ INR); phenobarbital, phenytoin (↑ metronidazole metabolism).

PI = package insert
PK = pharmacokinetic dose

Adverse Effects: Encephalopathy, metallic taste, aseptic meningitis, seizures, peripheral neuropathy. With oral formulation, nausea, vomiting, GI upset. May discolor urine brown.

Allergic Potential: Low

Safety in Pregnancy: B (avoid in 1st trimester)

Comments: For intra-abdominal/pelvic sepsis (**plus anti-aerobic GNB drug**). **q24h dosing is preferred to q6h/q8h dosing because of long half-life** ($t_{1/2}$ = 8 h).

C. difficile diarrhea dose: 250 mg (PO) q6h.

C. difficile colitis dose: 500 mg (IV/PO) q6-8h or 1 gm (IV) q24h.

For severe C. difficile colitis, add anti-GNB coverage, e.g., ertapenem or meropenem (for microscopic/macroscopic perforation/peritonitis). Use increases VRE prevalence. *Metronidazole misses some anerobes eg, Propionibacteria, Actinobacillus, Eikinella, and limited activity against Actinomyces, Mobiluncus and Clostridium ramosum.*

Meningeal dose = usual dose.

Cerebrospinal Fluid Penetration:

Non-Inflamed meninges = 30%

Inflamed meninges = 100%

(also see *Antibiotic Pearls & Pitfalls* p. 519).

REFERENCES:

Bouza E, Burillo A, Munoz P, Antimicrobial therapy of Clostridium difficile-associated diarrhea. Med Clin N Am 90:1141-63, 2006.

Canete R, Rodriguez P, Mesa L, et al. Albendazole versus metronidazole in the treatment of adult giardiasis: a randomized, double-blind, clinical trial. Curr Med Res Opin 28:149-54, 2012.

Clay PG, Graham MR, Lindsey CC, et al. Clinical efficacy, tolerability, and cost savings associated with the use of open-label metronidazole plus ceftriaxone once daily compared with ticarcillin/clavulanate every 6 hours as empiric treatment for diabetic lower-extremity infections in older males. Am J Geriatr Pharmacother 2:181-9, 2004.

Cunha BA.Oral Antibiotic Therapy of Serious Systemic Infections. Med Clin N Am 90:1197-1222, 2006.

Desai JA, Dobson J, Melanson M, et al. Metronidazole-induced encephalopathy: case report and review of MRI findings. Can J Neurol Sci 38:512-513, 2011.

Falagas ME, Gorbach SL. Clindamycin and metronidazole. Med Clin North Am 79:845-67, 1995.

Freeman CD, Klutman NE. Metronidazole: A therapeutic review and update. Drugs 54:679-708, 1997.

Freeman CD, Nightingale CH, Nicolau DP, et al. Serum bactericidal activity of ceftriaxone plus metronidazole against common intra-abdominal pathogens. Am J Hosp Pharm 51:1782-7, 1994.

Garbino J, Villiger P, Caviezel A, et al. A randomized prospective study of cefepime plus metronidazole with imipenem-cilastatin in the treatment of intra-abdominal infections. Infection 35:161-166, 2007.

Ishikawa T, Okamura S, Oshimoto H, et al. Metronidazole plus ciprofloxacin therapy for active Crohn's disease. Intern Med 42:318-21, 2003.

Metzger R, Swenson BR, Bonatti H, et al. Identification of risk factors for the development of Clostridium difficile-associated diarrhea following treatment of polymicrobial surgical infections. Ann Surg 251:722-727, 2010.

Musher DM, Aslam S, Logan N, et al. Relatively poor outcome after treatment of Clostridium difficile colitis with metronidazole. Clinical Infectious Disease 40:1586-90, 2005.

Vasa CV, Glatt AE. Effectiveness and appropriateness of empiric metronidazole for Clostridium difficile diarrhea. Am J Gastroenterol 98:354-8, 2003.

Wang S, Cunha BA, Hamid NS, et al. Intravenous metronidazole: once daily vs. multiple dosing in intra-abdominal infections. Journal of Chemotherapy 19:410-416, 2007.

"Usual dose" assumes normal renal/hepatic function. * For renal insufficiency, give usual dose × 1 followed by maintenance dose per CrCl. For dialysis patients, dose the same as for CrCl < 10 mL/min and give supplemental (post-HD/PD dose) immediately after dialysis. CrCl = creatinine clearance; CVVH = continuous veno-venous hemofiltration; HD/PD = hemodialysis/peritoneal dialysis.

Mezlocillin (Mezlin)

Drug Class: Anti-pseudomonal penicillin.
Usual Dose: 3 gm (IV) q6h.
Resistance Potential: Low
Pharmacokinetic Parameters:
Peak serum level: 300 mcg/ml
Bioavailability: Not applicable
Excreted unchanged (urine): 65%
Serum half-life (normal/ESRD): 1.1/4 hrs
Plasma protein binding: 30%
Volume of distribution (V_d): 0.18 L/kg
Primary Mode of Elimination: Renal
Dosage Adjustments*

CrCl > 30 mL/min	No change
CrCl 10–30 mL/min	3 gm (IV) q8h
CrCl < 10 mL/min	2 gm (IV) q8h
Post–HD dose	3 gm (IV)
Post–PD dose	None
CVVH/CVVHD/CVVHDF dose	3 gm (IV) q8h
Moderate hepatic insufficiency	No change
Severe hepatic insufficiency	3 gm (IV) q12h

Drug Interactions: Aminoglycosides (inactivation of mezlocillin in renal failure); warfarin (↑ INR); oral contraceptives (↓ oral contraceptive effect); cefoxitin (↓ mezlocillin effect).
Adverse Effects: Drug fever/rash, E. multiforme/Stevens–Johnson Syndrome, anaphylactic reactions (hypotension, laryngospasm, bronchospasm), hives; serum sickness. **Dose-dependent inhibition of platelet aggregation is minimal/absent** (usual dose is less than carbenicillin).
Allergic Potential: Low
Safety in Pregnancy: B
Comments: Dose-dependent half-life ($t_{1/2}$). Na^+ content = 1.8 mEq/g.
Cerebrospinal Fluid Penetration: < 10%
Bile Penetration: 3000%
(also see ***Antibiotic Pearls & Pitfalls*** p. 508).

REFERENCES:
Wright AJ. The penicillins. Mayo Clin Proc 74:290–307, 1999.

Micafungin (Mycamine)

Drug Class: Echinocandin antifungal.
Usual Dose:
<u>Candidemia:</u>
      100 mg (IV) q24h.
<u>Esophageal candidiasis:</u>
      150 mg (IV) q24h.
<u>Prophylaxis of candidal infections in stem cell transplants:</u>
      50 mg (IV) q24h.
Pharmacokinetic Parameters:
Peak serum level: 5.1 mcg/ml (50 mg); 11.2 mcg/ml (100 mg); 16.4 mcg/ml (150 mg)
Bioavailability: Not applicable
Excreted unchanged (urine): 11%
Serum half-life (normal/ESRD): 10–15 hrs/no change
Plasma protein binding: > 99%
Volume of distribution (V_d): 0.39 L/kg
Primary Mode of Elimination: Liver
Dosage Adjustments

CrCl < 10 mL/min	No change
Post–HD dose	None
Post–PD dose	None

"Usual dose" assumes normal renal/hepatic function. * For renal insufficiency, give usual dose × 1 followed by maintenance dose per CrCl. For dialysis patients, dose the same as for CrCl < 10 mL/min and give supplemental (post-HD/PD dose) immediately after dialysis. CrCl = creatinine clearance; CVVH = continuous veno-venous hemofiltration; HD/PD = hemodialysis/peritoneal dialysis.

CVVH/CVVHD/CVVHDF dose	No change
Mild or Moderate hepatic insufficiency	No change
Severe hepatic insufficiency	Use with caution

Drug Interactions: Sirolimus AUC ↑ by 21% with no change in Cmax (monitor for sirolimus toxicity), nifedipine AUC, and Cmax ↑ by 18% and 42%, respectively (monitor for nifedipine toxicity).

Adverse Effects: Nausea, vomiting, leukopenia, anemia, thrombocytopenia, ↑ SGOT/SGPT, rash.

Allergic Potential: Low

Safety in Pregnancy: C

Comments: Administer by IV infusion over one hour—do not give as a bolus as more rapid infusions may result in more frequent histamine mediated reactions. Do not mix or co-use with other medications; flush intravenous line with 0.9% saline prior to infusion.

Highly active against Candida albicans and non-albicans Candida (↓ susceptibility to C. parasilosis), and Hansenula.

Some activity against Aspergillus. No activity against Cryptococcus, Fusarium, Pseudoallescheria/Scedosporium, Trichosporon, Rhodotorula or Mucor.

Most cost effective parenteral antifungal for empiric therapy of systemic Candida/Aspergillus infections.

Cerebrospinal Fluid Penetration: < 1%

REFERENCES:

Andes D, Safdar N. Efficacy of micafungin for the treatment of candidemia. Eur J Clin Microbiol Infect Dis 24:662–664, 2005.

Chandraseka PH, Sobel JD. Micafungin: A New Echinocandin. Clin Infect Dis 42:1171–78, 2006.

Cornely OA, Marty FM, Stucker F, et al. Efficacy and safety of micafungin for treatment of serious Candida infections in patients with or without malignant disease. Mycoses 54:838–47, 2011

Denning DW, Marr KA, Lau WM, et al. Micafungin (FK463), alone or in combination with other systemic antifungal agents, for the treatment of acute invasive aspergillosis. Journal of Infection 53:337–349, 2006.

Higashiyama Y, Kohno S. Micafungin: a therapeutic review. Expert Rev Anti Infect Ther 2:345–55, 2004.

Ikeda F, Tanaka S, Ohki H, et al. Role of micafungin in the antifungal armamentarium. Curr Med Chem 14:1263–1275, 2007.

Isumikawa K, Ohtsu Y, Kawabata M, et al. Clinical efficacy of micafungin for chronic pulmonary aspergillosis. Med Mycol 45:273–278, 2007.

Joseph JM, Jain R, Danziger LH. Micafungin: a new echinocandin antifungal. Pharmacotherapy 27:53–67, 2007.

Kofia G, Ruhnke M. Pharmacology and metabolism of anidalafungin, caspofungin, and micafungin in the treatment of invasive candidosis: review of the literature. Eur J Med Res 16:159–166, 2011.

Kohno S, Izumikawa K, Ogawa K, et al. Intravenous micafungin versus voriconazole for chronic pulmonary aspergillosis. J Infect 61:410–418, 2011.

Kuse ER, Chetchotisakd P, da Cunha CA, et al. Micafungin versus liposomal amphotericin B for candidaemia and invasive candidosis: a phase III radomised double-blind trial. Lancet 369:1519–1527, 2007.

Nakagawa Y, Ichii Y, Saeki Y, et al. Plasma concentration of micafungin in patients with hematologic malignancies. J Infect Chemother 13:39–45, 2007.

Okugawa S, Ota Y, Tatsuno K, et al. A case of invasive central nervous system aspergillosis treated with micafungin with monitoring of micafungin concentrations in the cerebrospinal fluid. Scand J Infect Dis 39:344–346, 2007.

Ostrosky-Zeichner L, Kontoyiannis D, Raffalli J, et al. International, open-label, noncomparative, clinical trial of micafungin alone and in combination for treatment of newly diagnosed and refractory candidemia. Eur J Clin Microbiol Infect Dis 24: 654–661, 2005.

Pappas PG, Rotstein CM, Betts RF, et al. Micafungin versus caspofungin for treatment of candidemia and

"Usual dose" assumes normal renal/hepatic function. * For renal insufficiency, give usual dose × 1 followed by maintenance dose per CrCl. For dialysis patients, dose the same as for CrCl < 10 mL/min and give supplemental (post-HD/PD dose) immediately after dialysis. CrCl = creatinine clearance; CVVH = continuous veno-venous hemofiltration; HD/PD = hemodialysis/peritoneal dialysis.

other forms of invasive candidiasis. Clin Infect Dis 45:883–893, 2007.

Pawlitz D, Young M, Klepser M. Micafungin. Formulary 38:354–67, 2003.

Pettengell K, Mynhardt J, et al. Successful treatment of oesophageal candidiasis by micafungin: a novel systemic antifungal agent. Aliment Pharmacol 20:475–481, 2004.

Toubai T, Tanaka J, Ota S, et al. Efficacy and safety of micafungin in febrile neutropenic patients treated for hematological malignancies. Intern Med 46:3–9, 2007.

Wiederhold NP, Lewis JS 2nd. The echinocandin micafungin: a review of the pharmacology, spectrum of activity, clinical efficacy and safety. Expert Opin Pharmacother 8:1155–1166, 2007.

Yamaguchi M, Kurokawa T, Ishiyama K, et al. Efficacy and safety of micafungin as an empirical therapy for invasive fungal infections in patients with hematologic disorders: a multicenter, prospective study. Ann Hematol 90:1209–17, 2011.

Yoshida M, Tamura K, Imamura M, et al. Efficacy and safety of micafungin as an empirical antifungal therapy fir suspected fungal infection in neutropenic patients with hematological disorders. Ann Hematol 91:449–57, 2012.

Wilke M. Treatment and prophylaxis of invasive candidiasis with anidulafungin, caspofungin, and micafungin and its impact on use and costs: review of the literature. Eur J Med Res 16:180–186, 2011.

Website: www.mycamine.com

Minocycline (Minocin)

Drug Class: 2nd generation IV/PO tetracycline.
Usual Dose: 100 mg (IV/PO) q12h or 200 mg (IV/PO) q24h (see comments).
Spectrum: (see *Susceptibility Profiles* pp. 186–190).
Resistance Potential: Low
Pharmacokinetic Parameters:
Peak serum level: 4 mcg/mL
Bioavailability: 95%
Excreted unchanged (urine): 10%

Serum half-life (normal/ESRD): 15/18–69 hrs
Plasma protein binding: 75%
Volume of distribution (V_d): 1.5 L/kg
Primary Mode of Elimination: Hepatic
Dosage Adjustments*

CrCl < 10 mL/min	No change
Post–HD/PD dose	None
CVVH/CVVHD/ CVVHDF dose	No change
Moderate hepatic insufficiency	No change
Severe hepatic insufficiency	100 mg (IV/PO) q24h

Drug Interactions: Antacids, Al^{++}, Ca^{++}, Fe^{++}, Mg^{++}, Zn^{++}, multivitamins, sucralfate (↓ minocycline absorption); isotretinoin (pseudotumor cerebri); warfarin (↑ INR).
Adverse Effects: Nausea, GI upset if not taken with food, hyperpigmentation of skin with prolonged use, vestibular toxicity (dizziness), photosensitivity (rare), drug induced SLE.
Allergic Potential: Low
Safety in Pregnancy: D
Comments: Infuse slowly over 1 hour. Also *effective against Nocardia.*
One of only two oral antibiotics effective against serious systemic MSSA/ MRSA infections, e.g., MSSA/MRSA ABE, osteomyelitis, or meningitis.
Even if MRSA strains susceptible to doxycycline, minocycline more effective clinically. Minocycline may be preferable to doxycycline for neuroborreliosis. Meningeal dose = usual dose.
Cerebrospinal Fluid Penetration:
Non-inflamed meninges = 50%
Inflamed meninges = 50%

"Usual dose" assumes normal renal/hepatic function. * For renal insufficiency, give usual dose × 1 followed by maintenance dose per CrCl. For dialysis patients, dose the same as for CrCl < 10 mL/min and give supplemental (post-HD/PD dose) immediately after dialysis. CrCl = creatinine clearance; CVVH = continuous veno-venous hemofiltration; HD/PD = hemodialysis/peritoneal dialysis.

Bile Penetration: 1000%
(also see ***Antibiotic Pearls & Pitfalls***
p. 512).

REFERENCES:

Bouza E. New therapeutic choices for infections caused by methicillin-resistant Staphylococcus aureus. Clin Microbiol Infect Dis 15:44–52, 2009.

Copeland KFT, Brooks JI. A Novel use for an old drug: the potential for minocycline as anti-HIV adjuvant therapy. J Infect Dis 201:1115–1117, 2010.

Cukras CA, Petrou P, Chew EY, et al. oral minocycline for the treatment of diabetic macular edema (DME): results of a phase I/II clinical study. Invest Opthalmol Vis Sci 53:3865–74, 2012.

Cunha BA. Minocycline vs. doxycycline for the antimicrobial therapy of lyme neuroborreliosis. Clin Infect Dis 30:237–238, 2000.

Cunha BA. New uses for older antibiotics: nitrofurantoin, amikacin, colistin, polymyxin B, doxycycline and minocycline revisited. Med Clin North Am 90:1089–107, 2006.

Cunha BA. Minocycline versus doxycycline for CA-MRSA: in vitro versus in vivo differences. International Journal of Antimicrobial Agents 35:517–518, 2010.

Cunha BA, Schoch PE, Hage JR. Nitrofurantoin: preferred empiric therapy for community-acquired-lower urinary tract infections. Mayo Clin Proc 86:1243–4, 2011.

Cunha BA. Minocycline versus doxycycline for methicillin-resistant Staphylococcus aureus (MRSA): in vitro susceptibility versus in vivo effectiveness. Int J Antimicrob Agents 35:517–8, 2012.

Elkayam O, Yaron M, Caspi D. Minocycline-induced autoimmune syndromes: an overview. Semin Arthritis Rheum 28:392–397, 1999.

Ferule GE, Moos V, Schneider T, et al. The combination of chloroquine and minocycline, a therapeutic option in Whipple's disease refractory to treatment with ceftriaxone, meropenem and co-trimoxazole. J Antimicrob Chemother 67:1295–6, 2012.

Padma Srivastava MV, Bhasin A, Bhatia R, et al. Efficacy of minocycline in acute ischemic stroke: a single-blinded, placebo-controlled trial. Neurol India 60:23–8, 2012.

Schwartz BS, Graber CJ, Diep BA, et al. Doxycycline, not minocycline, induces Its own resistance in multidrug-resistant community-associated methicillin-resistant Staphylococcus aureus clone USA300. Clin Infect Dis 48:1483–1484, 2009.

Tsai CC, Lay CJ, Ho YH, et al. Intravenous minocycline versus oral doxycycline for the treatment of noncomplicated scurb typhus. J Microbiol Infect 44:33–38, 2011.

Website: www.pdr.net

Moxifloxacin (Avelox)

Drug Class: Respiratory fluoroquinolone.
Usual Dose: 400 mg (IV/PO) q24h (see comments).
Spectrum: (see ***Susceptibility Profiles*** pp. 198–202).
Resistance Potential: Low
Pharmacokinetic Parameters:
Peak serum level: 4.4 (IV)/4.5 (PO) mcg/mL
Bioavailability: 90%
Excreted unchanged (urine): 20%
Serum half-life (normal/ESRD): 12/12 hrs
Plasma protein binding: 50%
Volume of distribution (V_d): 2.2 L/kg
Primary Mode of Elimination: Hepatic
Dosage Adjustments*

CrCl < 10 mL/min	No change
Post–HD dose	None
Post–PD dose	None
CVVH/CVVHD/CVVHDF dose	No change
Moderate hepatic insufficiency	No change
Severe hepatic insufficiency	No change

Drug Interactions: Al⁺⁺, Fe⁺⁺, Mg⁺⁺, Zn⁺⁺
antacids, citrate/citric acid, dairy products

"Usual dose" assumes normal renal/hepatic function. * For renal insufficiency, give usual dose × 1 followed by maintenance dose per CrCl. For dialysis patients, dose the same as for CrCl < 10 mL/min and give supplemental (post-HD/PD dose) immediately after dialysis. CrCl = creatinine clearance; CVVH = continuous veno-venous hemofiltration; HD/PD = hemodialysis/peritoneal dialysis.

(↓ absorption of fluoroquinolones only if taken together); amiodarone, procainamide, sotalol (may ↑ QT_c interval, torsade de pointes), rifampicin (↓ moxifloxacin levels).

Adverse Effects: C. difficile diarrhea/ colitis. May ↑ QT_c interval; avoid taking with medications, e.g., amiodarone that prolong the QT_c interval, and in patients with cardiac arrhythmias/heart block. Does not cause seizures. FQ use has an increased risk of tendinitis/tendon rupture. Risk in highest in the elderly, those on steroids, and those with heart, lung or renal transplants.

Allergic Potential: Low

Safety in Pregnancy: C

Comments: *Only quinolone with anti-B. fragilis activity.* **FQ with the highest activity against S. pneumoniae, VSE, and MSSA.** Metabolized to microbiologically-inactive glucuronide (M1)/sulfate (M2) conjugates. Take 4 hours before or 8 hours after calcium or magnesium containing antacids or didanosine. No interactions with oral hypoglycemics. C8-methoxy group increases activity and decreases resistance potential. **TB dose** (*alternate drug in MDR TB drug regimens*): 400 mg (PO) q24h. ↑ incidence of C. difficile diarrhea/colitis with PPIs (for patients on PPIs during FQ therapy, D/C PPIs or switch to H_2 blocker for duration of FQ therapy).

Cerebrospinal Fluid Penetration: < 10%

Bile Penetration: 93%

(also see *Antibiotic Pearls & Pitfalls* p. 516).

REFERENCES:

Al-Nawas B, Walter C, Morbach T. Clinical and microbiological efficacy of moxifloxacin versus amoxicillin/clavulanic acid in severe odontogenic abscesses: a pilot study. Eur J Clin Microbiol Infect Dis 28:75–82, 2009.

Arrieta JR, Galgano AS, Sakano E, et al. Moxifloxacin vs. amoxicillin/clavulanate in the treatment of acute sinusitis. Am J Otolaryngol 28:78–82, 2007.

Balfour JA, Wiseman LR. Moxifloxacin. Drugs 57:363–73, 1999.

Bassetti M, Rosso R, Tosi C, et al. Moxifloxacin in the treatment of hospitalized community acquired pneumonia in HIV-infected subjects. J Chemother 19:104–105, 2007.

Brunkhorst FM, Oppert M, Marx G, et al. Effect of empirical treatment ith moxifloxacin and meropenem vs meropenem on sepsis-related organ dysfunction in patients with severe sepsis: a randomized trial. JAMA 307:2309–9, 2012.

Cheadle W, Lee JT, Napolitano LM, et al. Clinical update on the use of moxifloxacin in the treatment of community-acquired complicated intra-abdominal infections. Surg Infect 11:487–494, 2010.

Cheon JH, Kim N, Lee DH, et al. Efficacy of moxifloxacin-based triple therapy as second-line treatment for Helicobacter pylori infection. Helicobacter 11:46–51, 2006.

Cox H, Ford N, Keshavjee S, et al. Rational use of moxifloxacin for tuberculosis treatment. Lancet Infect Dis 11: 259–260, 2011.

Cunha BA. Oral antibiotic therapy of serious systemic infections. Med Clin N Am 90:1197–1222, 2006.

Drummond MF, Becker DL, Hux M, et al. An economic evaluation of sequential i.v./po moxifloxacin therapy compared to i.v./po co-amoxiclav with or without clarithromycin in the treatment of community-acquired pneumonia Chest 124:526–35, 2003.

Ewig S, Hecker H, Suttorp N, et al. Moxifloxacin monotherapy versus B-lactam mono or combination therapy in hospitalized patients with community-acquired pneumonia. J Infect 62: 218–225, 2011.

Fouad M, Gallagher JC. Moxifloxacin as an alternative or additive therapy for treatment of pulmonary tuberculosis. Ann Pharmacother, 45:1439–1444, 2011.

Giordano P, Song J, Pertel P, et al. Sequential intravenous/oral moxifloxacin versus intravenous piperacillin-tazobactam followed by oral amoxicillin-clavulanate for the treatment of complicated skin and skin structure infection. Int J Antimicrob Agents 26:357–65, 2005.

"Usual dose" assumes normal renal/hepatic function. * For renal insufficiency, give usual dose × 1 followed by maintenance dose per CrCl. For dialysis patients, dose the same as for CrCl < 10 mL/min and give supplemental (post-HD/PD dose) immediately after dialysis. CrCl = creatinine clearance; CVVH = continuous veno-venous hemofiltration; HD/PD = hemodialysis/peritoneal dialysis.

Goldstein EJ, Citron DM, Warren YA, et al. In vitro activity of moxifloxacin against 923 anaerobes isolated from human intra-abdominal infections. Antimicrob Agents Chemother 50:148–55, 2006.

Haggerty CL, Ness RB. Newest approaches to treatment of pelvic inflammatory disease: a review of recent randomized clinical trials. Clin Infect Dis 44:953–960, 2007.

Hariprasad SM, Shah GK, Mieler WF, Feiner L, Blinder KJ, et al. Vitreous and aqueous penetration of orally administered moxifloxacin in humans. Arch Opthamol 124:178–82, 2006.

Hoeffken G, Talan D, Larsen LS, et al. Efficacy and safety of sequential moxifloxacin for treatment of community-acquired pneumonia associated with atypical pathogens. Eur J Clin Microbiol Infect Dis 23:772–5, 2004.

Katz E, Larsen LS, Fogarty CM, et al. Safety and efficacy of sequential I.V. to P.O. moxifloxacin versus conventional combination therapies the treatment of community-acquired pneumonia in patients requiring initial I.V. therapy. J Emerg Med 27:554–9, 2004.

Klutman NE, Culley CM, Lacy ME, et al. Moxifloxacin. Antibiotics for Clinicians 5:17–27, 2001.

Lapi F, Wilchesky M, Abbas K, et al. Fluoroquinolones and the risk of serious arrhythmia: A population-based study. Clin Infect Dis 55:1457–65, 2012.

Lode H, Grossman C, Choudhri S, et al. Sequential IV/PO moxifloxacin treatment of patients with severe community-acquired pneumonia. Respir Med 97:1134–42, 2003.

Lobera T, Audicana MT, Alarcon E, et al. Allergy to quinolones: low cross-reactivity to levofloxacin. J Investig Allergol Clin Immunol 20: 607–611, 2010.

Malincarne L, Ghebtegzabher M, Moretti MV, et al. Penetration of moxifloxacin into bone in patients undergoing total knee arthroplasty. J Antimicrob Chemother 57:950–4, 2006.

Malingoni MA, Song J, Herrington J, et al. Randomized controlled trial of moxifloxacin compared with piperacillin-tazobactam and amoxicillin-clavulanate for the treatment of complicated intra-abdominal infections. Ann Surg 244:204–11, 2006.

Mendel C, Springsklee M. Moxifloxacin for tuberculosis. Lancet Infect Dis 176–17, 2012.

Mu YP, Liu RL, Wang LQ, et al. Moxifloxacin monotherapy for treatment of complicated intro-abdominal infections : a meta-analysis of randomized controlled trials. Int J Clin 66:210–7, 2012.

Nguyen HA, Grellet J, Dubois V, et al. Factors compromising the activity of moxifloxacin against intracellular Staphylococcus aureus. J Antimicrob Chemother 59:755–758, 2007.

Nijland HM, Ruslami R, Suroto AJ, et al. Rifampicin reduces plasma concentrations of moxifloxacin in patients with tuberculosis. Clin Infect Dis 45:1001–1007, 2007.

Pranger AD, Van Altena R, Aarnoutse RE, et al. Evaluation of moxifloxacin for the treatment of tuberculosis: 3 years of experience. Eur Respir J. 38: 884–894, 2011.

Rijnders BJ. Moxifloxacin for community-acquired pneumonia. Antimicrob Agents Chemother 47:444–445, 2003.

Singh KP, Brown M, Murphy ME, et al. Moxifloxacin for tuberculosis. Lancet Infect Dis 12:176, 2012.

Schlossberg D. Treatment of multi-drug resistant tuberculosis. Antibiotics for Clinicians 9:317–321, 2005.

Schulze MH, Keller C, Müller A, et al. Rickettsia ryphi infection with interstitial pneumonia in a traveler treated with moxifloxacin. J Clin Microb 49: 741–743, 2011.

Solnick, JV. Treatment with moxifloxacin versus standard therapy for community-acquired pneumonia. 10 Clinics 41:1697–1705, 2005.

Stass, H, Rink AD, Delesen H, et al. Pharmacokinetics and peritoneal penetration of moxifloxacin in peritonitis. J Antimicrob Chemother 58:693–6, 2006.

Torres A, Muir JF, Corris P, et al. Effectiveness of oral moxifloxacin in standard first-line therapy in community-acquired pneumonia. Eur Respir J 21:135–43, 2003.

Walter S, Kuchenbecker J, Banditt P, et al. Concentration of moxifloxacin in serum and human aqueous humor following a single 400 mg oral dose. J Cataract Refract Surg 33:553–555, 2007.

Welte T, Petermann W, Schurmann D, et al. Treatment with sequential intravenous or oral moxifloxacin was associated with faster clinical improvement that the standard therapy for hospitalized patients with community-acquired pneumonia who received initial parenteral therapy. Clin Infect Dis 41:1697–705, 2005.

"Usual dose" assumes normal renal/hepatic function. * For renal insufficiency, give usual dose × 1 followed by maintenance dose per CrCl. For dialysis patients, dose the same as for CrCl < 10 mL/min and give supplemental (post-HD/PD dose) immediately after dialysis. CrCl = creatinine clearance; CVVH = continuous veno-venous hemofiltration; HD/PD = hemodialysis/peritoneal dialysis.

Zervos M, Martinez FJ, Amsden GW, et al. Efficacy and safety of 3-day azithromycin versus 5-day moxifloxacin for the treatment of acute bacterial exacerbations of chronic bronchitis. Int J Antimicrob Agents 29:56–61, 2007.
Website: www.avelox.com

Nafcillin (Unipen)

Drug Class: Anti-staphylococcal penicillin.
Usual Dose: 2 gm (IV) q4h.
Spectrum: (see *Susceptibility Profiles* pp. 186–190).
Resistance Potential: Low
Pharmacokinetic Parameters:
Peak serum level: 80 mcg/ml
Bioavailability: Not applicable
Excreted unchanged (urine): 10–30%
Serum half-life (normal/ESRD): 0.5/4 hrs
Plasma protein binding: 90%
Volume of distribution (V_d): 0.24 L/kg
Primary Mode of Elimination: Hepatic
Dosage Adjustments*

CrCl < 10 mL/min	No change
Post–HD/PD dose	None
CVVH/CVVHD/CVVHDF dose	No change
Moderate—severe hepatic insufficiency	No change

Drug Interactions: Cyclosporine (↓ cyclosporine levels); nifedipine, warfarin (↓ interacting drug effect).
Adverse Effects: Not hepatotoxic. Drug fever/rash, leukopenia, interstitial nephritis.
Allergic Potential: High
Safety in Pregnancy: B
Comments: Avoid oral formulation (not well absorbed/erratic serum levels).

Meningeal dose = usual dose.
Cerebrospinal Fluid Penetration:
Non-Inflamed meninges = 1%
Inflamed meninges = 20%
Bile Penetration: 100%
(also see *Antibiotic Pearls & Pitfalls* p. 509).

REFERENCES:
Donowitz GR, Mandell GL. Beta-lactam antibiotics. N Engl J Med 318:419–26 490–500, 1993.
Wright AJ. The penicillins. Mayo Clin Proc 74:290–307, 1999.
Website: www.pdr.net

Nelfinavir (Viracept) NFV

Drug Class: Antiretroviral protease inhibitor.
Usual Dose: 1250 mg (PO) q12h (two 625-mg tablets per dose) with meals, or five 250-mg tabs or 750 mg (three 250-mg tabs) (PO) q8h.
Pharmacokinetic Parameters:
Peak serum level: 35 mcg/mL
Bioavailability: 20–80%
Excreted unchanged (urine): 1–2%
Serum half-life (normal/ESRD): 4 hrs/no data
Plasma protein binding: 98%
Volume of distribution (V_d): 5 L/kg
Primary Mode of Elimination: Hepatic
Dosage Adjustments*

CrCl < 10 mL/min	No change
Post–HD dose	None
Post–PD dose	None
CVVH/CVVHD/CVVHDF dose	No change

"Usual dose" assumes normal renal/hepatic function. * For renal insufficiency, give usual dose × 1 followed by maintenance dose per CrCl. For dialysis patients, dose the same as for CrCl < 10 mL/min and give supplemental (post-HD/PD dose) immediately after dialysis. CrCl = creatinine clearance; CVVH = continuous veno-venous hemofiltration; HD/PD = hemodialysis/peritoneal dialysis.

Mild hepatic insufficiency	No change
Moderate—severe hepatic insufficiency	Use with caution

Antiretroviral Dosage Adjzustments

Delavirdine	No data (monitor for neutropenia)
Efavirenz	No change
Indinavir	Limited data for nelfinavir 1250 mg q12h + indinavir 1200 mg q12h
Lopinavir/ritonavir	Nelfinavir 1000 mg q12h or lopinavir/r 600/150 mg q12h
Nevirapine	No data
Ritonavir	No data
Saquinavir	Saquinavir 1200 mg q12h
Rifampin	Avoid
Rifabutin	Nelfinavir 1250 mg q12h; rifabutin 150 mg q24h or 300 mg 2–3x/week

Drug Interactions: Antiretrovirals, rifabutin, rifampin (see dose adjustment grid, above); amiodarone, quinidine, astemizole, terfenadine, benzodiazepines, cisapride, ergot alkaloids, statins, St. John's wort (avoid if possible); carbamazepine, phenytoin, phenobarbital (↓ nelfinavir levels, ↑ anticonvulsant levels; monitor); caspofungin (↓ caspofungin levels,

may ↓ caspofungin effect); clarithromycin, erythromycin, telithromycin (↑ nelfinavir and macrolide levels); didanosine (dosing conflict with food; give nelfinavir with food 2 hours before or 1 hour after didanosine); itraconazole, voriconazole, ketoconazole (↑ nelfinavir levels); lamivudine (↑ lamivudine levels); methadone (may require ↑ methadone dose); oral contraceptives, zidovudine (↓ zidovudine levels); sildenafil (↑ or ↓ sildenafil levels; do not exceed 25 mg in 48 hrs, tadalafil (max. 10 mg/72 hrs, vardenafil (max. 2.5 mg/72 hrs).

Adverse Effects: Impaired concentration, nausea, abdominal pain, secretory diarrhea, ↑ SGOT/SGPT, rash, ↑ cholesterol/triglycerides (evaluate risk for coronary disease/pancreatitis), fat redistribution, hyperglycemia (including worsening diabetes, new-onset diabetes, DKA), possible increased bleeding in hemophilia.

Allergic Potential: Low

Safety in Pregnancy: B

Comments: Take with food (absorption increased 300%). 625-mg tablet available.

Cerebrospinal Fluid Penetration: Undetectable

REFERENCES:

Albrecht MA, Bosch RJ, Hammer SM, et al. Nelfinavir, efavirenz, or both after the failure of nucleoside treatment of HIV infection. N Engl J Med 345:398–407, 2001.

Go J, Cunha BA. Nelfinavir: a review. Antibiotics for Clinicians 4:17–23, 2000.

Hughes PJ, Cretton-Scott E, Teague A, et al. Protease inhibitors for patients with HIV-1 infection. Pharm Ther 36:332–344, 2011.

Panel on Antiretroviral Guidelines for Adults and Adolescents. Department of Health and Human Services. Guidelines for the use of antiretroviral agents in HIV-infected adults and adolescents.

"Usual dose" assumes normal renal/hepatic function. * For renal insufficiency, give usual dose × 1 followed by maintenance dose per CrCl. For dialysis patients, dose the same as for CrCl < 10 mL/min and give supplemental (post-HD/PD dose) immediately after dialysis. CrCl = creatinine clearance; CVVH = continuous veno-venous hemofiltration; HD/PD = hemodialysis/peritoneal dialysis.

http://aidsinfo.nih.gov/ConsentFiles/
AdultandAdolescentGL.pdf, 2012.

Perry CM, Benfield P. Nelfinavir. Drugs 54:81–7, 1997.

Saberi P, Ranatunga DK, Quesenberry CP, et al.
Clinical implications of the nelfinavir-proton pump
inhibitor drug interaction in patients with human
immunodeficiency virus. Pharmacotherapy 31:253–61,
2011.

Simpson KN, Luo MP, Chumney E, et al. Cost-effective
of lopinavir/ritonavir versus nelfinavir as the first-line
highly active antiretroviral therapy regimen for HIV
infection. HIV Clin Trials 5:294–304, 2004.

Thompson MA, Aberg JA, Cahn P, et al. Antiretroviral
treatment of adult HIV infection: 2012 recommendations of the International Antiviral Society — USA
panel. JAMA 308:387–402, 2012.

Walmsley S, Bernstein B, King M, et al. Lopinavir-
ritonavir versus nelfinavir for the initial treatment
of HIV infection. N Engl J Med 346:2039–46,
2002.

Website: www.viracept.com

Nevirapine (Viramune) NVP

Drug Class: Antiretroviral NNRTI (non-
nucleoside reverse transcriptase inhibitor).
Usual Dose: 200 mg (PO) q24h × 2 weeks,
then 200 mg (PO) q12h.

Pharmacokinetic Parameters:
Peak serum level: 0.9–3.6 mcg/mL
Bioavailability: 90%
Excreted unchanged (urine): 5%
Serum half-life (normal/ESRD): 40 hrs/no data
Plasma protein binding: 60%
Volume of distribution (V_d): 1.4 L/kg

Primary Mode of Elimination: Hepatic
Dosage Adjustments*

CrCl 10–50 mL/min	No change
CrCl < 20 mL/min	Use with caution
Post–HD dose	200 mg (PO)

Post–PD dose	None
CVVH/CVVHD/ CVVHDF dose	No change
Moderate hepatic insufficiency	Use with caution
Severe hepatic insufficiency	Avoid

Antiretroviral Dosage Adjustments

Delavirdine	No data
Efavirenz	No data
Indinavir	Indinavir 1000 mg q8h
Lopinavir/ritonavir (l/r)	Consider l/r 600/150 mg q12h in PI-experienced patients
Nelfinavir	No data
Ritonavir	No change
Saquinavir	No data
Rifampin	Avoid
Rifabutin	Use with caution

Drug Interactions: Antiretrovirals, rifabutin,
rifampin (see dose adjustment grid, above);
carbamazepine, phenobarbital, phenytoin
(monitor anticonvulsant levels); caspofungin
(↓ caspofungin levels), itraconazole
(↓ itraconazole/↑ nevirapine levels), voriconazole
(↑ nevirapine levels); ethinyl estradiol
(↓ ethinyl estradiol levels; use additional/
alternative method); methadone (↓ methadone
levels; titrate methadone dose to effect);
tacrolimus (↓ tacrolimus levels) clarithromycin
(↓ clarithromycin levels), rifapentine (avoid).

Adverse Effects: Severe, life-threatening, and
in some cases fatal hepatotoxicity, particularly
in the first 18 weeks, has been reported in

"Usual dose" assumes normal renal/hepatic function. * For renal insufficiency, give usual dose × 1 followed by maintenance dose per CrCl. For dialysis patients, dose the same as for CrCl < 10 mL/min and give supplemental (post-HD/PD dose) immediately after dialysis. CrCl = creatinine clearance; CVVH = continuous veno-venous hemofiltration; HD/PD = hemodialysis/peritoneal dialysis.

patients treated with nevirapine. In some cases, patients presented with non-specific prodromal signs or symptoms of hepatitis and progressed to hepatic failure. These events are often associated with rash. Female gender and higher CD_4 counts at initiation of therapy place patients at increased risk; women with CD_4 counts > 250 cells/mm^3, including pregnant women receiving nevirapine in combination with other antiretrovirals for the treatment of HIV infection, are at the greatest risk. However, hepatotoxicity associated with mevirapine use can occur in both genders, all CD_4 counts and at any time during treatment. Severe, life-threatening skin reactions, including fatal cases, have occurred in patients treated with nevirapine. These have included cases of Stevens-Johnson Syndrome, toxic epidermal necrolysis, and hypersensitivity reactions characterized by rash, constitutional findings, and organ dysfunction. Extra vigilance is warranted during the first 6 weeks of therapy, which is the period of greatest risk of these events. Do not repeat nevirapine following severe hepatic, skin or hypersensitivity reactions. Take out all the rest under adverse reactions.

Allergic Potential: High

Safety in Pregnancy: B

Comments: Absorption not affected by food. Not to be used for post-exposure prophylaxis because of potential for fatal hepatitis.

Cerebrospinal Fluid Penetration: 45%

REFERENCES:

Bogner JR. Nevirapine extended-release for the treatment of HIV-1 infection. Expert Rev Anti Infect Ther 10:21–30, 2012.

Coster LO, Kumar PN. Contemporary role of nevirapine in HIV treatment. AIDS Rev 14:132–44, 2012.

Herzmann C, Karcher H. Nevirapine plus zidovudine to prevent mother-to-child transmission of HIV. N Engl J Med 351:2013–5, 2004.

Milinkovic A, Martinez E. Nevirapine in the treatment of HIV. Expert Rev Anti Infect Ther 2:367–73, 2004.

Nachman S, McIntyre J. Nevirapine-based therapy after suppression: can we switch? Lancet Infect Dis 12:498–9, 2012.

Panel on Antiretroviral Guidelines for Adults and Adolescents. Department of Health and Human Services. Guidelines for the use of antiretroviral agents in HIV-infected adults and adolescents. http://aidsinfo.nih.gov/ConsentFiles/AdultandAdolescentGL.pdf, 2012.

Schafer JJ, Ravi S, Rowland EV, et al. The expanding class of non-nucleoside reverse transcriptase inhibitors for the treatment of HIV-1 infection. Pharm Ther 36:46–364, 2011.

Thompson MA, Aberg JA, Cahn P, et al. Antiretroviral treatment of adult HIV infection: 2012 recommendations of the International Antiviral Society — USA panel. JAMA 308:387–402, 2012.

Urial A, Lewthwaite P. Malaria therapy in HIV: drug interactions between nevirapine and quinine. Int J STD AIDS 22:768, 2011.

Website: www.viramune.com

Nitazoxanide (Alinia)

Drug Class: Antiprotozoal; anti-C. difficile antibiotic.

Usual Dose: 500 mg (PO) q12h.

Pharmacokinetic Parameters:

Peak serum level: 9.1–10.6 mcg/mL; tizoxanile/tizoxanile glucuronide (metabolites)

Bioavailability: No data

Excreted unchanged (urine): < 10%

Serum half-life (normal/ESRD): No data

Plasma protein binding: 99%

Volume of distribution (V_d): No data

Primary Mode of Elimination: Hepatic (66%); renal (34%)

Dosage Adjustments*

"Usual dose" assumes normal renal/hepatic function. * For renal insufficiency, give usual dose × 1 followed by maintenance dose per CrCl. For dialysis patients, dose the same as for CrCl < 10 mL/min and give supplemental (post-HD/PD dose) immediately after dialysis. CrCl = creatinine clearance; CVVH = continuous veno-venous hemofiltration; HD/PD = hemodialysis/peritoneal dialysis.

CrCl 50–80 mL/min	No change
CrCl 10–50 mL/min	No change
CrCl < 10 mL/min	Use with caution
Post–HD dose	None
Post–PD dose	None
CVVH/CVVHD/ CVVHDF dose	No change
Mild/moderate	No change
Mild hepatic insufficiency	No change
Moderate–severe hepatic insufficiency	Use with caution

Drug Interactions: Avoid in patients with hypersensitivity to salicylates.
Adverse Effects: Dizziness, headache, nausea/vomiting, abdominal pain, flu-like syndrome, yellow discoloration of sclera/urine.
Allergic Potential: Low
Safety in Pregnancy: B
Comments: Nitazoxanide concentrates in GI tract but is not present in serum. **Give with food**; absorption greatly increased with food (↑ plasma levels of metabolites ~ 50%). Contains 1.4 gm sucrose/5 mL of reconstituted suspension. **Preferred therapy for *Cryptosporidia* and giardiasis. Also effective against *Cyclospora* and *Iospora*. Effective for severe *C. difficile* diarrhea/colitis (including metronidazole / vancomycin failures). Also useful for *H. pylori* or *B. hominis* and Norovirus diarrhea.**

REFERENCES:

Aslam S, Hamill RJ, Musher DM. Treatment of Clostridium difficile-associated disease: old therapies and new strategies. Lancet Infect Dis 5:549–57, 2005.

Basu PP, Rayapudi K, Pacana T, et al. A randomized study comparing levofloxacin, omeprazole, nitazoxanide, and doxycycline versus triple therapy for the eradication of Helicobacter pylori. AM J Gastoroent 106:1970–5, 2011.

Bouza E, Burillo A, Munoz P. Antimicrobial therapy of Clostridium difficile-associated diarrhea. Med Clin N Am 90:1141–63, 2006.

Freeman J, Baines SD, Todhunter SL, et al. Nitazoxanide is active against Clostridium difficile strains with reduced susceptibility to metronidazole. J Antimicrob Chemother 66:1407–1408, 2011.

Gilles HM, et al. Treatment of intestinal parasitic infections: a review of nitazoxanide. Trends in Parasitology 18:95–7, 2002.

Gurgen J, Hogan D, Grace E, et al. Nitazoxanide in the treatment of chronic cutaneous leishmaniasis resistant to traditional sodium stidogluconate. J Am Acad Dermatol 64: 202–203, 2011.

Jung KS, Park JJ, Chon YE, et al. Risk factors for treatment failure and recurrence after metronidazole treatmet for Clostridium difficile-associated diarrhea. Gut Liver 4:332–337, 2011.

Musher DM, Logan N, Hamill RJ, et al. Nitazoxanide for the treatment of Clostridium difficile colitis. Clin Infect. Dis 43:421–30, 2006.

White CA Jr. Nitazoxanide: a new broad spectrum antiparasitic agent. Expert Rev Anti Infect Ther 2:43–9, 2004.

Web site: www.romark.com

Nitrofurantoin (Macrodantin, Macrobid)

Drug Class: Urinary antiseptic.
Usual Dose: 100 mg (PO) q12h.
Spectrum: (see *Susceptibility Profiles* pp. 198–202).
Resistance Potential: Low
Pharmacokinetic Parameters:
Peak serum level: 1 mcg/mL
Bioavailability: 80%
Excreted unchanged (urine): 25%
Serum half-life (normal/ESRD): 0.5/1 hrs
Plasma protein binding: 40%

"Usual dose" assumes normal renal/hepatic function. * For renal insufficiency, give usual dose × 1 followed by maintenance dose per CrCl. For dialysis patients, dose the same as for CrCl < 10 mL/min and give supplemental (post-HD/PD dose) immediately after dialysis. CrCl = creatinine clearance; CVVH = continuous veno-venous hemofiltration; HD/PD = hemodialysis/peritoneal dialysis.

Volume of distribution (Vd): 0.8 L/kg
Primary Mode of Elimination: Renal
Dosage Adjustments*

CrCl 50–80 mL/min	100 mg (PO) q12h
CrCl 30–50 mL/min	100 mg (PO) q24h
CrCl < 30 mL/min	Avoid
Post–HD dose	Avoid
Post–PD dose	Avoid
CVVH/CVVHD/CVVHDF dose	Avoid
Moderate hepatic insufficiency	No change
Severe hepatic insufficiency	No change

Drug Interactions: Antacids, magnesium (↓ nitrofurantoin absorption); probenecid (↑ nitrofurantoin levels).
Adverse Effects:
Acute hypersensitivity reactions (reversible): pneumonitis.
Chronic reactions (irreversible): chronic hepatitis, peripheral neuropathy, interstitial fibrosis.
Allergic Potential: Moderate
Safety in Pregnancy: B
Comments: For CAB/lower UTIs only, not systemic infection. GI upset minimal with microcrystalline preparations. **Useful for asymptomatic bacteriuria of pregnancy;** no transplacental transfer. Chronic toxicities associated with prolonged use/renal insufficiency; optimal effectiveness if CrCl > 60 mL/min. Avoid if CrCl < 30 mL/min. **Active against most aerobic GNB uropathogens, except P. aeruginosa, Serratia marcesens, and Proteus sp. Effective for VSE/VRE catheter-associated bacteriuria (CAB)/lower UTIs**

(also see **Antibiotic Pearls & Pitfalls** p. 516).

REFERENCES:
Auer S, Wojna A, Hell M. Oral treatment options for ambulatory patients with urinary tract infections caused by extended-spectrum-beta-lactamase-producing Escherichia coli. Antimicrob Agents Chemother 54:4006–4008, 2010.

Cunha BA. Nitrofurantoin: Bioavailability and therapeutic equivalence. Adv Ther 5:54–63, 1988.

Cunha BA. Nitrofurantoin: An update. OB/GYN 44:399–406, 1989.

Cunha BA. New uses for older antibiotics: nitrofurantoin, amikacin, colistin, polymyxin B, doxycycline, and minocycline revisited. Med Clin North Am 90:1089–107, 2006.

Cunha BA. Nitrofurantoin: Preferred Empiric Therapy for Community Acquired and Nosocomial Lower Urinary Tract Infections (UTIs). Mayo Clinic Proceedings 86: 1243–1244, 2011.

Cunha BA, Schoch PE, Hage JR. Nitrofurantoin: preferred empiric therapy for community-acquired-lower urinary tract infections. Mayo Clin Proc 86:1243–4, 2011.

Cunha BA. Prophylaxis for Recurrent Urinary Tract Infections (UTIs): Nitrofurantoin, Not TMP-SMX or Cranberry Juice. Archives of Internal Medicine 172:82, 2012.

Cunha BA, Schoch P, Hage JE. Oral therapy of catheter-associated bacteriuria (CAB) in the ear of antibiotic resistance: nitrofurantoin revisited. J Chemother 24:122–4, 2012.

Cunha BA. Prophylaxis for recurrent urinary tact infections: nitrofurantoin, not trimethoprim-sulfamethoxazole or cranberry juice. Arch Intern Med 172:82–3, 2012.

Livermore DM, Warner M, Mushtaq S, et al. What remains against carbapenem-resistant Enterobacteriaceae? Evaluation of chloramphenicol, ciprofloxacin, colistin, fosfomycin, minocycline, nitrofurantoin, temocillin and tigecycline. Int J Antimicrob Agents 37:415–9, 2011.

McKinnel JA, Stollenwerk NS, Jung CW, et al. Nitrofurantoin compares favorably to recommended

---

"Usual dose" assumes normal renal/hepatic function. * For renal insufficiency, give usual dose × 1 followed by maintenance dose per CrCl. For dialysis patients, dose the same as for CrCl < 10 mL/min and give supplemental (post-HD/PD dose) immediately after dialysis. CrCl = creatinine clearance; CVVH = continuous veno-venous hemofiltration; HD/PD = hemodialysis/peritoneal dialysis.

agents as empirical treatment of uncomplicated urinary tract infections in a decision and cost analysis. Mayo Clin Proc 86:480–8, 2011.

Mendoza-Valdes A, Rosete A, Rios Bueno E, Frentzel A, et al. Antimicrobial and clinical efficacy of nitrofurantoin in the treatment of acute lower urinary tract infections in adults. Med Klin 105:698–704, 2010.

Ofloxacin (Oflox)

Drug Class: Fluoroquinolone.
Usual Dose: 400 mg (IV/PO) q12h (see comments).
Spectrum: (see *Susceptibility Profiles* pp. 198–202).
Resistance Potential: Low
Pharmacokinetic Parameters:
Peak serum level: 5.5–7.2 mcg/ml
Bioavailability: 95%
Excreted unchanged (urine): 90%
Serum half-life (normal/ESRD): 6/40 hrs
Plasma protein binding: 32%
Volume of distribution (V_d): 2 L/kg
Primary Mode of Elimination: Renal
Dosage Adjustments*

CrCl 20–50 mL/min	400 mg (IV/PO) q24h
CrCl < 20 mL/min	200 mg (IV/PO) q24
Post-HD dose	200 mg (IV/PO)
Post-PD dose	200 mg (IV/PO)
CVVH/CVVHD/ CVVHDF dose	300 mg (IV/PO) q24h
Mild-moderate hepatic insufficiency	No change
Severe hepatic insufficiency	400 mg (IV/PO) q24h

Drug Interactions: Al^{++}, Ca^{++}, Fe^{++}, Mg^{++}, Zn^{++} antacids, citrate/citric acid, dairy products (↓ absorption of ofloxacin only if taken together); cimetidine (↑ ofloxacin levels); cyclosporine (↑ cyclosporine levels); NSAIDs (CNS stimulation); probenecid (↑ ofloxacin levels); warfarin (↑ INR).
Adverse Effects: Drug fever/rash, mild neuroexcitatory symptoms. C. difficile diarrhea/colitis. FQ use has an increased risk of tendinitis/tendon rupture. Risk in highest in the elderly, those on steroids, and those with heart, lung or renal transplants.
Allergic Potential: Low
Safety in Pregnancy: C
Comments: H_2 antagonist increases half-life by ~ 30%. Levofloxacin has improved pharmacokinetics/pharmacodynamics and greater antimicrobial activity. Take ofloxacin 2 hours before or after calcium/magnesium containing antacids. **PPNG dose:** 400 mg (PO) × 1 dose. **NGU/cervicitis dose:** 300 mg (PO) q12h × 1 week.
Cerebrospinal Fluid Penetration: < 10%
Bile Penetration: 1500%
(also see *Antibiotic Pearls & Pitfalls* p. 516).

REFERENCES:

Absalon J, Domenico PD, Ortega AM, Cunha, BA. The antibacterial activity of ofloxacin versus ciprofloxacin against Pseudomonas aeruginosa in human urine. Adv Ther 13:191–4, 1996.

Fuhrmann V, Schenk P, Thalhammer F. Ofloxacin clearance during continuous hemofiltration. Am J Kidney Dis 42:1327–8, 2003.

Monk JP, Campoli-Richards DM. Ofloxacin: A review of its antibacterial activity, pharmacokinetics properties, and therapeutic use. Drugs 33:346–91, 1987.

Website: www.pdr.net

"Usual dose" assumes normal renal/hepatic function. * For renal insufficiency, give usual dose × 1 followed by maintenance dose per CrCl. For dialysis patients, dose the same as for CrCl < 10 mL/min and give supplemental (post-HD/PD dose) immediately after dialysis. CrCl = creatinine clearance; CVVH = continuous veno-venous hemofiltration; HD/PD = hemodialysis/peritoneal dialysis.

Oseltemavir (Tamiflu)

Drug class: Neuraminidase inhibitor.
Usual dose: Treatment: 75 mg (PO) q12h × 5 days; Prophylaxis: 75 mg (PO) q24h × 10 days.

Pharmacokinetic Parameters:
Peak serum level: 65.2 mcg/L
Bioavailability: 75%
Excreted unchanged: 1%
Serum half-life (normal/ESRD): 1–3 hours/no data
plasma protein binding: 42%
Volume of distribution (V_d): 23–26 L
Primary Mode of Elimination: Renal (oseltamivir carboxylate)
Dosage Adjustments*

CrCl ~ 30–49 mL/min	No adjustment
CrCl ~ 10–29 mL/min	75 mg (PO) q24h (treatment) 75 mg (PO) q48h or 30 mg (PO) q24h (prophylaxis)
CrCl < 10 mL/min	No data
Post-HD dose	30 mg (PO)
Post-PD dose	30 mg (PO) q week
CVVH/CVVHD/CVVHDF dose	75 mg (PO) q24h (treatment) 75 mg (PO) q48h or 30 mg (PO) q24h (prophylaxis)
Moderate—severe hepatic insufficiency	Use with caution

Drug Interactions: Live attenuated influenza vaccine 2 weeks before or 2 days after oseltemavir.

Adverse Effects: nausea, vomiting, serious skin reactions, diplopia, visual disturbances, palpitations, atrial fibrillation, supraventricular/ventricular tachycardias neuropsychiatric events.
Allergic Potential: Low
Safety in Pregnancy: C
Comments: Begin prophylaxis within 3 days of exposure. **Pediatric treatment doses:** ≤ 15 kg = 30 mg (PO) q12h, 16–23 kg = 45 mg (PO) q12h, 24–40 kg = 60 mg (PO) q12h, > 40 kg = 75 mg (PO) q12h. **Pediatric prophylaxis dose** ≤ 15 kg = 30 mg (PO) q24h, 16–23 kg = 45 mg (PO) q24h, 24–40 kg = 60 mg (PO) q24h, > 40 kg = 75 mg (PO) q24h. Available as 30, 45 and 75 mg capsules and 300 mg oral suspension.

REFERENCES:

Agrawal R, Rewatkar PV, Kokil GR, et al. Oseltamivir: a first line defense against swine flu. Med Chem 6:247–251, 2010.

Chen H, Cheung CL, Tai H, et al. Oseltamivir-Resistant Influenza A Pandemic (H1N1) 2009 Virus, Hong Kong, China. Emerg Infect Dis 15:1970–1972, 2009.

Cho D, Hossain M, Liew P, et al. Side effects of oseltamivir in end-stage renal failure patients. Nephrol Dial Transplant 26:2339–2344, 2011.

Couch RB, Davis BR. Has oseltamivir been shown to be effective for treatment of H5N1 influenza? J Infect Dis 202:1149–1151, 2010.

Jackson RJ, Cooper KL, Tappenden P, et al. Oseltamivir, zanamivir and amantadine in the prevention of influenza: A systematic review. J Infect 62:14–25, 2011.

Lee VJ, Yap J, Maurer-Stroh S, et al. Investigation causes of oseltamivir chemoprophylaxis failures during influenza A (HINI-2009) outbreaks. J Clin Virology 50:104–108, 2011.

Sophia NG, Cowling BJ, Fang VJ, et al. Effects of oseltamivir treatment on duration of clinical illness and viral shedding and household transmission of influenza virus. Clin Infect Dis 50:707–714, 2010.

"Usual dose" assumes normal renal/hepatic function. * For renal insufficiency, give usual dose × 1 followed by maintenance dose per CrCl. For dialysis patients, dose the same as for CrCl < 10 mL/min and give supplemental (post-HD/PD dose) immediately after dialysis. CrCl = creatinine clearance; CVVH = continuous veno-venous hemofiltration; HD/PD = hemodialysis/peritoneal dialysis.

Sotos JG. Emergence of Oseltamivir-Resistant Pandemic H1N1 Virus during Prophylaxis. N Engl J Med 361:2296–2298, 2009.

Oxacillin (Prostaphlin)

Drug Class: Anti-staphylococcal penicillin.
Usual Dose: 1–2 gm (IV) q4h.
Spectrum: (see *Susceptibility Profiles* pp. 186–190).
Resistance Potential: Low
Pharmacokinetic Parameters:
Peak serum level: 43 mcg/ml
Bioavailability: Not applicable
Excreted unchanged (urine): 39–66%
Serum half-life (normal/ESRD): 0.5/1 hrs
Plasma protein binding: 94%
Volume of distribution (V_d): 0.2 L/kg
Primary Mode of Elimination: Renal
Dosage Adjustments* (based on 2 gm q4h)

CrCl 10–80 mL/min	No change
CrCl < 10 mL/min	No change
Post–HD dose	None
Post–PD dose	None
CVVH/CVVHD/CVVHDF dose	No change
Moderate hepatic insufficiency	No change
Severe hepatic insufficiency	No change

Drug Interactions: Cyclosporine (↓ cyclosporine levels); nifedipine, warfarin (↓ interacting drug effect).
Adverse Effects: Drug fever/rash, leukopenia, ↑ SGOT/SGPT, hepatitis.
Allergic Potential: High
Safety in Pregnancy: B

Comments: Avoid oral formulation (not well absorbed/erratic serum levels).
Meningeal dose = 2 gm (IV) q4h.
Cerebrospinal Fluid Penetration:
Non-inflamed meninges = 1%
Inflamed meninges = 10%
Bile Penetration: 25%
(also see *Antibiotic Pearls & Pitfalls* p. 509).

REFERENCES:

Al-Homaidhi H, Abdel-Haq NM, El-Baba M, et al. Severe hepatitis associated with oxacillin therapy. South Med J 95:650–2, 2002.

Donowitz GR, Mandell GL. Beta-lactam antibiotics. N Engl J Med 318:419–26 and 318:490–500, 1993.

Wright AJ. The penicillins. Mayo Clin Proc 74:290–307, 1999.

Website: www.pdr.net

Pegylated Interferon alfa-2a (Pegasys)

Drug Class: Interferon/antiviral.
Usual Dose: Pegasys: 180 mcg (SQ) once weekly × 48 weeks; Ribavirin: 500 mg (< 75 kg) or 800 mg (> 75 mg) (PO) q12h × 48 weeks (see comments).
Pharmacokinetic Parameters:
Trough level: 16 ng/ml
Bioavailability: No data
Excreted unchanged (urine): No data
Serum half-life (normal/ESRD): 80/100–120 hrs
Plasma protein binding: No data
Volume of distribution (V_d): 8–12 L/kg
Primary Mode of Elimination: Renal
Dosage Adjustments*

CrCl 10–50 mL/min	Pegasys: 180 mcg (SQ); avoid ribavirin
CrCl < 10 mL/min	Pegasys: 135 mcg (SQ) q week; avoid ribavirin

---

"Usual dose" assumes normal renal/hepatic function. * For renal insufficiency, give usual dose × 1 followed by maintenance dose per CrCl. For dialysis patients, dose the same as for CrCl < 10 mL/min and give supplemental (post-HD/PD dose) immediately after dialysis. CrCl = creatinine clearance; CVVH = continuous veno-venous hemofiltration; HD/PD = hemodialysis/peritoneal dialysis.

Post–HD dose	Pegasys: 135 mcg (SQ) q week; avoid ribavirin
Post–PD dose	Pegasys: 135 mcg (SQ); avoid ribavirin
CVVH/CVVHD/ CVVHDF dose	Avoid ribavirin
Moderate hepatic insufficiency	135 mcg if ALT ↑; Avoid ribavirin
Severe hepatic insufficiency	Avoid
Moderate depression	↓ Pegasys to 135 mcg (90 mcg in some); evaluate once weekly
Severe depression	Discontinue Pegasys; immediate psychiatric consult

Pegasys Adjustment for Hematologic Toxicity

Absolute neutrophil count < 750/mm³	↓ Pegasys to 135 mcg
Absolute neutrophil count < 500/mm³	Discontinue Pegasys until neutrophils > 1000/mm³. Reinstitute at 90 mcg and monitor neutrophil count
Platelets < 50,000/ mm³	↓ Pegasys to 90 mcg
Platelets < 25,000/ mm³	Discontinue Pegasys

Ribavirin Adjustment for Hematologic Toxicity

Hgb < 10 gm/dL and no cardiac disease	↓ Ribavirin to 600 mg/day†
Hgb < 8.5 gm/dL and no cardiac disease	Discontinue ribavirin

Hgb ≥ 2 gm/dL ↓ during 4-week treatment period and stable cardiac disease	↓ Ribavirin to 600 mg/day*
Hgb < 12 gm/dL despite 4 weeks at reduced dose and stable cardiac disease	Discontinue ribavirin

* One 200-mg tablet in a.m. and two 200-mg tablets in p.m.

Drug Interactions: Inhibits CYP IA2. May ↑ theophylline levels.

Adverse Effects: Flu-like symptoms, neuropsychiatric disturbances, bone marrow toxicity, nausea/vomiting/diarrhea, alopecia, hypothyroidism, ARDS.

Allergic Potential: Low

Safety in Pregnancy: Pegasys: C (ribavirin: X; also avoid in partners of pregnant women)

Comments: Ribavirin dose with Pegasys for HCV (genotypes 2, 3) is 800 mg/d. The optimal ribavirin dose for HCV (genotype 1) has not been determined but 800–1400 mg/d has been used. Combination therapy is more effective than monotherapy. Avoid in autoimmune hepatitis and decompensated cirrhosis. Check CBC weekly. For genotypes 2 and 3, duration of therapy is 24 weeks and ribavirin dose is 400 mg (PO) bid (rather than q12h). Ribavirin should be taken with breakfast and dinner to ↑ bioavailability/↓ nausea. Ribavirin taken after dinner may cause insomnia. Ribavirin's long serum half-life allows q24h dosing, but ↑ nausea.

Cerebrospinal Fluid Penetration: No data
Bile Penetration: No data

REFERENCES:

Davis GL. Combination treatment with interferon and ribavirin for chronic hepatitis C. Clin Liver Dis 1:811–26, 1999.

Ferenci P. Peginterferon alfa-2a (40KD) (Pegasys) for the treatment of patients with chronic hepatitis C. Int J Clin Pract 57:610–5, 2003.

- -
"Usual dose" assumes normal renal/hepatic function. * For renal insufficiency, give usual dose × 1 followed by maintenance dose per CrCl. For dialysis patients, dose the same as for CrCl < 10 mL/min and give supplemental (post-HD/PD dose) immediately after dialysis. CrCl = creatinine clearance; CVVH = continuous veno-venous hemofiltration; HD/PD = hemodialysis/peritoneal dialysis.

Fried MN, et al. Peg-interferon alfa-2a plus ribavirin for chronic hepatitis C virus infection. N Engl J Med 347:975–82, 2002.

Kamal SM, et al. Peg-interferon alone or with ribavirin enhances HCV-specific CD_4 T-helper responses in patients with chronic hepatitis C. Gastroenterology 123:1070–83, 2002.

Liu C-H, Liang C-C, Liu C-J, et al. Pegylated interferon alfa-2a monotherapy for hemodialysis patients with acute hepatitis c. Clin Infect Dis 51:541–549, 2010.

Plosker GL, Keating GM. Peginterferon-alpha-2a (40kD) plus ribavirin: a review of its use in hepatitis C virus and HIV co-infection. Drugs 64:2823–43, 2004.

Rasenack J, Zeuzem S, Feinman SV, et al. Peginterferon alpha-2a (40kD) [Pegasys] improves HR-QOL outcomes compared with unmodified interferon alpha-2a [Roferon-A]: in patients with chronic hepatitis C. Pharmacoeconomics 21:341–9, 2003.

Torriani FJ, Rodriguez-Torres M, Rockstroh JK, et al. Peginterferon alfa-2a plus ribavirin for chronic hepatitis C virus infection in HIV-infected patients. N Engl J Med 351:438–50, 2004.

Website: www.pegasys.com

Pegylated Interferon alfa-2b (Peg-Intron)

Drug Class: Interferon/antiviral.
Usual Dose: See pp. 97–98.
Pharmacokinetic Parameters:
Peak serum level: 30 IU/ml / 3680 ng/ml
Bioavailability: No data/64%
Excreted unchanged (urine): No data/17%
Serum half-life (normal/ESRD): [40 hrs/no data] / [298 hrs/no data]
Plasma protein binding: No data
Volume of distribution (V_d): 0.99 L/kg
Primary Mode of Elimination: Renal/renal
Dosage Adjustments*

CrCl 30–50 mL/min	give 75% of Peg-Intron dose; avoid ribavirin
CrCl < 30 mL/min	give 50% of Peg-Intron dose; avoid ribavirin
Post–HD dose	Avoid ribavirin
Post–PD dose	Avoid ribavirin
CVVH/CVVHD/CVVHDF dose	Avoid ribavirin
Moderate hepatic insufficiency	None
Severe hepatic insufficiency	Avoid
Moderate depression	↓ Peg-Intron by 50%; evaluate once weekly
Severe depression	Discontinue both drugs; immediate psychiatric consult

Dosage Adjustments for Hematologic Toxicity

Hgb < 10 gm/dL	↓ ribavirin by 200 mg/day
Hgb < 8.5 gm/dL	Permanently discontinue both drugs
WBC < 1.5×10^9/L	↓ Peg-Intron by 50%
WBC < 1.0×10^9/L	Permanently discontinue both drugs
Neutrophils < 0.75 $\times 10^9$/L	↓ Peg-Intron by 50%
Neutrophils < 0.5 $\times 10^9$/L	Permanently discontinue both drugs
Platelets < 80 $\times 10^9$/L	↓ Peg-Intron by 50%

"Usual dose" assumes normal renal/hepatic function. * For renal insufficiency, give usual dose × 1 followed by maintenance dose per CrCl. For dialysis patients, dose the same as for CrCl < 10 mL/min and give supplemental (post-HD/PD dose) immediately after dialysis. CrCl = creatinine clearance; CVVH = continuous veno-venous hemofiltration; HD/PD = hemodialysis/peritoneal dialysis.

Platelets < 50 × 10⁹/L	Permanently discontinue both drugs
Hgb ≥ 2 gm/dL ↓ during 4-week treatment period and stable cardiac disease	↓ Peg-Intron by 50% and ribavirin by 200 mg/day
Hgb < 12 gm/dL despite ribavirin dose reduction	Permanently discontinue both drugs

Drug Interactions: Nucleoside analogs: fatal/non-fatal lactic acidosis. May ↑ levels of theophylline. Overlapping toxicity with other bone marrow suppressants.

Adverse Effects: Hemolytic anemia, psychological effects, cytopenias, pulmonary symptoms, pancreatitis, hypersensitivity reactions, ↑ triglycerides, flu-like symptoms, nausea/vomiting, alopecia, rash, hypothyroidism.

Allergic Potential: Low

Safety in Pregnancy: Peg-Intron: C (ribavirin: X; also avoid in partners of pregnant women)

Comments: Avoid in autoimmune hepatitis. Check CBC pretreatment and at 2 and 4 weeks (must adjust doses for ↓ WBC, ↓ neutrophils, ↓ platelets, ↓ hemoglobin). Poorly tolerated in decompensated cirrhosis or recurrent hepatitis C after transplant. Be alert for severe depression/psychiatric changes.

Cerebrospinal Fluid Penetration: No data

Bile Penetration: No data

REFERENCES:

Alfaleh FZ, Hadad Q, Khuroo MS, et al. Peginterferon alpha-2b plus ribavirin compared with interferon alpha-2b plus ribavirin for initial treatment of chronic hepatitis C in Saudi patients commonly infected with genotype 4. Liver Int 24:568–74, 2004.

Fried MN. Side effects of therapy of hepatitis C and their management. Hepatology 36:S237–44, 2002.

Jaeckel E, Cornberg M, Wedemeyer H, et al. Treatment of acute hepatitis C with interferon alfa-2b. N Engl J Med 345:1452–7, 2001.

Wright TL. Treatment of patients with hepatitis C and cirrhosis. Hepatology 36:S185–91, 2002.

Website: www.pegintron.com

Penicillin G (various)

Drug Class: Natural penicillin.
Usual Dose: 2–4 mu (IV) q4h (see comments).
Spectrum: (see *Susceptibility Profiles* pp. 186–190).
Resistance Potential: Low
Pharmacokinetic Parameters:
Peak serum level: 20–40 mcg/ml
Bioavailability: Not applicable
Excreted unchanged (urine): 80%
Serum half-life (normal/ESRD): 0.5/5.1 hrs
Plasma protein binding: 60%
Volume of distribution (V_d): 0.3 L/kg
Primary Mode of Elimination: Renal
Dosage Adjustments*

CrCl 50–80 mL/min	2–4 mu (IV) q4h
CrCl 10–50 mL/min	1–2 mu (IV) q4h
CrCl < 10 mL/min	1 mu (IV) q8h
Post–HD dose	2 mu (IV)
Post–PD dose	0.5 mu (IV)
CVVH/CVVHD/CVVHDF dose	2 mu (IV) q6h
Moderate hepatic insufficiency	No change
Severe hepatic insufficiency	No change

"Usual dose" assumes normal renal/hepatic function. * For renal insufficiency, give usual dose × 1 followed by maintenance dose per CrCl. For dialysis patients, dose the same as for CrCl < 10 mL/min and give supplemental (post-HD/PD dose) immediately after dialysis. CrCl = creatinine clearance; CVVH = continuous veno-venous hemofiltration; HD/PD = hemodialysis/peritoneal dialysis.

Drug Interactions: Probenecid (↑ penicillin G levels).

Adverse Effects: Drug fever/rash, E. multiforme/ Stevens–Johnson Syndrome; anaphylactic reactions (hypotension, laryngospasm, bronchospasm), hives, serum sickness.

Allergic Potential: High

Safety in Pregnancy: B

Comments: Incompatible in solutions containing erythromycin, aminoglycosides, calcium bicarbonate, or heparin. Penicillin G (potassium): K^+ content = 1.7 mEq/g; Na^+ content = 0.3 mEq/g. Penicillin G (sodium): Na^+ content = 2 mEq/g.

1°, 2°, early latent syphilis dose: PCN benzathine 2.4 mu (IM) × 1 dose. **Late latent syphilis dose:** PCN benzathine 2.4 mu (IM) q8h once weekly × 3. **Neurosyphilis dose:** PCN G 4 mu (IV) q4h × 2 weeks. Meningeal dose = 4 mu (IV) q4h.

Cerebrospinal Fluid Penetration:
Non-inflamed meninges ≤ 1%
Inflamed meninges = 5%

Bile Penetration: 500%
(also see *Antibiotic Pearls & Pitfalls* p. 508).

REFERENCES:

Falco V, Almirante B, Jordano Q, et al. Influence of penicillin resistance of outcome in adult patients with invasive pneumococcal pneumonia. Is penicillin useful against intermediately resistant strains? J Antimicrob Chemother 54:481–8, 2004.

Giachetto G, Pirez MC, Nanni L, et al. Ampicillin and penicillin concentration in serum and pleural fluid of hospitalized children with community-acquired pneumonia. Pediatr Infect Dis J 7:625–9, 2004.

Steininger C, Allerberger F, Gnaiger E. Clinical significance of inhibition kinetics for Streptococcus pyogenes in response to penicillin. J Antimicrob Chemother 50:517–23, 2002.

Wendel Jr GD, Sheffield JS, Hollier LM, et al. Treatment of syphilis in pregnancy and prevention of congenital syphilis. Clin Infect Dis 35(Suppl2):S200–9, 2002.

Wright AJ. The penicillins. Mayo Clin Proc 74:290–307, 1999.

Penicillin V (various)

Drug Class: Natural penicillin.

Usual Dose: 500 mg (PO) q6h. (Take without food).

Spectrum: (see *Susceptibility Profiles* pp. 186–190).

Resistance Potential: Low

Pharmacokinetic Parameters:
Peak serum level: 5 mcg/ml
Bioavailability: 60%
Excreted unchanged (urine): 80%
Serum half-life (normal/ESRD): 0.5/8 hrs
Plasma protein binding: 70%
Volume of distribution (V_d): 0.5 L/kg

Primary Mode of Elimination: Renal

Dosage Adjustments*

CrCl 10–50 mL/min	No change
CrCl < 10 mL/min	250–500 mg (PO) q6h
Post–HD dose	250 mg (PO)
Post–PD dose	250 mg (PO)
CVVH/CVVHD/ CVVHDF dose	500 mg (PO) q6h
Moderate hepatic insufficiency	No change
Severe hepatic insufficiency	No change

Drug Interactions: Probenecid (↑ penicillin V levels).

"Usual dose" assumes normal renal/hepatic function. * For renal insufficiency, give usual dose × 1 followed by maintenance dose per CrCl. For dialysis patients, dose the same as for CrCl < 10 mL/min and give supplemental (post-HD/PD dose) immediately after dialysis. CrCl = creatinine clearance; CVVH = continuous veno-venous hemofiltration; HD/PD = hemodialysis/peritoneal dialysis.

Adverse Effects: Drug fever/rash,
E. multiforme/Stevens-Johnson Syndrome,
anaphylactic reactions (hypotension,
laryngospasm, bronchospasm), hives, serum
sickness C. difficile diarrhea/colitis.
Allergic Potential: High
Safety in Pregnancy: B
Comments: Jarisch–Herxheimer reactions
when treating spirochetal infections, e.g., Lyme
disease, syphilis, yaws.
Cerebrospinal Fluid Penetration: < 10%
(also see *Antibiotic Pearls & Pitfalls*
p. 508).

REFERENCES:
Bisno AL, Gerber MA, Swaltney JM, et al. Practice
    guidelines for the diagnosis and management of
    group A streptococcal pharyngitis. Infectious Diseases
    Society of America. Clin Infect Dis 35:113–25, 2002.
Chiou CC, Does penicillin remain the drug of choice for
    pneumococcal pneumonia in view of emerging in
    vitro resistance? Clin Infect Dis 42:234–7, 2006.
Donowitz GR, Mandell GL. Beta-lactam antibiotics.
    N Engl J Med 318:419–26 and 490–500, 1993.
Klugman KP, Yu VL. No Impact of Penicillin Resistance
    on Mortality. Clin Infect Dis 43:261, 2006.
Peterson LR. Penicillin for treatment of pneumococcal
    pneumonia: does in vitro resistance really matter?
    Clin Infect Dis 42:224–33, 2006.
Portier H, Filipecki J, Weber P, et al. Five day
    clarithromycin modified release versus 10 day
    penicillin V for group A streptococcal pharyngitis:
    a multi-centre, open-label, randomized study.
    J Antimicrob Chemother 49:337–44, 2002.
Wright AJ. The penicillins. Mayo Clin Proc 74:290, 1999.

Pentamidine (Pentam 300, NebuPent)

Drug Class: Antiparasitic.
Usual Dose: 4 mg/kg (IV) q24h (see comments).
Pharmacokinetic Parameters:
Peak serum level: 0.6–1.5 mcg/mL

Bioavailability: Not applicable
Excreted unchanged (urine): 50%
Serum half-life (normal/ESRD): 6.4/90 hrs
Plasma protein binding: 69%
Volume of distribution (V_d): 5 L/kg
Primary Mode of Elimination: Metabolized
Dosage Adjustments*

CrCl < 10 mL/min	No change
Post–HD dose	None
Post–PD dose	None
CVVH/CVVHD/CVVHDF dose	No change
Moderate—severe hepatic insufficiency	No change

Drug Interactions: Alcohol, valproic acid,
didanosine, (↑ risk of pancreatitis); foscarnet
(severe hypocalcemia reported; do not
combine); amphotericin B, aminoglycosides,
capreomycin, cis-platinum, colistin,
methoxyflurane, polymyxin B, vancomycin,
other nephrotoxic drugs (↑ nephrotoxicity).
Adverse Effects: Severe hypotension,
hypocalcermia, hypoglycemia, increase in
creatinine, pancreatitis, severe leukopenia,
anemia and thrombocytopenia. May increase
the QT interval with IV administration and cause
ventricular tachycardia. Severe hypoglycemic
episodes may result in later diabetes mellitus.
IV extravasation may cause severe skin necrosis
and IM injections can be severely painful and
should be avoided if possible. The following
tests should be carried out at regular intervals;
Daily blood urea nitrogen and serum creatinine,
blood glucose, complete blood count and
platelet count as well as every other day
bilirubin, alkaline phosphatase, AST (SGOT,
and ALT (SGPT). An electrocardiogram should
be done at regular intervals to calculate the

"Usual dose" assumes normal renal/hepatic function. * For renal insufficiency, give usual dose × 1 followed by maintenance dose per CrCl. For dialysis patients, dose the same as for CrCl < 10 mL/min and give supplemental (post-HD/PD dose) immediately after dialysis. CrCl = creatinine clearance; CVVH = continuous veno-venous hemofiltration; HD/PD = hemodialysis/peritoneal dialysis.

QT$_c$ interval. If creatinine starts to rise the dose should be cut back to 3 or 2 mg/kg. The medication should be held if hypoglycemia occurs and or if the QT$_c$ interval increases.

Allergic Potential: High

Safety in Pregnancy: C

Comments: Well absorbed IM, but painful. Administer IV slowly in D$_5$W over 1 hour, not saline/may be used at a dose of 300 mg aerosol q month to prevent aerosol pentamine. Caution should be used with inhalent pentamidine especially around pregnant employees as it can induce spontaneous abortion. Special attention should be made to the proper aerosolization of medication so that it is distributed evenly through the lung. Adverse effects with aerosolized pentamidine include chest pain, arrhythmias, dizziness, wheezing, coughing, dyspnea, headache, anorexia, nausea, diarrhea, rash, pharyngitis. **If PCP patient also has pulmonary TB, aerosolized pentamidine treatments may expose medical personnel to TB via droplet inhalation**. Nebulizer dose: Inhaled pentamidine isethionate (NebuPent) 300 mg monthly via Respirgard II nebulizer can be used for PCP prophylaxis. **Nebulized pentamidine less effective than IV/IM pentamidine and is not effective against extrapulmonary PCP**. Use with caution in renal disease. Subtle creatinine changes may be associated with severe toxicity.

Cerebrospinal Fluid Penetration: < 10%

REFERENCES:

Chan C, Montaner J, LeFebvre BA, et al. Atovaquone suspension compared with aerosolized pentamidine for prevention of Pneumocystis carinii pneumonia in human immunodeficiency virus infected subsets intolerant of trimethoprim or sulfamethoxazole. J Infect Dis 180:369–376, 1999.

Goa KL, Campoli-Richards DM. Pentamidine isethionate: A review of its antiprotozoal activity, pharmacokinetic properties and therapeutic use in Pneumocystis carinii pneumonia. Drugs 33:242–58, 1987.

Guerin PJ, Alar P, Sundar S, et al. Visceral leishmaniasis: current status of control, diagnosis, and treatment, and a proposed research and development agenda. Lancet Infect Dis 2:494–501, 2002.

Lionakis MS, Lewis RE, Samonis G, et al. Pentamidine is active in vitro against Fusarium species. Antimicrob Agents Chemother 47:3252–9, 2003.

Monk JP, Benfield P. Inhaled pentamidine: An overview of its pharmacological properties and a review of its therapeutic use in Pneumocystis carinii pneumonia. Drugs 39:741–56, 1990.

Rodriquez M, Fishman JA. Prevention of infection due to Pneumocystis spp. in human immunodeficiency virus-negative immunocompromised patients. Clin Microbiol Rev 17:770–82, 2004.

Sattler FR, Cowam R. Nielsen DM, et al. Trimethoprim-sulfamethoxazole compared with pentamidine for treatment of Pneumocystis carinii pneumonia in the acquired immunodeficiency syndrome. Ann Intern Med 109:280–7, 1988.

Website: www.pdr.net

Peramivir

Drug class: Neuroaminidase inhibitor.

Usual dose: 400 mg (IV) q24h or 10 mg/kg (IV) q24h, maximum dose 600 mg/day (IV) over 30 minutes.

Pharmacokinetic Parameters:

Peak serum level: 17–44 mcg/mL/13 mcg/mL

Bioavailability: not applicable

Excreted unchanged: no data

Serum half-life (normal/ESRD): 7–20 hrs/no data

Plasma protein binding: no data

Volume of distribution (V$_d$): no data

Primary Mode of Elimination: Renal

Dosage Adjustments*

"Usual dose" assumes normal renal/hepatic function. * For renal insufficiency, give usual dose × 1 followed by maintenance dose per CrCl. For dialysis patients, dose the same as for CrCl < 10 mL/min and give supplemental (post-HD/PD dose) immediately after dialysis. CrCl = creatinine clearance; CVVH = continuous veno-venous hemofiltration; HD/PD = hemodialysis/peritoneal dialysis.

CrCl > 49 mL/min	600 mg (IV) q24h
CrCl 31–49 mL/min	150 mg (IV) q24h
CrCl 10–30 mL/min	100 mg (IV) q24h
CrCl < 10 mL/min	15 mg (IV) q24h
Post-HD dose	15 mg (IV) q24h
Post-PD dose	15 mg (IV)
CVVH/CVVHD/CVVHDF dose	600 mg (IV) q24h
Moderate–severe hepatic insufficiency	No change

Drug Interactions: No data.

Adverse Effects: Diarrhea, nausea, vomiting, neutropenic fever, rare cause of anaphylaxis.

Allergic Potential: Low (do not use if severely allergic to other neuroaminidase inhibitors)

Safety in Pregnancy: No data

Comments: Emergency use authorization (EUA) for the investigational antiviral drug peramivir intravenous (IV) in certain adult and pediatric patients with confirmed or suspected H1N1 influenza infection who are admitted to a hospital. **IV peramivir is for hospitalized adult and pediatric patients for whom therapy with an IV drug is clinically appropriate, based on one or more of the following reasons: 1. the patient is not responding to either oral or inhaled antiviral therapy, or 2. when drug delivery by a route other than an intravenous route—eg., enteral (absorbed by the intestines) or 3. for adults only, when the clinician judges IV therapy is appropriate due to other circumstances**. To obtain peramivir go to www.cdc.gov/h1niflu/eua. Should be used within 72 of symptom onset. **Do not use if oseltamivir resistance**. Do not exceed 40 mg/minute infusion rate.

Highly active against swine influenza (H1N1).

Cerebrospinal Fluid Penetration: No data

REFERENCES:

Arya V, Carter WW, Robertson SM. The role of clinical pharmacology in supporting the emergency use authorization of an unapproved anti-influenza drug, peramivir. Clin Pharmacol Ther 88:587–589, 2010.

Bazan JA, Bauer KA, Hollister AS, et al. Peramivir pharmacokinetics in two critically ill adults with 2009 H1N1 influenza A concurrently receiving continuous renal replacement therapy. Pharacotherapy 30:1016–1020, 2010.

Castillo R, Holland LE, Bolz DA. Peramivir and its use in H1N1 influenza. Drugs Today (Barc) 46:399–408 2010.

Hernandez JE, Adiga R, Armstrong R, et al. Clinical experience in adults and children treated with intravenous peramivir for 2009 influenza A (H1N1) under an emergency IND program in the United States. Clin Infect Dis 52:695–706, 2011.

Kohno S, Kida H, Mizuguchi M, et al. Efficacy and safety of intravenous peramivir for treatment of seasonal influenza virus infection. Antimicrob Agents Chemother 54:4568–4574, 2010.

Kohno S, Kida H, Mizuguchi M, et al. Intravenous peramivir for treatment of influenza A and B virus infection in high-risk patients. Antimicrob Agents Chemother 55:2803–2812, 2011.

Mancuso CE, Gabay MP, Steinke LM, et al. Peramivir: an intravenous neuraminidase inhibitor for the treatment of 2009 H1N1 influenza. Ann Pharmacother 44:1240–1249, 2010.

Moss RB, Davey RT, Steigbigel RT, et al. Targeting pandemic influenza: a primer on influenza antivirals and drug resistance. J Antimicrob Chemother 65:1086–1093, 2010.

Nasu T, Ogawa D, Wada J, et al. Peramivir for severe influenza infection in a patient with diabetic nephropathy. Am J Respir Crit Care Med 182:1209–1210, 2010.

Nguyen HTm, Sheu TG, Mishin VP, et al. Assessment of pandemic and seasonal influenza A (H1N1) virus susceptibility to neuraminidase inhibitors in three

---

"Usual dose" assumes normal renal/hepatic function. * For renal insufficiency, give usual dose × 1 followed by maintenance dose per CrCl. For dialysis patients, dose the same as for CrCl < 10 mL/min and give supplemental (post-HD/PD dose) immediately after dialysis. CrCl = creatinine clearance; CVVH = continuous veno-venous hemofiltration; HD/PD = hemodialysis/peritoneal dialysis.

enzyme activity inhibition assays. Antimicrob Agents Chemother 54:3671–3677, 2010.

Thomas B, Hollister AS, Muczynski KA. Peramivir clearance in continuous renal replacement therapy. Hemodial Int 14:339–340, 2010.

Website: www.cdc.gov

Website: www.fda.gov

Piperacillin (Pipracil)

Drug Class: Anti-pseudomonal penicillin.
Usual Dose: 3 gm (IV) q4-6h (see comments).
Spectrum: (see *Susceptibility Profiles* pp. 186–190).
Resistance Potential: Low
Pharmacokinetic Parameters:
Peak serum level: 412 mcg/ml
Bioavailability: Not applicable
Excreted unchanged (urine): 50–70%
Serum half-life (normal/ESRD): 1/3 hrs
Plasma protein binding: 16%
Volume of distribution (V_d): 0.24 L/kg
Primary Mode of Elimination: Renal
Dosage Adjustments* (based on 4 gm q8h)

CrCl 20–50 mL/min	3 gm (IV) q8h
CrCl < 20 mL/min	3 gm (IV) q12h
Post–HD dose	1 gm (IV)
Post–PD dose	2 gm (IV)
CVVH/CVVHD/CVVHDF dose	3 gm (IV) q8h
Moderate or severe hepatic insufficiency	No change

Drug Interactions: Aminoglycosides (inactivation of piperacillin in renal failure); warfarin (↑ INR); oral contraceptives (↓ oral contraceptive effect); cefoxitin (↓ piperacillin effect).

Adverse Effects: Drug fever/rash, anaphylactic reactions (hypotension, laryngospasm, broncho-spasm), hives, serum sickness, leukopenia, hemolytic anemia, C. difficile diarrhea/colitis.
Allergic Potential: High
Safety in Pregnancy: B
Comments: 75% absorbed when given IM. Do not mix/administer with aminoglycosides. **Most active antipseudomonal penicillin against P. aeruginosa. Nosocomial pneumonia/P. aeruginosa dose:** 3 gm (IV) q4h. Meningeal dose = usual dose.
Cerebrospinal Fluid Penetration:
Non-Inflamed meninges = 1%
Inflamed meninges = 30%
Bile Penetration: 1000%
(also see *Antibiotic Pearls & Pitfalls* p. 509).

REFERENCES:
Donowitz GR, Mandell GL. Beta-lactam antibiotics. N Engl J Med 318:419–26 and 318:490–500, 1993.

Kim MK, Capitano B, Mattoes HM, et al. Pharmacokinetic and pharmacodynamic evaluation of two dosing regimens for piperacillin-susceptible organisms. Pharmacotherapy 22:569–77, 2002.

Peacock JE, Herrington DA, Wade JC, et al. Ciprofloxacin plus piperacillin compared with tobramycin plus piperacillin as empirical therapy in febrile neutropenic patients. A randomized, double-blind trial. Ann Intern Med 137:120, 2002.

Tan JS, File TM, Jr. Antipseudomonal penicillins. Med Clin North Am 79:679–93, 1995.

Website: www.pdr.net

Piperacillin/Tazobactam (Zosyn, Tazocin)

Drug Class: Anti-pseudomonal penicillin/ β-lactamase inhibitor.
Usual Dose: 3.375 gm (IV) q6h (see comments).

"Usual dose" assumes normal renal/hepatic function. * For renal insufficiency, give usual dose × 1 followed by maintenance dose per CrCl. For dialysis patients, dose the same as for CrCl < 10 mL/min and give supplemental (post-HD/PD dose) immediately after dialysis. CrCl = creatinine clearance; CVVH = continuous veno-venous hemofiltration; HD/PD = hemodialysis/peritoneal dialysis.

Spectrum: (see *Susceptibility Profiles* pp. 186–190).

Resistance Potential: Low

Pharmacokinetic Parameters:

Peak serum level: 298/34 mcg/ml
Bioavailability: Not applicable
Excreted unchanged (urine): 60/80%
Serum half-life (normal/ESRD): [1.5/8] / [1/7] hrs
Plasma protein binding: 30/30%
Volume of distribution (V_d): 0.3/0.21 L/kg

Primary Mode of Elimination: Renal

Dosage Adjustments* (also see comments)

CrCl 20–40 mL/min	2.25 gm (IV) q6h 3.375 (IV) q6h for NP
CrCl < 20 mL/min	2.25 gm (IV) q8h 2.25 (IV) q6h for NP
CrCl < 10 mL/min	2.25 gm (IV) q8h
Post–HD dose	0.75 gm (IV)
Post–PD dose	None
CVVH/CVVHD/ CVVHDF dose	3.375 gm (IV) q6h
Moderate—severe hepatic insufficiency	No change

Drug Interactions: Aminoglycosides (↓ aminoglycoside levels); vecuronium (↑ vecuronium effect); probenecid (↑ piperacillin/tazobactam levels); methotrexate (↑ methotrexate levels).

Adverse Effects: Drug fever/rash, eosinophilia, ↓/↑ platelets, leukopenia (with prolonged use > 21 days), ↑ PT/PTT, mild transient ↑ SGOT/SGPT, insomnia, nausea, headache, constipation, hypertension, hemolytic anemia, C. difficile diarrhea/colitis.

Allergic Potential: High

Safety in Pregnancy: B

Comments: For P. aeruginosa/nosocomial pneumonia (normal CrCl) use 4.5 g (IV) q6h *plus* amikacin 1 g (IV) q24h. P. aeruginosa/ nosocomial pneumonia doses (↑ CrCl):

    CrCl > 40 mL/min: 4.5 gm (IV) q6h.
    CrCl 20–40 mL/min: 3.375 gm (IV) q6h.
    CrCl < 20 mL/min: 2.25 gm (IV) q6h.

Hemodialysis (HD) doses: 2.25 gm (IV) q8h; give 0.75 gm (IV) Post–HD on HD days.

Cerebrospinal Fluid Penetration:

Non-Inflamed meninges = 1%
Inflamed meninges = 30%

Bile Penetration: 6000%

(also see *Antibiotic Pearls & Pitfalls* pp. 509, 512).

REFERENCES:

Bauer SR, Salem C, Connor MJ Jr, et al. Pharmacokinetics and pharmacodynamics of piperacillin-tazobactam in 42 patients treated with concomitant CRRT. Clin J Am Soc Nephrol 7:452–457, 2012.

Gin A, Dilay L, Karlowsky JA, et al. Piperacillin-tazobactam: a beta-lactam/beta-lactamase inhibitor combination. Expert Rev Anti Infect Ther 5:365–383, 2007.

Hayashi Y, Roberts JA, Paterson DL, et al. Pharmacokinetic evaluation of piperacillin-tazobactam. Expert Opin Drug Metab Toxicol 6:1017–1031, 2010.

Jones RN, Stilwell MG, Rhomberg PR, et al. Antipseudomonal activity of piperacillin/tazobactam: more than a decade of experience from the SENTRY Antimicrobial Surveillance Program (1997–2007). Diagn Microbiol Infect Dis 65:331–334, 2009.

Kang CL, Park SY, Chung DR, et al. Piperacillin-tazobactam asan initial empirical therapy of bacteremia caused by extended-spectrum ß-lactamase-producing Escherichia coli and Klebsiella pneumoniae. J Infect 64:533–534, 2012.

Lau WK, Mercer D, Itani KM, et al. Randomized, open-label, comparative study of piperacillin-tazobactam administered by continuous infusion versus intermittent infusion for treatment of hospitalized

---

"Usual dose" assumes normal renal/hepatic function. * For renal insufficiency, give usual dose × 1 followed by maintenance dose per CrCl. For dialysis patients, dose the same as for CrCl < 10 mL/min and give supplemental (post-HD/PD dose) immediately after dialysis. CrCl = creatinine clearance; CVVH = continuous veno-venous hemofiltration; HD/PD = hemodialysis/peritoneal dialysis.

patients with complicated intra-abdominal infection. Antimicrob Agents and Chemother 50:3556–61, 2006.

Mah GT, Mabasa VH, Chow I, et al. Evaluating outcomes associated with alternative dosing strategies for piperacillin/tazobactam: a qualitative systematic review. Ann Pharmacother 46:265–267, 2012.

Mikulska M, Furfaro E, Del Bono V, et al. Piperacillin/tazobactam seems to be no longer responsible for false-positive results of the galactomannan assay. J Antimicrob Chemother 67:1746–1748, 2012.

Mattoes HM, Capitano B, Kim MK, et al. Comparative pharmacokinetic and pharmacodynamic profile of piperacillin/tazobactam 3.375 G Q4H and 4.5 G Q6H. Chemotherapy 458:59–63, 2002.

Minnaganti VR, Cunha BA. Piperacillin/tazobactam. Antibiotics for Clinicians 3:101–8, 1999.

Saltoglu N, Dalkiran A, Tetiker T, et al. Piperacillin/tazobactam versus imipenem/cilastatin for severe diabetic foot infections: a prospective, randomized clinical trial in a university hospital. Clin Microbiol Infect 16:1252–1257, 2010.

Yamagishi Y, Terada M, Ohki E, et al. Investigation of the clinical breakpoints of piperacillin-tazobactam against infections caused by Pseudomonas aeruginosa. J Infect Chemother 18:127–129, 2012.

Website: www.zosyn.com

Polymyxin B

Drug Class: Cell membrane-altering antibiotic.
Usual Dose: 1–1.25 mg/kg (IV) q12h (1 mg = 10,000 units) (see comments).
Spectrum: (see *Susceptibility Profiles* pp. 198–202).
Pharmacokinetic Parameters:
Peak serum level: 8 mcg/ml
Bioavailability: Not applicable
Excreted unchanged (urine): 60%
Serum half-life (normal/ESRD): 6/48 hrs
Plasma protein binding: < 10%
Volume of distribution (V_d): No data
Primary Mode of Elimination: Renal

Dosage Adjustments*

CrCl 20–50 mL/min	1 mg/kg (IV) q12h
CrCl 5–20 mL/min	0.5 mg/kg (IV) q12h
CrCl < 5 mL/min	0.2 mg/kg (IV) q12h
Post–HD/PD dose	No information
CVVH/CVVHD/ CVVHDF dose	0.5 mg/kg (IV) q12h
Moderate—severe hepatic insufficiency	No change

Drug Interactions: Amphotericin B, amikacin, gentamicin, tobramycin, vancomycin (↑ nephrotoxicity).
Adverse Effects: Renal failure. Neurotoxicity associated with very prolonged/high serum levels; neuromuscular blockade potential with renal failure/neuromuscular disorders.
Resistance Potential: Low
Allergic Potential: Low
Safety in Pregnancy: B
Comments: Inhibits endotoxin release from gram-negative bacilli. Avoid intraperitoneal infusion due to risk of neuromuscular blockade. Increased risk of reversible non-oliguric renal failure (ATN) when used with other nephrotoxic drugs. No ototoxic potential. May be given IM with procaine, but painful. **Nebulizer dose for multidrug resistant P. aeruginosa in cystic fibrosis/bronchiectasis:** 80 mg in saline via aerosol/nebulizer q8h (for recurrent infection use 160 mg). **Intrathecal (IT) polymyxin B dose:** 5 mg (50,000 u) q24h × 3 days, then q48h × 2 weeks. Dissolve 50 mg (500,000 u) into 10 ml for IT administration.
Cerebrospinal Fluid Penetration: < 10% (also see *Antibiotic Pearls & Pitfalls* p. 520).

"Usual dose" assumes normal renal/hepatic function. * For renal insufficiency, give usual dose × 1 followed by maintenance dose per CrCl. For dialysis patients, dose the same as for CrCl < 10 mL/min and give supplemental (post-HD/PD dose) immediately after dialysis. CrCl = creatinine clearance; CVVH = continuous veno-venous hemofiltration; HD/PD = hemodialysis/peritoneal dialysis.

REFERENCES:

Cavaillon JM. Plymyxin B for endotoxin removal in sepsis. Lancet Infect Dis 11:426–7, 2011.

Falagas ME, Kasiakou SK. Colistin: the revival of polymyxins for the management of multidrug-resistant gram-negative bacterial infections. Clin Infect Dis 40:1333–41, 2005.

Kunin CM. The Pharmacokinetics of Polymyxin B are Dependent on Binding and Release from Deep-Tissue Compartments. Clin Infect Dis 48:842–844, 2009.

Kwa AL, Abdelraouf K, Low JG, et al. Pharmacokinetics of polymyxin B in a patient with renal insufficiency: a case report. Clin Infect Dis 52:1280–1, 2011.

Li J, Nation RL. Old Polymyxins are Back: Is Resistance Close? Clin Infect Disease 43:663–64, 2006.

Menzies D, Minnaganti VR, Cunha BA. Polymyxin B. Antibiotics for Clinicians 4:33–40, 2000.

Pankey GA, Ashcraft DS. Detection if synergy using the combination of polymyxin B with either meropenem or rifampin against carbapenemase-producing Klebsiella pneumoniae. Diagn Microbiol Infect Dis 70:561–4, 2011.

Parchuri S, Mohan S, Young S, Cunha BA. Chronic ambulatory peritoneal dialysis associated peritonitis ESBL producing Klebsiella pneumoniae successfully treated with polymyxin B. Heart & Lung 34:360, 2005.

Satlin MJ, Kubin CJ, Blumenthal JS, et al. Comparative effectiveness of aminoglycosides, polymyxin B, and tigecycline for clearance of carbapenem-resistant Klebsiella pneumoniae from urine. Antimicrob Agents Chemother 55:5893–9, 2011.

Segal-Maurer S, Mariano N, Qavi A, et al. Successful treatment of ceftazidime-resistant Klebsiella pneumoniae ventriculitis with intravenous meropenem and intraventricular polymyxin B: Case report and review. Clin Infect Dis 28:1134–8, 1999.

Wareham DW, Bean DC. In vitro activities of polymyxin B, imipenem and rifampin against multidrug-resistant Acinetobacter baumannii. Antimicrob Agents Chemother 50:825–26, 2006.

Posaconazole (Noxafil)

Drug Class: Antifungal (triazole).
Usual Dose: <u>Prophylaxis of invasive Aspergillus and Candida infections in high-risk patients:</u>[†]
200 mg (PO) q8h; <u>oropharyngeal candidiasis</u>; 100 mg (PO) q12h × 1 day, then 100 mg (PO) q24h × 13 days; for fluconazole- and/ or itraconazole-resistant strains, use 400 mg (PO) q12h with duration of therapy based on underlying condition and clinical response.

Pharmacokinetic Parameters:
Peak serum level: 3 mcg/mL
Bioavailability: Absorption is ↑ 2–6-fold by food
Excreted unchanged (urine): < 1%
Excreted unchanged (feces): 66%
Serum half-life (normal/ESRD): 35/35 hrs
Plasma protein binding: 98.2%
Volume of distribution (V_d): 1774 L
Primary Mode of Elimination: Hepatic
Dosage Adjustments*

CrCl < 10 mL/min	No change
Post-HD dose	None
Post-PD dose	None
CVVH/CVVHD/ CVVHDF dose	None
Moderate—severe hepatic insufficiency	No change

Drug Interactions: Posaconazole is metabolized by hepatic glucuronidation. Inducers (e.g., rifampin, phenytoin) may alter disposition. Amiodarone, rifabutin, phenytoin, cimetidine (↓ posaconazole levels 50%). Posaconazole inhibits hepatic CYP3A4 and can increase levels of drugs metabolized by this enzyme. QT prolonging drugs terfenadine, astemizole, cisapride, pimozide, halofantrine, quinidine (↑ interacting drug levels, ↑ risk of cardiac arrhythmias); ergot (↑ ergot levels); statins (↑ statin levels and risk of rhabdomyolysis); vinca alkaloids (↑ vinca alkaloid levels and risk of neurotoxicity); cyclosporine, tacrolimus, sirolimus, midazolam and other benzodiazepines metabolized by CYP3A4,

---

"Usual dose" assumes normal renal/hepatic function. * For renal insufficiency, give usual dose × 1 followed by maintenance dose per CrCl. For dialysis patients, dose the same as for CrCl < 10 mL/min and give supplemental (post-HD/PD dose) immediately after dialysis. CrCl = creatinine clearance; CVVH = continuous veno-venous hemofiltration; HD/PD = hemodialysis/peritoneal dialysis.
† (graft-vs-host disease, prolonged neutropenia from chemotherapy) ≥ 13 years of age.

calcium channel blockers metabolized by CYP3A4 (diltiazem, verapamil, nifedipine, nisoldipine); digoxin, sulfonylureas, ritonavir, indinavir (↑ interacting drug levels); rifampin, omperazole (↓ posaconazole levels).

Adverse Effects: Nausea, vomiting, diarrhea, headache, ↑ SGOT/SGPT; ↑ QTc.

Allergic Potential: Low

Safety in Pregnancy: C

Comments: Available as a 40 mg/mL oral suspension. Take with a meal or 240 mL of a nutritional supplement. ***Highly active against Candida albicans, most non-albicans Candida, Aspergillus, Crypotococcus, Histoplasmosis, Blastomycocis, Sporotrichosis, Paracoccidiomycosis. Some activity against Coccidiomycosis, Fusarium and C. glabrata. No activity against Pseudollescheria/ Scedosporium or Mucor***. Blood levels not increased with higher dosages.

Cerebrospinal Fluid Penetration: > 10%

Bile Penetration: 76%

REFERENCES:

Alffenaar JWC, van Assen S, van der Werf TS. Omeprazole significantly reduces poconazole serum through level. Clin Infect Dis 48:839–840, 2009.

Bruggemann RJM, Alffenaar JWC, Blijlevens NMA, et al. Clinical relevance of the pharmoacokinetic interactions of azole antifungal drugs with coadministered agents. Clin Infect Dis 48: 1441–1458, 2009.

Cornely OA Helfgott D, Langston A, et al. Pharmacokinetics of different dosing strategies of oral posaconazole in patients with compromised gastrointestinal function and who are at high risk for invasive fungal infection. Antimicrob Agents Chemother 56:2652–8, 2012.

Cornely OA, Maertens J, Winston DJ, et al. Posaconazole vs. fluconazole or itraconazole prophylaxis in patients with neutropenia. N Engl J Med 356:348–59, 2007.

Courtney R, Sansone A, Smith W, et al. Posaconazole pharmacokinetics, safety, and tolerability in subjects with varying degrees of chronic renal disease. J Clin Pharmacol 45:185–192, 2005.

Dodds Ashley ES, Alexander BD. Posaconazole. Drugs Today 41:393–400, 2005.

Ezzet F, Wexler D, Courtney R, et al. Oral bioavailability of posaconazole in fasted healthy subjects- comparison between three regimens and basis for clinical dosage recommendations. Clin Pharmacokinet 44:211–220, 2005.

Felton TW, Baxter C, Moore CB, et al. Efficacy and safety of posaconazole for chronic pulmonary aspergillosis. Clin Infect Dis 51:1383–1391, 2010.

Girmenia C, Frustaci AM, Gentile G, et al. Posaconazole prophylaxis during front-line chemotherapy of acute myeloid leukemia: a single-center real-life experience. Haematologica 97:560–7, 2012.

Green MR, Woolery JE. Optimising absorption of posaconazole. Mycoses 54:775–779, 2011.

Greenberg RN, Mullane K, van Burik JA, et al. Posaconazole as salvage therapy for zygomycosis. Antimicrob Agents Chemother 50:126–33, 2006.

Gubbins PO, Krishna G, Sansone-Parsons A, et al. Pharmacokinetics and safety of oral posaconazole in neutropenic stem cell transplant recipients. Antimicrob Agents Chemother 50:1993–9, 2006.

Herbrecht R, Nivoix Y, Fohrer C, et al. Management of systemic fungal infections: alternatives to itraconazole. J Antimicrob Chemother 56:139–148, 2005.

Hoenigl M, Raggam RB, Salzer HJ, et al. Posaconazole plasma concentrations and invasive mould infections in patients with haematological malignancies. Int J Antimicrob Agents 39:510–3, 2012.

Hohmann C, Kang EM, Jancel T: Rifampin and posaconazole coadministration leads to decreased serum posaconazole concentrations. Clin Infect Dis 50:939–940, 2010.

Howard SJ, Lestner JM, Sharp A, et al. Pharmacokinetics and pharmacodynamics of posaconazole for invasive pulmonary aspergillosis: clinical implications for antifungal therapy. J Infect Dis 203:1324–1332, 2011.

Karthaus M. Prophylaxis and treatment of invasive aspergillosis and voriconazole, posaconazole, and caspofungin: review of the literature. Eur J Med Res 16:145–152, 2011.

Keating GM, Posaconazole. Drugs 65:1553–69, 2005.

Kim MM, Vikram HR, Kusne S, et al. Treatment of refractory coccidioidomycosis with voriconazole or posaconazole. Clin Infect Dis, 53:1060–6, 2011.

Kontoyiannis DP, Lewis RE. Posaconazole prophylaxis in hematologic cancer. N Engl J Med 24:2214–2215, 2007.

Lipp HP. Posaconazole: clinical pharmacokinetics and drug interactions. Mycoses 54:32–38, 2011.

Miceli MH, Diaz JA, Lee SA. Emerging opportunistic yeast infections. Lancet Infectious Diseases 11: 142–151, 2011.

Mehta AK, Langston AA. Use of posaconazole in the treatment of invasive fungal infections. Expert Rec Hematol 2:619–630, 2009.

Pound MW, Townsend ML, Dimondi V, et al. Overview of treatment options for invasive fungal infections. Med Mycol 49:561–580, 2011.

Raad II, Graybill JR, Bustamante AB, et al. Safety of long-term oral posaconazole use in the treatment of refractory invasive fungal infections. Clin Infect Dis 42:1726–34, 2006.

Raad II, Hachem RY, Herbrecht R, et al. Posaconazole as salvage treatment for invasive fusariosis in patients with underlying hematologic malignancy and other conditions. Clin Infect Dis 42:1398–403, 2006.

Restrepo A, Tobon A, Clark B, et al. Salvage treatment of histoplasmosis with posaconazole. Salvage treatment of histoplasmosis with posaconazole. J Infect 54:319–327, 2007.

Ullmann AJ, Cornely OA, Burchardt A, et al. Pharmacokinetics, safety, and efficacy of posaconazole in patients with persistent febrile neutropenia or refractory invasive fungal infection. Antimicrob Agents Chemother 50:658–66, 2006.

Ullmann AJ, Lipton JH, Vesole DH, et al. Posaconazole or fluconazole for prophylaxis in severe graft-versus-host disease. N Engl J Med 356:335–47, 2007.

Walsh TJ, Raad I, Patterson TF, et al. Treatment of invasive Aspergillosis with posaconazole in patients who are refractory to or intolerant of conventional therapy: an externally controlled trial. Clin Infect Dis 44:2–12, 2007.

Website: www.noxafil.com

Primaquine

Drug Class: Antimalarial/Anti-PCP.

Usual Dose: **Antimalarial dose:** 15 mg (base 26.3 mg) (PO) q24h. **PCP dose:** 15–30 mg (PO) q24h plus clindamycin 600 mg (IV) or 300 mg (PO) q6h.

Pharmacokinetic Parameters:

Peak serum level: 30–100 mcg/ml
Bioavailability: 90%
Excreted unchanged (urine): 3.6%
Serum half-life (normal/ESRD): 3.7–9.6/3.7–9.6 hrs
Plasma protein binding: 75%
Volume of distribution (V_d): No data

Primary Mode of Elimination: Hepatic

Dosage Adjustments*

CrCl < 80 mL/min	No change
Post–HD/Post–PD dose	None
CVVH/CVVHD/ CVVHDF dose	No change
Hepatic insufficiency	No change

Drug Interactions: Avoid in patients receiving bone marrow suppressive drugs

---

"Usual dose" assumes normal renal/hepatic function. * For renal insufficiency, give usual dose × 1 followed by maintenance dose per CrCl. For dialysis patients, dose the same as for CrCl < 10 mL/min and give supplemental (post-HD/PD dose) immediately after dialysis. CrCl = creatinine clearance; CVVH = continuous veno-venous hemofiltration; HD/PD = hemodialysis/peritoneal dialysis.

(↑ risk of agran-ulocytosis), alcohol (↑ GI side effects), quinacrine (↑ primaquine levels/toxicity).

Adverse Effects: Nausea/vomiting, headache, abdominal pain, leukopenia (dose dependent), agranulocytosis, pruritus. Hemolytic anemia in G6PD deficiency; methemoglobinemia in NADH reductase deficiency.

Allergic Potential: Low

Safety in Pregnancy: D

Comments: Take with food to ↓ GI side effects. Use with caution in G6PD deficiency. Use with caution in NADH reductase deficiency.

Cerebrospinal Fluid Penetration: No data

REFERENCES:

Baird JK. Effectiveness of antimalarial drugs. N Engl J Med 352:1565–77, 2005.

Chen LH, Keystone JS. New strategies for the prevention of malaria in travelers. Infect Dis Clin North Am 19:185–210, 2005.

Korraa H, Saadeh C. Options in the management of pneumonia caused by Pneumocystis carinii in patients with acquired immune deficiency syndrome and intolerance to trimethoprim/sulfamethoxazole. South Med J 89:272–7, 1996.

Safrin S, Finkelstein DM, Feinberg J, et al. Comparison of three regimens for treatment of mild to moderate Pneumocystis carinii pneumonia in patients with AIDS. A double-blind randomized trial of oral TMP–SMX, dapsone-TMP & clinda-primaquine. Ann Intern Med 124:792–802, 1996.

Warren E, George S, You J, Kazanjian P. Advances in the treatment and prophylaxis of Pneumocystis carinii pneumonia. Pharmacotherapy 17:900–16, 1997.

Pyrazinamide (PZA)

Drug Class: Anti-TB drug.
Usual Dose: 25 mg/kg (PO) q24h (max. 2 gm) (see comments).

Pharmacokinetic Parameters:
Peak serum level: 30–50 mcg/ml
Bioavailability: 90%
Excreted unchanged (urine): 10%
Serum half-life (normal/ESRD): 9/26 hrs
Plasma protein binding: 10%
Volume of distribution (V_d): 0.9 L/kg

Primary Mode of Elimination: Hepatic

Dosage Adjustments*

CrCl < 30 mL/min	25 mg/kg (PO) 3×/week
Post–HD dose	25 mg/kg (PO) or 1 gm (PO)
Post–PD dose	None
CVVH/CVVHD/CVVHDF dose	25 mg/kg (PO) 3×/week
Moderate hepatic insufficiency	Use with caution
Severe hepatic insufficiency	Avoid

Drug Interactions: INH, rifabutin, rifampin (may ↑ risk of hepatotoxicity).

Adverse Effects: Drug fever/rash, malaise, nausea, vomiting, anorexia, ↑ SGOT/SGPT, ↑ uric acid, sideroblastic anemia.

Allergic Potential: Low

Safety in Pregnancy: C

Comments: Avoid in patients with gout (may precipitate acute attacks). **TB D.O.T. dose:** 4 gm (PO) 2x/week or 3 gm (PO) 3x/week. Meningeal dose = usual dose.

Cerebrospinal Fluid Penetration: 100%

REFERENCES:

Ahn C, Oh KH, Kim K, et al. Effect of peritoneal dialysis on plasma and peritoneal fluid concentrations of isoniazid, pyrazinamide, and rifampin. Perit Dial Int 23:362–7, 2003.

"Usual dose" assumes normal renal/hepatic function. * For renal insufficiency, give usual dose × 1 followed by maintenance dose per CrCl. For dialysis patients, dose the same as for CrCl < 10 mL/min and give supplemental (post-HD/PD dose) immediately after dialysis. CrCl = creatinine clearance; CVVH = continuous veno-venous hemofiltration; HD/PD = hemodialysis/peritoneal dialysis.

Davidson PT, Le HQ. Drug treatment of tuberculosis 1992. Drugs 43:651–73, 1992.

[No authors listed.] Drugs for tuberculosis. Med Lett Drugs Ther 35:99–101, 1993.

Furin J, Nardell EA. Multidrug-resistant tuberculosis: An update on the best regimens. J Respir Dis 27:172–82, 2006.

Iseman MD. Treatment of multidrug-resistant tuberculosis. N Engl J Med 329:784–91, 1993.

Ijaz K, McElroy PD, Navin TR. Short course rifampin and pyrazinamide compared with isoniazid for latent tuberculosis infection: a cost-effectiveness analysis based on a multicenter clinical trial. Clin Infect Dis 39:289, 2004.

McIllerson H, Wash P, Burger A, et al. Determinants of rifampin, isoniazid, pyrazinamide and ethambutol pharmacokinetics in a cohort of tuberculosis patients. Antimicrob Agents Chemother 50:1170–77, 2006.

Schlossberg D: An approach to drug-induced liver injury during tuberculosis therapy. Infect Dis Clin Pract 18:107–108, 2010.

Van Scoy RE, Wilkowske CJ. Antituberculous agents. Mayo Clin Proc 67:179–87, 1992.

Pyrimethamine (Daraprim)

Drug Class: Antiparasitic.
Usual Dose: 75 mg (PO) q24h (see comments).
Pharmacokinetic Parameters:
Peak serum level: 0.4 mcg/ml
Bioavailability: 90%
Excreted unchanged (urine): 25%
Serum half-life (normal/ESRD): 96/96 hrs
Plasma protein binding: 87%
Volume of distribution (V_d): 2.5 L/kg
Primary Mode of Elimination: Hepatic
Dosage Adjustments*

CrCl < 10 mL/min	Use with caution
Post–HD dose	None
Post–PD dose	25 mg (PO)

CVVH/CVVHD/ CVVHDF dose	No change
Moderate hepatic insufficiency	No change
Severe hepatic insufficiency	Use with caution

Drug Interactions: Folic acid (↓ pyrimethamine effect); lorazepam (↑ risk of hepatotoxicity); sulfamethoxazole, trimethoprim, TMP–SMX (↑ risk of thrombocytopenia, anemia, leukopenia).
Adverse Effects: Megaloblastic anemia, leukopenia, thrombocytopenia, ataxia, tremors, seizures.
Allergic Potential: Low
Safety in Pregnancy: C
Comments: Antacids decrease absorption.
Toxoplasmosis dose: 200 mg (PO) × 1 dose, then 50–75 mg/kg (PO) q24h (with folinic acid 20 mg PO q24h plus either sulfadiazine or clindamycin).
Cerebrospinal Fluid Penetration: 10–25%

REFERENCES:

[No authors listed.] Drugs for Parasitic Infections. Med Lett Drugs Ther 40: 1–12, 2000.

Lemnge MM, Ali AS, Malecela EK, et al. Therapeutic efficacy of sulfadoxine pyrimethamine and amodiaquine among children with uncomplicated Plasmodium falciparum malaria in Zanzibar, Tanzania. Am. J. Trop. Med Hyg 73:681–5, 2005.

Podzamczer D, Salazar A, Jiminez J, et al. Intermittent trimethoprim-sulfamethoxazole compared with dapsone-pyrimethamine for the simultaneous primary prophylaxis of Pneumocystis pneumonia and toxoplasmosis in patients infected with HIV. Ann Intern Med 122:755–61, 1995.

Porter SB, Sande MA. Toxoplasmosis of the central nervous system in the acquired-immunodeficiency syndrome. N Engl J Med 327:1643–8, 1992.

Website: www.pdr.net

"Usual dose" assumes normal renal/hepatic function. * For renal insufficiency, give usual dose × 1 followed by maintenance dose per CrCl. For dialysis patients, dose the same as for CrCl < 10 mL/min and give supplemental (post-HD/PD dose) immediately after dialysis. CrCl = creatinine clearance; CVVH = continuous veno-venous hemofiltration; HD/PD = hemodialysis/peritoneal dialysis.

Quinine sulfate

Drug Class: Antimalarial.
Usual Dose: 650 mg (PO) q8h (see comments).
Pharmacokinetic Parameters:
Peak serum level: 3.8 mcg/ml
Bioavailability: 80%
Excreted unchanged (urine): 5%
Serum half-life (normal/ESRD): 7/14 hrs
Plasma protein binding: 95%
Volume of distribution (V_d): 3 L/kg
Primary Mode of Elimination: Renal/hepatic
Dosage Adjustments*

CrCl 10–50 mL/min	650 mg (PO) q12h
CrCl < 10 mL/min	650 mg (PO) q24h
Post–HD dose	None
Post–PD dose	650 mg (PO)
CVVH/CVVHD/ CVVHDF dose	650 mg (PO) q24h
Mild-moderate hepatic insufficiency	No change
Severe hepatic insufficiency	325 mg (PO) q12h; use caution

Drug Interactions: Amiodarone, aluminum-based antacids (↓ quinidine absorption); astemizole, cisapride, terfenadine (↑ interacting drug levels, torsade de pointes; avoid); cimetidine, ritonavir (↑ quinidine toxicity: headache, deafness, blindness, tachycardia); cyclosporine (↓ cyclosporine levels); digoxin (↑ digoxin levels); dofetilide, flecainide (arrhythmias); mefloquine (seizures, may ↑ QT interval, torsade de pointes, cardiac arrest, ↓ mefloquine efficacy); metformin (↑ risk of lactic acidosis); pancuronium, succinylcholine, tubocurarine (neuromuscular blockade); warfarin (↑ INR).

Adverse Effects: Drug fever/rash, ↑ QT_c interval, arrhythmias, drug-induced SLE, lightheadedness, diarrhea, abdominal discomfort, nausea, vomiting, cinchonism with chronic use. Avoid in patients with G6PD deficiency.
Allergic Potential: High
Safety in Pregnancy: C
Comments: PO malaria dose: 650 mg (PO) q8h (*plus doxycycline* 100 mg PO q12h) × 3–7 days). IV malaria dose: quinine hydrochloride 600 mg (IV) q8h × 3–7 days, or quinidine gluconate 10 mg/kg (IV) × 1 dose (infuse over 1–2 hours) then 0.02 mg/kg/min (IV) × 72 hours or until parasitemia < 1%.
Cerebrospinal Fluid Penetration: 2–5%

REFERENCES:
Corpelet C, Vacher P, Coudor F, et al. Role of quinine in life-threatening Babesia divergens infection successfully treated with clindamycin. Eur J Clin Microbiol Infect Dis 24:74–75, 2005.
Croft AM, Herxheimer A. Tolerability of antimalaria drugs. Clin Infect Dis 34:1278; discussion 1278–9, 2002. Drugs for Parasitic Infections. Med Letter. March, 2000.
Panisko DM, Keystone JS. Treatment of malaria. Drugs 39:160–89, 1990.
Wyler DJ, Malaria: Overview and update. Clin Infect Dis 16:449–56, 1993.

Quinupristin/dalfopristin (Synercid)

Drug Class: Streptogramin.
Usual Dose: 7.5 mg/kg (IV) q8h.
Spectrum: (see *Susceptibility Profiles* pp. 198–202).
Resistance Potential: Low
Pharmacokinetic Parameters:
Peak serum level: 3.2/8 mcg/ml

"Usual dose" assumes normal renal/hepatic function. * For renal insufficiency, give usual dose × 1 followed by maintenance dose per CrCl. For dialysis patients, dose the same as for CrCl < 10 mL/min and give supplemental (post-HD/PD dose) immediately after dialysis. CrCl = creatinine clearance; CVVH = continuous veno-venous hemofiltration; HD/PD = hemodialysis/peritoneal dialysis.

Bioavailability: Not applicable
Excreted unchanged: 20% (urine); 80% (feces)
Serum half-life (normal/ESRD): [3.1/1]/[3.1/1] hrs
Plasma protein binding: 55/15%
Volume of distribution (V_d): 0.45/0.24 L/kg
Primary Mode of Elimination: Hepatic
Dosage Adjustments*

CrCl < 10 mL/min	No change
Post–HD dose	None
Post–PD dose	None
CVVH/CVVHD/CVVHDF dose	No change
Moderate hepatic insufficiency	No change
Severe hepatic insufficiency	Use with caution

Drug Interactions: Amiodarone, amlodipine (↑ amlodipine toxicity); astemizole, cisapride (may ↑ QT interval, torsades de pointes); carbamazepine (↑ carbamazepine toxicity: ataxia, nystagmus, diplopia, headache, seizures); cyclosporine, delavirdine, indinavir, nevirapine (↑ interacting drug levels); diazepam, midazolam (↑ interacting drug effect); diltiazem, felodipine, isradipine (↑ interacting drug toxicity: dizziness, hypotension, headache, flushing); disopyramide (↑ disopyramide toxicity: arrhythmias, hypotension, syncope); docetaxel (↑ interacting drug toxicity: neutropenia, anemia, neuropathy); lidocaine (↑ lidocaine toxicity: neurotoxicity, arrhythmias, seizures); methylprednisolone (↑ methylprednisolone toxicity: myopathy, diabetes mellitus, cushing's syndrome); nicardipine, nifedipine, nimodipine (↑ interacting drug toxicity: dizziness,

hypotension, flushing, headache); statins (↑ risk of rhabdomyolysis).
Adverse Effects: Pain, inflammation, and swelling at infusion site (dose related), severe/prolonged myalgias, hyperbilirubinemia. Hepatic insufficiency increases concentration (AUC) of metabolites by 180%/50%.
Allergic Potential: Low
Safety in Pregnancy: B
Comments: Administer in D_5W or sterile water, not in saline. Requires central IV line for administration. ***Not effective against E. faecalis (VSE). May be useful for daptomycin resistant MSSA/MRSA infections.***
Cerebrospinal Fluid Penetration: < 10% (also see ***Antibiotic Pearls & Pitfalls*** p. 518).

REFERENCES:
Blondeau JM, Sanche Se. Quinupristin/dalfopristin. Expert Opin Pharmacother 3:1341–64, 2002.
Bouza E. New therapeutic choices for infections caused by methicillin-resistant Staphylococcus aureus. Clin Microbiol Infect Dis 15:44–52, 2009.
Bryson HM, Spencer CM. Quinupristin/dalfopristin. Drugs 52:406–15, 1996.
Chant C, Ryback MH. Quinupristin/dalfopristin (RP 59500): A new streptogramin antibiotic. Ann Pharmacother 29:1022–7, 1995.
Goff DA, Sierawski SJ. Clinical experience of quinupristin-dalfopristin for the treatment of antimicrobial-resistant gram-positive infections. Pharmacotherapy 22:748–58, 2002.
Griswold MW, Lomaestro BM, Briceland LL. Quinupristin-dalfopristin (RP 59500): An injectable streptogramin combination. Am J Health Syst Pharm 53:2045–53, 1996.
Kim MK, Nicolau DP, Nightingale CH, et al. Quinupristin/dalfopristin: A treatment option for vancomycin-resistant enterococci. Conn Med 64:209–12, 2000.
Klastersky J. Role of quinupristin/dalfopristin in the treatment of Gram-positive nosocomial infections in haematological or oncological patients. Cancer Treat Rev 29:431–40, 2003.

"Usual dose" assumes normal renal/hepatic function. * For renal insufficiency, give usual dose × 1 followed by maintenance dose per CrCl. For dialysis patients, dose the same as for CrCl < 10 mL/min and give supplemental (post-HD/PD dose) immediately after dialysis. CrCl = creatinine clearance; CVVH = continuous veno-venous hemofiltration; HD/PD = hemodialysis/peritoneal dialysis.

Nadler H, Dowzicky MJ, Feger C, et al. Quinupristin/
  dalfopristin: A novel selective-spectrum antibiotic
  for the treatment of multi-resistant and other
  gram-positive pathogens. Clin Microbiol Newslett
  21:103–12, 1999.

Nailor MD, Sobel JD. Antibiotics for gram-positive
  bacterial infection: vancomycin, teicoplanin,
  quinupristin/dalfopristin, oxazolidinones, daptomycin,
  telavancin, and ceftaroline fosamil. Med Clin North
  Am 95:723–742, 2011.

Scotton PG, Rigoli R, Vaglia A. Combination of quinupristin/
  dalfopristin and glycopeptide in severe methicillin-
  resistant staphylococcal infections failing previous
  glycopeptide regimen. Infection 30:161–3, 2002.

Website: www.synercid.com

Raltegravir (Isentress) RAL

Drug Class: HIV-1 integrase inhibitor.
Usual Dose: 400 mg (PO) q12h.
Pharmacokinetic Parameters:
Peak serum level: 6.5 μM
Bioavailability: ~ 32% (20–43%)
Excreted unchanged: 51% (feces); 9% (urine)
*Serum half-life (normal/ESRD): 9–12 hrs/
no data*
Plasma protein binding: 83%
Volume of distribution (V_d): not studied
Primary Mode of Elimination: Fecal/renal
Dosage Adjustments*

CrCl < 10 mL/min	No change
Post–HD dose	None
Post–PD dose	None
CVVH/CVVHD/ CVVHDF dose	No change
Mild/moderate hepatic insufficiency	No change
Severe hepatic insufficiency	Use with caution

Antiretroviral Dosage Adjustments

Atazanavir	No change
Atazanavir/ritonavir	No change
Efavirenz	No change
Rifampin	raltegravir 800 mg q12h
Ritonavir	No change
Tenofovir	No change
Tipranavir/ritonavir	No change

Drug Interactions: Rifampin (↓ raltegravir levels, use with caution). In-vitro, raltegravir does not inhibit CYP1A2, CYP2B6, CYP2C8, CYP2C9, CYP2C19, CYP2D6 or CYP3A and does not induce CYP3A4. In addition, raltegravir does not inhibit P-glycoprotein-mediated transport. Raltegravir is therefore not expected to affect the pharmacokinetics of drugs that are substrates of these enzymes or P-glycoprotein (e.g., protease inhibitors, NNRTIs, methadone, opioid analgesics, statins, azole antifungals, proton pump inhibitors, oral contraceptives, anti-erectile dysfunction agents).
Adverse Effects: Nausea, headache, diarrhea, pyrexia, rash, stevens-Johnson Syndrome, TEN.
Allergic Potential: Low
Safety in Pregnancy: C
Comments: May be taken with or without food. CPK elevations, myopathy and rhabdomyolysis have been reported—use with caution in patients at increased risk for myopathy or rhabdomyolysis, such as those receiving concomitant medications e.g., statins. Raltegravir is indicated for treatment-naive/experienced adult patients who have evidence of viral replication and HIV-1 strains resistant to

---

"Usual dose" assumes normal renal/hepatic function. * For renal insufficiency, give usual dose × 1 followed by maintenance dose per CrCl. For dialysis patients, dose the same as for CrCl < 10 mL/min and give supplemental (post-HD/PD dose) immediately after dialysis. CrCl = creatinine clearance; CVVH = continuous veno-venous hemofiltration; HD/PD = hemodialysis/peritoneal dialysis.

multiple antiretroviral agents. Slight increase in cancer in severly immunocompromised hosts.

Cerebrospinal Fluid Penetration: No data

REFERENCES:

Carey D, Pett SL, Bloch M, et al. A randomized study of pharmacokinetics, efficacy, and safety of 2 raltegravir plus atazanavir strategies in ART-treated adults. J Acquir Immune Defic syndr 60:143–9, 2012.

Hicks C, Gulick RM. Raltegravir: The First HIV Type 1 Integrase Inhibitor. Clin Infect Dis 48:931–940, 2009.

Iwamoto M, Wenning LA, Petry AS, et al. Safety, tolerability, and pharmacokinetics of raltegravir after single and multiple doses in healthy subjects. Clin Pharmacol Ther 83: 293–299,2008.

Palmisano L, Role of integrase inhibitors in the treatment of HIV disease. Expert Rev Anti Infect Ther 5:67–75, 2007.

Panel on Antiretroviral Guidelines for Adults and Adolescents. Department of Health and Human Services. Guidelines for the use of antiretroviral agents in HIV-infected adults and adolescents. http://aidsinfo.nih.gov/ConsentFiles/ AdultandAdolescentGL.pdf, 2012.

Thompson MA, Aberg JA, Cahn P, et al. Antiretroviral treatment of adult HIV infection: 2012 recommendations of the International Antiviral Society — USA panel. JAMA 308:387–402, 2012.

Website: www.isentress.com

Ribavirin (Rebetol) (Copegus)

Drug Class: RSV, HCV Antiviral; (see comments).

Usual Dose: 600 mg (PO) q12h (see comments).

Pharmacokinetic Parameters:

Peak serum level: 0.07–0.28 mcg/ml
Bioavailability: 64%
Excreted unchanged (urine): 40%
Serum half-life (normal/ESRD): 120 hrs/no data
Plasma protein binding: 0%

Volume of distribution (V_d): 10 L/kg

Primary Mode of Elimination: Hepatic

Dosage Adjustments*

CrCl 50–80 mL/min	No change
CrCl < 50 mL/min	Avoid
Post–HD dose	Avoid
Post–PD dose	Avoid
CVVH/CVVHD/CVVHDF dose	Avoid
Mild-moderate hepatic insufficiency	No change
Severe hepatic insufficiency	Avoid

Drug Interactions: Ribavirin may antagonize the *in vitro* antiviral activity of stavudine and zidovudine against HIV. Pegylated interferon (Pegasys) in HIV patients ($\downarrow$ CD_4 counts).

Adverse Effects: Hemolytic anemia. The *anemia* associated with ribavirin therapy may result in worsening of cardiac disease that has led to fatal and non-fatal myocardial infarctions. Patients with a history of significant cardiac disease should not be treated with ribavirin. If hemoglobin level falls < 10 g/dL reduce ribavirin dose to 600 mg daily. If hemoglobin falls < 8.5 g/dL discontinue ribavirin. When combined with interferon adverse effects includes severe depression and suicidal ideation, bone marrow suppression, autoimmune/infectious disorders, pulmonary dysfunction, pancreatitis, and diabetes. Drug fever/rash, nausea, vomiting, GI upset, leukopenia, hyperbilirubinemia, hemolytic anemia, $\uparrow$ uric acid.

Allergic Potential: Low

Safety in Pregnancy: X (avoid pregnancy during therapy and for 6 months after

---

"Usual dose" assumes normal renal/hepatic function. * For renal insufficiency, give usual dose × 1 followed by maintenance dose per CrCl. For dialysis patients, dose the same as for CrCl < 10 mL/min and give supplemental (post-HD/PD dose) immediately after dialysis. CrCl = creatinine clearance; CVVH = continuous veno-venous hemofiltration; HD/PD = hemodialysis/peritoneal dialysis.

completion of therapy in both female patients and male partners of taking ribavirin)

Comments: Nebulizer dose for RSV: 20 mg/ml aerosolized over 12 hours administered once daily × 3–7 days. Also as activity against Lassa fever and HPS. **Transplant Dose:**

Loading Dose: 30 mg/kg (IV) (not to exceed 2g), then 16 mg/kg (IV) q6h × 4 days (not to exceed 1g); ***Maintenance Dose:*** 8 mg/kg (IV) (not to exceed 500 mg) x 3–6 days. *Highly active against HCV and RSV. Some activity against, HEV, adenoviruses and arboviral hemorrhagic fever viruses. No activity against EBV, CMV, HBV, HDV.* For Crimean-Congo hemorrhagic fever give ribavirin initial ***Loading Dose*** 30 mg/kg (PO) × 1 then ***Maintenance Dose:*** 15 mg/kg (PO) q6h × 4 days, then give 7.5 mg/kg (PO) q8h × 6 days.

Cerebrospinal Fluid Penetration: 70%

REFERENCES:

Khalid O, Bacon BR. Management of the treatment-experienced patient infected with Hepatitis C virus genotype 1: options and considerations. Clin Liver Dis 15:573–583, 2011.

Razonable RR. Antiviral drugs for viruses other than human immunodeficiency virus. Mayo Clin Proc 86:1009–1026, 2011.

Vanpouille C, Lisco A, Introini A, et al. Exploiting the anti-HIV-1 activity of acyclovir: suppression of primary and drug-resistant HIV isolates and potentiation of the activity by ribavirin. Antimicrob Agents Chemother 56:2604–2611, 2012.

Website: www.rocheusa.com/products/

Rifabutin (Mycobutin)

Drug Class: Anti-MAI drug.

Usual Dose: 5 mg/kg or 300 mg (PO) q24h (see comments).

Pharmacokinetic Parameters:

Peak serum level: 0.38 mcg/ml
Bioavailability: 20–50%

Excreted unchanged (urine): 10%
Serum half-life (normal/ESRD): 45/45 hrs
Plasma protein binding: 85%
Volume of distribution (V_d): 9.3 L/kg

Primary Mode of Elimination: Hepatic

Dosage Adjustments*

CrCl < 30 mL/min	150 mcg (PO) q24h
CrCl < 10 mL/min	No change
Post–HD dose	None
Post–PD dose	None
CVVH/CVVHD/CVVHDF dose	None
Moderate hepatic insufficiency	No change
Severe hepatic insufficiency	No change

Drug Interactions: Atovaquone, amprenavir, indinavir, nelfinavir, ritonavir, clarithromycin, erythromycin, telithromycin, fluconazole, itraconazole, ketoconazole (↓ interactg drug levels, ↑ rifabutin levels); beta-blockers, clofibrate, cyclosporine, enalapril, oral contraceptives, quinidine, sulfonylureas, tocainide, warfarin (↓ interacting drug effect); corticosteroids (↑ corticosteroid requirement); delavirdine (↓ delavirdine levels, ↑ rifabutin levels; avoid); digoxin, phenytoin, propafenone, theophylline, zidovudine (↓ interacting drug levels); methadone (↓ methadone levels, withdrawal); mexiletine (↑ mexiletine clearance); protease inhibitors (↓ protease inhibitor levels, ↑ rifabutin levels; caution).

Adverse Effects: Headache, nausea, vomiting. ↑ SGOT/SGPT, leukopenia, anemia, thrombocytopenia, drug

---

"Usual dose" assumes normal renal/hepatic function. * For renal insufficiency, give usual dose × 1 followed by maintenance dose per CrCl. For dialysis patients, dose the same as for CrCl < 10 mL/min and give supplemental (post-HD/PD dose) immediately after dialysis. CrCl = creatinine clearance; CVVH = continuous veno-venous hemofiltration; HD/PD = hemodialysis/peritoneal dialysis.

fever/rash. Brown/orange discoloration
of body fluids.
Allergic Potential: High
Safety in Pregnancy: B
Comments: Avoid in leukopenic patients
with WBC ≤ 1000 cells/mm^3. Always use
as part of a multi-drug regimen, never as
monotherapy. **Rifabutin doses when
co-administered with antiretrovirals:** 450
mg (PO) q24h with EFV; 150 mg (PO) q24h
with AVP, IDV, NFV, FPN; 150 mg (PO) q48h
with RTV/LPV combination.
Meningeal dose = usual dose.
Cerebrospinal Fluid Penetration: 50–70%

REFERENCES:

Benson CA, Williams PL, Cohn DL, and the ACTG
196/CPCRA 009 Study Team. Clarithromycin or
rifabutin alone or in combination for primary
prophylaxis of Mycobacterium avium complex
disease in patients with AIDS: A randomized,
double-blinded, placebo-controlled trial. J Infect Dis
181:1289–97, 2000.

Centers for Disease Control and Prevention. Notice to
readers: Updated guidelines for the use of rifabutin
or rifampin for the treatment and prevention of
tuberculosis among HIV-infected patients taking
protease inhibitors or nonnucleoside reverse
transcriptase inhibitors. MMWR 49:183–189, 2000.

Choong K, Looke D. Cross-reaction to rifabutin
after rifampicin induced flu-liked syndrome and
thrombocytopenia. Scand J Infect Dis 43:238, 2011.

Finch CK, Chrisman CR, Baciewicz AM, et al. Rifampin
and rifabutin drug Interactions: an update. Arch
Intern Med 162:985–92, 2002.

Horne DJ, Spitters C Narita M. Experience with rifabutin
replacing rifampin in the treatment of tuberculosis.
Int J Tuberc Lung Dis 15:1485–9, 2011.

Hoy J, Mijch A, Sandland M, et al. Quadruple-drug therapy
for Mycobacterium avium-intracellulare bacteremia in
AIDS patients. J Infect Dis 161:801–5, 1990.

Nightingale SD, Cameron DW, Gordin FM, et al. Two
controlled trials of rifabutin prophylaxis against
Mycobacterium avium complex infection in AIDS.
N Engl J Med 329:828–33, 1993.

Nishizawa T, Suzuki H, Matsuzaki J, et al. Helicobacter
pylori resistance to rifabutin in the last 7 years.
Antimicrob Agents Chemother 55:5374–5, 2011.

Sax PE, Cohen CJ, Kuritzkes DR. HIV Essentials, 5th
edition, Jones & Bartlett, Sudbury, MA, 2011.
pp. 123–125.

Zhang J, Shu L, Stonier M, et al. Determination of
rifabutin dosing regimen when administered in
combination with ritonavir-boosted atazanavir.
J Antimicrob Chemother 66:2075–82, 2011.

Website: www.pdr.net

Rifampin (Rifadin, Rimactane)

Drug Class: Antibiotic/anti-TB drug.
Usual Dose: 600 mg (PO) q24h
(see comments).
Spectrum: (see *Susceptibility Profiles*
pp. 186–190).
Resistance Potential: High (aerobic GNBs with
non-TB monotherapy)
Pharmacokinetic Parameters:
Peak serum level: 7 mcg/ml
Bioavailability: 95%
Excreted unchanged (urine): 15%
Serum half-life (normal/ESRD): 3.5/11 hrs
Plasma protein binding: 80%
Volume of distribution (V_d): 0.93 L/kg
Primary Mode of Elimination: Hepatic
Dosage Adjustments*

CrCl < 10 mL/min	No change
Post–HD dose	None
Post–PD dose	None
CVVH/CVVHD/CVVHDF dose	No change

"Usual dose" assumes normal renal/hepatic function. * For renal insufficiency, give usual dose × 1 followed by maintenance dose per CrCl. For dialysis patients, dose the same as for CrCl < 10 mL/min and give supplemental (post-HD/PD dose) immediately after dialysis. CrCl = creatinine clearance; CVVH = continuous veno-venous hemofiltration; HD/PD = hemodialysis/peritoneal dialysis.

Moderate hepatic insufficiency	No change; use caution
Severe hepatic insufficiency	Avoid

Drug Interactions: Amprenavir, indinavir, nelfinavir (↑ rifampin levels); beta-blockers, clofibrate, cyclosporine, oral contraceptives, quinidine, sulfonylureas, tocainamide, warfarin (↓ interacting drug effect); caspofungin (↓ caspofungin levels, may ↓ caspofungin effect); clarithromycin, ketoconazole (↑ rifampin levels, ↓ interacting drug levels); corticosteroids (↑ corticosteroid requirement); delavirdine (↑ rifampin levels, ↓ delavirdine levels; avoid); disopyramide, itraconazole, phenytoin, propafenone, theophylline, methadone, nelfinavir, ritonavir, tacrolimus, drugs whose metabolism is induced by rifampin, e.g., ACE inhibitors, dapsone, diazepam, digoxin, diltiazem, doxycycline, fluconazole, fluvastatin, haloperidol, nifedipine, progestins, triazolam, tricyclics, zidovudine (↓ interacting drug levels); fluconazole, rifampin (↓ posaconazole levels) TMP–SMX (↑ rifampin levels); INH (INH converted into toxic hydrazine); mexiletine (↑ mexiletine clearance); nevirapine (↓ nevirapine levels; avoid).

Adverse Effects: Dizziness, Flu–like symptoms, ↑ SGOT/SGPT, drug fever/rash, thrombocytopenia. Red/orange discoloration of body secretions.

Allergic Potential: Moderate

Safety in Pregnancy: C

Comments: Potent CYP 3A4 inducer. Contraindicated in HIV. For anti–TB prophylaxis/therapy, monitor potential hepatotoxicity with serial SGOT/SGPTs weekly × 3, then monthly × 3. Take 1 hour before or 2 hours after meals. **TB D.O.T. dose:** 10 mg/kg or 600 mg (PO) 2–3x/week. **Do not use as monotherapy for S. aureus. Of no proven clinical advantage when combined with another anti–MSSA/MRSA antibiotic. With another anti-staphylococcal drug dose:** 300 mg (PO) q12h. 300 mg (PO) q8h may be used for S. aureus PVE.

Nasal carriage dose: 600 mg (PO) q12h × 72 hours.

Meningeal dose = usual dose.

Cerebrospinal Fluid Penetration:

Non-Inflamed meninges = 50%

Inflamed meninges = 50%

Bile Penetration: 7000%

REFERENCES:

Cascio A, Scarlata F, Giordano S, et al. Treatment of human brucellosis with rifampin plus minocycline. J Chemother 15:248–52, 2003.

Castahneira D, Rifampin. Antibiotics for Clinicians 6:89–100, 2001.

Curry SR, Marsh JW, Shutt KA, et al. High frequency of rifampin resistance identified in an epidemic clostridium difficile clone from a large teaching hospital. Clin Infect Dis 48:425–430, 2009.

Czekaj J, Dinh A, Moldovan A, et al. Efficacy of a combined oral clindamycin-rifampicin regimen for therapy of staphylococcal osteoarticular infections. Scand J Infect Dis 43:962-967, 2011.

Davidson PT, Le HQ. Drug treatment of tuberculosis 1992. Drugs 43:651–73, 1992.

Ena J, Valls V. Short-course therapy with rifampin plus isoniazid compared with standard therapy with isoniazid, for latent tuberculosis infection: a meta-analysis. Clin Infect Dis 40:670–6, 2005.

Euga G, Murillo O, Fernandez-Sabe N, et al. Treatment of chronic staphylococcal osteomyelitis: intravenous or oral? how long? Antimicrob Agents Chemother 53:2672–2676, 2009.

Giamarellos-Bourboulis EJ, Sambatakou H, Galani I, et al. In vitro interaction of colistin and rifampin on multidrug-resistant Pseudomonas aeruginosa. J Chemother 15:235–8, 2003.

Gomez J, Canovas E, Banos V, et al. Linezolid plus rifampin as a salvage therapy in prosthetic joint infections treated without removing the implant. Antimicrob Agents Chemother 55:4308–4310, 2011.

"Usual dose" assumes normal renal/hepatic function. * For renal insufficiency, give usual dose × 1 followed by maintenance dose per CrCl. For dialysis patients, dose the same as for CrCl < 10 mL/min and give supplemental (post-HD/PD dose) immediately after dialysis. CrCl = creatinine clearance; CVVH = continuous veno-venous hemofiltration; HD/PD = hemodialysis/peritoneal dialysis.

Hohmann C, Kang EM, Jancel T: Rifampin and posaconazole coadministration leads to decreased serum posaconazole concentrations. Clin Infect Dis 50:939–940, 2010.

Hoyo I, Martinez-Pastor J, Garcia-Ramiro S, et al. Decreased serum linezolid concentrations in two patients receiving linezolid and rifampicin due to bone infections. Scand J Infect Dis 44:548-50, 2012.

Ijaz K, Jereb JA, Lambert LA, et al. Severe or fatal injury in 50 Patients in the United States taking rifampin and pyrazinamide for latent tuberculosis infection. Clin Infect Dis 42:346–56, 2006.

Ijaz K, McElroy PD, Navin TR. Short course rifampin and pyrazinamide compared with isoniazid for latent tuberculosis infection: a cost-effectiveness analysis based on a multicenter clinical trial Clin Infect Dis 39:289, 2004.

Johnson JR. Rifampin and methicillin-resistant Staphylococcus aureus bone and joint infections. Clin Infect Dis 53:98–99, 2011.

Krause PJ, Corrow CL, Bakken JS. Successful treatment of human granulocytic ehrlichiosis in children using rifampin. Pediatrics. 112:e252–3, 2003.

Lundstrom TS, Sobel JD. Vancomycin, trimethoprim - sulfamethoxazole, and rifampin. Infect Dis Clin North Am 91:747–67, 1995.

McIllerson H, Wash P, Burger A, et al. Determinants of rifampin, isoniazid, pyrazinamide and ethambutol pharmacokinetics in a cohort of tuberculosis patients. Antimicrob Agents Chemother 50: 1170–77, 2006.

Nguyen S, Pasquet A, Legout L, et al. Efficacy and tolerance of rifampin-linezolid compared with rifampin-cotrimoxazole combinations in prolonged oral therapy for bone and joint infections. Clin Microbiol Infect Dis 15:1163–1169, 2009.

Perlman DC, Segal Yoniah, Rosenkranz S, et al. The clinical pharmacokinetics of rifampin and ethambutol in HIV-infected persons with tuberculosis. Clin Infect Dis 41:1638–47, 2005.

Sax PE, Cohen CJ, Kuritzkes DR. HIV Essentials, 5th edition Jones & Bartlett, Sudbury, MA, 2012.

Schlossberg D: An approach to drug-induced liver injury during tuberculosis therapy. Infect Dis Clin Pract 18:107–108, 2010.

Schlossberg D, Treatment of multi-drug resistant tuberculosis. Antibiotics for Clinicians 9:317–321, 2005.

Van Scoy RE, Wilkowske CJ. Antituberculous agents. Mayo Clin Proc 67:179–87, 1992.

Vesely JJ, Pien FD, Pien BC. Rifampin, a useful drug for nonmycobacterial infections. Pharmacotherapy 18:345–57, 1998.

Wareham DW, Bean DC. In vitro activities of polymyxin B, imipenem and rifampin against multidrug-resistant Acinetobacter baumannii. Antimicrob Agents Chemother 50:825–26, 2006.

Website: www.pdr.net

Rilpivirine (Edurant) RPV

Drug class: NNRTI.
Usual dose: 25 mg (PO) q24h (with meal).
Pharmacokinetic Parameters:
Peak serum level: 1 mcg/L
Bioavailability: unknown
Excreted unchanged: 1%
Serum half-life (normal/ESRD): 50/50 hrs
Plasma protein binding: 99%
Volume of distribution (V_d): unknown
Primary Mode of Elimination: Hepatic
Dosage Adjustments*

CrCl <10 mL/min	No change
Post-HD dose	None
Post-PD dose	None
CVVH/CVVHD/ CVVHDF dose	No change
Mild to moderate hepatic insufficiency	No change
Severe hepatic insufficiency	Use with caution

Drug Interactions: Clarithromycin (↓ clarithromycin levels). Any drug that induces or inhibits CYP3A may ↑/↓ rilpivirine levels.

"Usual dose" assumes normal renal/hepatic function. * For renal insufficiency, give usual dose × 1 followed by maintenance dose per CrCl. For dialysis patients, dose the same as for CrCl < 10 mL/min and give supplemental (post-HD/PD dose) immediately after dialysis. CrCl = creatinine clearance; CVVH = continuous veno-venous hemofiltration; HD/PD = hemodialysis/peritoneal dialysis.

Contraindications: carbamazepine, oxycarbamazepine, phenobarbital, phenytoin, rifabutin, rifampin, rifapentine, proton pump inhibitors, dexamethasone (*except* single dose), St. John's Wort.

Adverse Effects: Nausea, vomiting, abdominal pain, fatigue, headache, dizziness, depressive disorders, insomnia, abnormal dreams, rash, ↑ QTc.

Allergic Potential: Low

Safety in Pregnancy: B

Comments: Antacid and H2 blockers should be separated. **Do not administer with other NNRTI's.** Use only if benefit outweighs risk.

REFERENCES:

Miller CD, Crain J, Tran V, et al. Rilipivirine: A new addition to the anti-HIV-1 armamentarium. Drugs Today 47:5–15, 2011.

Molina JM, Cahn P, Grinsztejn B, et al. Rilipivirine versus efavirenz with tenofovir and emtricitabine in treatment- naïve adults infected with HIV-1 (ECHO): A phase 3 randomised double- blind active-controlled trail. Lancet ID 16:238–246, 2011.

Schrijvers R, Desimmie BA, Debyser Z. Rilipivirine: A step forward in tailored HIV treatment. Lancet ID 16:201–203, 2011.

Rimantadine (Flumadine)

Drug Class: Antiviral.

Usual Dose: 100 mg (PO) q12h (see comments).

Pharmacokinetic Parameters:

Peak serum level: 0.7 mcg/ml
Bioavailability: 90%
Excreted unchanged (urine): 25%
Serum half-life (normal/ESRD): 25/38 hrs
Plasma protein binding: 40%
Volume of distribution (V_d): 4.5 L/kg

Primary Mode of Elimination: Hepatic

Dosage Adjustments*

CrCl 10–50 mL/min	No change
CrCl < 10 mL/min	100 mg (PO) q24h
Post-HD dose	None
Post-PD dose	None
CVVH/CVVHD/ CVVHDF dose	No change
Moderate hepatic insufficiency	No change
Severe hepatic insufficiency	100 mg (PO) q24h

Drug Interactions: Alcohol (↑ CNS effects); benztropine, trihexyphenidyl, scopolamine (↑ interacting drug effect: dry mouth, ataxia, blurred vision, slurred speech, toxic psychosis); cimetidine (↓ rimantadine clearance); CNS stimulants (additive stimulation); digoxin (↑ digoxin levels); trimethoprim (↑ rimantadine and trimethoprim levels).

Adverse Effects: Dizziness, headache, insomnia, anticholinergic effects (blurry vision, dry mouth, orthostatic hypotension, urinary retention, constipation).

Allergic Potential: Low

Safety in Pregnancy: C

Comments: Less anticholinergic side effects than amantadine. Patients ≥ 60 years old or with a history of seizures should receive 100 mg (PO) q24h. **Influenza dose (prophylaxis):** 100 mg (PO) q12h for duration of exposure/ outbreak. **Influenza dose (therapy):** 100 mg (PO) q12h × 7 days. **May improve peripheral airway function/oxygenation in severe influenza pneumonia.** *Highly active against influenza A. No activity against other viruses.*

Cerebrospinal Fluid Penetration: < 10%

"Usual dose" assumes normal renal/hepatic function. * For renal insufficiency, give usual dose × 1 followed by maintenance dose per CrCl. For dialysis patients, dose the same as for CrCl < 10 mL/min and give supplemental (post-HD/PD dose) immediately after dialysis. CrCl = creatinine clearance; CVVH = continuous veno-venous hemofiltration; HD/PD = hemodialysis/peritoneal dialysis.

REFERENCES:

[No authors listed.] Antiviral drugs for prophylaxis and treatment of influenza. Med Lett Drugs Ther 46:85–7, 2004.

Dolin R, Reichman RC, Madore HP, et al. A controlled trial of amantadine and rimantadine in the prophylaxis of Influenza A infection. N Engl J Med 307:580–4, 1982.

Gravenstein S, Davidson HE. Current strategies for management of influenza in the elderly population. Clin Infect Dis 35:729–37, 2002.

Jefferson T, Deeks JJ, Demicheli V, et al. Amantadine and rimantadine for preventing and treating influenza A in adults. Cochrane Database Syst Rev 3:CD001169, 2004.

Keating MR, Antiviral agents. Mayo Clin Proc 67:160–78, 1992.

Schmidt AC, Antiviral therapy for influenza: a clinical and economic comparative review. Drugs 64:2031–46, 2004.

Wintermeyer SM, Nahata MC. Rimantadine: A clinical perspective. Ann Pharmacotherapy 29:299–310, 1995.

Website: www.pdr.net

Ritonavir (Norvir) RTV

Drug Class: Antiretroviral protease inhibitor.
Usual Dose: 100–400 mg (PO) q12h–q24h (see comments).
Pharmacokinetic Parameters:
Peak serum level: 11 mcg/ml
Bioavailability: No data
Excreted unchanged (urine): 3.5%
Serum half-life (normal/ESRD): 4 hrs/no data
Plasma protein binding: 99%
Volume of distribution (V_d): 0.41 L/kg
Primary Mode of Elimination: Hepatic
Dosage Adjustments*

CrCl < 10 mL/min	No change
Post–HD dose	None
Post–PD dose	None
CVVH/CVVHD/CVVHDF dose	None
Mild-moderate hepatic insufficiency	No change
Severe hepatic insufficiency	Avoid

Antiretroviral Dosage Adjustments

Atazanavir	Ritonavir 100 mg q24h + atazanavir 300 mg q24h (with food)
Delavirdine	Delavirdine: no change; ritonavir: No data
Efavirenz	Ritonavir 600 mg q12h (500 mg q12h for intolerance)
Fosamprenavir	Fosamprenavir 1400 mg + ritonavir 200 mg q24h
Indinavir	Ritonavir 100–200 mg q12h + indinavir 800 mg q12h, or 400 mg q12h of each drug
Nelfinavir	Ritonavir 400 mg q12h + nelfinavir 500–750 mg q12h
Nevirapine	No change
Saquinavir	Ritonavir 400 mg q12h + saquinavir 400 mg q12h
Ketoconazole	Caution; do not exceed ketoconazole 200 mg q24h
Rifampin	Avoid
Rifabutin	Rifabutin 150 mg q48h or 3x/week

"Usual dose" assumes normal renal/hepatic function. * For renal insufficiency, give usual dose × 1 followed by maintenance dose per CrCl. For dialysis patients, dose the same as for CrCl < 10 mL/min and give supplemental (post-HD/PD dose) immediately after dialysis. CrCl = creatinine clearance; CVVH = continuous veno-venous hemofiltration; HD/PD = hemodialysis/peritoneal dialysis.

Drug Interactions: Antiretrovirals, rifabutin, rifampin (see dose adjustment grid, above); saquinavir (↑ QTc/torsades de pointes, ↑ PR intervals) alprazolam, diazepam, estazolam, flurazepam, midazolam, triazolam, zolpidem, meperidine, propoxyphene, piroxicam, quinidine, amiodarone, encainide, flecainide, propafenone, astemizole, bepridil, bupropion, cisapride, clorazepate, clozapine, pimozide, St. John's wort, terfenadine (avoid); alfentanil, fentanyl, hydrocodone, tramadol, disopyramide, lidocaine, mexiletine, erythromycin, clarithromycin, warfarin, dronabinol, ondansetron, metoprolol, pindolol, propranolol, timolol, amlodipine, diltiazem, felodipine, isradipine, nicardipine, nifedipine, nimodipine, nisoldipine, nitrendipine, verapamil, etoposide, paclitaxel, tamoxifen, vinblastine, vincristine, loratadine, tricyclic antidepressants, paroxetine, nefazodone, sertraline, trazodone, fluoxetine, venlafaxine, fluvoxamine, cyclosporine, tacrolimus, chlorpromazine, haloperidol, perphenazine, risperidone, thioridazine, clozapine, pimozide, methamphetamine (↑ interacting drug levels); voriconazole (↓ voriconazole levels); telithromycin (↑ ritonavir levels); codeine, hydromorphone, methadone, morphine, ketoprofen, ketorolac, naproxen, diphenoxylate, oral contraceptives, theophylline (↓ interacting drug levels); carbamazepine, phenytoin, phenobarbital, clonazepam, dexamethasone, prednisone (↓ ritonavir levels, ↑ interacting drug levels; monitor anticonvulsant levels); metronidazole (disulfiram-like reaction); tenofovir, tobacco (↓ ritonavir levels); sildenafil (do not exceed 25 mg in 48 hrs); tadalafil (max. 10 mg/72 hrs); vardenafil (max. 2.5 mg/72 hrs).

Adverse Effects: Anorexia, anemia, leukopenia, hyperglycemia (including worsening diabetes, new-onset diabetes, DKA), ↑ cholesterol/ triglycerides (evaluate risk for coronary disease/ pancreatitis), fat redistribution, ↑ CPK, nausea, vomiting, diarrhea, abdominal pain, circumoral/ extremity paresthesias, ↑ SGOT/SGPT, pancreatitis, taste perversion, possible increased bleeding in hemophilia, ↑ incideuce of renal stones with ritonavir boosted atazanavir.

Allergic Potential: Low

Safety in Pregnancy: B

Comments: Usually used at low dose (100–400 mg/day) as pharmacokinetic "booster" of other PI's. GI intolerance decreases over time. Take with food if possible (serum levels increase 15%, fewer GI side effects). Separate dosing from ddI by 2 hours.

Cerebrospinal Fluid Penetration: < 1%

REFERENCES:

Cameron DW, Japour AJ, Xu Y, et al. Ritonavir and saquinavir combination therapy for the treatment of HIV infection. AIDS 13:213–224, 1999.

DeJeus E, Rockstroh JK, Henry K, et al. Co-Formulated elvitegravir, cobicistat, emtricitabine and tenofovir disoproxil fumarate versus ritonavir-boosted atazanavir plus co-formulated emtricitabine and tenofovir disoproxil fumarate for initial treatment of HIV-infection: a randomized, double-blind, phase 3, non-inferiority trial. Lancet 379–2429–38, 2012.

Diaz-Brito V, Leon A, Knobel H, et al. Post-exposure prophylaxis for HIV-infection: a clinical trail comparing lopinavir/ritonavir versus atazanavir each with zidovudine/lamivudine. Antivir Ther 17:337–46, 2012.

Kaul DR, Cinti SK, Carver PL, et al. HIV protease inhibitors: Advances in therapy and adverse reactions, including metabolic complications. Pharmacotherapy 19:281–98, 1999.

Lea AP, Faulds D. Ritonavir. Drugs 52:541–6, 1996.

McDonald CK, Kuritzkes DR. Human immunodeficiency virus type 1 protease inhibitors. Arch Intern Med 157:951–9, 1997.

McDonald C, Uy J, Hu W, et al. Clinical significance of hyperbilirubinemia among HIV-1-infected patients treated with atazanavir/ ritonavir through 96 weeks in the CASTLE study. AIDS patient care STDS 26–259–64, 2012.

"Usual dose" assumes normal renal/hepatic function. * For renal insufficiency, give usual dose × 1 followed by maintenance dose per CrCl. For dialysis patients, dose the same as for CrCl < 10 mL/min and give supplemental (post-HD/PD dose) immediately after dialysis. CrCl = creatinine clearance; CVVH = continuous veno-venous hemofiltration; HD/PD = hemodialysis/peritoneal dialysis.

Nishijima T, Tsukada K, Teruya K, et al. Efficacy and safety of once-daily ritonavir-based antiretroviral therapy in low-body weight treatment-naïve patients with HIV infections. AIDS 13;26:649–51 2012.

Panel on Antiretroviral Guidelines for Adults and Adolescents. Department of Health and Human Services. Guidelines for the use of antiretroviral agents in HIV-infected adults and adolescents. http://aidsinfo.nih.gov/ConsentFiles/AdultandAdolescentGL.pdf, 2012.

Piliero PJ. Interaction between ritonavir and statins. Am J Med 112:510–1, 2002.

Rockwood N, Mandalia S, Bower M, et al. Ritonavir-boosted atazanavir exposure is associated with an increased rate of renal stones compared with efavirenz, ritonavir-boosted lopinavir and ritonavir-boosted darunavir. AIDS 25:1671–3, 2011.

Thompson MA, Aberg JA, Cahn P, et al. Antiretroviral treatment of adult HIV infection: 2012 recommendations of the International Antiviral Society — USA panel. JAMA 308:387–402, 2012.

Saquinavir (Invirase) SQV

Drug Class: Antiretroviral protease inhibitor.
Usual Dose: 1000 mg (PO) q12h (see comments) with ritonavir 100 mg (PO) q12h.
Pharmacokinetic Parameters:
Peak serum level: 0.07 mcg/mL
Bioavailability: hard-gel (4%)
Excreted unchanged (urine): 13%
Serum half-life (normal/ESRD): 13 hrs/no data
Plasma protein binding: 98%
Volume of distribution (V_d): 10 L/kg
Primary Mode of Elimination: Hepatic
Dosage Adjustments*

CrCl < 10 mL/min	No change
Post–HD dose	None
Post–PD dose	None
CVVH/CVVHD/CVVHDF dose	No change
Moderate hepatic insufficiency	Use with caution
Severe hepatic insufficiency	Avoid

Antiretroviral Dosage Adjustments

Darunavir	Avoid
Delavirdine	No data
Efavirenz	Avoid use as sole PI
Indinavir	No data
Lopinavir/ritonavir 2 capsules q12h	Saquinavir 1 gm q12h
Nelfinavir	Saquinavir 1 gm q12h or 1200 mg q12h
Nevirapine	No data
Ritonavir	Ritonavir 100 mg q12h + saquinavir 1 gm q12h
Rifampin	Avoid
Rifabutin	Avoid

Drug Interactions: Antiretrovirals, rifabutin, rifampin (see dose adjustment grid, above); astemizole, terfenadine, benzodiazepines, cisapride, ergotamine, statins, St. John's wort (avoid if possible); carbamazepine, phenytoin, phenobarbital, dexamethasone, prednisone (↓ saquinavir levels, ↑ interacting drug levels; monitor anticonvulsant levels); clarithromycin, erythromycin, telithromycin (↑ saquinavir and macrolide levels); grapefruit juice, itraconazole, voriconazole, ketoconazole (↑ saquinavir levels); sildenafil (do not give > 25 mg/48 hrs); tadalafil (max. 10 mg/72 hrs), vardenafil (max. 2.5 mg/72 hrs), ritonavir (↑ QTc, ↑ PR intervals), PPIs(↑ saquinavir leves). Atovaquone/proguanil (↑ saquinavir levels).

Contraindications: Rifapentine, trazodone.

Adverse Effects: Anorexia, headache, anemia, leukopenia, hyperglycemia (including worsening diabetes, new-onset diabetes, DKA), ↑ cholesterol/triglycerides (evaluate risk for coronary disease/pancreatitis), ↑ SGOT/SGPT, hyperuricemia, fat redistribution, night sweats, possible increased bleeding in hemophilia.

Allergic Potential: Low

Safety in Pregnancy: B

Comments: Take with food. Avoid garlic supplements, which ↓ saquinavir levels ~ 50%. Boosted dose: 1 gm saquinavir/100 mg ritonavir (PO) q12h. Preferred formulation is 500 mg hard-gel capsule (Invirase 500). Soft-gel capsules (Fortovase) no longer available.

Cerebrospinal Fluid Penetration: < 1%

REFERENCES:

Cameron DW, Japour AJ, Xu Y, et al. Ritonavir and saquinavir combination therapy for the treatment of HIV infection. AIDS 13:213–224, 1999.

Hughes PJ, Cretton-Scott E, Teague A, et al. Protease inhibitors for patients with HIV-1 infection. Pharm Ther 36:332–344, 2011.

Panel on Antiretroviral Guidelines for Adults and Adolescents. Department of Health and Human Services. Guidelines for the use of antiretroviral agents in HIV-infected adults and adolescents. http://aidsinfo.nih.gov/ConsentFiles/AdultandAdolescentGL.pdf, 2012.

Perry CM, Noble S. Saquinavir soft-gel capsule formation: A review of its use in patients with HIV infection. Drugs 55:461–86, 1998.

Thompson MA, Aberg JA, Cahn P, et al. Antiretroviral treatment of adult HIV infection: 2012 recommendations of the International Antiviral Society — USA panel. JAMA 308:387–402, 2012.

Tomassi C, Bellagamba R, Tempestilli M, et al. Marked increase in etravirine and saquinavir plasma concentrations during atovaquone/proguanil prophylaxis. Malar J 10:141, 2011.

Website: www.fortovase.com

Spectinomycin (Spectam, Trobicin)

Drug Class: Aminocyclitol.
Usual Dose: 2 gm (IM) × 1 dose.
Pharmacokinetic Parameters:
Peak serum level: 100 mcg/ml
Bioavailability: Not applicable
Excreted unchanged (urine): 80%
Serum half-life (normal/ESRD): 1.6/16 hrs
Plasma protein binding: 20%
Volume of distribution (V_d): 0.25 L/kg
Primary Mode of Elimination: Renal
Dosage Adjustments*

CrCl < 10 mL/min	No change
Post–HD dose	None
Post–PD dose	None
CVVH/CVVHD/CVVHDF dose	None
Moderate hepatic insufficiency	No change
Severe hepatic insufficiency	No change

Drug Interactions: None.
Adverse Effects: Local pain at injection site.
Allergic Potential: Low
Safety in Pregnancy: B
Comments: Ineffective in pharyngeal GC (poor penetration into secretions).
Cerebrospinal Fluid Penetration: < 10%

REFERENCES:

Fiumara NJ. The treatment of gonococcal proctitis: An evaluation of 173 patients treated with 4 gm of spectinomycin. JAMA 239:735–7, 1978.

Holloway WJ. Spectinomycin. Med Clin North Am 66:169–173, 1995.

"Usual dose" assumes normal renal/hepatic function. * For renal insufficiency, give usual dose × 1 followed by maintenance dose per CrCl. For dialysis patients, dose the same as for CrCl < 10 mL/min and give supplemental (post-HD/PD dose) immediately after dialysis. CrCl = creatinine clearance; CVVH = continuous veno-venous hemofiltration; HD/PD = hemodialysis/peritoneal dialysis.

McCormack WM, Finland M. Spectinomycin. Ann Intern Med 84:712–16, 1976.

Tapsall J. Current concepts in the management of gonorrhoea. Expert Opin Pharmacother 3:147–57, 2002.

Website: www.pdr.net

Stavudine (Zerit) d4T

Drug Class: Antiretroviral NRTI (nucleoside reverse transcriptase inhibitor).

Usual Dose: ≥ 60 kg: 40 mg (PO) q12h; < 60 kg: 30 mg (PO) q12h.

Pharmacokinetic Parameters:
Peak serum level: 4.2 mcg/mL
Bioavailability: 86%
Excreted unchanged (urine): 40%
Serum half-life (normal/ESRD): 1.0/5.1 hrs
Plasma protein binding: 0%
Volume of distribution (V_d): 0.5 L/kg

Primary Mode of Elimination: Renal

Dosage Adjustments* ≥ 60 kg/[≤ 60 kg]

CrCl 50–80 mL/min	40 mg (PO) q12h [30 mg (PO) q12h]
CrCl 25–50 mL/min	20 mg (PO) q12h [15 mg (PO) q12h]
CrCl ~ 10–25 mL/min	20 mg (PO) q24h [15 mg (PO) q24h]
Post–HD dose	20 mg (PO) [15 mg (PO)]
Post–PD dose	No data
CVVH/CVVHD/ CVVHDF dose	20 mg (PO) q24h [15 mg (PO) q24h]
Moderate hepatic insufficiency	No change
Severe hepatic insufficiency	No change

Drug Interactions: Ribavirin (↓ stavudine efficacy, ↑ risk of lactic acidosis); dapsone, INH, other neurotoxic agents (↑ risk of neuropathy), didanosine (↑ risk of neuropathy, lactic acidosis). Avoid combining zidovudine with stavudine.

Adverse Effects: Lactic acidosis and severe hepatomegaly with steatosis, including fatal cases, have been reported with the use of nucleoside analogues alone or in combination, including stavudine and other antiretrovirals. Fatal lactic acidosis has been reported in pregnant women who reveived the combination of stavudine and didanosine with other antiretroviral agents. The combination of stavudine and didanosine sould be used with great caution during pregnancy and only when necessary. Drug fever/rash, nausea, vomiting, GI upset, diarrhea, headache, insomnia, dose dependent peripheral neuropathy, myalgias, pancreatitis, ↑ SGOT/SGPT, ↑ cholesterol, facial fat pad wasting, lipodystrophy, thrombocytopenia, leukopenia, lactic acidosis with hepatic steatosis. There is an increased risk of hepatotoxicity may occur in patients treated with stavudine in combination with didanosine and hydroxyurea. Immune reconstitution syndrome can occur.

Allergic Potential: Low

Safety in Pregnancy: C

Comments: Pancreatitis may be severe/fatal. Avoid coadministration with AZT or ddC. Decrease dose in patients with peripheral neuropathy to 20 mg (PO) q12h. Pregnant women may be at increased risk for lactic acidosis/liver damage when stavudine is used with didanosine (ddI). WHO recommends 30 mg q12h regardless of body weight.

Cerebrospinal Fluid Penetration: 30%

"Usual dose" assumes normal renal/hepatic function. * For renal insufficiency, give usual dose × 1 followed by maintenance dose per CrCl. For dialysis patients, dose the same as for CrCl < 10 mL/min and give supplemental (post-HD/PD dose) immediately after dialysis. CrCl = creatinine clearance; CVVH = continuous veno-venous hemofiltration; HD/PD = hemodialysis/peritoneal dialysis.

REFERENCES:

Berasconi E, Boubaker K, Junghans C, et al. Abnormalities of body fat distribution in HIV-infected persons treated with antiretroviral drugs: The Swiss HIV Cohort Study. J Acquir Immune Defic Syndr 31:50–5, 2002.

Dudley MN, Graham KK, Kaul S, et al. Pharmacokinetics of stavudine in patients with AIDS and AIDS-related complex. J Infect Dis 166:480–5, 1992.

Miller KD, Cameron M, Wood LV, et al. Lactic acidosis and hepatic steatosis associated with use of stavudine: Report of four cases. Ann Intern Med 133:192–196, 2000.

Panel on Antiretroviral Guidelines for Adults and Adolescents. Department of Health and Human Services. Guidelines for the use of antiretroviral agents in HIV-infected adults and adolescents. http://aidsinfo.nih.gov/ConsentFiles/AdultandAdolescentGL.pdf, 2012.

Thompson MA, Aberg JA, Cahn P, et al. Antiretroviral treatment of adult HIV infection: 2012 recommendations of the International Antiviral Society — USA panel. JAMA 308:387–402, 2012.

Website: www.zerit.com

Streptomycin

Drug Class: Anti-TB aminoglycoside.
Usual Dose: 15 mg/kg (IM) q24h or 1 gm (IM) q24h (see comments).
Pharmacokinetic Parameters:
Peak serum level: 25–50 mcg/ml
Bioavailability: Not applicable
Excreted unchanged (urine): 90%
Serum half-life (normal/ESRD): 2.5/100 hrs
Plasma protein binding: 35%
Volume of distribution (V_d): 0.26 L/kg
Primary Mode of Elimination: Renal
Dosage Adjustments*

CrCl 10–50 mL/min	15 mg/kg (IM) q72h or 1 gm (IM) q72h
CrCl < 10 mL/min	15 mg/kg (IM) q72h or 1 gm (IM) q96h

Post–HD dose	15 mg/kg (IM) or 1 gm (IM) 2–3 x/week
Post–PD dose	15 mg/kg (IM) or 1 gm (IM) or 20–40 mg/ml in dialysate q24h
CVVH/CVVHD/CVVHDF dose	15 mg/kg (IM) or 1 gm (IM) q96h
Mild-moderate hepatic insufficiency	No change
Severe hepatic insufficiency	No change

Drug Interactions: Amphotericin B, cephalothin, cyclosporine, enflurane, methoxyflurane, NSAIDs, polymyxin B, radiographic contrast, vancomycin (↑ nephrotoxicity); cis-platinum (↑ nephrotoxicity, ↑ ototoxicity); loop diuretics (↑ ototoxicity); neuromuscular blocking agents (↑ apnea, prolonged paralysis); non-polarizing muscle relaxants (↑ apnea).
Adverse Effects: Most ototoxic aminoglycoside (usually vestibular ototoxicity); least nephrotoxic aminoglycoside.
Allergic Potential: Low
Safety in Pregnancy: D
Comments: May be given IV slowly over 1 hour. **TB D.O.T. dose:** 20–30 mg/kg (IM) 2–3x/week. **Tularemia dose:** 1 gm (IV/IM) q12h. **Plague dose:** 2 gm (IV/IM) q12h.
Cerebrospinal Fluid Penetration: 20%

REFERENCES:

Akaho E, Maekawa T, Uchinashi M. A study of streptomycin blood level information of patients undergoing hemodialysis. Biopharm Drug Dispos 23:47–52, 2002.

Davidson PT, Le HQ. Drug treatment of tuberculosis 1992. Drugs 43:651–73, 1992.

"Usual dose" assumes normal renal/hepatic function. * For renal insufficiency, give usual dose × 1 followed by maintenance dose per CrCl. For dialysis patients, dose the same as for CrCl < 10 mL/min and give supplemental (post-HD/PD dose) immediately after dialysis. CrCl = creatinine clearance; CVVH = continuous veno-venous hemofiltration; HD/PD = hemodialysis/peritoneal dialysis.

Kim-Sing A, Kays MB, Vivien EJ, et al. Intravenous streptomycin use in a patient infection with high-level gentamicin-resistant Streptococcus faecalis. Ann Pharmacother 27:712–4, 1993.

Morris JT, Cooper RH. Intravenous streptomycin: A useful route of administration. Clin Infect Dis 19:1150–1, 1994.

Roushan MRH, Mohraz M, Hajiahmadi M, et al. Efficacy of gentamicin plus doxycycline versus streptomycin plus doxycycline in the treatment of brucellosis in humans. Clin Infect Dis 42:1075–80, 2006.

Van Scoy RE, Wilkowske CJ. Antituberculous agents. Mayo Clin Proc 67:179–87, 1992.

Ormerod P. The clinical management of the drug-resistant patient. Ann NY Acad Sci 953:185–91, 2001.

Telaprevir (Incivek)

Drug class: NS3/4A PI for HCV (genotype 1).
Usual dose: 750 mg PO q 7–9h with food, not low fat (+ ribavirin and peginterferon alfa).
Pharmacokinetic Parameters:
Peak serum level: 3510 mcg/L
Bioavailability: no data
Excreted unchanged: 1%
Serum half-life (normal/ESRD): 4.5/4–5 hrs
Plasma protein binding: 60–76%
Volume of distribution (V_d): 252 L/kg
Primary Mode of Elimination: Hepatic through CYP3A4/5
Dosage Adjustments*

CrCl <10 mL/min	No change
Post-HD dose	None
Post-PD dose	None
CVVH/CVVHD/CVVHDF dose	No change
Moderate to severe hepatic insufficiency	Avoid

Drug Interactions: Strong inhibitor of and metabolized through CYP3A4/5. Digoxin, carbamazapine, trazodone, itraconazole, posiconazole, colchicine, alprazolan, midazolam, calcium channel blockers, prednisone, methylprednisone, inhaled/nasal steroids, atazanavir, tenofovir, immunosupressants, inhaled salmeterol, PDE5 inhibitor (↑ levels). Warfarin, phenytoin, phenobarbital and voriconazole (↑/↓ levels). ↓ ethinyl estradilol, efavirenz (↓ levels). ↑ telaprevir to 1125 mg q8h.
Contraindications: alfuzosin, rifampin, rifabutin, ergot derivatives, cisapride, St. John's Wort, darunavir, fosamprenavir, lovastatin, simvastatin, drosperinone, Revatio or Adcirca, pimozide, triazolam, inhaled salmeterol.
Adverse Effects: Rash (drug rash with eosinophilia, Stevens-Johnson Syndrome), pruritis, dysgeusia, dausea, vomiting, diarrhea, anorectal discomfort, fatigue, anemia.
Allergic Potential: High
Safety in Pregnancy: B for Incivek, X for ribavirin, (See Ribavirin Drug Summary)
Comments: Do not use as monotherapy, only use with ribavirin and peginterferon alfa. No data for Child-Pugh class B and C, organ transplant, HIV, HBV coninfection or children < 18 yo. Discontinue for severe or progressive rash. If missed dose is within 4 hours of usual dose time to take the missed dose and resume the normal dosing schedule. If the missed dose is noted more than 4 hours after the usual dose time, skip the missed dose and continue with the next dose. Hormonal contraceptives may not be reliable during Incivek and for 2 weeks after discontinuation. Adjust dose for decrease in hemoglobin (See Ribavirin Drug Summary).

"Usual dose" assumes normal renal/hepatic function. * For renal insufficiency, give usual dose × 1 followed by maintenance dose per CrCl. For dialysis patients, dose the same as for CrCl < 10 mL/min and give supplemental (post-HD/PD dose) immediately after dialysis. CrCl = creatinine clearance; CVVH = continuous veno-venous hemofiltration; HD/PD = hemodialysis/peritoneal dialysis.

REFERENCES:

Jacobson IM, McHutchinson JG, Dusheiko G. Telaprevir for previously untreated chronic Hepatitis C virus infection. N Eng Journal of Medicine 23:2405–2416, 2011.

Kilbanov OM, Williams SH, Smith LS, et al. Telaprevir: a novel NS3/4 protease inhibitor for the treatment of hepatitis C. Pharmacotherapy 31:951–974, 2011.

Kumada H, Toyota J, Okanoue T, et al. Telaprevir with peginterferon and ribacirin for treatment-naïve patients chronically infected with HCV of genotype 1 in Japan, J Hepatol 2011.

Leise MD, Kim WR, Canterbury KM, et al. Drug therapy: telaprevir. Hepatology 54:1463–1469, 2011.

Razonable R. Antiviral drug for viruses other than human immunodeficiency virus. Mayo Clinic Proceedings 86:1009–1026, 2011.

Zeuzem S, Androneo P, Pol S. Telaprevir for retreatment of HCV infection. N Eng Journal of Medicine 23:2471–2428, 2011.

Telavancin (Vibativ)

Drug class: Lipolycopeptide.
Usual dose: 10 mg/kg (IV) q24h.
Spectrum: (see *Susceptibility Profiles* pp. 198–202).
Resistance Potential: Low
Pharmacokinetic Parameters:

Peak serum level: 93–108 mcg/mL
Bioavailability: not applicable
Excreted unchanged: 76%
Serum half-life (normal/ESRD): 6–9 hrs/no data
Plasma protein binding: 93%
Volume of distribution (V_d): 0.133-0.145 mL/kg

Primary Mode of Elimination: Renal
Dosage Adjustments*

CrCl > 50 mL/min	No change
CrCl 30–50 mL/min	7.5 mg/kg (IV) q24h
CrCl 10–29 mL/min	10 mg/kg (IV) q48h
CrCl < 10 mL/min	Avoid
Post–HD dose	None
Post–PD dose	None
CVVH/CVVHD/ CVVHDF dose	7.5 mg/kg (IV) q24h
Mild-moderate hepatic insufficiency	No change
Severe hepatic insufficiency	Use with caution

Drug Interactions: Drugs that prolong QT_c (additive effect); PT, INR, PTT (↑ levels); other interactions unlikely because is not metabolized through CYP450 system.
Adverse Effects: Headache, taste disturbance, nausea, vomiting, diarrhea, nephrotoxicity, "red-man syndrome."
Allergic Potential: Low
Safety in Pregnancy: C
Comments: Infuse over at least 60 minutes to minimize infusion-related reactions. Effective for MSSA/MRSA cSSSIs. Efficacy may be decreased with CrCl < 50 ml/min.
Cerebrospinal Fluid Penetration:
Inflamed meninges: 2%
Non-inflamed meninges: 1%
(also see *Antibiotic Pearls & Pitfalls* p. 519).

REFERENCES:

Damodaran SE, Madhan S. Telavancin: A novel lipoglycopeptide antibiotic. J Pharmacother 2: 135–137, 2011.

Joson J, Grover C, Downer C, et al. Successful treatment of methicillin-resistant Staphylococcus aureus mitral valve endocarditis with sequential linezolid and telavancin monotherapy following

---

"Usual dose" assumes normal renal/hepatic function. * For renal insufficiency, give usual dose × 1 followed by maintenance dose per CrCl. For dialysis patients, dose the same as for CrCl < 10 mL/min and give supplemental (post-HD/PD dose) immediately after dialysis. CrCl = creatinine clearance; CVVH = continuous veno-venous hemofiltration; HD/PD = hemodialysis/peritoneal dialysis.

daptomycin failure. J Antimicrob Chemother 66:2186–2188, 2011.

Leonard SN, Szeto YG, Zolotarev M, et al. Comparative in vitro activity of telavancin, vancomycin, and linezolid against heterogeneously vancomycin-intermediate Staphylococcus aureus (hVISA). Int J Antimicrob 37:558–561, 2011.

Marcos LA, Camins BC. Successful treatment of vancomycin-intermediate Staphylococcus aureus pacemaker lead infective endocarditis with telavancin. Antimicrob Agents Chemother 54:5376–5378, 2010.

Nailor MD, Sobel JD. Antibiotics for gram-positive bacterial infection: vancomycin, teicoplanin, quinupristin/dalfopristin, oxazolidinones, daptomycin, telavancin, and ceftaroline fosamil. Med Clin North Am 95:723–742, 2011.

Plotkin P, Patel K, Uminski A, et al. Telavancin (Vibativ), a new option for the treatment of gram-positive infections. Pharm Ther 36:127–138, 2011a.

Plotkin P, Patel K, Uminski A, et al. Telavancin for the treatment of methicillin-resistant staphylococcus aureus J Antimicrob Chemother 66:2675–2677, 2011b.

Saravolatz LD, Stein GE, Johnson LB. Telavancin: a novel lipoglycopeptide. Clin Infect Dis 49:1908–1914, 2009.

Shams W, Walker ES, Levy F, et al. Comparative activity of telavancin and other antimicrobial agents against methicillin-resistant Staphylococcus aureus isolates collected from 1991 to 2006. Chemotherapy 56:411–416, 2010.

Stryjewski ME, Graham DR, Wilson SE, et al. Telavancin versus vancomycin for the treatment of complicated skin and skin-structure infections caused by gram-positive organisms. Clin Infect Dis 46:1683–1693, 2008.

Twilla JD, Gelfand MS, Cleveland KO, et al. Telvancin for the treatment of methicillin-resistant Staphylococcus aureus osteomyelitis. J Antimicrob Chemother 66:2675–2677, 2011.

Wilson SE, O'Rierdan W, Hopkins A, et al. Telavancin versus vancomycin for the treatment of complicated skin and skin-structure infections associated with surgical procedures. Am J Surg 197:791–796, 2009.

Website: www.vibativ.com

Telbivudine (Tyzeka)

Drug class: HBV antiviral.

Usual dose: 600 mg (PO) q24h.

Pharmacokinetic Parameters:

Peak serum level: 3.69 mcg/mL

Bioavailability: high

Excreted unchanged: 42%

Serum half-life (normal/ESRD): 20 h/32 h

Plasma protein binding: 3%

Volume of distribution (V_d): no data

Primary Mode of Elimination: Renal

Dosage Adjustments*

CrCl 30–49 mL/min	600 mg tablet (PO) q48h or 400 mg solution (PO) q24h
CrCl < 30 mL/min	600 mg tablet (PO) q72h or 200 mg solution (PO) q24h
CrCl < 10 mL/min	600 mg tablet (PO) q96h or 120 mg solution (PO) q24h
Post–HD dose	600 mg tablet (PO) q96h or 120 mg solution (PO) q24h
Post–PD dose	No data
CVVH/CVVHD/ CVVHDF dose	600 mg tablet (PO) q72h or 200 mg solution (PO) q24h
Moderate—severe hepatic insufficiency	No change

Drug Interactions: Interferon (↑ risk of peripheral neuropathy) nephrotoxic drugs (↑ nephrotoxicity).

Adverse Effects: myopathy; peripheral neuropathy; fatigue; dizziness; headache; throat pain; cough; diarrhea; abdominal pain; abdominal distension; nausea; arthralgias;

"Usual dose" assumes normal renal/hepatic function. * For renal insufficiency, give usual dose × 1 followed by maintenance dose per CrCl. For dialysis patients, dose the same as for CrCl < 10 mL/min and give supplemental (post-HD/PD dose) immediately after dialysis. CrCl = creatinine clearance; CVVH = continuous veno-venous hemofiltration; HD/PD = hemodialysis/peritoneal dialysis.

rash; fever; myalgias; insomnia. ↑ CPK, ↑ SGOT/ SGPT.

Comments: Lactic acidosis and hepatomegaly, some cases fatal.

Allergic Potential: Low

Safety in Pregnancy: B

Highly active against HBV.

REFERENCES:

Liaw YF, et al. 2-year GLOBE trial results: telbivudine is superioir to lamivudine in patients with crhonic hepatitis B. Gastroenterology 136:486–95, 2009.

Zhou X, et al. Pharmacokinetics in telbivudine in subjects with various degrees of renal impairment. Antimicrob Agents Chemother 51:4231–35, 2007.

Telithromycin (Ketek)

Drug Class: Ketolide.

Usual Dose: Acute sinusitis/AECB: 800 mg (PO) q24h × 5 days. Community-acquired pneumonia: 800 mg (PO) q24h × 7–10 days. 800 mg (PO) dose taken as two 400-mg tablets (PO) at once.

Spectrum: (see *Susceptibility Profiles* pp.186–190).

Resistance Potential: Low.

Pharmacokinetic Parameters:

Peak serum level: 2.27 mcg/ml

Bioavailability: 57%

Excreted unchanged (urine): 13%

Serum half-life (normal/ESRD): 9.8/11 hrs

Plasma protein binding: 65%

Volume of distribution (V_d): 2.9 L/kg

Primary Mode of Elimination: Hepatic

Dosage Adjustments*

CrCl < 30 mL/min	600 mg (PO) q24h
CrCl < 30 mL/min + hepatic impairment	400 mg (PO) q24h

Post–HD/Post–PD dose	400 mg (PO)
CVVH/CVVHD/ CVVHDF dose	400 mg (PO) q24h

Drug Interactions: Digoxin (↑ interacting drug levels); ergot derivatives (acute ergot toxicity); itraconazole, ketoconazole (↑ telithromycin level); midazolam, triazolam (↑ interacting drug levels, sedation); oral anticoagulants (may ↑ anticoagulant effects; monitor PT/INR); simvastatin (↑ risk of rhabdomyolysis; giving simvastatin 12h after telithromycin decreases the ↑ in simvastatin levels ~ 50%); theophylline (additive nausea). CYP 3A4 inhibitor/substate. Telithromycin is contraindicated with cisapride and pimozide.

Adverse Effects: Nausea, diarrhea, dizziness, syncope, eye accomodation difficulties. *Contraindicated in patients with history of hepatitis/jaundice* (rarely fatal acute/ fulminant hepatitis or acute liver failure in those with pre-existing liver disease). Avoid with myasthenia gravis (↑ risk of respiratory failure).

Allergic Potential: Low

Safety in Pregnancy: C

Comments: May take with or without food. New smaller tablets minimize potential GI upset.

REFERENCES:

Aubier M, Aldons PM, Leak A, et al. Telithromycin is as effective as amoxicillin/clavulanate in acute exacerbations of chronic bronchitis. Respir Med 96:862–71, 2002.

Brown SD, Farrell DJ. Antibacterial susceptibility among Streptococcus pneumoniae isolated from paediatric and adult patients as part of the PROTECT US study in 2001–2002. Journal of Antimicrobial Chemotherapy 54 (Suppl. S1):23–29, 2004.

"Usual dose" assumes normal renal/hepatic function. * For renal insufficiency, give usual dose × 1 followed by maintenance dose per CrCl. For dialysis patients, dose the same as for CrCl < 10 mL/min and give supplemental (post-HD/PD dose) immediately after dialysis. CrCl = creatinine clearance; CVVH = continuous veno-venous hemofiltration; HD/PD = hemodialysis/peritoneal dialysis.

Brown SD, Rybak MJ. Antimicrobial susceptibility of Streptococcus pneumoniae, Streptococcus pyogenes and Haemophilus influenzae collected from patients across the USA, in 2001–2002, as part of the PROTECT US study. Journal of Antimicrobial Chemotherapy 54 (Suppl. S1):7–15, 2004.

Carbon C, Moola S, Velancsics I, et al. Telithromycin 800 mg once daily for seven to ten days is an effective and well-tolerated treatment for community-acquired pneumonia. Clin Microbiol Infect 9:691–703, 2003.

Dunbar LM, Carbon C, van Rensburg D, et al. Efficacy of telithromycin in community-acquired pneumonia caused by atypical and intracellular pathogens. Infect Dis Clin Pract 13:10–16, 2005.

Ferguson BJ, Guzzetta RV, Spector SL, et al. Efficacy and safety of oral telithromycin once daily for 5 days versus moxifloxacin one daily for 10 days in the treatment of acute bacterial rhinosinusitis. Otolaryngol Head Neck Surg 131:207–14, 2004.

Hagberg L, Torres A, van Rensburg D, et al. Efficacy and tolerability of once-daily telithromycin compared with high-dose amoxicillin for treatment of community-acquired pneumonia. Infection 30:378–386, 2002.

Jacobs MR. In vivo veritas: in vitro macrolide resistance in systemic S. pneumoniae infections does result in clinical failure. Clin Infect Dis 35:565–9, 2002.

Kim, DM, Yu KD, Lee JH, et al. Controlled trial of 5-day course of telithromycin versus doxycycline for treatment of mild to moderate scrub typhus. Antimicrob Agents Chemother 51:2011–2015, 2007.

Klugman KP, Lonks JR. Hidden epidemic of macrolide-resistant pneumococci. Emerg Infect Dis 11:802–807, 2005.

Low DE, Brown S, Felmingham D. Clinical and bacteriology efficacy of the ketolide telithromycin against isolates of key respiratory pathogens: a pooled analysis of phase III studies. Clin Microbiol Infect 10:27–36, 2004.

Ortega M, Marco F, Almela M, et al. Activity of telithromycin against erythromycin-susceptible resistant Streptococcus pneumoniae is from adults with invasive infections. Int J Antimicrob Agents 24:616–8, 2004.

Tellier G, Niederman MS, Nusrat R, et al. Clinical and bacteriological efficacy and safety of 5 and 7 day regimens of telithromycin once daily compared with a 10 day regimen of clarithromycin twice daily in patients with mild to moderate community-acquired pneumonia. Journal of Antimicrobial Chemotherapy 54:515–523, 2004.

van Rensburg D, Fogarty C, De Salvo MC, et al. Efficacy of oral telithromycin in community-acquired pneumonia caused by resistant Streptococcus pneumoniae. Journal of Infection 51:201–5, 2005.

Zervos MJ, Heyder AM, Leroy B. Oral telithromycin 800 mg once daily for 5 days versus cefuroxime axetil 500 mg twice daily for 10 days in adults with acute exacerbations of chronic bronchitis. J Int Med Res 31:157–69, 2003.

Website: www.ketek.com

Tenofovir disoproxil fumarate (Viread) TDF

Drug Class: Antiretroviral (nucleotide analogue).

Usual Dose: 300 mg (PO) q24h.

Pharmacokinetic Parameters:

Peak serum level: 0.29 mcg/mL

Bioavailability: 25%/39% (fasting/high fat meal)

Excreted unchanged (urine): 32%

Serum half-life (normal/ESRD): 17 hrs/no data

Plasma protein binding: 0.7–7.2%

Volume of distribution (V_d): 1.3 L/kg

Primary Mode of Elimination: Renal

Dosage Adjustments*

CrCl 30–49 mL/min	300 mg (PO) q48h
CrCl 10–29 mL/min	300 mg (PO) 2x/week
CrCl < 10 mL/min	Avoid
Post–HD dose	300 mg q7 days

"Usual dose" assumes normal renal/hepatic function. * For renal insufficiency, give usual dose × 1 followed by maintenance dose per CrCl. For dialysis patients, dose the same as for CrCl < 10 mL/min and give supplemental (post-HD/PD dose) immediately after dialysis. CrCl = creatinine clearance; CVVH = continuous veno-venous hemofiltration; HD/PD = hemodialysis/peritoneal dialysis.

Post–PD dose	No data
CVVH/CVVHD/CVVHDF dose	300 mg (PO) 2x/week
Moderate hepatic insufficiency	No change
Severe hepatic insufficiency	No change

Drug Interactions: Not a substrate/inhibitor of cytochrome P-450 enzymes. Didanosine (if possible, avoid concomitant didanosine due to impaired CD$_4$ response and increased risk of virologic failure); valganciclovir (↑ tenofovir levels); atazanavir, lopinavir/ritonavir (↓ atazanavir levels; use atazanavir 300 mg/ritonavir 100 mg with tenofovir); telaprevir (↑ tenofovir levels).

Adverse Effects: Lactic acidosis and severe hepatomegaly with steatosis, including fatal cases, with nucleoside analogs. Severe acute exacerbations of hepatitis in HBV who have discontinued HBV therapy, including teonofovir. Mild nausea, vomiting, GI upset, asthenia, headache, diarrhea renal tubular acidosis, decrease bone density occur. It is recommended that creatinine clearance be calculated in all patients prior to initiating therapy and as clinically appropriate during therapy with tenofovir. Fanconi-like Syndrome routine monitoring of calculated creatinine clearance and serum phosphorus should be performed in patients at risk for renal impairment. Immune constitution syndrome can occur.

Allergic Potential: Low
Safety in Pregnancy: B

Comments: Eliminated by glomerular filtration/tubular secretion. May be taken with or without food. If possible, avoid concomitant didanosine (see drug interactions). ***Active against HBV.***
Cerebrospinal Fluid Penetration: No data

REFERENCES:
Choi AL, Vittinghoff E, Deeks SG, et al. Cardiovascular risks associated with abacavir and tenofovir exposure in HIV-infected persons. AIDS 19;25:1289–98, 2011.

Cooper RD, Wiebe N, Smith N, et al. Systematic review and Meta-analysis: Renal safety of tenovovir disoproxil fumarate in HIV-infected patients. Clin Infect Dis 51:496–505, 2010.

Daudé M, Rostaing L, Sauné K, et al. Tenofovir therapy in hepatitis B virus-positive solid-organ transplant recipients. Transplantation 91:916–920, 2011.

Dupouey J, Gerolami R, Solas C, et al. Adefovir and tenofovir therapy. Clin Res Hepatol Gastroenterol 36:e26–28, 2012.

Gallant JE, Deresinski S, Tenofovir disoproxil furnarate. Clin Infect Dis 37:944–50, 2003.

Hall AM, Hendry BM, Nitsch D, et al. Tenofovir-associated kidney toxicity in HIV-infected patients: A review of new evidence. Am J Kidney Dis 57:773–80, 2011.

Maggi P, Montinaro V, Bellacosa C, et al. Tenofovir versus abacavir. AIDS Patient Care STDS 26:5–11, 2012.

Panel on Antiretroviral Guidelines for Adults and Adolescents. Department of Health and Human Services. Guidelines for the use of antiretroviral agents in HIV-infected adults and adolescents. http://aidsinfo.nih.gov/ConsentFiles/AdultandAdolescentGL.pdf, 2012.

Ratcliffe L, Beadsworth MD, Pennell A, et al. Managing hepatitis B/HIV co-infected: adding entecavir to truvada (tenofovir disoproxil/emtricitabine) experienced patients. AIDS 25:1051–1056, 2011.

Sax PE, Tierney C, Collier AC, et al. Abacavir/lamivudine versus tenofovir DF/emtricitabine as part of combination regimens for initial treatment of HIV: final results. AIDS clinical trials group study A5202 team 204:1191–1201, 2011.

"Usual dose" assumes normal renal/hepatic function. * For renal insufficiency, give usual dose × 1 followed by maintenance dose per CrCl. For dialysis patients, dose the same as for CrCl < 10 mL/min and give supplemental (post-HD/PD dose) immediately after dialysis. CrCl = creatinine clearance; CVVH = continuous veno-venous hemofiltration; HD/PD = hemodialysis/peritoneal dialysis.

Sax PE, Tierney C, Collier AC, et al. Abacavir/lamivudine versus tenofovir DF/emtricitabine as part of combination regimens for initial treatment of HIV: final results. J Infect Dis 204:1191–201, 2011.

Scotto G, D'Addiego G, Giammario A, et al. Tenofovir plus entecavir as rescue therapy for multidrug-resistant chronic hepatitis B. Liver Int 32:171–2, 2012.

Si-Ahmen SN, Pradat P, Soutendijik R, et al. Efficacy and tolerance of a combinatory tenofovir disoproxil fumarate plus emtricitabine in patients with chronic hepatitis B: A European multicenter study 92: 90–95, 2011.

Thompson MA, Aberg JA, Cahn P, et al. Antiretroviral treatment of adult HIV infection: 2012 recommendations of the International Antiviral Society — USA panel. JAMA 308:387–402, 2012.

Website: www.viread.com

Terbinafine (Lamisil, Daskil)

Drug Class: Antifungal.
Usual Dose: 250 mg (PO) q24h.
Pharmacokinetic Parameters:
Peak serum level: 1 mcg/ml
Bioavailability: 70%
Excreted unchanged (urine): < 1%
Serum half-life (normal/ESRD): 24 hrs/no data
Plasma protein binding: 99%
Volume of distribution (V_d): 13.5 L/kg
Primary Mode of Elimination: Renal/hepatic
Dosage Adjustments*

CrCl ~ 50–60 mL/min	No change
CrCl < 50 mL/min	Avoid
Post–HD dose	Avoid
Post–PD dose	Avoid
CVVH/CVVHD/CVVHDF dose	Avoid
Moderate–severe hepatic insufficiency	Avoid

Drug Interactions: Cimetidine (↓ terbinafine clearance, ↑ terbinafine levels); phenobarbital, rifampin (↑ terbinafine clearance, ↓ terbinafine levels).
Adverse Effects: Drug fever/rash, lymphopenia, leukopenia, ↑ SGOT/SGPT, visual disturbances, nausea, vomiting, GI upset.
Allergic Potential: Low
Safety in Pregnancy: B
Comments: May cause green vision and changes in the lens/retina.
Cerebrospinal Fluid Penetration: < 10%

REFERENCES:

Abdel-Rahman SM, Nahata MC. Oral terbinafine: A new antifungal agent. Ann Pharmacother 31:445–56, 1997.

Amichai B, Grunwald MH. Adverse drug reactions of the new oral antifungal agents – terbinafine, fluconazole, and itraconazole. Int J Dermatol 37:410–5, 1998.

Darkes MJ, Scott LJ, Goa KL. Terbinafine: a review of its use in onychomycosis in adults. Am J Clin Dermatol 4:39–65, 2003.

Jain S, Sehgal VN. Itraconazole versus terbinafine in the management of onychomycosis: an overview. J Dermatolog Treat 14:30–42, 2003.

Mosquera J, Shartt A, Moore CB, et al. In vitro interaction of terbinafine with itraconazole, fluconazole, amphotericin B and 5-flucytosine against Aspergillus spp. J Antimicrob Chemother 50:189–94, 2002.

Salo H, Pekurinen M. Cost effectiveness or oral terbinafine (Lamisil) compared with oral fluconazole (Diflucan) in the treatment of patients with toenail onychomycosis. Pharmacoeconomics 20:319–24, 2002.

Trepanier EF, Amsden GW. Current issues in onychomycosis. Ann Pharmacother 32:204–14, 1998.

Website: www.pdr.net

Tetracycline (various)

Drug Class: Tetracycline.
Usual Dose: 500 mg (PO) q6h (Take without food).
Spectrum: (see *Susceptibility Profiles* pp. 186–190).

"Usual dose" assumes normal renal/hepatic function. * For renal insufficiency, give usual dose × 1 followed by maintenance dose per CrCl. For dialysis patients, dose the same as for CrCl < 10 mL/min and give supplemental (post-HD/PD dose) immediately after dialysis. CrCl = creatinine clearance; CVVH = continuous veno-venous hemofiltration; HD/PD = hemodialysis/peritoneal dialysis.

Resistance Potential: High (S. pneumoniae, MSSA)

Pharmacokinetic Parameters:

Peak serum level: 1.5 mcg/ml

Bioavailability: 60%

Excreted unchanged (urine): 60%

Serum half-life (normal/ESRD): 8/108 hrs

Plasma protein binding: 5%

Volume of distribution (V_d): 0.7 L/kg

Primary Mode of Elimination: Renal

Dosage Adjustments*

CrCl 50–80 mL/min	500 mg (PO) q12h
CrCl 10–50 mL/min	500 mg (PO) q24h
Post–HD/Post–PD dose	None
CVVH/CVVHD/ CVVHDF dose	500 mg (PO) q12h
Moderate hepatic insufficiency	No change
Severe hepatic insufficiency	≤ 1 gm (PO) q24h

Drug Interactions: Antacids, Al⁺⁺, Ca⁺⁺, Fe⁺⁺, Mg⁺⁺, Zn⁺⁺, multivitamins, sucralfate (↓ absorption of tetracycline); barbiturates, carbamazepine, phenytoin (↓ half-life of tetracycline); bicarbonate (↓ absorption and ↑ clearance of tetracycline); digoxin (↑ digoxin levels); insulin (↑ insulin effect); methoxyflurane (↑ nephrotoxicity).

Adverse Effects: Nausea, vomiting, GI upset, diarrhea, hepatotoxicity, vaginal candidiasis, photosensitizing reactions, benign intracranial hypertension (pseudotumor cerebri).

Allergic Potential: Low

Safety in Pregnancy: D

Comments: Take without food. *Hepatotoxicity dose dependent (≥ 2 gm/day), especially in pregnancy/renal failure. Avoid prolonged sun exposure. Doxycycline or minocycline preferred for all tetracycline indications.*

Cerebrospinal Fluid Penetration:

Non-Inflamed meninges = 5%

Inflamed meninges = 5%

Bile Penetration: 1000% (also see ***Antibiotic Pearls & Pitfalls*** p. 512).

REFERENCES:

Agwuh KN, MacGowan A. Pharmacokinetics and pharmacodynamics of the tetracyclines including glyclcyclines. J of Antimicrob Chemotherapy 58:256–265, 2006.

Cunha BA, Comer J, Jonas M. The tetracyclines. Med Clin North Am 66:293–302, 1982.

Dahl EL, Shock JL, Shenai BR, et al. Tetracyclines specifically target the apicoplast of the malaria parasite Plasmodium falciparum. Antimicrob Agents Chemother 50:3124–31, 2006.

Malfertheiner P, Bazzoli F, Delchier JC, et al. Helicobacter pylori eradication with a capsule containing bismuth subcitrate potassium, metronidazole, and tetracycline given with omeprazole versus clarithromycin-based triple therapy: a randomized, open-label, non-inferiority, phase 3 trial. Lancet 33:905–913, 2011.

Pugliese A, Cunha BA. Tetracyclines. Int J Urogyn 5:221–7, 1994.

Smilack JD, Wilson WE, Cocerill Fr 3rd. Tetracycline, chloramphenicol, erythromycin, clindamycin, and metronidazole. Mayo Clin Proc 66:1270–80, 1991.

Ticarcillin (Ticar)

Drug Class: Anti-pseudomonal penicillin.

Usual Dose: 3 gm (IV) q6h.

Spectrum: (see ***Susceptibility Profiles*** pp. 186–190).

Resistance Potential: Low

Pharmacokinetic Parameters:

Peak serum level: 118–300 mcg/ml

"Usual dose" assumes normal renal/hepatic function. * For renal insufficiency, give usual dose × 1 followed by maintenance dose per CrCl. For dialysis patients, dose the same as for CrCl < 10 mL/min and give supplemental (post-HD/PD dose) immediately after dialysis. CrCl = creatinine clearance; CVVH = continuous veno-venous hemofiltration; HD/PD = hemodialysis/peritoneal dialysis.

Bioavailability: Not applicable
Excreted unchanged (urine): 95%
Serum half-life (normal/ESRD): 1/5 hrs
Plasma protein binding: 45%
Volume of distribution (V_d): 0.2 L/kg
Primary Mode of Elimination: Renal
Dosage Adjustments*

CrCl 50–80 mL/min	No change
CrCl 10–50 mL/min	2 gm (IV) q8h
CrCl < 10 mL/min	2 gm (IV) q12h
Post–HD dose	2 gm (IV)
Post–PD dose	3 gm (IV)
CVVH/CVVHD/CVVHDF dose	2 gm (IV) q8h
Moderate hepatic insufficiency	No change
Severe hepatic insufficiency	No change

Drug Interactions: Aminoglycosides (inactivation of ticarcillin in renal failure); warfarin (↑ INR); oral contraceptives (↓ oral contraceptive effect); cefoxitin (↓ ticarcillin effect).
Adverse Effects: Drug fever/rash; E. multiforme/Stevens-Johnson Syndrome, anaphylactic reactions (hypotension, laryngospasm, bronchospasm), hives, serum sickness. Dose-dependent inhibition of platelet aggregation is minimal/absent (usual dose is less than carbenicillin). C. difficile diarrhea/colitis.
Allergic Potential: High
Safety in Pregnancy: B
Comments: Administer 1 hour before or after aminoglycoside. Na$^+$ content = 5.2 mEq/g. Meningeal dose = usual dose.
Cerebrospinal Fluid Penetration:
Non-Inflamed meninges = 1%

Inflamed meninges = 30%
(also see **Antibiotic Pearls & Pitfalls** p. 509).

REFERENCES:
Donowitz GR, Mandell GL. Beta-lactam antibiotics. N Engl J Med 318:419–26 and 318:490–500, 1993.
Tan JS, File TM, Jr. Antipseudomonal penicillins. Med Clin North Am 79:679–93, 1995.
Wright AJ. The penicillins. Mayo Clin Proc 74:290–307, 1999.

Ticarcillin/Clavulanate (Timentin)

Drug Class: Anti-pseudomonal penicillin.
Usual Dose: 3.1 gm (IV) q6h.
Spectrum: (see **Susceptibility Profiles** pp. 186–190).
Resistance Potential: Low
Pharmacokinetic Parameters:
Peak serum level: 330 mcg/ml
Bioavailability: Not applicable
Excreted unchanged (urine): 95/45%
Serum half-life (normal/ESRD): [1/13]/[1/2] hrs
Plasma protein binding: 45/25%
Volume of distribution (V_d): 0.2/0.3 L/kg
Primary Mode of Elimination: Renal
Dosage Adjustments*

CrCl 30–60 mL/min	3.1 gm (IV) q8h
CrCl 10–30 mL/min	3.1 gm (IV) q12h
CrCl < 10 mL/min	2 gm (IV) q12h
Post–HD dose	3.1 gm (IV)
Post–PD dose	3.1 gm (IV)

"Usual dose" assumes normal renal/hepatic function. * For renal insufficiency, give usual dose × 1 followed by maintenance dose per CrCl. For dialysis patients, dose the same as for CrCl < 10 mL/min and give supplemental (post-HD/PD dose) immediately after dialysis. CrCl = creatinine clearance; CVVH = continuous veno-venous hemofiltration; HD/PD = hemodialysis/peritoneal dialysis.

CVVH/CVVHD/CVVHDF dose	3.1 gm (IV) q8h
Moderate hepatic insufficiency	If CrCl < 10 mL/min: 2 gm (IV) q24h
Severe hepatic insufficiency	If CrCl < 10 mL/min: 2 gm (IV) q24h

Drug Interactions: Aminoglycosides (↓ aminoglycoside levels); methotrexate (↑ methotrexate levels); vecuronium (↑ vecuronium effect).

Adverse Effects: Drug fever/rash, E. multiforme/Stevens-Johnson Syndrome, anaphylactic reactions (hypotension, laryngospasm, bronchospasm), hives, serum sickness. C. difficile diarrhea/colitis.

Allergic Potential: High

Safety in Pregnancy: B

Comments: 20% of clavulanate removed by dialysis. Na^+ content = 4.75 mEq/g. K^+ content = 0.15 mEq/g.

Cerebrospinal Fluid Penetration: < 10%

Bile Penetration:

Without obstruction = 100%

With obstruction = 10%

(also see *Antibiotic Pearls & Pitfalls* p. 509).

REFERENCES:

Donowitz GR, Mandell GL. Beta-lactam antibiotics. N Engl J Med 318:419–26 and 318:490–500, 1993.

Graham DR, Talan DA, Nichols RL, et al. Once-daily, high-dose levofloxacin versus ticarcillin-clavulanate alone or followed by amoxicillin-clavulanate for complicated skin and skin-structure infections: a randomized, open-label trial. Clin Infect Dis 35: 381–9, 2002.

Itokazu GS, Danziger LH. Ampicillin-sulbactam and ticarcillin-clavulanic acid: A comparison of their in vitro activity and review of their clinical efficacy. Pharmacotherapy 11:382–414, 1991.

Winston LG, Charlebois ED, Pang S, et al. Impact of a formulary switch from ticarcillin-clavulanate to piperacillin-tazobactam on colonization with vancomycin-resistant enterococci. Am J Infect Control 32:462–9, 2004.

Website: www.timentin.com

Tigecycline (Tygacil)

Drug Class: Glycylcycline.

Usual Dose: *Loading Dose:* **100 mg (IV) × 1 dose, (PI dose) or 200 mg (IV) × 1 dose, then 100 mg (IV) q24h (PK dose)** then *Maintenance Dose:* **50 mg (IV) q12h (PI dosing) or 100 mg (IV) q24h (PK dosing) (see comments†).**

Spectrum: (see *Susceptibility Profiles* pp. 198–202).

Resistance Potential: Low (Acinetobacter baumanii)

Pharmacokinetic Parameters:

Peak serum level: 1.45 mcg/ml (100 mg dose); 0.87 mcg/ml (50 mg dose)

Bioavailability: Not applicable

Excreted unchanged (urine): 22%

Serum half-life (normal/ESRD): 42/42 hrs

Plasma protein binding: 89%

Volume of distribution (V_d): 8 L/kg

Primary Mode of Elimination: Biliary

Dosage Adjustments*

CrCl < 10 mL/min	No change
Post–HD dose	None
Post–PD dose	None
CVVH/CVVHD/CVVHDF dose	No change

Mild-moderate hepatic insufficiency	No change
Severe hepatic insufficiency (Child Pugh C)	100 mg (IV) × 1 dose, then 25 mg (IV) q12h

Drug Interactions: Warfarin (↑ INR). Does not inhibit and is not metabolized by CYP450.
Adverse Effects: N/V, dyspepsia, diarrhea, dizziness, asthenia, thrombocytosis, ↑ SGOT, ↑ alkaline phosphatase, pancreatitis, (↑ amylase/lipase), ↑ LDH, ↑ BUN, ↓ total protein.
Allergic Potential: Low
Safety in Pregnancy: D
Comments: Effective for cSSSIs/cIAIs. *Higher loading/maintenance doses may be necessary for serious systemic infections or MDR Klebsiella pneumoniae or MDR Acinetobacter baumanii.*[*§†] *Following the initial Loading Dose* based on PK parameters, *Tigecycline may also be given q24h as a single daily Maintenance Dose.* Safe to use in penicillin/sulfa-allergic patients. *Tigacycline rarely causes N/V if sufficiently diluted and slowly infused.* If N/V occurs, ↑ infusion volume and infusion time as shown

Tigecycline Dose[†]	Volume	Infusion Time
100 mg	100 ml	30 min
200 mg[*]	250 ml	60 min
400 mg[§]	500 ml	120 min

* For serious systemic infections.
§ For GNB, serious systemic infections, or UTIs due to susceptible MDR GNBs.
† Maintence dose half of the loading dose.

Cerebrospinal Fluid Penetration: No data
Bile Penetration: 3800%
(also see *Antibiotic Pearls & Pitfalls* p. 518).

REFERENCES:
Babinchak T, Ellis-Grosse E, Dartois N, et al. The efficacy and safety of tigecycline for the treatment of complicated intra-abdominal infections: analysis of pooled clinical trial data. Clin Infect Dis 41(Suppl 5:S3):54–67, 2005.
Baines SD, Saxton K, Freeman K, et al. Tigecycline does not induce proliferation or cytotoxin production by epidemic Clostridium difficile strains in a human gut model. J Antimicrob Chemother 58:1062–1065, 2006.
Bendu C, Culebras E, Gomez M, et al. In vitro activity of tigecycline against Bacteroides species. J Antimicrob Chemother 56:349–52, 2005.
Bergallo C, Jasovich A, Teglia O, et al. Safety and efficacy of intravenous tigecycline in Treatment of community-acquired pneumonia: results from a double-blind randomized Phase 3 comparison study with levofloxacin. Diagn Microbiol Infect Dis 63:52–61, 2009.
Bolmstrom A, Karlsson A, Engelhardt A, et al. Validation and reproducibility assessment of tigecycline MIC determinations by Etest. J Clin Microbiol 45:2474–2479, 2007.
Bopp LH, Baltch AL, Ritz WJ, et al. Activities of tigecycline and comparators against Legionella pneumophila and Legionella micdadei extracellularly and in human monocytederived macrophages. Diagn Microbiol Infect Dis 69:86–93, 2011.
Bouza E. New therapeutic choices for infections caused by methicillin-resistant Staphylococcus aureus. Clin Microbiol Infect Dis 15:44–52, 2009.
Bradford PA, Weaver-Sands DT, Petersen PJ. In vitro activity of tigecycline against isolates from patients enrolled in phase 3 clinical trials of treatment for complicated skin and skin-structure infections and complicated intra-abdominal infections. Clin Infect Dis 41(Suppl 5):S315–32, 2005.

"Usual dose" assumes normal renal/hepatic function. * For renal insufficiency, give usual dose × 1 followed by maintenance dose per CrCl. For dialysis patients, dose the same as for CrCl < 10 mL/min and give supplemental (post-HD/PD dose) immediately after dialysis. CrCl = creatinine clearance; CVVH = continuous veno-venous hemofiltration; HD/PD = hemodialysis/peritoneal dialysis.

Bulik CC, Wiskirchen DE, Shepard A, et al. Tissue penetration and pharmacokinetics of tigecycline in diabetic chronic wound infections described by using in vivo microdialysis. Antimicrob Agents Chemother 54:5209–4213, 2010.

Cai Y, Wang R, Liang B, et al. Systematic review and meta-analysis of the effectiveness and safety of tigecycline for treatment of infectious disease. Antimicrob Agents Chemother 55:1162–1172, 2011.

Cheong EY, Gottlieb T. Intravenous tigecycline in the treatment of severe recurrent Clostridium difficile colitis. Med J. Aust 4:374–375, 2011.

Conde-Estévez D, Grau S, Horcajada JP, et al. Off-label prescription of tigecycline: clinical and microbiological characteristics and outcomes. Int J Antimicrob Agents 36:471–472, 2010.

Cunha BA, McDermott B, Nausheen S. Single once daily high dose therapy of tigecycline in a urinary tract infection due to multi-drug resistant (MDR) Klebsiella pneumoniae and MDR Enterobacter agglomerans. Journal of Chemotherapy 19:753–754, 2008.

Cunha BA. Once daily tigecycline therapy of multidrug-resistant and non-multidrug resistant gram-negative bacteremias. J of Chemother 19:232–33, 2007.

Cunha BA. Antimicrobial therapy of multidrug-resistant Streptococcus pneumoniae, vancomycin-resistant enterococci, and methicillin-resistant Staphlycoccus aureus. Med Clin N Am 90:1165–82, 2006.

Daly MW, Riddle DJ, Ledeboer NA, et al. Tigecycline for treatment of pneumonia and empyema caused by carbapenems-producing Klebsiella pneumoniae. Pharmacotherapy 27:1052–1057, 2007.

Dandache P, Nicolau DP, Sakoulas G. Tigecycline for the treatment of multidrug-resistant Klebsiella pneumoniae meningitis. Infect Dis in Clin Practice 17:66–68, 2009.

Dartois N, Castiang N, Gandjini H, et al. Tigecycline versus levofloxacin for the treatment of community-acquired pneumonia: European experience. J Chemother 20:28–35, 2008.

Dizbay M, Kilic S, Hizel K, et al. Tigecycline: its potential for treatment of brucellosis. Scand J Infect Dis 39:432–434, 2007.

Dominguez EA. Single agent therapy with tigecycline in the treatment of complicated skin and skin structure and complicated intraabdominal infections. Infectious Diseases in Clinical Practice 17:144–149, 2009.

Ellis-Grosse EJ, Babinchak T, Dartois N, et al. The efficacy and safety of tigecycline in the treatment of skin and skin-structure infections: results of 2 double-blind phase 3 comparison studies with vancomycin-aztreonam. Clin Infect Dis 41(Suppl 5): S341–53, 2005.

Fraise AP. Tigecycline: The answer to beta-lactam and fluoroquinolone resistance? Journal of Infection 53:293–300, 2006.

Gardiner D, Dukart G, Cooper A, et al. safety and efficacy of intravenous tigecycline in subjects with secondary bacteremia: pooled results from 8 phase III clinical trials. Clin Infect Dis 50:229–238, 2010.

Geerlings SE, van Donselaar-van der Pant KA, Keur I. Successful treatment with tigecycline of two patients with complicated urinary tract infections caused by extended-spectrum betalactamase-producing Escherichia coli. J Antimicrob Chemother 65:2048–2049, 2010.

Hawkey P, Finch R. Tigecycline: in-vitro performance as a predictor of clinical efficacy. Clin Microbiol Infect 13:354–362, 2007.

Hawser SP. Activity of tigecycline against recent European clinical isolates of Clostridium difficile. Int J Antimicrob Agents 35:97–98, 2010.

Herpers BL, Vlaminckx B, Burkhardt O, et al. Intravenous tigecycline as adjunctive or alternative therapy for severe refractory Clostridium difficile infection. Clin Infect Dis 48:1732–1735, 2009.

Hoban DJ, Bouchillon SK, Dowzicky MJ. Antimicrobial susceptibility of extended-spectrum beta-lactamase producers and multidrug-resistant Acinetobacter baumannii throughout the United States and comparative in vitro activity of tigecycline, a new glycylcycline antimicrobial. Diagn Microbiol Infect Dis 57:423–428, 2007.

Hope R, Mushtaq S, James D, et al. Tigecycline activity: low resistance rates but problematic disc breakpoints revealed by a multicentre sentinel survey in the UK. J Antimicrob Chemother 65:2602–2609, 2010.

Huang V, Cheung CM, Kaatz GW, et al. Evaluation of dalbavancin, tigecycline, minocycline, tetracycline,

---

"Usual dose" assumes normal renal/hepatic function. * For renal insufficiency, give usual dose × 1 followed by maintenance dose per CrCl. For dialysis patients, dose the same as for CrCl < 10 mL/min and give supplemental (post-HD/PD dose) immediately after dialysis. CrCl = creatinine clearance; CVVH = continuous veno-venous hemofiltration; HD/PD = hemodialysis/peritoneal dialysis.

teicoplanin and vancomycin against community-associated and multidrug-resistant hospital-associated meticillin-resistant Staphylococcus aureus. Int J Antimicrob Agents 35:25–29, 2010.

Hunte CA, Abbo LM. Skin and soft tissue infections due to methicillin-resistant Staphylococcus aureus: Role of tigecycline. Clin Infect Dis 52:1468–1467, 2011.

Humphries RM, Kelesidis T, Dien Bard J, et al. Successful treatment of pan-resistant Klebsiella pneumoniae pneumonia and bacteraemia with a combination of high-dose tigecycline and colistin. J Med Microbiol 59:1383–1386, 2010.

Insa R, Cercenado E, Goyanes MJ, et al. In vitro activity of tigecycline against clinical isolates of Acinetobacter baumannii and Stenotrophomonas maltophilia. J Antimicrob Chemother 59:583–585, 2007.

Jenkins I. Linezolid- and vancomycin-resistant Enterococcus faecium endocarditis: successful treatment with tigecycline and daptomycin. J Hosp Med 2:343–344, 2007.

Jump RL, Li Y, Pultz, JF, et al. Tigecycline exhibits inhibitory activity against Clostridium difficile in the colon of mice and does not promote growth or toxin production. Antimicrob. Agents Chemother 55:546–549, 2011.

Kuo SC, Wang FD, Fung CP, et al. Clinical experience with tigecycline as treatment for serious infections in elderly and critically ill patients. J Microbiol Immunol Infect 44:45–51, 2011.

Larson KC, Belliveau PP, Spooner LM. Tigecycline for the treatment of severe Clostridium difficile infection. Ann Pharmacother 45:1005–10, 2011.

Lengerke C, Haap M, Mayer F, et al. Low tigecycline concentrations in the cerebrospinal fluid of a neutropenic patient with inflamed meninges. Antimicrob Agents Chemother 55:449–450, 2011.

Lu CL, Liu CY, Liao CH, et al. Severe and refractory Clostridium difficile infection successfully treated with tigecycline and metronidazole. Int J Antimicrob Agents 35:311–312, 2010.

McKeage K, Keating GM. Tigecycline: in community-acquired pneumonia. Drugs 68:2633–2644, 2008.

Meagher AK, Ambrose PG, Grasela TH, et al. The pharmacokinetic and pharmacodynamic profile of tigecycline. Clin Infect Dis 41(Suppl 5):S333–40, 2005.

Mendes RE, Farrell DJ, Sader HS, et al. Comprehensive assessment of tigecycline activity tested against a worldwide collection of Acinetobacter spp. (2005–2009). Diagn Microbiol Infect Dis 68:307–311, 2010.

Metan G, Alp E, Yildiz O, et al. Clinical experience with tigecycline in the treatment of carbapenem-resistant Acinetobacter infections. J Chemother 22:110–114, 2010.

Muralidharan G, Micalizzi M, Speth J, et al. Pharmacokinetics of tigecycline after single and multiple doses in healthy subjects. Antimicrob Agents Chemother 49:220–9, 2005.

Nagy E, Dowzicky MJ. In vitro activity of tigecycline and comparators against a European compilation of anaerobes collected as part of the Tigecycline Evaluation and Surveillance Trial (TEST). Scand J Infect Dis 42:33–38, 2010.

Nillson LE, Frimodt-Moller N, Vaara M, et al. Comparative activity of tigecycline and tetracycline on Gram-negative and Gram-positive bacteria revealed by a multicentre study in four North European countries. Scand J Infect Dis 43:707–713, 2011.

Nix DE, Matthias KR. Should tigecycline be considered for urinary tract infections? A pharmacokinetic re-evaluation. J Antimicrob Chemother 65:1311–1312, 2010.

Nord CE, Sillerstrom E, Wahlund E. Effect of Tigecycline on Normal Oropharyngeal and Intestinal Microflora. Antimicrob Agents Chemother 50:3375–80, 2006.

Noskin GA. Tigecycline: a new glycylcycline for treatment of serious infections. Clin Infect Dis 41(Suppl 5):S303–14, 2005.

Noviello S, Ianniello F, Leone S, et al. In vitro activity of tigecycline: MICs, MBCs, time-kill curves and post-antibiotic effect. J Chemotherapy 20:577–580, 2008.

Ozbek B, Sentruk A. Postantibiotic effects of tigecycline, colistin sulfate, and levofloxacin alone or tigecycline-colistin sulfate and tigecycline-levofloxacin combinations against Acinetobacter baumannii. Chemotherapy 56:466–471, 2010.

Pankey GA. Tigecycline. J Antimicrob Chemother 53:470–80, 2005.

"Usual dose" assumes normal renal/hepatic function. * For renal insufficiency, give usual dose × 1 followed by maintenance dose per CrCl. For dialysis patients, dose the same as for CrCl < 10 mL/min and give supplemental (post-HD/PD dose) immediately after dialysis. CrCl = creatinine clearance; CVVH = continuous veno-venous hemofiltration; HD/PD = hemodialysis/peritoneal dialysis.

Pavan M, Chaudhari AP, Ranganth R. Altered bioavailability of tacrolimus following intravenous administration of tigecycline. Am J Kidney Dis57:345, 2011.

Peleg AY, Potoski BA, Rea R, et al. Acinetobacter baumannii bloodstream infection while receiving tigecycline: a cautionary report. J Antimicrob Chemother 59:128–31, 2007.

Polidori M, Nuccorini A, Tascini C, et al. Vancomycin-resistant Enterococcus faecium (VRE) bacteremia in infective endocarditis successfully treated with combination daptomycin and tigecycline. J Chemother 23:240–241, 2011.

Qvist N, Warren B, Leister-Tebbe H, et al. Efficacy of tigecycline versus ceftriaxone plus metronidazole for the treatment of complicated intra-abdominal infections: results from a randomized, controlled trail. Surg Infect 13:102–3, 2012.

Raad I, Hanna H, Jiang Y, et al. Comparative activities of daptomycin, linezolid, and tigecycline against catheter-related methicillin-resistant Staphylococcus bacteremic isolates embedded in biofilm. Antimicrob Agents Chemother 51:1656–1660, 2007.

Rodvold KA, Gotfried MH, Cwik M, et al. Serum, tissue and body fluid concentrations of tigecycline after a single 100 mg dose. J Antimicrob Chemother 58:1221–1229, 2006.

Rubinstein E, Vaughan D. Tigecycline: a novel glycylcycline. Drugs 65:1317–36, 2005.

Sands M, McCarter Y, Sanchez W. Synergy testing of multidrug resistant Acinetobacter baumannii against tigecycline and polymyxin using an E-test methodology. Eur J Clin Microbiol Infect Dis 26: 521–522, 2007.

Scheetz MH, Q Chao, Warren JR, et al. In vitro activities of various antimicrobials alone and in combination with tigecycline against carbapenem-intermediate or -resistant Acinetobacter baumannii. Antimicrob Agents Chemother 51:1621–1626, 2007.

Slover CM, Rodvold KA, Danziger LH. Tigecycline: a novel broad-spectrum antimicrobial. Ann Pharmacother 41:965–972, 2007.

Stein GE, Craig WA. Tigecycline: A Critical Analysis. Clin Infect Dis 43:518–24, 2006.

Swoboda S, Ober M, Hainer C, et al. Tigecycline for the treatment of patients with severe sepsis of septic shock: a drug use evaluation in a surgical intensive care unit. J Antimicrob Chemother 61:729–733, 2008.

Taccone FS, Rodriguez-Villalobos H, DeBacker D, et al. Successful treatment of septic shock due to pan-resistant Acinetobacter baumannii using combined antimicrobial therapy including tigecycline. Eur J Clin Microbiol Infect Dis 25:257–60, 2006.

Tanaseanu C, Bergallo C, Teglia O, et al. Integrated results of 2 phase studies comparing tigecycline and levofloxacin in community-acquired pneumonia. Diagn Microbiol Infect Dis 61:329–338, 2008.

Valve K, Vaalasti A, Anttila VJ, et al. Disseminated Legionella pneumophila infection in an immunocompromised patient treated with tigecycline. Scand J Infect Dis 42:152–155, 2010.

Vardakas KZ, Rafailidis PL, Falagas ME. Effectiveness and safety of tigecycline: focus on use for approved indications. Clin Infect Dis 54:4672–4, 2012.

Wilcox MH. Evidence for low risk of Clostridium difficile infection associated with tigecycline. Clin Microbiol Infect 13:949–952, 2007.

Woodford N, Hill RL, Livermore DM. In vitro activity of tigecycline against carbapenem-susceptible and resistant isolates of Klebsiella spp. and Enterobacter spp. J Antimicrob Chemother 59:582–583, 2007.

Yaha D, Lador A, Paul M, et al. Tigecycline and overall mortality. Clin Infect Dis 55:1739, 2012.

Zinner SH. Overview of antibiotic use and resistance: setting the stage for tigecycline. Clin Infect Dis 41(Suppl 5):S289–92, 2005.

Website: www.tygacil.com

Tipranavir (Aptivus) TPV

Drug Class: Protease inhibitor.

Usual Dose: 500 mg (PO) q12h with ritonavir 200 mg (PO) q12h.

Pharmacokinetic Parameters:

Peak serum level: 77–94 mcg/mL

Bioavailability: No data

Excreted unchanged (urine): 44%

"Usual dose" assumes normal renal/hepatic function. * For renal insufficiency, give usual dose × 1 followed by maintenance dose per CrCl. For dialysis patients, dose the same as for CrCl < 10 mL/min and give supplemental (post-HD/PD dose) immediately after dialysis. CrCl = creatinine clearance; CVVH = continuous veno-venous hemofiltration; HD/PD = hemodialysis/peritoneal dialysis.

Serum half-life (normal/ESRD): 5.5–6/5.5–6 hrs
Plasma protein binding: 99.9%
Volume of distribution (V$_d$): 7–10 L/kg
Primary Mode of Elimination: Hepatic
Dosage Adjustments*

CrCl < 10 mL/min	No change
Post–HD dose	No change
Post–PD dose	No change
CVVH/CVVHD/ CVVHDF dose	No change
Mild hepatic insufficiency	No change
Moderate–severe hepatic insufficiency	Avoid

Drug Interactions: Metabolized via CYP3A4
rifabutin (↑ levels), clarithromycin (↑ levels),
loperamide (↓ levels), statins (↑ risk of
myopathy); abacavir, saquinavir, tenofovir,
zidovudine, amprenavir/RTV, lopinavir/RTV
(↓ levels). Aluminum/magnesium antacids
(↓ absorption 25–30%). Ritonavir (↑ risk of
hepatitis). St. John's Wort (↓ tipranavir levels).
Fluconazole (↑ tipranavir levels).
Contraindications: simvastatin, atorvastatin,
lovastatin, rifapentine
Adverse Effects: Contraindicated in
moderate/severe hepatic insufficiency. ↑ risk of
hepatotoxicity in HIV patients co-infected with
HBV/HCV. Intracerebral hemorrhage–use with
caution in patients with coagulopathies.
Allergic Potential: High. Tipranavir is a
sulfonamide; use with caution in patients with
sulfonamide allergies
Safety in Pregnancy: C
Comments: Should be taken with food. Keep
refrigerated 2–8°C.

**simvastatin, atorvastatin, lovastatin,
rifapentine** Increased bioavailability when
taken with meals. Must be co-administered
with 200 mg ritonavir. Tipranavir contains
a sulfa moiety (as do darunavir and
fosamprenavir).
Cerebrospinal Fluid Penetration: No data

REFERENCES:

Croom KF, Keam SJ. Tipranavir: a ritonavir-boosted
    protease inhibitor. Drugs 65:1669–79, 2005.
Kandula VR, Khanlou H, Farthing C. Tipranavir: a novel
    second-generation nonpeptidic protease inhibitor.
    Expert Rev Anti Infect Ther 3:9–21, 2005.
Kashuba AD. Drug-drug interactions and the
    pharmacotherapy of HIV infection. Top HIV Med
    13:64–9, 2005.
Panel on Antiretroviral Guidelines for Adults and
    Adolescents. Department of Health and Human
    Services. Guidelines for the use of antiretroviral
    agents in HIV-infected adults and adolescents.
    http://aidsinfo.nih.gov/ConsentFiles/
    AdultandAdolescentGL.pdf, 2012.
Plosker GL, Figgitt DP. Tripanavir. Drugs 63:1611–8, 2003.
Thompson MA, Aberg JA, Cahn P, et al. Antiretroviral
    treatment of adult HIV infection: 2012 recommen-
    dations of the International Antiviral Society — USA
    panel. JAMA 308:387–402, 2012.
Website: www.aptivus.com

Tobramycin (Nebcin)

Drug Class: Aminoglycoside.
Usual Dose: 240 mg or 5 mg/kg (IV) q24h
(preferred over q8h dosing) (see comments).
Spectrum: (see *Susceptibility Profiles*
pp. 198–202).
Resistance Potential: High (P. aeruginosa,
aerobic GNBs)
Pharmacokinetic Parameters:
Peak serum levels: 4–8 mcg/ml (q8h dosing);
16–24 mcg/ml (q24h dosing)
Bioavailability: Not applicable
Excreted unchanged (urine): 95%

"Usual dose" assumes normal renal/hepatic function. * For renal insufficiency, give usual dose × 1 followed by
maintenance dose per CrCl. For dialysis patients, dose the same as for CrCl < 10 mL/min and give supplemental
(post-HD/PD dose) immediately after dialysis. CrCl = creatinine clearance; CVVH = continuous veno-venous
hemofiltration; HD/PD = hemodialysis/peritoneal dialysis.

Serum half-life (normal/ESRD): 2.5/56 hrs
Plasma protein binding: 10%
Volume of distribution (V_d): 0.24 L/kg
Primary Mode of Elimination: Renal
Dosage Adjustments*

CrCl 50–80 mL/min	120 mg (IV) q24h or 2.5 mg/kg (IV) q24h
CrCl 10–50 mL/min	120 mg (IV) q48h or 2.5 mg/kg (IV) q48h
CrCl < 10 mL/min	60 mg (IV) q48h or 1.25 mg/kg (IV) q48h
Post–HD dose	80 mg (IV) or 1 mg/kg (IV)
Post–HFHD dose	120 mg (IV) or 2.5 mg/kg (IV)
Post–PD dose	40 mg (IV) or 0.5 mg/kg (IV) or 2–4 mg/L in dialysate q24h
CVVH/CVVHD/ CVVHDF dose	120 mg (IV) q48h or 2.5 mg/kg (IV)
Mild-moderate hepatic insufficiency	No change
Severe hepatic insufficiency	No change

Drug Interactions: Amphotericin B, cyclosporine, enflurane, methoxyflurane, NSAIDs, polymyxin B, radiographic contrast, vancomycin (↑ nephrotoxicity); cis-platinum (↑ nephrotoxicity, ↑ ototoxicity); loop diuretics (↑ ototoxicity); neuromuscular blocking agents (↑ apnea, prolonged paralysis); non-polarizing muscle relaxants (↑ apnea).
Adverse Effects: Neuromuscular blockade with rapid infusion/absorption. Nephrotoxicity

only with prolonged/extremely high serum trough levels; may cause reversible non-oliguric renal failure (ATN). Ototoxicity associated with prolonged/extremely high peak serum levels (usually irreversible): Cochlear toxicity (1/3 of ototoxicity) manifests as decreased high frequency hearing, but deafness is unusual. Vestibular toxicity (2/3 of ototoxicity) develops before ototoxicity, and typically manifests as tinnitus.
Allergic Potential: Low
Safety in Pregnancy: D
Comments: Single daily dosing greatly reduces nephrotoxic/ototoxic potential.
Incompatible with solutions containing β–lactams, erythromycin, chloramphenicol, furosemide, sodium bicarbonate. IV infusion should be given slowly over 1 hour. May be given IM. ***Avoid intraperitoneal infusion due to risk of neuromuscular blockade. Avoid intratracheal/ aerosolized intrapulmonary instillation, which predisposes to antibiotic resistance***.
V_d increases with edema/ascites, trauma, burns, cystic fibrosis; may require ↑ dose. V_d decreases with dehydration, obesity; may require ↓ dose.
Renal cast counts are the best indicator of aminoglycoside nephrotoxicity, not serum creatinines. Dialysis removes ~ 1/3 of tobramycin from serum. Tobramycin nebulizer dose: 300 mg via nebulizer q12h ***(not recommended due to ↑ risk of resistance)***.
CAPD dose: 2–4 mg/L in dialysate (I.P.) with each exchange.
Therapeutic Serum Concentrations
(for therapeutic efficacy, *not toxicity*):
  Peak (q24h/q8h dosing) = 16–24/8–10 mcg/ ml
  Trough (q24h/q8h dosing) = 0/1–2 mcg/ml
Synergy dose: 120 mg (IV) q24h or 2.5 mg/kg (IV) q24h
Intrathecal (IT) dose: 5 mg (IT) q24h

"Usual dose" assumes normal renal/hepatic function. * For renal insufficiency, give usual dose × 1 followed by maintenance dose per CrCl. For dialysis patients, dose the same as for CrCl < 10 mL/min and give supplemental (post-HD/PD dose) immediately after dialysis. CrCl = creatinine clearance; CVVH = continuous veno-venous hemofiltration; HD/PD = hemodialysis/peritoneal dialysis.

Cerebrospinal Fluid Penetration:
Non-inflamed meninges = 0%
Inflamed meninges = 20%
Bile Penetration: 30%
(also see *Antibiotic Pearls & Pitfalls*
p. 514).

REFERENCES:

Begg EJ, Barclay ML. Aminoglycosides - 50 years on.
Br J Clin Pharmacol 39:597–603, 1995.

Buijk SE Mouton JW, Gyssens IC, et al. Experience with a
once-daily dosing program of aminoglycosides in critically
ill patients. Intensive Care Med 28:936–42, 2002.

Cheer SM, Waugh J, Noble S. Inhaled tobramycin
(TOBI): a review of its use in the management
of Pseudomonas aeruginosa infections in patients with
cystic fibrosis. Drugs 63:2501–20, 2003.

Cunha BA. Aminoglycosides: Current role in antimicrobial
therapy. Pharmacotherapy 8:334–50, 1988.

Dupuis LL, Sung L, Taylor T, et al. Tobramycin
pharmacokinetics in children with febrile neutropenia
undergoing stem cell transplantation once-daily
versus thrice-daily administration. Pharmacotherapy
24:564–73, 2004.

Edson RS, Terrel CL. The aminoglycosides. Mayo Clin
Proc 74:519–28, 1999.

Geller DE, Pistlick WH, Nardella PA, et al.
Pharmacokinetics and bioavailability of aerosolized
tobramycin in cystic fibrosis. Chest 122:219–26, 2002.

Gilbert DN. Once-daily aminoglycoside therapy.
Antimicrob Agents Chemother 35:399–405, 1991.

Hustinx WN, Hoepelman IM. Aminoglycoside dosage
regimens: Is once a day enough? Clin Pharmacokinet
25:427–32, 1993.

Kahler DA, Schowengerdt KO, Fricker FJ, et al. Toxic serum
trough concentrations after administration of nebulized
tobramycin. Pharmacotherapy 23:543–5, 2003.

Lortholary O, Tod M, Cohen Y, et al. Aminoglycosides.
Med Clin North Am 79:761–87, 1995.

McCormack JP, Jewesson PJ. A critical reevaluation of
the "therapeutic range" of aminoglycosides. Clin
Infect Dis 14:320–39, 1992.

Moss RB. Long-term benefits of inhaled tobramycin
in adolescent patients with cystic fibrosis. Chest
121:55–63, 2002.

Whitehead A, Conway SP, Etherington C, et al. Once-
daily tobramycin in the treatment of adult patients
with cystic fibrosis. Eur Respir J 19:303–9, 2002.

Wood GC, Chapman JL, Boucher BA, et al. Tobramycin
bladder irrigation for treating a urinary tract
infection in a critically ill patient. Ann Pharmacother
38:1318–9, 2004.

Website: www.pdr.net

Trimethoprim (Proloprim, Trimpex) TMP

Drug Class: Folate antagonist.
Usual Dose: 100 mg (PO) q12h (see comments).
Spectrum: (see *Susceptibility Profiles*
pp. 186–190).
Resistance Potential: High (S. pneumoniae,
E. coli)
Pharmacokinetic Parameters:
Peak serum level: 2–8 mcg/ml
Bioavailability: 98%
Excreted unchanged (urine): 67%
Serum half-life (normal/ESRD): 8/24 hrs
Plasma protein binding: 44%
Volume of distribution (V_d): 1.8 L/kg
Primary Mode of Elimination: Renal
Dosage Adjustments*

CrCl 10–30 mL/min	50 mg (PO) q12h
CrCl < 10 mL/min	Avoid (except for PCP, see TMP–SMX)
Post–HD dose	Avoid (except for PCP, see TMP–SMX)
Post–PD dose	100 mg (PO)
CVVH/CVVHD/ CVVHDF dose	50 mg (PO) q12h
Moderate—severe hepatic insufficiency	No change

"Usual dose" assumes normal renal/hepatic function. * For renal insufficiency, give usual dose × 1 followed by maintenance dose per CrCl. For dialysis patients, dose the same as for CrCl < 10 mL/min and give supplemental (post-HD/PD dose) immediately after dialysis. CrCl = creatinine clearance; CVVH = continuous veno-venous hemofiltration; HD/PD = hemodialysis/peritoneal dialysis.

Drug Interactions: Azathioprine (leukopenia); amantadine, dapsone, digoxin, methotrexate, phenytoin, rifampin, zidovudine (↑ interacting drug levels, nystagmus with phenytoin); diuretics (↑ serum K⁺ with K⁺-sparing diuretics, ↓ serum Na⁺ with thiazide diuretics); warfarin (↑ INR, bleeding).
Adverse Effects: Folate deficiency, hyperkalemia.
Allergic Potential: Low
Safety in Pregnancy: C
Comments: Useful in sulfa-allergic patients unable to take TMP–SMX. PCP dose: 5 mg/kg (PO) q8h plus dapsone 100 mg (PO) q24h.
Meningeal dose: 300 mg or 5 mg/kg (PO) q6h.
Cerebrospinal Fluid Penetration: 40%
Bile Penetration: 100%
(also see *Antibiotic Pearls & Pitfalls* p. 515).

REFERENCES:

Brogden RN, Carmine AA, Heel RC, et al. Trimethoprim: A review of its antibacterial activity, pharmacokinetics and therapeutic use in urinary tract infections. Drugs 23:405–30, 1982.

Friesen WT, Hekster YA, Vree TB. Trimethoprim: clinical use and pharmacokinetics. Drug Intelligence & Clinical Pharmacy 15:325–30, 1981.

Neu HC. Trimethoprim alone for treatment of urinary tract infection. Rev Infect Dis 4:366–71, 1982.

Website: www.pdr.net

Trimethoprim–Sulfamethoxazole (Bactrim, Septra) TMP–SMX

Drug Class: Folate antagonist/sulfonamide.
Usual Dose: 2.5–5 mg/kg (IV/PO) q6h.
Spectrum: (see *Susceptibility Profiles* pp. 186–190).

Resistance Potential: High (S. pneumoniae, E. coli)
Pharmacokinetic Parameters:
Peak serum level: 2–8/40–80 mcg/ml
Bioavailability: 98%
Excreted unchanged (urine): 67/85%
Serum half-life (normal/ESRD): (10/8)/40–80 hrs
Plasma protein binding: 44–70%
Volume of distribution (V_d): 1.8/0.3 L/kg
Primary Mode of Elimination: Renal
Dosage Adjustments*

CrCl 15–30 mL/min	1.25–2.5 mg/kg (IV/PO) q6h
CrCl < 15 mL/min	Avoid (except for PCP use 1.25–2.5 mg/kg [IV/PO] q8h)
Post–HD dose	2.5 mg/kg (IV/PO)
Post–PD dose	0.16 mg/kg (IV/PO)
CVVH/CVVHD/ CVVHDF dose	2.5 mg/kg (IV/PO) q6h
Moderate–severe hepatic insufficiency	No change

Drug Interactions: *TMP component:* Azathioprine (leukopenia); amantadine, dapsone, digoxin, methotrexate, phenytoin, rifampin, zidovudine (↑ interacting drug levels, nystagmus with phenytoin); diuretics (↑ serum K⁺ with K⁺-sparing diuretics, ↓ serum Na⁺ with thiazide diuretics); warfarin (↑ INR, bleeding). *SMX component:* Cyclosporine (↓ cyclosporine levels); phenytoin (↑ phenytoin levels, nystagmus, ataxia); methotrexate (↑ antifolate activity); sulfonylureas, thiopental (↑ interacting drug effect); warfarin (↑ INR, bleeding).
Adverse Effects: Common cause of drug induced aseptic meningitis.

"Usual dose" assumes normal renal/hepatic function. * For renal insufficiency, give usual dose × 1 followed by maintenance dose per CrCl. For dialysis patients, dose the same as for CrCl < 10 mL/min and give supplemental (post-HD/PD dose) immediately after dialysis. CrCl = creatinine clearance; CVVH = continuous veno-venous hemofiltration; HD/PD = hemodialysis/peritoneal dialysis.

TMP: Folate deficiency, hyperkalemia.

SMX: Leukopenia, thrombocytopenia, hemolytic anemia ± G6PD deficiency, aplastic anemia, ↑ SGOT/SGPT, severe hypersensitivity reactions (E. multiforme/Stevens–Johnson Syndrome), ↑ risk of hypoglycemia in chronic renal failure.

Allergic Potential: Very high (SMX); none (TMP)

Safety in Pregnancy: C

Comments: Drug fever/rash
Excellent bioavailability (IV = PO).

TMP-SMX IV and PO Equivalence:

TMP-SMX (TMP component) **10 mg/kg (IV) q24h** (70 kg patient)

$$= 2 \ SS^† \ \text{tablets (PO) q6h}$$

or

$$= 1 \ DS^{††} \ \text{tablet (PO) q6h}$$

TMP-SMX (TMP component) **20 mg/kg (IV) q24h** (70 kg patient)

$$= 4 \ SS \ \text{tablets (PO) q6h}$$

or

$$= 2 \ DS \ \text{tablets (PO) q6h}$$

---

†   1 SS tablet = TMP 80 mg + SMX 400 mg.

†† 1 DS tablet = TMP 160 mg + SMX 800 mg.

In sulfa allergic patients, use TMP (SMX is the allergic component) which is equally effective as TMP-SMX.

Meningeal dose = 5 mg/kg (IV/PO) q6h.

Cerebrospinal Fluid Penetration:

Non-Inflamed meninges = 40%

Inflamed meninges = 40%

Bile Penetration: 100%

(also see ***Antibiotic Pearls & Pitfalls*** p. 515).

REFERENCES:

Cockerill FR, Edson RS. Trimethoprim-sulfamethoxazole. Mayo Clin Proc 66:1260–9, 1991.

Cunha BA. Oral antibiotic therapy of serious systemic infections. Med Clin N Am 90:1197–1222, 2006.

Cunha BA. Prophylaxis for recurrent urinary tract infections: nitrofurantoin, not trimethoprim-sulfamethoxazole or cranberry juice. Arch Intern Med 172:82–3, 2012.

Euga G, Murillo O, Fernandez-Sabe N, et al. Treatment of chronic staphylococcal osteomyelitis: intravenous or oral? how long? Antimicrob Agents Chemother 53:2672–2676, 2009.

Francis P, Patel VB, Bill PL, et al. Oral trimethoprim-sulfamethoxazole in the treatment of cerebral toxoplasmosis in AIDS patients-a prospective study. S Afr Med J 94:51–3, 2004.

Giannakopoulos G Johnson ES. TMP–SMX. Antibiotics for Clinicians 1:63–9, 1997.

Hooton TM, Besser R, Foxman B, et al. Acute uncomplicated cystitis in an era of increasing antibiotic resistance: a proposed approach to empirical therapy. Clin Infect Dis 39:75–80, 2004.

Masters PA, O'Bryan TA, Zurlo JM, et al. Trimethoprim-sulfamethoxazole revisited. Arch Intern Med 163:402–10, 2003.

Nguyen S, Pasquet A, Legout L, et al. Efficacy and tolerance of rifampin-linezolid compared with rifampin-cotrimoxazole combinations in prolonged oral therapy for bone and joint infections. Clin Microbiol Infect Dis 15:1163–1169, 2009.

Nicolle LE. Urinary tract infection: traditional pharmacologic therapies. Am J Med 113(Suppl 1A):35S–44S, 2002.

Sanchez GV, Master RN, Bordon J. Trimethoprim-sulfamethoxazole may no longer be acceptable for the treatment of acute uncomplicated cystitis in the United States. Clin Infect Dis 53:316–7, 2011.

Schaffer AJ. Empiric use of trimethoprim-sulfamethoxazole (TMP–SMX) in the treatment of women with uncomplicated urinary tract infections, in a geographic area with a high prevalence of TMP–SMX-resistance uropathogens. J Urol 168 (Pt 1):1652–3, 2002.

Soeter HM, Von Gottberg A, Cohen C, et al. Trimethoprim-sulfamethoxazole prophylaxis and antibiotic non-susceptibility invasive pneumococcal disease. Anitimicrob Agents Chemother 56:1602–5, 2012.

Website: www.pdr.net

"Usual dose" assumes normal renal/hepatic function. * For renal insufficiency, give usual dose × 1 followed by maintenance dose per CrCl. For dialysis patients, dose the same as for CrCl < 10 mL/min and give supplemental (post-HD/PD dose) immediately after dialysis. CrCl = creatinine clearance; CVVH = continuous veno-venous hemofiltration; HD/PD = hemodialysis/peritoneal dialysis.

Valacyclovir (Valtrex)

Drug Class: HSV, VZV antiviral (see comments).
Usual Dose:
HSV-1/2: <u>Herpes labialis:</u> 2 gm (PO) q12h × 1 day. <u>Genital herpes:</u> *Initial therapy:* 1 gm (PO) q12h × 3 days. *Recurrent/intermittent therapy* (< 6 episodes/year): normal host: 500 mg (PO) q24h × 5 days; HIV-positive: 1 gm (PO) q12h × 7–10 days. *Chronic suppressive therapy* (> 6 episodes/year): normal host: 1 gm (PO) q24h × 1 year; HIV-positive: 500 mg (PO) q12h × 1 year. <u>HSV-1 late onset VAP:</u> 1 gm (PO) q8h × 10 days. <u>Meningitis/encephalitis:</u> 1 gm (PO) q8h × 10 days.
VZV: <u>Chickenpox:</u> 1 gm (PO) q8h × 5 days. <u>VZV pneumonia:</u> 1–2 gm (PO) q8h × 10 days. <u>Herpes zoster (shingles) (dermatomal/ disseminated):</u> 1 gm (PO) q8h × 7–10 days. <u>VZV meningitis/encephalitis:</u> 2gm (PO) q6h × 10 days.

Pharmacokinetic Parameters:
Peak serum level: 3.7–5 mcg/ml
Bioavailability: 55%
Excreted unchanged (urine): 1%
Serum half-life (normal/ESRD): 3/14 hrs
Plasma protein binding: 15%
Volume of distribution (V_d): 0.7 L/kg
Primary Mode of Elimination: Renal
Dosage Adjustments* (based on 1 gm q8h)

CrCl 30–50 mL/min	1 gm (PO) q12h
CrCl 10–30 mL/min	1 gm (PO) q24h
CrCl < 10 mL/min	500 mg (PO) q24h
Post–HD dose	1 gm (PO)
Post–PD dose	500 mg

CVVH/CVVHD/ CVVHDF dose	500 mg (PO) q24h
Moderate hepatic insufficiency	No change
Severe hepatic insufficiency	No change

Drug Interactions: Cimetidine, probenecid (↑ acyclovir levels).
Adverse Effects: Headache, nausea, diarrhea, abdominal pain, weakness. Rarely, HUS/TTP (only in HIV).
Allergic Potential: Low
Safety in Pregnancy: B
Comments: Converted to acyclovir in liver. ***Highly active against HSV > VZV. Some activity against CMV. No activity against EBV, RSV or adenoviruses.***
VZV IC_{90} (mean) ~ 2 × HSV.
Meningeal dose = VZV: 2 gm (PO) q6h
　　　　　　　　HSV: 1 gm (PO) q8h
Cerebrospinal Fluid Penetration: 54%

REFERENCES:
Acost EP, Fletcher CV. Valacyclovir. Ann Pharmacotherapy 31:185–91, 1997.

Jacobsen T, Sipointis N. Drug interactions and toxicities associated with the antiviral management of cytomegalovirus infection. Am J Health Syst Pharm 67:1417–1425, 2010.

Kotton CN, Kumar D, Caliendo AM, et al. International consensus guidelines on the management of cytomegalovirus in solid organ transplantation. Transplantation 89:779–795, 2010.

Mugwanya K, Baeten JM, Mugo NR, et al. High-dose valacyclovir HSV-2 suppression results in greater reduction in plasma HIV-1 levels compared with standard dose acyclovir among HIV-1/HSV-2 coinfected persons: a randomized, crossover trial. J Infect Dis 204:1912–1017, 2011.

"Usual dose" assumes normal renal/hepatic function. * For renal insufficiency, give usual dose × 1 followed by maintenance dose per CrCl. For dialysis patients, dose the same as for CrCl < 10 mL/min and give supplemental (post-HD/PD dose) immediately after dialysis. CrCl = creatinine clearance; CVVH = continuous veno-venous hemofiltration; HD/PD = hemodialysis/peritoneal dialysis.

Pouplin T, Pouplin JN, Van Toi P, et al. valacyclovir for Herpes simplex encephalitis. Antimicrob Agents Chemother 55:3624–3626, 2011

Vigil KJ, ChemalyRF. Valacyclovir: approved and off-label uses for the treatment of herpes virus infections in immunocompetent and immunocompromised adults. Expert Opin Pharmacother 11:1901–1913, 2010.

Website: www.valtrex.com

Valganciclovir (Valcyte)

Drug Class: CMV, HSV, HHV-6 antiviral (see comments).
Usual Dose: *Induction Dose:* 900 mg (PO) q12h × 21 days, then **Maintanance Dose:** 900 mg (PO) q24h (Normal hosts: until cured; Compromised hosts: chronic suppressive therapy). 900 mg dose taken as two 450-mg tablets once daily with food.
Pharmacokinetic Parameters:
Peak serum level: 5.6 mcg/ml
Bioavailability: 59.4%
Excreted unchanged (urine): 90%
Serum half-life (normal/ESRD): 4.1/67.5 hrs
Plasma protein binding: 1%
Volume of distribution (V_d): 15.3 L/kg
Primary Mode of Elimination: Renal
Dosage Adjustments*

CrCl 40–60 mL/min	450 mg (PO) q12h (induction), then 450 mg (PO) q24h (maintenance)
CrCl 25–40 mL/min	450 mg (PO) q24h (induction), then 450 mg (PO) q48h (maintenance)
CrCl 10–25 mL/min	450 mg (PO) q48h (induction), then 450 mg (PO) 2x/ week (maintenance)
CrCl < 10 mL/min	Avoid
Post–HD dose	Avoid
Post–PD dose	Use same dose as CrCl 25–40 mL/min
CVVH/CVVHD/ CVVHDF dose	Use same dose as CrCl 25–50 mL/min
Mild-moderate hepatic insufficiency	No change
Severe hepatic insufficiency	Use with caution

Drug Interactions: Cytotoxic drugs (may produce additive toxicity: stomatitis, bone marrow depression, alopecia); imipenem (↑ risk of seizures); probenecid (↑ valganciclovir levels); zidovudine (↓ valganciclovir levels, ↑ zidovudine levels, possible neutropenia); didanosine (↑ didanosine); cyclosporine amphotericin, (↑ nephrotoxicity); mycophenolate mofetil (↑ mycophenolate mofetil and gangcyclovir levels in renal insufficiency); tenofovir (↑ tenofovir, gangcyclovir levels).
Adverse Effects: Drug fever/rash, diarrhea, nausea, vomiting, GI upset, leukopenia, anemia, thrombocytopenia, paresthesias/peripheral neuropathy, retinal detachment, aplastic anemia.
Allergic Potential: Low
Safety in Pregnancy: C
Comments: Valganciclovir exposures (AUC) larger than for IV ganciclovir. Tablets should be taken with food. Valganciclovir is rapidly hydrolyzed to ganciclovir. Not interchangeable on a tablet-to-tablet basis with oral ganciclovir. Much

---

"Usual dose" assumes normal renal/hepatic function. * For renal insufficiency, give usual dose × 1 followed by maintenance dose per CrCl. For dialysis patients, dose the same as for CrCl < 10 mL/min and give supplemental (post-HD/PD dose) immediately after dialysis. CrCl = creatinine clearance; CVVH = continuous veno-venous hemofiltration; HD/PD = hemodialysis/peritoneal dialysis.

higher bioavailability than ganciclovir capsules; serum concentration equivalent to IV ganciclovir. Indicated for induction/maintenance therapy of CMV infection. Preferred to ganciclovir for all indications except for CMV prophylaxis in liver transplants. **Highly active against CMV, HHV-6, and HSV. Some activity against VZV, EBV and adenoviruses. No activity against RSV.** Meningeal dose = usual dose.

Cerebrospinal Fluid Penetration: 70%

REFERENCES:

Avery RK. Low-dose valganciclovir for cytomegalovirus phylaxis in organ transplantation: is less really more? Clin Infect Dis 52:322–324, 2011.

Asberg A, Rollag H, Hartmann A. Valganciclovir for the prevention and treatment of CMV in solid organ transplant recipients. Expert Opin Pharmacother 11:1159–1166, 2010.

Boillat Blanco N, Pascual M, Venetz JP, et al. Impact of preemptive strategy after 3 months of valganciclovir cytomegalovirus prophylaxis in kidney transplant recipients. Transplantation 91:251–255, 2011.

Czock D, Scholle C, Rasche FM, et al. Pharmacokinetics of valganciclovir and ganciclovir in renal impairment. Clin Pharmacol Ther 72:142–50, 2002.

Humar A, Limaye AP, Blumberg EA, et al. Extended valganciclovir prophylaxis in D+/R- kidney transplant recipients is associated with long-term reduction in cytomegalovirus disease: two-year results of the IMPACT study. Transplantation 90:1427–1431, 2010.

Jacobsen T, Sipointis N. Drug interactions and toxicities associated with the antiviral management of cytomegalovirus infection. Am J Health Syst Pharm 67:1417–1425, 2010.

Kalil AC, Midru C, Florescu DF. Effectiveness of valganciclovir 900 mg versus 450 mg for cytomegalovirus prophylaxis in transplantation: direct and indirect treatment comparison meta-analysis. Clin Infect Dis 52:313–321, 2011.

Kotton CN, Kumar D, Caliendo AM, et al. International consensus guidelines on the management of cytomegalovirus in solid organ transplantation. Transplantation 89:779–795, 2010.

Lopau K, Greser A, Wanner C. Efficacy and safety of preemptive anti-CMV therapy with valganciclovir after kidney transplantation. Clin Transplant 21:80–85, 2007.

Luan, FL, Kommareddi M, Ojo AO. Impact of cytomegalovirus disease in D+/R- kidney transplant patients receiving 6 months low-dose valganciclovir prophylaxis. Am J Transplant 11:1936–1942, 2011.

Razonable RR, Paya CV. Valganciclovir for the prevention and treatment of cytomegalovirus disease in immunocompromised hosts. Expert Rev Anti Infect Ther 2:27–41, 2004.

Slifkin M, Doron S, Snydman DR. Viral prophylaxis in organ transplant patients. Drugs 64:2763–92, 2004.

Website: www.rocheusa.com/products/

Vancomycin (Vancocin)

Drug Class: Glycopeptide.
Usual Dose: 1 gm (IV) q12h (see comments).
Spectrum: (see **Susceptibility Profiles** pp. 198–202).
Resistance Potential: Low (MSSA, MRSA VSE; ↑ prevalence of VRE)
Pharmacokinetic Parameters:
Peak serum level: 63 mcg/ml
Bioavailability: IV (not applicable)/PO (0%)
Excreted unchanged (urine): 90%
Serum half-life (normal/ESRD): 6/180 hrs
Plasma protein binding: 55%
Volume of distribution (V_d): 0.7 L/kg
Primary Mode of Elimination: Renal
Dosage Adjustments*

CrCl 50–80 mL/min	1 gm (IV) q12h
CrCl 10–50 mL/min	1 gm (IV) q24h
CrCl < 10 mL/min	1 gm (IV) q week
Post–HD dose	None
Post–HFHD dose	500 mg (IV)

"Usual dose" assumes normal renal/hepatic function. * For renal insufficiency, give usual dose × 1 followed by maintenance dose per CrCl. For dialysis patients, dose the same as for CrCl < 10 mL/min and give supplemental (post-HD/PD dose) immediately after dialysis. CrCl = creatinine clearance; CVVH = continuous veno-venous hemofiltration; HD/PD = hemodialysis/peritoneal dialysis.

Post–PD dose	None
CVVH/CVVHD/ CVVHDF dose	1 gm (IV) q24h
Moderate hepatic insufficiency	No change
Severe hepatic insufficiency	No change

Drug Interactions: Aminoglycosides, amphotericin B, polymyxin B (↑ nephrotoxicity).
Adverse Effects: "Red man/neck syndrome" with rapid IV infusion (histamine mediated), leukopenia, thrombocytopenia, cardiac arrest, hypotension.
Allergic Potential: Low
Safety in Pregnancy: C
Comments: Not nephrotoxic. "Red man/ neck syndrome" can be prevented/minimized by infusing IV vancomycin slowly over 1–2 hours. Intraperitoneal absorption = 40%. **IV vancomycin increases VRE prevalence. C. difficile diarrhea dose:** oral vancomycin 250 mg (PO) q6h. *If no response in 72 hours ↑ dose to 500 mg (PO) q6h to complete therapy.* **C. difficile diarrhea relapse dose:** 500 mg (PO) q6h × 1 month and reevaluate. **Do *not* taper dose.** Should C. difficile recur, treat × 2 or 3 months with 500 mg (PO) q6h. **C. difficile colitis: *Oral vancomycin ineffective for C. difficile colitis*.** Vancomycin doesn't penetrate well into the CSF with non-inflamed meninges. For therapeutic CSF concentrations, use IV vancomycin *plus* IT vancomycin.
Therapeutic Serum Concentrations (for therapeutic efficacy, *not toxicity*):
  Peak = 25–40 mcg/ml
  Trough = 5–12 mcg/ml

There are **no convincing data that vancomycin is ototoxic or nephrotoxic. CrCl, not serum levels, should be used to adjust vancomycin dosing**. Prolonged/high dose vancomycin (60 mg/kg/day or 2 gm [IV] q12h) has been useful in treating S. aureus osteomyelitis, S. aureus infections with high MICs (VISA), and infections in difficult-to-penetrate tissues without toxicity. In bone or CSF, vancomycin tissue concentrations are ~ 15% of serum levels.
Intrathecal (IT) dose: 20 mg (IT) in preservative free NaCl.
Cerebrospinal Fluid Penetration:
Non-Inflamed meninges = <1%
Inflamed meninges = 15%
Bile Penetration: 50%
(also see *Antibiotic Pearls & Pitfalls* p. 517).

REFERENCES:
Ajao AO, Harris AD, Roghmann MC, et al. Systematic review of measurement and adjustment for colonization pressure in studies of methicillin-resistant Staphylococcus aureus, vancomycin-resistant enterococci, and clostridium difficile acquisition. Infect Control Hosp Epidemiol 32:481–489, 2011.
Black E, Lau TT, Ensom MH. Vancomycin-induced neutropenia: is it dose- or duration-related? Ann Pharmacother 45:629–638, 2011.
Bhavnani SM, Prakhya A, Hammel JP, et al. Cost-Effectiveness of daptomycin versus vancomycin and gentamicin for patients with methicillin-resistant Staphylococcus aureus bacteremia and/or endocarditis. Clin Infect Dis 49:691–698, 2009.
Bouza E. New therapeutic choices for infections caused by methicillin-resistant Staphylococcus aureus. Clin Microbiol Infect Dis 15:44–52, 2009.
Cantu TG, Yamanaka-Yuen NA, Lietman PS. Serum vancomycin concentrations: Reappraisal of their clinical value. Clin Infect Dis 18:533–43, 1994.

Cosgrove SE, Carroll KC, Perl TM. Staphylococcus aureus with reduced susceptibility to vancomycin. Clin Infect Dis 39:539–45, 2004.

Cruciani M, Gatti G, Lazzarini L, et al. Penetration of vancomycin into human lung tissue. Journal of Antimicrobial Chemotherapy 38:865–69, 1996.

Cunha BA, Mohan SS, Hamid N, McDermott GP, Daniels P. Cost ineffectiveness of serum vancomycin levels. Eur J Clin Microbiol Infect Dis 13:509–511, 2007.

Cunha BA. Vancomycin revisisted: a reappraisal of clinical use. Critical Care Clinics of North America 24:394–420, 2008.

Cunha BA. Vancomycin. Med Clin North Am 79:817–31, 1995.

Cunha BA. Vancomycin serum levels: unnecessary, unhelpful, and costly. Antibiotics for Clinicians 8:273–77, 2004.

Cunha BA, Deglin J, Chow M, et al. Pharmacokinetics of vancomycin in patients undergoing chronic hemodialysis. Rev Infect Dis 3:269–72, 1981.

DelDot ME, Lipman J, Tett SE. Vancomycin pharmacokinetics in critically ill patients receiving continuous venovenous haemodiafiltration. Br J Clin Pharmacol 58:259–68, 2004.

del Mar Fernandez de Gatta Garcia, Revilla N, Calvo MV, et al. Pharmacokinetic/pharmacodynamic analysis of vancomycin in ICU patient. Intensive Care Med 33:279–285, 2007.

Deresinski S. Vancomycin: does it still have a role as an antistaphylococcal agent? Expert Rev Anti Infect Ther 5:393–401, 2007.

El Amari EB, Vuagnat A, Stern R, et al. High versus standard dose vancomycin for osteomyelitis. Scand J Infect Dis 36:712–7, 2004.

Hidayat LK, Hsu DI, Quist R, et al. High-dose vancomycin therapy for methicillin-resistant Staphylococcus aureus infections. Arch Inter Med 166:2138–44, 2006.

Huttner A, Harbarth S: Guidelines for vancomycin use. Clin Infect Dis 50:616, 2010.

Johnson JR. Vancomycin levels, efficacy, and toxicity. Arch Intern Med 167:1207–1209, 2007.

Leonard SN, Szeto YG, Zolotarev M, et al. Comparative in vitro activity of telavancin, vancomycin, and linezolid against heterogeneously vancomycin-intermediate Staphylococcus aureus (hVISA). Int J Antimicrob 37:558–561, 2011.

Menzies D. Goel K, Cunha BA. Vancomycin. Antibiotics for Clinicians 2:97–9, 1998.

Moellering RC Jr. Monitoring serum vancomycin levels: climbing the mountain because it is there? Clin Infect Dis 18:544–6, 1994.

Okamoto H. Vancomycin-induced immune thrombocytopenia. N Engl J Med 356:2537–2538, 2007.

Patanwala AE, Erstad BL, Nix DE. Cost-effectiveness of linezolid and vancomycin in the treatment of surgical site infections. Curr Med Res Opin 23:185–193, 2007.

Patel N, Lubanski P, Ferro S, et al. Correlation between vancomycin MIC values and those of other agents against gram-positive bacteria among patients with bloodstream infections caused by methicillin-resistant Staphylococcus aureus. Antimicrob Agents Chemother 53:5141–5144, 2009.

Pope SD, Roecker A. Vancomycin for treatment of invasive, multi-drug resistant Staphylococcus aureus infections. Exp Opin Pharmacother 8:1245–1261, 2007.

Ricard JD, Wolff M, Lacerade JC, et al. Levels of vancomycin in cerebrospinal fluid of adult patients receiving adjunctive corticosteroids to treat pneumococcal meningitis: a prospective multicenter observational study. Clin Infect Dis 44:250–255, 2007.

Rybak MJ. The pharmacokinetic and pharmacodynamic properties of vancomycin. Clin Infect Dis 42:S35–9, 2006.

Rybak MJ, Lomaestro BM, Rotschafer JC, et al. Vancomycin therapeutic guidelines: a summary of consensus recommendations from the infectious diseases Society of America, the American Society of Health-System Pharmacists, and the Society of Infections Diseases Pharmacists. Clin Infect Dis 49:325–327, 2009.

Saribas S, Bagdatli Y. Vancomycin tolerance in enterococci. Chemotherapy 50:250–4, 2004.

Smith DL. Vancomycin way of administration: Where is the evidence? Clin Infect Dis 53:308–309, 2011.

Stevens DL. The role of vancomycin in the treatment paradigm. Clin Infect Dis 42:S51–7, 2006.

"Usual dose" assumes normal renal/hepatic function. * For renal insufficiency, give usual dose × 1 followed by maintenance dose per CrCl. For dialysis patients, dose the same as for CrCl < 10 mL/min and give supplemental (post-HD/PD dose) immediately after dialysis. CrCl = creatinine clearance; CVVH = continuous veno-venous hemofiltration; HD/PD = hemodialysis/peritoneal dialysis.

Stryjewski ME, Szczech LA, Benjamin DK Jr, et al. Use
of vancomycin or first-generation cephalosporins
for the treatment of hemodialysis-dependent
patients with methicillin-susceptible Staphylococcus
aureus bacteremia. Clin Infect Dis 44:190–196,
2007.

Tenover FC, Moellering RC. The rationale for revising
the clinical and laboratory standards institute
vancomycin minimal inhibitory concentration
interpretive criteria for staphylococcus aureus. Clin
Infect Dis 44:1208–1215, 2007.

Vandecasteele SJ, De Vriese AS. Vancomycin dosing
in patients on intermittent hemodialysis. Semin Dial
24:50–55, 2011.

Von Drygalski A, Curtis BR, Bougie DW, et al.
Vancomycin-induced immune thrombocytopenia.
N Engl J Med 356:904–10, 2007.

Wang G, Hindler JF, Ward KW, et al. Increased
vancomycin MICs for Staphylococcus aureus clinical
isolates from a university hospital during a 5-year
period. Journal of Clinical Microbiology 44:3883–86,
2006.

Website: www.pdr.net

Voriconazole (Vfend)

Drug Class: Triazole antifungal.
Usual Dose: IV dosing: **Loading dose:**
6 mg/kg (IV) q12h × 1 day, then
maintenance dose: 4 mg/kg (IV) q12h. Can
switch to weight-based PO maintenance dosing
anytime while on maintenance IV dose (see
comments).

PO dosing: Weight ≥ 40 kg: Loading dose of
400 mg (PO) q12h × 1 day, then maintenance
dose of 200 mg (PO) q12h. If response is
inadequate, the dose may be increased
to 300 mg (PO) q12h. Weight < 40 kg:
Loading dose of 200 mg (PO) × 1 day, then
maintenance dose of 100 mg (PO) q12h.
If response is inadequate, the dose may be
increased to 150 mg (PO) q12h. For chronic/

non-life-threatening infections, loading dose
may be given PO (see comments).
Pharmacokinetic Parameters:
Peak serum level: 2.3–4.7 mcg/ml
Bioavailability: 96%
Excreted unchanged (urine): 2%
Serum half-life (normal/ESRD): 6/6 hrs
Plasma protein binding: 58%
Volume of distribution (V_d): 4.6 L/kg
Primary Mode of Elimination: Hepatic
Dosage Adjustments*

CrCl 50–80 mL/min	No change
CrCl 10–50 mL/min	No change PO; avoid IV
CrCl < 10 mL/min	No change PO; avoid IV
Post–HD dose	Usual dose PO; avoid IV
Post–PD dose	No data
CVVH/CVVHD/ CVVHDF dose	4 mg/kg (PO) q12h; avoid (IV)
Mild-Moderate hepatic insufficiency	6 mg/kg (IV) q12h × 1 day or 200 mg (PO) q12h × 1 day, then 2 mg/kg (IV) q12h or 100 mg (PO) q12h (> 40 kg)
Severe hepatic insufficiency	Use with caution

Drug Interactions: Benzodiazepines,
vinca alkaloids (↑ interacting drug levels);
carbamazepine, ergot alkaloids, rifampin,
rifabutin, sirolimus, long-acting barbiturates
(contraindicated with voriconazole);
cyclosporine, ↓ (cyclosporine by 1/2 and
monitor); efavirenz (↑ maintence dose of

"Usual dose" assumes normal renal/hepatic function. * For renal insufficiency, give usual dose × 1 followed by
maintenance dose per CrCl. For dialysis patients, dose the same as for CrCl < 10 mL/min and give supplemental
(post-HD/PD dose) immediately after dialysis. CrCl = creatinine clearance; CVVH = continuous veno-venous
hemofiltration; HD/PD = hemodialysis/peritoneal dialysis.

voriconazole to 400 mg (PO) q12h and decrease efavirenz dose to 300mg (PO) q12h while on voriconazole); omeprazole (↑ interacting drug levels, ↓ interacting drug dose by 50%); tacrolimus (↑ tacrolimus levels, ↓ tacrolimus dose by 66%); phenytoin (↓ voriconazole levels); ↑ voriconazole dose from 4 mg/kg [IV] to 5 mg/kg [IV] and from 200 mg [PO] to 400 mg [PO]; warfarin (↑ INR); statins (↑ risk of rhabdomyolysis); dihydropyridine calcium channel blockers (hypotension); tacrolimus (reduce tacrolimus dose by 1/3 and monitor while on voriconazole); sulfonylureas (hypoglycemia). Voriconozole has not been studied with protease inhibitors or NNRTIs, but ↑ voriconazole levels are predicted (↑ hepatotoxicity/adverse effects).

Adverse Effects: ↑ SGOT/SGPT; visual events (blurring vision, ↑ brightness, pain; occurs soon after ingestion and usually resolves quickly (~ ½ hour), hallucinations, hypoglycemia, dose-dependent arrhythmias, ↑ QT_c interval; rash, including Stevens-Johnson Syndrome; photosensitivity reactions (avoid direct sunlight); melanoma (↑ risk of with chronic therapy).

Allergic Potential: High

Safety in Pregnancy: D

Comments: If intolerance to therapy develops, the IV maintenance dose may be reduced to 3 mg/kg and the PO maintenance dose may be reduced in steps of 50 mg/d to a minimum of 200 mg/d q12h (weight ≥ 40 kg) or 100 mg q12h (weight < 40 kg). Non-linear kinetics (doubling of oral dose = 2.8-fold increase in serum levels). 10–15% of patients have serum levels > 6 mcg/ml. Food decreases bioavailability; take 1 hour before or after meals. Do not use IV voriconazole if CrCl < 50 mL/min to prevent accumulation of voriconazole IV vehicle, sulphobutyl ether cyclodextrin (SBECD); instead use oral formulation, which has no SBECD. Loading dose may be given PO for chronic/non-life-threatening infections. Because of visual effects, do not drive or operate machinery. Monitor LFTs before and during therapy. Take without food; suspension contains sucrose.

Highly active against C. albicans, non-albicans Candida, Aspergillus, Cryptococcus, Hansenula and Pseudoallescheria/ Scedosporium. Some activity against Fusaria, Fluconazole/Itraconazole resistant C. albicans, Coccidiomycosis, and Penicillium marneffei. No activity against Rhizopus or Mucor.
Meningeal dose = usual dose.

Cerebrospinal Fluid Penetration: 90%

REFERENCES:

Aypar E, Kendirli T, Tutar E, et al. Voriconazole-induced QT interval prolongation and torsades de pointes. Pediatr Int 53: 761–763, 2011.

Bruggemann RJM, Alffenaar JWC, Blijlevens NMA, et al. Clinical relevance of the pharmacokinetic interactions of azole antifungal drugs with coadministered agents. Clin Infect Dis 48:1441–1458, 2009.

Camuset J, Nunes H, Dombret MC, et al. Treatment of chronic pulmonary aspergillosis by voriconazole in nonimmunocompromised patients. Chest 131:1435–1441, 2007.

Capitano B, Potoski BA, Husain S, et al. Intrapulmonary penetration of voriconazole in patients receiving an oral prophylactic regimen. Antimicrob Agents Chemother 50:1878–80, 2006.

Cowen EW, Nguyen JC, Miller DD, et al. Chronic phototoxicity and aggressive squamous cell carcinoma of the skin in children and adults during treatment with voriconazole. J Am Acad Dermatol 62:31–37, 2010.

den Hollander JG, van Arkel C, Rijnders BJ, et al. Incidence of voriconazole hepatotoxicity during intravenous and oral treatment for invasive fungal infections. J Antimicrob Chemother 57:1248–50, 2006.

"Usual dose" assumes normal renal/hepatic function. * For renal insufficiency, give usual dose × 1 followed by maintenance dose per CrCl. For dialysis patients, dose the same as for CrCl < 10 mL/min and give supplemental (post-HD/PD dose) immediately after dialysis. CrCl = creatinine clearance; CVVH = continuous veno-venous hemofiltration; HD/PD = hemodialysis/peritoneal dialysis.

Denes E, Boumediene A, Durox H, et al. Voriconazole concentrations in synovial fluid and bone tissues. J Antimicrob Chemother 59:818–819, 2007.

Denning DW, Ribaud P, Milpied N, et al. Efficacy and safety of voriconazole in the treatment of acute invasive aspergillosis. Clin Infect Dis 34:563–71, 2002.

Dickmeyer NJ, Kiel PJ. Dosing voriconazole in an obese patient. Clin Infect Dis 53:745, 2011.

Elter T, Sieniawski M, Gossmann A, et al. Voriconazole brain tissue levels in rhinocerebral aspergillosis in a successfully treated young woman. Int J Antimicrob Agents 28:262–5, 2006.

Hicheri Y, Cook G, Cordonnier C. Antifungal prophylaxis in haematology patients: the role voriconazole. Clin Microbiol Infect 18:1–15, 2012.

Ho DY, Lee JD, Rosso F, et al. Treating disseminated fusariosis: amphotericin B, voriconazole or both? Mycoses 50:227–231, 2007.

Hoffman HL, Rathbun RC. Review of the safety and efficacy of voriconazole. Expert Opin Investig Drugs 11:409–29, 2002.

Jurkunas UV, Langston DP, Colby K. Use of voriconazole in the treatment of fungal keratitis. Int Ophthalmol Clin 47:47–59, 2007.

Keirns J, Sawamoto T, Holum M, et al. Steady-state pharmacokinetics of micafungin and voriconazole after separate and concomitant dosing in healthy adults. Antimicrob Agents Chemother 51:787–790, 2007.

Kim MM, Vikram HR, Kusne S, et al. Treatment of refractory coccidioidomycosis with voriconazole or posaconazole. Clin Infect Dis, 53:1060–6, 2011.

Leveque D, Nivoix Y, Jehl F, Herbrecht R. Clinical pharmacokinetics of voriconazole. Int J Antimicrob Agents 27:274–84, 2006.

Masomoto Y, Nannya Y, Kurokawa M. Voriconazole is effective as secondary antifungal prophylaxis in leukemia patients with prior pulmonary fungal disease: case series and review of literature. J Chemother 23:17–23, 2011.

Miceli MH, Diaz JA, Lee SA. Emerging opportunistic yeast infections. Lancet Infectious Diseases.11: 142–151, 2011.

Miller DD, Cown EW, Ngugen JC, et al. Melanoma associated with long-term voriconazole therapy: a new manifestation of chronic photosensitivity. Arch Dermatol 146:300–304, 2010.

Oude Lashof AM, Sobel JD, Ruhnke M, et al. Safety and tolerability of voriconazole in patients with baseline renal insufficiency and candidemia. Antimicrob Agents Chemother 56:3133–7, 2012.

Pagano L, Valentini CG, Fianchi L, et al. Treatment strategies for invasive aspergillosis in neutropenic patients: voriconazole or liposomal amphotericin- B J Chemother 23:5–8, 2011.

Poza G, Montoya J, Redondo C, et al. Meningitis caused by Pseudallescheria boydii treated with voriconazole. Clin Infect Dis 30:981–2, 2000.

Radaj J, Krouzecky A, Stehlik P, et al. Pharmacokinetic evaluation of voriconazole treatment in critically ill patients undergoing continuous venovenous hemofiltration. Ther Drug Monit 33:393–397, 2011.

Rondeau S, Couderu L, Dominique S, et al. High Frequency of voriconazole-related phototoxicity in cystic fibrosis patients. Eur Respir J 39:782–4, 2012.

Sambatakou H, Dupont B, Lode H, Denning DW. Voriconazole treatment for subacute invasive and chronic pulmonary aspergillosis. Am J Med 119:527, 2006.

Schwartz S, Ruhnke M, Ribaud P, et al. Improved outcome in central nervous system aspergillosis, using voriconazole treatment. Amer Soc of Hematology 106:2641–5, 2006.

Scott LJ, Simpson D. Voriconazole: a review of its use in the management of invasive fungal infections. Drugs 67:269–98, 2007.

Shehab N, DePestel DD, Mackler ER, et al. Institutional experience with voriconazole compared with liposomal amphotericin B as empiric therapy for febrile neutropenia. Pharmacotherapy 27:970–979, 2007.

Smith J, Safdar N, Knasinski V, et al. Voriconazole Therapeutic Drug Monitoring. Antimicrob Agents Chemother 50:1570–72, 2006.

Supparatpinyo K, Schlamm HT. Voriconazole as therapy for systemic Penicillium marneffei infections in AIDS patients. Am J Trop Med Hyg 77:350–353, 2007.

Tan K, Brayshaw N, Tomaszewski K, et al. Investigation of the potential relationships between plasma

---

"Usual dose" assumes normal renal/hepatic function. * For renal insufficiency, give usual dose × 1 followed by maintenance dose per CrCl. For dialysis patients, dose the same as for CrCl < 10 mL/min and give supplemental (post-HD/PD dose) immediately after dialysis. CrCl = creatinine clearance; CVVH = continuous veno-venous hemofiltration; HD/PD = hemodialysis/peritoneal dialysis.

voriconazole-concentrations and visual adverse events or liver function test abnormalities. J Clin Pharmacol 46:235–43, 2006.

Walsh TJ, Anaissie EJ, Denning DW, et al. Treatment of Aspergillosis: Clinical Practice Diseases Society of America. Clin Infect Dis 46:327–360, 2008.

Website: www.vfend.com

Zalcitabine (HIVID) ddC

Drug Class: Antiretroviral NRTI (nucleoside reverse transcriptase inhibitor).
Usual Dose: 0.75 mg (PO) q8h.
Pharmacokinetic Parameters:
Peak serum level: 0.08 mcg/ml
Bioavailability: 80%
Excreted unchanged (urine): 75%
Serum half-life (normal/ESRD): 2/8.5 hrs
Plasma protein binding: 0%
Volume of distribution (V_d): 0.54 L/kg
Primary Mode of Elimination: Renal
Dosage Adjustments*

CrCl 10–50 mL/min	0.75 mg (PO) q12h
CrCl < 10 mL/min	0.75 mg (PO) q24h
Post–HD dose	No data
Post–PD dose	No data
CVVH/CVVHD/CVVHDF dose	0.75 mg (PO) q12h
Moderate hepatic insufficiency	No change
Severe hepatic insufficiency	No change

Drug Interactions: Cimetidine, probenecid, TMP–SMX (↑ zalcitabine levels); dapsone, didanosine, stavudine, INH, phenytoin, metronidazole, other neurotoxic agents or history of neuropathy (↑ risk of peripheral neuropathy); magnesium/aluminum containing antacids, metoclopramide (↓ bioavailability of zalcitabine); pentamidine IV, valproic acid, alcohol, other agents known to cause pancreatitis (↑ risk of pancreatitis).

Adverse Effects: Drug fever/rash, leukopenia, anemia, thrombocytopenia, hepatomegaly, hepatotoxicity/hepatic necrosis, peripheral neuropathy, pancreatitis, stomatitis, oral/genital ulcers, dysphagia, arthritis, hyperglycemia, lipotrodystrophy, wasting, night sweats, lactic acidosis with hepatic steatosis (rare, but potentially life-threatening toxicity with use of NRTIs).

Allergic Potential: High
Safety in Pregnancy: C
Comments: Foscarnet may increase toxicity. Do not use with stavudine, didanosine, or lamivudine to avoid additive toxicities. Food decreases absorption by 39%. Effective antiretroviral therapy consists of at least 3 antiretrovirals (same/different classes).
Cerebrospinal Fluid Penetration: 25%

REFERENCES:
Panel on Antiretroviral Guidelines for Adults and Adolescents. Department of Health and Human Services. Guidelines for the use of antiretroviral agents in HIV-infected adults and adolescents. http://aidsinfo.nih.gov/ConsentFiles/AdultandAdolescentGL.pdf, 2011.

Shelton MJ, O'Donnell AM, Morse GD. Zalcitabine. Ann Pharmacotherapy 27:480–9, 1993.

Thompson MA, Aberg JA, Cahn P, et al. Antiretroviral treatment of adult HIV infection: 2012 recommendations of the International Antiviral Society — USA panel. JAMA 308:387–402, 2012.

Website: www.rocheusa.com/products/

Zidovudine (Retrovir) ZDV Azidothymidine AZT

Drug Class: Antiretroviral NRTI (nucleoside reverse transcriptase inhibitor).

Usual Dose: 300 mg (PO) q12h or 200 mg (PO) q8h (see comments). IV solution 10 mg/mL (dose 1 mg/kg 5–6 x/day).

Pharmacokinetic Parameters:
Peak serum level: 1.2 mcg/mL
Bioavailability: 64%
Excreted unchanged (urine): 16%
Serum half-life (normal/ESRD): 1.1/1.4 hrs
Plasma protein binding: < 38%
Volume of distribution (V_d): 1.6 L/kg

Primary Mode of Elimination: Hepatic

Dosage Adjustments*

CrCl < 15 mL/min	100 mg (PO) q8h or 300 mg (PO) q24h
Post–HD/PD dose	100 mg or 300 mg
CVVH/CVVHD/CVVHDF dose	300 mg (PO) q24h
Moderate–severe hepatic insufficiency	Use with caution

Drug Interactions: Acetaminophen, atovaquone, fluconazole, methadone, probenecid, valproic acid (↑ zidovudine levels); clarithromycin, nelfinavir, rifampin, rifabutin (↓ zidovudine levels); dapsone, flucytosine, ganciclovir, interferon alpha, bone marrow suppressive/cytotoxic agents (↑ risk of hematologic toxicity); indomethacin (↑ levels of zidovudine toxic metabolite); phenytoin (↑ zidovudine levels, ↑ or ↓ phenytoin levels); ribavirin (↓ zidovudine effect; avoid).

Adverse Effects: Zidovudine, has been associated with hematologic toxicity including neutropenia and severe anemia. Prolonged use of zidovudine has been associated with symptomatic myopathy as well as lactic acidosis and severe hepatomegaly with steatosis, including fatal cases. May cause nausea, vomiting, GI upset, diarrhea, malaise, anorexia, macrocytosis, headachese, insomnia, blue/black nail discoloration and asthenia. Nausea, vomiting, GI upset, diarrhea, malaise, anorexia, leukopenia, severe anemia, macrocytosis, thrombocytopenia, headaches, ↑ SGOT/SGPT, hepatotoxicity, myalgias, myositis, symptomatic myopathy, insomnia, blue/black nail discoloration, asthenia, lactic acidosis with hepatic steatosis (rare, but potentially life-threatening toxicity with use of NRTI's).

Allergic Potential: Low

Safety in Pregnancy: C

Comments: Antagonized by ganciclovir or ribavirin. Also a component of Combivir and Trizivir. Patients on IV therapy should be switched to PO as soon as able to take oral medication. For IV administration, dilute in D5W to a concentration no greater than 4 mg/mL and infuse over 1 hour.

Cerebrospinal Fluid Penetration: 60%

REFERENCES:

Barry M, Mulcahy F, Merry C, et al. Pharmacokinetics and potential interactions amongst antiretroviral agents used to treat patients with HIV infection. Clin Pharmacol 36:289–304, 1999.

Been-Tiktak AM, Boucher CA, Brun-Vezinet F, et al. Efficacy and safety of combination therapy with delavirdine and zidovudine: A European/Australian phase II trial. Intern J Antimcrob Agents 11:13–21, 1999.

Diaz-Brito V, Leon A, Knobel H, et al. Post-exposure prophylaxis for HIV-infection: a clinical trail comparing lopinavir/ritonavir versus atazanavir each with zidovudine/lamivudine. Antivir Ther 17:337–46, 2012.

McDowell JA, Lou Y, Symonds WS, et al. Multiple-dose pharmacokinetics and pharmacodynamics

---

"Usual dose" assumes normal renal/hepatic function. * For renal insufficiency, give usual dose × 1 followed by maintenance dose per CrCl. For dialysis patients, dose the same as for CrCl < 10 mL/min and give supplemental (post-HD/PD dose) immediately after dialysis. CrCl = creatinine clearance; CVVH = continuous veno-venous hemofiltration; HD/PD = hemodialysis/peritoneal dialysis.

of abacavir alone and in combination with zidovudine in human immunodeficiency virus-infected adults. Antimicrob Agents Chemother 44:2061–7, 2000.

Panel on Antiretroviral Guidelines for Adults and Adolescents. Department of Health and Human Services. Guidelines for the use of antiretroviral agents in HIV-infected adults and adolescents.

http://aidsinfo.nih.gov/ConsentFiles/AdultandAdolescentGL.pdf, 2012.

Thompson MA, Aberg JA, Cahn P, et al. Antiretroviral treatment of adult HIV infection: 2012 recommendations of the International Antiviral Society — USA panel. JAMA 308:387–402, 2012.

Website: www.TreatHIV.com

REFERENCES AND SUGGESTED READINGS

TEXTBOOKS

Ambrose P, Nightingale AT (eds). Principles of Pharmacodynamics. Marcel Dekker, Inc., New York, 2001.

Baddour L, Gorbach SL (eds). Therapy of Infectious Diseases. Saunders, Philadelphia, 2003.

Bennet WM, Aronoff GR, Golper TA, Morrison G, Brater DC, Singer I (eds). Drug Prescribing in Renal Failure, 2nd Edition, American College of Physicians, Philadelphia, 2000.

Bowden RA, Ljungman P, Snydman DR (eds). Transplant Infections 3rd Edition, Lippincott Williams & Wilkins, Philadelphia, PA, 2010.

Bryskier A (ed). Antimicrobial Agents. ASM Press, Washington, D.C., 2005.

Finch RG, Greenwood D, Norrby SR, Whitley RJ (eds). Antibiotic and Chemotherapy. Churchill Livingstone, United Kingdom, 2003.

Gorbach SL, Bartlett JG, Blacklow NR (eds). Infectious Diseases, 4th Edition, Lippincott Williams Wilkins, Philadelphia, 2004.

Grayson ML (ed). Kucers' The Use of Antibiotics, 6th Edition, ASM Press, Washington, DC, 2010.

Koff RS, Hepatitis Essentials. Jones & Bartlett, Sudbury, MA, 2011.

Mandell GL, Bennett JE, Dolin R (eds). Mandell, Douglas and Bennett's Principles and Practice of Infectious Disease, 7th Edition. Elsevier, Philadelphia, 2010.

Pai MP, Momary KM, Rodvold KA. Antibiotic Drug Interactions. Med Clin N Am 90:1223–55, 2006.

Physicians' Desk Reference, 66th Edition, Thompson PDR, Montvale, NJ, 2012.

Piscitelli SC, Rodvold KE (eds). Drug Interactions in Infectious Diseases. Humana Press, Totowa, 2001.

Ristuccia AM, Cunha BA (eds). Antimicrobial Therapy. Raven Press, New York, 1984.

Sax PE, Cohen CJ, Kuritzkes DR. HIV Essentials. 5th Edition, Jones & Bartlett, Sudbury, MA, 2012.

Schlossberg D (ed). Current Therapy of Infectious Disease, 3rd Edition. Mosby-Yearbook, St. Louis, 2008.

Schlossberg D (ed). Tuberculosis and Non-Tuberculous Mycobacterial Infections, 7th Edition, McGraw-Hill, New York, 2011.

Scholar EM, Pratt WB (eds). The Antimicrobial Drugs, 2nd Edition, Oxford University Press, New York, 2000.

Wormser GP (ed). AIDS, 4th Edition, Elsevier, Philadelphia, 2004.

Yoshikawa TT, Rajagopalan S (eds). Antibiotic Therapy for Geriatric Patients. Taylor & Francis, New York, 2006.

Yu VL, Merigan, Jr. TC, Barrier SL (eds). Antimicrobial Therapy and Vaccines, 2nd Edition, Williams & Wilkins, Baltimore, 2005.

Zinner SH, Young LS, Acar JF, Ortiz-Neu C (eds). New Considerations for Macrolides, Azalides, Streptogramins, and Ketolides. Marcel Dekker, New York, 2000.

"Usual dose" assumes normal renal/hepatic function. * For renal insufficiency, give usual dose × 1 followed by maintenance dose per CrCl. For dialysis patients, dose the same as for CrCl < 10 mL/min and give supplemental (post-HD/PD dose) immediately after dialysis. CrCl = creatinine clearance; CVVH = continuous veno-venous hemofiltration; HD/PD = hemodialysis/peritoneal dialysis.

APPENDIX

Malaria in Adults (United States)

Clinical Diagnosis/ *Plasmodium* species	Region Acquired	Recommended Adult Drug Doses
Severe malaria[1,2,3,4]	All regions	**Quinidine gluconate[2] *plus* either: Doxycycline or Clindamycin** **Quinidine gluconate:** 6.25 mg base/kg (=10 mg salt/kg) (IV over 1–2 hrs) then 0.0125 mg base/kg/min (=0.02 mg salt/kg/min) continuous infusion for at least 24 hours. An alternative regimen is 15 mg base/kg (=24 mg salt/kg) loading dose IV infused over 4 hours, followed by 7.5 mg base/kg (=12 mg salt/kg) infused over 4 hours q8h, starting 8 hours after the loading dose. Once parasite density <1% and patient can take oral medication, complete treatment with oral quinine, dose as above. Quinidine/quinine course = 7 days in Southeast Asia; = 3 days in Africa or South America. **Doxycycline:** Treatment as above, give 100 mg (IV/PO) q12h × 7 days. **Clindamycin:** Treatment as above. If patient not able to take oral medication, give 10 mg base/kg (IV) then 5 mg base/kg (IV/PO) q8h × 7 days.
Uncomplicated malaria/ *P. falciparum* or Species not identified (If "species not identified" is subsequently diagnosed as *P. vivax* or *P. ovale*: see *P. vivax* and *P. ovale* treat with primaquine)	**Chloroquine-resistant or unknown resistance[5]** (Middle Eastern countries with chloroquine-resistant *P. falciparum* include Iran, Oman, Saudi Arabia, and Yemen. Malaria acquired in the newly independent states of the former Soviet Union and Korea to date have been uniformly caused by *P. vivax* and should therefore be treated as chloroquine-sensitive infections.)	**A. Atovaquone-proguanil (Malarone)[6]** *Adult tab = 250 mg atovaquone/ 100 mg proguanil* 4 adult tabs (PO) q24h × 3 days **or**

Malaria in Adults (United States) (cont'd)

Clinical Diagnosis/ *Plasmodium* species	Region Acquired	Recommended Adult Drug Doses
Uncomplicated malaria/ *P. falciparum* (cont'd)	**Chloroquine-resistant or unknown resistance** (cont'd)	**B. Artemether-lumefantrine (Coartem)[6]** *1 tablet = 20 mg artemether/120 mg lumefantrine* A 3-day treatment schedule with a total of 6 oral doses is recommended based on weight. The patient should receive the initial dose, followed by the second dose 8 hours later, then 1 dose (PO) q12h × 2 days. ≥35 kg: 4 tablets per dose **or** **C. Quinine sulfate** *plus* **either: Doxycycline[9] or Clindamycin** **Quinine sulfate[8]:** 542 mg base (=650 mg salt)[7] (PO) q8h × 3 or 7 days **Doxycycline:** 100 mg (PO) q12h × 7 days **Clindamycin:** 20 mg base/kg/day (PO) divided q8h × 7 days **or** **D. Mefloquine (Lariam)[10]** 684 mg base (=750 mg salt) (PO) as initial dose, followed by 456 mg base (=500 mg salt) (PO) given 6–12 hours after initial dose Total dose = 1,250 mg salt
Uncomplicated malaria/ *P. falciparum* or *Species not identified*	**Chloroquine-sensitive** (Central America west of Panama Canal; Haiti; the Dominican Republic; and most of the Middle East)	**Chloroquine phosphate (Aralen)** 600 mg base (=1,000 mg salt) (PO) immediately, followed by 300 mg base (=500 mg salt) (PO) at 6, 24, and 48 hours Total dose: 1,500 mg base (=2,500 mg salt) **or** **Hydroxychloroquine (Plaquenil)** 620 mg base (=800 mg salt) (PO) immediately, followed by 310 mg base (=400 mg salt) (PO) at 6, 24, and 48 hours Total dose: 1,550 mg base (=2,000 mg salt)

Malaria in Adults (United States) (cont'd)

Clinical Diagnosis/ *Plasmodium* species	Region Acquired	Recommended Adult Drug Doses
Uncomplicated malaria/ P. malariae or **P. knowlesi**	**All regions**	**Chloroquine phosphate:** Treatment as above **or** **Hydroxychloroquine:** Treatment as above
Uncomplicated malaria/ P. vivax or **P. ovale**	**All regions** (for suspected chloroquine-resistant *P. vivax*, see below)	**Chloroquine phosphate** *plus* **Primaquine phosphate**[11] **Chloroquine phosphate:** Treatment as above **Primaquine phosphate:** 30 mg base (PO) q24h × 14 days **or** **Hydroxychloroquine** *plus* **Primaquine phosphate**[11] **Hydroxychloroquine:** Treatment as above **Primaquine phosphate:** 30 mg base (PO) q24h × 14 days
Uncomplicated malaria/ P. vivax	**Chloroquine-resistant**[12] (Papua New Guinea and Indonesia)	**A. Quinine sulfate** *plus* **either: Doxycycline** *plus* **Primaquine phosphate**[11] **Quinine sulfate:** Treatment as above **Doxycycline:** Treatment as above **Primaquine phosphate:** Treatment as above **or** **B. Atovaquone-proguanil** *plus* **Primaquine phosphate** **Atovaquone-proguanil:** Treatment as above **Primaquine phosphate:** Treatment as above **or** **C. Mefloquine**[10] *plus* **Primaquine phosphate**[11] **Mefloquine:** Treatment as above **Primaquine phosphate:** Treatment as above

Malaria in Adults (United States) (cont'd)

Clinical Diagnosis/ Plasmodium species	Region Acquired	Recommended Adult Drug Doses
Uncomplicated malaria: alternatives for pregnant women[13,14,15,16]	**Chloroquine-sensitive** (see uncomplicated malaria sections above for chloroquine-sensitive species by region)	**Chloroquine phosphate:** Treatment as above **or** **Hydroxychloroquine:** Treatment as above
Uncomplicated malaria: alternatives for pregnant women (cont'd)	**Chloroquine resistant P. falciparum**[1] (see sections above for regions with chloroquine resistant P. falciparum)	**Quinine sulfate** *plus* **Clindamycin** **Quinine sulfate:** Treatment as above **Clindamycin:** Treatment as above
	Chloroquine-resistant P. vivax (see uncomplicated malaria sections above for regions with chloroquine-resistant P. vivax)	**Quinine sulfate** **Quinine sulfate**[7]: 650 mg salt (PO) q8h × 7 days

1. Persons with a positive blood smear or history of recent possible exposure and no other recognized pathology who have one or more of the following clinical criteria (impaired consciousness/coma, severe normocytic anemia, renal failure, pulmonary edema, acute respiratory distress syndrome, circulatory shock, disseminated intravascular coagulation, spontaneous bleeding, acidosis, hemoglobinuria, jaundice, repeated generalized convulsions, and/or parasitemia of >5%) are considered to have manifestations of more severe disease. Severe malaria is most often caused by P. falciparum.

2. Patients diagnosed with severe malaria should be treated aggressively with parenteral antimalarial therapy. Treatment with IV quinidine should be initiated as soon as possible after the diagnosis has been made. Patients with severe malaria should be given an intravenous loading dose of quinidine unless they have received more than 40 mg/kg of quinine in the preceding 48 hours or if they have received mefloquine within the preceding 12 hours. Consultation with a cardiologist and a physician with experience treating malaria is advised when treating malaria patients with quinidine. During administration of quinidine, blood pressure monitoring (for hypotension) and cardiac monitoring (for widening of the QRS complex and/or lengthening of the QTc interval) should be monitored continuously and blood glucose (for hypoglycemia) should be monitored periodically. Cardiac complications, if severe, may warrant temporary discontinuation of the drug or slowing of the intravenous infusion.

3. Consider exchange transfusion if the parasite density (i.e. parasitemia) is >10% OR if the patient has altered mental status, non-volume overload pulmonary edema, or renal complications. The parasite density can be estimated by examining a monolayer of red blood cells (RBCs) on the thin smear under oil immersion magnification. The slide should be examined where the RBCs are more or less touching (approximately 400 RBCs per field). The parasite density can then be estimated from the percentage of infected RBCs and should be monitored every 12 hours. Exchange transfusion should be continued until the parasite density is <1% (usually requires 8–10 units). IV quinidine administration should not be delayed for an exchange transfusion and can be given concurrently throughout the exchange transfusion.

4. Pregnant women diagnosed with severe malaria should be treated aggressively with parenteral antimalarial therapy.

5. There are 4 options (A, B, C, or D) available for treatment of uncomplicated malaria caused by chloroquine-resistant P. falciparum. Options A, B, and C are equally recommended. Because of a higher rate of severe neuropsychiatric reactions seen at treatment doses, option D (mefloquine) not recommend

unless the other options cannot be used. For option C, because there is more data on the efficacy of quinine in combination with doxycycline, these treatment combinations preferred to quinine with clindamycin.

6. Take with with food or whole milk. If patient vomits within 30 minutes of taking a dose, then they should repeat the dose.

7. US manufactured quinine sulfate capsule is in a 324 mg dosage; therefore 2 capsules should be sufficient for adult dosing. Pediatric dosing may be difficult due to unavailability of non-capsule forms of quinine.

8. For infections acquired in Southeast Asia, quinine treatment should continue for 7 days. For infections acquired elsewhere, quinine treatment should continue for 3 days.

9. Doxycycline are not indicated for use in children less than 8 years old. For children less than 8 years old with chloroquine-resistant *P. falciparum*, atovaquone-proguanil and artemether-lumefantrine are recommended treatment options; mefloquine can be considered if no other options are available. For children less than 8 years old with chloroquine-resistant *P. vivax*, mefloquine is the recommended treatment. If it is not available or is not being tolerated and if the treatment benefits outweigh the risks, atovaquone-proguanil or artemether-lumefantrine should be used instead.

10. Treatment with mefloquine is not recommended in persons who have acquired infections from Southeast Asia due to drug resistance.

11. Primaquine is used to eradicate any hypnozoites in the liver, to prevent relapses, in *P. vivax* and *P. ovale* infections. Because primaquine can cause hemolytic anemia in G6PD-deficient persons, G6PD screening must occur prior to starting treatment with primaquine. For persons with borderline G6PD deficiency or as an alternate to the above regimen, primaquine may be given 45 mg orally one time per week for 8 weeks; consultation with an expert in infectious disease and/or tropical medicine is advised if this alternative regimen is considered in G6PD-deficient persons. Primaquine must not be used during pregnancy.

12. There are three options (A, B, or C) available for treatment of uncomplicated malaria caused by chloroquine-resistant *P. vivax*. High treatment failure rates due to chloroquine-resistant *P. vivax* have been well documented in Papua New Guinea and Indonesia. Rare case reports of chloroquine-resistant *P. vivax* have also been documented in Burma (Myanmar), India, and Central and South America. Persons acquiring *P. vivax* infections outside of Papua New Guinea or Indonesia should be started on chloroquine. If the patient does not respond, the treatment should be changed to a chloroquine-resistant *P. vivax* regimen and CDC should be notified (Malaria Hotline number listed below). For treatment of chloroquine-resistant *P. vivax* infections, options A, B, and C are equally recommended.

13. For pregnant women diagnosed with uncomplicated malaria caused by chloroquine-resistant *P. falciparum* or chloroquine-resistant *P. vivax* infection, treatment with doxycycline is generally not indicated. However, doxycycline may be used in combination with quinine (as recommended for non-pregnant adults) if other treatment options are not available or are not being tolerated, and the benefit is judged to outweigh the risks.

14. Atovaquone-proguanil and artemether-lumefantrine are generally not recommended for use in pregnant women, particularly in the first trimester due to lack of sufficient safety data. For pregnant women diagnosed with uncomplicated malaria caused by chloroquine-resistant *P. falciparum* infection, atovaquone-proguanil or artemether-lumefantrine may be used if other treatment options are not available or are not being tolerated, and if the potential benefit is judged to outweigh the potential risks.

15. Because of a possible association with mefloquine treatment during pregnancy and an increase in stillbirths, mefloquine is generally not recommended for treatment in pregnant women. However, mefloquine may be used if it is the only treatment option available and if the potential benefit is judged to outweigh the potential risks.

16. For *P. vivax* and *P. ovale* infections, primaquine phosphate for radical treatment of hypnozoites should not be given during pregnancy. Pregnant patients with *P. vivax* and *P. ovale* infections should be maintained on chloroquine prophyla_ ._ 'or the duration of their pregnancy. The chemoprophylactic dose of chloroquine phosphate is 300 mg base (=500 mg salt) orally once per week. After delivery, pregnant patients who do not have G6PD deficiency should be treated with primaquine.

Based on CDC Recommendations for Malaria in the US
CDC Malaria Hotline: weekdays 8 am – 4:30 pm EST: (770) 488-7788
after hours, weekends and holidays: (770) 488-7100

Malaria in Children (United States)

Clinical Diagnosis/ *Plasmodium* species	Region Acquired	Recommended Drugs and Pediatric Dose (*pediatric dose should not exceed adult dose*)
Severe malaria[1,2,3]	**All regions**	**Quinidine gluconate**[2] **plus either: Doxycycline**[8] **or Clindamycin** **Quinidine gluconate:** Same mg/kg dosing and recommendations as for adults. **Doxycycline:** Treatment as above. For children <45 kg, give 2.2 mg/ kg (IV) q12h and then switch to (PO) doxycycline (dose as above) as soon as patient can take oral medication. For children ≥45 kg, use same dosing as for adults. Treatment × 7 days. **Clindamycin:** Treatment as above. 10 mg base/kg loading dose (IV) followed by 5 mg base/kg (IV/PO) q8h. Treatment × 7 days.
Uncomplicated malaria/ *P. falciparum* or Species not identified[4]	**Chloroquine-resistant or unknown resistance**[11] (Middle Eastern countries with chloroquine-resistant *P. falciparum* include Iran, Oman, Saudi Arabia, and Yemen. Of note, infections acquired in the	**A. Atovaquone-proguanil (Malarone)**[5] *Adult tab = 250 mg atovaquone/ 100 mg proguanil* *Peds tab = 62.5 mg atovaquone/ 25 mg proguanil* 5–8 kg: 2 peds tabs (PO) q24h × 3d 9–10 kg: 3 peds tabs (PO) q24h × 3d 11–20 kg: 1 adult tab (PO) q24h × 3d 21–30 kg: 2 adult tabs (PO) q24h × 3d 31–40 kg: 3 adult tabs (PO) q24h × 3d >40 kg: 4 adult tabs (PO) q24h × 3d **or**

Malaria in Children (United States) (cont'd)

Clinical Diagnosis/ *Plasmodium* species	Region Acquired	Recommended Drugs and Pediatric Dose (*pediatric dose should not exceed adult dose*)
If "species not identified" is subsequently diagnosed as *P. vivax* or *P. ovale*: see *P. vivax* and *P. ovale* (below) re. treatment with primaquine	Newly Independent States of the former Soviet Union and Korea to date have been uniformly caused by *P. vivax* and should therefore be treated as chloroquine-sensitive infections.)	**B. Artemether-lumefantrine (Coartem)[5]** *1 tablet = 20 mg artemether/120 mg lumefantrine* A 3-day treatment schedule with a total of 6 oral doses is recommended for both adult and pediatric patients based on weight. The patient should receive the initial dose, followed by the second dose 8 hours later, then 1 dose (PO) q12h × 2 days. 5–<15 kg: 1 tablet per dose 15–<25 kg: 2 tablets per dose 25–<35 kg: 3 tablets per dose ≥35 kg: 4 tablets per dose **or** **C. Quinine sulfate[3] *plus* either: Doxycycline[8] or Clindamycin** **Quinine sulfate[6,7]:** 8.3 mg base/kg (=10 mg salt/kg) (PO) tid × 3 or 7 days **Doxycycline:** 2.2 mg/kg (PO) q12h × 7 days **Clindamycin:** 20 mg base/kg/day (PO) divided q8h × 7 days **or** **D. Mefloquine (Lariam)[9]** 13.7 mg base/kg (=15 mg salt/kg) (PO) as initial dose, followed by 9.1 mg base/kg (=10 mg salt/kg) (PO) given 6–12 hours after initial dose. Total dose = 25 mg salt/kg

Malaria in Children (United States) (cont'd)

Clinical Diagnosis/ Plasmodium species	Region Acquired	Recommended Drugs and Pediatric Dose (*pediatric dose should not exceed adult dose*)
Uncomplicated malaria/P. falciparum or *Species not identified*	**Chloroquine-sensitive** (Central America west of Panama Canal; Haiti; the Dominican Republic; and most of the Middle East)	**Chloroquine phosphate (Aralen)** 10 mg base/kg (PO) immediately, followed by 5 mg base/kg (PO) at 6, 24, and 48 hours Total dose: 25 mg base/kg **or** **Hydroxychloroquine (Plaquenil and generics)** 10 mg base/kg (PO) immediately, followed by 5 mg base/kg (PO) at 6, 24, and 48 hours Total dose: 25 mg base/kg
Uncomplicated malaria/ P. malariae or **P. knowlesi**	**All regions**	**Chloroquine phosphate:** Treatment as above **or** **Hydroxychloroquine:** Treatment as above
Uncomplicated malaria/ P. vivax or **P. ovale**	**All regions** For suspected chloroquine-resistant *P. vivax*, see below	**Chloroquine phosphate** *plus* **Primaquine phosphate**[10] **Chloroquine phosphate:** Treatment as above **Primaquine:** 0.5 mg base/kg (PO) qd × 14 days **or** **Hydroxychloroquine** *plus* **Primaquine phosphate**[10] **Hydroxychloroquine:** Treatment as above **Primaquine phosphate:** 0.5 mg base/kg (PO) qd × 14 days

Malaria in Children (United States) (cont'd)

Clinical Diagnosis/ *Plasmodium* species	Region Acquired	Recommended Drugs and Pediatric Dose (*pediatric dose should not exceed adult dose*)
Uncomplicated malaria/ *P. vivax*	**Chloroquine-resistant**[11] (Papua New Guinea and Indonesia)	**A. Quinine sulfate** *plus either* **Doxycycline**[8] *plus* **Primaquine phosphate**[10] **Quinine sulfate:** Treatment as above **Doxycycline** Treatment as above **Primaquine phosphate:** Treatment as above
		or
		B. Atovaquone-proguanil *plus* **Primaquine phosphate** **Atovaquone-proguanil:** Treatment as above **Primaquine phosphate:** Treatment as above
		or
		C. Mefloquine *plus* **Primaquine phosphate**[10] **Mefloquine:** Treatment as above **Primaquine phosphate:** Treatment as above

1. Persons with a positive blood smear or history of recent possible exposure and no other recognized pathology who have one or more of the following clinical criteria (impaired consciousness/coma, severe normocytic anemia, renal failure, pulmonary edema, acute respiratory distress syndrome, circulatory shock, disseminated intravascular coagulation, spontaneous bleeding, acidosis, hemoglobinuria, jaundice, repeated generalized convulsions, and/or parasitemia of >5%) are considered to have manifestations of more severe disease. Severe malaria is most often caused by *P. falciparum.*

2. Patients diagnosed with severe malaria should be treated aggressively with parenteral antimalarial therapy. Treatment with IV quinidine should be initiated as soon as possible after the diagnosis has been made. Patients with severe malaria should be given an intravenous loading dose of quinidine unless they have received more than 40 mg/kg of quinine in the preceding 48 hours or if they have received mefloquine within the preceding 12 hours. Consultation with a cardiologist and a physician with experience treating malaria is advised when treating malaria patients with quinidine. During administration of quinidine, blood pressure monitoring (for hypotension) and cardiac monitoring (for widening of the QRS complex and/or lengthening of the QTc interval) should be monitored continuously and blood glucose (for hypoglycemia) should be monitored periodically. Cardiac complications, if severe, may warrant temporary discontinuation of the drug or slowing of the intravenous infusion.

3. Consider exchange transfusion if the parasite density (i.e. parasitemia) is >10% OR if the patient has altered mental status, non-volume overload pulmonary edema, or renal complications. The parasite density can be estimated by examining a monolayer of red blood cells (RBCs) on the thin smear under oil immersion magnification. The slide should be examined where the RBCs are more or less touching (approximately 400 RBCs per field). The parasite density can then be estimated from the percentage

of infected RBCs and should be monitored every 12 hours. Exchange transfusion should be continued until the parasite density is <1% (usually requires 8–10 units). IV quinidine administration should not be delayed for an exchange transfusion and can be given concurrently throughout the exchange transfusion.

4. There are 4 options (A, B, C, or D) available for treatment of uncomplicated malaria caused by chloroquine-resistant *P. falciparum*. Options A, B, and C are equally recommended. Because of a higher rate of severe neuropsychiatric reactions seen at treatment doses, we do not recommend option D (mefloquine) unless the other options cannot be used. For option C, because there is more data on the efficacy of quinine in combination with doxycycline or tetracycline, these treatment combinations are generally preferred to quinine in combination with clindamycin.

5. Take with with food or whole milk. If patient vomits within 30 minutes of taking a dose, then they should repeat the dose.

6. US manufactured quinine sulfate capsule is in a 324 mg dosage; therefore 2 capsules should be sufficient for adult dosing. Pediatric dosing may be difficult due to unavailability of non-capsule forms of quinine.

7. For infections acquired in Southeast Asia, quinine treatment should continue for 7 days. For infections acquired elsewhere, quinine treatment should continue for 3 days.

8. Doxycycline is not indicated for use in children less than 8 years old. For children less than 8 years old with chloroquine-resistant *P. falciparum*, atovaquone-proguanil and artemether-lumefantrine are recommended treatment options; mefloquine can be considered if no other options are available. For children less than 8 years old with chloroquine-resistant *P. vivax*, mefloquine is the recommended treatment. If it is not available or is not being tolerated and if the treatment benefits outweigh the risks, atovaquone-proguanil or artemether-lumefantrine should be used instead.

9. Treatment with mefloquine is not recommended in persons who have acquired infections from Southeast Asia due to drug resistance.

10. Primaquine is used to eradicate any hypnozoites that may remain dormant in the liver, and thus prevent relapses, in *P. vivax* and *P. ovale* infections. Because primaquine can cause hemolytic anemia in G6PD-deficient persons, G6PD screening must occur prior to starting treatment with primaquine. For persons with borderline G6PD deficiency or as an alternate to the above regimen, primaquine may be given 45 mg orally one time per week for 8 weeks; consultation with an expert in infectious disease and/or tropical medicine is advised if this alternative regimen is considered in G6PD-deficient persons. Primaquine must not be used during pregnancy.

11. There are three options (A, B, or C) available for treatment of uncomplicated malaria caused by chloroquine-resistant *P. vivax*. High treatment failure rares due to chloroquine-resistant *P. vivax* have been well documented in Papua New Guinea and Indonesia. Rare case reports of chloroquine-resistant *P. vivax* have also been documented in Burma (Myanmar), India, and Central and South America. Persons acquiring *P. vivax* infections outside of Papua New Guinea or Indonesia should be started on chloroquine. If the patient does not respond, the treatment should be changed to a chloroquine-resistant *P. vivax* regimen and CDC should be notified (Malaria Hotline number listed above). For treatment of chloroquine-resistant *P. vivax* infections, options A, B, and C are equally recommended.

Based on CDC Recommendations for Malaria in the US

CDC Malaria Hotline: weekdays 8 am – 4:30 pm EST: (770) 488-7788
after hours, weekends and holidays: (770) 488-7100

INDEX

Note: Tables are noted with a *t*.